MW00590776

CARE OF THE COMBAT AMPUTEE

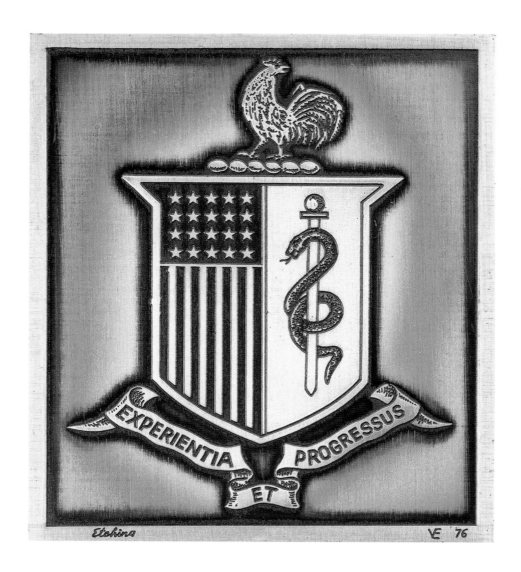

The Coat of Arms
1818
Medical Department of the Army

A 1976 etching by Vassil Ekimov of an
original color print that appeared in
The Military Surgeon, Vol XLI, No 2, 1917

This book is dedicated to the men and women of the armed forces who have been injured in their service to the United States, and to the men and women of the Department of Defense, Department of Veterans Affairs, and the civilian sector who have met the challenge to provide these heroes and their families with the highest quality of care, promoting unprecedented functional recovery and full participation in society.

Textbooks of Military Medicine

Published by the

Office of The Surgeon General
Department of the Army, United States of America

and

US Army Medical Department Center and School
Fort Sam Houston, Texas

Editor in Chief
Martha K. Lenhart, MD, PhD
Colonel, MC, US Army
Director, Borden Institute
Assistant Professor of Surgery
F. Edward Hébert School of Medicine
Uniformed Services University of the Health Sciences

For sale by the Superintendent of Documents, U.S. Government Printing Office
Internet: bookstore.gpo.gov   Phone: toll free (866) 512-1800;   DC area (202) 512-1800
Fax: (202) 512-2104 Mail: Stop IDCC, Washington, DC 20402-0001

ISBN 978-0-16-084077-7

The *TMM* Series

Published Textbooks

Medical Consequences of Nuclear Warfare (1989)

Conventional Warfare: Ballistic, Blast, and Burn Injuries (1991)

Occupational Health: The Soldier and the Industrial Base (1993)

Military Dermatology (1994)

Military Psychiatry: Preparing in Peace for War (1994)

Anesthesia and Perioperative Care of the Combat Casualty (1995)

War Psychiatry (1995)

Medical Aspects of Chemical and Biological Warfare (1997)

Rehabilitation of the Injured Soldier, Volume 1 (1998)

Rehabilitation of the Injured Soldier, Volume 2 (1999)

Medical Aspects of Harsh Environments, Volume 1 (2001)

Medical Aspects of Harsh Environments, Volume 2 (2002)

Ophthalmic Care of the Combat Casualty (2003)

Military Medical Ethics, Volume 1 (2003)

Military Medical Ethics, Volume 2 (2003)

Military Preventive Medicine, Volume 1 (2003)

Military Preventive Medicine, Volume 2 (2005)

Recruit Medicine (2006)

Medical Aspects of Biological Warfare (2007)

Medical Aspects of Chemical Warfare (2008)

Care of the Combat Amputee (2009)

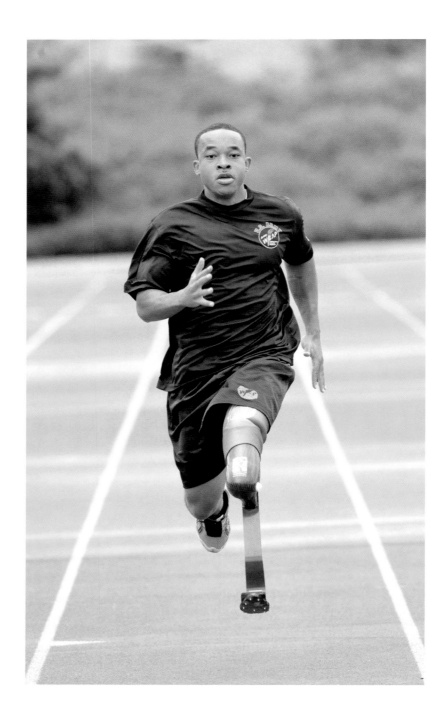

US Army World Class Athlete Program Paralympic sprinter hopeful Sergeant Jerrod Fields, seen here working out at the US Olympic Training Center in Chula Vista, California, won the 100 meters with a time of 12.15 seconds at the 2009 Endeavor Games in Edmond, Oklahoma, on June 13.

Photograph by Tim Hipps, US Army Family and Morale, Welfare and Recreation Public Affairs.

CARE OF THE
COMBAT AMPUTEE

Senior Editors

PAUL F. PASQUINA, MD
Colonel, MC, US Army
Chair, Integrated Department of Orthopaedics and Rehabilitation
Walter Reed Army Medical Center and National Naval Medical Center

and

RORY A. COOPER, PhD
Senior Career Scientist
US Department of Veterans Affairs
Distinguished Professor
University of Pittsburgh

Office of The Surgeon General
United States Army
Falls Church, Virginia

Borden Institute
Walter Reed Army Medical Center
Washington, DC

2009

Editorial Staff:	Joan Redding	Marcia Metzgar
	Senior Production Editor	*Technical Editor*
	Ronda Lindsay	Vivian Mason
	Technical Editor	*Technical Editor*
	Douglas Wise	Bruce Maston
	Senior Layout Editor	*Illustrator*

This volume was prepared for military medical educational use. The focus of the information is to foster discussion that may form the basis of doctrine and policy. The opinions or assertions contained herein are the private views of the authors and are not to be construed as official or as reflecting the views of the Department of the Army or the Department of Defense.

Dosage Selection:

The authors and publisher have made every effort to ensure the accuracy of dosages cited herein. However, it is the responsibility of every practitioner to consult appropriate information sources to ascertain correct dosages for each clinical situation, especially for new or unfamiliar drugs and procedures. The authors, editors, publisher, and the Department of Defense cannot be held responsible for any errors found in this book.

Use of Trade or Brand Names:

Use of trade or brand names in this publication is for illustrative purposes only and does not imply endorsement by the Department of Defense.

Neutral Language:

Unless this publication states otherwise, masculine nouns and pronouns do not refer exclusively to men.

CERTAIN PARTS OF THIS PUBLICATION PERTAIN TO COPYRIGHT RESTRICTIONS.
ALL RIGHTS RESERVED.

NO COPYRIGHTED PARTS OF THIS PUBLICATION MAY BE REPRODUCED OR TRANSMITTED IN ANY FORM OR BY ANY MEANS, ELECTRONIC OR MECHANICAL (INCLUDING PHOTOCOPY, RECORDING, OR ANY INFORMATION STORAGE AND RETRIEVAL SYSTEM), WITHOUT PERMISSION IN WRITING FROM THE PUBLISHER OR COPYRIGHT OWNER.

Published by the Office of The Surgeon General at TMM Publications
Borden Institute
Walter Reed Army Medical Center
Washington, DC 20307-5001

Library of Congress Cataloging-in-Publication Data

Care of the combat amputee / senior editors, Paul F. Pasquina and Rory A. Cooper.
       p. ; cm. -- (TMM series)
     Includes bibliographical references and index.
 1. War wounds--Patients--Care--United States. 2. Amputees--Care--United States.
3. Soldiers--Care--United States. I. Pasquina, Paul F. II. Cooper, Rory A. III.
United States. Dept. of the Army. Office of the Surgeon General. IV. Borden
Institute (U.S.) V. Series: Textbooks of military medicine.
     [DNLM: 1. Amputation--rehabilitation. 2. Amputation, Traumatic--therapy. 3.
Amputees--rehabilitation. 4. Military Medicine. 5. Military Personnel. 6.
Veterans. WE 170 C271 2009]
     RD156.C27 2009
     362.4'385--dc22

                                                        2009046218

PRINTED IN THE UNITED STATES OF AMERICA

16, 15, 14, 13, 12, 11, 10, 09   5 4 3 2 1

Contents

Contributors

JULIE A. AKE, MD, MSC
Captain, Medical Corps, US Army; Infectious Diseases Fellow, Walter Reed Army Medical Center, 6900 Georgia Avenue, NW, Washington, DC 20307; formerly, Chief of Medical Residents, Department of Medicine, Madigan Army Medical Center, Tacoma, Washington

MARK R. BAGG, MD
Chairman, Department of Orthopaedics and Rehabilitation, Brooke Army Medical Center, 3851 Roger Brooke Drive, Fort Sam Houston, Texas 78234

BRIAN BELNAP, DO
Major, Medical Corps, US Army; Medical Director, Amputee Program, Comprehensive Combat and Complex Casualty Care, Naval Medical Center, 34800 Bob Wilson Drive, San Diego, California 92134

KENDRA BETZ, MSPT, ATP
SCI Clinical Specialist, Veterans Health Administration, Prosthetic & Sensory Aids (113), 810 Vermont Avenue, NW, Washington, DC 20006

ANDREE BOUTERIE, MD
Staff Psychiatrist, Psychiatry Consultation Liaison Service, Department of Psychiatry, Department of Psychiatry, Walter Reed Army Medical Center, 6900 Georgia Avenue, NW, Building 2, Room 6237, Washington, DC 20307

JOHN C. BRADLEY, MD
Colonel, Medical Corps, US Army; Chief, Department of Psychiatry, Walter Reed Army Medical Center, 6900 Georgia Avenue, NW, Building 2, Room 6237, Washington DC, 20307

FRANK BRASILE, PhD
Professor, University of Nebraska, 6001 Dodge Street, Omaha, Nebraska 68182

STEPHEN P. BURNS, MD
Staff Physician, VA Puget Sound Health Care System, SCI (128), 1660 South Columbian Way, Seattle, Washington 98108; Associate Professor, Department of Rehabilitation Medicine, University of Washington, 1959 NE Pacific, Seattle, Washington 98195

CHARLOTTE CARNEIRO, RN, MS, COHN-S, CIC
Infection Control Nurse Specialist, Department of Infection Control and Epidemiology, Walter Reed Army Medical Center, 6900 Georgia Avenue, NW, Washington, DC 20307; formerly, Nurse Manager, Occupational Health, Marriott Wardman Park Hotel, 2660 Woodley Road, NW, Washington, DC

JAMES C. CASEY, MOT, OTR/L
Occupational Therapist, Burn Rehabilitation Department, US Army Burn Center, US Army Institute of Surgical Research, 3400 Rawley E. Chambers Avenue, Fort Sam Houston, Texas 78234

BRENDA L. CHAN
Research Analyst, CompTIA, 1815 South Meyers Road, Suite 300, Villa Park, Illinois 60181; Formerly, Research Assistant, Department of Physical Medicine and Rehabilitation, Walter Reed Army Medical Center, 6900 Georgia Avenue, NW, Washington, DC

KEVIN K. CHUNG, MD
Major, US Army, Medical Corps; Medical Intensivist, US Army Burn Center, US Army Institute of Surgical Research, 3400 Rawley E. Chambers Avenue, Fort Sam Houston, Texas 78234

VINCENT T. CODISPOTI, MD
Captain, Medical Corps, US Army; Resident Physician, Department of Physical Medicine and Rehabilitation, Walter Reed Army Medical Center, 6900 Georgia Avenue, NW, Washington, DC 20307

JENNIFER COLLINGER, BSE
Bioengineer, Department of Physical Medicine and Rehabilitation, University of Pittsburgh, Human Engineering Research Laboratories, 7180 Highland Drive, Building 4, Floor 2, 151R1-H, Pittsburgh, Pennsylvania 15206; formerly, Graduate Student Fellow, Bioengineering, University of Pittsburgh, Pittsburgh, Pennsylvania

JOHN J. COLTELLARO, MS, ATP
Clinical Instructor, Department of Rehabilitation Science and Technology, University of Pittsburgh Center for Assistive Technology, Forbes Tower, Suite 3010, 3600 Forbes Avenue, Pittsburgh, Pennsylvania 15213

DAN CONYERS, CPO
Upper Extremity Specialist, Advanced Arm Dynamics Incorporated, 10195 SW Egret Place, Beaverton, Oregon 97007

RORY A. COOPER, PhD
Senior Career Scientist, US Department of Veterans Affairs, and Distinguished Professor, Department of Rehabilitation Science and Technology, University of Pittsburgh, 5044 Forbes Tower, Pittsburgh, Pennsylvania 15260

ROSEMARIE COOPER, MPT, ATP
Assistant Professor, Department of Rehabilitation Science and Technology, University of Pittsburgh, Center for Assistive Technology, Forbes Tower, Suite 3010, 3600 Forbes Avenue, Pittsburgh, Pennsylvania 15213

MICAELA CORNIS-POP, PhD
Rehabilitation Planning Specialist, VA Central Office, 810 Vermont Avenue, NW, Washington, DC 20420

MICHAEL DEMARCO, DO
Major, Medical Corps, US Army; Director of Electrodiagnostic Medicine, Department of Orthopaedics and Rehabilitation, Walter Reed Army Medical Center, 6900 Georgia Avenue, NW, Washington, DC 20307

PETER A. DESOCIO, DO
Captain, US Army, Medical Corps; Anesthesiologist, US Army Burn Center, US Army Institute of Surgical Research, 3400 Rawley E. Chambers Avenue, Fort Sam Houston, Texas 78234

ERIC DESSAIN, MD
Lieutenant Colonel, Medical Corps, US Army; Physician, Chief, Physical Disability Evaluation Service, Walter Reed Army Medical Center, 6900 Georgia Avenue, NW, Washington, DC 20307

WILLIAM S. DEWEY, PT, CHT, OCS
Occupational Therapist, Burn Rehabilitation Department, US Army Burn Center, US Army Institute of Surgical Research, 3400 Rawley E. Chambers Avenue, Fort Sam Houston, Texas 78234

BRAD DICIANNO, MD
Assistant Professor, Human Engineering and Research Labs, VA Pittsburgh Healthcare System, 7180 Highland Drive, 151R1-H, Building 4, 2nd Floor East, Pittsburgh, Pennsylvania 15260

WILLIAM C. DOUKAS, MD
Colonel (Retired), Medical Corps, US Army; Chairman, Integrated Department of Orthopaedics and Rehabilitation, National Naval Medical Center and Walter Reed Army Medical Center, 6900 Georgia Avenue, NW, Washington, DC 20307

JAIME L. DROOK, OTR/L
Occupational Therapist, Burn Rehabilitation Department, US Army Burn Center, US Army Institute of Surgical Research, 3400 Rawley E. Chambers Avenue, Fort Sam Houston, Texas 78234

CHRISTOPHER EBNER, MS, OTR/L
Occupational Therapist, Department of Orthopaedics and Rehabilitation, Brooke Army Medical Center, Center for the Intrepid, 3851 Roger Brooke Drive, Fort Sam Houston, Texas 78234; formerly, Occupational Therapist, Department of Orthopaedics and Rehabilitation, Brooke Army Medical Center, Fort Sam Houston, Texas

ALBERT ESQUENAZI, MD
Chair, Physical Medicine and Rehabilitation, Chief Medical Officer, MossRehab/Einstein at Elkins Park, 60 East Township Line Road, Elkins Park, Pennsylvania 19027

STEPHEN A. FAUSTI, PhD
Director, National Center for Rehabilitative Auditory Research, Portland VA Medical Center, 3710 SW US Veterans Hospital Road, Portland, Oregon 97207; Professor, Department of Otolaryngology, Oregon Health & Science University, 3181 SW Sam Jackson Park Road, Portland, Oregon 97239

JOHN R. FERGASON, CPO
Chief Prosthetist, Department of Orthopaedics and Rehabilitation, Brooke Army Medical Center, 3851 Roger Brooke Drive, Fort Sam Houston, Texas 78234

JAMES R. FICKE, MD
Colonel, Medical Corps, US Army; Chairman, Department of Orthopaedics and Rehabilitation, Brooke Army Medical Center, 3851 Roger Brooke Drive, Fort Sam Houston, Texas 78234

STEVEN V. FISHER, MD
Chief, Department of Physical Medicine and Rehabilitation, Hennepin County Medical Center, Minneapolis, MN 55415; Associate Professor, Department of Physical Medicine and Rehabilitation, University of Minnesota Medical School

KEVIN F. FITZPATRICK, MD, CPT
Major, Medical Corps, US Army; Physiatrist, Department of Orthopaedics and Rehabilitation, Walter Reed Army Medical Center, 6900 Georgia Avenue, NW, Washington, DC 20307

JONATHAN A. FORSBERG, MD
Lieutenant Commander, Medical Corps, US Navy; Orthopaedic Surgeon, Department of Orthopaedic Surgery, National Naval Medical Center, 8901 Wisconsin Avenue, Bethesda, Maryland 20889

PAUL FOWLER, DO, JD
Senior Medical Evaluation Board Disability Advisor; Physician-Attorney, Command Group, Walter Reed Army Medical Center, 6900 Georgia Avenue, NW, Washington, DC 20307

ALLISON FRANKLIN, DO
Captain, Medical Corps, US Army; Director of Inpatient Rehabilitation, Department of Orthopaedics and Rehabilitation, Walter Reed Army Medical Center, 6900 Georgia Avenue, NW, Washington, DC 20307; formerly, Resident, Department of Physical Medicine and Rehabilitation, Walter Reed Army Medical Center, 6900 Georgia Avenue, NW, Washington, DC

LOUIS M. FRENCH, PsyD
Director, TBI Program, Department of Orthopaedics and Rehabilitation, Walter Reed Army Medical Center, Military Advanced Training Center, 6900 Georgia Avenue, NW, Washington, DC 20307, and Assistant Professor of Neurology, Uniformed Services University of the Health Sciences, 4301 Jones Bridge Road, Bethesda, Maryland 20814

ROBERT S. GAILEY, PhD, PT
Director, Functional Outcomes Research and Evaluation Laboratory, Miami Veterans Affairs Healthcare System, 1201 NW 16th Street, Miami, Florida 33125, and Associate Professor, Department of Physical Therapy, University of Miami Miller School of Medicine, 5915 Ponce de Leon Boulevard, Plumer Building, Coral Gables, Florida 33146

FREDERICK J. GALLUN, PhD
Research Investigator, National Center for Rehabilitative Auditory Research, Portland VA Medical Center, 3710 SW US Veterans Hospital Road, Portland, Oregon 97207; Assistant Professor, Department of Otolaryngology, Oregon Health & Science University, 3181 SW Sam Jackson Park Road, Portland, Oregon 97239

JEFF GAMBEL, MD
Colonel, Medical Corps, US Army; Physician, Department of Orthopaedics and Rehabilitation, Walter Reed Army Medical Center, 6900 Georgia Avenue, NW, Washington, DC 20307

OREN GANZ, MOT, OTR/L
Occupational Therapist, Department of Orthopaedics and Rehabilitation/Occupational Therapy Services, Amputee Section, Walter Reed Army Medical Center, 6900 Georgia Avenue, NW, Washington, DC 20307

BRANDON J. GOFF, DO
Major, Medical Corps, US Army; Assistant Chief, Amputee Service, Integrated Department of Orthopaedics and Rehabilitation, National Naval Medical Center, 8901 Rockville Pike, Bethesda, Maryland 20889 and Walter Reed Army Medical Center, 6900 Georgia Avenue, NW, Washington, DC 20307; formerly, Director of Inpatient Rehabilitation, Walter Reed Army Medical Center, 6900 Georgia Avenue, NW, Washington, DC

BARRY GOLDSTEIN, MD, PhD
Associate Chief Consultant, Spinal Cord Injury/Disorders Services, Department of Veterans Affairs; VA Puget Sound Health Care System, SCI (128N), 1660 South Columbian Way, Seattle, Washington 98108; Professor, Department of Rehabilitation Medicine, 1959 NE Pacific, Seattle, Washington 98195

ROBERT R. GRANVILLE, MD
Colonel, Medical Corps, US Army; Orthopaedic Surgeon, Department of Orthopaedics and Rehabilitation, Brooke Army Medical Center, 3851 Roger Brooke Drive, Fort Sam Houston, Texas 78234; formerly, Director of Amputee Service, Department of Orthopaedics and Rehabilitation, Brooke Army Medical Center, 3851 Roger Brooke Drive, Fort Sam Houston, Texas

GARTH T. GREENWELL, DO
Captain, Medical Corps, US Army; Staff Physiatrist, Department of Physical Medicine and Rehabilitation Services, MCHK-PT, Tripler Army Medical Center, One Jarrett White Road, Tripler Army Medical Center, Hawaii 96859; formerly, Resident, Department of Physical Medicine, Walter Reed Army Medical Center, 6900 Georgia Avenue, NW, Washington, DC

GARRETT G. GRINDLE, MS
Research Associate, Department of Rehabilitation Science and Technology, University of Pittsburgh, Human Engineering and Research Labs, 7180 Highland Drive, Building 4, Second Floor East Wing 151R7-H, Pittsburgh, Pennsylvania 15206

KRISTIN GULICK, OTR/L, BS, CHT
Occupational Therapist; formerly, Director of Therapy Services, Advanced Arm Dynamics, 123 West Torrance Boulevard, Suite 203, Redondo Beach, California 90277

MARGARET C. HAMMOND, MD
Chief Consultant, Spinal Cord Injury/Disorders Services, Department of Veterans Affairs; Chief, Spinal Cord Injury Service, VA Puget Sound Health Care System, SCI (128N), 1660 South Columbian Way, Seattle, Washington 98108; Professor, Department of Rehabilitation Medicine, University of Washington, 1959 NE Pacific, Seattle, Washington 98195

PETER D. HARSCH, CP
Chief Prosthetist, C5 Combat Care Center Prosthetics, Navy Medical Center, 34800 Bob Wilson Drive, Building 3, San Diego, California 92134

JOSHUA D. HARTZELL, MD
Captain, Medical Corps, US Army; Infectious Diseases Fellow, Department of Medicine, Walter Reed Army Medical Center, 6900 Georgia Avenue, NW, Washington, DC 20307; formerly, Chief of Medical Residents, Department of Medicine, Walter Reed Army Medical Center, 6900 Georgia Avenue, NW, Washington, DC

ALAN J. HAWK
Collections Manager, Historical Collections, National Museum of Health and Medicine, Armed Forces Institute of Pathology, Walter Reed Army Medical Center, 6900 Georgia Avenue, NW, Washington, DC 20306

ROMAN A. HAYDA, MD
Colonel, Medical Corps, US Army; Chief Orthopaedic Trauma, Residence Program Director, Department of Orthopaedic Surgery, Brooke Army Medical Center, 3851 Roger Brooke Drive, Fort Sam Houston, Texas 78234

TRAVIS L. HEDMAN, PT
Captain, US Army, Medical Corps; Chief, Burn Rehabilitation Department, US Army Burn Center, US Army Institute of Surgical Research, 3400 Rawley E. Chambers Avenue, Fort Sam Houston, Texas 78234

CHRISTINE HEINER, BA
Communications Specialist, Human Engineering Research Laboratories, VA Pittsburgh Healthcare System/University of Pittsburgh, 7180 Highland Drive, 151RI-HD, Building 4, 2nd Floor East, Pittsburgh, Pennsylvania 15206

SANDRA L. HUBBARD WINKLER, PhD
Research Health Scientist, Rehabilitation Outcome Research Center Research Enhancement Award Program, Malcolm Randall VA Medical Center, 1601 SW Archer Road, 151-B, Gainesville, Florida 32608, and Assistant Professor, Department of Occupational Therapy, University of Florida, College of Public Health and Health Professions, PO Box 100164, Gainesville, Florida 32610; formerly, Research Associate, Predoctoral Fellow, Department of Rehabilitation Science and Technology, University of Pittsburgh, 5044 Forbes Tower, Pittsburgh, Pennsylvania

BRADLEY IMPINK, BSE
Predoctoral Fellow, Human Engineering Research Laboratories, VA Pittsburgh Healthcare System, 7180 Highland Drive, 151R1-H, Building 4, 2nd Floor East, Pittsburgh, Pennsylvania 15206; formerly, Graduate Student Researcher, Department of Bioengineering, University of Pittsburgh, Pittsburgh, Pennsylvania

AENEAS JANZE, MD
Captain, Medical Corps, US Army; Resident Physician, Department of Physical Medicine and Rehabilitation, Walter Reed Army Medical Center, 6900 Georgia Avenue, NW, Washington, DC 20307

MELISSA JONES, PhD, OTR/L
Lieutenant Colonel (Retired), Medical Specialist Corps, US Army; formerly, Research Coordinator, Department of Orthopaedics and Rehabilitation, Walter Reed Army Medical Center, 6900 Georgia Avenue, NW, Washington, DC 20307

SUSAN KAPP, MEd, CPO, LPO
Associate Professor and Director, Prosthetic and Orthotic Program, University of Texas Southwestern Medical Center at Dallas, 5323 Harry Hines Boulevard, Suite V5.400, Dallas, Texas 75390

AMOL KARMARKAR, MS
Research Associate, Human Engineering Research Laboratories, VA Pittsburgh Healthcare System/University of Pittsburgh, 7180 Highland Drive, 151RI-H, Building 4, 2nd Floor East, Pittsburgh, Pennsylvania 15206; formerly, Research Assistant, Department of Rehabilitation Science, State University of New York at Buffalo, Buffalo, New York

JOHN J. KEELING, MD
Commander, Medical Corps, US Navy; Director, Orthopaedic Trauma and Foot and Ankle Division, Department of Orthopaedics, National Military Medical Center, Walter Reed National Military Medical Center, 8901 Rockville Pike, Bethesda, Maryland 20899

NICOLE M. KEESEE, MS
Colonel, US Army; Office of The Surgeon General/Veterans Affairs Central Office Seamless Transition Office, 810 Vermont Avenue, NW, VACO 10D1, Washington, DC 20420

KEVIN K. KING, DO
Major, Medical Corps, US Army; Resident Anesthesiologist, Department of Anesthesiology, Brooke Army Medical Center, 3851 Roger Brooke Drive, Fort Sam Houston, Texas 78234

ANDY KRIEGER
Director, Department of Sports and Recreation, Paralyzed Veterans of America, 801 18th Street, NW, Washington, DC 20006; formerly, Adapted Athletic Specialist, Wright State University, 3640 Colonel Glenn Highway, Dayton, Ohio

TODD KUIKEN, MD, PhD
Director of Amputee Services, Department of Physical Medicine and Rehabilitation, Rehabilitation Institute of Chicago, Room 1309, 345 East Superior Street, Chicago, Illinois 60611

SCOTT KULLA, MS, OTR
Captain, Medical Specialist Corps, US Army; Chief, Department of Occupational Therapy, HHC 121 Combat Support Hospital, Box 238, APO AP 96205; formerly, Chief, Amputee Services, Department of Occupational Therapy, Center for the Intrepid, Brooke Army Medical Center, 3851 Roger Brooke Drive, Fort Sam Houston, Texas

WILLIAM LAKE
Colonel (Retired), US Marine Corps; Associate, Department of IT Strategy, Booz Allen Hamilton Incorporated, 4040 North Fairfax Drive, Arlington, Virginia 22203

MacJULIAN LANG, CPO
Clinical Specialist, Advanced Arm Dynamics, 123 West Torrance Boulevard, Suite 203, Redondo Beach, California 90277

NICOLE J. LEHNERZ, OTR/L
Occupational Therapist, Burn Rehabilitation Department, US Army Burn Center, US Army Institute of Surgical Research, 3400 Rawley E. Chambers Avenue, Fort Sam Houston, Texas 78234

M. SAMANTHA LEWIS, PhD
Research Investigator, National Center for Rehabilitative Auditory Research, Portland VA Medical Center, 3710 SW US Veterans Hospital Road, Portland, Oregon 97207; Assistant Professor, Department of Otolaryngology, Oregon Health & Science University, 3181 SW Sam Jackson Park Road, Portland, Oregon 97239

JAMES W. LITTLE, MD, PhD
Assistant Chief, VA Puget Sound Health Care System, SCI (128), 1660 South Columbian Way, Seattle, Washington 98108; Professor, Department of Rehabilitation Medicine, University of Washington, 1959 NE Pacific, Seattle, Washington 98195

CHRISTOPHER V. MAANI, MD
Major, US Army, Medical Corps; Chief, Anesthesiology, US Army Burn Center, US Army Institute of Surgical Research, 3400 Rawley E. Chambers Avenue, Fort Sam Houston, Texas 78234

JAMES M. MacAULAY
Chief of Vocational Rehabilitation, Department of Physical Medicine and Rehabilitation Services, James A. Haley Veterans' Hospital, 13000 Bruce B. Downs Boulevard, Tampa, Florida 33612; formerly, Vocational Rehabilitation Specialist, James A. Haley Veterans' Hospital, 13000 Bruce B. Downs Boulevard, Tampa, Florida

RANDALL J. MALCHOW, MD
Colonel, Medical Corps, US Army; Chief, Regional Anesthesia and Acute Pain Management, Department of Anesthesia and Operative Services, Brooke Army Medical Center, 3851 Roger Brooke Drive, Fort Sam Houston, Texas 78234; formerly, Chief of Anesthesia, Brooke Army Medical Center, 3851 Roger Brooke Drive, Fort Sam Houston, Texas, and Program Director, Anesthesiology, Brooke Army Medical Center-Wilford Hall Medical Center, Fort Sam Houston, Texas

RAUL MARIN, MD
Colonel (Retired), Medical Corps, US Army; Physician, Center for the Intrepid, Brooke Army Medical Center, 3851 Roger Brooke Drive, Fort Sam Houston, Texas 78234; formerly, Medical Director, GaitLab, Physical Medicine and Rehabilitation Teaching Staff, and Chair, Internal Review Board, Department of Orthopaedics and Rehabilitation, Walter Reed Army Medical Center, 6900 Georgia Avenue, NW, Washington, DC

LUIS J. MARTINEZ, MD
Major, Medical Corps, US Army; Infectious Diseases Fellow, Infectious Diseases Clinic, Walter Reed Army Medical Center, 6900 Georgia Avenue, NW, Washington, DC 20307

MARIA MAYORGA, MD
Colonel (Retired), Medical Corps, US Army; Physician, Past Chief, Physical Disability Evaluation Service, Walter Reed Army Medical Center; Currently, PhD Candidate, Sweden

CAIBRE McCANN, MD
Physiatrist-in-Chief (Retired), Department of Rehabilitation Medicine, Maine Medical Center, Portland, Maine

THANE D. McCANN, MD
Major, Medical Corps, US Army; Staff Physiatrist, Department of Orthopaedics and Rehabilitation, Brooke Army Medical Center, Center for the Intrepid, 3851 Roger Brooke Drive, Fort Sam Houston, Texas 78234; formerly, Resident Physician, Department of Orthopaedics and Rehabilitation, Walter Reed Army Medical Center, 6900 Georgia Avenue, NW, Washington, DC

MICHAEL McCUE, PhD
Associate Professor, Department of Rehabilitation Science and Technology, University of Pittsburgh, 5050 Forbes Tower, Pittsburgh, Pennsylvania 15260

SHANE McNAMEE, MD
Medical Director, Polytrauma, Assistant Professor, Department of Physical Medicine and Rehabilitation, Virginia Commonwealth University, 1201 Broadrock Boulevard, Richmond, Virginia 23249

JOHN MIGUELEZ, CP, FAAOP
President and Senior Clinical Director, Advanced Arm Dynamics, 123 West Torrance Boulevard, Suite 203, Redondo Beach, California 90277

JOSEPH A. MILLER, MS, CP, CPT
Captain, Medical Service Corps, US Army; Chief Prosthetic and Orthotic Service, Integrated Department of Orthopaedics and Rehabilitation, Walter Reed Army Medical Center, 6900 Georgia Avenue, NW, Building 2, RM3H, Washington, DC 20307, and the National Naval Medical Center, 8901 Rockville Pike, Bethesda, Maryland 20889; formerly, Deputy Chief, Prosthetic and Sensory Aids Service, Department of Veterans Affairs, Central Office, 50 Irving Street, NW, Washington, DC 20422

RUPAL M. MODY, MD
Captain, Medical Corps, US Army; Physician, Department of Infectious Diseases, Walter Reed Army Medical Center, 6900 Georgia Avenue, NW, Washington, DC 20307

ALFREDO E. MONTALVO, MSN, BSN, APN
Lieutenant Colonel, US Army, Medical Corps; Psychiatric Clinical Nurse Specialist, US Army Burn Center, US Army Institute of Surgical Research, 3400 Rawley E. Chambers Avenue, Fort Sam Houston, Texas 78234

MARIA MOURATIDIS, PsyD
Command Consultant and Subject Matter Expert for Traumatic Brain Injury and Psychological Health, National Naval Medical Center, 8901 Wisconsin Avenue, Bethesda, Maryland 20889

PAULA J. MYERS, PhD
Chief, Audiology Section, Department of Audiology and Speech Pathology, James A. Haley Veterans Hospital, 13000 Bruce B. Downs Boulevard, Tampa, Florida 33612; formerly, Pediatric Audiologist, All Children's Hospital, St. Petersburg, Florida

MARVIN OLESHANSKY, MD
Staff Psychiatrist, Department of Psychiatry, Tripler Army Medical Center, 1 Jarrett Hite Road, Honolulu, Hawaii 96859

PAUL F. PASQUINA, MD
Colonel, Medical Corps, US Army; Chair, Integrated Department of Orthopaedics and Rehabilitation, Walter Reed Army Medical Center and National Naval Medical Center, Section 3J, 6900 Georgia Avenue, NW, Washington, DC 20307

CINDY E. POORMAN, MS
Rehabilitation Planning Specialist, Department of Veterans Affairs, Denver Veterans Affairs MVA Central Office, US Department of Veterans Affairs, 810 Vermont Avenue, NW, Washington, DC 20420

BENJAMIN K. POTTER, MD
Major, Medical Corps, US Army; Musculoskeletal Oncology Fellow, Department of Orthopaedics and Rehabilitation, University of Miami School of Medicine, (D-27), PO Box 016960, Miami, Florida 33101; formerly, Chief Resident, Integrated Department of Orthopaedics and Rehabilitation, Walter Reed Army Medical Center, Washington, DC

MICHAEL PRAMUKA, PhD
Assistant Professor, Department of Rehabilitation Science and Technology, University of Pittsburgh, 5044 Forbes Tower-Atwood, Pittsburgh, Pennsylvania 15260; formerly, Neuropsychologist, Henry M. Jackson Foundation/San Diego Naval Medical Center, 34800 Bob Wilson Drive, San Diego, California

CHARLES D. QUICK OTR/L
Major, US Army, Medical Corps; Chief, Occupational Therapy Service, Burn Rehabilitation Department, US Army Burn Center, US Army Institute of Surgical Research, 3400 Rawley E. Chambers Avenue, Fort Sam Houston, Texas 78234

ROBERT RADOCY, MSC
Chief Executive Officer and President, TRS Incorporated, 3090 Sterling Circle, Studio A, Boulder, Colorado 80301

EVAN M. RENZ, MD
Lieutenant Colonel, US Army, Medical Corps; Director, US Army Burn Center, US Army Institute of Surgical Research, 3400 Rawley E. Chambers Avenue, Fort Sam Houston, Texas 78234

JEFFREY S. REZNICK, PhD
Director, Institute for the Study of Occupation and Health, American Occupational Therapy Foundation, 4720 Montgomery Lane, Bethesda, Maryland 20824

ANDREW RHODES, DO
Captain, Medical Corps, US Army; Physician, Medical Evaluation Board, Physical Disability Evaluation Service, Walter Reed Army Medical Center, 6900 Georgia Avenue, NW, Washington, DC 20307

REGINALD L. RICHARD, MS, PT
Clinical Research Coordinator, Burn Rehabilitation Department, US Army Burn Center, US Army Institute of Surgical Research, 3400 Rawley E. Chambers Avenue, Fort Sam Houston, Texas 78234

ELIZABETH A. RIVERS, OTR, RN
Burn Rehabilitation Specialist (Retired), Burn Center, Regions Hospital, formerly known as St. Paul Ramsey Medical Center, 640 Jackson Street, Saint Paul, Minnesota 55101

MATTHEW SCHERER, PT, MPT, NCS
Captain, Medical Specialist Corps, US Army; Doctoral Student, Department of Rehabilitation Science, University of Maryland at Baltimore, 111 South Greene Street, Baltimore, Maryland 21212; formerly, Amputee Physical Therapy Section Chief, Physical Therapy Service, Department of Orthopaedics and Rehabilitation, Walter Reed Army Medical Center, 6900 Georgia Avenue, NW, Washington, DC

CHARLES R. SCOVILLE, DPT
Colonel (Retired), Medical Service Corps, US Army; Chief, Integrated Amputee Service, Walter Reed Army Medical Center, 6900 Georgia Avenue NW, Washington, DC 20307

JONATHAN SENSINGER, PhD
Assistant Research Professor, Neural Engineering Center for Artificial Limbs, Rehabilitation Institute of Chicago, Room 1309, 345 East Superior Street, Chicago, Illinois 60611

SCOTT B. SHAWEN, MD
Lieutenant Colonel, Medical Corps, US Army; Orthopaedic Surgeon, Integrated Department of Orthopaedics and Rehabilitation, National Naval Medical Center/Walter Reed Army Medical Center, 6900 Georgia Avenue, NW, Washington, DC 20307

BETH A. SHIELDS, RD, LD, CNSD, MS
Dietitian, US Army Burn Center, US Army Institute of Surgical Research, 3400 Rawley E. Chambers Avenue, Fort Sam Houston, Texas 78234

JOSEPH A. SHROUT, MD
Lieutenant Colonel (P), Medical Corps, US Army; Orthopaedic Hand Surgeon, Department of Orthopaedics and Rehabilitation, Walter Reed Army Medical Center, Building 2, 6900 Georgia Avenue, NW, Washington, DC 20307; formerly, Chief, Department of Surgery and Special Care, Kimbrough Ambulatory Care Center, Fort George Meade, Maryland

BARBARA SIGFORD, MD
National Director, Physical Medicine, and Rehabilitation Service, VA Central Office, 810 Vermont Avenue, NW, Washington, DC 20420

DOUGLAS G. SMITH, MD
Professor of Orthopaedic Surgery, Department of Orthopaedic Surgery, University of Washington, Harborview Medical Center, 325 Ninth Avenue, Seattle, Washington 98104

MELISSA Z. SMITH, MOT, OTR/L
Occupational Therapist, Burn Rehabilitation Department, US Army Burn Center, US Army Institute of Surgical Research, 3400 Rawley E. Chambers Avenue, Fort Sam Houston, Texas 78234

LISA M. SMURR, MS, OTR/L, CHT
Major, Medical Specialist Corps, US Army; Assistant Chief of Occupational Therapy, Brooke Army Medical Center and Officer in Charge of Occupational Therapy, Center for the Intrepid, Brooke Army Medical Center, 3851 Roger Brooke Drive, Fort Sam Houston, Texas 78234; formerly, Chief of Occupational Therapy, Orthopaedic Podiatry, Schofield Barracks Health Clinic, Tripler Army Medical Center, 1 Jarrett White Road, Tripler Army Medical Center, Hawaii

MICHELLE L. SPORNER, MS, CRC
Research Assistant, Human Engineering Research Laboratories, VA Pittsburgh Healthcare System/University of Pittsburgh, 7180 Highland Drive, Building 4, 2nd Floor, 151R1-H, Pittsburgh, Pennsylvania 15206

BARBARA A. SPRINGER, PhD, PT, OCS, SCS
Colonel, Medical Specialist Corps, US Army; Director, Propency Office for Rehabilitation & Reintegration, Office of The Surgeon General, Falls Church, Virginia 22041; formerly, Chief, Integrated Physical Therapy Service, National Naval Medical Center, 8901 Rockville Pike, Bethesda, Maryland, and Walter Reed Army Medical Center, 6900 Georgia Avenue, NW, Washington, DC

GRETCHEN STEPHENS, MPA
Polytrauma/TBI Coordinator, VA Central Office, 810 Vermont Avenue, NW, Washington, DC 20420

STEVEN STIENS, MD
Staff Physician, VA Puget Sound Health Care System, SCI (128), 1660 South Columbian Way, Seattle, Washington 98108; Associate Professor, Department of Rehabilitation Medicine, University of Washington, 1959 NE Pacific, Seattle, Washington 98195

JELENA SVIRCEV, MD
Staff Physician, Department of Veterans Affairs, Puget Sound Health Care System, 1660 South Columbian Way, SCI 128, Seattle, Washington 98108; Acting Instructor, Department of Rehabilitation Medicine, University of Washington, 1959 NE Pacific, Seattle, Washington 98195

CHARLES K. THOMPSON, PA-C
Physician Assistant, US Army Burn Center, US Army Institute of Surgical Research, 3400 Rawley E. Chambers Avenue, Fort Sam Houston, Texas 78234

RICHARD F. TROTTA, MD
Colonel, Medical Corps, US Army; Assistant Chief, Infectious Disease Service, Department of Internal Medicine, Walter Reed Army Medical Center, 6900 Georgia Avenue, NW, Washington, DC 20307

JACK W. TSAO, MD, DPhil
Commander, Medical Corps, US Navy; Associate Professor, Department of Neurology, Uniformed Services University of the Health Sciences, 4301 Jones Bridge Road, Room A1036, Bethesda, Maryland 20814; Traumatic Brain Injury Consultant, US Navy Bureau of Medicine and Surgery, 2300 E Street, NW, Washington DC

HAROLD J. WAIN, PhD
Chief, Psychiatry Consultation Liaison Service, Department of Psychiatry, Walter Reed Army Medical Center, 6900 Georgia Avenue, NW, Building 2, Room 6238, Washington, DC, 20307

PAIGE E. WATERMAN, MD
Major, Medical Corps, US Army; Infectious Disease Fellow, Department of Medicine, Walter Reed Army Medical Center, 6900 Georgia Avenue, NW, Washington, DC 20307

SHARON R. WEEKS
Research Assistant, Physical Medicine and Rehabilitation, Walter Reed Army Medical Center, 6900 Georgia Avenue NW, Washington, DC 20307

ALICIA F. WHITE, PT, DPT
Physical Therapist, Burn Rehabilitation Department, US Army Burn Center, US Army Institute of Surgical Research, 3400 Rawley E. Chambers Avenue, Fort Sam Houston, Texas 78234

JASON M. WILKEN, PhD, PT
Director, Military Performance Laboratory, Department of Orthopaedics and Rehabilitation, Center for the Intrepid, Brooke Army Medical Center, 3851 Roger Brooke Drive, Fort Sam Houston, Texas 78234

JAMES F. WILLIAMS, PA-C, MPAS
Physician Assistant, US Army Burn Center, US Army Institute of Surgical Research, 3400 Rawley E. Chambers Avenue, Fort Sam Houston, Texas 78234

DEBRA J. WILMINGTON, PhD
Research Investigator, National Center for Rehabilitative Auditory Research, Portland VA Medical Center, 3710 SW US Veterans Hospital Road, Portland, Oregon 97207; Assistant Professor, Department of Otolaryngology, Oregon Health & Science University, 3181 SW Sam Jackson Park Road, Portland, Oregon 97239

ERIK J. WOLF, PhD
Research Engineer, Department of Physical Medicine and Rehabilitation, Walter Reed Army Medical Center, Building 2A, Room 146, 6900 Georgia Avenue, NW, Washington, DC 20307

ROBERT N. WOOD-MORRIS, MD
Major, Medical Corps, US Army; Infectious Disease Fellow, Department of Infectious Diseases, Walter Reed Army Medical Center, 6900 Georgia Avenue, NW, Washington, DC 20307; formerly, Chief of Medicine, Wurzburg Medical Center, Wurzburg, Germany

KATHLEEN YANCOSCK, MS, OTR/L, CHT
Major, Medical Specialist Corps, US Army; Graduate Student, Department of Rehabilitation Science, University of Kentucky, 923 Forest Lake Drive, Lexington, Kentucky 40515; formerly, Chief of Amputee Section of Occupational Therapy Service, Walter Reed Army Medical Center, 6900 Georgia Avenue, NW, Washington, DC

ALAN W. YOUNG, DO
Physiatrist, Burn Rehabilitation Department, US Army Burn Center, US Army Institute of Surgical Research, 3400 Rawley E. Chambers Avenue, Fort Sam Houston, Texas 78234

GEORGE ZITNAY, PhD
Founder and Director, Defense and Veterans Brain Injury Center –Laurel Highlands, 727 Goucher Street, Johnstown, Pennsylvania 15905

Foreword

Our country's Warriors—Soldiers, Sailors, Airmen, and Marines—who are wounded or injured as a consequence of their service deserve the highest quality care available. The leadership of the Department of Defense and of the Army have firmly declared that aside from fighting and winning our current conflict, the comprehensive, state-of-the-art care of our wounded, ill, and injured Warriors is the most important mission of the US Military. Despite more destructive weapons and horrific wounds, the men and women of Military Medicine, as a whole, have continuously adapted to changing requirements and have developed comprehensive rehabilitative methods. This approach, combined with the goal of restoring our wounded service members to the highest possible functional level, is resulting in the optimal reintegration of our wounded Warriors and the best opportunity for return to uniformed service and/or productive civilian life. For example, even as this textbook goes to print, elements of the US Army Medical Command in its Warrior Transition Command are developing tools and processes ("Comprehensive Transition Plans") for tailoring this optimal reintegration for all Soldiers.

Today, service members with amputations receive rapidly progressive rehabilitation. To enhance recovery—and in some respect recapturing lessons learned from rehabilitative care in prior conflicts—three designated military facilities across the continental United States—Walter Reed Army Medical Center in Washington, DC; Brooke Army Medical Center in San Antonio, Texas; and Balboa Naval Medical Center in San Diego, California—maintain multidisciplinary teams of highly trained professionals, each contributing to a decisive continuum of care from the earliest phases of recovery and healing to reintegration into military or civilian life. Comprised of experts from more than a dozen specialties, these teams work together in addressing the rehabilitative, social, family, vocational, and spiritual needs of our service members, while simultaneously incorporating leading-edge technology, innovative research, and collaboration with Department of Veterans Affairs and civilian institutions. Excellent outcomes are being achieved, and the lessons learned from this young, athletic population are providing significant contributions to the healthcare of other service members, as well as civilians with major limb amputations.

More than a decade has elapsed since the previous *Textbook of Military Medicine* specifically addressed rehabilitative aspects of war injuries. It is fitting that knowledge of the evolution and application of our current approach to rehabilitation for the combat amputee—a collaborative and integrated team approach—be recorded in this latest volume of the series. The publication of this textbook, *Care of the Combat Amputee*, will serve as a valuable reference for healthcare practitioners in and out of uniform and will further facilitate establishment of best practices in the multidisciplinary spectrum of amputee care.

Accomplished through collaboration among the armed services, the VA, and the civilian sector with a common goal of achieving preeminent medical treatment, comprehensive training, and cutting-edge research, this volume will serve as a milestone in a long tradition of patient care. The book was completed through the tireless efforts of the authors, guided by the exceptional leadership of Colonel Paul F Pasquina, MD, and Rory A Cooper, PhD; the dedicated staff of the Borden Institute; and the Pittsburgh VA Rehabilitation Research and Development Center team, on behalf of service members, veterans, and their families. It is a tribute to the dedication of the men and women who serve our nation and to those who care for our wounded Warriors.

Lieutenant General Eric B. Schoomaker, MD, PhD
The Surgeon General and
Commanding General, US Army Medical Command

Washington, DC
November 2009

Preface

The Department of Veterans Affairs (VA) succeeded the Veterans Administration in 1989. VA operates the nation's largest integrated healthcare system, providing a broad spectrum of medical, surgical, and rehabilitative care. VA's vocational rehabilitation and employment programs help veterans with service-connected disabilities achieve maximum independence in daily living, and, to the greatest extent feasible, obtain and maintain employment. Additionally, VA manages the largest medical education and health professions training program in the United States, and VA research has earned an international reputation for excellence in areas such as aging, chronic disease, assistive devices, and mental health. Studies conducted within VA help improve medical care not only for veterans but also for the nation at large. Because 7 in 10 VA researchers are also clinicians, VA is uniquely positioned to translate research results into improved patient care. About 60% of VA employees are veterans, and more than 24% of these are disabled. Three hold the Medal of Honor.

Advances in body armor and battlefield medical care have helped to prevent damage to vital organs and stem blood loss, saving lives of service members injured in Iraq and Afghanistan. At the same time, increasing numbers of service members are experiencing traumatic injuries to their extremities that can result in amputation, followed by the fitting of a prosthetic limb and assistive devices. To meet the challenge of providing the best care possible to veterans with limb amputations at this critical time and for the remainder of their lives, VA and DoD have collaborated at unprecedented levels, as well as working with leading clinicians, prosthetists, and bioengineers from academia and industry.

A central theme of VA–DoD collaboration is the team approach to prosthetics care—in particular, engineers working closely with clinicians to ensure that devices are designed to fit the needs of veterans. Colonel Paul F Pasquina, MD, MC, USA, chair of the Integrated Department of Orthopaedics and Rehabilitation of Walter Reed Army Medical Center and National Naval Medical Center, and Rory A Cooper, PhD, director of the VA Rehabilitation Research & Development Center in Pittsburgh, have assembled experts throughout the diverse range of disciplines that work together to care for military and veteran amputees, from battlefield evacuation and surgery through therapy, rehabilitation, and community reintegration, to create this seminal work in the annals of military and VA medicine. Doctors Pasquina and Cooper are to be commended for their dedication to providing the highest quality of care to veterans with disabilities, and for compiling this outstanding record of the programs, processes, medical care, and technological advances that maximize the opportunities for our combat amputees from Iraq and Afghanistan to lead full and productive lives.

The addition of *Care of the Combat Amputee* to the *Textbooks of Military Medicine* series from the Borden Institute, an agency of the US Army Medical Department Center & School, provides comprehensive coverage of current and emerging care of combat amputations. The dedicated personnel working in our nation's military and veterans' organizations are making substantial medical, rehabilitative, technical, administrative, and social advances. We all strive to provide the best available care to those most seriously injured in Iraq and Afghanistan. Injuries can change the life of a service member in an instant, but the rebuilding process can take years. The veterans who have left their limbs on the battlefield have done so in the service of all of us. The resilience and spirit of these men and women serve as an inspiration to us all.

Hon. Michael J. Kussman, MD, Brigadier General, US Army (Retired)
Under Secretary for Health, Veterans Health Administration
US Department of Veterans Affairs

Washington, DC
May 2008

Prologue

"As we express our gratitude, we must never forget that the highest appreciation is not to utter words, but to live by them."

—John Fitzgerald Kennedy

This book represents the cumulative work of some of the world's best minds in medical, surgical, and rehabilitative care. Dozens of people gave freely of their time in preparing and editing chapters, adding up to thousands of hours of work over a period of about 4 years. Because of the criticality of the topic and its historical impact, the book was written with close collaboration among authors via both e-mail and the Internet. Because face-to-face communication is also essential, we assembled experts within the core topic areas to lead discussion groups in reviewing materials for each chapter in detail. This 3-day meeting was held in September 2007—the first scientific meeting held at the Center for the Intrepid at Brooke Army Medical Center. Throughout the period of Operation Enduring Freedom and Operation Iraqi Freedom, care of combat amputees has made tremendous progress, accompanied by growing collaboration among clinicians and scientists within the Department of Defense and Department of Veterans Affairs. Many individuals from academia, industry, veterans' service organizations, and the public at large have made important and lasting contributions.

We have attempted to cover the spectrum of issues involved in combat amputee care while remaining focused on the service member or veteran with major limb amputation. The book is intended to serve as a reference for experienced clinicians; a textbook for students, residents, and fellows; and a source for researchers, as well as a historical document for posterity. This work was completed during a time of war, when despite the arrival of new wounded on a nearly daily basis to military and veteran medical centers, new programs were established, benefits were expanded, and medical care improved at a rapid pace, as has been the case during times of war over the centuries.

Topics covered follow the course of care and community reentry of service members with combat-related major limb amputations, from surgical complications and treatments in theater through follow-up care and even multiple revisions. Acute and outpatient rehabilitation is described, including comorbidities, complications, and outcomes. Therapeutic interventions are detailed, and many breakthroughs in active rehabilitation are noted throughout the textbook. Emerging technologies and the processes of fitting prosthetics are presented to the reader. Opportunities for sports and recreation, a critical aspect of successful rehabilitation and community reintegration, are described. Learning to challenge one's perception of self and master new abilities is often accomplished through these activities. The complex systems and structures for providing medical care and the benefits earned by wounded and injured service members can be difficult to navigate; we have attempted to summarize and clarify these systems. The entire book is thoroughly referenced to the scientific, clinical, and public-policy literature. If successful, this book will serve as a guide for years to come.

It has taken an entire cadre of professionals to create this volume, and it has been completed with a great sense of commitment and honor. There is no greater calling than to help other people, especially those with debilitating injuries. In addition to the authors and editors, a number of other people were critical to seeing this product to completion: Christine Heiner, Joan Redding and other Borden Institute staff, Colonel Martha Lenhart, Paula Stankovic, Colonel (Retired) Charles Scoville, Troy Turner, Colonel (Retired) Rebecca Hooper, Lieutenant Colonel Rachel Evans, and Amy Donovan made critical contributions to keeping the book on track and of the highest quality. Brad Impink, Jen Collinger, Michelle Sporner, Amol Karmarkar, and Garrett Grindle, all graduate students at the University of Pittsburgh, and Sharon Weeks from Walter Reed Army Medical Center provided invaluable assistance in writing, editing, formatting, and coordinating chapters. Several of our colleagues also assisted with reviewing chapters and checking facts, for which we are grateful. We would like to acknowledge Kendra Betz, Cindy Poorman, Lucille Beck, Barbara Sigford, John Milani, and Billie Randolph for their comments. This book was conceptualized under the leadership of Lieutenant General (Retired) Kevin Kiley, MD, during his tenure as Surgeon General of the Army; it was wholeheartedly and seamlessly supported by his successor, Lieutenant General Eric Schoomaker, MD, PhD.

Brigadier General (Retired) Michael Kussman, MD, the Under Secretary for Veterans Health, provided his unwavering commitment to completion of this project. We are both especially very thankful to our wives and families for their love and support, allowing us to take time away from them to complete this volume and to care for wounded, injured, and ill veterans and active duty soldiers. We also owe a debt of gratitude to Arnold Fisher and the Intrepid Fallen Heroes Fund, for their private donations in support of the Center for the Intrepid, and to Congressional leaders who secured government funding to build the Military Advanced Training Center.

For us this has been a labor of love, and has afforded us a tremendous opportunity to learn, connect with other professionals, expand upon research efforts, and influence policy and practice. Most importantly, we share deeply in the commitment to improve outcomes for wounded service members and their families. It is with a great sense of satisfaction and humility that we present this volume to present and future generations of healthcare professionals.

Paul F. Pasquina, MD, Colonel, Medical Corps, US Army
Chief, Integrated Department of Orthopaedics and Rehabilitation
Walter Reed Army Medical Center, Washington, DC
National Naval Medical Center, Bethesda, Maryland

Rory A. Cooper, PhD
Director, VA Rehabilitation Research and Development Center, Pittsburgh
Distinguished Professor and FISA Foundation/Paralyzed Veterans of America Chair
University of Pittsburgh

Washington, DC, and Pittsburgh, Pennsylvania
October 2009

Chapter 1

INTRODUCTION: DEVELOPING A SYSTEM OF CARE FOR THE COMBAT AMPUTEE

PAUL F. PASQUINA, MD*; CHARLES R. SCOVILLE, DPT†; BRIAN BELNAP, DO‡; AND RORY A. COOPER, PhD§

*Colonel, Medical Corps, US Army; Chair, Integrated Department of Orthopaedics and Rehabilitation, Walter Reed Army Medical Center and National Naval Medical Center, Section 3J, 6900 Georgia Avenue, NW, Washington, DC 20307

† Colonel (Retired), Medical Service Corps, US Army; Chief, Integrated Amputee Service, Walter Reed Army Medical Center, 6900 Georgia Avenue, NW, Washington, DC 20307

‡ Major, Medical Corps, US Army; Medical Director, Amputee Program, Comprehensive Combat and Complex Casualty Care, Naval Medical Center, 34800 Bob Wilson Drive, San Diego, California 92134

§ Senior Career Scientist, US Department of Veterans Affairs, and Distinguished Professor, Department of Rehabilitation Science and Technology, University of Pittsburgh, 5044 Forbes Tower, Pittsburgh, Pennsylvania 15260

INTRODUCTION

For many Americans, the world changed forever on September 11, 2001, when Islamic extremists crashed hijacked commercial airliners into the World Trade Center in New York City, into the Pentagon, and over rural Pennsylvania. In response to these terrorist attacks the president of the United States launched a new war, the global war on terror (GWOT). Soon afterward, military operations were initiated in Afghanistan, on October 7, 2001 (Operation Enduring Freedom [OEF]), followed by the invasion of Iraq on March 19, 2003 (Operation Iraqi Freedom [OIF]). Conducting war against terrorism has proven extremely challenging for US military forces and costly for service members and their families. To date, thousands of young Americans' lives have been lost and even more have sustained serious physical, emotional, and psychological injury, although advances in military medicine have contributed greatly to reducing morbidity and mortality. Improved body armor, advanced capabilities of field medics, forward area resuscitation and surgery, and sophisticated and rapid medical evacuation have all contributed to widespread survival of injuries that would have been fatal in previous wars.

Caring for returning service members with complex polytrauma injuries necessitated flexibility within the Military Health System (MHS) and the Department of Veterans Affairs (VA). Multiple programs needed to be established or upgraded to ensure a well-coordinated system of care to address the needs of injured service members and their families across the entire continuum of care. In particular, given the large numbers of casualties with severe limb trauma and amputation, an amputee patient care program needed to be established within the Department of Defense (DoD). This chapter will document the need for this program within the framework of the core mission and values of the MHS. It will also highlight important lessons learned during OIF and OEF within the context of lessons from prior wars and examine the key components of a successful program.

Over the past decade, a cultural shift has occurred within the military giving individuals with major limb amputation the opportunity to stay in active duty service. Advances in medical, surgical, and rehabilitative care, as well as prosthetic design, are helping individuals achieve this goal. Whether or not the soldier desires or has the ability to remain in active duty service, DoD and VA programs are committed to helping all combat amputees reach their maximal function and return to the highest possible quality of life.

Traditionally a textbook of this nature would not be written until the completion of military operations. This schedule normally allows historians, scientists, and clinicians to formulate their thoughts collectively in a time of peace. Unfortunately, despite over 7 years of active combat, the GWOT continues, military service members remain in harm's way, and casualties continue presenting to the MHS. The DoD and VA leadership contributing to this textbook, therefore, saw the need to capture the lessons learned to date to facilitate ongoing care and planning.

THE MILITARY HEALTH SYSTEM

The MHS is entrusted by the DoD to accomplish five core missions in support of US service members, who are asked by their nation to risk their lives, whether in response to natural disasters or threats to national security. While each mission of the MHS may be distinct, they are interrelated and their synergistic effect contributes greatly to the overall strength and effectiveness of US fighting forces. These missions are summarized as follows:

1. **Combat casualty care.**[1] Unique to the MHS mission is the treatment of combat casualties. On the battlefield, care begins with basic first aid provided by well-trained nonmedical service members as well as trained combat lifesavers. The military has established five levels of care for wounded service members. For minor wounds, patients are treated and returned to duty. For injuries not conducive to immediate return to duty, evacuation to the next level of care is warranted. Depending on the nature and extent of the injury, service members may skip one or more levels of care to expedite immediate medical attention. Because of the capability to rapidly evacuate, medical care in theater is limited to life- and limb-saving procedures. Military surgeons focus their attention on stopping and preventing hemorrhage, debriding wounds to prevent infection, and preserving function. Often decisions about whether to reconstruct or amputate a limb are reserved for level V care within the continental United States treatment areas. The levels of care are categorized as follows:

- **Level I**: Immediate first aid and lifesaving measures are initiated in theater by Army combat medics, Navy corpsmen, and Air Force pararescuemen. Each service member carries a one-handed tourniquet, which may be applied by any member of the unit. Evacuation is then made to either an Army battalion aid station or Navy/Marine Corps shock trauma platoon, where initial resuscitation and advanced trauma life support is initiated. If an injured service member requires surgical resuscitation, he or she will often bypass the aid station and go directly to level II or III care.

- **Level II**: This is the first level of care where surgical resuscitation, basic laboratory, and radiographic capabilities exist. The Army forward surgical team is typically found at this level together with a medical company, which has two operating tables and holds up to 40 beds, with a holding capacity of approximately 72 hours. These medical units are 100% mobile and can provide up to 30 resuscitative surgical operations without resupply. The team is composed of one orthopaedic surgeon, three general surgeons, two nurse anesthetists, one critical care nurse, and additional nursing staff. Navy/Marine Corps level II care is provided by either a surgical company or a forward resuscitative surgical system. The surgical company can support ongoing operations without resupply to sustain four operating tables and a 60-bed capacity for up to 72 hours. The forward resuscitative surgical system is a smaller, more mobile unit, composed of only nine to ten personnel who can treat up to 18 casualties in 48 hours, but the system has no holding capacity. The US Air Force has several different level-II–capable units. The mobile field surgical team, which can provide up to 10 surgical stabilization procedures in 24 to 48 hours, is often combined with a small, portable, expeditionary aeromedical rapid response team composed of 10 members. The expeditionary medical support (EMEDS) basic is a 25-member team with one operating table and four holding beds. Lastly, the EMEDS+10 is a 56-person team with an additional 10 beds. Because of the high mobility of level II medical units, they are assigned to tactical units and are critical in a rapidly moving battlefield.

- **Level III**: This is the highest level of medical and surgical care available within the combat area of operation. Level III hospitals are modular, allowing adaptability to a given tactical situation. Army level III care is provided at the combat support hospital (CSH), which is composed of up to 248 beds, made up of a 164-bed unit combined with an 84-bed hospital company that can split off and act independently. The combined CSH has six operating tables, 48 intensive care unit beds, and 200 holding beds and covers up to 5.7 acres. In addition to laboratory and radiographic capabilities, the CSH also has a blood bank, a full complement of surgical subspecialties, and physical therapy capabilities. Level III care for the Navy and Marine Corps is provided by the fleet hospital. These hospitals comprise 1,000 personnel, six operating rooms, 80 intensive care unit beds, and 500 other beds. Fleet hospitals are also modular to accommodate various tactical situations. The Navy also has two hospital ships, which may act as level III or level IV facilities, with 100 intensive care unit beds, 1,000 other beds, and 12 operating rooms each. The US Air Force theater hospital is similar in capability to the Army CSH.

- **Level IV**: This echelon of care is located outside the combat zone and may be provided by a CSH, a fleet hospital, or a fixed medical facility. During OEF/OIF, most level IV care has been provided at Landstuhl Regional Medical Center in Germany. At Landstuhl, injuries are further assessed, irrigated, and debrided. Definitive surgeries, especially amputations, are still generally reserved for level V facilities. Patients with severe injuries are usually held less than 72 hours before proceeding to the next echelon of care. Casualties with less severe injuries may be able to return to the combat zone from this level.

- **Level V**: This echelon of care is provided within the continental United States at fixed military medical treatment facilities (MTFs). Although every effort is made to evacuate injured service members to an MTF closest to their home duty stations, it is more important for individuals to be sent to the facility capable of providing the most appropriate care. For example, all burn patients, regardless of military service, are evacuated to the burn center of excellence at Brooke Army Medical Center (BAMC) in San Antonio, Texas. For service members with amputations, centers of excellence have also been established at Walter Reed Army Medical Center (WRAMC) in Washington, DC, and Balboa Naval Medical Center in San Diego, California, to provide expert care more conducive to family and service member travel, and less disruptive of family life.

- **Level VI**: This echelon of care primarily refers to rehabilitation units within the VA system of care; however, the relationship between the VA and DoD continues to evolve, with increasing levels of collaboration as more and more injured service members receive care in both systems. It is important to note that prior to OIF and OEF the Veterans Health Administration had well-established rehabilitation centers for individuals with spinal cord injury, brain injury, blindness, and limb amputation. Over the past decade, however, most amputee care in the VA system involved disease-related amputations such as those seen with vascular disease or diabetes, in contrast to the traumatic amputations in younger service members currently returning from OEF and OIF. This situation, coupled with the desire of some service members to return to active duty following limb amputation, led DoD to create comprehensive amputee care programs within MTFs that cooperate with VA care, especially in the areas of long-term care, veterans' benefits, recreation therapy, and the VA prosthetics and sensory aides service.

2. **Healthcare services to active duty and military beneficiaries**. Despite the attention given to care of combat casualties, military healthcare professionals also provide state-of-the-art primary, secondary, and tertiary care to military beneficiaries in a variety of healthcare settings across the globe. Beneficiaries receive the highest quality of preventive, medical, surgical, and rehabilitative care independent of age or military rank. Pediatric services for dependent children as well as world-class healthcare options for dependent spouses and retirees are equally important missions in preserving the fighting strength and in attaining recruitment goals within the DoD. For service members deployed to remote locations, the security of knowing their loved ones will receive the best of care allows them to remain mission-focused no matter where they may be deployed. To provide these services, most MTFs are staffed with medical professionals in virtually all specialties ranging from pediatrics to geriatrics. In addition, the military has partnered with civilian organizations in forming the TRICARE network throughout the continental United States to augment medical services not available within the MTF.

3. **Military readiness**. In addition to ensuring that medical providers are available to deploy in support of military missions at a moment's notice across the globe, the MHS is also responsible for ensuring that military combat and combat-support personnel are in good health to deploy. These services include health maintenance, dental care, immunizations, and medical clearance and assessment during premobilization and postmobilization. This mission is particularly challenging for the relatively high number of National Guard and reserve soldiers currently being deployed overseas in support of GWOT. Various mobilization/demobilization centers have been established across the United States, which receive staff and logistical support from the MHS.

4. **Health education**. A robust educational program is a fundamental component of the MHS. High-quality training and continuing education are needed to ensure that the highest quality of care is delivered to military beneficiaries. Over a hundred accredited teaching programs exist within MTFs in nearly all medical specialties and across various healthcare disciplines (eg, physicians, nursing, therapists, field medics). Professional skills and expertise to optimally treat the unique healthcare needs of service members are taught. Experience during OEF and OIF has demonstrated the critical impact that graduate medical educational (GME) programs have had in providing the finest care to service members, particularly those with combat injuries. Ongoing educational programs that include military-specific curricula have allowed military facilities to stay current with state-of-the-art medical, surgical, and rehabilitative care.

Examples of this impact can be found throughout the DoD. Practitioners in surgical subspecialties such as orthopaedics and vascular, general, and plastic surgery, by continuing training in combat trauma care even in times of peace, were prepared to deliver life-saving care immediately upon the onset of operations in Afghanistan. The physical medicine and rehabilitation (PM&R) residency program at WRAMC and the National Naval Medical Center in Bethesda, Maryland, through its emphasis on teaching rehabilitation principles for severely injured service members with polytrauma, spinal cord injury, traumatic brain injury, and major limb amputation, produced graduates prepared to help create a system of care for the combat amputee. Air Force training programs and staffing of critical care air transport teams have revolutionized air medical evacuation during OIF/OEF.[2] Intense teaching programs to enhance the skills of combat medics offered through the Tactical Combat Casualty Course at the Army Medical Department's Center and School at Fort Sam Houston in San Antonio continue to help save lives on the battlefield. Furthermore, physical and occupational therapy programs at the Center and School have continued to produce leaders within these fields, enhancing the capacity of the MHS to deliver comprehensive care for wounded warriors and their families.

5. **Biomedical research.** The DoD's investment in biomedical research has made a major contribution to the current 90% survival rate for US service members wounded in Iraq and Afghanistan. Pioneering efforts such as Major Walter Reed's research to unravel the cause of yellow fever have paved the way for generations of military medical researchers, scientists, and engineers to explore ways to save lives and reduce morbidity. Transitioning research discoveries into clinical practice is an extremely challenging process, requiring rigorous studies to demonstrate safety and efficacy, while complying with the regulatory statues of such entities as institutional review boards and the Food and Drug Administration. Examples of the military's commitment to this achievement include the development and deployment of the smallpox and anthrax vaccines as well as recently developed clotting bandages to help control hemorrhage on the battlefield.[3,4] Even simple discoveries such as improved field dressings and tourniquets have revolutionized battlefield medicine and continue to save lives.[5] To keep pace with the technological advances on the battlefield, the MHS must continue to explore new technologies to meet the needs of not just today's injured soldiers but those of the future. This requires continued partnerships between DoD, VA, and civilian academic institutions and industries.

HISTORICAL LESSONS LEARNED IN COMBAT AMPUTEE CARE

As described in his 1972 autobiography, *A World to Care For: The Autobiography of Howard A. Rusk. MD,*[6] Dr Howard Rusk volunteered for military service in 1942, was commissioned as a major, and served as director of the Army Air Corps convalescent and rehabilitation services during World War II. Dr Rusk quickly recognized that a large number of soldiers in military hospitals did not need full-time medical care, but remained unready for the rigors of returning to their units. Therefore, he began a program of "constructive training" that included physical conditioning exercises, practical courses taught within the hospital (for example, he hung model aircraft from the ceilings in the wards and had patients practice recognizing various airplanes, and later introduced courses such as trigonometry, calculus, and American history), and preparing soldiers for return to duty either in their original military occupational specialty or a new one. Dr Rusk convinced President Franklin

D Roosevelt to create a comprehensive rehabilitation program within the Army, stating, "the country owed 'him' [the wounded soldier] more than just an artificial leg, a discharge and the Purple Heart." The program had the goals of

*   returning soldiers to physical and mental health,
*   finding ways for soldiers to function despite their disabilities,
*   helping the Army and Army Air Corps preserve all the personnel possible by sending soldiers back to duty in the best possible condition in the shortest time,
*   helping soldiers no longer capable of doing their previous military job to choose new jobs in the military and retraining them.

The Army and Army Air Corps initially created

two specialty amputee rehabilitation programs: one in Pawling, New York, and the other at Walter Reed Army Hospital.

In addition to the new rehabilitation program, World War II saw an improved military effort to provide advanced prostheses. Before the war, military policy had been to stabilize soldiers with major limb amputations and provide them with temporary limbs; after discharge from military service, they were fitted by the VA with durable permanent limbs. To preserve the fighting force, Henry ("Hap") Arnold, commanding general of the Army Air Corps, ordered the Army surgeon general to provide the highest quality artificial limbs available and to begin a prosthetics research program. With General Arnold's urging, Congress passed the first prosthetics research bill, in 1943, to develop scientifically sound and workable artificial arms. This was the beginning of the Army's formal rehabilitation clinical care and research program for soldiers with major limb amputations.

By the end of World War II, with 18,000 amputations across all branches of the military, full-scale efforts to create better prosthetic limbs and improve amputee care were in place. By 1945 engineers and physicians working together had created the best prosthetic arm up to that time, which was demonstrated by a group of soldiers for President Harry S Truman at the White House. In 1946 President Truman appointed General Omar Bradley to head the Veterans Administration and bring about its transformation so that veterans would receive high-quality care and the latest technology. One of General Bradley's accomplishments was to follow the National Research Council recommendation to locate VA hospitals near medical schools to share resources. Paul B Magnuson, MD, an Army physician in World War I, became medical director of the VA and was largely responsible for the current structure of VA medical care.[7]

The Vietnam War brought further advances to military amputee care. Paul W Brown, a retired colonel, had served as an enlisted soldier in World War II and then as a medical officer during the Korean War before becoming a senior orthopaedic surgeon at Fitzsimons General Hospital in Denver, Colorado, during the Vietnam War. His article, "Rehabilitation of the Combat-Wounded Amputee," published by the Army Surgeon General's Office in 1994, provided insights in the principles and practice of combat amputee care.[8] Dr Brown recognized that the key to a successful program lay in tapping into and facilitating the "motivation" of the soldier/patient. His observations and lessons learned during Vietnam can be summarized as follows:

- **Create centers of excellence**. It became clear during the Vietnam War that amputations occurring as a result of combat wounds required specialized care, which an institution could establish only by seeing a high volume of patients. This care was recognized as more important than expediting a soldier's return to his or her hometown. According to Dr Brown, "specialized treatment centers should be established, staffed, and supported to accomplish their clearly defined missions and the patient moved as quickly as his physical condition permits to a definitive hospital for the major portion of his treatment and recovery."[8(p209)] It was also observed that excellence in care could only be achieved with continuing education for practitioners, including active military GME training programs.

- **Incorporate rehabilitation principles early**. Orthopaedic surgeons observed during Vietnam that no matter how competent their surgical skills were, patient outcomes depended most on patient motivation, which was enhanced through early rehabilitation. The paradigm of waiting for all medical and surgical issues to be resolved before beginning rehabilitation was unsuccessful. Rather, rehabilitation principles needed to be incorporated into the treatment process as early as possible in the patient's continuum of care.

- **Limit convalescent leave**. Because of the long and protracted medical evacuation process during Vietnam, which often took several months, many injured service members immediately requested convalescent leave to return home to see their loved ones. This leave often created an unanticipated negative effect: injured service members who returned home prior to fully engaging in the rehabilitation process and not yet independent in many skills were observed to fall into a dependent role within their families, relying on others for bathing, feeding, mobility, and basic hygiene. Despite the families' best intentions, this dependency had a negative psychological impact on the soldiers, who often were never able to reengage in the rehabilitative process of achieving maximal independence, function, and dignity. As the Vietnam War progressed, medical teams at Fitzsimons learned to limit convalescent leave and began linking leave to achieved rehabilitation goals.

- **Introduce recreational/motivational activities.** What had been traditionally referred to as "recreational therapy" was recognized by Dr Brown and his staff as "motivational therapy." Military providers partnered with local and community groups to develop programs for amputee horseback riding, swimming, and skiing. These programs were observed to have some of the most dramatic positive effects on outcomes. The keys to success were not just getting patients out in the community, but also to challenge them beyond the typical paradigms seen in hospital-based rehabilitation programs. As these programs became more popular, press coverage brought further interest, resources, and opportunities for the injured service members. However, the programs were also scrutinized by many, including the orthopaedic consultant to the Army Surgeon General's Office as well as many Navy orthopaedic surgeons, who claimed that these activities were both "dangerous" and "inappropriate" because they "fostered prolonged relationships with other amputees for companionship deterring from rehabilitation." Fortunately, this criticism did not stop the programs, and many of the programs formed or expanded during Vietnam served as the catalyst for today's numerous national and international sports and recreational organizations for people with disabilities.

- **Better define the VA's role**. During the Vietnam War, transfer to a VA hospital was often viewed as a decrement in medical care and a significant interruption of rehabilitation services. Hospital staff at Fitzsimons were reluctant to send their patients to the local VA for fear of this degradation of services, even if in meant going against the policy dictating that if a patient could not be "made well" within

a certain period of time, he or she should be transferred to a VA hospital. If VA hospitals were going to play a significant role in caring for combat casualties, their services would need to improve, their role would need to be clearly articulated, and their staffing would need to be concordant with their mission. Furthermore, transfer to the VA should not have a negative financial or retirement impact on the injured service member.

- **Provide holistic care**. Concentrating on the surgical aspects of care only was not sufficient for optimal treatment outcomes. Practitioners needed also to treat other physical and psychological impairments of each patient, especially those with multiple comorbid injuries. Individualized care was best achieved through a team approach, with practitioners from each discipline working together under one service, enhanced by communication between members as well as with patients and their families. Additionally, it was noted that consistency of care was a key factor in delivering the highest quality of care. The career of General Fred Franks, Jr, whose combat wounds resulted in a leg amputation, illustrates the success of Vietnam-era amputee care programs.[9] During his rehabilitation at Valley Forge Army Hospital, General Franks decided he wanted to continue military service. Aided by his surgeon, Dr James Herndon, Franks remained on active duty. After an exemplary military career, he has served in retirement as a tireless advocate for wounded soldiers and their efforts to remain on active duty.

DEVELOPING AN AMPUTEE PROGRAM WITHIN THE DEPARTMENT OF DEFENSE

According to data obtained from the Centers for Disease Control and Prevention, an estimated 1,285,000 persons in the United States were living with the major limb amputation (excluding finger and toe amputation) in 1996. Despite better prevention and treatment programs, the number of individuals with major limb amputations continues to increase. Over 82% of US amputations occur as a result of complications from diabetes and vascular disease, mostly in individuals over the age of 65.[10] Additionally, the vast majority of amputations performed in civilian communities involve the lower rather than upper limbs.[11–14]

Data from OEF and OIF reveal a much different patient population. As of August 2009, over 900 service members had sustained a major limb amputation in support of GWOT. Approximately 21% of these individuals have had an upper limb amputated, and

over 23% have lost more than one limb. Nearly 90% of these service members were under the age of 35, an age group with unique psychosocial needs, generally seeking to return to a more active lifestyle than older individuals. Adding to the challenges posed by combat-related amputation, the majority of these injuries have not occurred in isolation. Over 50% of the amputees seen during OEF/OIF have a documented traumatic brain injury, many with impaired vision and/or hearing. Additionally, many amputees have multiple complex fractures, soft tissue wounds, paralysis from peripheral nerve injury or spinal cord injury, and mental health problems.

In response, the DoD and VA together created a specialized system of care for combat amputees addressing these unique needs. To ensure communication between DoD and VA, Colonel Paul F Pasquina,

MD, was appointed to the Advisory Committee of the Secretary of Veterans Affairs on Prosthetics and Special Disability Populations. The first step in creating a comprehensive amputee care program within the DoD, in consultation with leaders from academia, consumer organizations, and VA, was to establish a well-articulated mission and vision statement to communicate to military and civilian leaders, as well as medical providers and service members, the intent of the program:

Mission: *Provide the highest quality of care to our soldiers, marines, sailors and airmen who are willing to put their life in harm's way.*

Vision: *Through the collaboration of a multidisciplinary team, we will provide world-renowned amputee care, assisting our patients as they return to the highest levels of physical, psychological and emotional function.*

While these statements articulated the goals of the program, a functioning system of care required acquiring and realigning resources within institutions, forming multidisciplinary teams, establishing productive partnerships with key constituencies (eg, VA, academia, veteran service organizations, industry, and relevant federal agencies and laboratories), and establishing strong leadership at all levels of clinical and administrative processes. It also meant adhering to and building upon the lessons learned from previous wars.

KEY ELEMENTS OF A COMPREHENSIVE AMPUTEE CARE PROGRAM

In preparation for OEF and OIF, WRAMC was designated as the primary site for amputee care in the US Army, with plans to expand the program to BAMC as needed, depending on casualty numbers. At WRAMC, providing holistic care for amputees has been a significant challenge for the medical and administrative staff, who have also been charged with caring for the over 8,000 other injured OEF/OIF service members arriving through August 2009.

During the early phases of the war, amputees at WRAMC received their primary medical and surgical care from a variety of different medical specialties. Because of the complex nature of their injuries, each amputee was admitted to the service that best met their immediate medical or surgical needs. For example, those with cranial trauma were admitted to neurosurgery, those with primary extremity trauma were admitted to orthopaedics, abdominal trauma to general surgery, etc. While each of these patients received expert specialty care, their holistic and amputee-specific care was less than consistent. Additionally, with the constant arrival of new trauma patients, military surgeons found themselves in the difficult position of managing complex acute surgical issues in the operating room at all hours, while at the same time trying to remain attentive to patients on the ward with complex medical, pain, or psychosocial issues.

To help meet this challenge, specialists in orthopaedics and PM&R partnered to help share inpatient and outpatient responsibilities. The PM&R department was well positioned to adjust its practice patterns and residency training program to help create both an inpatient and outpatient amputee service, in which the physiatrist acted as the primary care physician for the patient with complex injuries, allowing medical and surgical subspecialists to continue to provide expert consultation services. This synergistic relationship allowed focused subspecialty care and added consistency to amputee pain management, early rehabilitation, patient and family education, psychological counseling, traumatic brain injury screening, and surveillance and prevention of secondary complications such as infection, deep venous thrombosis, and heterotopic bone formation. Eventually, all the subspecialties critical to the care of amputees (orthopaedics, PM&R, occupational therapy, physical therapy, and prosthetics and orthotics) were united within a single department, a new Department of Orthopaedics and Rehabilitation, under a competitively selected department chief. The new department greatly facilitated communication within the institution and helped establish a clearer clinical pathway for amputee care.

In the new department, the physiatrist, following a rehabilitation model, coordinates the recommendations and interventions of multiple medical and surgical subspecialists, therapists, nurses, prosthetics, psychologists, and social workers. This system best ensures that holistic care is provided and also helps improve the quality and standardization of care across the institution. Weekly interdisciplinary amputee clinics are held in conjunction with interdisciplinary team meetings. The interdisciplinary meetings offer an opportunity for team members to share their observations and help develop unified treatment plans for complex patient issues or bring in other specialists as needed. These meetings have proved especially helpful in identifying patients with problems, which can then be addressed earlier during the recovery process: patients often form closer relationships with certain team members, who identify patient issues as they develop and address them with the rest of the team. The patient flow diagram developed at WRAMC is depicted in Figure 1-1. Although this model may not be adaptable to all military sites, the principles of patient flow should remain consistent across healthcare systems.

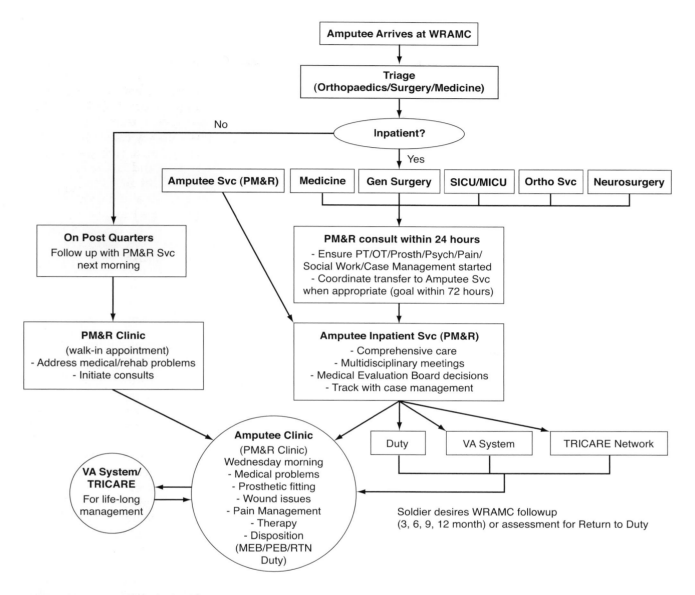

Figure 1-1. Patient flow chart at WRAMC's amputee service.
Gen: general
MEB: medical evaluation board
MICU: Medical Intensive Care Unit
Ortho: orthopaedics
OT: occupational therapy
Pain: Pain Management Service
PEB: physical evaluation board
PM&R: physical medicine and rehabilitation

Prosth: prosthetics
Psych: psychiatry / psychology
PT: physical therapy
RTN: return
SICU: Surgical Intensive Care Unit
Svc: service
VA: Department of Veterans Affairs
WRAMC: Walter Reed Army Medical Center

Organizational Structure

Standardizing medical care across different medical systems and geographic regions is dependent on multiple factors. Patient demographics, provider expertise and experience, and available resources greatly influence outcomes. To ensure that best practices are followed, it is essential to have a well-organized system in place. In addition, a model program should have adequate resources, support ongoing education and research, and incorporate continuous process improvement principles. Strong leadership is essential in implementing and sustaining such a program. The organizational structure of WRAMC's Department of Orthopaedics and Rehabilitation, described above, greatly facilitated the formation and execution of the

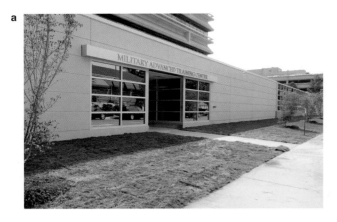

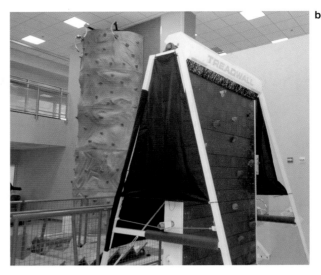

Figure 1-2. The Military Advanced Training Center at Walter Reed Army Medical Center, Washington, DC: **(a)** exterior view; **(b)** interior showing climbing wall.

amputee care program at both WRAMC and BAMC, and also contributed to the formation of two state-of-the-art rehabilitation facilities, WRAMC's Military Advanced Training Center (Figure 1-2) and BAMC's Center for the Intrepid (Figure 1-3). These two facilities were created with public and private funding after military, government, and civilian leaders recognized the need for additional support services at both locations.

Teamwork

Optimizing care for the individual with major limb loss is complex, and medical, surgical, and rehabilitative care has become subspecialized. In addition, the varieties of prosthetic components available on the market make prosthetic prescribing and fitting a complicated process. Whether providing inpatient or outpatient care, experts agree that formulating an interdisciplinary team is an essential feature of a successful program.

The "centers of excellence" concept developed in earlier conflicts[6-8] espoused the need for interaction of multiple specialties as well as incorporating basic rehabilitation principles to provide holistic care to the amputee. Critical specialties involved in caring for the amputee include physiatry, surgery, medicine, physical therapy, occupational therapy, recreation therapy, nursing, mental health, social work, and prosthetics. This type of teamwork has been shown to improve

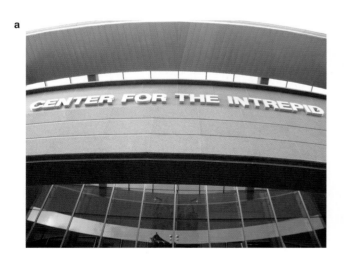

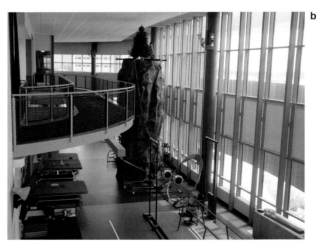

Figure 1-3. The Center for the Intrepid at Brooke Army Medical Center, San Antonio, Texas: **(a)** exterior view; **(b)** interior, third floor, showing track and climbing wall. Photograph (b) by Don Clinkscales.

short- and long-term outcomes.[15,16] Additionally, incorporating peer support, vocational rehabilitation, community reintegration, and assistive technology, as well as sports and recreational activities, greatly enhances a comprehensive program and improves the amputee's quality of life and ability to reintegrate with the community.[17] Finally, for a program to be successful, team members must recognize the importance of the patient and family members' participation in the entire treatment process, including the establishment of short- and long-term goals.

Staffing Ratios

As articulated by former Secretary of Defense Donald Rumsfeld, "you have to go to war with the Army you have, not the Army you want."[18] Although this may be true to a certain extent, the MHS strives to provide the best medical, surgical, and rehabilitation care achievable for wounded American service members. Essential to meeting this mission is establishing appropriate medical staffing ratios. Unfortunately, no standard matrix or formula exists to serve the complex needs of this unique patient population. Staffing ratios are dependent on factors such as patient acuity, experience and expertise of the provider, access to resources, and partnerships with other institutions and outside organizations. Table 1-1 presents ratios developed by expert consensus.

Graduate Medical Education and Research

Experience treating injured service members during OEF/OIF has demonstrated the critical impact GME has had on amputee care. Ongoing educational programs that include military-specific curricula help military facilities stay current with state-of-the-art medicine, surgical techniques, and rehabilitative approaches to care. WRAMC's PM&R residency program (the only one in the DoD) has greatly enhanced the incorporation of fundamental rehabilitation principles into the care of combat amputees. Even in times of peace, DoD surgical programs emphasized combat casualty care to ensure that today's surgeons are prepared to meet even the most complex trauma surgical issues. DoD-sponsored GME programs are vital to the strength of the MHS and ensure its capacity to meet current and future needs in military medicine.

An active research program is also an essential component of a successful amputee care center of excellence. To ensure that military-relevant clinical research is being conducted, active engagement of clinicians who care for the patients is paramount. Unfortunately,

TABLE 1-1

SUGGESTED STAFFING RATIOS FOR AMPUTEE CARE

Specialty	FTEs for 10 Ward Inpatients	FTEs for 20 Outpatients (Excluding TBI Impairment)
Orthopaedics	1	1
Physiatry	1	1
Physician Assistant	2	1
Physical Therapy	2	2
Physical Therapy Assistant	2	2
Occupational Therapy	2	2
Certified OT Assistant	2	2
Recreation Therapy	1	1
Nursing (RN)	1	0
Nursing (LPN)	2	0
Social Work	1	1.5
Case Management	.5	1
Administrative Assistant	.5	.5

FTE: full-time equivalent   RN: registered nurse
LPN: licensed practical nurse   TBI: traumatic brain injury
OT: occupational therapy

within most military clinical settings, a formal research infrastructure is not as robust as in most university programs. Despite the productivity of individual DoD clinicians and researchers, every opportunity should be taken to bring these groups together to collaborate on solving problems. Partnerships with the VA, universities, and industry have helped to build capacity in performing relevant research that can translate into clinical care.

Involving medical residents in research is also key. The partnership with the VA Rehabilitation Research and Development Service, which incorporates WRAMC residents into VA research activities, has resulted in military amputee care program successes. One such program, which included WRAMC PM&R residents in the Human Engineering Research Laboratories research team at the National Veterans Wheelchair Games and the National Disabled Veterans Winter Sports Clinic, cultivated residents responsive to research and encouraged some to become clinician scientists.

Continuing Education

In addition to GME, an ongoing educational program must be part of successful amputee care because of the varying levels of experience within DoD military treatment facilities and the high turnover of staff. Educational experiences must be comprehensive while at the same time targeting individual disciplines. Key leaders should be identified within each service (PM&R, nursing, orthopaedics, prosthetics, occupational and physical therapy, psychology, etc), who will first identify the educational needs of their services and then determine how these educational needs can best be met. A cost-effective way to meet these needs is bringing in outside experts or partnering with existing national organizations, such as VA, the Defense Advanced Research Projects Agency, and universities, as well as private companies and foundations. Issues of a cross-disciplinary nature, including pain management, wound management, and psychological adjustment, should be presented in a forum with all disciplines present to promote interdisciplinary discussion. The military amputee care program, in partnership with the VA, Human Engineering Research Laboratories, Paralyzed Veterans of America, and University of Pittsburgh, initiated a "state-of-the-science" symposium series in 2004 to bring the nation's best scientists and clinicians to WRAMC to facilitate communication, build collaborations, and accelerate the translation of research into clinical practice. Furthermore, collaborations were established with key universities, government agencies, and veteran service organizations to expand education opportunities, grand-rounds presentations, and clinical training.

Database

Any effective system of medical care requires accessible information on the patient population served; for military amputee care, a database is needed to track all patients as they enter the system. Important data elements include demographics, comorbidities, pathologic anatomy, and etiologic data, as well as interventions and outcomes. This database requires technological support and accurate data entry by employees (other than clinicians) skilled in these areas. Furthermore, the database must be secure, password-protected, and capable of removing all personal identifying information from the data. Data analysis such as prediction of outcomes, utilization of resources and equipment, and identification of areas in need of alternative interventions or approaches provides essential feedback to the clinical team.[19]

Prevention Programs

Preventative programs can help reduce the risk of both traumatic and nontraumatic amputation. Safety education and training have contributed to a significant decrease in trauma-related amputations.[20] The VA Preservation-Amputation Care and Treatment (PACT) program has contributed to an almost 40% reduction in nontraumatic amputations performed each year at VA medical centers. The program incorporates interdisciplinary coordination by the surgeon, rehabilitation physician, therapist, nurse, podiatrist, social worker, and prosthetic and/or orthotic personnel, as well as the primary care medical or diabetes team to track every patient with an amputation, or those at risk of limb loss, who enter the VA healthcare system.[21] Prevention of traumatic amputations from combat is also a priority of military forces. Medical teams have helped partner with military research teams in designing extremity protection armor as well as improving immediate medical aid to help save limbs.

Surgical Considerations

Standardizing surgical approaches to amputation is challenging, especially for combat victims whose wounds are not only extensive but also contaminated with dirt, bacteria, and fragments. With most amputees requiring comanagement of multiple surgical subspecialties, good communication between these services is essential. Limb-salvaging decisions remain complex and should be made in conjunction with the patient, as well as the entire medical and rehabilitation team. Tools such as the mangled extremity severity score are helpful in facilitating a decision (but may not be definitive). In addition to anatomic and physiologic factors, anticipated functional outcome should be considered, especially for this generally young and active patient population, many of them eager to return to high-level sporting and recreational activities. Similar considerations must be made when the rehabilitation team decides on amputation length and level. It is critical that the rehabilitation team, especially the prosthetist, be involved in these decisions preoperatively to ensure optimal length for prosthetic fitting and function.

Medical Management

Most service members with combat-related amputations have multiple comorbidities and a greater risk for secondary complications. Traumatic amputees are at increased risk for developing deep venous thrombosis in both their intact and residual limbs. For prophylaxis, all patients are started on low-molecular-weight heparin (enoxaparin), unless contraindicated. A high percentage of combat amputees also develop heterotopic ossification, although whether this incidence correlates with the nature of injury (typically, from a blast); patient demographics (age, race, genetic predisposition); wound management (vacuum dressings); or perhaps the presence of comorbid head injury is unclear. The secondary effects of heterotopic ossification can be significant pain, skin breakdown, and trouble with prosthetic fitting. All WRAMC patients receive a cyclooxygenase-2–selective nonsteroidal antiinflammatory agent, unless contraindicated, for both prophylaxis and treatment of heterotopic ossification.

Faculty have observed that in this patient population, signs of secondary complications such as deep venous thrombosis or heterotopic ossification are typically very subtle and may first appear only as a mild, low-grade fever; therefore, medical vigilance is imperative. Because of the high incidence of comorbid head injury, it is important that the medical staff have experience in managing patients with cognitive deficits. For posttraumatic seizure prophylaxis and treatment, levetiracetam has been very effective. Finally, because of the high incidence of multitrauma and blood loss, combat amputees have benefited from the use of epoetin alfa to stimulate red blood cell production. This treatment not only helps healing but also increases energy during rehabilitation. It should also be recognized that each patient has his or her own distinctive psychosocial needs, greatly affecting issues such as pain management, adjustment to disability and body image, ease with movement through the military disability system, and reintegration into the community or back to active-duty service.

Pain Management

An essential component to any successful inpatient or outpatient amputee program is expertise in pain management. Residual limb and phantom limb pain, reported in 55% to 85% of amputees, have a significant negative impact on long-term functional outcomes and quality of life.[22,23] The incidence of chronic pain may be reduced by aggressive preoperative and perioperative pain management. New Joint Commission on Accreditation of Healthcare Organizations standards, as well as the Accreditation Council for Graduate Medical Education, recognize pain medicine as a distinct medical subspecialty.[24] These organizations have helped establish institutional guidelines for appropriate pain management, as well as sensitizing medical institutions and clinicians to the patient's right to pain management. Furthermore, advances in medical and procedural interventions offer new ways to mitigate

pain associated with trauma care.

The entire medical and rehabilitation staff should be aware of the amputee's pain perception, incorporating questions about pain as part of routine evaluation. Team members who have subspecialty training in pain management contribute greatly to a successful outcome. Within the amputee care program, nurses, physicians, and therapists all play critical roles in monitoring patient pain complaints and optimizing treatment. WRAMC experience has shown that adequate pain control in most combat amputees requires multimodal medication. Nearly every patient is issued a patient-controlled anesthesia pump during the perioperative period and then quickly converted to long-acting opioids after definitive surgery. Short-acting opioids are also used for breakthrough pain or premedication prior to therapy.

Most patients are prescribed an anticonvulsant (gabapentin, oxcarbazepine, lamotrigine); a tricyclic antidepressant (nortriptyline, amitriptyline, desipramine); and a nonsteroidal antiinflammatory agent, typically one that is cyclooxygenase-2–selective, given the number and nature of comorbidities as well as frequent concurrent use of anticoagulation medication. Quetiapine fumarate is a very effective sleep aid, especially in cases when the soldier reports trouble with nightmares. In addition to pharmacological management, physical agent modalities (ice, heat), desensitization, and transcutaneous electrical nerve stimulation units have been helpful. Perhaps most effective, however, has been the support of the regional anesthesia team. The placement of peripheral infusion catheters to the brachial, lumbosacral plexus, or sciatic nerves has had a dramatic positive effect on pain control, reduction in medication use, and participation in therapy.

Cutting-edge programs should consider the use of topical agents, regional anesthesia, and multimodal pharmacological management, as well as complementary, integrative, or alternative measures such as biofeedback, hypnosis, relaxation techniques, and acupuncture. Physical and occupational therapists should be knowledgeable about both the indications and contraindications when applying modalities such as heat/cold, electrical stimulation, and desensitization techniques. The literature does not support clear evidence of a single agent as the treatment of choice for phantom or residual limb pain, but medications such as opioids, anticonvulsants, tricyclic antidepressants, botulinum toxin, and topical agents (lidocaine, capsaicin) may work synergistically along with mechanical stimuli modalities (eg, transcutaneous electrical nerve stimulation, tapping, massage) and mirror therapy to provide optimal pain relief. It is also generally accepted that the use of an appropriately fitted prosthetic socket reduces pain.

Advances in Prosthetics

Military amputee care providers believe that the technological advances in prosthetic design not only significantly improve patient satisfaction and functional outcomes, but also facilitate progression in rehabilitation.

Upper-Limb Prosthetics

Because of the complex nature of combat wounds, prosthetic fitting is often delayed to allow time for graft healing. Comorbid fractures, nerve plexus injuries, or soft tissue defects often prohibit the use of body-powered prostheses and suspension harnesses or cables. During the immediate postoperative period, myoelectric control sites should be identified. At WRAMC, occupational therapists work closely with the patients using preamplified electrodes over remaining intact muscles. These electrodes capture electromyograph signals that trigger audio and video feedback to the patient and therapist. These signals are also used to operate video games, which create a friendly and therapeutic competitive environment for the patients and quickly lead to mastering of certain skills. Once these skills are acquired, patients progress rapidly to operating myoelectric prostheses as soon as their limb is cleared for fitting. Body-powered prostheses are introduced later, as comorbid injuries permit. Today's advanced prosthetic components allow simultaneous operation and control of both the elbow and terminal device. The addition of a wrist control unit permits more useful upper-limb functioning in some patients. Newer terminal devices allow faster and more responsive opening and closing. They also have the ability to maintain constant grip force, utilizing built-in sensors within the fingertips.

Lower-Limb Prosthetics

Advances in technology have been applied to both prosthetic component design and socket fabrication. Traditional plaster casting, while still utilized, is augmented with computer-aided design and manufacture equipment, which has contributed to a more rapid and standardized approach to socket delivery for traumatic lower-limb amputees. The computerized system allows the fabrication of a custom-made socket in a fraction of the time needed for traditional casting. The shorter fabrication time is especially helpful in caring for the combat amputee, whose residual limbs have complex scar and suture lines and experience substantial rapid volume changes.

Advanced components, such as microprocessor knees and dynamic response feet, have not only enhanced function but also promote a more rapid progression through rehabilitation. The prosthetist's ability to program microprocessor knees to provide more or less stance or swing control assists advancement from early weight bearing to initial ambulation and, eventually, to stair and obstacle negotiation, without having to change prosthetic components or alignment. MHS and VA providers have also found that during initial ambulation, patients perform well with multi-axial feet and vertical compression pylons. As patients' confidence and activities increase, they perform better with lighter-weight feet that have vertical compression features built into the heel of the foot itself.

A fully equipped gait laboratory provides useful functional measures during the early phases of fitting to aid with prosthetic alignment and choice of components. Staff can also provide feedback to the patients and therapists on specific items to work on during therapy sessions.

Peer and Psychosocial Support Programs

An extremely important aspect of a comprehensive program includes professional behavioral health and amputee peer support. DoD amputee programs have formed partnerships with VA and the Amputee Coalition of America to find and train outstanding individuals with limb loss who volunteer their time to support combat amputees returning from war. It is ideal if these volunteers have military experience. In addition to the emotional support they provide patients, they also provide valuable feedback to the rehabilitation team as to how a patient is progressing in rehabilitation both physically and emotionally. Family members are also encouraged to be fully engaged in the rehabilitation program. The DoD has been proactive in supporting nonmedical attendants, often family members, who stay with injured service members during their recovery. DoD provides travel and housing allowances to nonmedical attendants, enabling them able to assist in the recovery of the injured service member and provide much needed emotional support through the process. The VA should consider adopting a similar model based on the success of this program and the positive impact it has had on veterans and their families. Communication among patients, their families, and their multiple providers is greatly facilitated by social workers and nurse case managers, who help to coordinate continued care, discharge planning, and equipment purchases.

Events such as the National Disabled Veterans Winter Sports Clinic, National Disabled Veterans Summer

Sports Clinic, National Veterans Wheelchair Games, and the Paralympics, sponsored by VA in coordination with public and private organizations including the Paralyzed Veterans of America, Disabled American Veterans, Disabled Sports USA, Wounded Warrior Project, US Paralympics, Achilles Track Club, Team River Runner, the Yellow Ribbon Fund, and numerous others, introduce patients to the variety of sports and recreational opportunities available for individuals with disabilities. Improving both access and awareness of these programs is essential to the success of the amputee program.

Military Medical Disability System

Navigation through the military medical disability system is complicated. A single amputee service promotes communication and standardization. Physicians should be well educated and experienced in writing medical evaluation boards. In addition, a physical evaluation board liaison officer should be assigned to each patient during his or her inpatient stay. VA counselors are also necessary to ensure that patients are aware their potential benefits. Educational programs must be tailored to the service member's needs, especially those with head injury, hearing loss, or vision loss.

Optimal disposition of patients is often complicated by the frequent geographical challenges created when the patient's duty station, home of record, and nearest military or VA medical facility are far apart. In these situations, medical follow-up must be coordinated through the TRICARE military healthcare system. Unfortunately, standards and availability of healthcare services vary in both the private and public sectors across the United States. Through partnerships between the DoD and VA, military amputee programs are committed to provide ongoing care to veterans with limb loss for the rest of their lives, as needed to supplement VA programs.

Outcome Measures

An essential element to developing a program focused on best practices is a mechanism for collecting and analyzing outcomes. New Joint Commission on Accreditation of Healthcare Organizations and Accreditation Council for Graduate Medical Education guidelines emphasize the importance of outcomes-based practices. A multitude of outcome measures are available for the amputee population. While numerous reliable and validated measurement tools have been reported in the literature, considerable debate continues as to which tool is best for the various populations of patients. Additionally, the success or failure of a particular intervention in amputee care is often the result of many factors. Therefore, several tools may need to be employed to adequately assess a particular patient population.

The most common outcome domains to be examined in various amputee populations include mobility, function, and quality of life. Tools employed to measure these domains are generally self-reporting (survey) or observation based. Several examples of measurement tools are listed below.

Self-reporting measures:

- the Medical Outcomes Study Short Form 36-Item Health Survey[25]
- Legro and colleagues' prosthesis evaluation questionnaire[26]
- the locomotor capabilities index[27]
- the sickness impact profile[28]
- the questionnaire for persons with a transfemoral amputation (Q-TFA)[29]
- the Trinity Amputation and Prosthetic Experience Scale (TAPES)[30]

Performance-based measurement tools and devices:

- the "get up and go" test[31,32]
- the 6-minute walk test[33]
- Gailey and colleagues' amputee mobility predictor[34]
- the disabilities of the arm, shoulder, and hand (DASH) questionaire[35]
- the box and block test[36]
- the Jebsen-Taylor hand function test[37]
- the step activity monitor[38]
- three-dimensional gait and motion analysis[39,40]
- energy consumption measurements[41,42]

New technologies and improved methods are being developed to record activity in unstructured environments within the home and community to measure community participation, provide further insight into the usage and effectiveness of technology, and assess the impact of various rehabilitation interventions.

CONCLUSION

Today, science, advanced technology, and improved material design are being brought together to revolutionize the care for individuals with amputation. Optimizing this care requires significant teamwork and partnership both across and within different disciplines. Current medical research must involve all areas of science, including those not traditionally associated with healthcare. Clinicians must clearly identify and communicate the functional needs of patients to engineers, biologists, computer scientists, and systems scientists to achieve common goals. Furthermore, a mutual sharing of ideas among public and private universities, federal agencies and laboratories, and industry is essential to further advancements in the field.

REFERENCES

1. Bagg MR, Covey DC, Powell ET 4th. Levels of medical care in the Global War on Terrorism. *J Am Acad Orthop Surg.* 2006;14:S7–S9.

2. Topley DK, Schmelz J, Henkenius-Kirschbaum J, Horvath KJ. Critical care nursing expertise during air transport. *Mil Med.* 2003;168:822–826.

3. Kennedy K. Shell-based blood clotter works without heat. *Army Times* [serial online]. February 10, 2007. Available at: http://www.armytimes.com/news/2007/02/TNScelox070209/. Accessed August 1, 2009.

4. HemCon Bandage. Hem Con Medical Technologies Inc Web site. Available at: http://www.hemcon.com/products/hemconbandageoverview.aspx. Accessed September 1, 2007.

5. Fleming-Michael K. New tourniquet named one of Army's 10 greatest inventions [press release]. Washington, DC: Army News Service; June 22, 2006. Available at: http://www.globalsecurity.org/military/library/news/2006/06/mil-060622-arnews03.htm. Accessed August 1, 2009.

6. Rusk HA. *A World to Care For: The Autobiography of Howard A. Rusk, MD.* New York, NY: Random House; 1972.

7. Magnuson PB. *Ring the Night Bell.* Boston, Mass: Little, Brown and Company; 1960.

8. Brown P. Rehabilitation of the combat-wounded amputee. In: Burkhalter WE, Ballard A, eds. *Orthopedic Surgery in Vietnam.* Washington, DC: Department of the Army, Office of the Surgeon General and Center for Military History; 1994:189–209.

9. Clancy T, Franks F Jr. *Into the Storm: A Study in Command.* New York, NY: GP Putnam Sons; 1997.

10. Dillingham TR, Pezzin LE, Mackenzie EJ. Limb amputation and limb deficiency: epidemiology and recent trends in the United States. *South Med J.* 2002;95:875–883.

11. Bethel MA, Sloan FA, Belsky D, Feinglos MN. Longitudinal incidence and prevalence of adverse outcomes of diabetes mellitus in elderly patients. *Arch Intern Med.* 2007;167(9):921–927.

12. Collins TC, Beyth RJ, Nelson DB, et al. Process of care and outcomes in patients with peripheral arterial disease. *J Gen Intern Med.* 2007;22(7):942–948.

13. Ephraim PL, Dillingham TR, Sector M, Pezzin L, MacKenzie EJ. Epidemiology of limb loss and congenital limb deficiency: a review of the literature. *Arch Phys Med Rehab.* 2003;84(5):747–761.

14. Kurichi JE, Stineman MG, Kwong PL, Bates BE, Reker DE. Assessing and using comorbidity measures in elderly veterans with lower extremity amputations. *Gerontology.* 2007;53(5):255–259.

15. MacKenzie EJ, Morris JA Jr, Jurkovich GJ, et al. Return to work following injury: the role of economic, social, and job-related factors. *Am J Public Health.* 1998;88:1630–1637.

16. Pezzin LE, Dillingham TR, MacKenzie EJ. Rehabilitation and the long-term outcomes of persons with trauma-related amputations. *Arch Phys Med Rehabil.* 2000;81:292–300.

17. Gerhards F, Florin I, Knapp T. The impact of medical, reeducational, and psychological variables on rehabilitation outcome in amputees. *Int J Rehabil Res.* 1984;7:379–388.

18. Mount M. Troops put thorny questions to Rumsfeld. CNN.com. Available at: http://www.cnn.com/2004/WORLD/meast/12/08/rumsfeld.troops/. Updated December 9, 2004. Accessed September 1, 2007.

19. Acosta JA, Hatzigeorgiou C, Smith LS. Developing a trauma registry in a forward deployed military hospital: preliminary report. *J Trauma.* 2006;61(2):256–260.

20. Dillingham TR, Pezzin LE, MacKenzie EJ. Incidence, acute care length of stay, and discharge to rehabilitation of traumatic amputee patients: an epidemiologic study. *Arch Phys Med Rehabil.* 1998;79:279–287.

21. Department of Veterans Affairs, Veterans Health Administration. *Preservation-Amputation Care and Treatment (PACT) Program.* Washington, DC: VA; 2006. VHA Directive 2006-050.

22. Woodhouse A. Phantom limb sensation. *Clin Exp Pharmacol Physiol.* 2005;32:132–134.

23. Sherman RA, Sherman CJ. Prevalence and characteristics of chronic phantom limb pain among American veterans. Results of a trial survey. *Am J Phys Med.* 1983;62(5):227–238.

24. Benzon HT, Rathmell JP, Huntoon MA. New ACGME requirements for fellowship training in pain medicine. *Am Pain Soc Bull* [serial online]. 2007;17(3). Available at: http://www.ampainsoc.org/pub/bulletin/fall07/training.htm. Accessed August 3, 2009.

25. Ware JE Jr, Sherbourne CD. The MOS 36-item short-form health survey (SF-36). I. Conceptual framework and item selection. *Med Care.* 1992;30:473–483.

26. Legro MW, Reiber GD, Smith DG, del Aguila M, Larsen J, Boone D. Prosthesis evaluation questionnaire for persons with lower limb amputations: assessing prosthesis-related quality of life. *Arch Phys Med Rehabil.* 1998;79:931–938.

27. Franchignoni F, Orlandini D, Ferriero G, Moscato TA. Reliability, validity, and responsiveness of the locomotor capabilities index in adults with lower-limb amputation undergoing prosthetic training. *Arch Phys Med Rehabil.* 2004;85:743–748.

28. Gilson BS, Gilson JS, Bergner M, et al. The sickness impact profile. Development of an outcome measure of health care. *Am J Public Health.* 1975;65:1304–1310.

29. Hagberg K, Branemark R, Hagg O. Questionnaire for persons with a transfemoral amputation (Q-TFA): initial validity and reliability of a new outcome measure. *J Rehabil Res Dev.* 2004;41:695–706.

30. Gallagher P, Maclachlan M. The Trinity Amputation and Prosthesis Experience Scales and quality of life in people with lower-limb amputation. *Arch Phys Med Rehabil.* 2004;85:730–736.

31. Fleming KC, Evans JM, Weber DC, Chutka DS. Practical functional assessment of elderly persons: a primary-care approach. *Mayo Clin Proc.* 1995;70:890–910.

32. Mourey F, Camus A, Pfitzenmeyer P. Posture and aging. Current fundamental studies and management concepts [in French]. *Presse Med.* 2000;29:340–344.

33. Enright PL. The six-minute walk test. *Respir Care.* 2003;48:783–785.

34. Gailey RS, Roach KE, Applegate EB, et al. The amputee mobility predictor: an instrument to assess determinants of the lower-limb amputee's ability to ambulate. *Arch Phys Med Rehabil.* 2002;83:613–627.

35. Amadio PC. Outcomes assessment in hand surgery. What's new? *Clin Plast Surg.* 1997;24:191–194.

36. Mathiowetz V, Volland G, Kashman N, Weber K. Adult norms for the Box and Block Test of manual dexterity. *Am J Occup Ther.* 1985;39:386–391.

37. Stern EB. Stability of the Jebsen-Taylor Hand Function Test across three test sessions. *Am J Occup Ther.* 1992;46:647–649.

38. Coleman KL, Smith DG, Boone DA, Joseph AW, del Aguila MA. Step activity monitor: long-term, continuous recording of ambulatory function. *J Rehabil Res Dev*. 1999;36:8–18.

39. Czerniecki JM. Rehabilitation in limb deficiency. 1. Gait and motion analysis. *Arch Phys Med Rehabil*. 1996;77:S3–S8.

40. Perry J, Burnfield JM, Newsam CJ, Conley P. Energy expenditure and gait characteristics of a bilateral amputee walking with C-leg prostheses compared with stubby and conventional articulating prostheses. *Arch Phys Med Rehabil*. 2004;85:1711–1717.

41. Schmalz T, Blumentritt S, Jarasch R. Energy expenditure and biomechanical characteristics of lower limb amputee gait: the influence of prosthetic alignment and different prosthetic components. *Gait Posture*. 2002;16:255–263.

42. Chin T, Sawamura S, Fujita H, et al. %VO2max as an indicator of prosthetic rehabilitation outcome after dysvascular amputation. *Prosthet Orthot Int*. 2002;26:44–49.

Chapter 2

HISTORICAL PERSPECTIVES ON THE CARE OF SERVICE MEMBERS WITH LIMB AMPUTATIONS

JEFFREY S. REZNICK, PhD[*]; JEFF GAMBEL, MD[†]; AND ALAN J. HAWK[‡]

[*]*Director, Institute for the Study of Occupation and Health, American Occupational Therapy Foundation, 4720 Montgomery Lane, Bethesda, Maryland 20824-1220*

[†]*Colonel, Medical Corps, US Army; Physician, Department of Orthopaedics and Rehabilitation, Walter Reed Army Medical Center, 6900 Georgia Avenue NW, Washington, DC 20307*

[‡]*Collections Manager, Historical Collections, National Museum of Health and Medicine, Armed Forces Institute of Pathology, Walter Reed Army Medical Center, 6900 Georgia Avenue, NW, Washington, DC 20306*

INTRODUCTION

Since the US Civil War, philanthropy and military medicine have gone hand-in-hand in various systems of care available to US military service members with limb amputations. As a new century brings changing methods of warfare, this partnership is continued by the major military amputee care centers located across the United States: the Center for the Intrepid (CFI) at Brooke Army Medical Center, San Antonio, Texas; the Comprehensive Combat and Complex Casualty Care at San Diego Naval Medical Center, California; and the Military Advanced Training Center at Walter Reed Army Medical Center, Washington, DC. Altruism helped establish each of these facilities, and it remains vital to their missions of rehabilitating service members with limb amputations and reintegrating these men and women into civilian society.

The CFI emerged chiefly through a fundraising campaign by private citizens Arnold Fisher and Ken Fisher, a father-and-son business team who established and currently oversee the nonprofit Intrepid Fallen Heroes Fund and the Fisher House Foundation. At the CFI and around the country, as explained in Chapter 1, Introduction: Developing a System of Care for the Combat Amputee, these charitable organizations work alongside others in close cooperation with military officials to provide financial, material, and peer support to service members with limb amputations and related injuries, and to the families of service members who have given their lives in current military operations.[1,2]

The other two centers resulted from philanthropy of a different form, namely that of US taxpayers displayed collectively through the US Congress.[3,4] At both sites, and no less at the CFI, nonprofit organizations like those described in Chapter 7, Military and Veteran Support Systems, cooperate with military officials to administer "peer visitor," recreational, and other psychosocial programs for service members with limb loss and other injuries and for their families and loved ones.[5]

This introduction provides historical perspective on these present-day connections between philanthropy and military medicine, defining philanthropy broadly as the altruistic concern for human welfare and advancement manifested by endowment or donations of money, property, or work. The chapter's chief purpose is to inform readers that today's partnership of civilian altruism and military medical rehabilitation has deep roots in the past, taking various forms since the mid-19th century and playing an influential, if underappreciated, role in the care of service members with limb amputations. Understanding this partnership is critical as care providers consider not only current and future surgical and medical care available to these men and women (as discussed in Chapters 8–16) but also the best therapeutic and technological means (as discussed in Chapters 17–27) to enable their best possible health outcome and participation in society despite their physical and psychological challenges.

BACKGROUND

As many historians and medical experts have documented at length in the professional literature, the past 2 centuries have marked significant changes in military technology, tactics, and injuries of service members.[6–11] As firepower on the battlefield evolved from the rifled musket and minié ball of the US Civil War to the explosive artillery and machine gun of World War I to the high-velocity rifle of the Vietnam conflict, surgeons faced ever more serious wounds requiring treatment. Paralleling these changes in firepower were various innovations that combined to increase the odds of surviving wounds in theater. These included technology of transportation, such as the locomotive, automobile, airplane, and helicopter, which separately and together improved evacuation from the front lines, as well as the field of materials science, as armor for individuals and vehicles helped reduce injury. Finally, technological innovations in the field of medicine, such as radiology, aseptic techniques, blood banking, and antibiotics helped improve initial

and long-term treatment.

Current military transport evacuates injured service members from the area of operations to the continental United States more rapidly than in any other time. Patient care during flight continues in the same comprehensive and aggressive manner as it does on the ground, a practice that was largely absent in the past because of technological limits. Upon arrival at a US military hospital, service members with injuries enter into treatment plans shaped by knowledge and practice gleaned from past conflicts and from the best standards of civilian care. For example, patients who have sustained blast injuries have contaminated and dirty wounds. If such wounds are not treated properly, gangrene, sepsis, and death can occur. Aggressive wound irrigation and debridement, placement of antibiotic beads in the wound, soft-tissue grafting, and vacuum-assisted closure are examples of current techniques to salvage injured limbs and maximize the length of residual limbs that require amputation.

Interdisciplinary approaches to care begin in the acute phase and continue through all stages of medical rehabilitation to help patients reach the highest level of recovery possible in subsequent years.

With unique perspectives drawn from the US Civil War to the current global war on terror, this chapter aims to enrich appreciation of the value of philanthropy for care of the combat amputee both today and in the past, as well as the history of medical specialities that constitute the rehabilitation team and philanthropic organizations engaged in the care of both injured service members and their families and loved ones. This historical knowledge puts into perspective the current and future care of injured service members, showing that while their immediate care is a response to wounds sustained in combat, their longer-term physical and psychological rehabilitation should involve critical thinking not only about treatment by the various branches of military and civilian medical science but also about the engagement of civilian philanthropy in renewing their health and social participation.

CIVIL WAR

During the Civil War, amputations constituted approximately 75% of all operations performed, and among Union forces over 21,000 service members survived amputation procedures. Because antiseptics and disinfectants were not yet widely recognized, and specific treatments involving alcohol and opiates had limited success, many patients survived amputations only to suffer devastating postsurgical infections.

The writings of Walt Whitman (Figure 2-1) provide a graphic description of Civil War amputation. In 1863 Whitman traveled from Boston, Massachusetts, to Washington, DC, in search of his brother, George, whose name was listed in a newspaper casualty roster from the battlefield at Fredericksburg. After searching nearly 40 Washington hospitals, Whitman traveled from Washington to Fredericksburg to find George alive with a superficial facial wound. However, Whitman's personal relief quickly turned to horror at the costs of battle (Figure 2-2). As he wrote in his notebook, "I notice a heap of amputated feet, legs, arms, hands, &c . . . human fragments, cut, bloody black and blue, swelled and sickening."[12] Moved by the human dev-

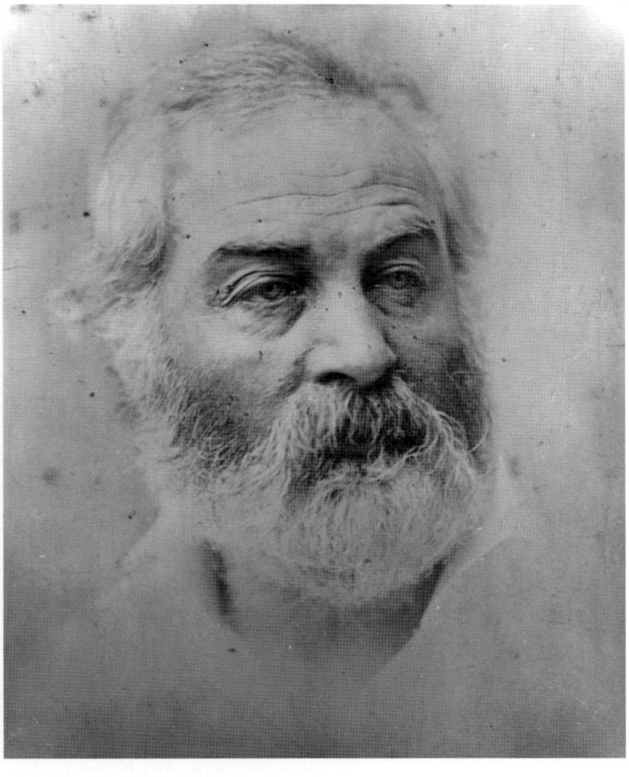

Figure 2-1. Walt Whitman (1819–1892), photographed in 1863, the same year he traveled from Boston to Washington, DC, in search of his brother, George.
Photograph: Courtesy of Library of Congress, Washington, DC. Feinberg-Whitman Collection, LOT 12017, box 1.

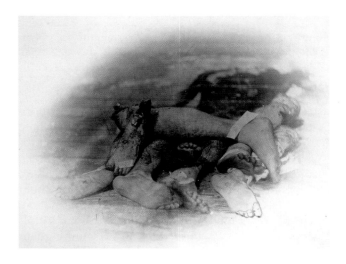

Figure 2-2. Amputations at Harewood Hospital, Washington, DC. This photograph by Dr Reed Bontecou, titled "Field Day," reflects a scene similar to that witnessed by Whitman in Fredericksburg, Virginia.
Photograph: Courtesy of Otis Historical Archives, National Museum of Health and Medicine, Armed Forces Institute of Pathology, Washington, DC. CP 1043.

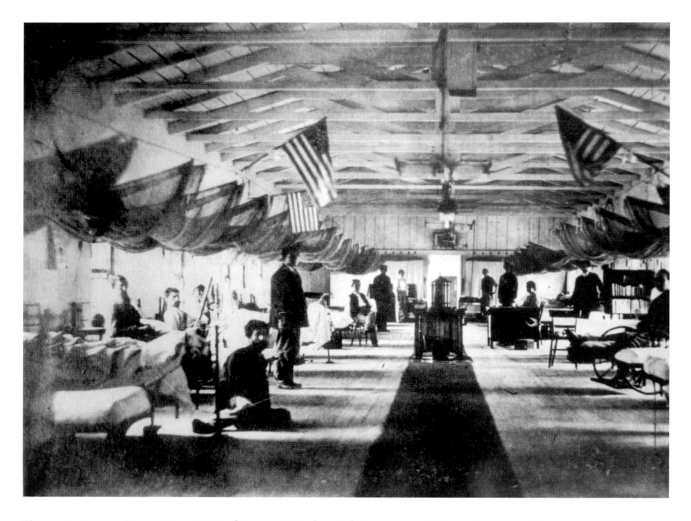

Figure 2-3. Armory Square Hospital, Washington, DC, where Whitman began defining his approach to wartime philanthropy. Photograph: Courtesy of Otis Historical Archives, National Museum of Health and Medicine, Armed Forces Institute of Pathology, Washington, DC. CP 2241.

astation he witnessed, Whitman traveled to Armory Square Hospital in Washington, DC (Figure 2-3), where he developed his own approach to wartime philanthropy by looking after many combat-wounded soldiers, recording their stories, composing letters for them, corresponding with their loved ones, giving them small gifts, and comforting them through conversation.

Hundreds of men benefited from Whitman's philanthropic spirit, including Private Oscar Cunningham of the 82nd Ohio Infantry, who, during the battle of Chancellorsville in May 1863, received a gunshot wound to the right thigh that resulted in a compound fracture. The bullet was extracted at Armory Square Hospital on June 15th by Dr D Willard Bliss (Figure 2-4), the hospital's chief surgeon, whom Whitman later described as "one of the best surgeons in the army."[13] Extensive abscesses formed following the procedure,

and on May 2nd, 1864, Bliss amputated Cunningham's leg and, shortly thereafter, forwarded a portion of it to the Army Medical Museum for preservation as a specimen that could teach future surgeons about military medicine of the day (Figures 2-5). Just after Cunningham's amputation Whitman stated in his journal that "he is in a dying condition—there is no hope for him—it would draw tears from the hardest heart to look at him—he is all wasted away to a skeleton, & looks like some one fifty years old—you remember I told you a year ago, when he was first brought in."[14] Whitman continued, describing Cunningham in his own way as "the noblest specimen of a young western man I had seen, a real giant in size, & always with a smile on his face—O what a change, he has long been very irritable, to every one but me, & his frame is all wasted away."[14]

Cunningham died on June 4, 1864. He was one of the first soldiers to be buried in what was then the new Arlington National Cemetery. His lower thigh bone remains preserved in the modern iteration of the Army Medical Museum, the National Museum of Health and Medicine, Armed Forces Institute of Pathology, as a reminder not only of surgical technique but also of the suffering endured by so many soldiers during the Civil War, as well as the comfort offered by Walt Whitman to hundreds of them.

Unlike Cunningham and thousands of other soldiers with limb amputations, thousands more survived the war with limb loss (Figures 2-6 through 2-8). Those who served the Union received prostheses from the federal government, and those who served

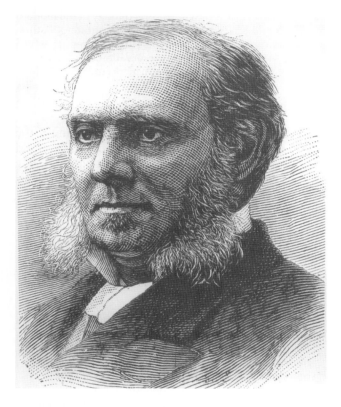

Figure 2-4. DW Bliss. At Armory Square Hospital, Whitman observed the work of Dr D Willard Bliss, the chief surgeon, whom Whitman described as "one of the best surgeons in the army." After the war, Bliss praised Whitman for his service to the nation's soldiers. "No one person who assisted in the hospitals during the war accomplished so much good to the soldier and for the Government as Mr. Whitman." Quotation from: Donaldson T. *Walt Whitman the Man*. New York, NY: Francis P Harper; 1896: 169.
Photograph: Courtesy of Otis Historical Archives, National Museum of Health and Medicine, Armed Forces Institute of Pathology, Washington, DC. NCP 1858.

the Confederacy received such technology from individual southern states. In both instances, however, many of the residual limbs produced by surgery were not conducive to fitting and wearing artificial limbs. Ragged tissue and protruding bones, or bones left close to the surface of the skin, caused immense pain and frustration for amputees who tried to use prostheses. Images of the period, in the form of photographs and paintings, fall short of conveying the difficulties faced by veterans with limb loss.

These challenges—combined with the sheer number of amputees produced by the war, and later by factories and railroad accidents—helped drive wartime and postwar entrepreneurialism in the nascent field of prosthetics.[15] In the 15 years before the war, 34 patents were issued for artificial limbs and assisting devices; during the 12 years from the beginning of the war to 1873, 133 patents for limbs were issued, nearly a 300% increase.[16] Among these was a patent held by James Edward Hanger, a Confederate soldier who, after losing his leg at the battle of Philippi, returned to his hometown of Churchville, Virginia. There, he developed what became known as the "Hanger limb" (Figure 2-9), which changed the so-called American leg by adding rubber bumpers to the ankle, and later a rubber foot, a forerunner of the solid-ankle, cushioned heel foot. Other patents of the day, often described prominently in advertising literature, included those held by George R Fuller of Rochester, New York (Figure 2-10), and AA Marks of New York, New York (Figure 2-11).

While Whitman exemplified individual philanthropy, contemporary voluntary aid organizations represented the philanthropy of communities in helping combat amputees acquire prostheses and other necessary aid, primarily because large numbers of combat casualties, and even larger numbers of sick soldiers, quickly overwhelmed the Army Medical Corps following the battle of Bull Run in 1861.[17,18] The acting Army Surgeon General, Colonel RC Wood, described the situation:

The pressure upon the Medical Bureau has been very great and urgent; and though all the means at its disposal have been industriously used, much remains to be accomplished by directing the intelligent mind of the country to practical results connected with the comforts of the soldier by preventive and sanitary means. The Medical Bureau would, in my judgment, derive important and useful aid from the counsels and well-directed efforts of an intelligent and scientific commission, to be styled 'A Commission of Inquiry and Advice in respect of the Sanitary Interests of the United States Forces,' and acting in co-operation with the Bureau, in elaborating and applying such facts as might be elicited from the experience

a

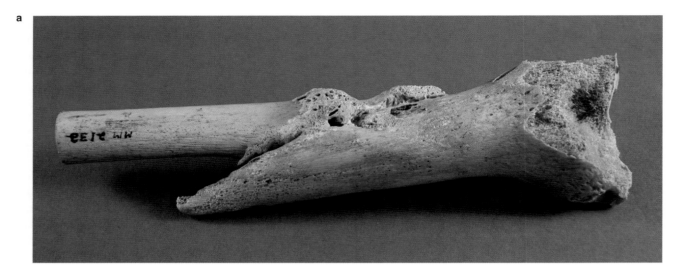

Figure 2-5. (a) Lower thigh bone of Private Oscar Cunningham, 82nd Ohio Infantry, which is preserved today in the modern iteration of the Army Medical Museum, the National Museum of Health and Medicine, Armed Forces Institute of Pathology, Washington, DC. **(b)** [*following page*] Description of Cunningham's injury by Dr Bliss, from his surgeon's report, which accompanied Cunningham's remains when Bliss sent them to the Army Medical Museum for preservation.
Photographs: Courtesy of Anatomical Collections, National Museum of Health and Medicine, Armed Forces Institute of Pathology, Washington, DC. Accession no. 1000755.

and more extended observation of those connected with armies, with reference to the diet and hygiene of troops, and the organization of Military Hospitals, etc. This Commission is not intended to interfere with, but to strengthen the present organization, introducing and elaborating such improvements as the advanced stage of Medical Science might suggest.[19]

Thus was born the US Sanitary Commission, which, alongside the US Christian Commission, mobilized thousands of volunteers in support of Union soldiers (Figure 2-12).

Different approaches initially emerged among these groups, but they were eventually resolved as both volunteers and military officers settled into appreciating their respective contributions.[20] The medical department, quartermasters corps, and various civilian relief agencies cooperated to evacuate the wounded after the battle of Gettysburg. Finding 2,000 wounded men awaiting transportation at the nearby railroad, Dr Edward P Vollum, a medical inspector with the office of the Surgeon General, immediately began organizing their evacuation to hospitals in New York, New York; Baltimore, Maryland; and York, Pennsylvania. Vollum described the collaborative effort: "Before leaving, the wounded were fed and watered by the Sanitary Commission, and often hundreds of wounded, laid over for a night or part of the day, were attended and fed by the commission whose agents placed them in the cars. At Hanover Junction, they were again refreshed and fed by the Christian Commission, at Baltimore the agents of several benevolent societies distributed food bountifully to the wounded in the cars immediately on their arrival; and at Harrisburg, the commissary department had made arrangements for feeding any number likely to pass that way."[21]

By the end of the war, the Sanitary Commission had played a central role in establishing programs and policies to help reintegrate disabled soldiers into postwar, civilian society. One of its representatives described the commission's work:

It seemed to us, that our pride, as a democratic nation ought to point . . . towards such a shaping of public opinion as would tend to reduce dependence among our returning soldiers to the lowest possible point; to quicken the local and family sense of responsibility, so as to make each neighborhood and each household, out of which a soldier had gone, and returned helpless and dependent, feel itself privileged and bound to take care of him . . . to encourage every community to do its utmost towards favoring the employment of returned soldiers, and especially, partially disabled ones in all light occupations . . . In short, we desired to favor in every way the proud and beneficent tendency of our vigorous American civilization, to heal its wounds by the first intention; to absorb the sick and wounded men into its ordinary life, providing for them through those domestic and neighborly sympathies, that local watchfulness and furtherance due to the weakness and wants of men well known to

b

No 2254

7-1-25

Amputation of Right Thigh

Oscar "HC" Cunningham" Private Co "I" 82" Ohio Vol. was wounded at the battle of Chancellorsville May 2" 1863" Entered Armory Square hospital June 15" 1863. with Gun Shot wound of right thigh." the ball Entered "on terior aspect of middle third passed backwards — producing a compound fracture of Femur the ball was Extracted by Surgeon in charge. the missle was a round or Conical ball subsequently Erysipelas of the cellulo cutaneous variety occured Involving the entire Extremity. Extensive Abscesses followed" the constitution became involved and suffered greatly from supperative and irritative fever" On the 2nd of May 1864" the thigh was amputated at the upper third. which Operation was performed by Surgeon In Charge" In the Operation the double lateral flaps were made by transfixion. hemorrhage was controlled by Compression of the artery underneath poupart's ligament" And but little blood lost. About the Usual number of vessels were tied in the flaps — which however were found to be unhealthy — affected by neighboring Abscesses. meeting at a projecting centre the flaps formed a very good but somewhat conical stump —

There was found Some necrosis indicated before Operation by the

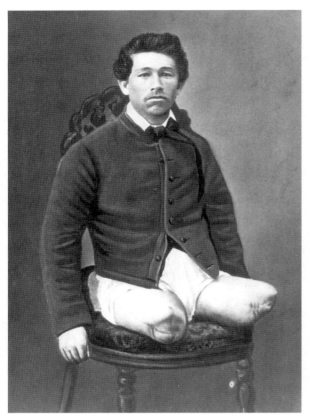

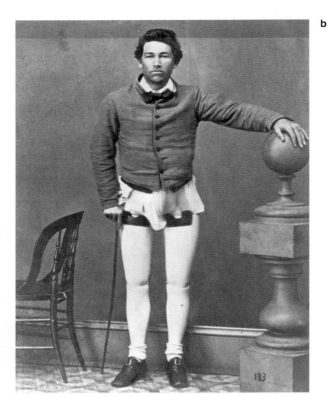

Figure 2-6. (a) Among the thousands who survived the US Civil War with limb loss was Private Columbus G Rush, Co C, 21st Georgia Regiment, who was wounded in an assault on Fort Sheridan, in the lines before Petersburg, Virginia, March 25, 1865, by a fragment of a shell. **(b)** Private Rush fitted with prostheses. Descriptive text on the reverse of this photo states that "with the aid of two canes he was enabled to walk about the wards of St. Luke's Hospital, New York, where he was transferred after amputation was completed at Lincoln Hospital, Washington, DC."
Photographs: Courtesy of Otis Historical Archives, National Museum of Health and Medicine, Armed Forces Institute of Pathology, Washington, DC. SP 132 (a); SP 133 (b).

their fellow citizens, and which is given without pride and received without humiliation; and this source of relief failing, then from the ordinary charities of the towns and counties from which they had sprung.[22]

More than rhetoric, these words represent an important opening chapter in the history of wartime and immediate postwar care for service members generally and those with limb amputations in particular.

WORLD WAR I

In May 1918 the French and Belgian ministries of war worked with their American and European counterparts to convene the second annual international conference and exhibition on the "after-care" of soldiers disabled in the ongoing war. Meeting in London, England, leading medical authorities, philanthropy representatives, labor leaders, and public figures exchanged views on two vital questions: (1) how could soldiers injured in the war be healed effectively, and (2) how could they be successfully reintegrated into civilian society after returning home? Officials at the

previous conference (held in Paris in May 1917) had examined these questions in detail, but the military campaigns of 1917 made efforts to rehabilitate the wounded all the more vital for the welfare of the soldiers as well as their families, communities, and nations.

Philanthropy was a key component of this conference. Its face was in part that of John Galsworthy (Figure 2-13), the British writer (and later a 1932 Nobel laureate in literature), who since the war began had donated time, writing talents, and thousands of dollars

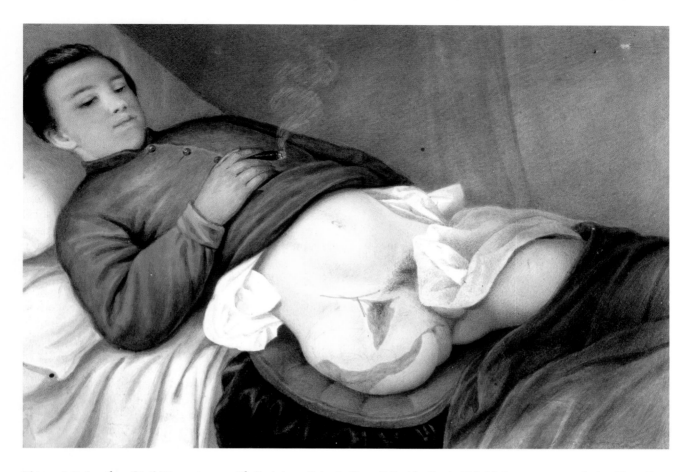

Figure 2-7. Another Civil War veteran with limb loss, Private Eben E Smith, Co A, 11th Maine, was wounded at Deep Bottom, Virginia, August 16, 1864, by a musket ball through the right leg. He survived the amputation of his right leg at the hip. Painting by Peter Baumgras.
Photograph: Courtesy of Otis Historical Archives, National Museum of Health and Medicine, Armed Forces Institute of Pathology, Washington, DC. CWMI 006.

of his literary earnings to support what he called "the sacred work": the rehabilitation of servicemen severely injured physically or psychologically in battle.[23] In the introduction to the official conference proceedings, Galsworthy characterized its goals:

> In special hospitals orthopaedic [sic], paraplegic, neurasthenic, we shall give him back functional ability, solidity of nerve or lung. The flesh torn away, the lost sight, the broken ear-drum, the destroyed nerve, it is true we cannot give back; but we shall so re-create and fortify the rest of him that he shall leave hospital ready for a new career. Then we shall teach him how to treat the road of it, so that he fits again into the national life, becomes once more a workman with pride in his work, a stake in the country and the consciousness that, handicapped though he be, he runs the race level with his fellows and is by that so much the better man than they.[24]

These observations encapsulate the contemporary work being undertaken in Britain's network of military orthopaedic hospitals, approaches that eventually informed US systems of care for service members with limb loss.

The flagship of Britain's network was Shepherd's Bush Military Orthopaedic Hospital, located in London, where rehabilitation before discharge involved not only prosthetics but also therapeutic work. In the "curative workshops" of Shepherd's Bush and its counterpart institutions throughout the United Kingdom, medical staff used water, weights, and electricity in an effort to repair both body and mind. At the same time, they promoted another form of rehabilitative work as a way to prepare disabled soldiers for reentry into civilian life. Vocational labor, medical authorities held, helped to return soldiers to civilian life as healthy individuals, as able-bodied breadwinners, and

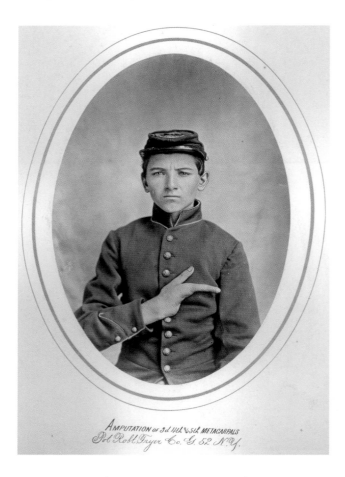

Figure 2-8. Another Civil War veteran with limb loss, Private Robert Fryer, Co G, 52nd New York, was wounded at Hatcher's Run, Virginia, and subsequently required amputation of his third, fourth, and fifth metacarpals.
Photograph: Courtesy of Otis Historical Archives, National Museum of Health and Medicine, Armed Forces Institute of Pathology, Washington, DC. CP 1041.

as productive citizens.[25,26] In achieving this objective, philanthropic support was critical, and it came chiefly in the form of the Joint War Committee of the British Red Cross and Order of St John. In October 1916, this entity awarded an initial £1,000 grant to Shepherd's Bush. This sum was followed by a £10,000 grant in 1918. Supplementing these funds throughout the war were thousands of pounds donated directly by the public to both Shepherd's Bush and its associated facilities across the country.[27]

By 1918 comparable rehabilitation programs had emerged in the United States, chiefly as a result of contact between British and American medical personnel. Among the surgeons at Shepherd's Bush was Joel Goldthwait, a Harvard-trained orthopaedic surgeon from

Boston General Hospital, who in late 1916 led a team of 2 dozen American orthopaedic surgeons in studying methods used by the Allies to heal combat-wounded soldiers. Goldthwait was particularly impressed with the organization and administration of the institution's curative workshops. The use of work as both treatment and retraining, Goldthwait believed during the closing months of 1917, could be implemented in the United States to help deal effectively with the increasing number of American disabled soldiers returning home, a number that eventually exceeded 4,000.

Goldthwait's recommendations to the surgeon general yielded plans to train teachers and medical aides to assist in the rehabilitation of America's service members disabled in the war. Called "reconstruction aides" (Figure 2-14), these individuals aimed to "to hasten the recovery of the patients . . . promote contentment and make the atmosphere of these hospitals such that the time spent in convalescence will pass most pleasantly because the minds and hands of the patients are properly occupied in profitable pursuits."[28] The work of these individuals received the support of most physicians and orthopaedic surgeons, and contributed greatly to the wartime and postwar expansion of the fields of occupational therapy and physical therapy.

A leading institution within America's network of rehabilitation centers was the Red Cross Institute for Crippled and Disabled Men in New York. In part through a $265,000 federal appropriation but largely through the generosity of wartime philanthropy directed to the Red Cross by the philanthropist Jeremiah Millbank, the institute offered a range of vocational training in constructing artificial limbs, welding, painting, business accounting, and mechanical drafting. It also included complementary departments of research, employment, surveys, and public education that, by October 1919, produced 7 million public-information pamphlets, sponsored 300 public lectures, and completed over 500 industrial surveys involving 1,500 factories and 100 trade associations, all to the end of empowering the disabled soldier to "win his own way to self-respect and self-support."[29,30]

Posters produced by the institution and displayed in its lobby, as well as in public spaces around New York City, incorporated images of physical reconstruction efforts being undertaken in US and Allied military hospitals (Figure 2-15). Conveying the philosophy of occupation as a vital means to helping the disabled reclaim participation in the fabric of postwar life, the images illustrate the historical roots of occupational therapy, physical therapy, and vocational rehabilitation (see Chapter 6).

INTERWAR PERIOD

Between World War I and World War II military "reconstruction centers" decreased in size substantially, and many disabled veterans found agencies like the Red Cross Institute ill-prepared to help them reenter civilian society. During this period Captain Robert S Marx (Figure 2-16), a wounded veteran, established an organization called Disabled American Veterans of the World War I. Under the leadership of Marx, the organization became a champion of the disabled veterans' cause. A year after he established the group, Marx called a national caucus of 250 disabled veterans, drawing together one of the first major associations to advocate for improved public services on behalf of disabled veterans. Disabled American Veterans remained active through World War II and continues its efforts today in cooperation with federal agencies and a constellation of other philanthropic organizations, including the American Legion, Paralyzed Veterans of America, and Vietnam Veterans of America Foundation.

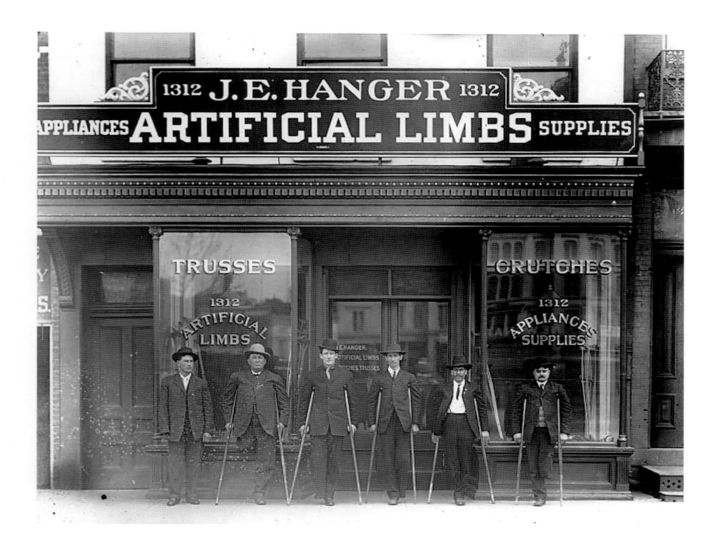

Figure 2-9. Six men, likely Civil War veterans, standing with the aid of their "Hanger limbs" near a JE Hanger storefront. Photograph commissioned by the JE Hanger Company. Undated but likely ca 1870–1880.
Photograph: Courtesy of Library of Congress, Washington, DC. CM Bell Collection of Glass Negatives.

WORLD WAR II AND THE IMMEDIATE POSTWAR ERA

By the Second World War, improvements in armor, aircraft, and radio communications that allowed for combined air/land operations tipped the scales in favor of offensive operations. Instead of the trench warfare that characterized World War I, combat tactics emphasized mobility. The new nature of combat changed the type of wounds sustained by soldiers. Lower extremity injuries involving bone and soft tissue represented 42% of the 20,747 battle casualties sustained by the Fifth US Army between August 1, 1944, and May 2, 1945, in contrast to 47% of casualties during the First World War. Upper extremity injuries accounted for 26% of the same sample during World War II, compared with 39% of World War I casualties.[31,32] Improvements in surgical technique, whole blood for transfusion, and antibiotics increased the chances of those wounded in the abdomen, while better methods for treating gunshot fractures, notably improved methods of traction and internal fixation of fractures, minimized the number of amputations performed.

Approximately 18,000 Americans sustained an amputation as a result of combat in World War II. However, the reason for loss of the limb had changed. One study concluded that 20% of the amputations resulted from arterial damage, while 80% were the result of "irreparable damage," usually from a land mine or artillery.[33] "When the limb was irretrievably shattered and mangled or was almost completely avulsed," reported Mather Cleveland, senior consultant in orthopaedic surgery in the European theater of operations during World War II, "the attending surgeon had no choice but to amputate it. In effect, a nearly complete traumatic amputation had already been performed, and it was his clear duty to complete it."[34] Germany's routine use of land mines as a defensive measure during the Italian campaign of 1944–1945 increased the number of US lower limb amputations. In 1943 land mines were responsible for approximately 15% of all amputations, but caused almost 36% in 1944–1945.[35]

By this period, rehabilitation of the combat-injured service member began in the combat zone. Military

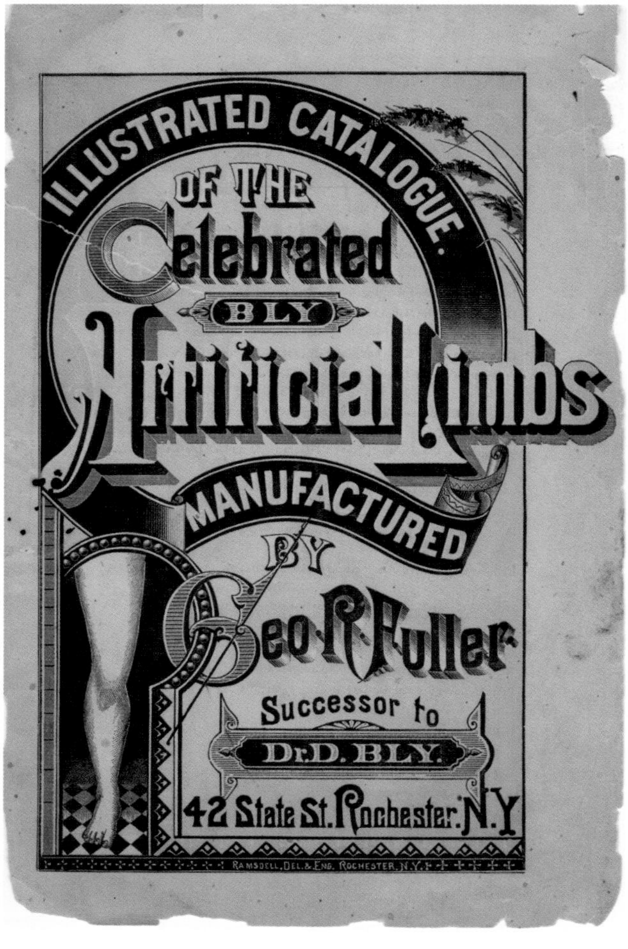

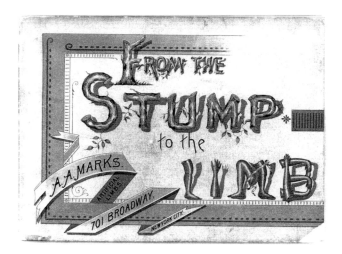

Figure 2-10. Advertising literature published by artificial limb manufacturer George R Fuller of Rochester, New York. Undated but likely 1870–1890.
Photograph: Courtesy of Warshaw Collection of Business Americana, National Museum of American History, Washington, DC.

Figure 2-11. Advertising literature published by artificial limb manufacturer AA Marks of New York, New York. Undated but likely ca 1900.
Photograph: Courtesy of Warshaw Collection of Business Americana, National Museum of American History, Washington, DC.

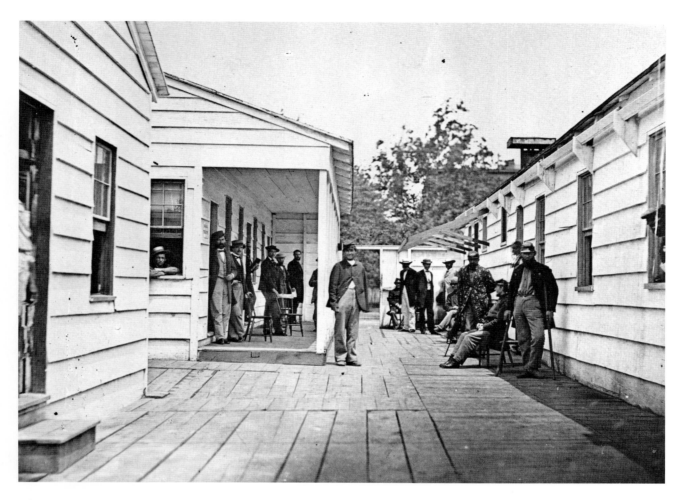

Figure 2-12. A US Sanitary Commission rest house in Washington, DC, where volunteers gathered in support of sick and wounded soldiers. Undated but likely 1863–1864.
Photograph: Courtesy of Prints and Photographs Division, Library of Congress, Washington, DC. Civil War Glass Negative Collection. LC-B811-1201.

medical authorities encouraged surgeons to focus on the whole patient as opposed to a single procedure. Circular letter no. 46, issued in August 1944 by Headquarters, North African Theater of Operations, contained details of this protocol, emphasizing "that casualties who required amputation should be told before operation, whenever their condition permitted, why this procedure was necessary. It was also suggested that, as soon as the patient was surgically comfortable and mentally receptive, an interview with a psychiatrist or chaplain might be useful. These instructions were based on the fact that about 1 in every 5 patients could be expected to exhibit psychic reactions, often depressive in type, a few days after operation." Additionally, the circular indicated that "particular attention was to be paid in this and other interviews to what the soldier might reasonably expect in the way

of aid. He was to be told of the amputation centers which had been established in the Zone of Interior, the prosthetic appliances which were available, and the economic and other aid which he could be assured of receiving. Fortification of this kind before the patient became the target of sympathetic family and friends," the circular letter pointed out, "might tip the scales in favor of rehabilitation, while its omission might result in lifelong disability and resentment."[36p328]

As in previous conflicts, philanthropy played an important role in the rehabilitation of World War II service members who suffered limb amputations. Dr Howard Rusk (Figure 2-17) embraced the "whole patient" concept in his techniques to help injured Air Force personnel. As he described the first Air Force rehabilitation center at Pawling, New York: "I guess you might describe [it] as a combination of a hospital,

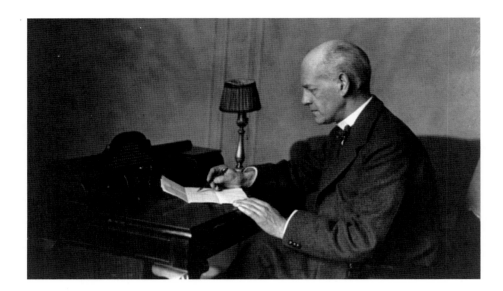

Figure 2-13. John Galsworthy (1867–1933), the British writer and later Nobel laureate who donated his time, writing talents, and thousands of dollars of literary earnings to support what he called "the sacred work": the rehabilitation of servicemen who were severely injured physically and psychologically in World War I. Photograph dated 1919.
Photograph: Courtesy of Prints and Photographs Division, Library of Congress, Washington, DC. George Grantham Bain Collection, Biography file.

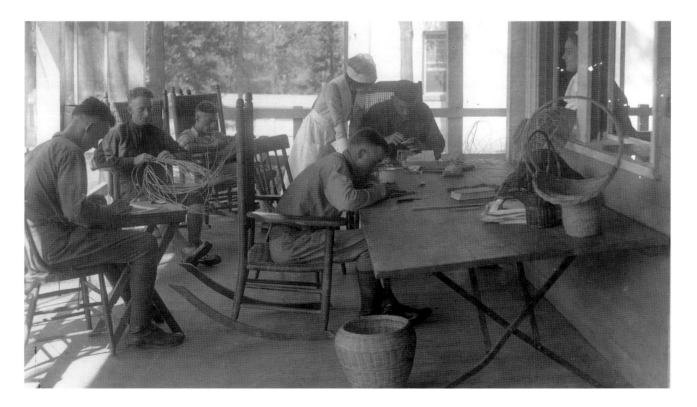

Figure 2-14. Occupational therapy at Walter Reed Hospital during the First World War. A reconstruction aide supervises the work of one soldier while her colleague observes the group.
Photograph: Courtesy of Otis Historical Archives, National Museum of Health and Medicine, Armed Forces Institute of Pathology, Washington, DC. Reeve 4272.

a country club, a school, a farm, a vocational training center, a resort, and a little bit of home as well. The discipline was minimal and the program informal. Old regular Army people would have shuddered, but fortunately General Arnold didn't have the traditional Army man's outlook [as he] reaffirmed his full support of the program and his conviction that it would prove its worth, not only by returning men to healthy lives, but by returning many of them to duty."[36] Rusk's approach helped establish many of the principles of rehabilitation later incorporated into the programs of the Institute of Rehabilitation at New York University, an institution that had a large impact nationally and internationally on the field.[37]

The efforts of Major General Norman Thomas Kirk (Figure 2-18) were also instrumental in the care of America's combat amputees during and after World War II. Based on his experiences in World War I, when he established himself chiefly at Walter Reed as a leading authority on amputations, Kirk helped establish multidisciplinary amputee centers around the country to provide up-to-date surgical, medical, prosthetic, and rehabilitative care. Later, as Army Surgeon General, Kirk asked the National Research Council to set up a committee on prosthetic devices to provide leadership and coordination of the emerg-

ing federal programs in the Army Surgeon General's Office of Scientific Research and Development and Veterans Administration.[38] According to historians and rehabilitation experts alike, these initiatives were dramatically successful, helping to make 1945 to 1975 one of the most productive periods in US prosthetics and rehabilitation research, benefiting both combat and civilian amputees.[39–41]

Philanthropy also joined military medicine through the activities of Dr Bernard Baruch (Figure 2-19), who funded the Baruch Committee on Physical Medicine in 1943. Chaired by Dr Ray Lyman Wilbur and composed of subcommittees on education, teaching, research, public relations, rehabilitation, hydrology, occupational therapy, prevention, and body mechanics, this group aimed to expand the medical specialty of physical medicine and rehabilitation and maximize its contribution to the care of injured soldiers and sailors. Baruch's generosity advanced the field of physical medicine as well as rehabilitative care for service members with limb amputations, paving the way to recognition that amputations are lifelong injuries, with sequelae requiring adequate support from federal agencies like the Veterans Administration as well as the philanthropic societies that are equally invested in the successful rehabilitation of veterans with disability.

KOREA AND VIETNAM

The Korean conflict was marked by extreme mobility during the 1st year of the war as North Korean and United Nations troops engaged along the Korean Peninsula. As the forces counterbalanced each other, 2 years of trench warfare followed. During this period medical authorities applied lessons learned from World War II in the form of helicopter ambulances and the mobile Army surgical hospital to help ensure that seriously wounded soldiers received prompt medical care and better odds of survival. The issuance of soft body armor complemented this effort. Of the final 7,200 United Nations soldiers wounded in Korea, 56% sustained injury to their extremities. As in the Second World War, surgeons performed amputations primarily on "extremities hopelessly destroyed by trauma or infection or both."[42] The number of cases requiring amputation decreased as a result of improved vascular surgery. Of the 16,890 simple and compound fractures sustained by soldiers during the war, only 1,477 amputations were performed, in addition to 1,120 traumatic amputations. Over 70% of the wounds resulting in amputations were caused by explosive projectiles, grenades, and land mines.[43] During the Second World War, one study found that 50% of 2,471 arterial wounds resulted in amputation. Vascular surgery was

attempted in 81 cases with a failure (and subsequent amputation) rate of 36%. A study during the Korean conflict reported that only 26 (13%) of the 194 vascular repairs failed, resulting in amputation.[44]

The Vietnam War brought a different style of warfare. Lighter weapons increased the amount of firepower that could be carried by infantry. New rifles such as the Colt M-16 and the Kalashnikov AK-47 fired high-velocity bullets that pulverized bone. US forces frequently operated from fixed firebases and sent patrols to monitor surrounding territory, and rather than risk direct contact, the Viet Cong preferred to deploy a wide variety of land mines, booby traps, and punji sticks along major paths and patrol routes. These weapons increased crippling wounds to the lower extremities by 300% compared to World War II and 70% compared to Korea. Over 5,200 US soldiers lost limbs in Vietnam.[9,10,45]

During the period ca 1950 to 1975 service members with limb loss had a much higher survival rate than in World War II and previous wars primarily because of improved resuscitation and surgical repair of damaged blood vessels, as well as better evacuation of soldiers from the frontlines to better equipped and more sanitary care facilities. However, as Colonel

a

GOOD USE OF TIME IN HOSPITAL

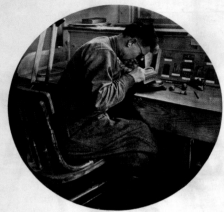

The period of treatment in hospital can be put to good use by men who will be discharged cured as well as by men who will be permanently disabled. This soldier at Walter Reed Hospital in Washington is enjoying instruction in the elements of engraving.

b

AT WORK AGAIN

A good substitute for a lost right arm enables this poilu to take up wood-turning at the School of Re-education at Montpellier, France.

BACK TO THE FARM

A double arm amputation did not keep this Frenchman from joining the army of workers after he was discharged from the army of fighters. He was taught farming at Lyons, France.

Physical handicaps are made up for so far as possible by modern artificial appliances—"Working Prostheses" they are called—which replace the missing limb. Men in the mechanical trades are fitted with chucks in which can be fitted interchangeably the various tools of their calling.

c

FIRST STEPS TO USEFULNESS

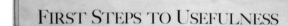

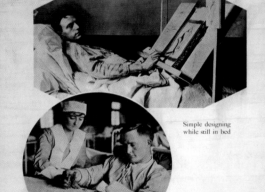

Simple designing while still in bed

An American soldier begins again to take an interest in life

Bedside and ward occupations serve to interest wounded men and keep their minds active and off their own troubles. Occupation is also one of the best curative agents at the command of the physician, and in most cases it does much to expedite recovery. Gone are the old days when men lay for months in a hospital bed gazing at the ceiling and brooding about the future.

d

Disabled Serbians Working in the Carpentry Shop at Lyons, France

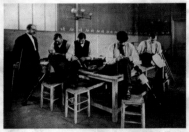

A Tailoring Class in Paris Taught by a One-legged Instructor

In France, Two Popular Trades Taught Disabled Soldiers Are Cabinet-making and Tailoring

Figure 2-15 *(preceding page).* Wartime exhibition posters developed and used by the Red Cross Institute for Crippled and Disabled Men and the Red Cross Institute for the Blind during World War I. **(a)** A soldier recovering from war wounds at Walter Reed Hospital and learning the craft of engraving. **(b)** Disabled French soldiers using "working prostheses" to perform manual labor in a woodworking shop and on a farm. **(c)** Two scenes of men in hospitals recovering from war wounds through occupational therapy. **(d)** Two scenes in which disabled French and Serbian soldiers are being taught useful skills to enable them to find employment upon discharge from military service.
Photographs: Courtesy of Prints and Photographs Division, Library of Congress, Washington, DC. POS – WWI – US, no. 43 (a); no. 30 (b); no. 44 (c); no. 46 (d).

Paul W Brown observed in his history of Vietnam-era amputee care that until the early years of Vietnam, the approach to wartime amputee care had changed little from that of World Wars I and II and the Korean War: heal the stump, fit it with a prosthesis, train the patient in its use, and discharge him to civilian life. Although advances in prosthetics and orthotics contributed to better function, and the addition of vocational counseling and driver education to some degree rendered the adjustment to civilian life easier, progress in programs to help amputees live lives as normal as possible had not been significant. All management programs had been directed toward what was lost, not toward what had been retained. Only when the number of amputees began climbing rapidly in 1967 were methods explored to expand their total rehabilitation through motiva-

tional therapeutic programs. Such an initiative was described by Dr Timothy Dillingham in the previous edition of this textbook:

a unique aspect of care at the Fitzsimons General Hospital was the amputee skiing program. Over 100 amputees treated during 1968 and 1969 learned to ski using adaptive aids. These casualties gained confidence and an enhanced sense that even with their disabilities they could find challenges and enjoyment through skiing and other recreational activities. [One contemporary] described the incredible psychological trauma involved with amputation, and the Fitzsimons program stressed treatment of the whole

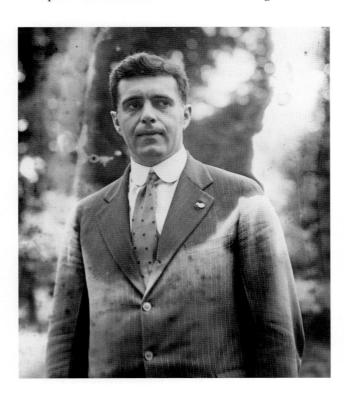

Figure 2-16. Judge Robert S Marx, National Commander, Disabled American Veterans of the World War, ca 1921.
Photograph: Courtesy of Library of Congress, Washington, DC. National Photo Company Collection, LC-F8-14813.

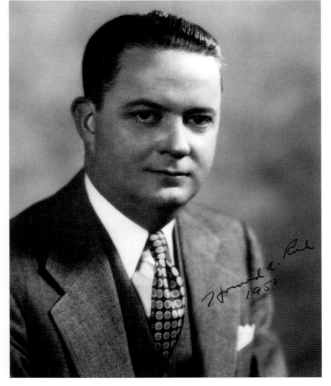

Figure 2-17. Dr Howard Rusk, who embraced the "whole patient" in his techniques to help injured Air Force personnel during World War II. Photograph ca 1950.
Photograph: Courtesy of History of Medicine Division, National Library of Medicine, Bethesda, Maryland.

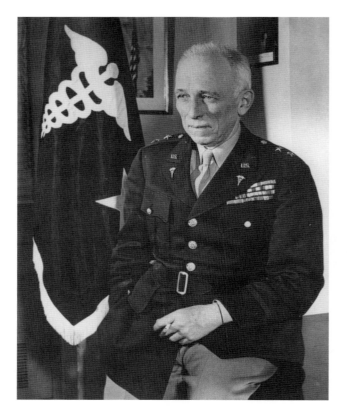

Figure 2-18. Norman Kirk, who, during World War II, used his experiences in World War I to help establish multidisciplinary amputee centers around the country to provide up-to-date surgical, medical, prosthetic, and rehabilitative care.
Photograph: Courtesy of Otis Historical Archives, National Museum of Health and Medicine, Armed Forces Institute of Pathology, Washington, DC. Medical Illustration Service Library. MIS57-07732-33.

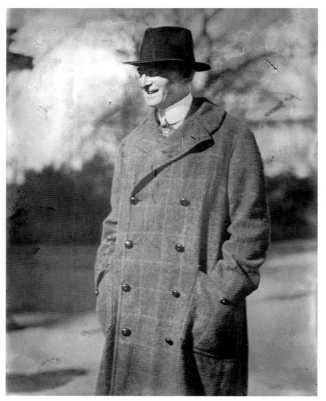

Figure 2-19. Bernard Baruch, who generously funded the Baruch Committee on Physical Medicine in 1943.
Photograph: Courtesy of Library of Congress, Washington, DC. George Grantham Bain Collection, LC-B2-4110-12.

individual with the goal of returning the soldier to an optimal level of function. The recreational activities had a positive impact on the mental well being of the soldier and were a vital part of the rehabilitation plan.[46]

The roots of rehabilitative athletics can be traced in part to the years immediately following World War II, when the English neurologist Sir Ludwig Guttmann organized a sports competition for veterans with spinal cord injuries. This competition eventually became known as the Stoke Mandeville Games. In 1952 competitors from the Netherlands took part in these games, giving an international character to the initiative and paving the way to the first Paralymic Games, held in Rome, Italy, in 1960.[47] Today the Paralympics are one of the greatest influences on the development of prostheses and their use by people with amputations. Whereas the 1960 games involved 400 athletes from 23

countries and limited, if any, media coverage or support by the prosthetics field, the Athens Games of 2004 involved 3,806 athletes from 136 countries competing under the eye of major media coverage—broadcast by the CBS television network and sponsored by Getty Images among other companies—as well as corporate support of Visa, Otto Bock HealthCare, Samsung, and Edelman, the world's largest independent public relations firm.[48] The Paralymics have also become one of the largest and most important showcases of the physical potential of people with disabilities and the power of prosthetic technology. In conjunction with affiliated nonprofit organizations, including the Challenged Athletes Foundation, Disabled Sports USA, and Orthotic and Prosthetic Assistance Fund (among many others described in Chapter 25), and with federal initiatives such as the National Veterans Winter Sports Clinic and National Disabled Veterans Wheelchair Games, both sponsored by the Department of Veterans Affairs and Paralyzed Veterans of America, the Paralympics help promote opportunities for disabled veterans and others to participate in competitive sports, at local, national, and international levels. And as an opportunity for the prosthetic industry to sponsor individual athletes as well as entire teams, the Paralympics help advance developments in prosthetic design and function. Today, dozens if not hundreds of disability-focused nonprofit organizations complement the mission of the Paralympics, which, in addition to providing athletic opportunities and advancing the field, expands public awareness of ability despite limb loss. The charitable work of these organizations is a current chapter in the history of philanthropy and military medical care working in tandem toward the rehabilitation of the service members with limb amputations.

CURRENT CONFLICTS

Current conflicts have reversed this declining trend of amputations among wounded service members, and recent studies have shown that major limb amputation rates for the current US engagements are similar to those of previous conflicts.[49] The nature of combat has changed as sensors, precision-guided munitions, and robotic weapons have made military formations of the opposing forces, even those taking advantage of the civilian population for cover and concealment, increasingly vulnerable. Suicide bombers and mechanical ambushes have proven to be a deadly tactic against a highly mobile military force. The land mine of World War II and punji stick of the Vietnam War have given way to the improvised explosive device. To treat the wounds caused by these new weapons military surgeons are using new medical technology such as hemostatic bandages that stop massive bleeding and miniaturized resuscitation devices that place the technology of an intensive care unit near or on the frontlines of battle. Emerging prosthetic technology holds greater promise than ever before. But so too does the altruism of private citizens and civilian organizations involved in providing rehabilitation and support programs to service members with limb loss and other injuries, and to their families and loved ones.

SUMMARY

If history is any guide, the partnership of US military medicine and the generosity of citizens will take on new forms as researchers follow the "roadmap for future research" described in Chapter 28, and assess its outcomes both for individuals with amputations and those with polytrauma and related conditions of 21st century warfare. History helps put this research and practice into perspective, showing that rehabilitation should involve critical thinking not only about medicine but also about the role of society in caring for military service members with limb amputations and in defining renewed occupations, social participation, and overall health of service members despite their physical and psychological challenges. This role is reflected by the diversity of professionals on the rehabilitation team, including anthropologists, economists, demographers, historians, psychologists, sociologists, and statisticians, and the current and potential future contributions of social scientists to rehabilitation research and to the reintegration into society of men and women who have sustained severe injury in service to the nation.

The history surveyed here is valuable in much the same way as taking a medical history is central to care of an individual with limb loss. That process involves discovery of the past, or as one physician described it, "acceptance of the truth that to care for the patient today, the patient of the past must be examined too."[50] This history reveals how today's service members with limb amputations receive care within systems with roots as much in past medical lessons learned as in the altruism of individuals and communities who care deeply about the rehabilitation of these veterans and their renewed health and participation in postwar, civilian society.

REFERENCES

1. Wilson E. America supports you: Army vice chief awards medals at new rehab center. US Department of Defense, American Forces Press Service Web site. Available at: www.defenselink.mil/news/newsarticle.aspx?id=2844. Accessed April 23, 2008.

2. Wilson E. $50 million rehabilitation center opens on Fort Sam Houston. US Army, Army.mil/News Web site. Available at: www.army.mil/-news/2007/01/30/1570-50-million-rehabilitation-center-opens-on-fort-sam-houston/. Accessed April 23, 2008.

3. Baker FW. New amputee care center opens at Walter Reed. Department of Defense, American Forces Press Service Web site. Available at: www.defenselink.mil/news/newsarticle.aspx?id=47432. Accessed April 23, 2008.

4. Coleman C. Military advanced training center opens at WRAMC. US Army, Army.mil/News Web site.Available at: www.army.mil/-news/2007/09/13/4849-military-advanced-training-center-opens-at-wramc/. Accessed April 23, 2008.

5. Liewer S. Talking to the guys who have been through it. *San Diego Union-Tribune*. August 28, 2007. Available at: www.signonsandiego.com/uniontrib/20070828/news_1n28amputee.html. Accessed April 23, 2008.

6. Dougherty PJ. Wartime amputations. *Mil Med*. 1993;158(12):755–763.

7. Hardaway RM. Wound shock: a history of its study and treatment by military surgeons. *Mil Med*. 2004;169(4):iv,265–269.

8. Trunkey DD. History and development of trauma care in the United States. *Clin Orthop Relat Res*. 2000;(374):36–46.

9. Dougherty PJ. Transtibial amputees from the Vietnam War. Twenty-eight-year follow-up. *J Bone Joint Surg Am*. 2001;83-A(3):383–389.

10. Dougherty PJ. Long-term follow-up study of bilateral above-the-knee amputees from the Vietnam War. *J Bone Joint Surg Am*. 1999;81(10):1384–1390.

11. Potter BK, Scoville CR. Amputation is not isolated: An overview of the US Army amputee patient care program and associated amputee injuries. *J Am Acad Orthop Surg*. 2006;14(10 suppl):S188–190.

12. Whitman W. Falmouth, Virginia, opposite Fredericksburgh, December 21, 1862. In: *Memoranda During the War*. Facsimile ed. Bloomington, Ind: Indiana University Press; 1962: 6.

13. Whitman W. *Specimen Days in America*. London, England: Walter Scott; 1887: 111.

14. Miller EH, ed. *Walt Whitman: The Correspondence*. Vol 1. New York, NY: New York University Press; 1961–1977: 229–230.

15. Reznick JS. Beyond war and military medicine: social factors in the development of prosthetics. *Arch Phys Med Rehabil*. 2008;89(1):188–193.

16. Figg L, Farrell-Beck J. Amputation in the Civil War: physical and social dimensions. *J Hist Med Allied Sci*. 1993;48(4):454–475.

17. Freemon F. Lincoln finds a Surgeon General: William A Hammond and the transformation of the Union Army Medical Bureau. *Civil War History*. 1987;33:6–7.

18. Phalen J. Clement Alexander Finley. *Army Med Bull*. 1940;52:38–14.

19. *The US Sanitary Commission of the United States Army: A Succinct Narrative of Its Works and Purposes*. New York, NY: US Sanitary Commission; 1864: 3–4.

20. Bremner RH. *The Public Good: Philanthropy and Welfare in the Civil War Era*. New York, NY: Knopf; 1980.

21. US Surgeon General's Office. *The Medical and Surgical History of the War of the Rebellion, 1861–1865*. Part I. Washington, DC: US Government Printing Office; 1870–1888: 143.

22. Bellows HW. *Sanitary Commission Report, No. 95: Provision Required for the Relief and Support of Disabled Soldiers and Sailors and Their Dependents*. New York, NY: US Sanitary Commission; 1865. Available at: www.disabilitymuseum.org/lib/docs/488.htm. Accessed April 23, 2008.

23. Reznick JS. *John Galsworthy, Disabled Soldiers, and the Great War*. Manchester, United Kingdom: Manchester University Press. In press.

24. Galsworthy J. Forward. *Reports Presented to the Second Annual Inter-Allied Conference on the After-Care of Disabled Men, London, England 20–25 May 1918.* London, England: Her Majesty's Stationery Office; 1918: 14–15.

25. Reznick J. Work-therapy and the disabled British soldier in Britain in the First World War: the case of Shepherd's Bush Military Hospital, London. In: Gerber D, ed. *Disabled Veterans in History.* Ann Arbor, Mich: University of Michigan Press; 2000: 185–203.

26. Cooter R. *Surgery and Society in Peace and War: Orthopaedics and the Organization of Modern Medicine.* New York, NY: Macmillan; 1993.

27. *Reports by the Joint War Committee and the Joint War Finance Committee of The British Red Cross Society and The Order of St. John of Jerusalem in England on Voluntary Aid Rendered to the Sick and Wounded at Home and Abroad and to British Prisoners of War, 1914–1919, With Appendices.* London, England: Her Majesty's Stationery Office; 1921: 733.

28. Devine ET. *Disabled Soldiers and Sailors Pensions and Training.* New York, NY: Oxford University Press; 1919: 318.

29. American Red Cross. *Work of the American Red Cross During the War: A Statement of Finances and Accomplishments for the Period July 1, 1917 to February 28, 1919.* Washington, DC: American Red Cross; 1919.

30. Davison HP. *The American Red Cross in the Great War.* New York, NY: Macmillan; 1919.

31. Beyer JC, ed. *Wound Ballistics.* Washington, DC: Department of the Army, Medical Department, Office of The Surgeon General; 1962: 482.

32. Love AG. War casualties. *Army Med Bull.* 1930;24. Available at: www.vlib.us/medical/stats/warcasTC.htm. Accessed April 23, 2008.

33. Hurwitt ES. A blood vessel bank under military conditions. *Mil Surg.* 1950;106(1):19–27.

34. Cleveland M, ed. *Orthopedic Surgery in the European Theater of Operations.* In: Coates JB Jr, ed. *Surgery in World War II.* Washington, DC: Department of the Army, Medical Department, Office of The Surgeon General; 1956: 157.

35. Hampton OP Jr. *Orthopedic Surgery in the Mediterranean Theater of Operations.* In: Coates JB Jr, Cleveland M, eds. *Surgery in World War II.* Washington, DC: Department of the Army, Medical Department, Office of The Surgeon General; 1957.

36. Rusk H. *A World to Care For.* New York, NY: Random House; 1972.

37. Brandt EN Jr, Pope AM, eds. *Enabling America: Assessing the Role of Rehabilitation Science and Engineering.* Washington, DC: National Academies Press; 1997: 32.

38. Reswick JB. How and when did the rehabilitation engineering center program come into being? *Jrn RR&D.* 2002;39:11–16. Available at: www.rehab.research.va.gov/jour/02/39/6/sup/reswick.html. Accessed April 23, 2008.

39. Daniel EH. *Amputation Prosthetic Service.* Baltimore, Md: Williams and Wilkins Company; 1950: 280–282.

40. Klopsteg PE, Wilson PD. *Human Limbs and Their Substitutes: Presenting Results of Engineering and Medical Studies of the Human Extremities and Application of the Data to the Design and Fitting of Artificial Limbs and to the Care and Training of Amputees.* New York, NY: McGraw-Hill Book Company; 1954: 797–798.

41. Ott K, Serlin D, Mihm S, eds. *Artificial Parts, Practical Lives: Modern Histories of Prosthetics.* New York:, NY: New York University Press; 2002.

42. Salyer J, Esslinger J. Specific considerations in primary surgery of the extremities. Paper presented at: Course on Recent Advances in Medicine and Surgery, Army Medical Service Graduate School, Walter Reed Army Medical Center; April 22, 1954; Washington, DC. Available at: http://history.amedd.army.mil/booksdocs/korea/recad1/ch7-3.htm. Accessed April 23, 2008.

43. Reister FA. *Battle Casualties and Medical Statistics, United States Army Experience in the Korean War.* Washington, DC: Department of the Army, Office of The Surgeon General; 1973. Available at: http://history.amedd.army.mil/booksdocs/korea/reister/. Accessed May 4, 2008.

44. Hughes C. The primary repair of wounds of major arteries. An analysis of experience in Korea in 1953. *Ann Surg.* 1955;141(3):297–303.

45. Mayfield G. Vietnam War amputees. In: Burkhalter W. *Orthopedic Surgery.* Washington, DC: Department of the Army, Medical Department, Office of The Surgeon General and Center of Military History; 1994: 131.

46. Dillingham TR, Belandres PV. Physiatry, physical medicine, and rehabilitation: historical development and military roles. In: *Rehabilitation of the Injured Combatant.* Vol 1. In: Zajtchuk R, Bellamy RF, eds. *Textbook of Military Medicine.* Washington, DC: Department of the Army, Office of The Surgeon General, Borden Institute; 1998: Chap 1.

47. Peterson C, Steadward R. *Paralympics: Where Heroes Come.* Edmonton, Alberta, Canada: One Shot Holdings Ltd; 1997.

48. International Paralympic Committee, Worldwide Partners Web site. Available at: www.paralympic.org/release/Main_Sections_Menu/Partners_and_Patrons/worldwide_corporate_partners/index.html. Accessed May 4, 2008.

49. Stansbury LG, Lalliss SJ, Branstetter JG, Bagg MR, Holcomb JB. Amputations in US military personnel in the current conflicts in Afghanistan and Iraq. *J Orthop Trauma.* 2008;22(1):43–46.

50. Morens DM. Thoughts on the relevance of medical history. *Hawaii Med J.* 1995;54(11):768–769.

Chapter 3

DEPARTMENT OF VETERANS AFFAIRS SYSTEM OF CARE FOR THE POLYTRAUMA PATIENT

CINDY E. POORMAN, MS*; MICHELLE L. SPORNER, MS, CRC†; BARBARA SIGFORD, MD‡; MICAELA CORNIS-POP, PhD§; GRETCHEN STEPHENS, MPA¥; GEORGE ZITNAY, PhD¶; AND MICHAEL PRAMUKA, PhD**

INTRODUCTION

DEVELOPMENT OF THE POLYTRAUMA SYSTEM OF CARE

COMPONENTS OF THE POLYTRAUMA SYSTEM OF CARE

SCOPE OF SERVICES
The Interdisciplinary Team
Specialized Programs

COORDINATION OF CARE AND CASE MANAGEMENT

FAMILY AND CAREGIVER SUPPORT

RESEARCH AND COLLABORATIONS

OUTCOME MEASURES

SUMMARY

* Rehabilitation Planning Specialist, VA Central Office, US Department of Veterans Affairs, 810 Vermont Avenue, NW, Washington, DC 20420
† Research Assistant, Human Engineering Research Laboratories, VA Pittsburgh Healthcare System/University of Pittsburgh, 7180 Highland Drive, Building 4, 2nd Floor, 151R1-H, Pittsburgh, Pennsylvania 15206
‡ National Director, Physical Medicine, and Rehabilitation Service, VA Central Office, 810 Vermont Avenue, NW, Washington, DC 20420
§ Rehabilitation Planning Specialist, VA Central Office, 810 Vermont Avenue, NW, Washington, DC 20420
¥ Polytrauma/TBI Coordinator, VA Central Office, 810 Vermont Avenue, NW, Washington, DC 20420
¶ Founder and Director, Defense and Veterans Brain Injury Center –Laurel Highlands, 727 Goucher Street, Johnstown, Pennsylvania 15905
** Assistant Professor, Department of Rehabilitation Science and Technology, University of Pittsburgh, 5044 Forbes Tower-Atwood, Pittsburgh,Pennsylvania 15260; formerly, Neuropsychologist, Henry M. Jackson Foundation/San Diego Naval Medical Center, 34800 Bob Wilson Drive, San Diego, California

INTRODUCTION

Since the beginning of the global war on terror (GWOT), many combat veterans have been exposed to some type of blast explosion, with the most prevalent and devastating injuries resulting from improvised explosive devices (IEDs). Service members with devastating injuries resulting from blasts often have unique clinical presentations that affect multiple organ systems and physical structures of the body, including traumatic brain injury (TBI), amputations, complex orthopaedic injuries, burns, spinal cord injuries (SCIs), and injuries to the sensory organs, as well as post-traumatic stress disorder (PTSD) and other mental health disorders. The combination of multiple injuries sustained as a result of the same traumatic event was termed "polytrauma" by the Department of Veterans Affairs (VA) for the purpose of characterizing these injuries and defining the system of rehabilitation services required for treatment.

The term polytrauma, used to describe the complexity of GWOT injuries, has helped define the unique needs of the military and veteran healthcare systems that drive optimal treatment for these patients. Polytrauma is defined as "two or more injuries to physical regions or organ systems, one of which may be life threatening, resulting in physical, cognitive, psychological, or psychosocial impairments and functional disability."[1] Advances in body armor, field medical care, and rapid evacuation during Operation Enduring Freedom (OEF) and Operation Iraqi Freedom (OIF) have led to a dramatic reduction in mortality from combat injuries, resulting in common survival of injuries that were fatal in previous wars.

In response to the high number of service members returning from Iraq and Afghanistan with unique injuries, including polytrauma, the VA developed the Polytrauma System of Care (PSC). Because of the high association between polytrauma and TBI, expertise in treating TBI was critical for the system's successful development. The PSC is an integrated system of specialized interdisciplinary services designed to meet the complex medical, psychological, rehabilitation, and prosthetic needs of veterans with polytrauma, TBI, and other injuries.

DEVELOPMENT OF THE POLYTRAUMA SYSTEM OF CARE

The PSC grew out of established expertise in specialized VA rehabilitation programs including TBI, amputation care, and blindness and low vision. These programs have been supported through congressional legislation as well as collaboration with the Department of Defense (DoD). In 1986 the VA and DoD established a Memorandum of Agreement for the referral and treatment of active duty service members with TBI, SCI, and blindness.[2] This agreement provided authority for the VA to provide rehabilitative services for active duty service members with these impairments. In 1992 the VA designated four TBI lead centers in coordination with the Defense and Veterans Brain Injury Center (DVBIC). These centers were located at Minneapolis, Minn; Palo Alto, Calif; Richmond, Va; and Tampa, Fla.[3] Their role was to provide specialized acute rehabilitation services for active duty service members and veterans with TBI. In 1996 Congress mandated that the VA maintain capacity for specialized services for veterans with special disabilities including TBI, SCI, and blindness, which require specialized rehabilitation services.[4] This mandate was followed by the 1997 designation of a TBI network of care to support and coordinate services for veterans and service members with TBI across the VA system of healthcare.[5]

The VA has been a leader in amputation rehabilitation since World War II and has continued to develop this expertise through special teams and programs. Public Law 102-405, Veterans' Medical Programs Amendments, passed in 1992, identified veterans with amputations as a special disability group.[6] The current Preservation Amputation Care and Treatment program provides a model of care focused on the prevention of amputations through early identification of veterans at risk of limb loss. It also provides comprehensive care for those with an amputation through interdisciplinary care management.[7] In addition, the VA currently has 62 prosthetic laboratories accredited by the Board for Orthotist/Prosthetist Certification or American Board for Certification in Orthotics and Prosthetics, and 76 outpatient amputation clinics throughout the VA system, 95% of which are headed by rehabilitation physicians. All of these programs are designed to improve the function of veterans with amputations. Amputation is often part of the polytrauma spectrum and, as a result, expertise in amputation rehabilitation in the VA has been emphasized through specialized training in state-of-the-art rehabilitation techniques and technology for polytrauma and amputation care teams.

In 1997 the VA established an agreement with the Commission on Accreditation of Rehabilitation Facilities (CARF)[8] demonstrating the VA's commitment to providing excellent care to veterans. All VA inpatient rehabilitation programs maintain accreditation by CARF for comprehensive interdisciplinary inpatient rehabilitation.

The 2005 Consolidated Appropriations Act (Public Law 108-447)[9] charged the VA to develop a system of specialized expertise to provide the best available medical care and integrative rehabilitation. PL 108-422 charged the VA to establish centers for research, education, and clinical activities on complex multitrauma associated with combat injuries.[10] The PSC was developed to address these requirements. In February 2005, four polytrauma rehabilitation centers (PRCs) were designated at the four sites of the existing VA TBI lead centers.[1] These sites are tertiary care medical centers that also have established amputation care programs and services for veterans with visual impairment and SCI. Further development of this system of care came in December 2005 when 21 polytrauma network sites (PNSs) were designated. The polytrauma telehealth network (PTN), which established state-of-the-art connectivity among PRCs and PNSs for the purposes of telemedicine and videoconferencing, was added in July 2006.

In March 2007, the remaining PSC components were established with the designation of 76 polytrauma support clinic teams (PSCTs) and 54 polytrauma points of contact (PPOCs) across the country. When the need for an additional PRC was recognized in 2007, the Audie L Murphy VA Medical Center in San Antonio, Texas, was selected due to its geographic location and proximity to major military facilities. Additional PSCTs are in continuous development as veterans with polytrauma and TBI enter the Veterans Health Administration for care. Also in 2007, President George W Bush formed the Dole-Shalala Commission to examine existing processes and find ways to improve care across the DoD and VA system and optimize outcomes. The commission made several recommendations applicable to the PSC[11]:

1. Immediately create comprehensive recovery plans for every seriously injured service member.
2. Aggressively prevent and treat PTSD and TBI.
3. Significantly strengthen support for families.
4. Rapidly transfer patient information between the DoD and VA.

These recommendations were added to the programs already in place within the VA to ensure quality of care to veterans.

COMPONENTS OF THE POLYTRAUMA SYSTEM OF CARE

In recognition of the wide range in the type and severity of injuries sustained in combat, and that veterans desire to receive care at locations close to their homes, the four components of the PSC were developed to balance access and expertise. The regional centers have the capability to provide care for the most seriously injured and require the greatest distance in travel, and local facilities, developed to provide ongoing, lifelong care, are located in closest proximity to the veteran's home. Depending on the severity of the injury, the veteran may enter the PSC via any component and move from one to another based on assessed needs. Details of each component are as follows:

1. PRCs serve as regional referral centers for acute medical and rehabilitation care, and as hubs for research and education on polytrauma and TBI. The PRC mission is to provide comprehensive inpatient rehabilitation services for individuals with complex physical, cognitive, and mental health sequelae

of severe and disabling trauma, to provide medical and surgical support for ongoing and/or new conditions, and to provide support to their families. These centers have the necessary expertise to provide the coordinated interdisciplinary care required for all patients who have sustained varied patterns of severe and disabling injuries.

PRCs provide a continuum of rehabilitation services that include comprehensive acute rehabilitation care for complex and severe polytraumatic injuries, inpatient evaluation and treatment planning, specialized emerging consciousness programs for individuals with severe disorders of consciousness, and residential transitional rehabilitation programs. The centers maintain a full staff of dedicated rehabilitation specialists and medical and surgical consultants. They are able to manage high levels of medical acuity. PRCs serve as resources for other PSC facilities and spearhead the development of educational programs and best practice models of care. In addition to the PSC's CARF accreditation, the PRCs maintain additional accreditation for comprehensive interdisciplinary brain injury rehabilitation.

2. PNSs were established to manage the post-acute phase of polytrauma rehabilitation and coordinate rehabilitation services for patients within their service network. PNSs have a dedicated interdisciplinary team of rehabilitation professionals who provide a high level of expert care, perform a full range of clinical and ancillary services, and serve as resources for other facilities within their network. Due to many referrals for care and treatment of service members and veterans not so seriously injured as to require inpatient rehabilitation, PNSs also evaluate and treat new referrals with polytrauma and TBI. The PNS sites are geographically dispersed across the country with one in each veterans integrated service network, which organize the medical care and services to veterans within their geographic area.

3. PSCTs have been established in smaller Veterans Affairs medical centers across the country to deliver and coordinate the care of veterans with stable polytrauma or TBI sequelae. These local teams of rehabilitation professionals provide services in, or close to, the veteran's home communities. PSCTs provide the lifelong care and follow-up for veterans with moderate to severe injuries requiring regular assessment and reassessment to maintain an optimal state of functioning, take

advantage of new technology and advances in rehabilitation care, and address changes in developmental stage or goals. The teams also evaluate and provide treatment for new referrals not requiring inpatient rehabilitation services.

4. PPOCs provide case management services to veterans with polytrauma and/or TBI and make referrals to programs that provide the level of rehabilitation care required. A PPOC is located at every VA medical center that is not designated as one of the above three components.

All components of the VA PSC have shared characteristics, making them a unique system of care. These characteristics include a deep commitment and respect for the military mission and those who have served their country. In addition, each facility has taken steps to maintain a military identity and connectedness for those who seek care. The facilities in the PSC have a shared system of managing medical information and communication, an integrated system of care management, including several unique innovations such as transition patient advocates who can travel with veterans to their points of care as needed, an in-depth knowledge of veteran and military benefits, and a diverse array of services to meet an individual's need across the full continuum of care. Extensive support to families is also available, and the environment of care is modified to meet the needs of young patients and their families. This comprehensive and coordinated system of care, in addition to the special programs found within the various components of the system, make the rehabilitation services provided unique to the VA.

SCOPE OF SERVICES

The Interdisciplinary Team

Each service delivery component of the PSC has at its core an interdisciplinary team (IDT). These interdisciplinary teams are characterized by a variety of disciplines working together in the assessment, planning, and implementation of each patient's care plan. The core IDT is responsible for the major therapeutic interventions of the rehabilitation program. To avoid fragmented care, continuous communication, collaboration, and coordination are critical. The IDT functions as a unit, ensuring cooperation among disciplines to achieve maximum patient and family outcomes. The membership of the team is determined by assessing the individual's rehabilitation needs, predicted outcomes,

and medical needs.

VA rehabilitation professionals have specialized skills and knowledge based upon education, clinical training, and experience. They are certified or licensed according to their specific discipline requirements and receive additional training in specific treatment areas relevant to polytrauma and TBI. These areas include, but are not limited to, neurorehabilitation, cognitive rehabilitation, visual rehabilitation, and state-of-the-art prosthetics and equipment. As well as having specialized training, new therapists receive mentoring by experienced therapists. They also attend training conferences sponsored by VA and DoD focusing on state-of-the-art practices in polytrauma rehabilitation. In addition, team members establish local, regional, and national collaborations within the disciplines to share new and emerging best practices.

The patient and the patient's family, or other support system, are crucial members of the IDT and are included in all phases of the rehabilitation process. Their input is actively solicited by team members and is essential to the development of an individualized plan of care based on goals that are patient-centered and relevant. Goals and progress are continually reviewed with the patient and family and modified as needed to remain centered on the patient's needs. Goals addressed include the full spectrum of function from basic skills to community reentry, including return to work, return to school, sports, and other leisure and recreational activities.

Members of the IDT include, but are not limited to, a physician specializing in physical medicine and rehabilitation (physiatrist), rehabilitation nurse, neuropsychologist, rehabilitation psychologist, physical therapist, kinesiotherapist, occupational therapist, speech language pathologist, social worker, recreational therapist, and a military liaison.[12] Each member contributes to the interdisciplinary team goals individualized to the specific patient.

- The **physiatrist** is a medical doctor who serves as the IDT leader to direct and coordinate the patient's care. Physiatrists specialize in the treatment of conditions associated with impairments of function due to disease or injury.
- A **rehabilitation nurse** combines traditional patient care skills with training in care of individuals who are experiencing an illness or disability that alters normal functioning. The rehabilitation nurse works to assist the family and individuals in implementing the different treatments and therapies to complete the treatment plan. The rehabilitation nurse also educates the patient and family about the patient's condition.
- An **occupational therapist** is on staff to help service members or veterans with motor function, basic, and instrumental activities of daily living (ADLs), as well as making recommendations for environmental modifications that allow the individual to function more independently after discharge. Occupational therapists also help to address cognitive impairment and assist with compensatory strategies.
- A **case manager** is made available and is responsible for ensuring that all components of the plan of care are implemented thoroughly and efficiently and according to the desires of

the patient and family. Case managers help to answer questions and locate needed services for the service member or veteran. The social worker case manager collects background information about financial resources, education level, work history, living situation, and level of social support to help with treatment and discharge planning. A case manager is also part of the postdischarge team to ensure that follow-up plans are implemented.

- A **speech language pathologist** addresses communication deficits and evaluates and treats cognitive deficits such as problems with attention, memory, reading comprehension, and planning and sequencing. The speech language pathologist may also help if there are deficits in swallowing.
- **Physical therapists** and **kinesiotherapists** work to aid in the restoration of function, improve mobility, relieve pain, and prevent or limit permanent physical disability. These therapists also teach service members or veterans how to use assistive devices such as gait aides, prostheses, and wheelchairs.
- A **recreational therapist** assists the individual with community reintegration by applying practical skills to real-life situations and ensuring safety in environments with various barriers such as curbs, stairs, and uneven surfaces. Recreational therapists also assess and assist with adaptations for leisure activities such as sports.
- A **rehabilitation psychologist** is a specialist with an advanced degree in psychology who works with clients in coping and adjusting to traumatic injury. The rehabilitation psychologist works with the patient and family to recognize and address specific issues that may occur after injury, in areas such as mood and emotions, stress management, body image, quality of life, and role changes.
- The **neuropsychologist** has a similar education to a rehabilitation psychologist, but specializes in the relationship between the brain and behavior. A neuropsychologist may administer cognitive or emotional assessments to identify strengths and weaknesses after injury.
- The **DoD military liaison** provides support to service members as they transition from military healthcare to the VA healthcare system in areas such as processing travel vouchers and claims. The military liaison also serves as a connection between the service member and his or her chain of command and consults with the IDT on military matters.[12]

Specialized Programs

Acute Rehabilitation

This phase typically occurs directly following initial medical and surgical stabilization and provides high-intensity rehabilitation care while optimizing the patient's medical condition. During this stage, typically occurring at the PRCs, active duty service members and veterans frequently continue to require significant medical and surgical support, unlike patients admitted to many private sector rehabilitation facilities. Thus, these medical and surgical services are available on an emergent basis at all four PRCs. Data collected at the PRCs reveal that approximately 90% of polytrauma patients in the acute rehabilitation setting have TBI as one of their impairments. Therefore, the environment of care and the expertise of the treating professionals are adapted to the specialized techniques required for neurological and particularly TBI rehabilitation, unlike many generalized rehabilitation units, which may have a very low census of TBI patients and limited experience with their rehabilitation.

Acute rehabilitation includes treatment planning, based upon medical stability, types of impairment, level of consciousness, and current cognitive and functional status. The focus may initially be on alertness and responsiveness and progress through developing basic skills such as bowel and bladder control, communication, mobility, basic hygiene, orientation, and basic ADLs, and advance to higher level ADLs such as meal preparation, managing money, community safety, and driving. Acute rehabilitation in the PSC requires the expertise of multiple healthcare professionals who work as an IDT, as well as dedicated medical and surgical consultants available around the clock, every day of the week.

Emerging Consciousness Program

This is a unique, specially developed program, based on the most up-to-date evidence, that is operational at the four PRCs. It is designed to optimize long-term functional outcomes after severe brain injury in patients who are not yet ready to participate in acute rehabilitation. It promotes return to consciousness, and facilitates progress to the next level of rehabilitation care. Individuals who benefit from this program have suffered severe polytraumatic injuries leading to ongoing impaired consciousness. The program encompasses nursing and rehabilitation medical services, an individualized therapy program, intensive case management, and psychological support services and education for families and caregivers.

Residential Transitional Rehabilitation Program

This program is for veterans and active duty service members with polytrauma and/or TBI who have physical, cognitive, and/or behavioral impairments that delay or inhibit their effective reintegration into the community or return to duty after the acute phase of rehabilitation. It was developed based on a thorough review of research on the effective components of existing transitional rehabilitation models. Transitional rehabilitation offers a progressive return to independent living through a milieu-based, structured program focused on restoring home, community, leisure, psychosocial, and vocational skills in a controlled, therapeutic setting. Services provided typically include group therapies, individual therapies, case management and care coordination, medical care, vocational and educational rehabilitation services, discharge planning, and follow-up. Services are often provided in community settings. These programs have been implemented at the PRCs.

Subacute Rehabilitation

This program provides services for persons with polytrauma who are medically stable and need a less intensive level of rehabilitation services, over a longer period of time than provided in the acute setting. In the PSC, patients typically are admitted to a subacute rehabilitation program after a period of acute rehabilitation. Subacute rehabilitation programs are often utilized for persons who have made progress in the acute rehabilitation setting and are still progressing, but are not making rapid functional gains and wish to be closer to their home community. The programs are also utilized during the transition home, providing education to families and caregivers, identifying community resources available for transitional support, and acquiring any necessary equipment. Subacute TBI rehabilitation is typically provided at the VA PNSs, where continued interdisciplinary treatment to meet patient and family goals is provided.

Outpatient Therapy

Following acute or subacute rehabilitation, a person with a traumatic injury may continue to receive outpatient therapies to meet ongoing goals. Additionally, a person with polytrauma or a brain injury that was not severe enough to require inpatient hospitalization may attend outpatient therapies to address their functional impairments. Outpatient therapies are typically provided at PNS and PSCT facilities. The outpatient interdisciplinary rehabilitation team addresses basic functional impairments, basic and advanced ADLs, and return to work, return to school, and community reintegration including driving and leisure skills. Therapies are geared to both restoration of function

and compensation for fixed impairments.

Day Treatment

This program provides rehabilitation therapies in a structured group setting during the day and allows the participant to return home at night. Several PNSs offer day treatment programs for veterans with polytrauma and TBI.

COORDINATION OF CARE AND CASE MANAGEMENT

Case management, an integral part of services provided throughout the PSC, plays a crucial role in ensuring lifelong coordination of services for patients with polytrauma and TBI. Several processes have been established to facilitate the transition of patients from DoD to VA care at the appropriate time, under optimal conditions of safety and convenience for the patients and their families. These processes address continuity of medical care and psychosocial support for patients and families.

Families of injured service members require particular assistance with transitioning from the acute medical setting of the military medical treatment facility (MTF) to the VA rehabilitation setting at the PRCs. Multiple levels of clinical, psychosocial, and logistical support have been put into place to ensure a smooth transition and continuity of care. At Walter Reed Army Medical Center (Washington, DC) and Bethesda (Maryland) National Naval Medical Center the process begins with the VA polytrauma rehabilitation nurse liaison, who meets the active duty members and their families while they are still in the acute treatment phase of care. The nurse liaison provides education about TBI, the rehabilitation process, and the PRC environment of care. Additionally, VA social workers at the MTFs provide logistical and psychosocial support during the transition process from DoD to the VA. At the same time, the admission case manager from the

PRC maintains personal contact with the family prior to transfer to provide additional support and further information about the expected plan of care. PRCs also schedule video teleconferences with the MTFs to discuss the referral with the transferring team, and to meet the patient and family members "face-to-face" whenever feasible.

Social worker case managers at the PRCs assess the psychosocial needs of each patient and family, and match treatment and support services to meet identified needs, coordinate services, and oversee the discharge planning process. As the veteran moves to the next level of care, the social worker case manager is responsible for a "warm hand-off" of care to the case manager at the receiving facility closer to the veteran's home. This is accomplished via personal communication through a phone call or through the PTN's state-of-the-art video conferencing capability. The case manager continues to follow the patient until transfer of care is complete, and services recommended in the discharge plan of care are fully implemented.

The PTN provides a reliable, easily accessible tool to further support care coordination and case management. The PTN was expanded during fiscal year 2007 to include all PRCs and PNSs and several DoD MTFs, ensuring that the polytrauma and TBI expertise available at the PRCs is readily accessible to locations closer to the veteran's home community.

FAMILY AND CAREGIVER SUPPORT

PSC programs are responsible for ensuring that patients and their families, or other caregivers, receive all necessary support services to enhance the rehabilitation process and minimize the inherent stress of recovery from a severe injury. The PRCs and PNSs strongly advocate involvement of families and caregivers throughout the rehabilitation process. Family members and caregivers actively engage in treatment and treatment decisions. They are invited to join therapy sessions and to participate in interdisciplinary

team meetings where treatment plans are discussed. Support groups and individual counseling for family members are available at all PRC sites.

Within the PSC, each service member or veteran identifies those individuals whom they consider family members, caregivers, or members of their social support network. Services described in this section would be provided to anyone identified by the patient as part of this extended network. For patients without good family or social support, the case manager tries to identify the best support available and provide the necessary education and training to enhance these connections. The designated polytrauma case manager (social worker and/or nurse) assigned to every veteran and active duty service member receiving care in the PSC coordinates the core needs and support efforts to match the needs of each family or caregiver. At the PRCs in particular, where patients and families spend extended periods of time away from home, an entire support system has been implemented that includes, but is not limited to, dedicated social worker case managers advocating for needs and interests throughout the rehabilitation process; access to a VA social worker 24 hours a day, 7 days a week; and counseling, education, and logistical support such as transportation, housing, nutrition, and child care.

Education and training for family caregivers are provided throughout the rehabilitation process. The goal of education is to empower families to support their loved one through the recovery process, and to provide strategies that will facilitate reintegration into the home community. VA services provided directly to families of polytrauma and TBI veterans include screening, assessment, education, and treatment for marital and family related problems. Family members may also receive respite care, home health services, education about the care of the veteran, referral to community resources, limited bereavement counseling, and support group services.

Resources have also been assembled nationally and locally to meet the special needs of families who accompany the seriously injured service members to the PRCs. Several educational products for patients and families were developed at the PRCs and distributed nationally in fiscal year 2007, including a TBI family education manual, a TBI information brochure, and a TBI screening brochure. A new PSC Web site is being planned.

Generous donations from VA Voluntary Services, Operation Helping Hand, Fisher House Foundation, other foundations and agencies, and local businesses frequently provide free housing, free or discounted meals, transportation, and entertainment for veterans' family members at or near the PRC sites. Additional donations have included laptop computers, media equipment, telephone cards, and gift cards for meals and entertainment. Voluntary Services at each PRC facility guide donations to meet the families' specific needs.

The PSC is committed to supporting the military identity of the wounded service members served at its facilities. Each of the PRCs has an Army and Marine liaison assigned full time. Their role is to help all active duty military and their families with invitational travel orders, medical boards, and access to military benefits. Additionally, several sites have a representative from the Military Severely Injured Service Center and Army Wounded Warriors available to provide information and assistance. While these professionals often work with patients independently, their interventions are integrated through collaboration with the social work case manager.

VA also spports GWOT veterans through the OEF/OIF program, a coordinated program that offers case management to all veterans transitioning into civilian life who have served in combat. Since 2003, VA has collaborated with DoD and MTFs to seamlessly transition the healthcare of injured or ill combat veterans and active duty service members from MTFs to VHA facilities. VA social worker liaisons are assigned to major MTFs to assist with transfers and to provide information to active duty patients and families about VA healthcare services. OEF/OIF case managers, both social workers and nurses, are also at the VA healthcare facilities to aid with the transition once the veteran or active duty service member presents for care. Services include helping veterans obtain the appropriate information about their healthcare benefits and eligibility.[13] PSC case managers work closely with this program.

RESEARCH AND COLLABORATIONS

The Polytrauma and Blast-Related Injuries (PT/BRI) Quality Enhancement Research Initiative (QUERI), located at the Minneapolis VA Medical Center, is the coordinating center for collaborative research activities for the PSC. The mission of the PT/BRI QUERI is to promote the successful rehabilitation, psychological adjustment, and community reintegration of individuals who have sustained polytraumatic and blast-related injuries. Based on needs assessment studies conducted in fiscal year 2006, and input from stakeholders, PT/BRI QUERI has identified four priority areas for research: (1) database development, (2) screening/evaluation of high-frequency comorbidities, (3) caregiver family members, and (4) care coordination. In addition, individual sites in the PSC have their own research programs funded through VA research offices, such as rehabilitation research and development and health services research and development, DoD research programs, and the DVBIC. These programs utilize the standard methodologies for applications for research grants.

The VA PSC actively collaborates with multiple

DoD and civilian sector programs and agencies. One of the most prominent and long-standing is that with the DVBIC. Collaboration with the DVBIC, even before GWOT, helped to lay the foundation for the system. DVBIC, then known as the Defense and Veterans Head Injury Program, was established in 1992 to help coordinate efforts across the VA, DoD, and the civilian sector in diagnosing and treating TBI. DVBIC is a congressionally supported program charged with developing military-relevant research to increase understanding of how TBI impacts troop readiness and improve outcomes, leading to return to active duty or productive community reintegration. Its mandate also calls for innovative rehabilitation for TBI, utilizing emerging technology, and the development of educational materials and programs for professionals, providers, and family members. Since its founding, DVBIC's role has expanded to include screening for mild TBI in the DoD, development of practice guidelines, data collection, and analysis and care coordination and case management.[14] These efforts are apparent in the four PRCs.

The PSC has also established collaborative relationships with other rehabilitation organizations. VA works closely with CARF to help identify and promote quality rehabilitation programs within the VA, utilizing CARF's directory of rehabilitation providers to ensure that care provided outside the VA system meets an established benchmark for quality rehabilitation. Leadership in VA rehabilitation also works closely with other national professional rehabilitation organizations such as the American Medical Rehabilitation Providers Association and the American Academy of Physical Medicine and Rehabilitation for the common goal of improved rehabilitation services to the nation's service members and veterans. A new collaboration has recently been established with the TBI Model Systems Program, a long-standing research consortium of private sector TBI treatment facilities that have established a common database and support joint research initiatives, to share in data collection for outcomes and joint research ventures. PSC facilities are also encouraged to form local collaborations with providers in their communities to ensure the best care without gaps as close to home as possible.

Many of the programs in the PSC have affiliations and collaborative relationships with academic medical centers. VA rehabilitation providers are often part of the academic medical rehabilitation community for training and affiliations, and share VA and affiliated positions in medical rehabilitation. VA clinicians are also frequently invited lecturers on polytrauma and TBI rehabilitation.

OUTCOME MEASURES

Rehabilitation programs in the VA utilize a standardized outcomes measurement system, the Functional Status Outcomes Database. This system allows tracking of functional outcomes in motor, self care, and cognitive domains across the continuum of care. Standardized reports are provided on a quarterly basis to inpatient rehabilitation units by the US Department of Health and Human Services' Uniform Data System program, which tracks information on the operation and performance of health centers. In addition, facilities can create their own customized reports based on their individualized data. Data can be utilized to measure change in function, length of the rehabilitation stay, discharge destination, and various demographic variables. With the establishment of the PSC, the Functional Status Outcomes Database was modified to include new variables relevant to polytrauma and the military experience. Reports of outcomes are presented in educational meetings as well as used to inform the development of the system.

The PSC also collaborates with the DVBIC in collection of outcome data. The DVBIC has primarily focused on ensuring the best practices for service members and veterans with TBI. Although data on the long-term consequences of TBI are not yet available, DVBIC has established a national database of individuals who have received care within the program. The database includes such descriptive information as mechanism of injury (blast or other type of injury), severity of injury, and measurements of neurologic function. These descriptive points are collected to make comparisons of outcomes based upon mechanism of injury, severity, and other injury types (closed or penetrating). This database is currently being used to allow longer follow-up of individuals receiving services to examine and address issues related to long-term outcomes (up to 10 years). The DVBIC also funds specific research endeavors at the PRCs. One important activity often associated with long-term outcomes is an individual's ability to return to independent driving. PRCs and military treatment facilities have utilized driving simulators to assist in retraining individuals to drive. These driving simulators are not only used for skills training, but also provide valid predictive measures of long-term performance in the community for individuals with TBI.[15]

VA medical care in general has achieved significant recognition for quality of care; in 2005, VA achieved a satisfaction score of 83 out of 100 for inpatient care and 80 out of 100 for outpatient care as rated by the American Customer Satisfaction Index. These scores were recognized as higher than the private sector, which scored 73 and 75, respectively.[16] VA also continually tracks its service quality using Clinical Practice Guidelines and the Prevention Index II. Clinical Practice Guidelines help to ensure that all healthcare professionals follow a nationally recognized standard of care, and Prevention Index II tracks compliance with the Guidelines for preventative care, which is associated with better health and well-being. In 2006 the mean scores of these measures were reported at 87% for the Clinical Practice Guidelines and 90% for the Prevention Index II.[16]

SUMMARY

The VA PSC was created to provide comprehensive care to severely injured service members, especially those presenting with unique injury patterns and complex rehabilitation needs associated with blast exposure. This network of care is committed to providing veterans access to the highest quality of care and helping them regain the functional skills to successfully return to active duty military service or reenter the community. In pursuing these goals, the PSC has achieved an unprecedented level of integration and coordination among the many DoD, VA, civilian, national, regional, and local facilities and systems involved in rehabilitation services for veterans. The standard of care in the PSC meets or exceeds that of the private sector.

REFERENCES

1. Department of Veterans Affairs, Veterans Health Administration. *Polytrauma Rehabilitation Procedures*. Washington DC: VA; 2005. VHA Handbook 1172.1. Available at: http://www1.va.gov/vhapublications/ViewPublication.asp?pub_ID=1317. Accessed January 5, 2008.

2. VA/DoD Health Executive Councils. *Department of Veterans Affairs (VA) and Department of Defense Memorandum of Agreement (MoA) Regarding Referral of Active Duty Military Personnel Who Sustain Spinal Cord Injury, Traumatic Brain Injury, or Blindness to Veterans Affairs Medical Facilities for Health Care and Rehabilitative Services*. Washington DC: DoD, VA: 2004. Available at: http://vadodrs.amedd.army.mil/legislation/MOA_DoD_Refera_SCI_TBI_Blindness_to_VA.pdf. Accessed July 15, 2008.

3. Schwab KA, Warden D, Lux WE, Shupenko LA, Zitnay G. Guest editorial: Defense and Veterans Brain Injury Center: peacetime and wartime missions. *J Rehabil Res Dev*. 2007;44(7):xiii–xxi.

4. Veterans' Health Care Eligibility Reform Act of 1996. Public Law 104-262. 9 October 1996. Available at: http://frwebgate.access.gpo.gov/cgi-bin/getdoc.cgi?dbname=104_cong_public_laws&docid=f:publ262.104. Accessed September 19, 2008.

5. Department of Veterans Affairs Employee Education System. *Traumatic Brain Injury*. Washington DC: VA; 2004. Available at: http://www1.va.gov/vhi/docs/TBI.pdf. Accessed July 15, 2008.

6. Veterans' Medical Programs Amendments of 1992. Public Law 102-405. 9 October 1992. Available at: http://uscode.house.gov/download/pls/38C73.txt. Accessed July 15, 2008.

7. Department of Veterans Affairs, Veterans Health Administration. *Preservation-Amputation Care and Treatment (PACT) Program*. Washington DC: VA; 2006. VHA Directive 2006-050. Available at: http://www1.va.gov/vhapublications/ViewPublication.asp?pub_ID=1483. Accessed June 15, 2008.

8. Commission on Accreditation of Rehabilitation Facilities. CARF Connection Web site. Available at: http://www.carf.org/Providers.aspx?content=content/Publications/Online/eConnection/JanFeb05/VA.htm. Accessed January 31, 2008.

9. Consolidated Appropriations Act, 2005. Public Law 108-447. 8 December 2004. Available at: http://www.dsca.osd.mil/programs/LPA/2005/getdoc.cgi_dbname=108_cong_public_laws&docid=f_publ447.108.pdf. Accessed July 15, 2008.

10. Veterans Health Programs Improvement Act of 2004. Public Law 108-422. 30 November 2004. Available at: http://thomas.loc.gov/cgi-bin/bdquery/z?d108:HR03936:@@@D&summ2=m&. Accessed July 15, 2008.

11. Dole R, Shalala D. A duty to the wounded: our newest veterans need help now. *Washington Post.* July 26, 2007. A11.

12. Department of Veterans Affairs Employee Education System. *Polytrauma Rehabilitation Family Education Manual.* Washington, DC: VA; 2007. Available at: http://dva.state.wi.us/Docs/TBI/Family_Ed_Manual112007.pdf. Accessed July 16, 2008.

13. Department of Veterans Affairs. *Operation Iraqi Freedom/Operation Enduring Freedom Program.* Washington, DC: VA; 2007.

14. Zitnay G. Defense and Veterans Brain Injury Center. Paper presented at: Hiram G Andrews Center Returning Veterans Symposium; July 24, 2007; Johnstown, Pa.

15. Lew HL, Poole JH, Lee EH, Jaffe DL, Huang HC, Brodd E. Predictive validity of driving-simulator assessments following traumatic brain injury: a preliminary study. *Brain Injury.* 2005;19(3):177–188.

Chapter 4

RETURNING TO DUTY AFTER MAJOR LIMB LOSS AND THE US MILITARY DISABILITY SYSTEM

JEFF GAMBEL, MD*; ERIC DESSAIN, MD[†]; PAUL FOWLER, DO, JD[‡]; ANDREW RHODES, DO[§]; AND MARIA MAYORGA, MD[¥]

*Colonel, Medical Corps, US Army; Physician, Department of Orthopaedics and Rehabilitation, Walter Reed Army Medical Center, 6900 Georgia Avenue, NW, Washington, DC 20307

[†]Lieutenant Colonel, Medical Corps, US Army; Physician, Chief, Physical Disability Evaluation Service, Walter Reed Army Medical Center, 6900 Georgia Avenue, NW, Washington, DC 20307

[‡]Senior Medical Evaluation Board Disability Advisor; Physician-Attorney, Command Group, Walter Reed Army Medical Center, 6900 Georgia Avenue, NW, Washington, DC 20307

[§]Captain, Medical Corps, US Army; Physician, Medical Evaluation Board, Physical Disability Evaluation Service, Walter Reed Army Medical Center, 6900 Georgia Avenue, NW, Washington, DC 20307

[¥]Colonel (Retired), Medical Corps, US Army; Physician, Past Chief, Physical Disability Evaluation Service, Walter Reed Army Medical Center; Currently, PhD Candidate, Sweden

INTRODUCTION

In recent decades, returning to duty after major limb loss has been a rare event in the US military. Today's military service member who wishes to remain on active duty after major limb loss commonly finds a more receptive atmosphere, if not strong encouragement from his or her chain of command. This support is well-founded given advances in amputee care that make it possible for such service members to effectively meet and exceed rigorous performance standards for a wide range of military occupations. This chapter will describe some of the key factors that service members with major limb loss and their families might consider when deciding whether to pursue return to duty or transition into civilian life. The military disability system, with the US Army's system as the prime example, will also be described.

RETURNING TO DUTY

Factors Involved

The severity of limb loss, as well as the nature and extent of associated injuries, has a dramatic impact on an injured service member's ability to return to active military duty. History has many examples of soldiers with major limb loss returning to active duty, including the Invalid Corps of the Union Army during the US Civil War[1] and approximately 1,500 World War II veterans who were recalled to active duty to support the Korean War.[2] While serving as junior officers in Vietnam, General (Retired) Eric Shinseki (a partial foot amputee) and General (Retired) Frederick Franks (a transtibial [below-knee] amputee) suffered major limb loss, yet retired after full active duty, reaching the highest positions of leadership in the US Army.[3] Despite these examples, a study by Kishbaugh et al[4] found that only 11 of 469 US soldiers with limb loss (2.3%) returned to duty in the 1980s, with amputation levels including partial foot, partial hand, and transtibial. More recently, during the global war on terror (GWOT), injured service members from Afghanistan and Iraq with more proximal levels of amputations, including transfemoral (above-knee) and transradial (below-elbow), have remained on active duty and continue to serve successfully.[5] From the onset of GWOT through 2008, approximately 17% to 20% of injured service members with major limb loss, across all US military services, have completed their respective medical board process and been retained on active duty or reserve status.[6,7]

Many factors associated with the traumatic event (commonly a blast injury) responsible for the amputation can make healing and realistic decision-making about return to duty more complex. Some of these factors include complications with the healing limb,[8] multiple limb loss, ongoing residual limb (stump) pain, uncomfortable and limited prosthetic use, decreased functional abilities,[9] traumatic brain injury, delayed psychological adjustment to limb loss,[10] and impaired confidence in one's ability to resume normal-life activities (self-efficacy).[11]

Traits characteristic of amputees who seek to remain on active duty include strong individual motivation for continued military service, anticipated ability to meet the performance standards of their military occupational specialty (MOS), solid support from close family members and friends, and possession of highly valued military-specific skills. In addition, service members most likely to return to duty are those who had strong service records prior to injury and can expect robust unit and command backing, especially after a trial of duty with their previous unit. It is particularly helpful if the unit has special MOS-related needs that the service member can fill. Also, service members are usually wise to remain flexible, with the willingness to consider the possibility of training in another MOS that can better match their current abilities with a valued military job. Amputee service members report that speaking with peer amputee visitors and veterans who have personal experience with the return-to-duty process provides helpful information to guide their own decision making.[12] The Web addresses of organizations with useful resources for injured service members are listed in Table 4-1.

US Army Process

In the US Army, many injured soldiers, especially those returning from overseas, are either assigned or attached to a medical holding company such as the one at Walter Reed Army Medical Center while recovering from their injuries. More recently, such units have been called warrior transition units (WTUs). The WTU acts as the medical and administrative facilitator between the hospital clinicians and the physical evaluation board liaison officer. The WTU further ensures administrative accountability for all soldiers receiving care by assigning a case manager or social worker to support them and their families. The range of support

TABLE 4-1

WEB SITE ADDRESSES OF ORGANIZATIONS HELPFUL TO INJURED SERVICE MEMBERS

Activity	Internet Address
US Army Publication Directorate	www.apd.army.mil
Walter Reed Army Medical Center	www.wramc.amedd.army.mil
Amputee Coalition of America	www.amputee-coalition.org
Department of Veterans Affairs	www.index.va.gov
Disabled Soldier Support System	www.ArmyDS3.org
Disabled American Veterans	www.dav.org
Paralyzed Veterans of America	www.pva.org
Veterans of Foreign Wars	www.vfw.org
American Legion	www.legion.org
Military Order of the Purple Heart of the USA	www.purpleheart.org
American Veterans	www.amvets.org
National Amputation Foundation	www.nationalamputation.org
National Military Family Association	www.nmfa.org
Combat Related Special Compensation	www.crsc.org
Physical Disability Agency	www.hrc.army.mil/site/active/tagd/pda/pdapage.htm

provided includes logistics (lodging), pay and allowances, convalescent and ordinary leave, and military orders. The WTU team of professionals makes certain that patients receive timely clinical appointments and that all required administrative documentation is properly processed.

The WTU also serves as a coordinator between the soldier and the transition office. The transition office prepares the discharge document, DD214, which verifies all periods of military service and character of discharge. The DD214 is required for Department of Veterans Affairs (VA) benefits to begin. In most situations, the soldier's transition out of the unit, and ultimately out of the Army, involves an administrative process that may take weeks, up to several months. For those who are able to return to duty, new orders will direct the soldiers to their next duty station. The length of time a soldier remains with the WTU depends upon his or her unique healthcare situation, individual resources, support system, and administrative needs.

PHYSICAL DISABILITY EVALUATION SYSTEM

Overview

Each branch of the Department of Defense (DoD) has specific standards by which it determines whether or not an injured or ill member will be continued on active duty, based upon the severity of the condition and the imposed functional limitations. The ensuing text will focus on the US Army physical disability evaluation system (PDES), and specifically the active duty soldier with major limb loss who must navigate the system. The rules and regulations for the reserve soldier, in relation to disability compensation, are different than those for the active duty soldier. However, in terms of the medical evaluation mechanics, once entered into the PDES, active duty, reserve, and National Guard soldiers all flow through the Army disability system in the same manner.

For example, soldiers with major limb loss may be medically retired from the US Army for a physical impairment if it renders them physically unfit for duty.

Fitness for duty is evaluated as a function of the reasonably expected ability to perform the duties of the soldier's primary MOS.[13(p14)] To get to this point, the Army must utilize the medical evaluation board (MEB) and physical evaluation board (PEB). The MEB determines "retention," per Army Regulation (AR) 40-501, Chapter 3.[14] The PEB determines "fitness," based upon MOS. This distinction is extremely important, because the medical treatment facility (MTF) does not and should not comment on the "fitness" of a soldier, but rather whether the amputee meets retention standards, regardless of MOS, based solely on AR 40-501, Chapter 3.[14]

If the soldier's medical condition could potentially be found to not meet the medical retention standards, as outlined in AR 40-501, Chapter 3, it is the treating physician's responsibility to refer the soldier to the MEB. The MEB physician, who receives specialized disability training, then reviews all clinical and administrative evaluations. The MEB physician (civilian or military) is directly employed by or assigned to the MTF, working under the authority of the MTF commander, through the deputy commander for clinical services. The MEB physician's key role is to determine whether or not the referred soldier's medical conditions meet the retention standards of AR 40-501, Chapter 3, regardless of MOS. If the soldier fails to meet retention standards and cannot satisfactorily perform his or her military duties, he or she is referred to the PEB. The PEB, under the authority of the US Army Physical Disability Agency, which manages the Army's PDES and acts on behalf of the secretary of the Army, will consider the recommendations of the MEB and make the determination of fitness or unfitness, rendered with the soldier's MOS in mind.[14]

Developing and implementing a system to best benefit the soldier, while providing for the overall good of the Army, whose "paramount mission is to maintain a fit fighting force," is a difficult and daunting endeavor.[15] A pilot program was established in November 2007 to streamline the process, improve overall customer satisfaction, and rely on the VA for disability rating purposes.[16] This joint effort was born out of the President's Commission on Care for America's Returning Wounded Warriors [Dole-Shalala], which provided an "agenda for moving forward."[17] The goal of the pilot is to streamline and improve the disability evaluation process by providing one medical examination and a single-sourced (VA) disability rating, making for a seamless transition from the care, benefits, and services of the DoD to the VA system, measured by customer satisfaction (Figure 4-1).[16] The PDES Joint Pilot Program was first put into practice at the three Washington, DC-area triservice facilities: Walter Reed Army Medical Center, National Naval Medical Center, and Malcolm Grow Medical Center. The plan has been to expand the pilot program throughout the DoD, worldwide. Army-wide rollout of the pilot has begun with Fort Meade, Maryland, and Fort Belvoir, Virginia, on October 1, 2008.

Medical Evaluation Board

Current Legacy System

To understand the Army's proposed changes to the PDES, a closer look at the legacy system is necessary. Currently, an Army infantry soldier with major limb loss found by the MEB to not meet retention standards is referred to the PEB for a fitness determination. When the PEB determines that the limb loss renders the soldier unfit for his or her infantry MOS, a disability rating is generated by the PEB using the VA Schedule for Rating Disabilities (VASRD).[15] Soldiers who receive at least a 30% disability rating from the Army, which is often the case with major limb loss, and do not want to continue in service are medically retired, either temporarily or permanently.[15]

For the now retired soldier to receive disability compensation from the VA with the same limb loss diagnosis already rated by the Army, he or she must restart the medical evaluation process with a new set of clinical examinations by the VA medical providers. After reexamination, the VA, using the same VASRD criteria used by the Army, rates the soldier's service-connected disability, often at a higher percentage. Soldiers may be left wondering (*a*) why they received two separate and different ratings, one from the Army and one from the VA, for the same impairment, and (*b*) why the process takes so long. These two problems with the legacy system deserve further discussion.

First and foremost, the legacy system allows for a discrepancy in the final disability rating, rendered by both the Army and the VA, irrespective of one another, on the exact same diagnoses. The primary reason for this discrepancy is that the two departments follow different rules. The Army is tasked with rating each diagnosis that the MEB found "unacceptable" or "not meeting retention standards" and the PEB also found "unfitting," preventing the soldier's performance within his or her specific military job training.[15] Furthermore, the Army rates an "unfitting condition for present level of severity," much like a snapshot of the soldier's condition, at the time the MEB is conducted.[15] The VA, on the other hand, rates any and all "service-connected conditions," keeping in mind future progression of the disease or injury process,

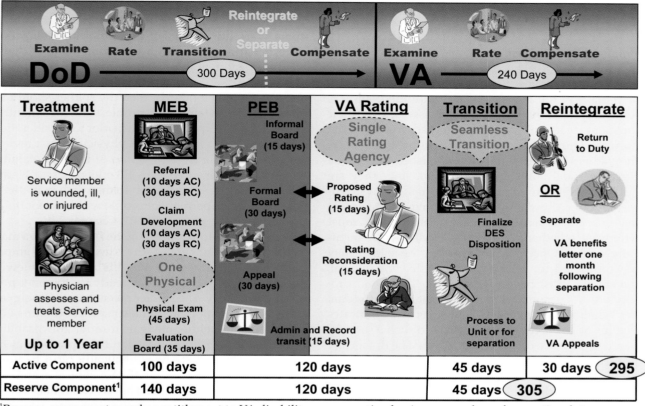

Active Component	100 days	120 days	45 days	30 days	295
Reserve Component¹	140 days	120 days	45 days	305	

¹Reserve component member entitlement to VA disability compensation begins upon release from active duty or separation.

Figure 4-1. Disability evaluation system Joint Pilot Program timeline overview. This graphic is part of the mass briefing provided to WTU members at Walter Reed Army Medical Center by the physical evaluation board liaison officer. Note that the treating physician, who generates the permanent "3" or "4" profile, which initiates the PDES, is distinct from the MEB physician, who administratively helps process the MEB.
AC: active component
DES: disability evaluation system
DoD: Department of Defense
MEB: medical evaluation board
PDES: physical disability evaluation system
PEB: physical evaluation board
RC: reserve component
VA: Veterans Administration

with respect to the condition's "adverse impact on employability within the civilian job sector."[15] These distinctions in laws and regulations allow for significantly different rating values. The final disability rating is expressed as a percentage rating between 0% and 100%, resulting from all types of diseases and injuries encountered as a result of, or incident to, military service.[18]

Second, the legacy MEB/PEB process may involve considerable delays for soldiers and their families. For soldiers suffering from multiple and complex "unacceptable" conditions, each requiring a disabil-

ity evaluation from a separate MTF specialty clinic, delays become inevitable. US Army Physical Disability Agency guidance requires that the disability evaluations of unacceptable conditions be performed no more than 6 months (30–45 days for psychiatric conditions) before submission to the PEB.[19] If the MTF disability evaluation of an unacceptable condition extends beyond the 6-month window before the case reaches the PEB, the soldier needs to be seen again by the particular MTF specialty clinic for an updated assessment and comment on whether or not the condition remains unacceptable. This reevaluation, a repeat of clinical work, places a tremendous strain on the specialty clinics.

Proposed Pilot System

Regardless of whether they enter the pilot program or remain in the legacy system, wounded soldiers returning from the battlefield are assessed by their inpatient treatment team prior to discharge from the hospital. During transition to the outpatient setting, the soldiers are placed into an established WTU to be cared for safely outside the hospital, since they are not well enough to return to their units. A physician-member of each soldier's interdisciplinary treatment team, serving as a competent medical authority, must determine whether the soldier's conditions are medically stable.[20] Once medically stable, the soldier may be considered for referral to the MEB. For referral, the soldier must have a permanent "3" or "4" profile.[20] A "3" designator signifies that the individual has "significant limitations"; whereas a "4" indicates that his or her "physical defects are to such a severity that performance of military duty must be drastically limited."[14(ch7)] For PDES purposes, the "3" and "4" designators are synonymous, meaning the soldier will not receive additional disability benefit in having a permanent "4" versus a permanent "3."

Once the permanent profile has been generated by the treating physician and signed by the designated approving authority, the soldier is recommended for referral into the Joint Pilot Program.[21]

An MEB physician reviews the permanent profile and ultimately determines if the soldier is a suitable candidate for entry into the pilot program, based on a completely new referral standard:

> When a competent medical authority determines a service member has one or more condition(s) which is suspected of not meeting medical retention standards, he or she will refer the service member into the DES at the point of hospitalization or treatment when a member's progress appears to have medically stabilized (and the course of further recovery is relatively predictable) and when it can be reasonably determined that the member is most likely not capable of performing the duties of his office, grade, rank, or rating. Referral will be within 1 year of being diagnosed with a medical condition(s) that does not appear to meet medical retention standards, but may be earlier if the examiner determines that the member will not be capable of returning to duty within 1 year.[20]

A condition is unstable when it has the potential, within 1 year of treatment intervention, to improve to such a degree that the soldier meets medical reten-

tion standards.[19] Examples of treatment interventions are condition-improving surgery or medication titrations, warranting a trial of duty prior to stabilization determination. If the MEB physician believes that a medical treatment intervention may improve the soldier's condition to such a degree that he or she will meet retention standards, then the soldier should be maintained on a temporary profile, valid for 3 months, and extendable up to 12 months, prior to consideration of permanency.[14(ch7)] The MEB physician must review all conditions for determination of medical stability before the soldier enters the MEB pilot program. Under no circumstances should any soldier with major limb loss be issued a permanent profile within 4 months of the amputation, per AR 40-501, Chapter 3.[14]

In a hypothetical example of the DES process, a male soldier with a right above-knee (transfemoral) amputation has had his permanent "3" profile reviewed by the MEB physician, and is ready for the pilot program MEB entry. The soldier meets with his assigned physical evaluation board liaison officer (Figure 4-2), who helps the soldier navigate through the disability process, helping him understand the procedural intricacies of the PDES. Next, the soldier is scheduled for medical evaluation with the VA clinical examiners at the regional VA facility. The VA examiners evaluate all conditions claimed by the soldier as well as all chronic conditions and those that have the potential to render the soldier militarily unfit.[22] After the VA clinical examinations, VA worksheets are generated to

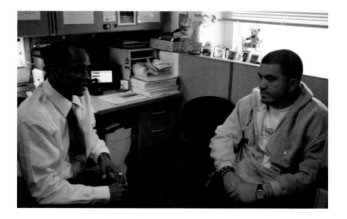

Figure 4-2. PEBLO counseling session: Mr Aaron Clemmons (left), Senior PEBLO, meets with SSG Juan Roldan to review all MEB administrative documents and answer procedural questions, prior to forwarding MEB case file to the PEB.
MEB: medical evaluation board
PEB: physical evaluation board
PEBLO: physical evaluation board liaison officer

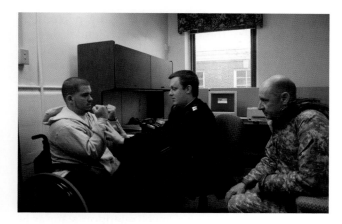

Figure 4-3. MEB physician encounter: Dr Andrew Rhodes, CPT, MC, USA (center), resolves discrepancy in soldier's medical record by examining SSG Juan Roldan (left), with consultation from Dr Eric Dessain, LTC, MC, USA (right), Disability Evaluation Service Chief, before finalizing the DoD/VA consolidated narrative summary.
DoD: Department of Defense
MEB: medical evaluation board
VA: Department of Veterans Affairs

document focused subjective complaints and objective findings, resulting in a final diagnosis for each claimed condition. The worksheets are returned to the MEB physician, who then prepares a consolidated narrative summary (NARSUM). The NARSUM must resolve any inconsistencies between the soldier's electronic medical record and the VA worksheets (Figure 4-3). The NARSUM also provides the physician with the opportunity to comment on each VA-generated diagnosis, with respect to whether or not the soldier meets retention standards, per AR 40-501, Chapter 3.

In generating the consolidated NARSUM, it is important that the MEB physician is knowledgeable about retention standards.[14] In the case of the soldier with an above-knee amputation, the MEB has no discretion; it must find that the soldier does not meet retention standards, per AR 40-501, Chapter 3, paragraph 13a(1b).[14] Paragraph 12a lists the specific impairment criteria for upper extremity limb loss.[14]

After the soldier with the above-knee amputation has returned from the VA and met with the MEB physician to review his consolidated NARSUM, his case is then officially referred to the MEB, an all-physician panel of at least two doctors, who review the entire case and make the final determination as to whether or not the soldier's conditions meet retention standards, per AR 40-501, Chapter 3.[14,23] The membership composition of the MEB, PEB, and medical MOS retention board (MMRB) is the same, regardless of whether the MTF

is involved in the pilot program. Soldiers found by the MEB to have conditions that do not meet retention standards are referred to the PEB for determination of fitness.

Soldiers who do not agree with MEB findings have a new option for further evaluation. A policy memorandum, issued by the under secretary of defense on October 14, 2008, describes the possibility of an independent medical review of MEB findings, prior to submission to the PEB:

> E3.P1.2.6.1.2. Upon request of a Service member referred into the DES, an impartial physician or other appropriate health care professional (not involved in the Service member's MEB process) is assigned to the Service member to offer a review of the medical evidence presented by the narrative summary or MEB findings. In most cases, this impartial health professional should be the Service member's primary care manager (PCM). The impartial health professional will have no more than 5 calendar days to advise the Service member on whether the findings of the MEB adequately reflect the complete spectrum of injuries and illness of the Service member.

. . .

> E3.P1.2.6.1.3. After review of findings with the assigned impartial health care professional, a Service member shall be afforded an opportunity to request a rebuttal of the results of the MEB. A Service member shall be afforded 7 calendar days to prepare a rebuttal to the convening medical authority. The convening medical board authority shall be afforded 7 calendar days to consider the rebuttal and return the fully documented decision to the Service member…The fully documented rebuttal will be included with the MEB information sent to the PEB.[24]

Medical Military Occupational Specialty Retention Board

There are a few instances in which a soldier with limb loss can meet retention standards, including the loss of toes or fingers. In the case of amputated toes, to fail to meet retention standards, the impairment must preclude the soldier's "abilities to run or walk without a perceptible limp and to engage in fairly strenuous jobs," as listed under 3-13a(1a).[14] In the case of lost fingers, to be considered as not meeting retention standards, the loss must be greater than or equal to: "a) a thumb proximal to the interphalangeal joint; b) two fingers of one hand, other than the little finger, at the proximal interphalangeal joints; [or] c) one finger, other than the little finger, at the metacarpophalangeal joint and the thumb on the same hand at the interphalangeal joint," as defined under 3-12a(1a-c).[14] An infantry soldier missing the trigger and little fingers on the same hand, resulting from a traumatic blast injury, is by regulation, if no other impairments exist, still able to meet retention standards.[14] Since this soldier requires "significant functional limitations," specifically being unable to fire a weapon, the soldier is issued a permanent "3" profile. However, because the soldier meets retention standards, he or she should be referred to an MMRB.[14(ch7)]

Soldiers may be referred to an MMRB if they have at least a permanent "3" designator for a condition that meets retention standards.[14(ch7)] The MMRB has the option of returning the soldiers to their units, placing them on medical probationary status, reclassifying them into another MOS, or referring them to the MEB.[25] The MMRB consists of five members, some voting and some nonvoting. The voting members include a colonel, either in combat arms, combat support, or combat service-support, serving as president; a field grade Medical Corps officer or MTF commander-designated civilian medical doctor; and an additional voting member who, if possible, is in the same branch, specialty, or primary MOS as the soldier appearing before the board.[25] The nonvoting members are a personnel advisor and recorder.[25] Treating physicians should be familiar with the options available for their injured soldiers.

Physical Evaluation Board

The Army PEB is composed of three voting members: a colonel, serving as the board president; a field grade personnel management officer; and a senior physician, either a Medical Corps officer or an Army civilian doctor.[24] The PEB first meets informally, meaning the soldier is not present, and also that the recommendations made at this meeting may later be changed. The three board members determine fitness by majority vote, taking into consideration the following: clinical evidence presented in the soldier's MEB; performance standards of the soldier's primary MOS; and the soldier's personnel records, including but not limited to his or her record brief, evaluation reports, and commanders' statements.[15] Under the pilot program, the PEB records its informal factual findings for each diagnosis, along with its recommendation for fitness determination, on DA Form 199 (Election to Formal Physical Evaluation Board Proceedings).[15] No rating determinations appear on Form 199; rather, for those conditions labeled as unfitting, the form has an explanation of the condition followed by a qualifier, signifying that the rating generated for the unfitting condition is to be completed by the VA. The VA rating board then evaluates the soldier's referred and claimed conditions, providing a rating percentage with rationale to the PEB within 15 calendar days of notification by the PEB that a soldier is unfit.[22] At this time, the soldier must request a copy of his or her VA rating for each claimed condition (generated by a VA regional office).[22]

In the pilot program, the Army is bound by the VA rating for those conditions found to be unfitting. In other words, if the Army finds the soldier unfit for a particular condition, the rating for that condition is determined by the rating provided by the VA.[22] For example, the soldier with the right above-knee amputation, whose only condition is major limb loss, is found to not meet retention standards, per AR 40-501, Chapter 3, Paragraph 13a(1b).[14] The soldier's primary MOS is 11B, infantry. He is found unfit for service, based on his injury and inability to satisfactorily perform the duties within his primary MOS. A soldier is physically unfit when a medical impairment prevents reasonable performance of the duties required of the soldier's office, grade, rank, or rating.[15] In this example, the soldier's residual limb length, as measured from the perineum, is found to be one-third of the distance from perineum to knee joint, when compared to the left, unaffected side. Thus, the right above-knee amputation transects the upper third of the femur bone. Per disability code 5161, as found in the VASRD, the VA rates his condition at 80% disability.[18] Under the pilot program, the Army is now bound by this 80% disability rating, whereas in the legacy disability system, the Army provides a disability rating independent of the VA rating.

After the informal PEB has convened and rendered DA Form 199, the soldier is entitled to government-appointed legal counsel (if not already obtained[24]) and has the following election options: (*a*) concur with the informal findings and recommendations; (*b*) request a formal administrative hearing, either with or without a personal appearance; or (*c*) nonconcur and submit a written appeal in lieu of proceeding with a formal board.[15] The formal PEB is administrative, fact-finding, and nonadversarial, meaning no government representative appears to oppose or counter the soldier's position at the hearing.[15] Because the informal PEB recommendations may be changed, the soldier may be found fit with a condition previously considered unfitting. Soldiers typically request a formal hearing to argue that conditions found to be fitting should be reconsidered as unfitting. Also, some soldiers found unfit for service request a formal hearing to argue that they are fit for duty, based upon duty performance, as substantiated by their chain of command.[15] Thus, before a soldier requests a formal hearing, it is extremely important for him or her to understand the VA rating, which will ultimately drive the subsequent Army disability disposition.

The end result is that the soldier receives a disability rating from the VA and a disability disposition from the Army. The VA rates all claimed service-connected conditions based upon its evaluations. The Army renders a disposition of the soldier, based upon the VA rating, for those conditions found unfitting by the PEB. If the soldier has less than 20 years of active federal service and reaches at least a 30% disability rating, the Army may place the soldier on either permanent disability retirement (PDR) or the temporary disability retirement list (TDRL). PDR applies when the soldier's condition is stable and not expected to improve or deteriorate in the next 18 months. TDRL applies to those conditions where the converse is believed to be clinically true: the condition will likely change in the next 18 months.[15] Soldiers on the TDRL are reexamined at 12 to 18 months following Army discharge. The soldier can be maintained on TDRL for a maximum of 5 years, with reexaminations at the 3- and 5-year marks, if the condition remains unstable and continues to meet the minimum criteria for at least a 30% rating.[15] If the soldier's unfitting condition has not stabilized in 5 years, the PEB will provide a disability rating based upon the level of severity at that point in time.[15] The legacy disability system applies to the TDRL, in that the reevaluations are conducted at the MTF and the disability rating can be adjusted by the PEB, independent of the VA.

Soldiers who are found unfit by the PEB but receive a combined VA rating of less than 30% for their service-connected conditions are separated with a one-time, lump-sum, severance payment.[15] The exact disability rating, whether 0%, 10%, or 20%, makes no difference in the calculation of severance pay. The disability severance payment amount is calculated by doubling the soldier's monthly basic pay, multiplying it by the number of combined years of federal service (not to exceed 12 years), and then adding this number to the inactive duty points, per AR 635-40, Appendix C.

Continuation on Active Duty

The Army provides an administrative procedure—continuation on active duty (COAD)—to determine whether or not the unfit soldier suffering major limb loss should be continued on active duty. The study by Kishbaugh et al,[4] which found that only 2.3% of soldiers in the 1980s remained on active duty after

amputation, did not discern whether the soldiers remaining on active duty were found fit or were granted a continuation on active duty. However, it is important to note that none of the 79 soldiers with above-knee amputations were retained on active duty.[4] "Soldiers with hand and/or finger amputations (54.5%) constituted the majority of the return-to-duty group, with the remainder made up of foot and/or toe amputees (27.3%) and below-knee amputees (18.2%)."[4]

Over the past year, all soldiers with combat-related limb loss referred by the Walter Reed Army Medical Center MEB who failed to meet retention standards (per AR 40-501, Chapter 3) were found unfit. AR 635-40, Chapter 6, prescribes the criteria by which soldiers with major limb loss who have been found unfit by the PEB may be continued on active duty or on active reserve status.[13(ch6)]

In the example of the active duty soldier with above-knee amputation, to be considered for COAD, he must meet one of the following criteria:

- have 15, but less than 20, years of active federal service, or
- be qualified in a critical skill or shortage MOS, or
- possess a disability resulting from combat or terrorism.[13(ch6)]

Per Army Regulation, the soldier does not have an inherent or vested right to continuation on active duty; the primary objective of the COAD program is to conserve personnel by effective use of needed skills or experience.[13(ch6)] If approved by the Human Resources Command, the COAD for soldiers with major limb loss lasts for any period of time up to the last day of the month in which they obtain 20 years of active federal service.[13(ch6)] If the disability precludes continuation in a limited duty status within the soldier's current primary MOS, the soldier may request reclassification into another MOS, listing three alternatives, in order of preference.[13(ch6)] A soldier approved for COAD longer than 6 months is referred to the PDES before the continuance expires.[13(ch6)] During the final PDES evaluation, soldiers whose disabilities have healed or improved to such a degree that they are capable of performing their primary MOS may be found fit; however, the ability to perform duties with prostheses does not constitute healing or improvement of a soldier's condition for purposes of a fit finding.[13(ch6)]

RETIREMENT AND DISABILITY COMPENSATION

Soldiers considering a return to duty should clearly understand the nuances of a COAD and reaching regular/longevity retirement after a minimum of 20 years

of active duty service. If a COAD is approved and the soldier retires after at least 20 years, the soldier must be reevaluated with a new MEB at the time of retirement or separation. The same applies for soldiers with an approved continuation on active reserve (COAR) and 20 qualifying years for reserve retirement. The final MEB/PEB does not affect longevity retirement benefits, to which every soldier with over 20 years of service is entitled. However, the percentage of retirement pay may be increased because of a disability causing unfitness for duty, and receipt of additional VA disability compensation as well as potential tax-free military retirement monies may be affected, as described below.

Retired amputee service members *may* be eligible to receive both military retirement and VA disability compensation (known as concurrent receipt [CR]), if they are found by a PEB to have at least 30% disability, or if their COAD or COAR is approved and they qualify for longevity retirement. A longevity retirement, which requires completion of at least 20 years of active duty service, or 20 years of accumulated required retirement points for reserve or National Guard service, is the basis for either CR or combat-related special compensation (CRSC). Service members may also be eligible for CR if they have over 20 years of active duty service and are retiring because of disability, without ever having a COAD or COAR.

Military retirement pay is taxable income unless the soldier's injuries are combat-related as determined by the PEB. All VA benefits are nontaxable. Current law requires that military retirement pay (taxable income) be reduced dollar-for-dollar for each dollar of VA compensation (nontaxable income) paid. However, CR and CRSC are designed to replace that offset. To qualify for CR, a veteran must retire with 20 or more years of service and be rated with a 50% or more service-connected disability by the VA. CR increases taxable retirement pay, but not nontaxable VA compensation. Payment of CR is automatic for qualified retirees; however, the benefit is being phased-in over a 10-year period, and full CR will not be achieved until January 2014. CRSC is a DoD program designed to correct the offset when all or some of the service-connected conditions are the result of combat or combat-type injuries or illnesses. Veterans must apply to their service for CRSC after they receive a disability rating from the VA. CRSC does not increase or replace retirement pay; it is a special nontaxable compensation. Qualifying veterans have the choice of either CR or CRSC, and both programs are capped at the amount equal to full retirement pay. Service members and veterans should contact the Defense Finance and Accounting service or a VA benefits counselor for specific information about their situation. Amputee service members who do not qualify for longevity retirement still qualify for VA benefits.

Reserve component amputee service members whose COAR is approved face unique challenges with benefits. While in inactive status, they have no personal or family TRICARE benefits or military income. Healthcare can be received at any MTF, but only with a line-of-duty statement. Travel to and from an MTF is generally not reimbursed. COAR-approved amputee service members can apply for VA benefits and receive VA compensation and medical care, but their monthly VA disability compensation is offset by their monthly military compensation.

VETERANS AFFAIRS BENEFITS

Besides understanding the PDES, service members with major limb loss should also be familiar with the range of potential VA benefits available to them as they consider whether or not to remain on active or reserve duty (see Chapter 3, Department of Veterans Affairs System of Care for the Polytrauma Patient). VA counselors are available to discuss each of the following benefits:

- compensation and pension payments,
- home loan guaranty (VA loan funding fee waived for disabled veterans),
- life insurance,
- tuition assistance,
- vocational rehabilitation and employment opportunities,
- medical care for all service-connected conditions,
- civil service preference, and
- special grants (some available to active duty disabled service members and retired veterans alike), such as:

- a special adaptive housing grant (up to $50,000),
- an automobile grant (up to $11,000),
- automobile adaptive equipment,
- annual clothing allowance, and
- aide and attendant's care.

Vocational rehabilitation benefits (see Chapter 6, Vocational Rehabilitation of the Combat Amputee) are especially important, for service members with major limb loss will at some time likely transition to the civilian workforce. Assessment of service members' vocational aptitudes and interests, as well as individual training services, can start while they are still on active duty; however, the financial stipend cannot be paid until a DD214 is issued and a VA service-connected disability rating is obtained. Specific training benefits include tuition, books, fees and supplies, a monthly stipend, transportation support, and any necessary adaptive equipment.

WAY FORWARD

According to the Armed Forces Amputee Care Program database at the time of this writing, the US Army retained over 15% of soldiers with major limb loss in uniform. Further research is required to more fully assess this cohort and the significant factors that influenced their decisions to stay in the military, the duration and quality of their subsequent military service, and their eventual transition to civilian life. In addition, studies to compare the amputee care treatment and policies related to military retention between US military personnel with major limb loss and their counterparts in allied militaries may lead to further improvements in US military healthcare and personnel systems.

The PDES pilot program is the first attempt to merge complicated and separate military and VA disability systems across the entire DoD. Soldiers in the pilot program no longer have to repeat Army disability evaluations at the VA. This relieves some of the burden of the MTF specialty clinics; without sole responsibility for providing the disability evaluation, they are able to focus more on soldiers' treatment and continuity of care.

Challenges remain, including differences in VA and military disability terminology and the responsibilities assigned to an already overburdened VA disability system. The pilot program has not yet reformed the compensation system. The Dole-Shalala Commission recommended that service members found unfit because of their combat-related injuries should receive comprehensive healthcare for themselves and their dependents through the DoD TRICARE program, regardless of rating percentage.[17] The Commission also recommended that the VA reform the VASRD to reflect current understanding of the impact of disability on quality of life, such as described in the civilian American Medical Association *Guides to Evaluation of Permanent Impairment*.[17]

Another proposed idea is to shorten the time soldiers remain on TDRL by having the VA clinicians, rather than MTF physicians, provide the medical determination of whether a condition is stable, once, at 18 months after retirement, as opposed to numerous times. In October 2008 a change was made to TDRL policy for service members found unfit secondary to a mental disorder sustained from a traumatic stress, the prime examples being posttraumatic stress disorder and traumatic brain injury with its resultant sequelae; a rating of not less than 50% is assigned and the soldier is automatically placed into TDRL, with reevaluation within 6 months.[24] Reworking the entire TDRL policy will allow for greater efficiency, consistency, and overall patient-provider satisfaction.

Customer satisfaction is the driving force behind the PDES pilot program, as evidenced by the *Report to Congress on the Current Status of the Department of Defense and Department of Veterans' Affairs Disability Evaluation System Pilot Program*, prepared by the Wounded, Ill, and Injured Overarching Integrated Product Team on November 20, 2008.[26] This team was established by an oversight committee cochaired by the deputy secretaries of DoD and VA, which also developed eight workgroups to focus on specific care areas for wounded, injured, or ill service members entering the PDES, within each service. The care areas ranged from case management and disability evaluation of service members to compensation and benefits to overall collaboration between the DoD and VA. Process and outcome measures were established, with the evaluation and assessment of the pilot program based on a balanced score card approach, focusing on four dimensions: (1) process improvement, (2) customer satisfaction, (3) financial management, and (4) learning and growth. To determine measurable results that can be used to assess the program's success, specific parameters have been established, including a continuing process improvement effort, a cost-benefit analysis, participant and stakeholder surveys, and a mechanism to track the duration of the process for service members, in relation to their location and DoD/VA regional treatment facilities. Feedback initiatives that provide service members and their families a voice throughout the disability process are intended to improve the overall satisfaction and understanding of the process. An online data-capturing tool has been implemented to track each service member through the process, allowing for management review and oversight. Preliminary indications are favorable that the pilot program is improving the disability system, yet data is limited and further efforts to collect information are needed.[26]

SUMMARY

Soldiers who sustain traumatic injuries, including major limb loss, are challenged with a complex recovery process that unfolds over weeks to years. The personal decision of whether to pursue return-to-duty or transition into civilian life requires a realistic appraisal of one's clinical, psychological, and functional progress, in light of the demands of self, family, and ultimate reentry into a military or civilian occupation. Effectively navigating the PDES requires an awareness of the military and VA disability systems.

Through military and VA counseling, self-education, and early involvement of military-appointed legal counsel or other soldier advocate groups, injured soldiers can best understand the options afforded to them and their families. With the commitment of support from the highest levels of the DoD and VA, more service members with amputations can be expected to successfully return to duty.

REFERENCES

1. Pelka F, ed. *The Civil War Letters of Colonel Charles F. Johnson, Invalid Corps*. Amherst, Mass: University of Massachusetts Press, 2004: 336.

2. Callison L. Army will call back amputees back to active duty: regulation is break for handicapped. *Washington Times-Herald*. November 11, 1951:13.

3. Greve F. 50% of Walter Reed amputees want to return to active duty. *McClatchy Newspapers*. June 22, 2007.

4. Kishbaugh D, Dillingham TR, Howard RS, Sinnott MW, Belandres PV. Amputee soldiers and their return to active duty. *Mil Med*. 1995;160:82–84.

5. Rozelle D. *Back in Action: An American Soldier's Story of Courage, Faith, and Fortitude*. Washington, DC: Regnery Publishing Inc; 2005.

6. US Army Military Amputee Care Data Base. Washington, DC: Walter Reed Army Medical Center.

7. Wingert P, Gegax T. Back to the front: soldiers who lost limbs in Iraq and Afghanistan are doing the unthinkable, going back to battle. *Newsweek*. 2005;145(11):38–41.

8. Dougherty PJ. Transtibial amputees from the Vietnam War: twenty-eight year follow-up. *J Bone Joint Surg Am*. 2001;83A:383–389.

9. Steinbach T. Total rehabilitation for amputees in special conditions. *Prosthet Orthot Int*. 1977;1:125–126.

10. Pasquina PF, Gambel J, Foster LS, Kim A, Doukas WC. Process of care for battle casualties at the Walter Reed Army Medical Center: Part III. Physical Medicine and Rehabilitation Service. *Mil Med*. 2006;171:206–208.

11. Mackenzie EJ, Bosse MJ. Factors influencing outcome following limb-threatening lower limb trauma: lessons learned from the Lower Extremity Assessment Project (LEAP). *J Am Acad Orthop Surg*. 2006;14:S205–210.

12. Gambel J, Mayer J, Lourake A, Downs F. Peer visitor support of recent U.S. military amputees. *inMotion*. 2004;Nov–Dec:26–27.

13. US Department of the Army. *Personnel Separations: Physical Evaluation for Retention, Retirement, or Separation*. Washington, DC: DA, 2006. Army Regulation 635-40.

14. US Department of the Army. *Standards of Medical Fitness*. Washington, DC: DA; 2008. Army Regulation 40-501, Chapter 3.

15. Webb RE, White DC. Physical disability separation. Louisville Law, Kentucky Legal Resources on the Internet. Available at: http://louisvillelaw.com/federal/physical_disbility_sep_1.htm. Accessed June 2006.

16. Mansfield GH, Deputy Secretary of Veterans Affairs; England G, Deputy Secretary of Defense. *Department of Defense (DoD) and Department of Veterans' Affairs (DVA) Implementation of Recommendations of the President's Commission on Care for America's Returning Wounded Warriors (Dole/Shalala Report)*. DoD/VA Wounded, Ill, and Injured Senior Oversight Committee Memorandum, 07 August 2007.

17. Dole R, Shalala D. *Serve, Support, Simplify: Report of the President's Commission on Care for America's Returning Wounded Warriors*. Washington, DC: President's Commission on Care for America's Returning Wounded Warriors; 2007.

18. 38 CFR, Part 4, § 4.71a.

19. US Department of the Army. US Army Physical Disability Agency. Guidance for medical evaluation board (MEB) physicians, guidance for MEB examiners. Available at: https://www.hrc.army.mil/site/Active/TAGD/Pda/pdapage.htm. Updated November 25, 2008. Accessed January 15, 2009.

20. Chu DSC, Under Secretary of Defense. *Policy Memorandum on Implementing Disability-Related Provisions of the National Defense Authorization Act of 2008 (Pub L. 110-181).* Memorandum for Secretaries of the Military Departments, Chairman of the Joint Chiefs of Staff, General Counsel of the Department of Defense, Inspector General of the Department of Defense, 14 October 2008.

21. Chu DSC, Under Secretary of Defense. *Policy Guidance for the Disability Evaluation System and Establishment of Recurring Directive-Type Memoranda.* Memorandum for Secretaries of the Military Departments, Chairman of the Joint Chiefs of Staff, General Counsel of the Department of Defense, Inspector General of the Department of Defense, and Director, Administration and Management, 03 May 2007.

22. Under Secretary of Defense. *Policy and Procedural Directive-Type Memorandum (DTM) for the Disability Evaluation System (DES) Pilot Program.* Washington, DC: DoD; 21 November 2007.

23. US Department of the Army. *Medical Services: Patient Administration.* Washington, DC: DA; 2008. Army Regulation 40-400: Chap 7.

24. Under Secretary of Defense. *Policy Memorandum on Implementing Disability-Related Provisions of the National Defense Authorization Act of 2008 (Pub L. 110-181).* Washington, DC: DoD; 14 October 2008.

25. US Department of the Army. *Physical Performance Evaluation System.* Washington, DC: DoD; 2008. Army Regulation 600-60: Chap 4.

26. Wounded, Ill, and Injured Overarching Integrated Product Team. *Report to Congress on the Current Status of the Department of Defense and Department of Veterans' Affairs Disability Evaluation System Pilot Program.* Washington, DC: Department of Defense, Department of Veterans Affairs; 2008.

Chapter 5

OVERVIEW OF THE DEPARTMENT OF VETERANS AFFAIRS

NICOLE M. KEESEE, MS*

*Colonel, US Army; Office of The Surgeon General/Veterans Affairs Central Office Seamless Transition Office, 810 Vermont Avenue, NW, VACO 10D1, Washington, DC 20420

INTRODUCTION

The Plymouth colony Pilgrims enacted the first veteran's benefit over 300 years ago, providing pecuniary pensions for their disabled war veterans in the 1636 war with the Pequot Indians. Over 100 years later, to increase the ranks of the Continental Army over the course of the Revolutionary War, the 1776 Continental Congress enacted the first pension law granting half pay for life in cases of loss of limb or other serious disability. However, the Continental Congress did not have the authority or financial backing to fund the new law, so states paid the pensions and provided public land grants to veterans.

On July 21, 2005, the US Department of Veterans Affairs (VA) celebrated its 75th anniversary. With a budget of $63.5 billion,[1] the VA is the most comprehensive veterans' benefits system in the world, serving over 26 million veterans of the US armed services (Army, Navy, Marine Corps, Air Force, Coast Guard) and other beneficiary populations. About one third of Americans (70 million) are eligible for VA benefits.[1] Slightly less than half of all Americans who ever served during wartime are alive today, and nearly 80% of today's veterans served during a period of war.

The VA is a Cabinet-level, government-run, single-payer healthcare system responsible for administering benefits programs whose beneficiaries are active duty service personnel, veterans, their family members, and survivors. On October 13, 1987, Representative Jack B Brooks introduced HR 3471 declaring the VA an executive department. A little over a year later, President Ronald Reagan signed the bill, which became Public Law 100-527. President George Bush heralded the new department's activation on March 15, 1989, declaring, "There is only one place for the veterans of America, in the Cabinet Room, at the table with the President of the United States of America."[2] Of the 14 Cabinet departments, the VA is the second largest, surpassed only by the Department of Defense. The president, with the Senate's advice and consent, appoints the VA secretary.

Navigating the VA system in pursuit of legislated benefits and entitlements can be a daunting task. No instructional "VA 101" course is available to educate service members, and the majority of military healthcare providers have no knowledge of veteran and service member benefits, let alone how to apply for them. Today all service members should be made aware of the VA's transformation: no longer is the VA caring only for the nation's veterans, but it is also providing benefits to active duty service members and starting initiatives to serve family members. This chapter provides an overview of VA benefits and programs.

DEPARTMENT DESCRIPTION

The VA has the federal government's second largest civilian work force, including approximately 15,000 physicians, 4,500 pharmacists, 1,000 dentists, 38,000 nurses, and 4,800 master's prepared social workers. The department operates in all 50 states, Puerto Rico, the Philippines, Guam, and Washington, DC, and owns more than 4,000 buildings and 27,000 acres of land. Of approximately 198,000 employees, 30% are veterans and 15,000 are members of the reserve and National Guard forces.

Mission

The VA draws its mission statement from President Abraham Lincoln's second inaugural address: "to care for him who shall have borne the battle and for his widow and his orphan."[3] Veteran benefits are determined by a number of variables over any given period of time. Benefits one veteran receives may not be the same as those another veteran receives.

Organization

The VA comprises a central office (VACO) located in Washington, DC; facilities throughout the nation and abroad; and three administrations that provide for the delivery of services and benefits: the Veterans Health Administration (VHA), the Veterans Benefits Administration (VBA), and the National Cemetery Administration (NCA). The head of each administration reports to the secretary through the deputy secretary. These administrations give centralized program direction to field facilities that provide diverse program services to their beneficiaries. Furthermore, each administration has central office components supporting operations. Seven assistant secretaries advise and support the secretary and the administrations, and 11 staff offices provide specific assistance to the secretary (Figure 5-1).[4] The VA structure uses a centralized policy-directed/decentralized execution approach to govern daily operations.

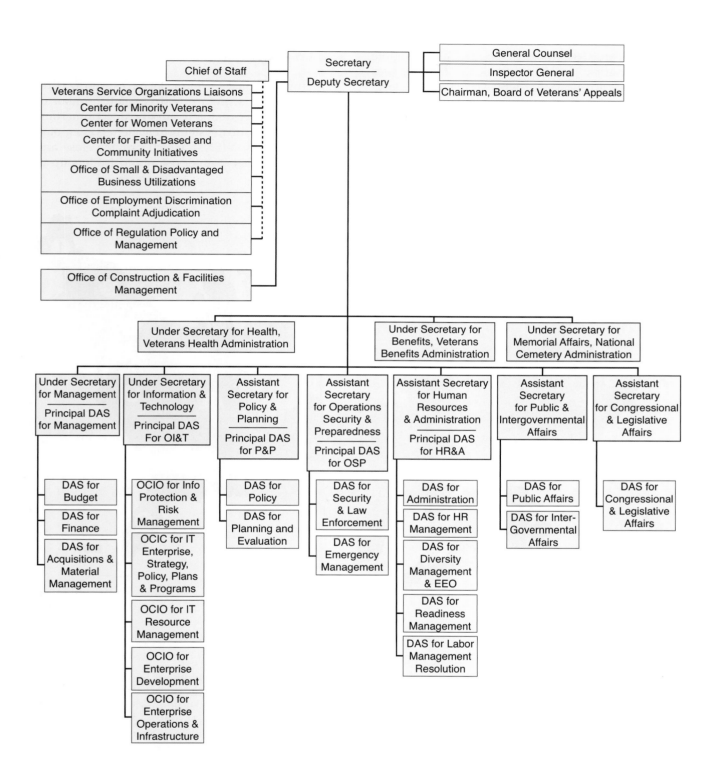

Figure 5-1. Department of Veterans Affairs organizational chart.
Reproduced from: Department of Veterans Affairs. *2007 Organizational Briefing Book*. Washington, DC: VA Office of Human Resources and Administration; 2007.

VETERANS HEALTH ADMINISTRATION

US Code title 38 authorizes medical care to eligible VA beneficiaries. The VHA administers and operates the VA medical care system, which is the nation's largest integrated healthcare system, providing care to over 5.6 million (FY 2007) unique patients and handling 54 million outpatient visits in 2006. The VA's 2007 healthcare budget was more than $34 billion, and the 2008 budget was expected to be almost $40 billion.[5]

Veterans Integrated Service Networks

During the past 7 years, VHA's organization changed from a structure with a small number of regional directors remotely supervising numerous, complex activities, to a system of 21 veterans integrated service networks (VISNs), which provide close and continuing hands-on supervision and leadership to

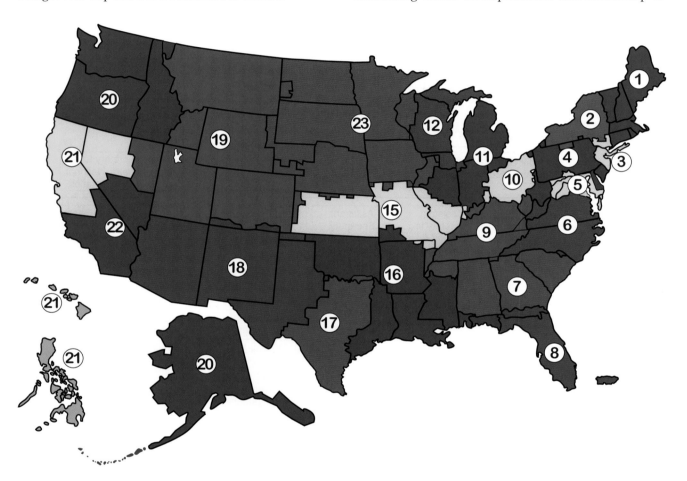

Figure 5-2. Veterans integrated service network (VISN) map. Note: VISNs 13 and 14 do not exist.

VISN 1: VA New England Healthcare System
VISN 2: VA Healthcare Network Upstate New York
VISN 3: VA NY/NJ Veterans Healthcare Network
VISN 4: VA Healthcare
VISN 5: VA Capitol Healthcare Network
VISN 6: VA Mid-Atlantic Healthcare Network
VISN7: VA Southeast Network
VISN 8: VA Sunshine Healthcare Network
VISN 9: VA Mid South Healthcare Network
VISN 10: VA Healthcare System of Ohio
VISN 11: Veterans in Partnership

VISN 12: VA Great Lakes Healthcare System
VISN 15: VA Heartland Network
VISN 16: South Central VA Healthcare Network
VISN 17: VA Heart of Texas Healthcare Network
VISN 18: VA Southwest Healthcare Network
VISN 19: Rocky Mountain Network
VISN 20: Northwest Network
VISN 21: Sierra Pacific Network
VISN 22: Desert Pacific Healthcare Network
VISN 23: VA Midwest Healthcare Network

Reproduced from: Media Net. Veterans Affairs intranet site. Available at: http://vaww.mam.lrn.va.gov/MediaNet04. Accessed May 16, 2008.

local VA facilities (Figure 5-2).[6] The current system's goal is to deliver the right care in the right place at the right time. The transformation resulted in a change in the ratio of outpatient visits to inpatient admissions from 29:1 in 1995 to more than 100:1 in 2006.

Mission

The VHA's mission is to serve the needs of America's veterans by providing primary care, specialized care, and related medical and social support services. The VHA provides a broad spectrum of medical, surgical, and rehabilitative healthcare in all its forms, as well as conducting medical research. VHA manages the largest medical education and health profession training programs in the United States. VHA facilities are affiliated with more than 105 medical schools, 55 dental schools, and more than 1,200 other schools across the country. Each year VHA medical centers train about 83,000 health professionals. More than half of all physicians practicing in the United States had some of their professional education in the VA healthcare system.

As of June 2007, approximately 1.4 million service members have served in Iraq and Afghanistan since the beginning of hostilities. Of 837,458 veterans who became eligible for VA healthcare from fiscal year (FY) 2002 to FY 2008 (1st quarter), 39% (324,846) of the total separated veterans of operations Iraqi Freedom and Enduring Freedom (OIF/OEF) obtained VA healthcare (cumulative total). Of the 324,846 evaluated OIF/OEF patients, 96% (311,730) have been seen as outpatients and not hospitalized, and 4% (13,116) have been hospitalized at least once in a VA medical facility. Of 414,588 former active duty troops, 40% (165,578) have sought VA healthcare (cumulative total since FY 2002). Of 422,870 reserve/National Guard members, 38% (159,268) have sought VA healthcare. These 324,846 OIF/OEF veterans (Table 5-1) evaluated by VA over approximately 6 years represent about 6% of the 5.5 million individual patients who received VHA healthcare in any 1 year (the 2007 total VHA patient population was 5.5 million).[7]

Changes in the Veteran Population

The current OEF/OIF VA population is very different from the general VHA population. The median age of the general VA population is 65 (FY05), whereas the median age of the OIF/OEF population is 28.6 (active duty) and 35.0 (reserve/Guard). Of the general VA population, 95.2% are male and 4.8% are female. Of the OEF/OIF population, 87% are male and 13% are female. The five leading diagnoses of all VHA users

TABLE 5-1

CHARACTERISTICS OF OPERATIONS IRAQI FREEDOM AND ENDURING FREEDOM VETERANS

	Category	Percentage (%)
Sex	Male	88
	Female	12
Branch	Air Force	12
	Army	65
	Marine Corps	12
	Navy	11
Rank	Enlisted	92
	Officer	8
Unit Type	Active duty	51
	Reserve/Guard	49
Age	<20	7
	20–29	51
	30–39	23
	> or = 40	19

Total: 324,846

(2006) are hypertension; diabetes; lipids-related (ie, fatty acids, cholesterol, estrogen, and other related compounds); adjustment reaction; and ischemic heart disease. In contrast, the five leading diagnoses for OEF/OIF veterans are musculoskeletal, mental health, digestive (dental), ill-defined, and nervous system/sensory disorders. The VA is making adjustments to meet the new demands of the OEF/OIF beneficiary population: a major expansion of mental health services, implementation of a suicide hotline, development of a polytrauma care network, significant increase in women's health services, the addition of OEF/OIF care cooordination at each VA medical center, and, the addition of OEF/OIF polytrauma/traumatic brain injury individual care coordinators.[7]

Assistive Technology

The VA is dedicated to restoring the capabilities of disabled veterans to the greatest extent possible. VA has an integrated delivery system designed to provide medically prescribed prosthetic and sensory aids, devices, assistive aids, repairs, and services to disabled individuals to facilitate treatment of their medical conditions. The VA Prosthetic and Sensory Aids Service (PSAS) is the healthcare provider and case manager for assistive aids and prosthetic equipment needs of disabled veterans. The service's goal is to provide seamless service from prescription through procurement, delivery, training, replacement, and repair. Care providers who prescribe an aid or a device to veterans enrolled in the VA system are eligible for PSAS services.

Other products and services disabled veterans receive include wheelchairs and scooters; braces; shoes and orthotics; oxygen and respiratory equipment; other medical equipment and supplies (beds, lifts, computer equipment, telehealth products); adaptive sports and recreation equipment; and surgical implants (pacemakers, cardiac defibrillators, stents, dental devices). PSAS also has programs providing home improvements and structural changes, automobile adaptive equipment, and a clothing allowance to eligible veterans with service-connected disabilities. The Prosthetics Clinical Management Program coordinates national integrated product teams—interdisciplinary workgroups consisting of clinical and administrative subject-matter experts who develop clinical practice recommendations for prosthetic devices and national contracts to purchase them. As of April 2008, VA had 61 accredited orthotic-prosthetic laboratories staffed by 185 employees, 139 of whom are certified by either the American Board for Certification in Orthotics, Prosthetics and Pedorthotics or the Board of Orthotist and Prosthetist Certification. Additionally, 18 of these laboratories have also earned certification from the National Commission on Orthotic and Prosthetic Education, which enables them to participate in residency programs from the nine prosthetic and orthotic programs in US universities and colleges.

PSAS staff provide prescribed devices, consult in clinics, and custom fabricate, fit, and repair artificial limbs and braces or order them from commercial vendors. They and other medical specialists in various disciplines form amputee clinic teams who see the veteran regularly after fitting to ensure the proper functioning of the artificial limb as well as the integration of body, mind, and machine. VA PSAS staff work alongside Army healthcare providers at the Center for the Intrepid, Fort Sam Houston, Texas. At Walter Reed Army Medical Center in Washington, DC, VA's vocational rehabilitation and employment program provides voice-recognition computers so Iraq war soldiers who have lost a hand can learn computer skills. Continuing to increase collaboration and implement resource-sharing initiatives, both DoD and VA can further improve facility utilization, provide greater access to care, and reduce the federal cost of providing healthcare services to beneficiaries. VA also collaborates with non-DoD organizations. The VA Medical Center's Center for Restorative and Regenerative Medicine and Brown University, in Providence, Rhode Island, and the Massachusetts Institute of Technology

are collaborating to create artificial limbs that function almost like biological ones.

No less important than new prosthetic component technology is the overall care an amputee receives during rehabilitation. The model for care has changed over the years to improve services to VA patients that go beyond teaching amputees to walk or use a prosthetic arm and hand. Continuing care and long-term support from VA multidisciplinary teams enable patients to improve their functioning months or years after their injuries or amputation. To contact the VHA prosthetics central office, call (202) 254-0440, or go to the Web site: www.prosthetics.va.gov.

Healthcare Programs

The VA offers a spectrum of healthcare services to veterans enrolled in its healthcare system. Each program has specific admissions and eligibility requirements. To determine eligibility, contact the nearest VA medical facility. The following is a list with brief descriptions of VA programs.

Long-Term Care

More than 90% of VA's medical centers provide home- and community-based outpatient long-term care programs. This patient-focused approach supports the wishes of most patients who want to live at home in their own communities for as long as possible.[8]

Noninstitutional Care

Veterans can receive home-based primary care, contract home healthcare, adult day healthcare, homemaker and home health aide services, home respite care, home hospice care, and community residential care. VA's extended care patient population receives care in the following noninstitutional settings:

- **Home-based primary care**. Provides long-term primary medical care to chronically ill veterans in their own homes under the coordinated care of an interdisciplinary treatment team. This program has led to guidelines for medical education in home care, use of emerging technology in home care, and improved care for veterans with dementia and the families who support them.
- **Contract home healthcare**. Professional home care services, mostly nursing services, are purchased from private-sector providers at every VA medical center. The program is com-

monly called "fee basis" home care (when the VA cannot provide care within its healthcare system, the VA will pay for healthcare services obtained from local community providers, depending on eligibility criteria).

- **Adult day healthcare**. Provides health maintenance and rehabilitative services to veterans in a group setting during daytime hours.
- **Homemaker and home health aide program**. Provides health-related services for veterans with service-connected disabilities needing nursing home care in the community (public or private) but case managed directly by VA staff.
- **Community residential care.** Provides room, board, limited personal care, and supervision to veterans who do not require hospital or nursing home care but are not able to live independently because of medical or psychiatric conditions, and who have no family to provide care. Medical care is provided to the veteran primarily on an outpatient basis at VA facilities.
- **Respite care.** Temporarily relieves the spouse or other caregiver from the burden of caring for a chronically ill or disabled veteran at home. The 1999 Veterans Millennium Healthcare and Benefits Act expanded respite care to home and other community settings. Respite care is usually limited to 30 days per year.
- **Home hospice care.** Provides comfort-oriented and supportive services in the home for persons in the advanced stages of an incurable disease. The goal is to achieve the best possible quality of life through relief of suffering, control of symptoms, and restoration or maintenance of functional capacity. Services are provided by an interdisciplinary team of healthcare providers and volunteers. Bereavement care is available to the family following the death of the patient. Hospice services are available 24 hours a day, 7 days a week.
- **Telehealth**. For most of VA's noninstitutional care, this technology can play a major role in coordinating veterans' total care with the goal of maintaining independence. Telehealth offers the possibility of treating chronic illnesses in a cost-effective manner while contributing to the patient satisfaction generally found with care available at home.
- **Geriatric evaluation and management**. Older veterans with multiple medical, functional, or psychosocial problems and those with particular geriatric problems receive assessment

and treatment from an interdisciplinary team of VA health professionals. These services are provided on inpatient units, in outpatient clinics, and in geriatric primary care clinics.
- **Geriatric research, education, and clinical centers**. These centers increase basic knowledge of aging for healthcare providers and improve the quality of care through development of improved models of clinical services. Each center has an identified focus of research in the basic biomedical, clinical, and health services areas, such as the geriatric evaluation and management program. Medical and associated health students and staff in geriatrics and gerontology are trained at these centers.

Nursing Homes

VHA provides nursing home services to veterans through three national programs: homes owned and operated by VA, state veterans' homes owned and operated by the states, and the community nursing home program.

- **VA nursing homes**. Typically admit residents requiring short-term skilled care or those who have a 70% or greater service-connected disability.
- **State veterans' home program**. A cooperative venture between the states and VA whereby the states petition VA for matching construction grants and the state, the veteran, and VA pay a portion of the per diem. The per diem is set in legislation. State veterans' homes accept all veterans in need of long-term or short-term nursing home care. Specialized services offered are dependent upon the each home's capability.
- **Community nursing home program**. VA medical centers maintain contracts with community nursing homes though every VA medical center. The purpose of this program is to meet the nursing home needs of veterans who require long-term nursing home care in their own community, close to their families.

Domiciliary Care

Domiciliary care is a residential rehabilitation program that provides short-term rehabilitation and long-term health maintenance to veterans who require minimal medical care as they recover from medical, psychiatric, or psychosocial problems. Most domiciliary patients return to the community after a period of rehabilitation. Domiciliary care is provided by VA and state homes. VA also provides a number of psychiatric residential rehabilitation programs, including assistance for veterans coping with posttraumatic stress disorder and substance abuse, and compensated work therapy or transitional residences for homeless veterans with chronic mental illness and veterans recovering from substance abuse.

Community-Based Outpatient Clinics

Former Undersecretary for Health Kenneth W Kizer realigned the VA healthcare delivery system from a traditional acute care hospital system to an integrated delivery system employing principles of managed care. An important component of the realignment was the initiative to implement a nationwide system of community-based outpatient clinics to improve veterans' access to primary healthcare. In 2007 VA had 887 community-based outpatient clinics and plans to open 38 more in 22 states. The new facilities will become operational by October 2008. A complete listing of the community clinics can be found on the VA Web site or in the benefits booklet.

Emergency Medical Care in External Facilities

VA may reimburse or pay for medical care provided to enrolled veterans by non-VA facilities only in cases of medical emergencies where VA or other federal facilities were not feasibly available. Other conditions also apply. To determine eligibility or initiate a claim, contact the VA medical facility nearest to where the emergency service was provided.

National Rehabilitation Special Events

VA sponsors a number of special events as part of the comprehensive rehabilitation provided to veterans. For information on eligibility and participation, or to be a volunteer, contact the VA national advisor at the following Web site: www.va.gov/opa/speceven/index.asp.

Vet Centers

Vet Centers are VHA outreach offices located in communities where large veteran and family member populations reside. The VHA's Readjustment Counseling Service governs the Vet Center network, which consists of 232 centers (with plans for expansion). All centers have an OEF/OIF outreach specialist, and most have at least one combat veteran on staff.

Veterans who served in any combat zone (Vietnam,

Southwest Asia, OEF, OIF, etc) and received a military campaign ribbon, and their family members, are eligible for Vet Center services. Active duty service members are not eligible for services, but combat veteran family members are eligible for readjustment counseling services for military-related problems. Center staff specialize in readjustment counseling, providing a wide range of services to help combat veterans make a satisfying transition from military to civilian life. Services include individual counseling, group counseling, marital and family counseling, bereavement counseling, medical referrals, benefits application assistance, employment counseling, alcohol and drug assessments, information and referral to community resources, military sexual trauma counseling and referral, and outreach and community education.

Vet Center beneficiaries do not incur any fees for services. The VA Web site (www.va.gov) publishes a listing of all center locations and point of contact information. Vet Center information can also be found under government listings in the local telephone directory. Center staff are available toll free during normal business hours at 1-800-905-4675 (Eastern) and 1-866-496-8838 (Pacific).

Spinal Cord Injury

Nearly 44,000 veterans with spinal cord injuries (SCIs) are eligible for VA medical care. Many of these veterans are eligible not only for healthcare but also for monetary or other benefits because they have a service-connected disability, meaning a condition that occurred or worsened during military service. Veterans with SCI service-connected disabilities are also entitled to vocational counseling, grants for adapted housing and automobiles, a clothing allowance, and payment for home and attendant care. Veterans with spinal cord injury unrelated to their military service may still receive VA medical care because of their catastrophic disability.

Services

A study conducted by a major consulting firm in 2000 comparing VA's SCI services to those funded by several private and public health insurers showed that VA's coverage was more comprehensive. VA integrates vocational, psychological, and social services within a continuum of care that addresses changing needs throughout the veteran's life. VA provides supplies, offers preventive healthcare and education, and maintains medical equipment for veterans with SCI.

Services are delivered through a "hub and spoke" system of care, extending from 23 regional SCI centers (see Attachment) offering primary and specialty care by multidisciplinary teams to the 135 SCI primary care teams or support clinics at non-SCI local VA medical centers. Each primary care team has a physician, nurse, and social worker, and those with support clinics may have additional team members. Newly injured veterans and active duty members are referred to a VA SCI center for rehabilitation after being stabilized at a trauma center. Each year, approximately 400 newly injured veterans and active duty members receive rehabilitation at VA's SCI centers. The SCI center nearest to a veteran can provide the name of the SCI coordinator in the primary care team at the nearest VA facility.

National Recreational Events

Staying active is as important to the physical and emotional well-being of people with SCI as it is to other people. VA sponsors two annual athletic events that offer camaraderie with other SCI veterans and the opportunity to enjoy and participate in competitive sports. These are the National Veterans Wheelchair Games, which are cosponsored by Paralyzed Veterans of America, and the National Disabled Veterans Winter Sports Clinic, cosponsored by Disabled American Veterans.

Continuing Education

The Rehabilitation Accreditation Commission has accredited all 20 VA SCI centers that provide acute rehabilitation. Thirteen of these centers are training sites certified by the Accreditation Council on Graduate Medical Education, which accredits postgraduate medical training programs in the United States. All VA physicians can take an independent study course on medical care for patients with SCI, and two SCI training programs are held annually for VA healthcare professionals. A guide called *Yes, You Can!*, prepared by the VA and published by Paralyzed Veterans of America, explains how to handle problems and where to turn for help (available at VA SCI centers and from Paralyzed Veterans of America).

Blind Rehabilitation Service

The mission of Blind Rehabilitation Service is to coordinate a healthcare service delivery system that provides a continuum of care for blinded veterans extending from their home environment to the local VA facility and the appropriate rehabilitation setting. These services include adjustment to blindness counseling, patient and family education, benefits analysis, comprehensive residential inpatient training, outpatient rehabilitation services, provision of assistive technology, and research.

Blind Rehabilitation Center

The blind rehabilitation center, a residential inpatient program providing training in comprehensive adjustment to blindness, serves as a resource to a catchment area usually composed of multiple states. The centers offer a variety of skill courses designed to help blinded veterans achieve a realistic level of independence. These skill areas include orientation and mobility, communication skills, activities of daily living, manual skills, visual skills, computer access training, and social/recreational activities. The veteran is also assisted in making an emotional and behavioral adjustment to blindness through individual counseling sessions and group therapy meetings.

Visual Impairment Services Team Coordinator

The visual impairment services team coordinator is a case manager who coordinates all services for legally blind veterans and their families. Duties include providing or arranging for the provision of appropriate treatment modalities (eg, referrals to blind rehabilitation centers or specialists) to enhance a blinded veteran's functioning level. Other duties include identifying new cases of blindness, providing professional counseling, resolving problems, arranging annual healthcare reviews, and conducting education programs.

Visual Impairment Services Outpatient Program

The Visual Impairment Services Outpatient Program (VISOR) is an intermediate 9-day rehabilitation program located at the Lebanon VA medical center in Pennsylvania. It provides comfortable, safe, overnight accommodations for visually impaired beneficiaries requiring temporary lodging to access program services. VISOR offers skills training, orientation and mobility, and low-vision therapy. It is staffed with blind rehabilitation specialists and visual impairment service team coordinators who are either social workers or certified low-vision therapists. Veterans must be able to perform activities of daily living independently, including the ability to self-medicate, to qualify for the program.

Visual Impairment Center to Optimize Remaining Sight Program

VHA developed the Visual Impairment Center to Optimize Remaining Sight (VICTORS) concept to complement existing inpatient blind rehabilitation centers in caring for veterans with significant visual impairment (20/70 to 20/200 or worse visual acuity or significant visual field loss). In the VICTORS outpatient program, a multidisciplinary team consisting of specialists in optometry, ophthalmology, social work, psychology, and low-vision therapy provides rehabilitative care. VICTORS provides rehabilitation through definitive medical diagnosis, functional vision evaluation, prescription of low-vision aids and training in their use, counseling, and follow-up. Frequently, other necessary patient care services (eg, social work, psychology, audiology, and ophthalmology) are provided at the local station. There are currently four VICTORS programs, located in Kansas City, Missouri; Chicago, Illinois; Northport, New York; and Lake City, Florida.

Blind Rehabilitation Outpatient Specialists

Blind rehabilitation outpatient specialists with specialized training teach skills to veterans in their homes or in the local VA facility. The specialists have advanced technical knowledge and competencies in at least two of the following disciplines at the journeyman level: orientation and mobility, living skills, manual skills, and visual skills. They possess a broad range of knowledge in the aforementioned disciplines, including computer access training. The program is located in the following areas: Albuquerque, New Mexico; Ann Arbor, Michigan; Augusta, Georgia; Bay Pines/St Petersburg, Florida; Baltimore, Maryland; Boston, Massachusetts; Brooklyn, New York; Cleveland, Ohio; Dallas, Texas; Gainesville, Florida; Hines, Illinois; Houston, Texas; Greater Los Angeles, California; North Las Vegas, Nevada; Orlando, Florida; Palo Alto, California; Phoenix, Arizona; Portland, Oregon; Richmond, Virginia; San Antonio, Texas; San Diego, California; San Juan, Puerto Rico; Seattle, Washington; Tampa, Florida; Waco, Texas; Washington, DC; West Haven, Connecticut; and West Palm Beach, Florida. The blind rehabilitation outpatient specialist handbook is available at: www.va.gov/publdirec/health/handbook/1174-1.html.

Travel Expenses and Refunds

The VA will reimburse veterans for travel costs if they meet eligibility requirements. Reimbursement is paid and subject to a deductible for each one-way trip with a per-month maximum payment. Two exceptions to the deductible are travel for compensation and pension examinations and the need for special modes of transportation, such as an ambulance or a specially equipped van.

Homeless Veterans

VA has programs providing medical care, benefits assistance, and transitional housing to more than 100,000 homeless veterans. VA makes grants for transitional housing, service centers and vans for outreach and transportation to state and local governments, tribal governments, and nonprofit community and faith-based service providers.

Presumptive Conditions Considered for Disability Compensation

Certain veterans are eligible for disability compensation based on the presumption that their disability is service connected.

Prisoners of War

If the following conditions received a 10% disability rating anytime after military service, the conditions are presumed to be service connected for former prisoners of war: psychosis, anxiety states, dysthymic disorder, organic residuals of frostbite, posttraumatic osteoarthritis, heart disease or hypertensive vascular disease and their complications, and stroke and residuals of stroke. The VA also presumes additional conditions to be service connected for veterans imprisoned at least 30 days: avitaminosis, beriberi, chronic dysentery, helminthiasis, malnutrition (including optic atrophy), pellagra or other nutritional deficiencies, irritable bowel syndrome, peptic ulcer disease, peripheral neuropathy, and cirrhosis of the liver.

Veterans Exposed to Agent Orange and Other Herbicides

Veterans who served in the Republic of Vietnam between January 9, 1962, and May 7, 1975, regardless of length of service, were presumed to have been exposed to Agent Orange and other herbicides used in support of military operations. Presumptive conditions for service connection include chloracne or other acneform disease similar to chloracne; porphyria cutanea tarda; soft-tissue sarcoma (other than osteosarcoma, chondrosarcoma, Kaposi's sarcoma, or mesothelioma); Hodgkin's disease; multiple myeloma; respiratory cancers (lung, bronchus, larynx, trachea); non-Hodgkin's lymphoma; prostate cancer; acute and subacute peripheral neuropathy; diabetes mellitus (type 2); and chronic lymphocytic leukemia.

Veterans Exposed to Radiation

Presumptive service-connected conditions for

veterans exposed to radiation include all forms of leukemia (except for chronic lymphocytic leukemia); cancer of the thyroid, breast, pharynx, esophagus, stomach, small intestine, pancreas, bile ducts, gall bladder, salivary gland, urinary tract (renal pelvis, ureter, urinary bladder, and urethra), brain, bone, lung, colon, and ovary; bronchiolo-alveolar carcinoma; multiple myeloma; lymphomas (other than Hodgkin's disease); and primary liver cancer (unless cirrhosis or hepatitis B is indicated).

Gulf War Veterans

Presumptive service-connected conditions for Gulf War veterans are undiagnosed illnesses or medically unexplained chronic (existing for at least 6 months) multisymptom illnesses defined by a cluster of signs or symptoms such as chronic fatigue syndrome, fibromyalgia, skin disorders, headache, muscle pain, joint pain, neurological symptoms, neuropsychological symptoms, symptoms involving the respiratory system, sleep disturbances, gastrointestinal symptoms, cardiovascular symptoms, abnormal weight loss, and menstrual disorders.

Veterans With Amyotrophic Lateral Sclerosis

More commonly recognized as Lou Gehrig's disease, amyotrophic lateral sclerosis may be a presumptive condition for service connection for veterans who served in operations in Southwest Asia between August 2, 1990, and July 31, 1991. The Southwest Asia theater of operations includes Iraq, Kuwait, Saudi Arabia, the neutral zone between Iraq and Saudi Arabia, Bahrain, Qatar, the United Arab Emirates, Oman, the Gulf of Aden, the Gulf of Oman, the Persian Gulf, the Arabian Sea, the Red Sea, and the airspace above these locations.

Combat Veterans

The 2008 National Defense Authorization Act (Public Law 110-181) provides active duty, reserve, and National Guard service members deployed to a theater of combat operations eligibility for a 5-year, cost-free VA healthcare package including nursing home care. Eligibility requirements are as follows: (*a*) combat service against a hostile force during a period of hostilities after November 11, 1998; or (*b*) active duty service in a theater of combat operations during a period of war after the Persian Gulf War; and (*c*) discharge under other than dishonorable conditions; and (*d*) medical condition related to military service. The VA defines "hostilities" as a conflict that places armed forces members in harm's way comparable to

danger inherent in a period of war. Combat veterans discharged from active duty between November 11, 1998, and January 27, 2003, may apply for this benefit until January 27, 2011.

Documents to substantiate combat service include (*a*) service documentation that reflects service in a combat theater, (*b*) combat service medals, or (*c*) receipt of imminent danger or hostile fire pay or tax benefits. Active duty, reserve, and National Guard service members should register for VA healthcare prior to discharge, retirement, or removal from active duty. VA personnel assigned duty at military medical facilities or military installations can assist service members with the registration process.

After receiving DD form 214 (discharge certificate) and returning home, the service member or veteran must visit the nearest VA medical facility and enroll in VA healthcare to receive eligible medical care and services. *VA healthcare is not rendered until the service member or veteran is enrolled.* Upon completion of the 5-year healthcare package, veterans will continue to be enrolled although their assigned priority group may change based on their income, and they may be required to make applicable copayments. Unless exempted, veterans may need to disclose their previous year's gross household income. Disclosure is not required; however, disclosure may provide additional benefits such as eligibility for travel reimbursement, cost-free medication, or medical care for service unrelated to combat. Continued eligibility for subsequent care is determined by compensable service-connected disability, VA pension status, catastrophic disability determination, or the veteran's financial status. *Combat veterans are strongly encouraged to apply for enrollment to take advantage of the special combat veteran eligibility, even if no medical care is currently needed.*

Combat veterans may be eligible for a one-time treatment for dental conditions. Eligibility criteria for this dental benefit are as follows:

- Active duty of not less than 90 days.
- Discharge under conditions other than dishonorable.
- DD form 214 containing a statement the service member did not receive a complete dental examination including dental radiographs, and did not receive subsequent care dictated by the examination.
- Must be applied for within 90 days of discharge or release. Care can be rendered past the 90 days but not past 12 months.

Veterans discharged between August 1, 2007, and January 27, 2008, are eligible for the dental benefit by making application within 180 days of their discharge.[9]

Enrollment

Veterans must apply for enrollment into the VA healthcare system. Once enrolled, veterans can receive eligible care and services at any VA healthcare facilities and are afforded various privacy rights under federal law and regulations.[10] Exemptions from the enrollment process are as follows:

- Veterans with service-connected disability of 50% percent or more.
- Veterans seeking care for a disability the military determined was incurred or aggravated in the line of duty, but which VA has not yet rated, within 12 months of discharge.
- Veterans seeking care for a service-connected disability only.

Regardless of exemption, all veterans are advised to enroll (Exhibit 5-1).

Priority Groups

The VA uses a priority system as a way to meet healthcare needs within resource constraints. The VA assigns each veteran to a priority group based on a number of factors: amount of service-connected disability, income, private health insurance, and geographical location. The priority group is subject to change. Priority groups range from priority 1 (50% service-connected disability or more, or unemployable due to service-connected conditions) to priority 8 (indigent veterans).

Foreign Medical Program

Veterans traveling or residing abroad who have VA-rated service connected conditions can obtain healthcare services from the following foreign locations:

- In the Philippines: VA Outpatient Clinic, Pasay City 1300, Republic of the Philippines; e-mail: manlopc.inqry@vba.va.gov.
- All other countries: Foreign Medical Program, PO Box 65021, Denver, CO 80206-9021; telephone: 303-331-7590; e-mail: www.va.gov/hac/contact; Web site: www.va.gov/hac .

EXHIBIT 5-1

THINGS TO REMEMBER ABOUT VETERANS AFFAIRS HEALTHCARE

1. Veterans need to enroll to receive VA healthcare.
2. Registration is not enrollment; it is an intention to enroll.
3. Priority group assignment is subject to change based on the law of supply and demand and eligibility.
4. Veterans must provide supporting documents to substantiate enrollment eligibility.
5. Financial status can determine eligibility for specific benefits.
6. Veterans should enroll as soon after discharge or release from active duty as possible.
7. Learn more about VA healthcare programs and eligibility from the nearest VA medical facility. VA facilities including telephone numbers are listed online, at www.va.gov/directory, or in the local telephone directory under the US government listings. Veterans can also call the Health Benefit Service Center toll free at 1-877-222-VETS (8387), or visit the VA health eligibility Web site at www.va.gov/healtheligibility.

VETERANS BENEFITS ADMINISTRATION

The VBA is the VA's benefits delivery system. "*The mission of the Veterans Benefits Administration (VBA), in partnership with the Veterans Health Administration and the National Cemetery Administration, is to provide benefits and services to veterans and their families in a responsive, timely and compassionate manner in recognition of their service to the Nation.*"[11] VBA has four area offices, 57 regional offices, and 153 benefits delivery-at-discharge sites.

The VA dispenses a broad spectrum of benefits programs and services to eligible active duty, reserve, and National Guard service members and veterans. These benefits are legislated in title 38 of the US Code. Every year the VA publishes a booklet in English and Spanish containing a summary of veteran benefits for the calendar year (available at: www.va.gov). VBA is responsible for initial veteran registration, eligibility determination, and five key lines of benefits and entitlements: (1) compensation and pension, (2) vocational rehabilitation and employment, (3) insurance, (4) education (GI Bill), and (5) loan guaranty. In 2006 the VBA paid out $38.9 billion in claims (approximately half going for disability compensation, pension, education assistance, and medical care), $25.0 billion in guaranteed loans coverage, and $1.4 trillion in insurance coverage for service members and veterans.

Compensation and Pension Programs

These programs provide direct payments to veterans, dependents, and survivors as a result of the veteran's service-connected disability or because of financial need.[3]

- **Disability compensation.** A monetary benefit paid to veterans with disabilities resulting from a disease or injury incurred or aggravated during active military service. The benefit amount is graduated according to the degree of the veteran's disability on a scale from 0% to 100% (in 10% increments).
- **Dependency and indemnity compensation.** Benefits generally payable to the survivors of service members who died while on active duty or survivors of veterans who died from their service-connected disabilities.
- **Pension programs.** Provide income support to veterans with wartime service and their families for a nonservice-connected disability or death. These programs are for low-income veterans and survivors.
- **Burial and interment allowances.** Payable allowances for certain veterans. A higher rate of burial allowance applies if the veteran's death is service-connected.
- **Spina bifida monthly allowance.** This allowance under 38 USC 1805 provides for individuals born with spina bifida who are children of personnel who served in the Republic of Vietnam during the Vietnam War era or served in or near the demilitarization zone in Korea during the period September 1, 1967, through August 31, 1971. Payment is made at one of three levels based on the degree of disability suffered by the child.
- **Children of female Vietnam veterans born with certain defects.** This program provides a monetary allowance, healthcare, and vocational training benefits to eligible children born to women who served in the Republic of Vietnam during the period beginning February 28, 1961, and ending May 7, 1975, if they suffer from certain covered birth defects associated with the service of the mother in Vietnam that result in permanent physical or mental disability.

Vocational Rehabilitation and Employment Program

The vocational rehabilitation and employment program helps veterans with service-connected disabilities prepare for, find, and keep suitable jobs. For veterans with service-connected disabilities so severe that they cannot immediately consider work, the program offers services to improve their ability to live as independently as possible. Vocational rehabilitation services include a vocational evaluation (ie, assessment of interests, aptitudes, and abilities); vocational counseling and planning; employment services (ie, job-seeking skills and job placement assistance); training for suitable employment; supportive rehabilitation services; and independent living services. Generally, a veteran must complete a program of rehabilitation services within 12 years from the date of VA notification of entitlement to compensation. This period may be deferred or extended if a medical condition prevents the veteran from pursuing rehabilitation services for a period of time, or if the veteran has a serious employment handicap.

The vocational rehabilitation and employment program can also provide a wide range of vocational and educational counseling services to service members still on active duty, as well as veterans and dependents who are eligible for one of VA's educational benefit programs. These services are designed to help an individual choose a vocational direction and determine the course needed to achieve the goal. Assistance may include interest and aptitude testing, occupational exploration, setting occupational goals, locating the right type of training program, and exploring appropriate educational or training facilities.

Insurance Programs

VA insurance programs were created to provide life insurance at a "standard" premium rate to members of the armed forces who are exposed to the extra hazards of military service. Service members may maintain their VA life insurance following discharge, regardless of their health, and special programs were established for veterans with service-connected disabilities that may make them otherwise uninsurable. In general, a new program was created for each wartime period since World War I. Seven distinct VA life insurance programs have been created by legislation, and four of these programs, as well as a program of traumatic injury coverage, still issue coverage.

Servicemembers' Group Life Insurance

Servicemembers Group Life Insurance (SGLI) provides up to $400,000 of life insurance coverage to active duty members of the uniformed services, National Guard, Commissioned Corps of the National Oceanic and Atmospheric Administration, Public Health Service, and reserves and Reserve Officer Training Corps, as well as cadets and midshipmen of the four service academies and volunteers in the Individual Ready Reserve. In addition, all dependent children are automatically insured for $10,000 at no charge.

Family Service Members' Group Life Insurance

SGLI also offers insurance for up to $100,000 in coverage for a service member's spouse, if the service member is on active duty or a reserve member of a uniformed service. All dependent children are automatically insured for $10,000 at no charge.

Veterans' Group Life Insurance

Individuals who separate from service with SGLI coverage to Veterans' Group Life Insurance, regardless of health, by submitting an application with the first month's premium within 120 days of discharge. After 120 days, the individual may still be granted coverage if evidence of insurability is submitted within 1 year of the end of the 120-day period.

Service-Disabled Veterans Insurance

A veteran who has a VA service-connected disability rating but is otherwise in good health may apply for life insurance coverage of up to $10,000 within 2 years of the date of notification by VA of the service-connected status. This insurance is limited to veterans who left service after April 24, 1951. Totally disabled veterans may apply for an additional $20,000 of coverage under this program.

Veterans' Mortgage Life Insurance

Mortgage life insurance protection for up to $90,000 is available to severely disabled veterans who receive a specially adapted housing grant.

Service Members' Traumatic Injury Protection

This coverage program is a rider to basic SGLI coverage policies and provides automatic traumatic injury protection coverage to all service members covered under SGLI effective December 1, 2005. It provides for payments between $25,000 and $100,000 (depending on the type of injury) to insured SGLI members who sustain traumatic injuries that result in certain severe losses. The benefit paid depends on the nature of the loss, as defined by VA regulations. Benefits are also retroactive to October 7, 2001, if the loss was suffered while deployed outside the United States on orders in support of OEF/OIF or while on orders in a combat zone tax exclusion area from October 7, 2001, through November 30, 2005.

Education Programs

VA education programs provide veterans; active duty, reserve, and National Guard service members; and certain veterans' dependents with educational resources to supplement opportunities missed because of military service and to assist in the readjustment to civilian life. Currently there are six education programs (details may be found at: www. gibill.va.gov).

Post-Vietnam Era Veterans' Educational Assistance Program

This program is available for eligible veterans who entered active duty between January 1, 1977, and June 30, 1985. Benefits and entitlement are determined by the contributions paid while on active duty, and veterans have 10 years after separation to use the benefit.

Montgomery GI Bill—Active Duty

The Montgomery GI Bill for active duty personnel is a program of education benefits that may be used while on active duty or after separation. There are several distinct eligibility categories. Generally a veteran receives 36 months of entitlement and has 10 years after separation to use the benefit.

Post-9/11 GI Bill

A new benefit provides educational assistance to individuals who served on active duty on or after September 11, 2001. Service members may elect to receive benefits under the post-9/11 GI bill if, on August 1, 2009, they have met qualifying requirements; are eligible for Chapter 30, 1606, or 1607 of the Montgomery GI Bill (see below); or are serving in the armed forces. Eligibility for benefits are for 15 years from the last period of active duty of at least 90 consecutive days. Built into this new benefit is the opportunity for the service members to transfer benefits to their spouse or dependent children. The most current information can be found at: www. gibill.va.gov.[12]

Montgomery GI Bill—Selected Reserve

This version of the GI Bill is available to members of the Selected Reserve. VA administers this program, but DoD determines the member's eligibility. Generally a qualified member of the Reserve receives 36 months of entitlement and has 14 years in which to use the benefit.

Reservists Educational Assistance Program

This program funded and managed by DoD is available to members of the Selected or Ready Reserve who are called to active duty to support contingency operations. VA administers this program but DoD and the Department of Homeland Security determine the member's eligibility. Generally a qualified individual receives 36 months of entitlement and is able to use the benefit as long as he or she remains in the Selected or Ready Reserve.

National Call to Service

This educational benefit program may be used while on active duty or after separation. The person must have enlisted on or after October 1, 2003, under the National Call to Service program and selected one of the two education incentives provided. These are either (1) education benefits of up to 12 months of GI Bill benefits (the 3-year rate) or (2) education benefits of up to 36 months of the GI Bill benefits (half the 2-year rate).

Dependents Educational Assistance Program

This program assists dependents of veterans who (*a*) have been determined to be 100% permanently disabled because of a service-connected condition, (*b*) died from a service-connected condition, or (*c*) died while on active duty. Dependents typically receive 45 months of eligibility. The criteria for using this benefit as follows:

- Children have 8 years to use this benefit.
- A spouse of a living veteran has 10 years to use this benefit.
- A surviving spouse of a veteran who died with a 100% service-connected condition has 10 years to use this benefit.
- A surviving spouse of a veteran who died on active duty has 20 years to use this benefit.

Education benefits are available to children of active duty personnel who have served for at least 2 years and have contributed $1,200 under the Montgomery GI Bill (Chapter 30) or Selected Reserve and National Guards members certified as eligible under the Montgomery GI Bill—Selected Reserves (Chapter 1606). The Chapter 30 program is limited to payment for tuition and fees, and the Chapter 1606 program provides a monthly stipend.

Loan Guaranty Program

The VA home loan guaranty program helps eligible veterans and service members purchase and retain homes, in recognition of their service to the nation. Assistance is provided through VA's partial guaranty of loans made by private lenders in lieu of the substantial down payment and other investment safeguards required in conventional mortgage transactions. This protection means that in most cases qualified veterans can obtain a loan without making a down payment. Additionally, the program offers the benefits listed below.

Servicing Assistance

The loan guaranty program provides help for borrowers having difficulty in making their loan payments. The assistance ranges from financial counseling to direct intervention with the lender to obtain forbearance or arrange a reasonable repayment schedule. Whenever possible, the goal is to help the veteran retain ownership of his or her home and avoid foreclosure. In instances where homeownership retention is not possible, several alternatives to foreclosure are available that can somewhat mitigate the negative impact on the borrower.

Specially Adapted Housing Grants

Veterans who have specific service-connected disabilities can obtain specially adapted housing grants for constructing an adapted dwelling or modifying an existing dwelling. The program's goal is to provide disabled veterans a barrier-free living environment that affords a level of independent living not otherwise possible. The grant can be used up to three times, as long as the combined grant totals do not exceed the allowable grant maximum. Additionally, eligible veterans who are temporarily residing in a home owned by a family member may also use a portion of the grant maximum to assist in adapting the family member's home to meet his or her special needs.

Native American Direct Home Loans

These loans, made directly by the VA, are available to eligible Native American veterans who wish to purchase or construct a home on federal trust lands.

Benefits for Active Duty Personnel

The VA has a variety of associated or similar benefits available to active duty personnel.

Insurance Benefits

Service members and reserve forces are eligible for

up to a maximum of $400,000 in SGLI. Spousal coverage is available up to a maximum of $100,000, and children are automatically covered for $10,000 at no cost. Any member of the uniformed services covered by SGLI is automatically covered by a traumatic injury protection rider, which provides payments of between $25,000 and $100,000 to members who have a traumatic injury and suffer losses such as, but not limited to, amputations, blindness, and paraplegia.

Home Loan Guaranty Benefits

Persons on active duty are eligible for a VA home loan guaranty after serving on continuous active duty for 90 days. Service members going through the benefits delivery-at-discharge program who are found to have service-connected conditions are exempt from the loan guaranty funding fee.

Specially Adapted Housing Grants

Certain service members as well as veterans with service-connected disabilities may be entitled to a specially adapted housing grant from VA to help build a new specially adapted house or buy a house and modify it to meet their disability-related requirements. Eligible individuals may now receive up to three grants, with the total dollar amount of the grants not to exceed the maximum allowable amount. Previous grant recipients who had received assistance of less than the current maximum allowable amount may be eligible for an additional grant.

Financial Assistance for Purchasing a Vehicle

Veterans and service members may be eligible for a one-time payment of not more than $11,000 toward the purchase of an automobile or other conveyance if they have service-connected loss or permanent loss of use of one or both hands or feet, permanent impairment of vision of both eyes to a certain degree, or ankylosis (immobility) of one or both knees or one or both hips. They may also be eligible for adaptive equipment, and for repair, replacement, or reinstallation required be-cause of disability or for the safe operation of a vehicle purchased with VA assistance.

Healthcare Benefits

VA healthcare facilities are available to active duty service members in emergency situations and upon referral by military treatment facilities or TRICARE. VA provides a comprehensive medical benefits package to veterans enrolled in its healthcare program and is fully capable of meeting the treatment needs of those who are referred for care or who require emergency healthcare services. Service members may receive a one-time dental treatment up to 90 days from separation if they were not provided treatment within 90 days before separation from active duty.

Medal of Honor Pension Payments

Active duty personnel who have been awarded the Medal of Honor and determined to be eligible by one of the service departments are entitled to receive a special Medal of Honor pension from the VA.

Benefits Delivery at Discharge

Through this program, service members can file claims for disability compensation, pension, vocational rehabilitation, automobile allowance, and specially adapted housing prior to separation. VA employees will assist in the filing and preparation of the claim as well as adjudicate the claim within days following separation. Additionally, VA offers counseling and claims assistance to separating service members throughout the United States and around the world through the transition assistance program and disabled transition assistance program.

Vocational Rehabilitation and Employment

Service members pending medical separation from active duty may also apply if their disabilities are reasonably expected to be rated at least 20% following discharge. These service members must be referred to a VBA coordinator for application assistance.

NATIONAL CEMETERY ADMINISTRATION

On November 11, 1998, President Bill Clinton signed the Veterans Programs Enhancement Act, changing the name of the National Cemetery System to the National Cemetery Administration (NCA). The NCA operates 125 national cemeteries in the United States and territories, together with management of 33 soldiers' lots, Confederate cemeteries, and monument sites. The mission of NCA is to honor US veterans with a final resting place and commemorate their service. This mission is accomplished through four major program areas:

1. Providing for the interment of eligible service members, veterans, reserve and National Guard members, and certain family members

in national cemeteries. A total of 96,797 veterans and eligible family members were buried in national cemeteries in FY 2006. More than 3.2 million veterans, spouses, and dependents are buried in over 7,200 acres of NCA's developed land. NCA maintains these cemeteries and memorials as national shrines.

2. Furnishing headstones and markers for the 335,172 graves of veterans across the United States and the world. In national cemeteries, a headstone or marker is provided, including the cost of placement. The government does not provide for the cost of setting the headstone or marker in private cemeteries.

3. Administering the state cemetery grants program, which provides financial assistance to states for establishing, expanding, and improving state veterans' cemeteries. Since the program was established in 1978, 151 grants have been made, totaling over $264 million through FY 2006. The program provides federal funding for up to 100% of the cost of establishing, expanding, or improving state veterans' cemeteries that complement NCA. There are currently 65 state veterans' cemeteries in 35 states throughout the nation, Guam, and Saipan. In FY 2006, 22,434 veterans and dependents were buried in these cemeteries.

4. Providing presidential memorial certificates to veterans' loved ones to honor the service of honorably discharged deceased service members or veterans. In FY 2006, NCA issued 405,538 certificates on behalf of the president. Today, more than 24 million veterans, reservists, and National Guard members with 20 years of qualifying service (who are entitled to retirement pay or would be entitled, if at least 60 years of age), have earned the honor of burial in a national cemetery. Veterans with discharges other than dishonorable, their spouses, and dependent children may be eligible for burial in a VA national cemetery. Those who die on active duty may also be buried in a national cemetery.

BENEFITS PROVIDED BY OTHER AGENCIES

Department of Agriculture Loans for Farms and Homes

The US Department of Agriculture provides loans and guarantees to buy, improve, or operate farms. Loans and guarantees are available for housing in towns generally up to 20,000 in population. Applications from veterans have preference. For further information, contact Farm Service Agency or Rural Development, US Department of Agriculture, 1400 Independence Avenue, SW, Washington, DC 20250, or apply at local Department of Agriculture offices, usually located in county seats.

Housing and Urban Development Veteran Resource Center

US Department of Housing and Urban Development sponsors the Veteran Resource Center (HUD-VET), which works with national veterans' service organizations to serve as a general information center on all of the department's housing and community development programs and services. To contact HUD-VET, call 1-800-998-9999, TDD 800-483-2209, or visit the Web site: www.hud.gov/hudvet.

Naturalization Preference

Honorable active duty service in the US armed forces during a designated period of hostility allows an individual to naturalize without any required periods of residence or physical presence in the United States. A service member who was in the United States, certain territories, or aboard an American public vessel at the time of enlistment, reenlistment, extension of enlistment, or induction may naturalize even if he or she is not a lawful permanent resident.

On July 3, 2002, president George W Bush issued Executive Order 13269, establishing a new period of hostility for naturalization purposes beginning September 11, 2001, and continuing until a date designated by a future executive order. Qualifying members of the armed forces who have served at any time during a specified period of hostility may immediately apply for naturalization using the current form N-400, Application for Naturalization. Additional information about filing and requirement fees and designated periods of hostility are available on the US Citizenship and Immigration Services Web site: www.uscis.gov.

Individuals who served honorably in the US armed forces but were no longer on active duty status as of September 11, 2001, may still be naturalized without the usual residence and physical presence requirements if they filed form N-400 while still serving or within 6 months of termination of their active duty service. An individual who files the application after the 6-month period following termination of service is not exempt from the residence and physical presence requirements, but may count any period of active duty service toward the requirements. Individuals seeking naturalization under this provision must establish that they are lawful permanent residents (such status having not been lost, rescinded, or abandoned) and that they served honorably in the US armed forces for at least 1 year.

If a service member dies as a result of injury or disease incurred or aggravated by service during a time of combat, the service member's survivors can apply for the deceased service member to receive posthumous citizenship at any time within 2 years of death. The issuance of a posthumous certificate of citizenship does not confer US citizenship on surviving relatives; however, non-US citizen spouses or qualifying family members may file for certain immigration benefits and services based upon their relationship to a citizen service member who died during hostilities or a noncitizen service member who died during hostilities and was later granted posthumous citizenship (see www.uscis.gov for more information).

Small Business Administration Outreach to Veterans

The US Small Business Administration (SBA) Office of Veterans Business Development conducts comprehensive outreach to veterans, service-disabled veterans, and reserve component members of the US military. The office formulates, executes, and promotes policies and programs that provide assistance to veteran-owned small businesses. The SBA is the primary federal agency responsible for assisting veterans who own or are considering starting small businesses. The SBA also conducts research in veterans' entrepreneurship.

Among the services provided are business counseling and training through five veterans' outreach centers, more than 1,000 small business development centers, nearly 400 SCORE (Service Corps of Retired Executives) chapters with 11,000 volunteer counselors, 100 women's business centers, and various loan and loan guarantee programs ranging from micro loans to venture capital assistance. A special military reservist economic injury disaster loan is available for self-employed reservists whose small businesses may have been damaged through extended absences of the owner or essential employee as a result of activation to military duty. Veterans participate in all SBA federal procurement programs, and the SBA supports veterans and others in international trade. A veterans' business development officer is stationed at every SBA district office. Information about SBA's full range of services can be found at: www.sba.gov/vets or by calling 202-205-6773 or 1-800-U-ASK-SBA (1-800-827-5722).

Information on programs for reservists is available at: www.sba.gov/reservists.

Social Security Administration Benefits for Veterans and Dependents

Monthly retirement, disability, and survivor benefits under Social Security are payable to veterans and dependents if the veteran has earned enough work credits under the program. Upon the veteran's death, a one-time payment of $255 also may be made to the veteran's spouse or child. In addition, a veteran may qualify at age 65 for Medicare's hospital insurance and medical insurance. Medicare protection is available to people who have received Social Security disability benefits for 24 months, and to insured people and their dependents who need dialysis or kidney transplants, or who have amyotrophic lateral sclerosis (more commonly known as Lou Gehrig's disease). Since 1957 military service earnings for active duty (including active duty for training) have counted toward Social Security, and those earnings are already on Social Security records. Since 1988 inactive duty service in the reserve component (such as weekend drills) has also been covered by Social Security. Service members and veterans are credited with $300 in additional earnings for each calendar quarter in which they received active duty basic pay after 1956 and before 1978.

Veterans who served in the military from 1978 through 2001 are credited with an additional $100 in earnings for each $300 in active duty basic pay, up to a maximum of $1,200 a year. No additional Social Security taxes are withheld from pay for these extra credits. If veterans enlisted after September 7, 1980, and completed less than 24 months of active duty or their full tour of duty, they may not be able to receive the additional earnings. Check with Social Security for details. Additional earnings are no longer credited for military service periods after 2001. Also, noncontributory Social Security earnings of $160 a month may be credited to veterans who served after September 15, 1940, and before 1957, including attendance at service academies. For information, call 1-800-772-1213 or visit: www.socialsecurity.gov. (Note: Social Security cannot add these extra earnings to the record until an application is filed for Social Security benefits.)

Individuals age 65 or older and those who are blind or otherwise disabled may be eligible for monthly Supplemental Security Income payments if they have little or no income or resources. States may supplement the federal payments to eligible persons and may disregard additional income. Although VA compensation and pension benefits are counted in determining income for Supplemental Security Income purposes, some other income is not counted. Also, not all resources count in determining eligibility. For example, a person's home and the land it is on do not count. Personal effects, household goods, automobiles, and life insurance may not count, depending upon their value. Information and help is available at any Social Security office or by calling 1-800-772-1213.

Military service members can receive expedited processing of disability claims from Social Security. These claims are separate from VA claims and require separate application for benefits. This program is for military service members who become disabled while on active duty on or after October 1, 2001, regardless of disability location. Active duty status and receipt of military pay does not, in itself, prevent payment of disability benefits and should never stop a service member from making an application. The service member's actual work activity, not the amount of pay or military status, is the determining factor for benefits. Disability benefits are disbursed through two programs: (1) the Social Security disability insurance program, which pays benefits to those who worked long enough and paid Social Security taxes; and (2) the Supplemental Security Income program, which pays benefits based on financial need. For additional information see the Web site: www.socialsecurity.gov.[13]

Armed Forces Retirement Home

Veterans are eligible to live in the Armed Forces Retirement Home located in Washington, DC, if their active duty military service is at least 5% enlisted, warrant officer, or limited duty officer, and if they qualify under one of the following four categories:

1. At least 60 years of age and were discharged or released under honorable conditions after 20 or more years of active service.
2. Determined to be incapable of earning a livelihood because of a service-connected disability incurred in the line of duty.

3. Served in a war theater during a time of war declared by Congress or were eligible for hostile fire special pay and were discharged or released under honorable conditions, and are determined to be incapable of earning a livelihood because of injuries, disease, or disability.
4. Served in a women's component of the armed forces before June 12, 1948, and are determined to be eligible for admission due to compelling personal circumstances.

Eligibility determinations are based on rules prescribed by the home's chief operating officer. Veterans are not eligible if they have been convicted of a felony or have alcohol, drug, or psychiatric problems. Married couples are welcome, but both must be eligible in their own right. At the time of admission, applicants must be capable of living independently. The Armed Forces Retirement Home is an independent federal agency. For information, call 1-800-332-3527 or 1-800-422-9988, or visit the Web site: www.afrh.gov.

Commissary and Exchange Privileges

Unlimited exchange and commissary store privileges in the United States are available to honorably discharged veterans with a service-connected disability rated at 100%, un-remarried surviving spouses of members or retired members of the armed forces, recipients of the Medal of Honor, and the dependents and orphans of any of these individuals. Certification of total disability is done by VA. Reservists and their dependents also may be eligible. Privileges overseas are governed by international law and are available only if agreed upon by the local government. Though these benefits are provided by DoD, VA does provide assistance in completing DD form 1172, Application for Uniformed Services Identification and Privilege Card. For detailed information, contact the nearest military installation.

WHAT EVERY VETERANS AFFAIRS BENEFICIARY NEEDS TO KNOW

1. Benefits are always changing and are based on a number of variables—type of discharge, length of service, dates of service, number of family members, degree of disability, legislative actions, combat service, just to name a few. "May be eligible" does not mean "is eligible." Benefits can vary widely among beneficiaries.
2. VA beneficiaries **must apply** for VA benefits

to receive benefits.
3. VA beneficiaries should not apply for benefits alone. Applying is easier when the beneficiary is accompanied by a family member, power of attorney, veteran representative, or legal representation.
4. The following documents are needed for benefits application processing:
   • A copy of DD form 214, Certificate of

Release or Discharge from Active duty, if available.

- VA claim number or Social Security number if receiving benefits under prior service.
- A copy of all marriage certificates or divorce decrees (if any).
- A copy of each child's birth certificate (or adoption order).
- A copy of the beneficiary's certificate if he or she has dependent parents.
- A copy of any service medical records substantiating disabilities for compensation for military service-related injuries.
- A completed VA form 21-526, Veterans Application for Compensation or Pension (an online version is available, and paper versions are available from any VA regional office).
- If applicable, combat operations documentation:
  - o copy of leave and earnings statement showing receipt of hostile fire or imminent danger pay,
  - o receipt of the Armed Forces Expeditionary Medal,
  - o receipt of the Kosovo Campaign Medal,
  - o receipt of the Global War on Terrorism Expeditionary Medal,
  - o receipt of the Southwest Asia Campaign Medal,
  - o proof of exemption of federal tax status for hostile fire or imminent danger pay,
  - o orders to a theater of combat operations, and
  - o copy of other awarded medals associated with the combat operations or operations involving imminent danger.

5. Application for health and other benefits can be done many ways:
- Online by accessing the VA Web site: www.va.gov/1010EZ.htm.
- Using a paper version of VA form 10-10EZ, Application for Health Benefits. The form can be obtained several different ways:
  - o Calling VA's health benefits service center, toll free at 1-877-222-VETS (8387), Monday through Friday between 8:00 AM and 8:00 PM (Eastern Standard Time).
  - o Contacting any VA regional office at 1-800-827-1000 from any location in the United States or Puerto Rico. VA facilities also are listed in the federal govern-

ment section blue pages of the telephone directories under "Veteran Affairs."
  - o Contacting the VA liaison or VBA counselor colocated with the warrior transition unit's case managers.
  - o Contacting a Vet Center.

6. State, local, and national veterans' service organization representatives are available to assist with benefits counseling and claims processing. A list of such representatives can be found in the attachment to this chapter and online at: www.va/gov/vso.

7. The VHA (Veterans Health Administration) and VBA (Veterans Benefits Administration) are distinct, separate branches of the VA. These two VA branches engage in limited collaboration, interaction, and information exchange. Every step in the application process requires beneficiary action or oversight. Beneficiaries need to keep records of every action taken throughout the claim process; they should provide only copies of original documents (do not provide original documents unless absolutely required) and make a record of telephone contacts and personal visits, including date, time, name of VA employee and contact information, what transpired during the conversation or visit, follow-up action required, etc.

8. The Veterans Claims Act of 2000 and Duty to Assist, requires the VA to obtain any records in the VA's possession or within any other federal agency. The law also mandates that the VA tell the claimant what evidence is needed to support his or her claim. The VA now must make several efforts to obtain any evidence identified by the claimant.

9. By law, the burden of proof falls on the veteran or dependent. Even though the VA is now required to look for evidence, the process may take many months. Veterans can help their claim and speed up the process if they can obtain supporting evidence such as the following:
- personal statements, especially those of combat veterans claiming a "combat-related" injury or illness;
- statements from friends, relatives, or anyone who has knowledge of the veteran's disability and its relationship to service; and
- medical evidence.

However, any lay statements must fit certain criteria and are not always helpful. Some can be harmful to the veteran's claim. The veteran should discuss any statements with a veterans' benefits counselor.

10. Although the VA strives for standardization, not all VA medical facilities and regional offices are alike. VA and DoD medical facilities are similar in that they have a degree of autonomy, as do the VA regional offices—interpretation of regulations, policies, and procedures can vary from facility to facility, impacting beneficiary benefits.

WHAT MILITARY HEALTHCARE PROVIDERS NEED TO KNOW

1. DoD healthcare providers cannot underestimate the importance of proper medical record documentation for service members wounded, injured, or sickened in the line of duty. The more "who, what, when, where, and how" is documented in the medical record, the better the supporting documentation the service member or veteran will be able to present when filing a claim. For combat injuries, the medical record should contain as much information about the details of the injury as possible, including the service member's duty assignment, unit, location, name of witnesses, and other identifying information about the injury or illness and circumstances.

2. The partnership between DoD and VA will continue to strengthen over time. Providers must stay educated about VA benefits and develop professional relationships with VA personnel on the installation or assigned duty at the MTF.

3. It is better to refer service members, veterans, and other beneficiaries to VA personnel than to give out erroneous information about benefits.

4. States also provide veteran benefits, and benefits can vary from state to state.

5. Providers should learn the VA language, obtain copies of VA regulations governing disability rating, and write medical notes and reports in a manner that provides the necessary information for VA rating specialists to make appropriate rating decisions.

6. Key VA programs and personnel[14]:
   - VHA facilities provide appropriate health and mental healthcare services to active duty service members who served in OEF or OIF. Coordination of those services is to be ensured by the following personnel:
     - o **OEF/OIF program manager,** a designated nurse or social worker serving at each VA medical center to coordinate care provided to OEF or OIF service members and veterans; functions as the facility's point of contact for the VA liaisons at military treatment facilities.
     - o **OEF/OIF case managers,** nurses and social workers at each VHA facility who work with those who are severely injured, ill, and otherwise in need of case management services.
   - Between three and eight **transition patient advocates** for OEF and OIF service members and veterans serve at each VISN. Although the positions are distributed to the VISN offices, the duty stations are at designated medical centers within the VISN. These positions are funded by the VA central office.
   - The **VA liaison,** stationed at major MTFs nationwide, is considered the VHA representative to the military installation and represents the VA in all aspects of patient care, transfer, and outreach. The primary role of the VA liaison is to ensure the effective transfer of healthcare, both inpatient and outpatient, from the MTF to the appropriate VHA facility. The liaisons work with on-site staff, service members, and families to ensure priority access to needed healthcare services and education about VHA benefits. Service members returning from Iraq and Afghanistan may have severe and complex injuries, minor injuries, and/or mental health needs. VA liaisons obtain clear referral information and authorization for VHA to treat those still on active duty, as well as coordinating with VHA facility enrollment coordinators to initially register active duty OEF/OIF service members or enroll veterans. Registering service members in the computer system eases transfer of care to the VHA treatment facility. Although the liaisons report administratively to the VHA facility closest to the MTF, they report programmatically to the VHA Office of Care Management and Social Work. The VA liaison is an experienced clinical social worker, recognized as an independent practitioner who can demonstrate the ability to manage

and evaluate programs and policies.[15]

- **VA rehabilitation nurses** may be assigned duty at major MTFs. Nursing care in a rehabilitation setting focuses on helping individuals with impairments resulting from injuries, illness, or chronic disease reach their optimal level of health and function. Rehabilitation nurses have additional expertise in the sequelae and rehabilitation care of conditions such as amputation, brain injury, neuromuscular conditions, orthopaedic conditions, stroke, and visual impairment. As integral members of the patient's management team, rehabilitation nurses carry out the rehabilitation plan of care 24 hours a day, 7 days a week. Rehabilitation nurses are also involved in educating the patient and caregivers to facilitate optimal transition to the next level of care.

- **VBA military service coordinators** at key MTFs or VA medical facilities must meet with every injured OIF/OEF service member, when medically appropriate, to make them aware of all potential VA benefits and services, as well as other benefits and services available through other sources, and assist them in completing claims and gathering supporting evidence. Counselors must provide all their clients with a business card containing contact information, and routinely inform hospitalized service members about the status of their pending claims.[7]

- **VBA OIF/OEF coordinators** ensure that a liaison is established with military and VA medical facility staff, particularly discharge planners. For VBA outreach efforts and coordination to be effective, VBA must have access to admission and discharge information as seriously disabled service members are admitted, transferred to another medical facility, and finally released. VBA OIF/OEF coordinators are responsible for the duties of the case manager if one has not been assigned.[7]

- **VBA case managers** work out of the VBA's regional office as the primary VBA point of contact for claims processing. However, VBA counselors at the MTF may stay involved if the service member is still a patient at the facility. In those cases, coordination between the VBA counselor and case manager is essential.

- **Transition assistance advisors** work in each state or territory as the statewide point of contact to assist service members in accessing VA benefits and healthcare services. Advisors also provide assistance in obtaining entitlements through the TRICARE military health system and access to community resources. Staffed by 55 contract positions and two federal technicians, this program began in May 2005 with a memorandum of agreement between the National Guard Bureau and the VA.

- The **Army Medical Department VA polytrauma liaison program** facilitates the continuity of care between MTFs and VA treatment facilities. The Army polytrauma liaison serves as the interface between case management and administrative matters, while functioning as the primary point of contact in the transition process for injured soldiers and their family members. The presence of a uniformed liaison is required to ensure that all the soldier's needs, both clinical and administrative, are seamlessly addressed, retaining a military link and precluding potential feelings of abandonment during this critical transition period. Army liaisons should reach out to all soldiers in the VA treatment facilities. Liaisons are currently active in the four VA polytrauma centers listed below[16]:
  - o Minneapolis VA Medical Center, Minnesota (geographic responsibility for Great Plains Regional Medical Command).
  - o Hunter Holmes McGuire VA Medical Center, Richmond, Virginia (geographic responsibility for North Atlantic Regional Medical Command).
  - o Palo Alto VA Medical Center, California (geographic responsibility for Western Regional Medical Command).
  - o James A Haley VA Hospital, Tampa, Florida (geographic responsibility for South East Regional Medical Command).

An additional polytrauma center is scheduled to open at the Audie Murphy VA Medical Center in San Antonio, Texas.

SUMMARY

This overview of the VA veterans' benefits is intended to educate military healthcare providers to better care for and assist wounded, injured, and ill service members and their family members. Every person entering the armed forces must understand VA organization and the benefits they may become eligible for before and after separation or discharge. Additional details for benefits and services are available on the VA Web site: www.va.gov. The one constant factor about VA benefits is that benefits are constantly changing.

REFERENCES

1. Department fact sheet. Department of Veterans Affairs Web site. Available at: http://www1.va.gov/opa/fact/index.asp#health. Accessed November 1, 2007.

2. Office of Construction and Facilities Management: Historic Preservation. A brief history of the VA. Department of Veterans Affairs Web site. Available at: http://www.va.gov/facmgt/historic/Brief_VA_History.asp. Accessed November 1, 2007.

3. Department of Veterans Affairs. *Federal Benefits for Veterans and Dependents.* 2007 ed. Washington, DC: US Government Printing Office; 2007.

4. Department of Veterans Affairs. *2007 Organizational Briefing Book.* Washington, DC: VA Office of Human Resources and Administration; 2007.

5. Department of Veterans Affairs, Office of Policy and Planning, National Center for Veteran Analysis and Statistics, *VA Benefits & Health Care Utilization.* Washington, DC: VA; 2008.

6. Department of Veterans Affairs. VA Web site. Available at: http://www.va.gov/. Accessed November 1, 2007.

7. Department of Veterans Affairs. *Analysis of VA Healthcare Utilization Among US Global War on Terrorism (GWOT) Veterans: Operation Enduring Freedom, Operation Iraqi Freedom (OEF/OIF).* Washington, DC: VHA Office of Public Health and Environmental Hazards; 2008.

8. Fact sheet: VA long term care, January 2005. Department of Veterans Affairs Web site. Available at: http://www.va.gov. Accessed November 1, 2007.

9. Department of Veterans Affairs Web site. VA health care overview. March 2008. Available at: http://www.va.gov/healtheligibility/library/pubs/healthcareoverview/. Accessed October 14, 2008.

10. Department of Veterans Affairs. *Notice of Privacy Practices.* Washington, DC: VA: 2003. IB 10-163.

11. Veterans Benefits Administration. Department of Veterans Affairs Web site. Available at: http://www.vba.va.gov/org/vbaorg.htm. Accessed November 1, 2007.

12. Department of Veterans Affairs. *The Post-9/11 Veterans Education Assistance Act of 2008.* Washington, DC: VA; 2008. Factsheet 22-08-01.

13. Social Security Administration. *Disability Benefits for Wounded Warriors.* Washington, DC: SSA; 2007. SSA Publication No. 05-10030.

14. Department of Veterans Affairs. *Transition Assistance and Case Management of Operation Iraqi Freedom (OIF) and Operation Enduring Freedom (OEF) Veterans.* Washington, DC: VA; 2007. VHA Handbook 1010.01.

15. Department of Veterans Affairs. *Polytrauma Rehabilitation Procedures.* Washington, DC: VA; 2005. VHA Handbook 1172.1.

16. Office of the Surgeon General. *AMEDD Veterans Affairs (VA) Liaison Program*. Washington, DC: OTSG; 2006. OTSG/MEDOM Memorandum Policy 06-03.

ATTACHMENT: RESOURCES FOR VETERANS

Important Telephone Numbers

Program	Phone Number
VA Benefits	1-800-827-1000
Health Care	1-877-222-8387
Education	1-888-442-4551
Life Insurance	1-800-669-8477
Debt Management	1-800-827-0648
Mammography Hotline	1-888-492-7844
Telecommunication Device for the Deaf (TDD)	1-800-829-4833
Civilian Health and Medical Program of the Department of Veterans Affairs	1-800-733-8387
Headstones and Markers	1-800-697-6947
Special Health Issues: Gulf War, Agent Orange, Project 112/Shad	1-800-749-8387

Important Web Addresses

Activity	Internet Address
VA Home Page	http://www.va.gov
VA Health Care	http://www.va.gov/health/
Returning Veterans	http://www.seamlesstransition.va.gov/
Survivor Benefits	http://www.vba.va.gov/survivors/index.htm
VA Facilities	http://www.va.gov/directory/guide/home.asp
VA Forms	http://www.va.gov/vaforms/
VA Benefit Payment Rates	http://www.vba.va.gov/bln/21/Rates/
Education Benefits	http://www.gibill.va.gov/
Home Loan Guaranty	http://www.homeloans.va.gov/
Life Insurance	http://www.insurance.va.gov/
Vocational Rehabilitation	http://www.vba.va.gov/bln/vre/index.htm
Burial and Memorial Benefits	http://www.cem.va.gov/
Veterans Employment and Training	http://www.dol.gov/vets/
Federal Jobs	http://www.usajobs.opm.gov/
Veterans Preference	http://www.opm.gov/veterans/index.asp
Military Records	http://www.archives.gov/st-louis/military-personnel/
Department of Defense	http://www.defenselink.mil/

Organizations Chartered by Congress or Recognized by Veterans Affairs for Claim Representation

Air Force Sergeants Association
American Defenders of Bataan and Corregidor
American Ex-Prisoners of War
American GI Forum of the United States
American Gold Star Mothers, Inc.
American Legion
American Red Cross
American War Mothers
AMVETS
Armed Forces Services Corporation
Army and Navy Union, USA, Inc
Blinded Veterans Association
Blue Star Mothers of America, Inc
Catholic War Veterans, USA, Inc

Congressional Medal of Honor Society of the United States of America
Disabled American Veterans
Fleet Reserve Association
Gold Star Wives of America, Inc
Italian American War Veterans of the USA
Jewish War Veterans of the USA
Legion of Valor of the USA, Inc
Marine Corps League
Military Chaplains Association of the United States of America
Military Order of the Purple Heart of the USA, Inc
Military Order of the World Wars
National Amputation Foundation, Inc

National Association for Black Veterans, Inc
National Association of County Veterans Service Officers, Inc
National Association of State Directors of Veterans Affairs (NASDVA)
National Veterans Legal Services Program
Navy Club of the United States of America
Navy Mutual Aid Association
Non Commissioned Officers Association
Paralyzed Veterans of America
Pearl Harbor Survivors Association, Inc.

Polish Legion of American Veterans, USA
Swords to Plowshares: Veterans Rights Organization
The Retired Enlisted Association
United Spinal Association
US Submarine Veterans of World War II
Veterans Assistance Foundation, Inc
Veterans of Foreign Wars of the United States
Veterans of the Vietnam War, Inc/Vets Coalition
Veterans of World War I of the USA, Inc
Vietnam Veterans of America
Women's Army Corps Veterans Association

Nonchartered Veterans Service Organizations

African American Veterans and Families
Air Force Association
Air Force Women Officers Association
Air Warrior Courage Foundation, Inc
All Faith Consortium
Alliance of Women Veterans
Americal Division Veterans Association
American Coalition for Filipino Veterans
American Merchant Marine Veterans
American Military Retirees Association
American Military Society
American Retiree Association
American Veterans Alliance, Inc
American Veterans for Equal Rights Inc
American Volunteer Reserve
American WWII Orphans Network (AWON)
Arab American War Veterans, Inc
Army Aviation Association of America
Asian American Veterans Association
Association for Service Disabled Veterans
Association of Ex-POW of the Korean War, Inc
Association of Military Surgeons (AMSUS)
Association of the 199th Light Infantry Brigade
Association of the US Army, USA
Association of Veterans Education Certifying Office
Blinded American Veterans Foundation
Bureau of Maine Veterans Services
BVL Fund—Bowlers Serving America's Veterans
China Burma India Veterans Association, Inc
Cold War Veterans Association
Combined National Veterans Association of America
Congressional Black Caucus Veterans Braintrust
Chief Warrant Officer & Warrant Officer (CWO&WO) Association US Coast Guard
Daughters of Union Veterans of the Civil War
Destroyer Escort Sailors Association
Eighth Air Force Historical Society
Enlisted Association of the National Guard of the US
Florida Department of Veterans Affairs
Help Hospitalized Veterans
Hispanic War Veterans of America
Homeless & Disabled Veterans
Japanese American Veterans Association
Japanese American Veterans Counsel

Korea Veterans of America
Korean Defense Veterans of America
Korean Ex-Prisoners of War
Korean War Veterans Association of the USA, Inc
Marine Corps Reserve Association
Military Justice Clinic, Inc
Military Officers Association of America
Vietnam Era Prisoners of War (NAM-POWS), Inc
National 4th Infantry (IVY) Division Association
National Academy for Veterans Service Officers
National Alliance for the Mentally Ill
National American Indian Veterans
National Association for Society of Military Widow
National Association for Uniformed Services
National Association of American Veterans, Inc
National Association of Atomic Veterans
National Association of Black Military Women (NABMW)
National Association of Concerned Veterans
National Association of Fleet Tug Sailors, Inc
National Association of Radiation Survivors
National Association of State Veterans Homes
National Association of State Women Veterans Coordinators
National Association of Veterans Program Administrators
National Coalition for Homeless Veterans
National Congress of Puerto Rican Veterans, Inc
National Guard Association of the United States
National Gulf War Resource Center, Inc
National League of Families of American Prisoners and Missing in Southeast Asia
National Military Family Association
National Order of Battlefield Commissions
National Society Daughters of the American Revolution
National Society of New England Women
National Veterans Business Development Corporation
National Veterans Foundation
National Vietnam Veterans Coalition
Naval Enlisted Reserve Association
Naval Reserve Association
Navy League of the United States
Navy Nurse Corps Association
Navy Seabee Veterans of America
New Era Veterans, Inc (registered in NY and PA)

Office of Strategic Services (OSS)- 101 Veterans Association, (The American-Kachin Rangers"
P-38 (The Flying Bulls) National Association
Reserve Officers Association of the United States
Second Airborne Ranger Association, Inc
Supreme Headquarters Allied Expeditionary Force (SHAEF)/European Theater of Operations, United States Army (Etousa) Veterans Association
Society of Military Widows
The 2nd Airborne Ranger Association, Inc
The Center for Internee Rights, Inc
The Chosen Few
The Forty & Eight
The National Veterans Organization of America
The Red River Valley Fighter Pilot
The Women Marines Association
Thailand, Laos, Cambodia (TLC) Brotherhood, Inc
Tragedy Assistance Program for Survivors, Inc
US Merchant Marine Veterans of World War II
US Navy Veterans Association
United States Ship (USS) LSM-LSMR Association
United Armed Forces Association
United States Army Warrant Officers Association

United States Federation of Korea Veterans Organization
United States Merchant Marine Veterans of WWII
United States Merchant Marine Veterans of WWII
United States Navy Cruiser Sailors Association
United States Navy Veterans Association
United States Submarine Veterans, Inc
United States Volunteers
United States Coast Guard (USCG) Chief Petty Officers Association
Veterans and Military Families for Progress
Veterans Leadership Program of Western PA
Veterans of America
Veterans of the Battle of the Bulge
Veterans United for a Strong America
Veterans' Widows/ers International Network, Inc
Vietnam Veterans Institute
Vietnam Veterans Memorial Fund
Vietnam Women's Memorial Foundation, Inc
Women Accepted for Volunteer Emergency Services (WAVES) National
Women Airforce Service Pilots of World War II
Women In Military Service for America Memorial
Women's Overseas Service League

Chapter 6

VOCATIONAL REHABILITATION OF THE COMBAT AMPUTEE

MICHAEL PRAMUKA, PhD[*]; JAMES M. MacAULAY[†]; MICHELLE L. SPORNER, MS, CRC[‡]; AND MICHAEL McCUE, PhD[§]

[*]Assistant Professor, Department of Rehabilitation Science and Technology, University of Pittsburgh, 5044 Forbes Tower-Atwood, Pittsburgh, Pennsylvania 15260; formerly, Neuropsychologist, Henry M. Jackson Foundation/San Diego Naval Medical Center, 34800 Bob Wilson Drive, San Diego, California
[†]Chief of Vocational Rehabilitation, Department of Physical Medicine and Rehabilitation Services, James A. Haley Veterans' Hospital, 13000 Bruce B. Downs Boulevard, Tampa, Florida 33612; formerly, Vocational Rehabilitation Specialist, James A. Haley Veterans' Hospital, 13000 Bruce B. Downs Boulevard, Tampa, Florida
[‡]Research Assistant, Human Engineering Research Laboratories, VA Pittsburgh Healthcare System/University of Pittsburgh, 7180 Highland Drive, Building 4, 2nd Floor, 151R1-H, Pittsburgh, Pennsylvania 15206
[§]Associate Professor, Department of Rehabilitation Science and Technology, University of Pittsburgh, 5050 Forbes Tower, Pittsburgh, Pennsylvania 15260

INTRODUCTION

Vocational rehabilitation (VR) refers both to the overarching goal of returning an individual to gainful employment after he or she acquires a disability, and to a complex process of assessment, counseling, support services, and retraining that should begin, at least conceptually, shortly after the onset of disability. Cultural values of independence, self-sufficiency, and the importance of being able to contribute to the community provide a strong incentive for individuals to return to employment, and both local and national communities recognize the financial and humanitarian value of maximizing employment. In today's rapidly changing world, service members with amputation are more likely than ever to remain on active duty status in the same or a modified position, or to seek a job or retraining for competitive employment in the civilian sector.

This chapter summarizes the basic components of VR of the combat amputee, describing both the general process of preparing an individual with amputation to return to work and the issues related to vocational success specific to combat amputees. The structure and opportunities of Department of Veterans Affairs (VA) vocational rehabilitation are outlined. The chapter concludes with a description of a model system developed over several years via collaboration between the vocational rehabilitation service of the James A Haley VA Hospital and the Veterans Benefits Administration (VBA) staff at the St Petersburg, Florida, regional office.

BACKGROUND

Legislation

In the United States, systems of VR have been initiated primarily in response to wartime casualties, then mandated and broadened for civilian populations afterwards via federal legislation. The Soldiers Rehabilitation Act was passed in Congress in 1918 to require vocational education for returning World War I soldiers with disabilities. Additional legislation broadened the scope of VR services to individuals with blindness, mental retardation, and mental illness. World War II resulted in the 1943 Disabled Veterans Act, which authorized vocational support, and the 1944 Servicemen's Readjustment Act, which provided vocational training and education for those whose careers were cut short by military service. The 1952 Veterans Readjustment Assistance Act provided vocational education to Korean War veterans. Additionally, the shortage of traditional employees in World War II created an opportunity for individuals with disabilities to demonstrate their ability to participate competitively in the workforce, resulting in additional legislation broadening VR and education for civilians. The 1973 Rehabilitation Act resulted in significant infrastructure growth for VR; 25 years later the 1998 WorkForce Investment Act brought dramatic changes to the field.

Vocational Rehabilitation Professionals

VR services, particularly in terms of initiating support and developing employment plans, have primarily been provided in both the VA and the public sector by the discipline of rehabilitation counseling.

The field of rehabilitation counseling was developed as master's level education of professional counselors with specialty training in disability, medical aspects of disability, advocacy, career guidance and vocational assessment, and rehabilitation systems. Rehabilitation counselors have a national credential, the Certified Rehabilitation Counselor (CRC), and in many states are licensed as master's level counselors. Rehabilitation counseling is defined by recognized competencies expected of a CRC; some of these identified in the CRC Scope of Practice include career counseling, assessment and appraisal, case management, referral and service coordination, job analysis, job development, placement services including assistance with employment and job accommodations, and interventions to remove environmental, employment, and attitudinal barriers.[1]

The national credentialing body for master's programs in rehabilitation counseling, the Council on Rehabilitation Education, also specifies competencies for all graduates of rehabilitation counseling programs. A brief review of these competencies confirms that training and expertise in VR are essential aspects of rehabilitation counseling. Competencies include the following:

- utilize career and occupational materials and labor market information with the consumer to accomplish vocational planning;
- evaluate work activities through the use of job and task analyses and utilize the evaluation in facilitation of successful job placement;
- establish follow-up procedures to maximize an individual's independent function through the provision of postemployment services;

- use computerized systems for consumer job placement assistance; and
- identify and arrange educational and training resources that can be utilized by consumers to meet job requirements.

Other rehabilitation professions may also be involved with VR in some settings, particularly occupational therapy, psychology, or social work. Some aspects of the rehabilitation counseling profession may overlap with psychology and social work, particularly in the areas of individual or group counseling services, discharge planning, case management, and treatment team coordination. Occupational therapists, in particular, often participate in evaluation of return-to-work status through a work hardening trial or a functional capacities evaluation that operationalizes fitness and safety for specific occupational tasks.

Rehabilitation engineers often play essential roles in VR, identifying assistive technologies and providing training on how best to implement the technologies as an accommodation for either training or on the worksite. Rehabilitation engineers may also be involved with making worksite modifications, making recommendations for ease of computer accessibility, or prescribing and setting up an environmental control unit that allows the employee to remotely control numerous appliances or other electronic devices.

Outcomes

The professional literature describes vocational and psychosocial outcomes in individuals with amputation, although the heterogeneity of amputation and differences between the civilian population and the combat amputee render most findings unlikely to generalize to this group of individuals. Vocational rehabilitation has played an essential role in the rehabilitation and community reentry of other disability groups.

Vocational Rehabilitation and the Combat Amputee

VR is tailored to the characteristics of each individual who has experienced a disability. Given their active duty status before injury, combat amputees tend to be young, fit, healthy, and oriented to physical activity, competition, and independence. These individuals, at least since the end of the draft in 1973, have chosen a career path in the military knowing of its increased level of risk, as well as uncertainty about living conditions, job duties, and an ongoing need to reestablish new peer relationships. These preinjury characteristics imply a set of values and expectations for employment

and independent living that may differ significantly from other groups of amputees, such as sedentary, elderly persons with chronic medical conditions, who make up the largest group of amputees. In general, the characteristics of combat amputees imply significant motivation to return to employment and strength of character to tolerate the ambiguity of VR. However, these same characteristics may present some obstacles to VR. Many service members have had a hiatus from their academic discipline and may find it difficult to reengage in academics, reducing their interest or confidence in their ability to succeed in vocational retraining programs.

A unique characteristic of military service members is a shift in primary identity from an "I" to a "we" upon joining the military, placing service to the country and protection of fellow service members over their individual needs. This value greatly facilitates success in combat, but may be inconsistent with planning for individual goals; the combat amputee may need to reprioritize the self and personal needs over group needs to successfully engage in the VR plan. Many veterans maintain this core value for their entire lives.

An additional component of VR is to plan pragmatically for employment. In today's military population, some service members may have learned English as a second language, and may not have been formally educated in English. Concurrently, some service members may have joined the US armed forces from another country in the hopes of facilitating US citizenship for themselves, and are not currently US citizens. Both of these issues need to be considered in light of the demands of academically oriented vocational training programs, the requirements for employment, and the long-term opportunities for employment if the service member chooses to return to the home country to be closer to family and friends.

A third tenet of VR is evaluation of the individual's strengths and limitations, taken as a whole, after injury has stabilized. For combat amputees, the mechanism and context of amputation is therefore a significant factor for future VR. The current etiology of limb loss due to explosions and motor vehicle accidents often includes numerous additional injuries such as spinal cord injury, burns, orthopedic injuries, and head trauma (and resultant cognitive or other dysfunction). These additional injuries greatly challenge the VR process and may supersede amputation as the primary limitation or consideration in identifying future employment opportunities. However, the context of combat limb loss in the system of care provided by the Department of Defense (DoD) acutely and postacutely differs significantly from typical civilian amputee care. In the DoD, active duty personnel are very likely to be recuperating in the company of other service members with similar injuries, providing a built-in support network and an organizational structure oriented to optimal rehabilitation and access to cutting-edge prosthetics.

A fourth basic issue to consider in VR is the feasibility of transferring past work experience to future employment options. The employment circumstances of active duty personnel differ dramatically from civilians both in overall format and frequently in specific job duties. Although many of the tasks completed by service members have a parallel in civilian settings, other duties are much more specific to military needs and have no clear parallel position in civilian employment. However, some resources are available to assist in generalizing from military to civilian employment, which will be discussed in the next section.

In addition, many individuals with a combat amputation are young and may have joined the military due to a lack of other vocational direction; often they have not had other types of work experience. This group may require more evaluation and exploration to determine a future employment direction. Although the opportunity to remain on active duty has greatly increased and a formal return-to-duty process exists, some service members may be unwilling to pursue this route if they are unable to return to their previous military occupational specialty.

Finally, the VR process must include consideration of long-term needs and outcomes in determining type, location, and characteristics of employment. As previously stated, the literature on long-term outcomes for individuals with combat amputations has been scarce; however, individuals with amputations resulting from the current conflicts represent a unique population in which the complexity of injury mechanism along with polytrauma, access to rapid medical and rehabilitation services, and access to state-of-the-art prosthetics all combine to produce an individual with significantly greater opportunities for functional recovery than previously seen.

The vast majority of service members with amputations are rated by the VA system as having some level of disability, or percent of "service connection" for the amputation. This commits the VA healthcare system to lifelong medical and rehabilitative care for the service member for any needs related to the disability. Therefore, many service members with limb loss find proximity to a VA hospital or a military medical treatment facility (MTF) that offers these services, in addition to the ongoing needs for rehabilitation, therapy, and modifications with a VA prosthetics service, to be an important factor in choosing a location for long-term employment. For individuals considering retraining in new career fields, additional consideration will therefore need to be given to the "transferability" of employment from a current home to areas with access to VA rehabilitation services.

THE VOCATIONAL REHABILITATION PROCESS

This section summarizes various VA and DoD systems and potential paths to access VR services. For the service member with amputation as the primary injury, medical and rehabilitation services are most likely to be provided in an MTF with specialized amputee care resources. Military MTFs now have access to VR professionals, who may establish preliminary rapport with service members and determine when to make formal referral to initiate the VR process. Particularly for those service members who express interest and are likely to remain on active duty status, consultation with VR specialists occurs after stabilization and transfer to outpatient rehabilitation, when functional status is better known and return to employment ability can be assessed and discussed in a realistic manner.

The VA incorporates VR specialists in some hospital settings and in VBA offices. For service members sustaining polytrauma, transfer to a VA polytrauma center may occur early in rehabilitation. These individuals are treated by a transdisciplinary team that includes VR. The VR team member can begin to provide education to family members and to the service member about VR options. Depending on severity of disability, some of these individuals may become veterans and may in fact need access to VA VR benefits to assist in transition to community-based services upon discharge from the military.

For medical professionals working with a combat amputee, a brief overview of the basic components of VR is offered here. VR begins early in the rehabilitative process and must be understood, reinforced, and supported by all professionals providing services to the combat amputee. VR steps discussed below include assessment and career exploration, rehabilitation plan development, intervention and training, and ongoing follow-up.

Assessment and Career Exploration

VR involves a process of intake and referral to services within DoD, VA, and community settings that will ultimately support future efforts toward return to employment, as well as a process of individually oriented assessment and intervention. Both intake and preliminary assessment can begin early in the rehabilitation of the combat amputee, but these initial steps must lead to a rehabilitation plan developed in conjunction with the individual service member. It is critical to include an overall assessment of strengths that might contribute to future employment, not just an evaluation of ambulation or other motor and sensory skills presumed to have changed after amputation. Assessment should be conducted after the service member has had ample time to adapt to prostheses or any other compensatory strategies.

Individually oriented assessment uses a variety of interviews, observations, standardized questionnaires and tests, and techniques, not all of which are necessary or relevant for every individual. In general, the process follows this sequence: interview and background gathering, evaluation of transferability of previous employment, tests or other data gathered on current ability level, determination of current interests, functional or situational assessment to assist the individual in exploring fit to a position, matching of current personal attributes to potential jobs, and finally a market study to determine utility of career choices.

Assessment in VR includes current abilities and aptitudes, interests and preferences in type of work, and transferability of skills from previous employment or training to other jobs. Abilities and aptitudes may be identified via formal testing of intellectual, academic, motor, and sensory abilities; through informal interviews; and by observation in real world environments as the individual attempts various tasks. Numerous interest inventories, such as the Self-Directed Search, are available as written exercises.[2] Data on interests is gained in interviews with veterans about hobbies, avocational interests, and past successes, as well as interviews focused on why they have chosen previous employment and their subsequent subjective experiences with the work environment and work tasks. In determining transferable job skills, it may be useful to acquire a formal job description of the military occupational specialty as well as to conduct detailed interviews about daily function.

Numerous Internet-based programs are available to assist with career guidance, particularly to gain detailed information about the demands of specific jobs, educational requirements, and job prospects. These programs are often best used initially under the guidance of a VR counselor, but lend themselves well to further independent exploration by veterans. The most comprehensive Internet resource is ONET, available at www.onetcenter.org (previously available in hardcopy as the *Dictionary of Occupational Titles*[3]).

Several online resources can assist in comparing military occupational specialty with civilian sector employment, including a "crosswalk" page on ONET and Transition Assistance Online (at www.TAOnline.com). In addition, the American Council on Education offers a Web site that describes military training programs and compares them to educational training, assigning college credits to past military training (www.militaryguides.acenet/edu).

Development of the Rehabilitation Plan

Depending on residual abilities, interests, and the demands of employment, there are typically four possible directions for VR, in the following order of preference: (1) return to previous employment in active duty status; (2) remain in the military, but in another military occupational specialty; (3) leave the military and seek civilian employment using current skills; or (4) leave the military and seek retraining for new skills or a new environment. Each combat amputee may have specific opinions and preferences about which of these directions to pursue, but will also need to abide by military decisions and policy regarding retention of active duty personnel with limb loss.

As an individual moves closer to a specific vocational choice, an assessment of the impact of disability characteristics as he or she interacts with the environment is critical. This process of functional assessment can take many forms, but ultimately must address the day-to-day realities of employment and identify compensatory strategies and accommodations that the amputee may use to meet the demands of competitive employment.

Baseline Function

As an initial step in the rehabilitation plan, the service member must reestablish and achieve a baseline level of independent function that is robust enough to remain secure in the face of the demands of return to work or participation in retraining. For many service members, particularly those with comorbid conditions, this will entail the development and description of a "prevocational" phase of therapy and supports tailored to their specific needs. Areas to evaluate and support include basic activities of daily living, such as personal hygiene, dressing, and self-feeding; home and nutritional management; finances; ability to negotiate medical and rehabilitation appointments; and medication management.

A particular point of concern is the ability to maintain attention and endurance equivalent to a work-oriented daily schedule, and then return home to attend to other requirements of independent adult life. Emotional status is also a critical component of baseline coping—the demands on emotions escalate with increased responsibilities—and the attainment of adequate coping strategies may require ongoing counseling services, support groups, family education, or other supports. To address these issues, the VR plan often details a list of prevocational therapeutic activities involving ongoing outpatient medical rehabilitation, professional counseling, or participation in community-based reentry programs. These services are typically funded under VA independent living services.

Functional Assessment

A second aspect of developing a VR plan is functional assessment, to determine the veteran's current abilities in the everyday world.[4] This assessment may include functional capacity evaluations by occupational or physical therapists to identify specific levels of physical ability as related to work demands, work hardening programs that require individuals to return gradually to the demands of employment, functional interviews, and situational assessments (discussed below).

Interviewing individuals and collateral informants is another way of obtaining information about functional abilities and competencies in the everyday environment. Spouses, housemates, employers, coworkers, caregivers, and adult children can provide rich information on an individual's ability to perform a certain task, how an individual goes about performing a task, how the individual's environment is structured, what obstacles he or she encounters, and the supports the individual needs and has access to.

A functional interview is an extension of the information-gathering process that starts with collecting background information. The functional interview differs from the traditional clinical interview in its emphasis on the individual's current environment and relationships between that environment and current problems. It also differs in its emphasis on exploring the interface between cognitive strengths and limitations and everyday life. Its purpose is not to provide a historical view of social, vocational, educational, medical, or familial background; to conduct an interview that elicits truly functional information, it is critical to keep these two agendas separate. The goal of a functional interview is to provide specific information on what individuals can or cannot do. Examples of what might be obtained include a specific picture of daily life schedule and activities; statements detailing the impact of problems

on everyday life experiences; or a list of previously attempted remedies.

The manner of questioning is important because it may influence the response. For example, asking an informant whether an individual "can" perform a task may produce a different (and perhaps less accurate) response than asking if the person regularly "does" a task. Asking about *how* an individual goes about a task (the approach, strategies, and accommodations used) can provide the rehabilitation counselor with information to make generalizations about other functional skills and future behaviors. Systematic collection of information from both veterans and informants using rating scales or questionnaires may shed light on the problems that may not be apparent from test results. There are often dramatic differences in how individuals rate themselves versus how family or caretakers rate executive function.

Simulations and role-playing of real-life activities can be used to determine how an individual utilizes interpersonal and cognitive skills to resolve problems.[5] These activities require the individual to deal with multiple priorities, unforeseen circumstances, and interpersonal interactions—the real tests of effective executive function. Situational assessments are completed by putting the individual in a real-life environment and observing how he or she functions over a period of time. These short-term real-life experiences can be arranged through temporary employment, often through the use of a temporary personnel agency. Volunteer work or short-term employment arranged through family or friends can also be considered. Large institutional settings such as a VA hospital or MTF offer a protected setting to establish a wide variety of short-term employment-oriented simulations, given the wide range of professions and environmental demands in such places and the relative facility an inside employee may have in developing such a simulation.

Situational assessments can be arranged to match the demands of training environments if the individual's vocational goals include training. Arrangements can be made for individuals to sit in on classes on a time-limited basis, or they can attend professional seminars or continuing education courses to assess their response to training at this level. In any context, a situational assessment permits evaluation of executive function across time and in the face of real-life demands and conflicts that closely parallel the employment or educational settings in which the person will need to function.

Cognitive endurance, ability to adjust to new demands and learn from the environment, social interactions with coworkers and supervisors, and problem-solving with transportation can all be observed during a situational assessment, even in a field unrelated to the individual's expressed vocational goal. The individual's ability to perform in his or her own environment may be markedly different than performance in other settings would predict, and should be assessed through direct observation. Observations can be completed at the individual's job site, in the classroom, or in his or her home, depending on the individual's level of functioning

Individual Choice

A third aspect of career guidance and exploration is the issue of consumer choice, or empowerment, especially in relation to vocational goals and choices about future employment and training. An individual may not spontaneously propose a vocational path that a professional deems most feasible, or may decline to participate in formal VR efforts when initially approached. It may be tempting to impose vocational goals on an individual that from an outside perspective appear to be a good fit. Ultimately however, each individual will need to maintain the motivation and commitment to the training and employment outlined, and will not be able to do so unless the choice was made freely. These issues have been detailed in a 2005 Institute on Rehabilitation Issues paper.[6]

Intervention and Training

In general, opportunities for intervention in VR fall broadly into three categories: (1) enhance the person's abilities; (2) change or modify the environmental demands; or (3) both. In terms of ability, VR may provide funding for a training or educational program to prepare the veteran for a new career. VR may also provide counseling or learning supports to assist veterans with the challenges of the new learning environment, particularly if the disability has a cognitive or emotional component. VR may also make environmental modifications, such as purchasing modified work stations, assistive technology, or other strategies in an environment that facilitates employment.

VR uses numerous strategies to support veterans as they return to employment. Among these are assistance in finding employment (job development), on-the-job coaching that diminishes over time as the veteran becomes more capable (job coaching), temporary employment positions that provide an opportunity to improve work skills (transitional employment settings), and on-the-job development of compensatory strategies and accommodations that allow the veteran to work competitively. The concept

of supported employment using some version of a job coach has been a part of VR for individuals with significant disabilities since the 1980s.[7,8] Concurrent with outpatient rehabilitation, institutional settings such as warrior transition units (or medical holding companies) offer an opportunity to initiate return to work in a supported, safe environment without demands on the client to meet the level required of competitive employment.

The current use of structured and supervised employment with professional support in VA hospital settings, or compensated work therapy (CWT), is one version of a supported employment program. CWT is a recovery-oriented model of VR to assist veterans with disabilities in gaining prevocational and vocational skills through employment opportunities throughout the VA and with local businesses based upon the individual's goals. CWT offers supported employment services while providing vocational assistance and counseling for a predetermined amount of time. Veterans work a specified number of hours each week as part of the therapeutic process to develop appropriate work habits and to facilitate the transition into full-time employment. Some CWT programs also have a CWT/transitional residence program to offer additional support with housing while the veteran is using CWT services.[9] Service members with complex acquired disability, however, may need professional support on the job over an extended period of time, and the psychosocial model of CWT may not be able to provide the full complement of vocational supports necessary.

Follow-Up Services

The "endpoint" for successful VR is controversial. Each program involved in VR is likely to have defined for itself a measure of successful outcome, but in the interests of serving the combat amputee, successful rehabilitation should better be conceptualized as a path rather than an endpoint. Work environments are dynamic, with ongoing and unpredictable changes in supervisory practices, coworker relationships, and intensity of workload; concurrently, physical status and stamina after amputation may also change over the years due to chronic pain, prosthesis comfort and tolerance, or prosthesis functionality. It is critical that any time a service member is referred for some aspect of VR, follow-up contact is maintained to ensure that the requested services are provided and that they result in the intended consequence. Frequently, multiple barriers arise unexpectedly, and medical professionals working with a combat amputee may need to reassess or redefine the VR plan.

SUPPORTS AND SYSTEMS FOR VOCATIONAL REHABILITATION OF THE COMBAT VETERAN

Psychosocial Adaptation to Amputation

Early in the rehabilitation of the combat amputee, it is critical to facilitate psychosocial adaptation to disability. It is much less important who intervenes to accomplish this, and much more relevant that all medical professionals providing services to the combat amputee have a basic orientation to possible psychological responses and changes after amputation.

It is important to communicate to the combat amputee that rehabilitation is a learning process, requiring rehearsal of new skills and a willingness to try new ways to accomplish old tasks. Neither acute rehabilitation nor eventual return to employment comes without attention, effort, and motivation to acquire new strategies, sequences of movement, and new attitudes and values. At times, the VR process may seem distant or unclear, and in fact it requires tolerating a high degree of ambiguity. This rehabilitative process involves ongoing change and modifications to the individual's overall level of function. Consequently, amputees cannot rapidly make an internal determination about their ultimate level of function.

One goal of rehabilitation professionals is to facilitate coping with amputation. Livneh et al[10] examined coping responses in a group of 61 amputees, noting that coping styles of amputees are similar to other groups of people dealing with a variety of illness or other life stressors. Generally, individuals chose between active coping/problem-solving perspectives versus denial, optimism versus pessimism, and seeking external support (talking to others, asking advice) versus internally oriented acceptance.

A wide variety of personal factors may be involved in psychosocial changes after amputation. Shifts in body image and personal identity, phantom pain or residual limb pain, and emotional changes related to depression or anxiety have all been noted in other amputee populations as potential areas complicating recovery. Horgan and MacLachlan[11] reviewed a wide range of published studies on psychosocial outcomes after amputation, concluding that better adjustment was associated with active coping, optimism, good social support, increased time since amputation, and less pain. These characteristics make intuitive sense, but are often lost in considering a specific individual and where professional intervention may fit at the current stage of the rehabilitation process.

Service members with amputations will encounter a wide range of professionals as they traverse their rehabilitation paths, most of whom have an opportunity to provide some aspect of psychosocial support that ultimately will facilitate return to independence and employment. General themes that may appear in any contact with service members include distress over appearance, a shift in personal values and goals, and identifying personally relevant goals to maintain motivation and stamina throughout the long rehabilitation process. Professionals may also be able to support service members as they begin to compare strengths and limitations of their "new self" in comparison to their "old self," offering a sounding board as amputees rehearse new ways to explain their current circumstances and changes to others. Veterans are also faced with the need to rapidly absorb complex medical information, synthesize it with family needs and personal values, and make weighty decisions about return to active duty, surgical and other treatment options, and use of prosthetics. These topics are all best addressed in a supportive, nonconfrontational manner, with repeated discussion until the veteran has become comfortable with a decision.

The Veterans Affairs Vocational Rehabilitation System

The VBA and DoD now operate a complex and detailed system of benefits that support VR for service members with a service-connected disability. An overview is provided here along with a description of VR services that may also be found in some VA healthcare facilities. An excellent summary is also offered at www.vetsuccess.gov. It is critical to note that funding and overall direction of VR occurs not within the hospital system but in the veterans' benefits system.

The primary vehicle in the VA system to implement rehabilitation plans is in the VBA Office of Vocational Rehabilitation and Education (VR&E). The VR&E employs rehabilitation counselors, housed under the VBA in regional offices, to develop and implement rehabilitation plans for veterans with disabilities. Typically, veterans with at least a 20%-level of service-connected disability are eligible to apply for VR under Chapter 31 of Title 38 of the US Code. For many veterans with significant disabilities, however, prevocational programs including ongoing therapy and community reintegration are required as the initial step in the VR process. The VA system may provide these services under an independent living program.

VR&E rehabilitation counselors assist veterans in applying to the program using Form 1900. Once the veteran is found eligible, VR&E may provide services under a rehabilitation plan for extended evaluation, independent living, or education and training. The VA process includes significant opportunities to ensure that veterans with a disability are fully prepared before initiating a formal education/training process.

Services for VR within VA hospitals currently vary widely from facility to facility. Those with the greatest emphasis on rehabilitation, particularly the polytrauma centers, are best equipped to provide face-to-face direct VR evaluation and career guidance. Increasingly, VA hospitals also have implemented the CWT program.

The Public Vocational Rehabilitation System

Each state is required by the federal government to establish and maintain a public VR system for citizens with disabilities. Established in 1920, the funding stream for public VR is now a mix of federal and state monies. Eligibility for VR services is based on documentation of disability and the decision that the disability represents a significant obstacle to competitive employment. The public VR system can provide a wide variety of resources and supports for an individual, including counseling, assessment, job development, and job coaching, as well as financial support for tuition and other fees associated with vocational training programs. The public VR system defines itself as the "payor of last resort," meaning that services should always be funded first by any other resource. Hence, the veteran who incurred an amputation in combat may more likely receive VR services under the VA, but may still be eligible for some public benefits, such as reimbursement of transportation.

A MODEL SYSTEM FOR VETERANS WITH DISABILITIES

VR services for veterans under Chapter 31 involve an exchange of information and collaboration between the VBA VR&E counselor and a contractor. A model program to facilitate rapid entry into the VBA VR system and timely deployment of a rehabilitation plan has been developed and disseminated by the joint efforts of the VR service of the Tampa, Florida, VA and the local regional benefits office in St Petersburg.[12] An outline of this model is provided here.

The Tampa model requests consultation from all programs that serve veterans likely to qualify for or need VR services upon admission; this ensures that the veteran will be identified as a potential VR candidate early in the rehabilitation process. The model includes ongoing collaboration between a VA VR specialist, a VBA VR&E counselor, and the assigned contractor in the community brought in to facilitate the rehabilitation plan. This collaboration includes face-to-face meetings and participation, when feasible, in client staffing. The VA hospital staff facilitates any necessary medical appointments for evaluation, triaging the requests. VA staff initiate vocational evaluations with veterans when relevant and appropriate, and maintain ongoing cross-training between the two entities. Notably, the VR&E staff are considered primary stakeholders in the VR process, sharing common outcome measures in client satisfaction and effectiveness measures. The regional office also maintains an out-stationed VR&E counselor at the hospital, greatly facilitating the partnership. For service members who participate in inpatient rehabilitation services in a VA setting, this approach is critical to timely and coordinated benefits and access to appropriate services as they transition home or to other services.

SUMMARY

This short overview of the VR process for the combat amputee has reflected the complex nature of returning to employment after limb loss. The process requires assessment and involvement of the service member as well as knowledge, access, and coordination across numerous systems of support and institutional bureaucracies. Even for those individuals who experience a rapid and successful return to competitive employment, education, training, and follow-up to anticipate and manage changes in the work environment successfully are critical to long-term retention of employment. Initiating discussions and referrals related to VR is one of numerous preliminary steps in the rehabilitation of the combat amputee.

REFERENCES

1. Commission on Rehabilitation Counselor Certification. *Scope of practice for rehabilitation counseling.* Available at: http:// www.crccertification.com/downloads/35scope/scope_of_practice_%200307I.pdf. Published 2003. Accessed March 13, 2008

2. Holland JL. *Professional Manual for the Self-Directed Search.* Odessa, Fla: Psychological Assessment Resources; 1985.

3. *Dictionary of Occupational Titles*. 4th ed. 2 vols. Washington, DC: US Department of Labor, Employment and Training Administration, US Employment Service; 1991.

4. McCue M, Pramuka M. Functional assessment. In: Goldstein G, Beers S, eds. *Handbook of Human Brain Function*. 4th ed. New York, NY: Springer; 1998:113–129.

5. McCue M, Pramuka M, Chase SL, Fabry P. Functional assessment procedures for individuals with severe cognitive disabilities. *Am Rehabil*. 1995;20:17–27.

6. 29th Institute on Rehabilitation Issues. Promoting consumer empowerment through professional vocational rehabilitation counseling. Available at: http://www.rcep6.org/IRI/IRI/29th%20IRI/29th_iri.htm. Published March 31, 2005. Accessed November 1, 2007.

7. Wehman P, Moon MS, eds. *Vocational Rehabilitation and Supported Employment*. Baltimore, Md: Paul H Brookes Publishing Co; 1988.

8. Wehman P, Sale P, Parent W. *Supported Employment: Strategies for Integration of Workers With Disabilities*. Stoneham, Mass: Butterworth-Heinemann; 1992.

9. Department of Veterans Affairs. *Compensated Work Therapy Supported Employment Services Implementation Plan*. Washington DC: Veterans Health Administration; 2007. VHA Directive 2007-005. Available at: http://www1.va.gov/vhapublications/ViewPublication.asp?pub_ID=1531 Accessed Retrieved November 1, 2007.

10. Livneh H, Antonak RF, Gerhardt J. Multidimensional investigation of the structure of coping among people with amputations. *Psychosomatics*. 2000;41:235–244.

11. Horgan O, MacLachlan M. Psychosocial adjustment to lower-limb amputation: a review. *Disabil Rehabil*. 2004;26:837–850.

12. Best Practices Model Partnership: VHA and VBA Vocational Rehabilitation Program. In: Veterans Administration Rehabilitation and Employment Task Force. *Report to the Secretary of Veterans Affairs. The Vocational Rehabilitation and Employment Program for the 21st Century Veteran*. Washington DC: VA; 2004: Appendix 14-B. Available at: http://www1.va.gov/op3/docs/VRE_report.pdf. Accessed November 1, 2007.

Chapter 7

MILITARY AND VETERAN SUPPORT SYSTEMS

MICHELLE L. SPORNER, MS, CRC*; RORY A. COOPER, PhD†; AND WILLIAM LAKE‡

*Research Assistant, Human Engineering Research Laboratories, VA Pittsburgh Healthcare System/University of Pittsburgh, 7180 Highland Drive, Building 4, 2nd Floor, 151R1-H, Pittsburgh, Pennsylvania 15206
†Senior Career Scientist, US Department of Veterans Affairs, and Distinguished Professor, Department of Rehabilitation Science and Technology, University of Pittsburgh, 5044 Forbes Tower, Pittsburgh, Pennsylvania 15260
‡Colonel (Retired), US Marine Corps; Associate, Department of IT Strategy, Booz Allen Hamilton Incorporated, 4040 North Fairfax Drive, Arlington, Virgina 22203

Warrior Ethos

- I will always place the mission first.
- I will never accept defeat.
- I will never quit.
- I will never leave a fallen comrade.

INTRODUCTION

To augment and facilitate a wounded service member's journey through the rehabilitation process, and to ensure a seamless transition from injury to civilian life or return to active duty, the US military has initiated several programs. Through the efforts of fellow military personnel and veterans, these programs offer support to injured service members and their families.

The programs embrace the military philosophy that all service members are brothers and sisters, as expressed in the Army's "we will never leave a fallen comrade" and the Marine Corps' "once a Marine, always a Marine." This chapter will examine the different programs available to injured service members and discuss their benefits.

MILITARY SEVERELY INJURED SUPPORT SYSTEMS

Army Wounded Warrior Program

On April 30, 2004, the Department of the Army established the Disabled Soldier Support System program, which became the US Army Wounded Warrior (AW2) program on November 10, 2005. Serving over 2,400 soldiers today, AW2 provides a system of advocacy and personal support for severely wounded soldiers and their families as they transition from military service to the civilian community,[1] in phased progression from initial casualty notification until after the soldiers' return home. AW2 works to facilitate contact and coordination between the soldier and external supporting agencies such as the Department of Veterans Affairs (VA), veteran service organizations, and vocational rehabilitation. The goal of AW2 is to help soldiers receive full Army and VA benefits, continued healthcare after retiring from the Army, financial counseling, and all the services awarded for as long as needed.[1,2]

To be eligible to receive services from AW2, a soldier must have sustained injuries or illnesses after September 10, 2001, in support of the global war on terror (GWOT), or have received or be expected to receive a 30% rating for one or more injuries rated by the Physical Disability Evaluation System including, but not limited to, loss of limb, spinal cord injury/paralysis, severe burn, traumatic brain injury, or posttraumatic stress disorder. AW2 monitors and tracks these severely wounded soldiers for 5 years beyond their medical retirement, ensuring that they and their families have continued access to an array of nonmedical support services through rehabilitation and return to duty or separation/retirement.[1] AW2 can be reached through its toll-free number: 1-800-237-1336. The attachment to this chapter provides a list of soldier family management specialist locations by state, with contact numbers.

Marine Wounded Warrior Regiment

The Marine Wounded Warrior Regiment (MWWR) was created in 2007 from the Marine for Life (M4L) program (established in 2002 and expanded in 2005 to include the Injured Support System) to serve active duty or honorably discharged marines. The regiment's mission is "to provide and facilitate assistance to ill/injured Marines, sailors attached to or in direct support of Marine units, and their family members throughout the phases of recovery in order to assist in rehabilitation and transition." Transition refers to a return to active duty or separation from active duty with all possible benefits. The MWWR helps marines and sailors with disabilities remain on active duty or transition from military to civilian life. Marines and sailors who have sustained severe injuries (and their families) have support throughout all phases of recovery.[3] The other military services modeled their support programs on M4L.

The Marine Corps had been providing similar support prior to the establishment of the regiment; however, despite a "unity of effort," no "unity of command" existed. Under the MWWR one command is accountable for tracking and meeting the needs of wounded, injured, or severely ill marines and their families. Under the regiment's unity of command and the unity of effort, procedures are standardized, resources are shared, and transitions from Department of Defense (DoD) care to VA care are as seamless as possible.

The MWWR has two battalions, the Wounded Warrior Battalion East (WWBN-E), located at Marine

Corps Base Camp Lejeune, North Carolina, and the Wounded Warrior Battalion West (WWBN-W), at Marine Corps Base Camp Pendleton, California. WWBN-E was officially formed on July 1, 2007, and WWBN-W on August 1, 2007 (previously these units were the II Marine Expeditionary Force Injured Support Unit and the I Marine Expeditionary Force Injured Support Unit, respectively). The battalions are home to the wounded warrior barracks, where marines recuperate from their injuries with the support of fellow wounded marines in a cohesive unit that assembles for morning formations, performs tasks appropriate to capabilities, and provides transportation to medical appointments. Wounded warrior battalions are responsible for their respective geographical area: WWBN-E covers the area east of the Mississippi River and WWBN-W handles the area west of the Mississippi. Marines at Brooke Army Medical Center in Fort Sam Houston, Texas, are tracked by WWBN-W.

The MWWR also monitors marines at the VA's four polytrauma rehabilitation centers located in Richmond, Virginia; Tampa, Florida; Minneapolis, Minnesota; and Palo Alto, California. These facilities are designed to help veterans who have traumatic brain injury in addition to other severe injuries and require specialized intensive rehabilitation. When a marine is transferred to a VA facility, the Marine Corps facilitates the transfer via the VA Office of Seamless Transition, which includes a Marine colonel who monitors the marines leaving the care of the DoD system and entering the VA system. Through connections with both systems, the colonel can alert the VA of the movement timeline. The MWWR can request marines' orders to be adjusted if the VA is not ready to accept them.

The MWWR is aggressively reaching out to all injured marines to ensure that their needs are being met. Those identified as seriously ill, who require extensive treatment and therapy prior to returning to duty or processing through the disability evaluation system, are placed in a limited-duty status in excess of 30 days. The acute phase of recovery includes all critical care services provided in theater and in the level-IV treatment area in Landstuhl, Germany. Medical and rehabilitation services provided at the medical treatment facility (MTF) or a VA polytrauma center are typically a part of the rehabilitation phase.[3] As injured marines enter the acute and rehabilitation phases, they receive support from MWWR headquarters, and during the separation or retention phase, they receive support from MWWR district injured support cells, located regionally throughout the United States, along with local hometown links. Many hometown links cover an area in excess of 100 miles to reach as many marines as possible; for those areas that do not have a hometown link, M4L has partnered with the Marine Corps League

and other veteran volunteers to provide support.[4] The attachment to this chapter lists hometown link contacts by state.

As of April 2006, the US Marine Corps was averaging over 200 injuries a month,[5] and the entire M4L program had served 5,500 marines who served in Operation Enduring Freedom or Operation Iraqi Freedom, with 30 to 40 active support cases at any time.[5] Currently the Corps has more than 400 injured or ill marines and sailors on the regiment's rolls, with more expected as units transfer wounded personnel. The MWWR is expected to grow to 100 active duty, reserve, and civilian personnel, in addition to 150 individual mobilization augmentees. Marines take care of each other before, during, and after the battle. The MMWR is living its motto "taking care of our own" through unwavering support for wounded, injured, and ill marines.

Navy Safe Harbor

The mission of the Navy Safe Harbor program is to provide personalized support and assistance to wounded, ill, and injured sailors and their families. Sailors who incurred severe injuries after September 10, 2001, in support of GWOT are eligible for Safe Harbor benefits. The program establishes and maintains communication with the sailor's command and works to encourage active duty retention. Sailors with a disability rating of 30% or greater are provided continuing support for transitioning to civilian life as appropriate.[6] For sailors assigned to Marine units, Safe Harbor partners with MWWR to provide support.

Air Force Wounded Warrior Program

Air Force Wounded Warrior Program (formerly Palace HART) is available to all injured airmen with a combat-related disability, including Purple Heart recipients.[7] The program ensures that all ill and injured airmen receive appropriate services by providing a support system that includes a family liaison officer to assist them through all phases of the rehabilitation process and transition, including assistance with filing VA disability claims or potential temporary duty retirements listing. Airmen also receive case management for 5 years post injury, vocational counseling, and placement assistance.[7]

Military Severely Injured Center

In 2005 the DoD opened the Military Severely Injured Center to ensure that all severely injured men and women returning from Iraq and Afghanistan received a seamless transition back to military service or into the civilian community. At the time, each branch of the military had its own injured support program, but the DoD saw a need to reach across all service branches to fill any gaps in the delivery and continuity of care as these programs developed. Since 2005 the service injured support programs have grown in staff and scope to the point where the level of augmentation support provided by the center has significantly decreased. Today, the center provides back-up support as requested by the services, and in most cases, acts as a referral agent for injured service members or their families to the appropriate service injured support program.[8]

Operation Warfighter Program

The DoD also sponsors the Operation Warfighter (OWF) program, which provides temporary assignments in participating federal agencies in the Washington, DC, area to volunteer service members in a medical hold status at an MTF.[9] OWF's goal is to engage injured service members in outside activities to enhance their well-being. The number of hours worked per week and the duration of the assignment are determined by an individual treatment schedule on a strict, noninterference basis with the service member's military or medical obligations. Although not an employment program per se (many OWF "graduates" have gone on to continue military service or secure employment at their home or in another area), OWF exposes service members to an area within the federal government that interests them, where they can contribute and are valued for their experience and training. Although the program's primary purpose is to keep injured service members actively engaged in their recovery, many OWF participants have received mentoring at their federal agency, and some have received offers of permanent employment with the agency after completion of their military service.

Defense Department Computer and Electronic Accommodation Program

The federally funded Computer and Electronic Accommodation Program (CAP) was established in 1990 to provide assistive technology for DoD employees with disabilities. Currently 64 other federal agencies have adopted this program to provide appropriate accommodations to help injured service members and veterans return to the workplace. CAP representatives demonstrate assistive technology devices and capabilities to injured service members and introduce new career possibilities. CAP provides assistive technology to any federal employee who needs it. In fiscal 2005 CAP filled more than 3,000 requests for accommoda-

tions within the DoD and more than 2,000 in other federal agencies. Located at the Pentagon, the CAP center demonstrates assistive technology to visitors that allows individuals with loss of vision, hearing, or hand function to interface with a computer, telephone, and other aspects of their environment. CAP also provides equipment installation and training. In addition, CAP helps DoD agencies with workers' compensation processes, tele-work solutions, and equal employment opportunity complaints.

Labor Department Recovery and Employment Assistance Lifelines

Developed by the Department of Labor's Veterans' Employment and Training Service (VETS), the Recovery and Employment Assistance Lifelines (REALifelines) program provides information and access to one-on-one employment assistance and online resources to help wounded and injured transitioning service members and veterans reintegrate into the civilian workforce. VETS' mission is to provide veterans and transitioning service members with the resources and services to succeed in the 21st century workforce by maximizing their employment opportunities, protecting their employment rights, and helping them meet labor market demands. The REALifelines program provides veterans and transitioning service members wounded and injured as a result of GWOT, and their family members, with the resources they need to successfully transition to a rewarding career.

Life Insurance, Special Pay Programs, and Travel Benefits

Traumatic Servicemembers' Group Life Insurance (TSGLI) provides monetary support to individuals covered by Servicemembers' Group Life Insurance (SGLI) who have had an injury resulting in traumatic loss (eg, loss of limbs, sight, hearing, traumatic brain injury) and their families. This vital assistance, which enables family members to join injured service members during recovery, does not affect Army or VA disability compensation determinations. TSGLI coverage, available for a flat rate of $1 per month for most service members, can pay between $25,000 and $100,000 depending upon the traumatic loss.[10] TSGLI is intended to cover expenses that may not be compensated by other mechanisms, for example, loss of spouse or parent income, extended family travel, and equipment or services not available through the DoD or VA.

Combat-related injury and rehabilitation pay (CIP) is payable up to $430 a month. Eligible members already receiving hazardous fire or imminent danger pay are paid $205 month. Basic allowance for subsistence (BAS) entitlements continue for service members during hospitalization (BAS-authorized service members not hospitalized must pay for their own meals). The 2007 monthly rates for BAS were $279.88 for enlisted personnel and $192.74 for officers. Service members who were medically evacuated from a combat zone and considered hospitalized are entitled to CIP. For the purposes of CIP entitlement, service members are considered hospitalized if they are admitted as an inpatient or receive extensive rehabilitation as an outpatient while living in quarters affiliated with the military healthcare system, such as the Fisher House at Walter Reed Army Medical Center. CIP is nontaxable, and no forms must be filled out to receive it. The hospitalized service member is eligible for CIP starting the month after medical evacuation, and it terminates at the end of the first month during which any of the following apply:

- the member is paid a TSGLI benefit;
- 30 days have passed since the member received notification of eligibility for a TSGLI benefit; or
- the service member is no longer "hospitalized" (no longer an MTF inpatient or receiving extensive outpatient rehabilitation or other medical care while living in quarters affiliated with the military healthcare system).

Combat zone tax exclusion allows military members to exclude all or a portion of pay and entitlements earned while serving in designated combat areas from tax liabilities. The exclusion is also authorized for each month of inpatient hospitalization as a result of wounds, disease, or injury incurred while serving in a combat zone. Wounded, injured, or ill service members may qualify for the exclusion for up to 2 years if rehospitalized for the same injury.

Invitational travel authorizations are government orders authorizing travel for family members to an MTF where a wounded, injured, or ill service member is receiving care. Travel to and from the hospital, hotel costs, meals, and incidental expenses are reimbursed by the government. Family members are paid a daily rate (per diem) for meals and incidental expenses, which differ depending on the location of the MTF. The local wounded warrior pay support team, located at the installation's finance office, provides information on per diem and maximum lodging rates for various locations and assists family members in completing and submitting vouchers.

The Transportation Security Administration (TSA) has partnered with the Military Severely Injured Center to help ensure that severely injured military personnel and their families have a smooth and uneventful airport screening experience. Once flight arrangements are made with the airline, the service member, family members, or staff of service programs, MTFs, and VA hospitals can call the TSA operations center with details of the itinerary. The TSA liaison will then notify the appropriate federal security directors at the involved airports to ensure that required security screenings are conducted respectfully by TSA experts to make the overall experience as expeditious and pleasant for the service member as possible.

Heroes to Hometowns

The Military Severely Injured Center also sponsors Heroes to Hometowns (H2H), a program designed to engage local community and state support groups to organize and welcome home an injured service member and his or her family to the community. Through an official memorandum of understanding, the American Legion has partnered with the DoD to mobilize its nearly 20,000 legion posts worldwide to act as facilitators in local communities to connect returning service members with needed resources. States have formed H2H committees consisting of the state American Legion adjutants, state VA directors, and the National Guard state family program directors to help mobilize local community support.

The purpose of H2H is to help returning service members become active and contributing members of the community and help them understand their local, state, and federal benefits. Ways in which the community can be involved include organizing a welcome home celebration, helping secure temporary or permanent housing, assisting in adapting a home or vehicle to the injury, finding jobs and educational opportunities, and creating a carpool for hospital visits. A community can also provide childcare, financial support, entertainment options, counseling, spiritual support, and family support. More information about H2H can be found at: www.militaryhomefront.dod.mil.

Services Offered by Military Support Systems

All of the military support systems offer the following services to assist injured service members throughout their rehabilitation and for many years afterward:

- medical care and rehabilitation;
- case management;
- education, job training, and employment assistance;
- personal mobility and functioning;
- home, transportation, and workplace accommodations;

TABLE 7-1

MILITARY SUPPORT SYSTEMS INTERNET ADDRESSES

Program	Internet Address
US Army Wounded Warrior Program	https://www.aw2.army.mil/index.html
Marine For Life	https://www.m4l.usmc.mil/
Navy Safe Harbor	http://www.npc.navy.mil/CommandSupport/SafeHarbor/
Air Force PALACE HART	http://www.socom.mil/care_coalition/docs/Palace_Hearts.pdf
Military HOMEFRONT/Military Severely Injured Center	http://www.militaryhomefront.dod.mil
Traumatic Servicemembers' Group Life Insurance	http://www.insurance.va.gov/sgliSite/TSGLI/TSGLI.htm

- personal, couple, and family counseling;
- financial resources;
- TSGLI claims submissions;
- military liaisons;
- return to active duty transitioning;
- VA transitioning;
- child care;
- information on and resources for major injuries;
- injured support processes; and
- communication with veteran service and charitable organizations.

Table 7-1 provides a list of military support organizations and their Internet contact information. DisabilityInfo.gov is a user-friendly Web site that contains links to information for people with disabilities, their families, employers, service providers, and other community members.

VETERAN SERVICE ORGANIZATIONS AND OTHER OPPORTUNITIES

Paralyzed Veterans of America

Paralyzed Veterans of America (PVA) is a congressionally chartered service organization founded in 1946 to provide support and assistance to veterans with spinal cord injuries and dysfunction.[11] PVA advocates for all veterans with spinal cord injuries or dysfunctions for quality healthcare, performs research and provides education on spinal cord injury and dysfunction, protects civil rights, and provides opportunities to maintain independence and increase the quality of life of all PVA members.[11]

Helping veterans, especially those who served in Operation Iraqi Freedom and Operation Enduring Freedom, secure the benefits and healthcare they are entitled to is central to PVA's mission. Through its congressional charter as a veteran service organization, PVA members can be accredited to represent claimants before the VA. PVA has 34 chapters and many more service offices, including 24 offices in VA medical centers that provide spinal cord injury care. Service offices help veterans file claims for benefits, monitor their healthcare and the progress of their claims, and serve as advocates for veterans with the VA. PVA national service officers, available regionally across the United States and in Puerto Rico, provide no-cost representation to veterans with spinal cord

injury and their dependents to the VA, DoD, and other local agencies.

PVA has a number of programs to help veterans receive benefits and live healthy and productive lives. When necessary, the PVA appellate services program provides legal representation at the VA Board of Veterans Appeals in Washington, DC. Appellate services also prepares and presents cases before various military boards to ensure that PVA members receive maximum benefits from the military. Research and education supports investigations into the cure of spinal cord injury and dysfunction as well as the development of innovative treatments and critical new technologies. A key function of the research and education division is support for Clinical Practice Guidelines.

Formed to fight for the rights of paralyzed veterans, PVA remains involved in the creation of nearly every piece of influential disability legislation and federal regulation through the work of its legislative division. PVA is also involved in broader issues such as military retirement benefits. PVA maintains an office of the general counsel, which works closely with the PVA veterans' benefits department and also monitors overall trends in the VA's administration of benefits and healthcare. General counsel works to provide internal legal counsel for issues within PVA and its member chapters, but also provides critical legal interpretations of changes in legislation or regulations affecting veterans.

The PVA accessible design division works to ensure that veterans with disabilities have access to public facilities and housing for independent living, providing example home layouts for wheelchair accessibility and consulting on major public venues to ensure maximum usage by veterans with a wide range of disabilities. The sports and recreation division provides a wide variety of opportunities for veterans with disabilities to learn and participate in activities that promote a healthy lifestyle, including the annual National Veterans Wheelchair Games.[12]

Disabled American Veterans

After World War I, Disabled American Veterans (DAV) was formed to help wounded veterans receive the care and benefits they deserved. With over 1.2 million members, 52 state departments, and almost 2,000 chapters located throughout the United States today, DAV continues helping veterans receive benefits, and its active legislative department ensures that privileges earned by veterans are protected and relevant to the current environment.[13] DAV helps service members with disabilities acquired during military conflict to transition from active duty to veteran status, and cosponsors the National Veterans Winter Sports Clinic with VA.[14]

Wounded Warrior Project

"Putting veterans first in America" is the motto of the Wounded Warrior Project, a 501c(3) organization, originally partnered with the United Spinal Association, that provides free assistance to veterans in the process of applying for benefits from VA and other agencies. Goals of the organization are to give a new generation of veterans a voice as they enter the rehabilitation process, promote mutual assistance among service members as they reintegrate into communities, and let them know they are not forgotten.[15] Like the military support systems, the Wounded Warrior Project assists with housing, daycare, identifying services, vocational support, and peer counseling, but also offers funding and sponsorship for adaptive sports and recreation, ranging from skiing in Colorado in partnership with Disabled Sports USA to deep-sea fishing in Alaska. The organization has delivered "wounded warrior packs" containing items such as telephone calling cards, magazines, clothing, and personal CD players to over 2,500 service members at MTFs. In addition to support for newly injured service members, the Wounded Warrior Project offers continued services and events to alumni long after their service to establish and maintain camaraderie among current and former service members.[16]

Other Important Organizations

There are many veteran service organizations and similar groups available to help veterans with disabilities successfully reintegrate into society, such as Veterans of Foreign Wars, the American Legion, and the Marine Corps League. The National Veterans Foundation is a not-for-profit organization that helps all veterans and their families and children. Its mission is to continue the process of rehabilitating and integrating American veterans into productive roles in society, and to facilitate, maintain, and operate a toll-free crisis management, referral, and information hotline for veterans and their families. The Armed Forces Relief Trust is a nonprofit fund created by the National Association of Broadcasters and the military aid societies to collect and distribute donations and loans in support of troops and families in need.

Newer organizations such as the Semper Fi Fund and Iraq War Veterans were created during Operation Iraqi Freedom/Operation Enduring Freedom to assist veterans and their families. Iraq War Veterans supports veterans of the war and their families, and its Web site links to other assistance and support organizations. The Coalition to Salute America's Heroes was created to provide a way for individuals, corporations, and others to help severely wounded and disabled veterans and their families rebuild their lives.

The VA, in cooperation with the National Association of State Directors of Veterans Affairs, initiated the State Benefits Seamless Transition Program, which placed VA staff at 10 DoD medical facilities. VA staff identify injured military members who will be transferred to VA facilities and contact state veterans affairs offices on the patients' behalf. The state offices, in turn, contact the veterans to inform them about state benefits for them and dependent family members. Most states and territories offer a range of benefits to veterans.

The Red Cross offers assistance to military members on active duty and their families, as well as veterans. The Fisher House program is a private-public partnership that supports America's military in times of need, recognizing the special sacrifices of US men and women in uniform and the hardships of military service by offering humanitarian services beyond those normally provided by DoD and VA. Fisher Houses provide homelike settings where injured service members, veterans, and their families can stay while undergoing medical treatment and rehabilitation. Operation First Response provides sweatshirts, socks, underwear, toothbrushes, razors, and other essentials in backpacks, as well as assisting families of wounded service members with travel expenses and financial burdens incurred during rehabilitation or medical treatment.

SUMMARY

Many organizations are currently working to ensure wounded service members the support and assistance they need and deserve. These organizations have been established to give injured service members a voice and show them their sacrifice has not been forgotten. The attachment to this chapter lists several charitable organizations and useful resources for service members and their families.

REFERENCES

1. US Army Human Resources Command. US Army Wounded Warrior Program. Army Wounded Warrior Web site. Available at: https://www.aw2.army.mil/index.html /. Accessed December 12, 2007.

2. US Army Human Resources Command. Wounded Warrior Lifecycle of Care and AW2. Army Wounded Warrior Web site. Available at: https://www.aw2.army.mil/about/lifecycle.html. Accessed December 10, 2008.

3. US Marine Corps. Wounded Warrior Regiment Web site. Available at: http://www.woundedwarriorregiment.org/WWR.aspx. Accessed December 1, 2008.

4. US Marine Corps. Marine for Life. US Marine Corps Web site. Available at: https://www.m4l.usmc.mil/. Accessed December 14, 2007.

5. Shafer JR. Marine for Life injured support: hometown link conference. Paper presented at: Annual Marine For Life Hometown Link Conference; May 2, 2006; San Diego, Calif.

6. US Navy. Safe Harbor—severely injured support. US Navy Web site. Available at: www.npc.navy.mil/CommandSupport/SafeHarbor/. Accessed December 14, 2007.

7. US Air Force. *PALACE HART (Helping Airmen Recover Together)*. Washington, DC: USAF; 2006. Available at: www.socom.mil/care_coalition/docs/Palace_Hearts.pdf. Accessed December 14, 2007.

8. US Department of Defense. Military severely injured support. Military HOMEFRONT Web site. Available at: www.militaryhomefront.dod.mil/portal/page/mhf/MHF/MHF_HOME_1?section_id=20.40.500.393.0.0.0.0.0. Accessed December 14, 2007.

9. US Department of Defense. Be a part of Operation Warfighter. Military HOMEFRRONT Web site. Available at: www.militaryhomefront.dod.mil/dav/lsn/LSN/BINARY_RESOURCE/BINARY_CONTENT/1952741.pdf. Accessed December 15, 2007.

10. US Department of Veterans Affairs. Traumatic injury protection under Servicemembers' Group Life Insurance (TSGLI). Department of Veterans Affairs Web site. Available at: www.insurance.va.gov/sgliSite/TSGLI/TSGLI.htm. Accessed December 14, 2007.

11. Paralyzed Veterans of America Web site. Available at: www.pva.org/. Accessed December 21, 2007.

12. US Department of Veterans Affairs. National Veterans Wheelchair Games. Department of Veterans Affairs Web site. Available at: www1.va.gov/vetevent/nvwg/2008/default.cfm. Accessed December 21, 2007.

13. Disabled Veterans of America Web site. Available at: www.dav.org/. Accessed December 21, 2007.

14. US Department of Veterans Affairs. National Veterans Winter Sports Clinic. Department of Veterans Affairs Web site. Available at: www1.va.gov/vetevent/wsc/2007/default.cfm. Accessed December 21, 2007.

15. Walter Reed Army Medical Center. *Our Hero Handbook*. Washington, DC: WRAMC; 2004. Available at: www.wramc.army.mil/WarriorsInTransition/handbooks/WalterReedHeroHandbook.pdf. Accessed December 14, 2007.

16. Wounded Warrior Project Web site. Available at: https://www.woundedwarriorproject.org/. Accessed December 14, 2007.

ATTACHMENT: REGIONAL RESOURCES AND SUPPORT ORGANIZATIONS

Army Wounded Warrior Soldier Family Management Specialist Locations

State	Telephone Number	State	Telephone Number
Alabama	205-382-3353	Minnesota	612-467-3578 ext 64810 (Minneapolis VAPTC)
Alaska	703-325-9976		
Arizona	703-325-9976	Mississippi	703-325-9957
Arkansas	703-325-9959	Missouri	314-652-4100 ext 64810 (St Louis VAMC)
California	703-325-9980	Montana	703-325-9976
	703-325-9958	Nebraska	703-325-9982
	619-476-0226 (San Diego VAPTC)	Nevada	703-325-9976
	310-478-3711 ext. 40935 (Los Angeles VAMC)	New Hampshire	NA
		New Jersey	703-325-8452
	650-387-2435 (Palo Alto VAPTC)	New Mexico	703-325-9982
Colorado	719-238-0777 (Fort Carson)	New York	718-772-2332 (Bronx VA)
	719-338-5284 (Denver VAMC)	North Carolina	703-325-8452
Connecticut	NA		703-325-9966
Delaware	617-314-5104 (Boston VAMC)		910-907-7165 (Fort Bragg-Womack AMC)
District of Columbia	202-356-1012 ext 40380 (WRAMC Outpatient)		910-864-8768 (Fayetteville VAMC)
		North Dakota	703-325-9982
	202-782-9713 (WRAMC Inpatient)	Ohio	216-791-3800 ext. 6227 (Cleveland VAMC)
	202-341-0044 (Washington VAMC)	Oklahoma	703-325-9971
Florida	813-979-3638 (Tampa VAPTC)	Oregon	703-325-9958
Georgia	706-631-0411 (Augusta VAMC)	Pennsylvania	703-325-9993
	912-435-5750 (Fort Stewart MTF)	Rhode Island	NA
Guam	703-325-9980	South Carolina	703-325-9957
Hawaii	703-325-9980	South Dakota	703-325-9982
Idaho	703-325-9976	Tennessee	703-325-9966
Illinois	703-325-9070	Texas	703-325-9987
	708-408-2708 (Hines VAMC)		210-275-5966 (BAMC Outpatient)
Indiana	703-325-9070		210-916-6417 (BAMC Inpatient)
	708-408-2708 (Hines VAMC)		214-797-4921 (Dallas VAMC)
Iowa	703-325-9982		713-857-5823 (Houston VAMC)
Kansas	785-223-1297 (Fort Riley MTF)		254-288-8139 (Fort Hood–Darnall AMC)
Kentucky	270-562-1780 (Fort Campbell MTF)	Utah	703-325-9976
	270-985-8509 (Fort Campbell MTF)	Vermont	NA
Louisiana	703-325-9959	Virginia	703-325-9992 (AW2 Headquarters)
Maine	NA		804-399-8048 (Richmond VAPTC)
Maryland	703-325-9993	Washington	703-325-9958
	202-330-1281 (National Naval Medical Center)		206-764-2945 ext. 62945 (Fort Lewis–Madigan AMC and Seattle VAMC)
Massachusetts	617-314-5104 (Boston VAMC)		
Michigan	703-325-9070	West Virginia	703-325-9993
Micronesia	703-325-9980	Wisconsin	703-325-9070
		Wyoming	703-325-9976

Marine for Life Hometown Link Locations

State	City	Phone	E-mail
Alabama	Birmingham	334-826-6460	birmingham@m4l.usmc.mil
	Mobile	205-965-1927	mobile@m4l.usmc.mil
Alaska	Anchorage	206-793-9800	anchorage@m4l.usmc.mil
Arizona	Phoenix	NA	Phoenix@m4l.usmc.mil
	Tucson	480-226-6921	Tucson@m4l.usmc.mil
Arkansas	Little Rock	703-499-4118	LittleRock@m4l.usmc.mil
California	Bakersfield	661-326-3672	Bakersfield@m4l.usmc.mil
	Camp Pendleton	619-520-3836	CampPendleton@m4l.usmc.mil
	Fresno	559-213-8538	Fresno@m4l.usmc.mil
	Los Angeles	310-261-8538	LosAngeles@m4l.usmc.mil
	Sacramento	916-416-5994	Sacramento@m4l.usmc.mil
	San Bernardino	310-420-3306	SanBernardino@m4l.usmc.mil
	San Diego	310-420-3338	SanDiego@m4l.usmc.mil
	San Diego	619-250-7268	SanDiego@m4l.usmc.mil
	San Francisco	415-850-8385	sanfrancisco@m4l.usmc.mil
Colorado	Colorado Springs	719-491-1080	ColoradoSprings@m4l.usmc.mil
	Denver	719-491-1080	Denver@m4l.usmc.mil
Connecticut	New Haven	619-293-4102	NewHaven@m4l.usmc.mil
Delaware	NA	NA	NA
Florida	Jacksonville	904-338-5385	JacksonvilleFL@m4l.usmc.mil
	Miami	786-229-6442	miami@m4l.usmc.mil
	Orlando	NA	orlando@m4l.usmc.mil
	Pensacola	703-499-4168	Pensacola@m4l.usmc.mil
	Tampa	813-241-7201	tampa@m4l.usmc.mil
Georgia	Albany	703-296-0577	Albany@m4l.usmc.mil
	Atlanta	770-294-0677	Atlanta@m4l.usmc.mil
Hawaii	NA	NA	NA
Idaho	Boise	208-627-0053	Boise@m4l.usmc.mil
	Couer d'Alene	NA	CouerdAlene@m4l.usmc.mil
Illinois	Chicago	773-617-2228	chicago@m4l.usmc.mil
Indiana	Indianapolis	317-223-8899	Indianapolis@m4l.usmc.mil
Iowa	NA	NA	NA
Kansas	NA	NA	NA
Kentucky	Bowling Green	703-296-0405	bowlinggreen@m4l.usmc.mil
	Lexington	703-843-6060	Lexington@m4l.usmc.mil
	Louisville	502-432-7996	Louisville@m4l.usmc.mil
Louisiana	Shreveport	318-771-1512	Shreveport@m4l.usmc.mil
	New Orleans	504-915-1062	NewOrleans@m4l.usmc.mil
Maine	Augusta	617-892-5269	Augusta@m4l.usmc.mil
Maryland	Andrews Air Force Base	410-212-5608	andrewsafb@m4l.usmc.mil
	Baltimore	301-573-3018	Baltimore@m4l.usmc.mil
Massachusetts	Boston	508-326-3988	Boston@m4l.usmc.mil
Michigan	Detroit	586-630-7357	Detroit@m4l.usmc.mil
	Lansing	616-293-0527	Lansing@m4l.usmc.mil
Minnesota	Minneapolis	651-497-0066	Minneapolis@m4l.usmc.mil
		651-497-0105	
Mississippi	Gulf Port	703-843-5830	gulfport@m4l.usmc.mil
	Jackson	703-499-4109	JacksonMS@m4l.usmc.mil
Missouri	Kansas City	913-927-4042	KansasCity@m4l.usmc.mil
	St Louis	314-226-6120	stlouis@m4l.usmc.mil

Montana	NA	NA	NA
Nebraska	Omaha	703-499-4167	omaha@m4l.usmc.mil
Nevada	Las Vegas	702-349-9608	LasVegas@m4l.usmc.mil
New Hampshire	Manchester	703-296-6730	Manchester@m4l.usmc.mil
New Jersey	Newark	862-849-9683	Newark@m4l.usmc.mil
	Trenton	609-209-0843	trenton@m4l.usmc.mil
New Mexico	Albuquerque	505-975-6512	Albuquerque@m4l.usmc.mil
New York	Buffalo	585-356-9582	Buffalo@m4l.usmc.mil
	New York City	NA	M4l.nyc@gmail.com
	Rochester	703-296-6561	Rochester@m4l.usmc.mil
North Carolina	Camp Lejeune	910-237-5618	CampLejeune@m4l.usmc.mil
	Charlotte	803-389-7067	Charlotte@m4l.usmc.mil
	Raleigh	919-644-2296	Raleigh@m4l.usmc.mil
North Dakota	Central HTL	719-380-6731	CentralHTL@m4l.usmc.mil
	Grand Forks	NA	GrandForks@m4l.usmc.mil
Ohio	Cincinnati	513-200-8103	Cincinnati@m4l.usmc.mil
	Cleveland	216-214-6248	Cleveland@m4l.usmc.mil
	Columbus	614-402-7322	Columbus@m4l.usmc.mil
	Dayton	937-605-4506	Dayton@m4l.usmc.mil
	Toledo	419-574-2641	Toledo@m4l.usmc.mil
Oklahoma	Oklahoma City	405-409-7971	OklahomaCity@m4l.usmc.mil
Oregon	Portland	503-209-4613	Portland@m4l.usmc.mil
Pennsylvania	Allentown	347-234-3856	Allentown@m4l.usmc.mil
	Philadelphia	610-476-1609	Philadelphia@m4l.usmc.mil
	Pittsburgh	NA	Pittsburgh@m4l.usmc.mil
Rhode Island	Providence	508-326-3988	Providence@m4l.usmc.mil
South Carolina	Charleston	803-317-4933	CharlestonSC@m4l.usmc.mil
	Columbia	803-317-4933	NA
	Greenville	864-844-4433	greenville@m4l.usmc.mil
South Dakota	NA	NA	NA
Tennessee	Knoxville	615-414-4171	Knoxville@m4l.usmc.mil
	Memphis	901-301-4839	Memphis@m4l.usmc.mil
	Nashville	347-623-3408	Nashville@m4l.usmc.mil
Texas	Austin	512-748-2372	Austin@m4l.usmc.mil
	Dallas Ft. Worth	972-880-0779	DFW@m4l.usmc.mil
	El Paso	915-726-4250	ElPaso@m4l.usmc.mil
	Houston	281-802-8107	Houston@m4l.usmc.mil
	Houston	281-642-5696	Houston@m4l.usmc.mil
	San Antonio	210-389-7630	rudyleos22@aol.com
Utah	Salt Lake City	NA	SaltLakeCity@m4l.usmc.mil
Vermont	NA	NA	NA
Virginia	Charlottesville	540-295-9267	Charlottesville@m4l.usmc.mil
	Richmond	804-400-0871	Richmond@m4l.usmc.mil
	Roanoke	540-295-9267	Roanoke@m4l.usmc.mil
	Virginia Beach	757-435-9524	VirginiaBeach@m4l.usmc.mil
	Williamsburg	804-400-0871	Williamsburg@m4l.usmc.mil
	Woodbridge	703-296-6727	Woodbridge@m4l.usmc.mil
Washington	Seattle	206-281-7917	Seattle@m4l.usmc.mil
	Spokane	509-370-0109	Spokane@m4l.usmc.mil
Washington, DC	Washington, DC	202-207-7837	washingtondc@m4l.usmc.mil
West Virginia	NA	NA	NA
Wisconsin	Green Bay	920-392-1005	GreenBay@m4l.usmc.mil
	Milwaukee	414-236-1968	Milwaukee@m4l.usmc.mil
Wyoming	NA	NA	NA

Useful Resources and Organizations for Veterans

American Legion	www.legion.org
American Red Cross	www.redcross.org
America Supports You	www.americasupportsyou.mil
Fisher House	www.fisherhouse.org
Disabled American Veterans	www.dav.org
Fallen Patriot Fund	www.fallenpatriotfund.org
Helping Our Heroes Foundation	www.hohf.org
Homes for Our Troops	www.homesforourtroops.org
Injured Marine Corps Semper Fi Fund	www.semperfifund.org
Intrepid Museum/Intrepid Fallen Heroes Fund	www.intrepidmuseum.org/pages/intrepidfoundation
Iraq and Afghanistan Veterans of America	www.iava.org
Marine Corps Law Enforcement Foundation	www.mc-lef.org
Military OneSource	www.militaryonesource.com
National Veterans Wheelchair Games	www1.va.gov/vetevent/nvwg/2008/default.cfm
National Veterans Winter Sports Clinic	www1.va.gov/vetevent/wsc/2007/default.cfm
Navy-Marine Corps Relief Society	www.nmcrs.org
Operation Comfort	www.operationcomfort.com
Operation Hero Miles through Fisher House Foundation	www.fisherhouse.org/programs/heroMiles.shtml
Paralyzed Veterans of America	www.pva.org
Veterans and Families Homecoming Initiative	www.veteransandfamilies.org
Veterans of Foreign Wars Unmet Needs	www.unmetneeds.com
Wounded Warrior Fund	www.woundedwarriors.org

Resources at Walter Reed Army Medical Center

Soldier Family Assistance Center

The SFAC is a team consisting of enlisted soldiers and civilian employees appointed by the Garrison Commander to coordinate resources and act as a point of contact for patients and their family members.

The SFAC is open to assist patients who have been evacuated to Walter Reed Army Medical Center from Operation Iraqi Freedom (OIF) and Operation Enduring Freedom (OEF). The SFAC also assists the family members of those patients. The SFAC encourages family members to come to the SFAC after arriving at WRAMC. SFAC staff will attempt to answer any questions you may have during your stay.

Warrior Transition Brigade

The Warrior Transition Brigade provides command and control, primary care, and case management for service members receiving treatment for wounds suffered deployed in the war on terror. The unit works to "promote their timely return to the force or transition to civilian life."

Army Wounded Soldier and Family Hotline: 1 (800) 984-8523

The Army Wounded Soldier and Family Hotline provides wounded and injured soldiers and their family members another way to resolve medical issues. The hotline provides an information channel for soldiers' medical-related issues to go directly to senior Army leadership and is staffed 24 hours a day, 7 days a week.

Reproduced from: Walter Reed Army Medical Center Web site. Available at: www.wramc.amedd.army.mil/WarriorsIn-Transition/Pages/default.aspx. Accessed June 5, 2008.

Chapter 8

GENERAL SURGICAL PRINCIPLES FOR THE COMBAT CASUALTY WITH LIMB LOSS

SCOTT B. SHAWEN, MD[*]; WILLIAM C. DOUKAS, MD[†]; JOSEPH A. SHROUT, MD[‡]; JAMES R. FICKE, MD[§]; BENJAMIN K. POTTER, MD[¥]; ROMAN A. HAYDA, MD[¶]; JOHN J. KEELING, MD[**]; ROBERT R. GRANVILLE, MD[††]; AND DOUGLAS G. SMITH, MD[‡‡]

INTRODUCTION AND HISTORICAL PERSPECTIVE

WOUND MANAGEMENT AT POINT OF INJURY

INDICATIONS AND TIMING FOR DEFINITIVE CLOSURE

MANAGEMENT OF SOFT TISSUE AND MUSCLE

MANAGEMENT OF NERVES

DRESSINGS

UPPER LIMB

LOWER LIMB

MULTIPLE INJURED LIMB AMPUTEE

DELAYED AMPUTATION VERSUS LIMB SALVAGE

CONCLUSION

[*]Lieutenant Colonel, Medical Corps, US Army; Orthopaedic Surgeon, Integrated Department of Orthopaedics and Rehabilitation, National Naval Medical Center/Walter Reed Army Medical Center, 6900 Georgia Avenue, NW, Washington, DC 20307

[†]Colonel (Retired), Medical Corps, US Army; Chairman, Integrated Department of Orthopaedics and Rehabilitation, National Naval Medical Center/ Walter Reed Army Medical Center, 6900 Georgia Avenue, NW, Washington, DC 20307

[‡]Lieutenant Colonel(P), Medical Corps, US Army; Orthopaedic Hand Surgeon, Department of Orthopaedics and Rehabilitation, Walter Reed Army Medical Center, Building 2, 6900 Georgia Avenue, NW, Washington, DC 20307; formerly, Chief, Department of Surgery and Special Care, Kimbrough Ambulatory Care Center, Fort George Meade, Maryland

[§]Colonel, Medical Corps, US Army; Orthopaedic Consultant, US Army Surgeon General, Chairman, Department of Orthopaedics and Rehabilitation, Brooke Army Medical Center, 3851 Roger Brooke Drive, Fort Sam Houston, Texas 78234

[¥]Major, Medical Corps, US Army; Musculoskeletal Oncology Fellow, Department of Orthopaedics and Rehabilitation, University of Miami School of Medicine (D-27), PO Box 016960, Miami, Florida 33101; formerly, Chief Resident, Integrated Department of Orthopaedics and Rehabilitation, Walter Reed Army Medical Center, Washington, DC

[¶]Colonel, Medical Corps, US Army; Chief Orthopaedic Trauma, Residence Program Director, Department of Orthopaedic Surgery, Brooke Army Medical Center, 3851 Roger Brooke Drive, Fort Sam Houston, Texas 78234

[**]Commander, Medical Corps, US Navy; Director, Orthopaedic Trauma and Foot and Ankle Division, Department of Orthopaedics, National Military Medical Center, Walter Reed National Military Medical Center, 8901 Rockville Pike, Bethesda, Maryland 20899

[††]Colonel, Medical Corps, US Army; Orthopaedic Surgeon, Department of Orthopaedics and Rehabilitation, Brooke Army Medical Center, 3851 Roger Brooke Drive, Fort Sam Houston, Texas 78234; formerly, Director of Amputee Service, Department of Orthopaedics and Rehabilitation, Brooke Army Medical Center, Fort Sam Houston, Texas

[‡‡]Professor of Orthopaedic Surgery, Department of Orthopaedic Surgery, University of Washington, Harborview Medical Center, 325 Ninth Avenue, Seattle, Washington 98104

INTRODUCTION AND HISTORICAL PERSPECTIVE

As Hippocrates eloquently stated, "War is the only proper school for a surgeon." Surgeons following historical armies learned firsthand the care of complex, open orthopaedic injuries. Amputations have long been and remain common sequelae of warfare. During the US Civil War, nearly 20,000 amputations were performed on Union troops alone, with approximately 60% of these involving the lower extremities. World War II saw equally high numbers, leading the US Army to establish several "amputation centers" to provide longitudinal care to injured servicemen who had sustained major amputations. Because penetrating thoraco-abdominal and head injuries were almost universally lethal in earlier conflicts, survivable extremity injuries with open, contaminated wounds were often treated with amputation. Transosseous amputation proximal to the area of gangrene with the use of compression dressings and vessel ligation for hemostasis became commonplace, with cauterization used as a last resort. As surgical management of combat extremity injuries improved, circular amputation became popular during the Vietnam War and subsequently evolved to the currently recommended technique of length-preserving open amputations to aid with eventual coverage with traditional or atypical myofasciocutaneous flaps. With advances in both vascular and orthopaedic reconstructive surgery, limb salvage has frequently become an option for limbs that would previously have been amputated. The introduction of modern blood replacement, aseptic surgery, antibiotics, and primary vascular repair and external fixation techniques, in concert with rapid evacuation to well-equipped far forward surgical hospitals, has greatly improved opportunities for limb salvage. Nonetheless, amputation is still required in many cases of unsalvageable injury, and soldiers sustaining traumatic amputations often survive what might previously have been lethal injuries.

Most near amputation injuries sustained during the current conflict are secondary to blast injuries from improvised explosive devices (IEDs). These injuries are universally grossly contaminated and often involve neurovascular compromise, frequently including damage to other extremities in addition to traumatic brain injury and other multisystem comorbidities. The physiologic status of the whole patient, not merely the mangled limb, must therefore be considered in the initial medical resuscitation and surgical management of the combat-injured patient, always insuring the salvage of life over limb. As of early 2008, over 700 patients have sustained major limb loss (nearly a quarter of which involve the upper extremity) during Operations Iraqi Freedom/Enduring Freedom (OIF/OEF), with approximately 20% having multiple limb involvement. Surgical management, therefore, must be tailored toward initial limb preservation and the utilization of length-sparing amputations when amputation is required, maximizing possible future reconstructive options and potentially offering injured service members the greatest opportunity for choice and eventual informed consent.

The major amputation rate during the US Civil War was in excess of 12%; post-Vietnam, however, the rate in modern conflicts has remained fairly constant, ranging from 1.2% to 3.4%.[1] Even this rate has resulted in thousands of survivors requiring long-term care, including delayed surgical revision and prosthetic modification, which often evolves based on patient experience and expectation. In the near future, functional outcome analyses, both physical and psychological (ie, evaluation of soldier self-efficacy), will be critical to the ongoing improvement of surgical treatment and rehabilitation protocols.

WOUND MANAGEMENT AT POINT OF INJURY

Tourniquet Use

The combat surgeon frequently faces dramatic war wounds in multiply, and often extremely severely, wounded patients. In these situations, preservation of life must always take priority over salvage of a limb. Toward this end, the development of a practicable field tourniquet, its universal distribution, individual training in its application, and a paradigm shift away from considering the tourniquet as the last resort have greatly facilitated the survival of critically injured patients. Tourniquet use is a relatively safe and often critical adjunct in resuscitation with great potential to contribute to improved survival rates.[2] On the modern battlefield tourniquet application rapidly corrects compressible hemorrhage and can be safely used during timely patient transport to a forward surgical facility.

Limb Salvage Versus Amputation

When receiving a patient with a tourniquet, forward surgeons often face difficult choices with respect to limb salvage versus completion of an amputation. A variety of scoring systems have been developed to assist the surgeon in surgical decision-making. However, none of these have been shown to reliably predict the salvageability and functional viability of an injured limb.[3,4]

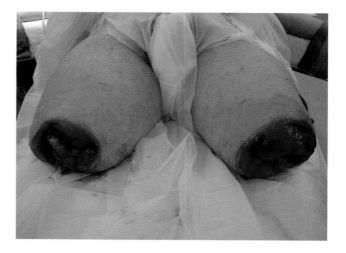

General Surgical Principles for the Combat Casualty With Limb Loss

On the modern battlefield, a variety of factors critically impact these difficult decisions. First and foremost among these is the individual patient. Most injured soldiers are young and previously healthy but now have severe, often life-threatening, injuries. In a hemodynamically unstable patient, amputation may be critical in saving the soldier's life. Additionally, when the limb is mangled, particularly if segmental concomitant vascular injury exists, provisional repair and reconstruction may be neither possible nor feasible with the available skill sets and resources in a combat theater. In the past, concomitant nerve injury had been considered an indication for early amputation. However, preliminary data from the Lower Extremity Assessment Project (LEAP) study (a multicenter study of severe lower extremity trauma in the US civilian population) recently demonstrated satisfactory 2-year results following tibial nerve injury and limb salvage with, in the absence of visualized transection, poor correlation between initial neurologic examination and final outcome.[5] Therefore, isolated nerve injury should no longer be considered an indication, in and of itself, for amputation. The final individual factor for amputation versus limb salvage is the extent of muscle and skeletal damage. Because even severe open and segmental fractures with bone loss can be provisionally stabilized with external fixation, recent advances in limb salvage have been remarkable. The goal of limb salvage thus remains to provide a functional limb with reasonable sensation and mobility. The challenge, then, is to predict those limbs that have the potential for achieving this goal. The degree of muscle loss appears to be the best predictor of function. Massive loss, involving multiple compartments or an extensive zone of injury, carries a grim prognosis, and primary amputation is most likely the best decision in such cases.

Another aspect of combat amputations and surgical decision-making involves the larger spectrum of limited hospital resources. The acutely injured patient, initially managed by buddy aid (level-I casualty care), receives a tourniquet, hemorrhage control, and rapid evacuation. Level-II facilities, a battalion aid station or possibly a forward surgical team, provide advanced trauma life support, possibly including damage-control surgery, stabilization or open amputation, and approximately 10 to 20 units of blood. It should be noted that in civilian settings, the average trauma resuscitation requires around 30 units of blood. Most Army combat support hospitals (level III) typically have enough equipment to perform two to four simultaneous surgical procedures and maintain less than 100 units of blood, enough for two or possibly three major trauma resuscitations. Therefore, lengthy and extensive procedures may lead to surgical delays, which could have devastating consequences for incom-

ing patients in dire need of surgical stabilization. The concept of "damage control surgery" in a combat zone or mass casualty situation demands brief, focused, initial stabilization for as many patients as possible. This applies to the soldier with a mangled limb as well. Often, salvage is questionable, and additional cases are waiting. This situation forces difficult choices: life must be favored over limb, and occasionally the decision-making process for an individual patient must also include assessment of patients in the holding area as well as those in the operating suite. Whenever possible, the optimal decision is to initially spare the limb, stabilize any surgical injuries, and establish conditions for subsequent reassessment and informed discussion.

Surgical Goals

Surgical goals during the initial treatment stage are to thoroughly excise contaminated wounds, retain viable tissue for subsequent reconstruction or amputation coverage, and ultimately leave the wounded warrior with the highest potential for a useful limb, either salvaged or with a prosthetic device. The three most critical principles to follow when combat wounds necessitate amputation are (1) to thoroughly debride the residual limb, (2) to preserve as much salvageable tissue as possible, and (3) to leave the wound open.[6] Historically, war surgery often meant a "guillotine" amputation, in which the blade sliced through all tissues at the same level (Figure 8-1). This antiquated technique leaves no residual tissue for later closure, coverage of the bone, or potential for modern pros-

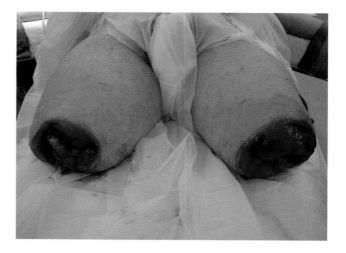

Figure 8-1. Open bilateral transfemoral guillotine amputations. The failure to leave any additional viable tissue for coverage limited subsequent reconstructive options, and the patient required substantial shortening of both residual limbs to achieve a functional myodesis and soft tissue coverage.

thesis management at the initially amputated level. Somewhat more recently, the concept of an open circular amputation has been advocated. This technique incises the skin, followed by skin retraction, then the muscle at a higher level, and, after muscle retraction, bone sectioning is conducted so that all planes roughly corresponded to a transverse amputation. Current consensus among war surgeons recommends removal of nonviable tissue at the lowest level, retaining irregular yet viable tissues (Figure 8-2). Rather than fashioning formal tissue flaps, this technique should include preservation of viable tissue to optimize later definitive closure and maximize ultimate residual limb length.

Orthopaedic surgeons often focus erroneously on the bone, whereas in most amputations the best predictor of length, final closure, and ultimate function is the soft tissue. A stable, well-padded residual limb with adequate soft tissue coverage is far more predictive of functional prosthetic use than simple residual limb length. In the immediate setting, preservation of bone length provides soft tissue support, minimizes edema, and seems to be least painful. It is not unreasonable to externally fixate fractures proximal to an amputation, as long as the nonviable soft tissue is completely debrided. In fact, when critical length can be maintained through proximal fracture fixation, this technique is warranted and should be advocated. All frankly devitalized skin, muscle, and fat must be removed. If there is question of viability, the authors recommend leaving skin, removing questionable fat and fascia, and applying the "four Cs" (developed during the Korean War) to muscle: color, consistency, circulation, and contractility.[7] Residual devitalized deep tissue, left for subsequent surgeons throughout the evacuation

chain, results in a risk of sepsis, myoglobinuria, and systemic inflammatory response, which can be fatal. If bone has periosteal attachments, it should be retained, and whenever possible externally stabilized.[8]

Nerve Management

The management of sectioned nerves remains a controversial aspect of amputation surgery. The free end of a divided nerve heals by forming a neuroma. Neuromas can frequently become symptomatic, and no described technique has been convincingly proven to prevent or ameliorate this process (neuroma preventative treatment and management is discussed later in this chapter). In the acute setting, even transected or injured nerves should be preserved in patients in whom limb salvage is attempted, potentially permitting later repair or reconstruction without creation of prohibitively large segmental defects. Transected nerve ends may be tagged with suture to assist in later identification for surgeons further up the evacuation chain.

For traumatic amputations or limbs deemed unsalvageable and undergoing amputation at the initial point of operative care, the surgeon's goal is to retain and employ as much useful nerve function in the residual limb as possible, just as with the conservation of muscle tissue in the residual limb. Nerves should be transected sharply under gentle tension and allowed to retract into viable soft tissues proximally. This process may prove to be definitive management of some nerves, and maximizes patient comfort during subsequent transport, dressing changes, or operative procedures. Sensory branches generally depart motor

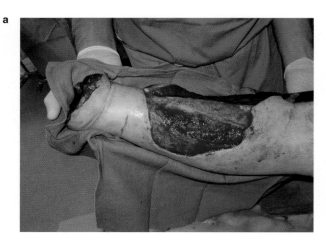 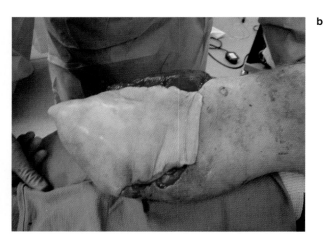

Figure 8-2. (a) Open, length-preserving transradial amputation. **(b)** The salvage of viable distal soft tissues permitted closure with an atypical flap of native tissues, not requiring flaps or grafts and retaining a functional transradial residual limb length.

nerves well proximal to their corresponding area of cutaneous innervation, but residual limb sensibility should not be compromised by overzealous nerve transection well proximal to the amputation. This consideration is important in segmentally injured limbs in which a nerve may be injured or exposed well proximal to the ostensible level of final amputation.

Care should be taken not to perform group ligation of vessels and adjacent nerves. Likewise, inadvertent deinnervation of remaining viable muscle groups, which can compromise residual limb control or result in eventual muscle atrophy and inadequate resulting soft tissue padding, should be avoided. This consideration is particularly critical in the upper extremity, where myoelectric prostheses are frequently desired and utilized. Furthermore, several investigators are currently evaluating reinnervation, nerve transfers, and even the potential for neural-prosthetic interfaces. Thus, in upper extremity amputations, particularly those proximal to the elbow, it is reasonable to forgo traction-assisted nerve transection and salvage transected nerve length by simply burying the cut nerve end within or deep to adjacent muscle.

Open Wound Management

Combat wounds must always be left open. A dry bulky gauze dressing, the historical standard, can be readily applied in all situations. Occasionally, skin traction can be applied, but the authors have not found this to be a strong contributor to accelerated functional limb closure. No strong evidence exists to support skin traction technique in contemporary war injuries subject to the stresses of evacuation. Rigid dressings or external fixation, as stated earlier, can stabilize soft tissue, and may assist with pain reduction during transport. Recent advances in open wound management have been applied to open amputations. Negative pressure wound therapy is an aggressive method to provide optimum wound-healing potential. This concept enhances vascularity, minimizes additional tissue necrosis and wound contamination, and has been widely used to temporize management between serial debridements.[6,9] Currently, protocols are underway to investigate the safety and effectiveness of negative pressure wound therapy as the patient traverses the air evacuation chain. If these prove successful, the therapy's application in theater is likely to eliminate any need for skin traction techniques.

Upper Versus Lower Extremity Considerations

The surgical considerations involving lower and upper extremity combat injuries are different. The weight-bearing nature of the lower extremity requires adequate soft tissue and a flexible and hopefully sensate residual limb, whereas the motion and intricate functional demands of the upper extremity are quite different. Additionally, prosthetic technology for upper and lower limb amputations is also vastly different. Lower limb prosthetic demands primarily involve durability and preserving energy expenditure during ambulation, whereas upper limb prosthetic demands are focused on lightweight devices that can adapt to multiple diverse functional activities. Therefore, in the upper extremity, surgical length often takes a higher priority than achieving robust soft tissue padding. In addition, definitive closure using partial thickness grafts is generally well tolerated for the upper limb. These differences in residual limb coverage and prosthetic management must be considered by the initial combat surgeon to maximize patient outcomes.

INDICATIONS AND TIMING FOR DEFINITIVE CLOSURE

Wound closure is undertaken only when strict criteria for residual tissue viability are met. In the absence of better indicators, military practitioners should use the four Cs to judge the viability of muscle.[7] Wounds cannot be closed over nonviable muscle, and it often takes several debridements for residual tissue to declare itself. This is particularly true in burn patients, who must have all nonviable and grossly contaminated tissue excised. In blast wounds, debris tracks proximally along fascial planes. This contamination may be masked by the elasticity of skin, and is easily missed in mass casualty situations. Once the patient arrives at a level-5 facility, the resources are available to ensure a calm, meticulous, and systematic surgical evaluation to determine the complete extent of the injury. Several additional debridements may be necessary to ensure that all nonviable tissue is excised. Fortunately, military resources allow for a less aggressive initial surgical approach than the treatment advocated by the International Committee of the Red Cross, which has published the most recent civilian discussion of treating war wounds, and is directed toward saving life over limb, especially in circumstances of limited resources.[10]

Negative pressure dressings are very useful during the period before wound closure, maintaining a favorable wound environment and promoting the formation of granulation tissue. When performing dressing changes using traditional bulky dry dressings, the presence of greenish drainage or some odor does not equate with infection, if the wound appears otherwise healthy. Similarly, growth on microbiologic cultures does not *per se* indicate infection. War wounds are often colonized without being "infected" and can be successfully closed when (*a*) the wound appears clean, (*b*) the patient shows no signs of systemic illness, and (*c*) no necrotic tissue remains. However, if the wound is colonized by multidrug-resistant organisms, antibiotic therapy is generally warranted. Empiric antibiotics should usually be continued for 72 hours after closure of wounds that are culture-negative or without gross evidence of infection. Topical wound care solutions can also decrease bacterial colonization for many severe open wounds. Although some topical solutions have fallen out of favor in most civilian wound care centers because they may slow granulation or epithelial cell growth, control of bacterial colonization must be achieved. In severe trauma, especially that seen in military combat, aggressive topical wound care solutions still have an important role.

Nutritional support plays a critical role in achieving successful wound closure and the ongoing resuscitation of wounded service members. The wound healing process has a catabolic effect on the individual, which combined with long transport times, sedating and nauseating medications, long periods of intubation, concurrent abdominal or facial injuries, and multiple returns to the operating room interrupting intake, nutritional deficits that impair wound healing develop rapidly and almost universally. Weight loss of 30 lb in 2 weeks is not uncommon. Serum albumin and pre-albumin levels should be monitored and maintained above 3.5 g/dL and 20 mg/dL, respectively, if at all possible. Gastric feeding is preferable to parenteral nutrition because it reduces the incidence of multisystem organ failure and parenteral nutrition-related complications.

Limbs that have sustained traumatic amputation in combat are frequently injured at multiple levels. Length and levels should be preserved whenever possible. The soft tissue injury dictates the final level of amputation, not the level of bony injury—a problematic transtibial amputation will likely function better than a long transfemoral amputation, and a long transfemoral amputation in the zone of injury usually functions better than a short transfemoral amputation above the zone of injury. It is important to keep an open mind, approaching each patient's situation unencumbered by traditional concepts of "appropriate" fracture fixation and "standard" closures. In accordance with International Committee of the Red Cross guidelines, the authors advocate length-preserving amputation techniques with closure by nontraditional flaps whenever possible (Figure 8-3).[11] Military surgeons have been successfully inventive in preserving length in the face of fractures and soft tissue defects. One example of this is the use of pediatric flexible intramedullary rods to fix fractures of the femoral diaphysis in transfemoral amputees (Figure 8-4).[12] Similarly, rotational and free tissue flaps are used whenever possible to retain an otherwise unsalvageable level or critical diaphyseal length. Especially in the multiple injury patient, preserving a viable, but unsalvageable, extremity until the time for definitive closure allows the amputated

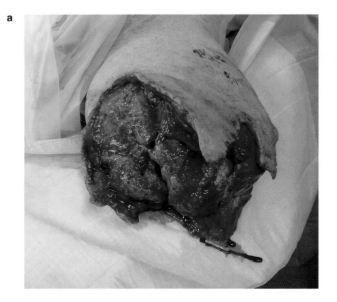

a

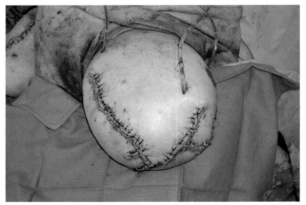

b

Figure 8-3. Open, length-preserving transfemoral amputation in a bilateral transfemoral amputee **(a)**, permitting eventual closure with atypical flaps **(b)** in an injury pattern that might otherwise have required hip disarticulation if a guillotine or open circular amputation had been performed in theater.

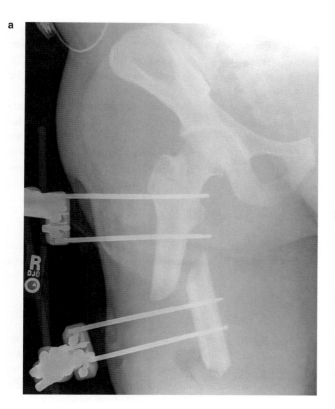

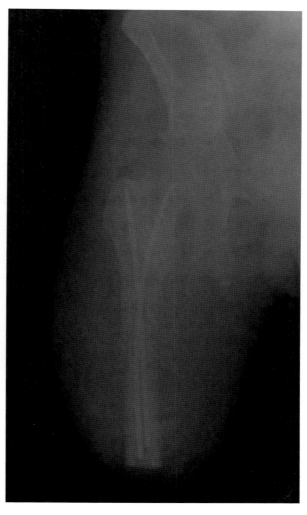

Figure 8-4. Radiographs of a transfemoral amputation with a proximal fracture provisionally stabilized with external fixation (**a**) and after definitive revision and closure following stabilization with flexible intramedullary nails (**b**).

part to serve as a source of autograft bone and skin to facilitate reconstruction of the other perhaps more functional residual limbs.

Retained bone must have soft tissue attachment and must bleed when ronguered. Exceptions are made if there is a large amount of articular cartilage on a dysvascular fragment, which may be initially retained in the interest of preserving articular congruity. However, in the face of deep wound infection, these fragments must be excised. Similarly, every attempt should be made to retain nerves and vessels, for without these structures, distal tissues will not survive with useful residual function.

Orthopaedic surgeons have long been taught, in treating civilian blunt trauma, that coverage must be achieved within 7 days to maximize patient outcome. This principle does not fully apply to combat wounds, where it is more important to have all nonviable tissue removed and no evidence of infection prior to definitive closure. Unfortunately, no objective criteria can reliably indicate the optimal timing for wound closure, so careful surgical judgment is needed.

The treatment of retained fragments or foreign bod-

ies also requires careful judgment. Injuries caused by explosively formed projectiles, IEDs, or antitank mines may lead to dozens of retained foreign bodies in the patient. Fragments may include pieces of the explosive device itself, spall from the interior of a vehicle, or soil and gravel from the surrounding site of the blast. Removal of every foreign body is often impractical due to the damage it would cause to the surrounding soft tissues. Many fragment wounds will heal uneventfully with only local wound care, and a scar will generally encapsulate the fragment. These wounds should generally be treated with "watchful waiting," debriding only those fragments that become infected, are painful, or negatively impair function. Exceptions to this principle include intraarticular fragments, which may damage the joint mechanically or by the toxicity of heavy metals, and large, superficial fragments that may interfere with prosthetic fit.

Heterotopic ossification (HO) has been a significant

problem for service members with an amputation from combat injuries sustained in OIF/OEF. It is believed that the greatest risk of HO formation occurs when the amputation is performed through the zone of injury. Revision surgery because of HO complications may occur in approximately 15% of patients.[13] The pathophysiology, prevention, and optimal treatment of HO is currently under investigation. A more complete discussion of this topic can be found in Chapter 9, Special Surgical Considerations for the Combat Casualty With Limb Loss.

In summary, decisions regarding definitive closure are guided by established general principles, but best executed with the gestalt gained by experience. The soldier who sustains an amputation is best served by the surgeon who follows accepted general tenets of debridement, who is experienced enough to differentiate the subtleties between infection and colonization, and who is skillful enough to employ inventive techniques for fracture fixation and soft tissue coverage—allowing preservation of functional length and levels to achieve a sound, painless, durable residual limb.

MANAGEMENT OF SOFT TISSUE AND MUSCLE

Muscle

In the treatment of extremities injured by the various implements of war, the surgeon is often forced to use what muscle and fasciocutaneous tissues remain and are viable. However, the basic principles of amputation surgery remain the same, with the goal of providing a functional residual limb that can be fit by a prosthetic socket. To achieve this goal, the residual limb is best covered with muscle to provide padding and sometimes aid in control of the terminal extremity. An important component of this principle is defined by how the muscle is treated when closing the amputation. A muscle that is not secured under physiologic tension and does not have fixed resistance will atrophy over time, becoming weaker and providing less padding over the bony prominences. Many of the muscles used in amputation surgery cross a proximal joint (eg, adductors, quadriceps, and hamstrings in transfemoral amputations or the gastrocnemius in transtibial amputations), providing function and stability. Several different techniques for maximal muscle treatment have been utilized, each with relative benefits and deficiencies.

Myofascial Closure

To provide a soft tissue envelope over the distal bone via myofascial closure, the outer fascial envelope over the top of the muscles is approximated. This technique approximates only loose tissues, providing minimal tension and stability to the underlying muscles. In dysvascular patients the absence of muscle and tissue tension provides a possible benefit,[14–16] and the technique is also thought to maximize the remaining blood flow to optimize healing. However, even in dysvascular and diabetic patients, the benefits of this technique are more theoretical than proven. Because of the loose attachment, myofascial closure alone does not generally provide a limb suitable for

prosthetic fitting and use. Therefore, muscle stabilization is critical to a successful surgery and is almost always possible.

Myoplasty

Most amputations seen in war surgery are diaphyseal (mid-bone) in nature. Whether the muscles are severed at this level by the blast, fragments, or other projectiles or surgically transected, the muscle belly is often encountered in cross-section without distal fascia, aponeuroses, or tendons. This is seen in most transhumeral, transradial, transfemoral, and transtibial amputations. To provide closure with the myoplasty technique, the muscle from the opposing muscle groups (quadriceps and hamstrings in a transfemoral amputation) are sewn to each other, covering the transected bone end. Although this is much easier than attaching the muscle to bone and provides more stabilization of the muscle than a myofascial closure, it is not recommended for routine amputation closure. Unless the muscle firmly adheres to the underlying bone and tissues, the myoplasty unit may move with contraction of either opposing muscle group, and a painful bursa can develop either between the muscle and bone or muscle and overlying soft tissues. Faulty adhesion can be detected on physical examination by palpating the muscle motion over the bone with the accompanying crepitus from the problematic bursa. Likewise, deliberate or inadvertent contraction of the involved muscle groups may lead to motion and shifting of the overlying skin within a prosthetic socket, leading to irritation and friction-related complications.

Myodesis

To avoid the complications associated with either myofascial closure or myoplasty, the muscle fascia of the padding or controlling muscle groups within a given residual limb should in most cases be attached to the end of the bone, a technique termed myodesis. Myodesis prevents motion over the bone end and provides padding between the bone and overlying prosthetic socket. One of two methods is utilized to perform this part of the amputation procedure: (1) connection of the muscle to bone through drill holes, or (2) connection of the muscle to the periosteum (Figure 8-5). Once the myodesis is performed, the remaining muscle fascia can be approximated using the techniques described above for myofascial and myoplasty stabilizations (Figure 8-6). In the typical transfemoral amputation the muscle bellies are transected and only the muscle and investing fascia may be available to attach to bone, and getting suture to hold in the muscle tissue and overlying fascia can be difficult.[17] In such cases, a muscle-grabbing suture technique can be used, achieving muscle-bone opposition under reasonable tension without undue tissue strangulation.

Tenodesis

Depending on the level of amputation, tendon may be associated with the muscle intended for attachment to bone. The presence of such tendon provides the ability to achieve good purchase with suture, allowing for the most effective type of muscle stabilization. Unfortunately, most amputations require transection of the muscle belly, leaving no tendon associated with the remaining muscle to allow bony attachment. However, in disarticulations and some transtibial and transradial amputations, tendon may still be present at the level of the amputation. This tendon can then be directly connected to the transected bone, as is the case

for knee disarticulations, where the patellar ligament may be sutured to the origin of the cruciate ligaments. Additionally, for long transtibial or Syme amputations the tendon of the gastrocnemius muscle may be connected to the posterior tibia.[18] Lastly, for transradial amputations, several muscle groups may be utilized to perform multiple myodeses to bone, maximizing distal soft tissue and residual limb control.

Muscle Tension

During stabilization, it is important to secure muscle under appropriate tension to ensure the maximum benefit. Appropriate tension may be difficult to determine in the operating room, because physiologic resting tension of the muscle is not studied in most surgical training programs. Experience gained from tendon transfers in the hand and foot can be a useful guide. Too much tension may cause pain because of persistent stretch on the muscle, and, in the absence of stable myodesis performed through robust, suture-holding tendon and fascia, lead to failure of suture fixation. Additionally, in instances where the muscle would normally cross two joints, proximal deformity and contractures may occur. For example, in transfemoral amputations overtensioning the quadriceps may lead to a hip flexion contracture because of the attachments above the hip joint. However, these instances are rare, and the surgeon should place a moderate amount of tension on all muscle attachments, especially when the muscle is important in stabilizing the residual limb (eg, adductor myodesis for transfemoral amputations). As a general rule, the surgeon should err on the side of too little rather than too much tension.

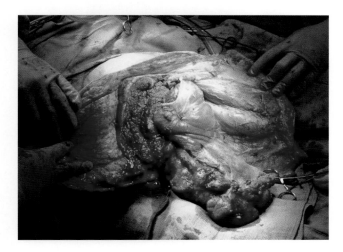

Figure 8-5. Transfemoral amputation with atypical skin flaps demonstrating use of the myodesis technique through drill holes in the femur to attach the adductor magnus muscle to the bone.

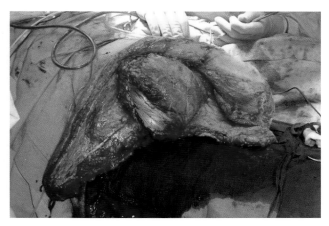

Figure 8-6. The amputation in Figure 8-5 after myoplasty of the quadriceps and hamstring muscles over the adductor muscle previously attached to bone (myodesis).

Skin Traction

One of the basic tenets of amputation surgery is that residual limb length directly correlates with patient function. Although this concept is generally true,[5] exceptions remain. For example, a very long transtibial amputation may limit the accommodation of advanced foot and ankle components. Similarly a very long transfemoral amputation may not accommodate more advanced knee components, thereby potentially limiting an individual's ultimate functional capacity. Despite these exceptions, it still remains the surgeon's goal to salvage as much of the limb as possible, especially when a joint is involved.

As previously stated, most traumatic amputations caused by explosive ordinance do not leave an abundance of viable tissue to work with. In past conflicts, it was commonplace to perform an open circular or guillotine amputation above the zone of injury, often followed by skin traction techniques to slowly pull the skin and dermal tissues over the end of the bone. The primary benefits of this technique included length preservation of the residual limb and low infection rates. Essentially, the limb was maintained in traction with daily dressing changes that allowed for application of various topical agents (eg, Dakin solution) and provided an environment inconducive to bacterial infection. The primary, and very important, downside to this technique, however, was the formation of an adherent, scarred, and thin covering over the distal residual limb, causing difficulty for prosthetic fitting. Therefore, this technique is currently not advocated for routine use.[19–21]

A newer variation on the use of skin traction is currently being applied to the treatment of residual limbs. As discussed previously, to preserve as much length as possible, circular amputations should be avoided. As much bone and soft tissue as possible should be left after the debridement is performed, even if only atypical muscle and fasciocutaneous flaps remain. A thorough debridement, typically performed through the entire zone of injury, is utilized to remove any devitalized tissue. After each debridement the tissues are partially closed over a vacuum-assisted closure device sponge (VAC; KCI, San Antonio, Tex) with vessel loops or no. 2 nylon, providing tension over the end of the bone (Figure 8-7). This technique prevents the muscle and fasciocutaneous tissues from retracting. Antibiotic beads may be placed in the deep tissues if infection is a significant concern. These beads may be tailored to the bacteria isolated in previous cultures. When operating within the zone of injury, it is often unclear which tissues will remain viable; therefore, multiple debridements must

be performed to ensure that all nonviable tissue is removed. When the amputation is ready for closure, typical myodesis and tenodesis techniques should be applied. Even when atypical skin flaps are present, the skin should be primarily closed, except when skin grafts are necessary.

Although the application of skin traction with the VAC saves length and amputation levels, it is not without complications or deficiencies. It is an extremely labor intensive technique, requiring multiple debridements and/or dressing changes under sedation every 2 to 3 days. Additionally, the formation of HO may be associated with amputations through the zone of injury and the use of pulsatile irrigation or VAC dressings. Traditional skin traction techniques permitted dressing changes at the bedside, infrequent visits to the operating room, and a less frequently reported incidence of HO formation, but did not offer the ability to save as much residual limb length as today's techniques.

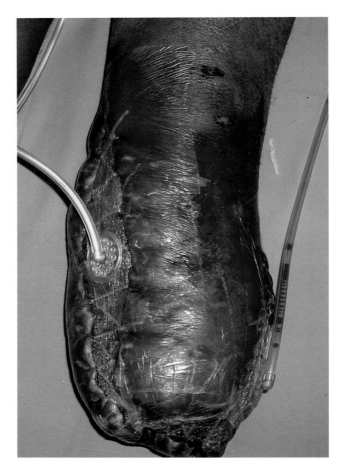

Figure 8-7. Technique using the vacuum-assisted closure (VAC) device and vessel loops for skin traction over the remaining bone.

MANAGEMENT OF NERVES

When performing an amputation at any level, the surgeon is faced with the decision of how to manage the transected nerves, with the primary goal of preventing a *symptomatic* neuroma. Every transected nerve will heal by forming a neuroma, which has the potential to become a source of pain in the residual limb with stimuli such as pressure, stretching, vascular pulsation, or other types of physical or physiologic irritation to the terminal neuroma bulb. Numerous techniques to minimize symptoms associated with neuroma formation have been described, but none have proven to be superior to any of the others, and the choice of technique remains a controversial aspect of amputation surgery.

Traction neurectomy involves identifying and isolating all major nerves in the limb, then applying moderate tension prior to dividing them. The nerves are then allowed to retract proximal to the wound into the muscles of the residual limb. This technique provides a technically simple way to move the eventual neuroma away from the expected areas of scarring, pressure, and pulsating blood vessels. Surgeons occasionally implant the end of the transected nerve into muscle or bone in an attempt to "give the nerve something to do."[22] Although both of these techniques have had good results reported when dealing with painful neuromas in nonamputated limbs,[23] their application in primary amputation surgery is not well documented. When performing an amputation, the latter technique, implanting the cut nerve into muscle or bone, involves transecting relatively less of the nerve so that the surgeon can perform a tensionless attachment of the nerve end into the muscle or bone, although usually still within the amputation wound. Because the nerve cannot retract as far proximally as it could with a well-done traction neurectomy, this technique may, in fact, contribute to the development of a painful postsurgical neuroma. Nerves within wounds are exposed to tension, pressure, anoxia, infection, and delayed wound healing, have been found to have increased amounts of connective tissue, and may be prone to painful neuroma formation.[24] Additionally, because of the nerve proximity to the end of the residual limb, they may be more prone to pressure, friction, and tension from a prosthetic socket.

Other described techniques for managing transected nerves include cauterization of the nerve end, ligation, nerve capping, and end loop anastomosis, but no definitive evidence exists demonstrating that these are more effective than a carefully performed traction neurectomy. Management of the sciatic nerve, however, is unique because of its own intrinsic large blood vessel. This nerve requires ligation prior to transaction to prevent significant bleeding, which may be associated with critical blood loss, hematoma formation, or wound breakdown.

Nerves frequently run parallel with major pulsating blood vessels, and the surgeon performing the amputation should take great care to prevent group ligation of nerves and blood vessels. Although no definitive proof exists, it seems logical that the presence of a pulsating vessel adjacent to a neuroma could lead to the throbbing pain reported by many amputees. In such situations, a revision surgery aimed at separating the nerve and artery vessel, re-ligating the vessel, and performing a better traction neurectomy, will allow the nerve to separate from the pulsating vessel and alleviate these symptoms.

A new and innovative technique in the management of nerves in amputation surgery, called targeted reinnervation, is now being investigated.[25–29] Preliminary results are very promising when the technique is applied to transhumeral and shoulder disarticulation amputees. The technique involves the dennervation of specific nonessential muscle bellies located within the residual limb, followed by the transfer of a freshly transected major mixed nerve of the upper extremity into the motor end point of the freshly dennervated muscle. Reinnervation of the muscle occurs very predictably with the transferred nerve, and the brain signals associated with the intuitive activation of that nerve lead to specific patterns of muscle contraction in the newly innervated muscle belly.

This procedure has been employed to achieve an increased number of surface myoelectric sites with more intuitive control. Thinning the adipose tissue under the skin also improves myoelectrical recording capability. Subsequent mapping of the contraction patterns associated with specific upper extremity functions, and wiring these surface electrodes to certain advanced myoelectric prosthetics, allows the use of an upper extremity prosthesis with multiple degrees of freedom at the shoulder, elbow, wrist, and digits. The end result can be far more efficient in performing fluid motion and manipulative tasks than previous generations of myoelectric prostheses. Although additional research is needed before this technique can be recommended for widespread application, the early results are promising and compelling.

DRESSINGS

Most surgeons are a product of their cumulative experiences, and when a clear standard has not been convincingly established through evidence-based medicine, multiple treatments are frequently recommended and rendered for any given condition. Such is the case with postoperative dressings after amputation surgery—while one surgeon may prefer a splint or cast, another would use padding and an elastic bandage on the same residual limb. The basic considerations for postoperative dressings are soft dressings, rigid dressings, and immediate postoperative prosthesis (IPOP). Each dressing technique has its own benefits and limitations.

Balanced compression of the residual limb is important, particularly in the early postoperative period. This helps to control swelling, which further minimizes postoperative pain and promotes a stable limb volume. Support of soft tissues is also important because the muscle and skin flaps require a tension-free environment for optimal healing. Some combination of compression and support is provided by each category of dressing.

Soft Dressings

A soft dressing is commonly applied in the care of the young combat amputee. Often first applied in the operating room, it provides a sterile dressing covered by an elastic bandage. The classic application of the elastic bandage is in the "figure 8" pattern. While using one hand to support the myofascial and fasciocutaneous flap, the bandage is applied with care taken to evenly distribute compression and to relieve tension on the flap and suture line (Figure 8-8). This type of dressing, with modifications, can be applied to any residual limb.

Careful application is paramount to avoid over-compression or a possible tourniquet effect, particularly near joints. With a transtibial or transradial amputation, the elastic bandage can act as a tourniquet, particularly at the joint level as the patient flexes and extends the joint immediately proximal to the amputation. In the perioperative phase, abundant padding with Webril (Kendall Company, Mansfield, Mass) or similar material under the elastic dressing, as well as extending the dressing well above the knee or elbow, helps to avoid this complication. Transition to a shrinker sock should be initiated as soon as possible.

Although soft dressings provide easy access to the wound, many surgeons feel that they do not provide sufficient compression or support to the residual limb to promote proper healing through soft tissue rest. No studies have shown a clear advantage of one type of dressing over another, but several have shown a trend toward better healing with rigid dressings.[30–36] However, soft dressings may facilitate unencumbered early mobilization of patients and allow focused early rehabilitation of more proximal muscles and joints within the residual limb. As stated above, dressing selection is very dependent on the surgeon as well as regional and hospital preferences.

Rigid Dressings

The dressing of choice for most surgeons for the transtibial amputation has traditionally been the rigid dressing, either in the form of a splint or cast. Early in its history this type of dressing was modified to include IPOP, which will be discussed in the next section. It is generally believed that injured tissues heal more consistently and with less pain when placed at rest. The three basic principles applied here are immobilization, application of gentle distal pressure, and infrequent dressing changes. These principles have

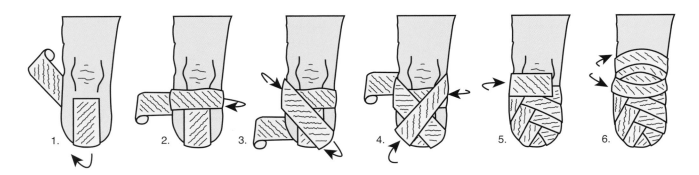

Figure 8-8. Application of a typical "figure 8" dressing. This provides support to the underlying tissues as well as compression.

been shown over time to be effective in the treatment of residual limbs.[37]

During the application of this type of dressing, several technical tips are warranted. Failure to follow the tenets of splint or cast application can lead to significant adverse complications. Extra padding should be placed over the patella when placing rigid dressing for transtibial amputations to prevent skin irritation and pressure necrosis in that area. Alternatively, the patella can be omitted entirely from the splint, with distal compression provided through a combination of plaster and soft dressing while the splint material assists in flexion contracture prevention (Figure 8-9). Although less of an issue and less frequently utilized for transradial amputations, the olecranon should also be meticulously padded for the same reason. The distal end should be well padded to maintain balanced pressure and gentle circumferential compression. Closed-cell foam or other similar material can be used for this purpose. A supracondylar mold is necessary to keep the dressing in place, avoiding distal migration of the cast or splint. With loss of distal-to-proximal pressure, unrelenting terminal edema can occur, resulting in severe wound complications. Patients and staff must be educated to avoid this situation and can assist by placing distal pressure with a looped towel or pulling up the dressing during straight leg raises.

One drawback of rigid dressing application actually contradicts one of the stated benefits, which is the need for infrequent dressing changes. In the combat amputee with an amputation performed through the zone of injury, the possibility of infection is a major concern. Many times the patient has undergone multiple thorough debridements, with healthy-appearing tissue prior to closure. Nonetheless, in these cases the authors have seen a high incidence of wound infections at 3 to 5 days after closure. Early detection of these cases is paramount to preventing tissue necrosis and salvaging soft tissue and possibly amputation level. Frequent dressing changes are therefore necessary, and rigid dressings have often been avoided for this reason. However, after the immediate postoperative period, soft dressings can be transitioned to rigid ones and wounds can generally be monitored via attentiveness to fluctuations in patient signs (eg, fever) and symptoms (eg, increasing pain).

Immediate Postoperative Prosthesis

A frequently cited source of controversy in amputee care has been the IPOP. The concept of early weight bearing through a rigid dressing was proposed by Wilson shortly after the end of First World War.[38] Many others have used and modified this technique over

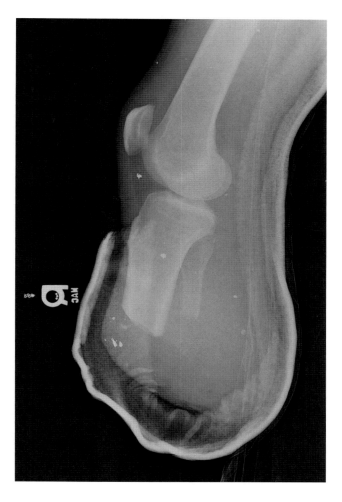

Figure 8-9. Lateral radiograph of a well-padded transtibial amputation in a posterior splint designed to prevent knee flexion contracture but avoid potential patella-related complications.

the years, especially following the Second World War, Korean War, and Vietnam War.[39–42] This evolution has included modifications ranging from casts with lower extremity components applied in the operating room to padded prefabricated sockets with distal components. This technique can be utilized with almost any level of amputation in either the upper or lower extremity.

Regardless of the type of IPOP used, many benefits have been demonstrated. These range from the psychological benefit of having a prosthesis in place immediately after the amputation, with less perceived loss of function, to shorter hospital stays, fewer revisions, and faster time to initial prosthetic fitting.[31,35,43,44] However, most of these studies have been performed in patients who have undergone amputation for nonreconstructible ischemia or infection.

Despite these reported benefits, this technique has

been infrequently used in the current treatment of combat amputees because of the extent of soft tissue and other remote injuries. Given the tenuous nature of zone-of-injury tissue damage and frequent use of flaps and skin grafts, early ambulation may compromise healing. Additionally, many of the other injuries sustained from combat, particularly blast injuries (eg, multiple other extremities, intra-abdominal) prohibit early mobilization. Most importantly, however, the authors have recognized that when the definitive amputation is performed in a setting where the patient will receive his or her rehabilitation, the patient has immediate contact with the rehabilitation team as well as other individuals going through amputee rehabilitation, making it much easier to see what the patient's potential function will be. This situation largely outweighs the potential psychological benefit of IPOP use.

UPPER LIMB

Amputations in the upper extremities from combat wounds generally involve massive trauma due to blast munitions, with a large resulting zone of injury. The decision to attempt limb salvage should be based on the technical feasibility of doing so and on the chance of providing a limb that maintains some useful function. Unlike the lower extremity, the upper extremity is nonweight bearing, generally allowing it to function very well despite decreased sensation. When addressing limb salvage versus amputation or residual limb length decisions in an individual with severe upper limb trauma, it is most important, however, to focus on the potential functional rehabilitation of the entire patient, especially giving significant considerations to the impact of other commonly associated severe injuries. In general, the goals of amputation surgery in the upper extremity should be the following: (*a*) preservation of functional length, (*b*) preservation of useful sensibility, (*c*) prevention of symptomatic neuromas, (*d*) prevention of adjacent joint contractures, (*e*) minimal and short morbidity, (*f*) early prosthetic fitting (where applicable), and (*g*) early return of patient to work and recreation.[45]

Hand and Carpus

The severity of amputations involving the hand ranges from single digit tip amputations to multiple digit amputations, loss of the thumb, and partial hand amputations. For most digital amputations distal to the flexor digitorum superficialis (FDS) insertion, skeletal shortening with primary closure or allowing the wound to heal secondarily will provide for early mobilization of the digit and yield a durable tip with excellent sensation and an acceptable appearance. Local advancement or pedicled soft-tissue flaps have limited application in the combat amputee for treatment of fingertip and distal amputations of digits. The adjacent tissue has usually also been injured to some extent by the blast, and attempting to mobilize it for wound coverage may lead to necrosis and further soft tissue loss. Additionally, these techniques usually require the restriction of adjacent joint and/or adjacent digit motion during the first 3 to 4 weeks following the flap procedure, risking the development of contracture and stiffness, and further limiting the use of the upper extremity in early phases of the patient's rehabilitation.

When a digit is severely injured proximal to the FDS insertion, the surgeon should make every attempt to salvage the important proximal interphalangeal joint. A stable skeletal core and functional arc of joint motion under active flexor/extensor control, with a viable, sensate, and durable soft tissue covering, are the desirable end points. However, when the degree of injury is too severe to salvage the proximal interphalangeal joint, the surgeon is faced with the decision of amputation through the proximal phalanx versus metacarpophalangeal joint (MCPJ) disarticulation or metacarpal ray amputation. Preservation of as much proximal phalanx as possible is desirable, because the remaining segment will be under the control of the intrinsic muscles and the extensor digitorum communis. Active flexion of the proximal phalanx up to 45° is possible with the intrinsics, and the remaining digit can participate in grasping and holding within those limitations.

If a relatively long portion of the proximal phalanx can be preserved, a flexor tendon tenodesis (FDS and/or flexor digitorum profundus) to the A2 pulley under normal resting tension of the muscle-tendon unit (if possible) can give extrinsic flexor control to the remaining proximal phalanx, and make MCPJ flexion up to 90° possible. This adds significant capability for grasping and holding small objects within the palm. If, however, the amputation occurs near the base of the proximal phalanx, the ability of the remaining segment to participate in meaningful grasp and hold is minimal, and the resulting gap (particularly when the long or ring finger is involved) often allows small objects to fall out of the palm. In this situation, consideration should be given to MCPJ disarticulation or more proximal metacarpal ray amputation.

The decision between MCPJ disarticulation and ray

amputation is more complex, involving factors such as which digit is injured, palm breadth and strength (particularly grip and pronation), cosmetic appearance, thumb web space impedance, and gap presence. This decision is individualized, and should be based on total rehabilitation needs (ie, other injuries), occupational demands, hand dominance, and psychological impact of hand appearance. It is important to remember that most metacarpal ray amputations are rarely indicated in the acute setting and are performed under elective conditions.

Because of the vital importance of the thumb in grip, pinch, and opposition, every attempt should be made to preserve as much length as possible in thumb amputation. For amputations distal to the interphalangeal joint, it is extremely important to attain sensate, durable, soft tissue and skin coverage. Failure to do so will result in a hypesthetic, dysesthetic, or tender thumb tip, which the patient would likely exclude in performing activities with the hand. For amputations distal to the interphalangeal joint where no bone is exposed, healing by secondary intent gives the most reliable outcome for the demands of the thumb. If this method cannot be used, then cross-finger flaps or radially innervated fasciocutaneous sensory flaps should be considered. For more proximal injuries, the surgeon should attempt preservation of thenar musculature and all remaining joints practicable for later reconstruction efforts, which may include metacarpal lengthening, index pollicization, or toe-to-thumb transfer.

Combat-related injuries to the hand almost always involve more than a single digit, however. In amputations involving multiple digits or partial hand amputations, it is extremely important to save all viable tissue by whatever means possible and preserve it for later reconstructive efforts. Similarly, when traumatic amputations occur through the carpus, the surgeon should preserve all viable tissue at the time of injury to maximize residual limb length and function. Although prosthetic socket design and terminal device availability for amputations at this level are problematic, many patients find the ability to flex and extend the wrist to be very useful for holding and carrying objects against the body, without the need for a prosthesis. Other patients experience significant frustration with the limited terminal devices available for carpus-level amputations and desire the ability to pinch and grasp with a standard terminal device available for transradial amputations. Patients rarely have the ability to make an informed decision about these issues at the time of injury. The surgeon should therefore preserve everything salvageable and allow the patient to evaluate his or her resulting function before proceeding to a more proximal amputation.

Wrist and Forearm

Wrist disarticulation continues to be a controversial procedure. Advantages include retention of most forearm pronation and supination, due to preservation of the distal radioulnar joint, and improved suspension of the prosthetic device, due to the radial styloid flare. Disadvantages include an excessively long and wide prosthetic socket, difficulty fitting in a wrist component, and fewer choices for the terminal device. Additionally, when myoelectric devices are used, there is little room at the distal end of the socket to conceal the electronics and batteries with wrist disarticulation compared to transradial amputations. In performing a wrist disarticulation, it is important to avoid injury to the triangular fibrocartilage and distal radioulnar joint, because preservation of these structures is vital to preserving the potential advantages of the disarticulation versus a transradial amputation.

When performing a transradial (below-elbow) amputation, attempts should be made to preserve as much length as possible because residual pronation and supination of the forearm is directly proportional to the length of remaining radius and ulna. Retaining as much of this function as possible can have a significant impact on the amputee's ability to position the prosthetic terminal device for functions involving pinch and grasp. For individuals with combat wounds, the level of amputation is dictated by the integrity of the soft tissue. Bony length should not be spared at the expense of providing a durable, stable, soft-tissue covering. In very proximal forearm amputations, all efforts should be made to preserve the elbow joint. In this situation, detaching the biceps tendon from the radius and reattaching it to the proximal ulna may allow the surgeon to excise the radius and gain a larger soft-tissue envelope for closure (Figure 8-10). At the very least, this technique preserves elbow flexion and may provide for easier prosthetic fitting at very proximal levels—even 5 cm of ulnar bone length is sufficient to permit transradial prosthetic fitting. Because of the significant advantage of retaining residual elbow flexion, the use of pedicle or free tissue transfers to provide durable soft tissue coverage over a preserved elbow joint is considered by most surgeons and prosthetists to be preferable to elbow disarticulation or transhumeral amputation.

Elbow and Humerus

Disarticulation of the elbow, like disarticulation of the wrist, is a controversial treatment option and amputation level. Its advantages include better suspension and control of the prosthesis, as well as improved

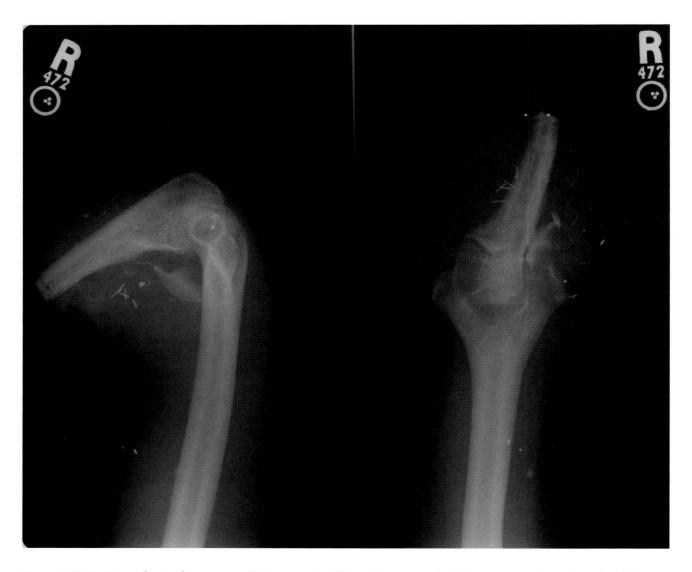

Figure 8-10. Radiograph of a short transradial amputation. The radius was excised due to a comminuted proximal fracture and inadequate available local soft tissue for closure, and the biceps tendon was transferred to the proximal ulna, providing the patient with satisfactory elbow flexion and extension.

function of the residual limb when not wearing the prosthesis due to the longer lever arm and preserved myotendinous units secured to the distal humerus with a tenodesis. The main disadvantages of elbow disarticulation involve prosthetic fitting and appearance. The prosthetic socket is larger than a traditional transhumeral prosthetic socket, and the placement of the prosthetic elbow joint is, by necessity, several centimeters distal to the anatomic joint, creating a disproportionate appearance to the upper extremities. This can be a difficult body image for some patients to accept. Despite the disadvantages of elbow disarticulation, better function and control with and without a prosthesis lends most surgeons and prosthetists to

prefer this level over the more proximal transhumeral amputation when adequate soft tissue coverage can be attained.

Transhumeral (above-elbow) amputations should be performed with the goal of preserving as much bone length as possible. The circumferential nature of muscle around the humerus, as well as the fact that it is not, generally, a weight-bearing extremity allows even the use of split-thickness skin grafting over adequate subcutaneous tissue to maintain humeral length. Traumatic amputations, particularly from blast-related wounds, generally have more proximal levels of skin and subcutaneous tissue loss than bone loss, but the surgeon should approach a more proximal bone transection to achieve primary closure with caution. The shorter the residual humeral length, the less control the amputee will have over the prosthesis.

Additionally, it is important to remember that the biceps and triceps both work across the glenohumeral joint, and a secure myodesis of these muscles distally is essential to retain their function in glenohumeral motion. Amputations at the level of the axillary fold and higher function effectively as shoulder disarticulations because essentially all useful glenohumeral motion is lost. At this level, it is important whenever possible to retain the humeral head, which can improve shoulder contour and the fit of clothing as well as prosthetic suspension systems. Some surgeons have even recommended arthrodesis of the glenohumeral joint in extremely short transhumeral amputations to prevent the abduction and flexion contracture that occurs in many of these patients and to provide further prosthesis stability. Although results of this procedure can be gratifying, internal fixation for formal arthrodesis is best performed in delayed, elective fashion in the setting of a contaminated, blast-related wound.

Shoulder disarticulations are generally performed in emergency situations when the patient's life is at stake due to severe proximal trauma. Once hemostasis is obtained and the patient's life is no longer in jeopardy, the clavicle and scapula should be retained if at all possible. Although not necessary or advocated at the initial point of care, the surgeon should strongly consider internally fixing fractures of the clavicle to retain the rigid strut suspending and supporting the scapula and maintain shoulder contour. Because the disfigurement of forequarter amputations is so severe and the fit of clothing so difficult for these patients, extreme measures to save the clavicle and scapula should be undertaken in this circumstance. These injuries, particularly in combat wounds, should not be closed primarily, and the abundance of muscle from the latissimus, deltoid, and pectoralis major make coverage and salvage of the clavicle and scapula possible in the vast majority of instances.

Handling of the median, radial, and ulnar nerves in transhumeral and shoulder disarticulation patients is gaining importance as research on targeted reinnervation definitively proves the potential of this technique in the management of shoulder disarticulation patients. If the surgeon, physiatrist, and prosthetist believe a particular patient to be a good candidate for this protocol, then it becomes important to leave adequate length of these nerves until the definitive transfer is performed. This approach does entail the risk of leaving the transected nerve ending relatively superficial within the scar, where a symptomatic neuroma may develop. However, this problem can be definitively addressed on an elective basis regardless of whether or not targeted nerve transfer is ultimately attempted. This approach at least preserves an alternative for the patient until that alternative can be discussed and an appropriate determination made.

LOWER LIMB

The location of the most severe injury sustained by a traumatized limb usually determines the level of amputation in extremity blast trauma.[46] Optimizing functional outcome is the goal when deciding upon definitive amputation or revision level. Improved function is usually associated with levels that require less energy consumption, which generally equates to preservation of length. Moreover, preservation of joint function should be attempted to improve a limb's mechanical advantages and preserve the benefits of articular and distal limb proprioception for the amputee. More proximal amputations are associated with increased energy consumption (Table 8-1).[47,48]

Traditionally, more functional amputation levels, in order of decreasing length, are transmetatarsal, Syme, transtibial, knee disarticulation, transfemoral amputation, hip disarticulation, and hemipelvectomy.[49] Lisfranc (tarsometatarsal) and Chopart (tarsotarsal) amputations may be the exception to improved outcome with preserving length. In many cases, these amputations have the disadvantage of causing progressive

TABLE 8-1

ENERGY EXPENDITURE FOR AMPUTATION

Amputation Level	Energy Above Baseline (%)	Oxygen Speed (m/min)	Cost (mL/kg/m)
Long transtibial	10	70	0.17
Average transtibial	25	60	0.20
Short transtibial	40	50	0.20
Bilateral transtibial	41	50	0.20
Transfemoral	65	40	0.28
Wheelchair	0–8	70	0.16

Data sources: (1) Waters RL, Perry J, Antonelli D, Hislop H. Energy cost of walking of amputees: the influence of level of amputation. *J Bone Joint Surg Am.* 1976;58(1):42–46. (2) Czerniecki JM. Rehabilitation in limb deficiency: gait and motion analysis. *Arch Phys Med Rehabil.* 1996;77:S3-S8.

equinus and inversion foot deformities that result from difficulties obtaining proper muscle balance and over-pull of the Achilles tendon. Additionally, difficulties can accompany fitting some energy storage feet for high-activity-level amputees who have received a very long transtibial or Syme amputation.

Closure

Because of the contaminated nature of traumatic extremity injury sustained in battle, most traumatic amputations are left open, preferably as a tissue-sparing and length-preserving amputation in which nontraumatized, viable soft tissue, muscle, and skin flaps are retained to aid in delayed definitive revision and closure. In either case, following serial irrigation and debridement, a plan for bony level and soft tissue closure should be formulated considering the local "flaps of opportunity." Because preservation of joint function is paramount, attempts to save an amputation level with use of skin grafting for local soft tissue coverage are warranted. Historically, skin grafts did not often withstand shear forces after prosthetic fitting in the lower extremity, and a plan for tissue expansion and eventual coverage with native skin was often required.[50,51] However, gel liners and improved prosthetic interface materials have improved the results of prosthetic fitting for amputated limbs with skin grafts in many individuals injured in the OIF/OEF conflicts.

Additional challenges in closure of traumatic blast wounds have been reported from the military centers treating returning blast victims. Amputation closure within the zone of injury approaches a 67% wound complication rate.[52] Additionally, approximately 63% of blast-related amputations are complicated by the formation of HO, which is most closely correlated with closure through the zone of injury.[13] These considerations must be factored into the decision-making process and included in patient and family counseling discussions.

Preoperative prophylactic antibiotics should be administered. In the absence of frank wound infection in which culture-specific antibiotics are preferred, antibiotic selection should be standard perioperative prophylaxis for a noninfected surgery. In an effort to prevent the formation of chronic postoperative phantom and stump pain, many centers continue to employ the techniques of preemptive epidurals and early regional nerve blocks, although these procedures are not completely supported by available controlled trials.[53]

The use of a pneumatic tourniquet has been shown to reduce blood loss and transfusion requirements during elective amputation and may have the extra benefit of a reduced rate of revision due to the resultant hemostasis and easier visualization.[54,55] In the manage-

ment of combat-related amputees, in whom multiple, repeated surgical procedures and multisystem trauma is the rule rather than the exception, judicious tourniquet use may further limit the need for serial transfusions with their attendant immunosuppression and other potential systemic complications. An assessment of perfusion without the tourniquet inflated should, however, be performed at least once before definitive closure to ensure both adequate hemostasis and residual tissue viability via capillary bleeding.

During secondary closure, the skin should be closed without tension. The scar should be placed to avoid adhesion to bone and trauma from pressure points in the prosthesis. Bone should be beveled distally to prevent a sharp end from causing discomfort or soft tissue breakdown with prosthetic wear. As mentioned previously, myodesis or myoplasty should be performed to provide better muscle balance and prevent atrophy.[56] Nerves should be sharply transected after gentle distal traction and allowed to retract into the deep padded soft tissue. Individual wound closure techniques will be discussed by section; however, all combat-related amputations should be managed with deep drains at the time of definitive closure to prevent postoperative hematoma formation and subsequent wound complications or infection.

Partial Foot Amputation

The transmetatarsal amputation can produce a highly acceptable functional and cosmetic amputation level. A healthy, durable soft tissue envelope is more important than a specific anatomic amputation level, so bone should be shortened to allow soft tissue closure without tension, rather than to a specific, described surgical level. Bone contouring to replicate the anatomic forefoot cascade is desirable for weight bearing, and the bone ends should be beveled to prevent bony prominence. A long plantar flap is preferable (Figure 8-11), but equal dorsal and plantar flaps can function

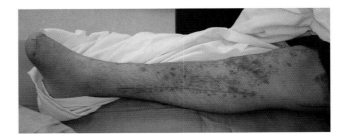

Figure 8-11. Healed transmetatarsal amputation with long plantar skin flap.

well when adequate viable plantar tissue is absent.

Lisfranc-level amputation (tarsometatarsal) can provide adequate functional outcomes as well. However, careful evaluation should be made of the muscle balance around the foot, with specific attention to heel cord tightness and function of the tibialis anterior and peroneal muscles. Midfoot amputations significantly shorten the lever arm of the foot, so prophylactic Achilles tendon lengthening should be considered intraoperatively. Furthermore, tibialis anterior and peroneal muscle insertions should be reattached under appropriate tension, if they are released during bone resection, to prevent muscle imbalance, which will inevitably lead to foot deformity followed by eventual difficulty with prosthetic fitting and decreased function. Postoperative casting can help prevent deformities by preventing Achilles tendon contractures, allowing tendon reattachments time to

heal, controlling residual limb edema, and preventing wound problems.

The Chopart (transverse tarsal) amputation removes the forefoot and midfoot while preserving the talus and calcaneus. Achilles tendon lengthening and tibialis and peroneal tendon reattachment and balancing are essential to prevent equinus and varus deformities at this level (Figure 8-12). Although described in the literature, tendon reattachment and balancing at this level can be quite humbling, with many patients progressing to hindfoot deformity necessitating further revision for functional limitations.[57] If available, plantar weight-bearing skin is best utilized as a flap for closure, with special attention paid to fastening the flap to bone to prevent shear and bursa formation. Postoperative casting is necessary to allow for tendon healing to bone. Although precise indications for revision to a Syme or transtibial amputation are

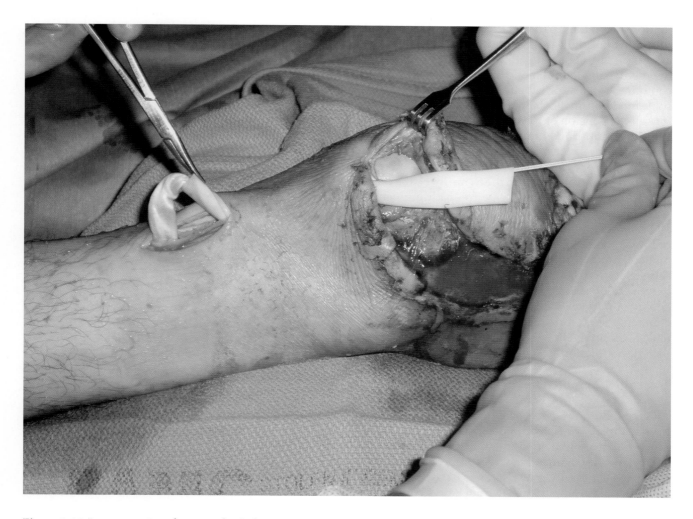

Figure 8-12. Intraoperative photograph of Chopart amputation. A Penrose drain is being utilized to pass the residual tibialis anterior tendon beneath a skin bridge to facilitate tenodesis distally.

lacking, a lengthy discussion with patients regarding rehabilitation and functional expectations is indicated prior to the decision to pursue a Lisfranc- or Chopart-level amputation.

Syme and Long Transtibial Amputation

Described by Syme[58] in 1843 and subsequently reviewed by Harris,[59] ankle disarticulation requires that the calcaneus and talus be removed. Care should be taken while dissecting out the calcaneus to preserve the heel skin and fat pad. The heel skin and fat pad are subsequently utilized as a durable end-bearing organ for ambulation, sometimes even without a prosthetic for short distances. It is important to stabilize the fat pad distally to prevent posterior and medial migration, which can compromise function. This can be accomplished several ways, including tenodesis of the Achilles tendon to the posterior margin of the tibia through drill holes, transfer of the tibialis anterior and extensor digitorum tendons to the anterior aspect of the fat pad, or removal of the cartilage and subchondral bone to allow scarring of the fat pad to bone.[18,60] Subsequently, the medial and lateral malleoli must be removed and contoured to allow prosthetic fitting. An effort to retain some moderate malleolar flare should be made to allow for self-suspension of the prosthesis.

A long transtibial amputation is an uncommonly used level for several reasons. Although it offers the potential advantages of improved lever arm and proproceptive control similar to the Syme level, the distal leg skin and lack of soft tissue for padding can be problematic. Patients with this amputation level generally cannot ambulate without a prosthesis, despite the putative benefits of a Syme amputation. Because the malleoli are absent, prosthetic fitting may not allow self-suspension. Moreover, similar to the Syme level, high-activity, athletic users often have difficulty fitting energy-storing feet typically used for running without cumbersome and heavy specialty attachments. This makes these levels less attractive in this particular patient population.

Transtibial Amputation

Arguably the most appealing level of amputation from a functional outcome perspective in the young active military population, the transtibial amputation (TTA) level has many advantages from a surgical perspective. Historically, many soldiers have been treated with this type of amputation. During World War II, from January 1, 1943, to May 1, 1944, five medical centers reported 627 TTAs and 550 transfemoral amputations, 35.7% and 31.3% of all amputations, respectively.[61]

Anteroposterior, lateral, and lateral oblique radiographs of the extremity should be obtained preoperatively. The lateral oblique radiograph allows assessment of preoperative tibiofibular distance to ensure that this distance remains constant during a bone-bridging procedure, if chosen. This view also allows for radiographic assessment of excessive distal tibiofibular diastasis, an indicator of proximal instability, which is an indication for either proximal stabilization or a distal bone-bridging procedure. A guideline of 2.5 cm for each 30 cm of height provides the appropriate residual limb length for the patient's stature. Typically, 12.5 to 17.5 cm below the tibiofemoral joint line is used as the final tibia length for nonischemic limbs.[62] For non-bone-bridging amputation, the fibula should be resected 1 to 2 cm proximal to the tibia. Definitive internal and external fixation of fractures has been used to preserve length in the traumatic amputee. Even segmental fractures can be stabilized to proximal segments, thereby preserving length. Amputation through the level of the highest fracture is not required, provided an adequate soft tissue envelope is present.[46]

Currently, most TTAs are performed utilizing a long posterior myocutaneous flap, which is based off the blood supply from the gastrocnemius muscle (Figure 8-13). A recent metaanalysis showed that the choice of

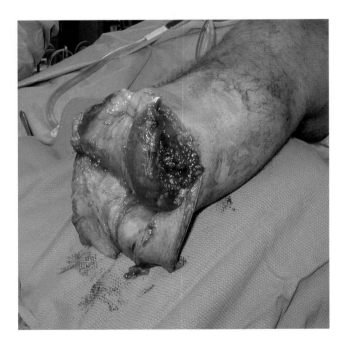

Figure 8-13. Gastrocnemius and soleus myodesis to the anterior tibia during definitive revision and closure of a transtibial amputation using conventional posterior myofascial and skin flaps.

amputation skin flap, including skew flaps and sagital flaps, had little impact on outcome when compared to the posterior myocutaneous flap.[63] A myodesis to bone holes of the gastrocnemius to the beveled distal tibia should be performed, with the knee in full extension to prevent flexion contracture. If the long posterior flap is compromised, available "flaps of opportunity" should be used to save length and level, including myodesis or myoplasty of anterior and/or lateral compartment musculature over the distal tibia to provide adequate distal soft tissue padding.

The distal bone bridge synostosis technique offers the theoretical advantage of providing a more end-bearing residual limb and has recently been shown to have some tangible benefits over traditional TTA in terms of prosthetic functional outcome.[64] Furthermore, the technique is valuable to treat a patient with tibiofibular instability, which can cause prosthetic fit issues from fibula widening and translation with weight bearing. For bone-bridging procedures, several modifications of the original Ertl technique can be performed to create a bone bridge between the tibia and fibula with either a fibula strut graft and/or a periosteal sleeve (Figure 8-14).[65,66] Distal bone bridging and modifications of the Ertl procedure are discussed

in greater detail in Chapter 9.

Contemporary prosthetic sockets and suspension systems allow fitting and function of even the shortest functional TTA, up to and including levels just below the tibial tubercle. Occasionally, however, these levels prove difficult to manage and patient frustration with an inability to regain adequate control of the prosthetic limb warrants additional strategies. Attempts at lengthening short residual limbs with either mono-planar or Ilizarov fixators have proven successful and should be discussed with the patient as an option prior to resorting to a higher level amputation.[67,68] Due to concerns about wound healing and infection, however, these techniques should generally not be employed until after wound healing is complete and initial prosthetic fitting and rehabilitation has been attempted. At present, there are no indications for salvaging a short TTA in the absence of the tibial tuberosity or, at least, a reconstructible extensor mechanism.

Postoperative care following TTA has traditionally been a rigid dressing in the form of a splint or cast. It is generally believed that injured tissues heal more consistently and with less pain when placed at rest. Furthermore, rigid immobilization affords the added benefit of preventing knee flexion contracture.[57] How-

a
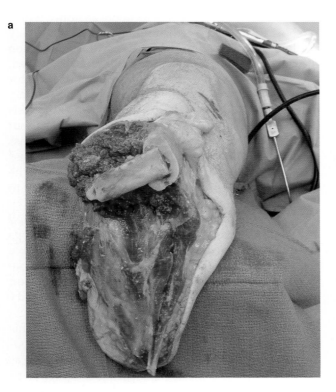

b
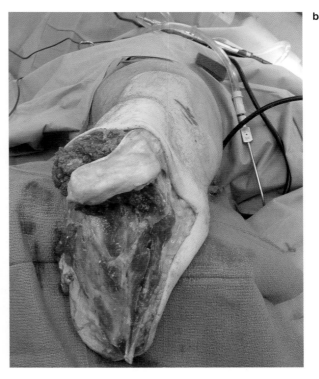

Figure 8-14. Demonstration of distal bone bridging technique for transtibial amputation utilizing a fibular autograft strut **(a)**, which is then covered with a periosteal sleeve from the anteromedial tibia **(b)**.

ever, as mentioned earlier, rigid dressings have not been widely utilized during the current conflict due to concerns about early postoperative infection and the need for frequent wound examination during the period when such dressings would be most beneficial. Early postoperative rehabilitation should emphasize full knee and hip range of motion, including prone lying and stretching. Avoidance of pillows under the knee or a chronically flexed hip is critical to prevent functional limb length discrepancy associated with contractures.

Through-Knee and Transfemoral Amputation

Above-knee amputation includes amputations through the knee (knee disarticulation) and transfemoral amputations (TFAs). Although knee disarticulation is often avoided due to the drawbacks of knee level disparity, unsatisfactory soft tissue padding and patient function, the procedure's putative advantages include a simpler surgical technique, which potentially lessens operating room time and blood loss. The thigh musculature is not disrupted during the procedure and all muscle attachments remain, resulting in better functional control and biomechanics for walking.[69] Additionally, this level can provide direct end-bearing characteristics for the residual limb and improved self-suspension, with a resulting decrease in socket length. Previously, knee disarticulation created problems for prosthetic components because of the knee height difference compared to the uninjured side, but newer components, especially in knee designs, have largely solved these problems. Particularly with bilateral through-knee or transfemoral amputees, knee height disparity is not an issue.[70]

A posterior skin flap has traditionally been described for wound closure; however, recently the use of a long posterior myocutaneous flap has become popular because of the added padding of the gastrocnemius muscle and its associated contributory blood supply to the skin flap.[71] Furthermore, the LEAP study[5] demonstrated that through-knee amputations may not function as well as conventional transfemoral amputations, particularly if the gastrocnemius padding is absent. Thus, for an optimal through-knee amputation, nearly as much intact posterior myocutaneous tissue is required as for a short transtibial amputation. If both adequate proximal tibial bone and posterior soft tissue are present, the patient may be better served with a short transtibial amputation, potentially salvaging a functional knee joint.

To complete a through-knee amputation, the distal extremity is removed sharply through the knee joint capsule. Care should be taken to resect the patellar tendon off the tibial tubercle. The patella should be sharply dissected from the encasing quadriceps mechanism to decrease the risk of future patella-femoral pain and patella prominence. Additionally, the remnants of the cruciate ligaments should be left attached to their femoral origins. Excessively bulbous lateral and medial femoral condyles may be modestly trimmed with a sagittal saw. Posterior condylectomy may be required to advance muscle coverage, but is not routinely needed. Finally, the patella ligament should be sutured to the remnants of the cruciate ligaments for quadriceps balance, and the posterior muscle flap brought forward and sutured to the thick anterior joint capsule, prior to tension-free skin closure.

Traumatic amputation through the femur can happen at any level. As the level migrates closer to the hip joint, function is compromised due to the decreased lever arm available for function and fitting, increasing disruption of the muscular attachments for thigh control and increasing the necessity for more complex proximal suspension systems for prosthetic use. When the skeletal muscle attachments are divided during amputation, muscle loses its mechanical abilities. Stabilization of the distal insertion of muscle can improve residual limb function. As noted, myodesis is the most effective technique to stabilize strong antagonistic muscle forces.

Care must be taken during transfemoral amputation to correctly identify the cross-sectional anatomy, which can be difficult because the thigh is usually externally rotated. A good reference point is the linea aspera on the posterior femur. Once the anatomy is identified, it is important to remember that the large adductor magnus inserts onto the femur as a direct posteromedial structure. The most critical step during myodesis is to place the femur across midline adduction without hip flexion while suturing the adductor muscle mass to the distal femur through bone holes. If this process is not performed correctly, postoperative control of the limb will be compromised during ambulation due to over-pull of the abductors.

The remaining muscle closure is usually performed as a series of myodeses or a hamstring-to-quadriceps myoplasty. Care must be taken to avoid excessive shortening of hip flexor musculature due to the position of the limb during surgery, which may result in a hip flexion contracture. The hamstrings and/or quadriceps may be further stabilized by adding a nonabsorbable suture to the adductor myodesis. This technique helps prevent shifting of the adductor myodesis over the distal femur with use, and can function as a myodesis-by-proxy of the hamstrings or quadriceps if additional attachments through drill holes for each muscle group are not made in the distal femur. At a minimum, the authors recommend formal myodesis of the semimembranosus, which is the strongest hamstring and typically the most robust muscle belly present at any transfemoral level. The quadriceps apron, if available, should be swung over the distal aspect of the remaining femur, for both stabilization and padding, as the last muscle layer closed.

Similar to length preservation in traumatic TTA, a proximal femur fracture can be stabilized to allow an eventual longer lever arm for TFA or knee disarticulation (Figure 8-15). Amputation through the level of the highest fracture is not required.[12] Additionally, lengthening of a particularly short TFA residual limb

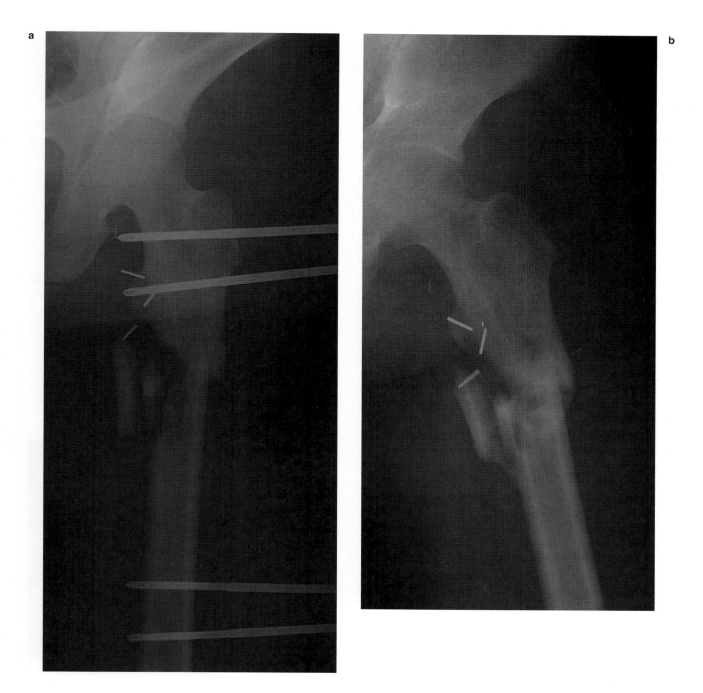

Figure 8-15. Radiographs of a through-knee amputation with external fixation of a proximal femur fracture. Due to soft tissue compromise and other injuries limiting potential early rehabilitation, the patient was treated definitively in this fashion until sufficient callous had formed to allow ambulation, with some additional support provided externally by the prosthetic socket.

can be accomplished with monoplanar fixation following corticotomy. If bone injury occurs proximal to the lesser trochanter, control of the limb is severely compromised and hip disarticulation or fusion of the short proximal femur to the acetabulum are usually the only remaining practicable options.

To avoid hip flexion contracture, postoperative rehabilitation with prone lying and stretching should begin early. Additionally, placement of pillows between the legs with abduction at the hip should be avoided to prevent less than optimal adductor control of the limb or early strain on the adductor myodesis.

Hip Disarticulation and Hemipelvectomy

Hip disarticulation and, in particular, hemipelvectomy, are amputations of last resort. Despite the historically dismal functional prognosis associated with these proximal levels, modern prosthetics and suction-fit suspension mechanisms have resulted in remarkable function in some of these patients. Therefore, attention to a few key points is warranted to maximize patient outcomes.

Hip disarticulation has traditionally been performed utilizing a posterior or posterolateral flap based on the gluteal musculature. The femoral and obturator vessels are identified, isolated, and double-ligated proximally as they exit the true pelvis. After removal or arthrodesis of the remaining (typically short or absent) proximal femur, the abductor musculature and/or pectineus can be sutured to the residual joint capsule or inserted directly into bone, filling the acetabular deadspace and reducing the risk of postoperative hematoma, seroma, and infection. Care is warranted to avoid dissection into the sciatic notch and violation of the gluteal vessels exiting there, which could compromise flap viability. The gluteus maximus tendon is then mobilized and sutured anteriorly to the inguinal ligament, resulting in a robust myofasciocutaneous flap over the residual hemipelvis.

Hemipelvectomy is rarely required in a posttraumatic or combat-related setting—most patients with traumatic amputations at this level do not survive, even on the modern battlefield, and in most surviving patients a hip disarticulation can be salvaged. When required, efforts to salvage as much of the residual ilium and ischium as possible are warranted, given the importance of these osseous supports for prosthetic support and sitting balance, respectively. The soft tissue management and techniques are essentially the same as those for hip disarticulation, except that greater vessel dissection is required. In males, all three blood supplies to the testicle travel within the spermatic cord, which should be salvaged, or a unilateral orchiectomy should be performed concurrently. The corresponding round ligament of the uterus in females can be sacrificed without sequelae.

For cases in which the gluteal musculature and skin are violated or absent, alternate coverage techniques are required. If possible, a femoral artery-based quadriceps anterior-posterior flap should be used.[72] The availability of this flap in a posttraumatic setting clearly relies on the initial performance of an open, length- and tissue-preserving amputation, which illustrates the critical importance of this technique. A modified abdominoplasty advancement fasciocutaneous flap can also be utilized for soft tissue coverage, although this flap lacks the muscle padding desired under optimal circumstances.[73] The authors have also had some success with rectus abdominus rotational flaps to augment soft tissue coverage in this region (Figure 8-16). Finally, in contradistinction to other lower extremity amputation levels, which are typically subjected to greater frictional and end-bearing forces with ambulation, split-thickness skin grafts can be utilized with relatively good anticipated results in this location.

Wound complication rates after either hip disarticulation or hemipelvectomy are quite high, even in an elective setting. Therefore, early rehabilitation consists largely of early patient mobilization to prevent secondary complications such as decubitus, thromboembolic phenomena, pulmonary dysfunction, and general deconditioning. Prosthetic fitting is typically delayed until wound healing is complete. However, as noted, recent advancements have made resultant function in some amputees at these levels quite surprising and gratifying.

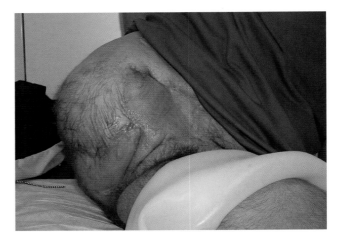

Figure 8-16. Clinical photograph of a hip disarticulation in which soft tissue closure and coverage of the femoral vessels was facilitated by use of a rectus abdominis flap and partial thickness skin grafting.

MULTIPLE INJURED LIMB AMPUTEE

The combat amputee often has injuries to multiple extremities as well as other organ systems, including eyesight. Additional injuries and more proximal levels of amputation can have a profoundly negative impact on functional capacity. Even in an era of great technologic and prosthetic advancements, the multiple limb amputee has challenges with prosthetic donning, fit, wear, and sustained use. In the traumatic amputee, the oxygen consumption of the bilateral transtibial amputee approaches that of a unilateral transfemoral amputee, while the bilateral transfemoral amputee requires double the oxygen consumption to maintain 60% of normal walking speed.[74]

A bilateral transfemoral amputee is difficult to fit effectively with bilateral ischial-bearing sockets. The high sockets impinge upon one another not only when walking but also when seated. For this reason, if it is possible to maintain one side at a through-knee level, the comfort of prosthetic wear may be greatly enhanced. An even more appealing alternative would be to maintain a single knee joint, even if it is a very short transtibial level, to obviate the need for a knee hinge[75,76]; balance and control are greatly enhanced in this circumstance. It is even reasonable to consider a free tissue transfer for coverage of a transtibial or through-knee amputation level to avoid bilateral transfemoral amputations, depending on the patient's condition.

Traumatic lower extremity injuries, especially in combat, often result in bilateral transtibial amputations. Fortunately, current prosthetic technology coupled with rehabilitative training has allowed for a high level of function in many patients. In fact, some unilateral lower extremity amputees with severe injuries of the contralateral limb have requested elective amputations of the remaining limb to improve functional level and reduce pain. The long-term outcomes of these individuals have not yet been determined, and it is still generally preferable in a patient with severe bilateral lower extremity injury to amputate the more severe limb and attempt salvage of the other through whatever means available (circular frames, free tissue transfer, etc). If function in the salvaged limb is not satisfactory after reconstructive and rehabilitative efforts are exhausted, consideration for elective amputation may be entertained in a careful, deliberate fashion.

The lower extremity amputee with severe upper extremity injury deserves special mention. Depending on the functional outcome of the lower extremity amputation, the upper extremities may be required for mobility and ambulation assistance in both the short and long terms. Although obviously desirable, regaining full function of the upper extremity is often not possible. In such a circumstance, stability and relatively painless upper extremity function become more important, because the upper limbs are required for transfers and wheelchair use. Deliberate arthrodesis or permissive ankylosis of the wrist, elbow, or shoulder may be preferred to an unstable or painful limb that is more mobile.

The blind upper extremity amputee presents particular and unique challenges. Due to the lack of tactile feedback, current prosthetic technology requires vision for control of the terminal devices of upper extremity prostheses. A Krukenberg procedure, despite its cosmetic limitations, may allow for improved upper extremity function in these patients because of the presence of sensation in the terminal limb. If desired, a cosmetic limb may be provided for patient use in social settings.

It is not possible to cover the complete array of injury combinations that may present as a result of wartime trauma. However, decisions can be made based on the specific injury and patient needs. The surgeon and the rehabilitation team, working cooperatively with the patient and family, must make careful and considerate individual decisions based on multiple factors to arrive at optimal solutions in each case.

DELAYED AMPUTATION VERSUS LIMB SALVAGE

The decision to proceed with limb salvage or amputation in the patient with a severely injured extremity or extremities will be a source of continued debate. Progress has been made every year in each of these areas, making it possible to save limbs that were previously unsalvageable as well as to provide more advanced prostheses with greater functional capacity. Another evolving concern is the cost of each treatment, although this factor may be a less significant consideration for the military amputee because of guaranteed lifelong care through military and Veterans Affairs healthcare systems. The most recent published cost analysis has demonstrated equivocal 2-year costs between the two groups, but a three-fold increase was shown for the lifetime cost of the amputee group.[77] Physicians have a responsibility to become knowledgeable about each of these areas to best advise patients and help them make these very difficult decisions. To be effective, physicians must learn to use a variety of tools and discussion points.

a

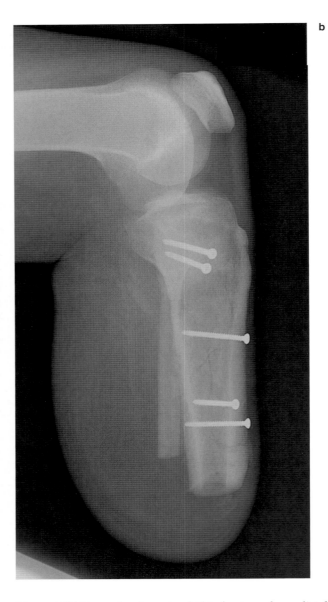

b

LEFT

Figure 8-17. Example of proximal tibia fracture above distal amputation. Limited internal fixation allowed preservation of a good length for the residual limb.

Partners/Mentors

Most surgeons have not managed every type of injury or situation during training or regular practice to prepare them for the patient facing limb salvage or amputation. Even among experienced trauma surgeons, a specific patient's injuries, dilemmas, and considerations are usually unique. The collective knowledge of peers and consultants is important when faced with treating this type of injury and patient. Fortunately, today's digital media and communication

allows advice to be sought quickly and securely, even across thousands of miles.

Amputee Counselors/Visitors

Peer visitors and certified counselors should be available at every major military treatment facility; they can be a tremendous assistance when treating patients in this situation. Many of these individuals have faced similar dilemmas and can provide specific insight that may not be readily apparent to the treating

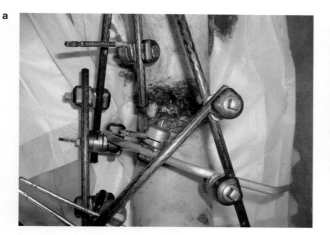

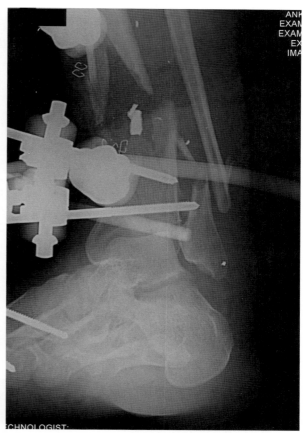

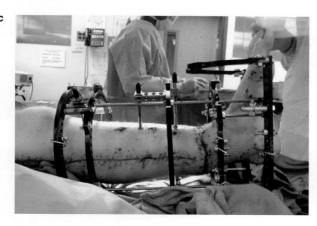

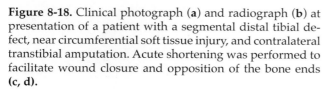

Figure 8-18. Clinical photograph (**a**) and radiograph (**b**) at presentation of a patient with a segmental distal tibial defect, near circumferential soft tissue injury, and contralateral transtibial amputation. Acute shortening was performed to facilitate wound closure and opposition of the bone ends (**c, d**).

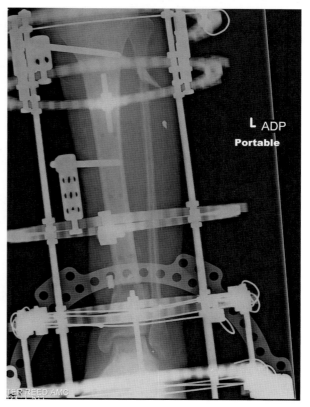

physician. Patients may discuss concerns with a fellow service member in similar circumstances that they may not express to the physician. Examples include how each treatment will affect the soldier's military career, relationships with spouses and family, recreational activities, and acceptance within society at large.

Surgical Considerations

When planning an amputation after attempted limb salvage, one of the most important considerations is the level at which the amputation should be performed. Multiple factors must be considered, including the condition of the soft tissues, presence of bone defects, injury to and function of proximal joints, vascular injury, and the presence of contralateral injuries. Each of these factors affects the level and type of amputation,

a

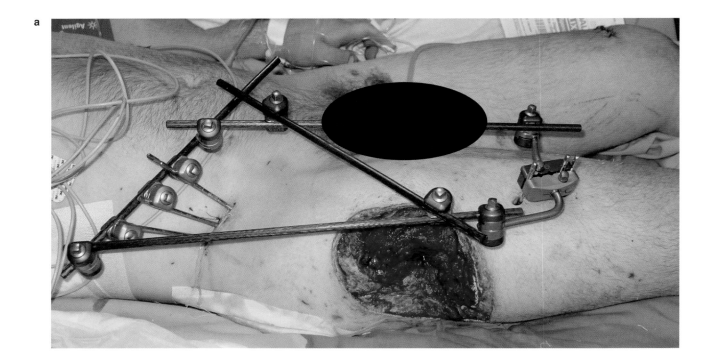

b

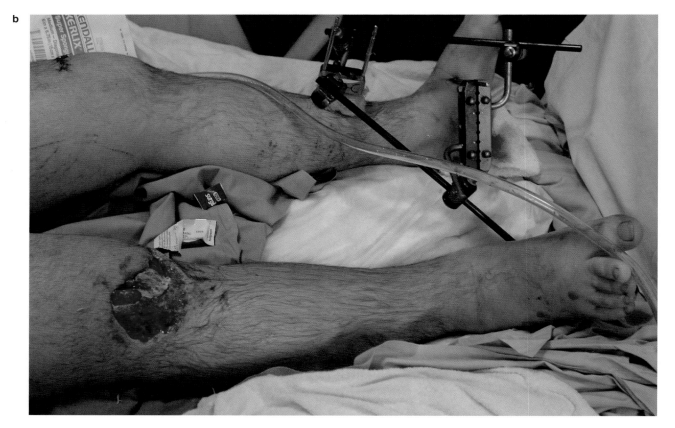

Figure 8-19. Open bilateral lower extremity injuries secondary to an improvised explosive device blast. (*c and d on opposite page*)

c

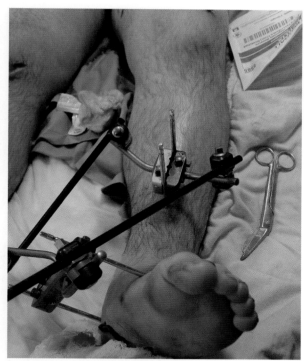

d

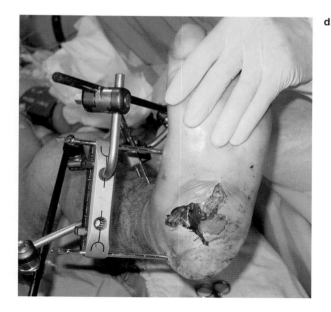

as well as the ultimate function anticipated.

The condition of soft tissue may have a dramatic effect on the level of amputation. If soft tissue is not adequate to cover the residual limb, or it is extremely tenuous, amputation at a higher level is likely warranted. For example, through-knee patients considered in a study by MacKenzie et al[78] did not function as well as either transtibial or transfemoral patients. Lesser function was primarily observed in patients with poor soft tissue coverage, whereas patients with a good soft tissue envelope did comparably well with their transfemoral and transtibial counterparts. Although the results of this study do not support avoiding through-knee amputations, they illustrate the importance of achieving the optimal level to enhance patient outcomes.

Bone defects or persistent nonunion of fractures can play a significant role in both upper and lower extremity amputations and limb salvage, particularly in the lower limb because of its requirement for weight bearing. Consideration should therefore be given to performing the amputation through the bone defect or higher, provided that this will give the patient an adequate amputation level. Fixation of fractures above the amputation can be done in many cases, providing length to the amputation (Figures 8-17 and 8-18). However, for late amputations after failed attempts at limb salvage, little evidence suggests that an unresolved bone or soft tissue problem will fare any better within the residual limb after amputation, despite the external support and soft tissue padding that a prosthetic component may afford.

Injuries to joints above the level of amputation should be evaluated closely. Reconstructible joints should always be salvaged with the amputation performed below. A functional joint will always be beneficial to the patient in the long run. Total knee arthroplasty has been performed successfully in transtibial amputees, with restoration of independent ambulation.[79] Salvaging joints is even more important in patients with above-knee amputations, because hip disarticulation is much more disabling than almost any length of functioning residual femur.

Vascular injury can easily preclude the salvage of the lower extremity. Every attempt should be made to assist the general and vascular surgeons with these patients. Given the almost inevitable future amputation in these patients if vascular injury is not resolved, the relative benefits of vascular reconstruction far outweigh the risks in this patient category, provided that the patient is physiologically stable.

Limb Salvage Versus Bilateral Amputation

Injury to the contralateral limb may have strong influences on decision-making for limb salvage versus amputation. When one limb has sustained a traumatic amputation, in most cases every effort should be made to salvage the contralateral limb. In these situations, acute shortening of the involved limb for closure of soft tissue defects may be necessary. Achieving equal limb lengths is not a concern in this situation, because the

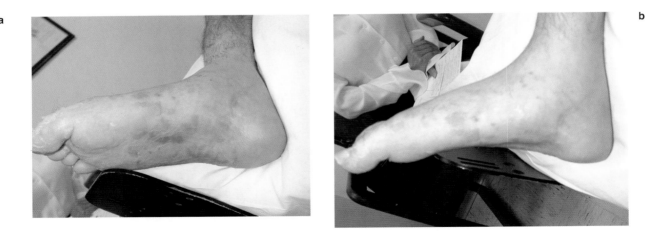

Figure 8-20. Right foot after reconstructive surgery for an open calcaneus fracture. The patient was unable to bear weight secondary to severe dysasthesias in the right foot, and elected to undergo late transtibial amputation.

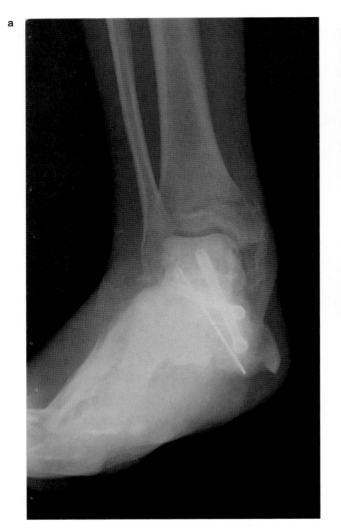

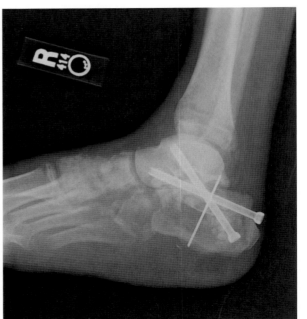

Figure 8-21. Follow-up radiographs of the foot and ankle of the patient in Figure 8-20 prior to elective late transtibial amputation.

prosthesis for the contralateral limb can be adjusted to compensate for any shortening. Today's soldiers may be eager to undergo elective amputation given the advances in prosthetics and their desire to return to functional independence and higher activity levels more rapidly.

Injury to bilateral lower extremities with traumatic amputation on one side strongly, and appropriately, influences the caregiver to recommend initial limb salvage. Surgeons are reticent to proceed directly to amputation when any possibility of limb salvage remains, even in the direst circumstances. Although contralateral salvage may prolong the hospital stay and rehabilitation course of the patient, it remains the recommended course of action. Some patients with severe injuries unpredictably go on to near full functionality with an amputation and a marginal contralateral limb, while others with a seemingly good limb and amputation are severely disabled. Each individual patient has impairments from his or her unique injuries, but the final level of residual disability depends on multiple physical, psychological, and social factors. Salvaging the remaining limb allows the patient the opportunity

and time to make an informed decision regarding future amputation. In the authors' experience, those who have attempted limb salvage and decide for late amputation have done very well.

A sample case is a 24-year-old patient who was sitting in the back of a Stryker combat vehicle when it was hit by a powerful IED. He sustained a right open subtrochanteric femur fracture, right open patella fracture, left tibial pilon fracture, bilateral open calcaneus and talar fractures, and multiple soft tissue wounds (Figure 8-19). Treatment of the right femur consisted of multiple debridements followed by intramedullary nail fixation, and skin grafting of the lateral thigh. The left lower extremity fractures were severe, requiring an early amputation. Multiple debridements were necessary to treat the right open calcaneus fracture and talar injuries. After several months, he remained unable to place weight on the right lower extremity secondary to severe neuropathic pain (Figures 8-20 and 8-21). A transtibial amputation was performed at the patient's request 9 months following the injury. Since that time he has returned to full activities including golf, work, and school.

CONCLUSION

Both early and late care of the combat casualty with limb loss remain challenging endeavors. Optimal early treatment, including initial decisions on limb salvage, open length-preserving amputations, thorough debridements, and provisional fracture stabilization techniques can dramatically influence reconstructive alternatives for surgeons at higher echelons of care as well as final patient outcomes. Subsequent treatment decisions are no

less difficult, but can often be made with the assistance of physiatrists, prosthetists, therapists, patients, and families, as well as peers and the medical literature. By making informed, systematic determinations regarding final amputation level, nerve handling, and soft tissue reconstruction and closure in this fashion, satisfactory and occasionally excellent outcomes can ultimately be achieved for even the most challenging patients.

Acknowledgment

The authors gratefully acknowledge Lieutenant Colonel Donald A Gajewski, MD, for his contributions to this chapter.

REFERENCES

1. Potter BK, Scoville CR. Amputation is not isolated: an overview of the U.S. Army amputee patient care program and associated amputee injuries. *J Am Acad Orthop Surg.* 2006;14:S188–S190.

2. Beekley AC, Sebesta J, Blackbourne L, et al. Pre-hospital tourniquet use in Operation Iraqi Freedom: effect on hemorrhage control and outcomes. *J Trauma.* In press.

3. Bonanni F, Rhodes M, Lucke JF. The futility of predictive scoring of mangled lower extremities. *J Trauma.* 1993;34:99–104.

4. Bosse MJ, MacKenzie EJ, Kellam JF, et al. A prospective evaluation of the clinical utility of the lower-extremity injury-severity scores. *J Bone Joint Surg Am.* 2001;83:3–14.

5. Bosse MJ, MacKenzie EJ, Kellam JF, et al. An analysis of outcomes of reconstruction or amputation after leg-threatening injuries. *N Engl J Med*. 2002;347(24):1924–1931.

6. Amputations. In: Burris DG, Dougherty PJ, Elliot DC, et al, eds. *Emergency War Surgery*. 3rd US Revision. Washington, DC: Department of the Army, Office of The Surgeon General, Borden Institute; 2004: Chapter 25.

7. Scully R, Hughes CW. The pathology of skeletal muscle ischemia in man: a description of early changes in extremity muscle following damage to major peripheral arteries on the battlefield. In: Howard JM, ed. *Battle Casualties in Korea: Studies of the Surgical Research Team. Vol. III*. Washington, DC: US Army Medical Service Graduate School; 1955.

8. VA/DoD Clinical practice guideline for rehabilitation of lower limb amputation. National Guideline Clearinghouse Web site. Available at: http://www.guideline.gov/summary/summary.aspx?ss=15&doc_id=11758&nbr=6060. Accessed September 12, 2008

9. Herscovici D Jr, Sanders RW, Scaduto DM, Infante A, DiPasquale T. Vacuum-assisted wound closure (VAC therapy) for the management of patients with high-energy soft tissue injuries. *J Orthop Trauma*. 2003;17(10):683–638.

10. Rowley DI. *War Wounds with Fractures: A Guide to Surgical Management*. Geneva, Switzerland: International Committee of the Red Cross; 1992.

11. Coupland RM. *Amputation for War Wounds*. Geneva, Switzerland: International Committee of the Red Cross; 1996.

12. Pickard-Gabriel CJ, Ledford CL, Gajewski DA, Granville RR, Robert R, Andersen RC. Traumatic transfemoral amputation with concomitant ipsilateral proximal femoral fracture: a report of two cases. *J Bone Joint Surg Am*. 2007;89(12):2764–2768.

13. Potter BK, Burns TC, Lacap AP, Granville RR, Gajewski DA. Heterotopic ossification following traumatic and combat-related amputations: prevalence, risk factors, and preliminary results of excision. *J Bone Joint Surg Am*. 2007;89A(3):476–486.

14. Burgess EM, Romano RL, Zettl JH, Schrock RD Jr. Amputations of the leg for peripheral vascular insufficiency. *J Bone Joint Surg Am*. 1971;53(5):874–890.

15. Pedersen HE. Treatment of ischemic gangrene and infection in the foot. *Clin Orthop*. 1960;16:199–202.

16. Pedersen HE. The problem of the geriatric amputee. *Artif Limbs*. 1968;12(suppl):1–3.

17. Konduru S, Jain AS. Trans-femoral amputation in elderly dysvascular patients: reliable results with a technique of myodesis. *Prosthet Orthot Int*. 2007;31(1):45–50.

18. Smith DG, Sangeorzan BJ, Hansen ST Jr, Burgess EM. Achilles tendon tenodesis to prevent heel pad migration in the Syme's amputation. *Foot Ankle Int*. 1994;15(1):14–17.

19. Schneider M, Nelson IJ. Ambulatory skin traction splint for the amputee. *Am J Surg*. 1965;109:684–685.

20. Serletti JC. An effective method of skin traction in A-K guillotine amputation. *Clin Orthop Relat Res*. 1981;157:212–214.

21. Vainio K. A portable apparatus for skin traction. *Ann Chir Gynaecol Fenn*. 1950;39(1):54–57.

22. Mackinnon SE, Dellon AL, Hudson AR. Alteration of neuroma formation by manipulation of its microenvironment. *Plast Reconstr Surg*. 1985;76:345–353.

23. Vernadakis AJ, Koch H, Mackinnon SE. Management of neuromas. *Clin Plast Surg*. 2003;30:247–268.

24. Davis L, Perret G, Hiler F. Experimental studies in peripheral nerve surgery. Effect of infection on regeneration and functional recovery. *Surg Gynecol Obstet*. 1945;81:302–308.

25. Kuiken T. Targeted reinnervation for improved prosthetic function. Review. *Phys Med Rehabil Clin N Am*. 2006;17(1):1–13.

26. Kuiken TA, Demanian GA, Lipschutz RD, Miller LA, Stubblefield KA. The use of targeted muscle reinnervation for improved myoelectric prosthesis control in a bilateral shoulder disarticulation amputee. *Prosthet Orthot Int.* 2004;28(3):245–253.

27. Kuiken TA, Miller LA, Lipschutz RD, et al. Targeted reinnervation for enhanced prosthetic arm function in a woman with a proximal amputation: a case study. *Lancet.* 2007;369(9559):371–380.

28. O'Shaughnessy KD, Dumanian GA, Lipschutz RD, Miller LA, Stubblefield K, Kuiken TA. Targeted reinnervation to improve prosthesis control in the transhumeral amputees. A report of three cases. *J Bone Joint Surg Am.* 2008;90(2): 393–400.

29. Zhou P, Lowery MM, Englehart KB, et al. Decoding a new neural machine interface for control of artificial limbs. *J Neurophysiol.* 2007;98(5):2974–2982.

30. Barber GG, McPhail NV, Scobie TK, Brennan MC, Ellis CC. A prospective study of lower limb amputations. *Can J Surg.* 1983;26(4):339–341.

31. Deutsch A, English RD, Vermeer TC, Murray PS, Condous M. Removable rigid dressings versus soft dressings: a randomized, controlled study with dysvascular, trans-tibial amputees. *Prosthet Orthot Int.* 2005;29(2):193–200.

32. Frogameni AD, Booth R, Mumaw LA, Cummings V. Comparison of soft dressing and rigid dressing in the healing of amputated limbs of rabbits. *Am J Phys Med Rehabil.* 1989;68(5):234–239.

33. Kane TJ 3rd, Pollak EW. The rigid versus soft postoperative dressing controversy: a controlled study in vascular below-knee amputees. *Am Surg.* 1980;46(4):244–247.

34. Nawijn SE, van der Linde LH, Emmelot CH, Hofstad CJ. Stump management after trans-tibial amputation: a systematic review. *Prosthet Orthot Int.* 2005;29(1):13–26.

35. Smith DG, McFarland LV, Sangeorzan BJ, Reiber GE, Czerniecki JM. Postoperative dressing and management strategies for transtibial amputations: a critical review. *J Rehabil Res Dev.* 2003;40(3):213–224.

36. Mooney V, Harvey JP Jr, McBride E, Snelson R. Comparison of postoperative stump management: plaster vs. soft dressings. *J Bone Joint Surg Am.* 1971;53(2):241–249.

37. Smith DG. General principles of amputation surgery. In: Smith DG, Michael JW, Bowker JH, eds. *Atlas of Amputations and Limb Deficiencies: Surgical, Prosthetic, and Rehabilitation Principles.* 3rd ed. Rosemont, Ill: American Academy of Orthopaedic Surgeons; 2004:21–30.

38. Wilson PD. Early weight-bearing in the treatment of amputations of the lower limbs. *J Bone Joint Surg.* 1922;4:224–227.

39. Berlemont M, Weber R. Temporary prosthetic fitting of lower limb amputees on the operating table. Technic and long-term results in 34 cases. *Acta Orthop Belg.* 1966;32(5):662–667.

40. Burgess EM, Romano RL. The management of lower extremity amputees using immediate postsurgical prostheses. *Clin Orthop Relat Res.* 1968;57:137–146.

41. Mooney V, Nickel VL, Snelson R. Fitting of temporary prosthetic limbs immediately after amputation. *Calif Med.* 1967;107(4):330–333.

42. Pinzur MS, Littooy F, Osterman H, Wafer D. Early post-surgical prosthetic limb fitting in dysvascular below-knee amputees with a pre-fabricated temporary limb. *Orthopedics.* 1988;11(7):1051–1053.

43. Schon LC, Short KW, Soupiou O, Noll K, Rheinstein J. Benefits of early prosthetic management of transtibial amputees: a prospective clinical study of a prefabricated prosthesis. *Foot Ankle Int.* 2002;23(6):509–514.

44. Weinstein ES, Livingston S, Rubin JR. The immediate postoperative prosthesis (IPOP) in ischemia and septic amputations. *Am Surg.* 1988;54(6):386–389.

45. Jebson PJ, Louis DS. Amputations. In: Green DP, ed. *Operative Hand Surgery.* 5th ed. St Louis, Mo: Elsevier; 2005: 1939–1982.

46. Bowker JH, Goldberg B, Poonekar PD. Transtibial amputation: surgical procedures and immediate postsurgical management. In: Bowker JH, Michael JW, eds. *Atlas of Limb Prosthetics: Surgical, Prosthetic, and Rehabilitation Principles.* 2nd ed. St Louis, Mo: Mosby Year Book; 1992: 429–452.

47. Waters RL, Perry J, Antonelli D, Hislop H. Energy cost of walking of amputees: the influence of level of amputation. *J Bone Joint Surg Am.* 1976;58(1):42–46.

48. Czerniecki JM. Rehabilitation in limb deficiency: gait and motion analysis. *Arch Phys Med Rehabil.* 1996;77:S3–S8.

49. Friedmann LW. Rehabilitation of the lower extremity amputee. In: Kottke FJ, Lehmann JF, eds. *Krusen's Handbook of Physical Medicine and Rehabilitation.* 4th ed. Philadelphia, Pa: WB Saunders; 1990: 1024–1069.

50. Anderson WD, Stewart KJ, Wilson Y, Quaba AA. Skin grafts for the salvage of degloved below-knee amputation stumps. *Br J Plast Surg.* 2002;55(4):320–323.

51. Watier E, Georgieu N, Manise O, Husson JL, Pailheret JP. Use of tissue expansion in revision of unhealed below-knee amputation stumps. *Scand J Plast Reconstr Surg Hand Surg.* 2001;35(2):193–196.

52. Gwinn DE, Keeling JJ, Froehner JA, McGuigan FX, Andersen RC. Perioperative differences between bone bridging and non-bone bridging transtibial amputations for wartime lower extremity trauma. *Foot Ankle Int.* In press.

53. Choksy SA, Lee Chong P, Smith C, Ireland M, Beard J. A randomized controlled trial of the use of a tourniquet to reduce blood loss during transtibial amputation for peripheral arterial disease. *Eur J Vasc Endovasc Surg.* 2006;31(6):646–650.

54. Halbert J, Crotty M, Cameron ID. Evidence for the optimal management of acute and chronic phantom pain: a systematic review. *Clin J Pain.* 2002;18(2):84–92.

55. Wolthuis AM, Whitehead E, Ridler BM, Cowan AR, Campbell WB, Thompson JF. Use of a pneumatic tourniquet improves outcome following trans-tibial amputation. *Eur J Vasc Endovasc Surg.* 2006;31(6):642–645.

56. Smith DG, Fergason JR. Transtibial amputations. *Clin Orthop Relat Res.* 1999;361:108–115.

57. Greene WB, Cary JM. Partial foot amputations in children. A comparison of the several types with the Syme amputation. *J Bone Joint Surg Am.* 1982;64(3):438–443.

58. Syme J. On amputation at the ankle joint. *London Edinbourough Monthly J Med Sci.* 1843;3(XXVI):93.

59. Harris RI. The history and development of Syme's amputation. *Artificial Limbs.* 1961;6:4–43.

60. Harris RI. Syme's amputation: the technique essential to secure a satisfactory end-bearing stump: Part I. *Can J Surg.* 1963;6:456–469.

61. Peterson LT. Administrative considerations in the amputation program. In: Mullins WS, Cleveland M, Shands AR, McFetridge EM, eds. *Surgery in World War II: Orthopedic Surgery in the Zone of the Interior.* Washington, DC: Department of the Army, Office of The Surgeon General; 1970.

62. Burgess EM, Matsen FA III. Determining amputation levels in peripheral vascular disease. *J Bone Joint Surg Am.* 1981;63:1493–1497.

63. Tis PV, Callum MJ. Type of incision for below knee amputation. *Cochrane Database Syst Rev.* 2004;(1):CD003749.

64. Pinzur MS, Pinto MA, Saltzman M, Batista F, Gottschalk F, Juknelis D. Health-related quality of life in patients with transtibial amputation and reconstruction with bone bridging of the distal tibia and fibula. *Foot Ankle Int.* 2006;27(11):907–912.

65. Keeling JJ, Schon LC. Tibiofibular bridge synostosis in below knee amputation. *Tech Foot Ankle Surg.* 2007;6(3):156–161.

66. Stewart JD, Anderson CD, Unger DV. The Portsmouth modification of the Ertl bone-bridge transtibial amputation: the challenge of returning amputees back to active duty. *Oper Tech Sports Med*. 2006;13:222–226.

67. Bowen RE, Struble SG, Setoguchi Y, Watts HG. Outcomes of lengthening short lower-extremity amputation stumps with planar fixators. *J Pediatr Orthop*. 2005;25(4):543–547.

68. Latimer HA, Dahners LE, Bynum DK. Lengthening of below-the-knee amputation stumps using the Ilizarov technique. *J Orthop Trauma*.1990;4(4):411–414.

69. Baumgartner RF. Knee disarticulation versus above-knee amputation. *Prosthet Orthot Int*. 1979;3(1):15–19.

70. Pinzur MS, Bowker JH. Knee disarticulation. *Clin Orthop Relat Res*. 1999;361:23–28.

71. Bowker JH, San Giovanni TP, Pinzur MS. North American experience with knee disarticulation with use of a posterior myofasciocutaneous flap. Healing rate and functional results in seventy-seven patients. *J Bone Joint Surg Am*. 2000;82–A(11):1571-1574.

72. Sugarbaker PH, Chretien PA. Hemipelvectomy for buttock tumors utilizing an anterior mycutaneous flap of quadriceps femoris muscle. *Ann Surg*. 1983;197:106–115.

73. Johnson ON, Potter BK, Bonnecarrere ER. Modified abdominoplasty advancement flap for coverage of trauma-related hip disarticulations complicated by heterotopic ossification: a report of two cases and description of surgical technique. *J Trauma*. In press.

74. Waters RL, Mulroy SJ. Energy expenditure of walking in individuals with lower limb amputations. In: Smith DG, Michael JW, Bowker JH, eds. *Atlas of Amputations and Limb Deficiencies: Surgical, Prosthetic, and Rehabilitation Principles*. 3rd ed. Rosemont, Ill: American Academy of Orthopedic Surgeons; 2004: 395–407.

75. Acikel C, Peker F, Akmaz I, Ulku E. Muscle transposition and skin grafting for salvage of below-knee amputation level after bilateral lower extremity thermal injury. *Burns*. 2001;27(8):849–852.

76. Yowler CJ, Patterson BM, Brandt CP, Fratianne RB. Osteocutaneous pedicle flap of the foot for salvage of below-knee amputation level after burn injury. *J Burn Care Rehab*. 2001;22(1):22–25.

77. MacKenzie EJ, Jones AS, Bosse MJ, et al. Health-care costs associated with amputation or reconstruction of a limb-threatening injury. *J Bone Joint Surg Am*. 2007;89(8):1685–1692.

78. MacKenzie EJ, Bosse MJ, Castillo RC, et al. Functional outcomes following trauma-related lower-extremity amputation. *J Bone Joint Surg Am*. 2004;86-A(8):1636–1645.

79. Crawford JR, Coleman N. Total knee arthroplasty in a below-knee amputee. *J Arthroplasty*. 2003;18(5):662–665.

Chapter 9

SPECIAL SURGICAL CONSIDERATIONS FOR THE COMBAT CASUALTY WITH LIMB LOSS

BENJAMIN K. POTTER, MD[*]; ROBERT R. GRANVILLE, MD[†]; MARK R. BAGG, MD[‡]; JONATHAN A. FORSBERG, MD[§]; ROMAN A. HAYDA, MD[¥]; JOHN J. KEELING, MD[¶]; JOSEPH A. SHROUT, MD[**]; JAMES R. FICKE, MD[††]; WILLIAM C. DOUKAS, MD[‡‡]; SCOTT B. SHAWEN, MD[§§]; AND DOUGLAS G. SMITH, MD[¥¥]

Major, Medical Corps, US Army; Musculoskeletal Oncology Fellow, Department of Orthopaedics and Rehabilitation, University of Miami School of Medicine, (D-27), PO Box 016960, Miami, Florida 33101; formerly, Chief Resident, Department of Orthopaedics and Rehabilitation, Walter Reed Army Medical Center, 6900 Georgia Avenue, NW, Washington, DC

†*Colonel, Medical Corps, US Army; Orthopaedic Surgeon, Department of Orthopaedics and Rehabilitation, Brooke Army Medical Center, 3851 Roger Brooke Drive, Fort Sam Houston, Texas 78234; formerly, Director of Amputee Service, Department of Orthopaedics and Rehabilitation, Brooke Army Medical Center, 3851 Roger Brooke Drive, Fort Sam Houston, Texas*

‡*Chairman, Department of Orthopaedics and Rehabilitation, Brooke Army Medical Center, 3851 Roger Brooke Drive, Fort Sam Houston, Texas 78234*

§*Lieutenant Commander, Medical Corps, US Navy; Orthopaedic Surgeon, Department of Orthopaedic Surgery, National Naval Medical Center, 8901 Wisconsin Avenue, Bethesda, Maryland 20889*

¥*Colonel, Medical Corps, US Army; Chief Orthopaedic Trauma, Residence Program Director, Department of Orthopaedic Surgery, Brooke Army Medical Center, 3851 Roger Brooke Drive, Fort Sam Houston, Texas 78234*

¶*Commander, Medical Corps, US Navy; Director, Orthopaedic Trauma and Foot and Ankle Division, Department of Orthopaedics, National Military Medical Center, Walter Reed National Military Medical Center, 8901 Rockville Pike, Bethesda, Maryland 20899*

**Lieutenant Colonel (P), Medical Corps, US Army; Orthopaedic Hand Surgeon, Department of Orthopaedics and Rehabilitation, Walter Reed Army Medical Center, Building 2, 6900 Georgia Avenue, NW, Washington, DC 20307; formerly, Chief, Department of Surgery and Special Care, Kimbrough Ambulatory Care Center, Fort George Meade, Maryland*

††*Colonel, Medical Corps, US Army; Orthopaedic Consultant, US Army Surgeon General; Chairman, Department of Orthopaedics and Rehabilitation, Brooke Army Medical Center, 3851 Roger Brooke Drive, Fort Sam Houston, Texas 78234*

‡‡*Colonel (Retired), Medical Corps, US Army; Chairman, Integrated Department of Orthopaedics and Rehabilitation, National Naval Medical Center/Walter Reed Army Medical Center, 6900 Georgia Avenue, NW, Washington, DC 20307*

§§*Lieutenant Colonel, Medical Corps, US Army; Orthopaedic Surgeon, Integrated Department of Orthopaedics and Rehabilitation, National Naval Medical Center/Walter Reed Army Medical Center, 6900 Georgia Avenue, NW, Washington, DC 20307*

¥¥*Professor of Orthopedic Surgery, Department of Orthopaedic Surgery, University of Washington, Harborview Medical Center, 325 Ninth Avenue, Seattle, Washington 98104*

INTRODUCTION

The operative treatment of the combat casualty with limb loss is challenging, but can also be immensely rewarding. The previous chapter discussed general surgical principles to guide early treatment, prevent complications, and optimize outcomes. This chapter discusses special surgical considerations for specific subgroups of amputees, with emphasis on late complications and patient complaints. Although no individual amputee will (hopefully) require operative intervention for all of the complaints, complications, and issues discussed herein, this chapter may serve as a guidepost in the long-term surgical management of the combat-related amputee.

EVALUATION OF THE LESS-THAN-SUCCESSFUL AMPUTEE

Even highly functioning posttraumatic amputees continue to suffer from perceived physical limitations and pain. Smith et al[1] retrospectively reviewed a large cohort of transtibial amputees, finding that short form 36 (SF-36) health status profile scores were significantly decreased from published normal aged-matched scores in the categories of physical function and role limitations because of physical health problems and pain. Similarly, Gunawardena and associates[2] found that differences in profiles for combat-injured soldiers with unilateral transtibial amputations were largest in scales sensitive to physical health as compared to uninjured, age-matched controls. More proximal levels of amputation and problems with the residual limb and sound leg were significantly associated with poor physical and mental health scores.

When considering the myriad potential causes of amputation-related disability, it is critical to remember that, regardless of how well the operative surgeon perceives the technical success of the surgery, a painful prosthesis will not be used by the patient.[3] To resolve this problem, a critical and systematic approach to the identification of residual disability, both real and perceived, is essential in the evaluation of amputees.

History

As in much of medicine, an adequate and complete history is the first step in the evaluation process. Patient age, comorbidities, and histories of original injury, infection, and revision operative procedures should be explored and documented in appropriate detail. A history of recent trauma or progressively increasing pain should be sought. Daily prosthetic usage, recreational activities, age of the prosthesis, and frequency and types of adjustments should be noted. Pain, perhaps one of the most nebulous areas in all of medicine, is by far the most common presenting problem for amputees. Nonetheless, elucidation of the intensity, onset, and character of the pain is often revealing of underlying cause. Medications, doses, and utilization patterns should be reviewed and discussed.

Numerous types of postamputation pain have been reported. However, three main categories are generally accepted: (1) phantom sensations, (2) phantom limb pain, and (3) residual limb or "stump" pain. Phantom sensations are defined as nonpainful sensations referred to the missing limb. These are estimated to be present in 4% to 20% of congenitally absent limbs and in 53% to 100% of traumatically or surgically removed limbs. Within the limb, sensations of tingling, itching, pins and needles, or numbness can occur. Additionally, "super-added" phenomena such as the sensation of wearing a ring or sock may be present. The phantom limb may "telescope" in size over time, leaving a relatively small area of foot or digits perceived on the stump. These sensations are generally more of a nuisance or curiosity than an overt problem and usually stabilize within the first year following amputation.[4]

Phantom limb pain is nociceptive afferent pain from the amputated limb. The quality of phantom limb pain varies but is generally described as either a burning or throbbing sensation, or a discomfort ranging from a mild ache to excruciating and intolerable pain.[5] Phantom limb pain occurs on some level in as many as 50% to 80% of amputees. Symptomatic neuroma may present with neuropathic pain of similar characteristics, but can frequently be localized and distinguished based on symptom onset, exacerbations, and physical examination.

Residual limb or stump pain is discomfort within, localized to, and identified with the residual limb itself. Although invariably present in the early postoperative period, chronic stump pain generally exhibits a characteristic dull and nagging nature. It has been reported in 6% to 76% of amputees and is not thought to be related to the central neural axis, but rather to organic issues within the residual limb itself.[4] Localized stump pain can be caused by skin disorders, delayed healing, infection, prosthetic fit and alignment issues, or fracture. Hirai et al[6] noted that residual limb problems were seen in about 37% of lower extremity amputees, and identified specific patterns of stump pain associated with different levels and methods of lower extremity amputation, including abnormal keratosis in Syme amputation, equinus deformity in Chopart amputation, reduced muscle power in transfemoral amputation, and knee joint dysfunction in transtibial amputation.

Physical Examination

Surgeons should attempt to develop a systematic approach to examination of a residual extremity that is efficient, complete, and reproducible to avoid over-looking potential problems. In general, examination should proceed gradually from benign maneuvers remote from the source of pain toward direct palpation of the source of discomfort to avoid "guarding" by the patient. Specifically, both passive and active range of motion of adjacent joints should be measured and recorded. Hip and knee flexion contractures are well-known problems associated with lower extremity amputation and may cause a functional limb length discrepancy and resulting problems. Stability, especially of the ankle, knee, shoulder, and elbow joints must be assessed with appropriate stress testing and provocative maneuvers. Strength of major muscle groups should be evaluated and documented as well as a complete sensory examination. Painful neuromas can sometimes be palpated directly, and reproducible symptoms can often be elicited during percussion testing for Tinel's sign.

The patient should be asked to don and doff the prosthesis under direct observation and point with a single digit to specific areas of discomfort or skin breakdown. Brief observation of static standing and ambulation in the prosthesis is essential to evaluate gait abnormalities and malaligned or malfunctioning prosthetic components. Hoagland et al[7] evaluated 251 veterans with major traumatic amputation-related problems. They found that approximately half of all patients had socket problems that caused or contributed to their symptoms. Among this group, 59% of the transtibial and 78% of the transfemoral prostheses had inadequate socket fitting. Improper shaping of socket margins was the most frequently observed deficiency. Moreover, 41% of transtibial and 22% of transfemoral residual limbs demonstrated signs of mechanical skin irritation or skin breakdown. Faulty suspension and alignment, in addition to improper socket fit and construction, contributed to these problems. Excessive stiffness of solid ankle cushion heels was the most common prosthetic foot problem and contributed to gait abnormalities. Socket-related skin complications are less frequently observed in upper extremity amputees, but prosthesis fit and utilization should be evaluated in these patients as well. One of the most important components of patient rehabilitation is the ability to consult with a prosthetist frequently and make pros-

thetic modifications as needed to ensure proper fitting and pressure relief. A more complete discussion of prosthetic alternatives and available modifications is presented elsewhere in this text (Chapters 20–24).

Skin disorders are frequent complaints among amputees due to the intimate and confined nature of the limb within the socket. Skin is challenged by both shear and loading forces delivered by the prosthesis to the residual limb during ambulation or prosthetic use. Furthermore, skin is taxed by the closed socket, which affects temperature regulation and creates a moist environment from sweat accumulation. When a socket is poorly fitted or an inadequate soft tissue envelope is present, chronic and recalcitrant skin changes may develop. Some of the more common skin disorders include verrucose hyperplasia, epidermoid inclusion cysts, contact dermatitis, stump edema, Marjolin's ulcers, and, infrequently, squamous cell carcinoma related to chronic infection. Skin disorders are usually easily identified on visual inspection of the limb.

Similarly, surgical scars may be symptomatic. The optimal surgical scar is linear and avoids bony prominences, the cut end of bone, and socket pressure points. Although ostensibly less of an issue with modern prosthetic liners and sockets, the scar or scars should ideally not lie directly over the terminal residual limb because of these problems. Unfortunately, achieving this scar position is not always possible or practicable in the setting of a posttraumatic or combat-related amputation. Nonetheless, the optimal scar should be freely moveable, soft, pliable, and insensitive. Scar adhesion to bone, in particular, renders the scar immobile and increases the risk of skin breakdown due to excessive shear forces at the skin-liner interface. The adherent scar thus often breaks down, necessitating discontinuance of the prosthesis until healing occurs. Frank wound dehiscence or inflammation, warmth, and persistent redness not relieved by rest and elevation around surgical scars usually heralds underlying infection and should be evaluated with routine laboratory testing of the white blood cell count with differential, erythrocyte sedimentation rate, and C-reactive protein, at a minimum.

Plain radiographic examination of the residual limb is simple and inexpensive and can reveal many problems unique to the traumatic blast-injured amputee. Posttraumatic or age-related arthritis in adjacent joints may be present. Fracture within the residual limb following subsequent trauma or minor falls has been noted by several authors.[8,9] Additionally, heterotopic ossification (HO) and bone spur formation complicate a large percentage of combat-related amputations and can be a disabling source of localized pain.[10] Likewise, nonunion of an attempted bone-bridging distal tibiofibular synostosis can be a potential source of continued pain. Both of these phenomena are discussed in greater detail in subsequent sections of this chapter.

Weight-bearing radiographs taken in the prosthesis can be extremely beneficial for analyzing complications related to myodesis failure and residual limb control or occult soft tissue envelope deficiencies. Xeroradiography is an excellent technique in evaluating the fit and alignment of extremity prostheses. With these tools, the degree of contact achieved and attendant pressure problems, if any, can be precisely determined.[11] More elusive problems thought to be associated with gait-related dynamic interface within the prosthesis can be further investigated in a gait laboratory or using videofluoroscopy, if available.[12]

Magnetic resonance imaging (MRI) has increased in popularity to aid in identification of inflammation-related pathology including bursitis, localized soft tissue inflammation, and bone marrow edema.[13] It is a sensitive tool for evaluation of infection and has demonstrated some utility in evaluation of neuroma formation in amputees.[14] Local lidocaine and steroid injections can be both diagnostic and therapeutic in evaluating and treating these frequently encountered problems.

HETEROTOPIC OSSIFICATION

HO is the formation of lamellar bone in nonosseous tissue. Although infrequently reported in previous modern conflicts, known reports of HO in combat-related amputations date back to World War I[15] and the US Civil War.[16] Because of its apparently increased prevalence following injuries sustained in the recent conflicts in Iraq and Afghanistan, HO is now recognized as a common and not infrequently problematic development in the residual limbs of traumatic and combat-related amputees.[10]

HO formation is thought to require cellular elements capable of osteogenesis, an inciting event, and an environment supportive of bone formation.[17] The most accepted theory about this dysplastic process regards mesenchymal stem cells present in muscle, periosteum, and soft tissue as the cells of origin, with the inciting event in these cases being a blast injury or combat-related trauma.[18] It is now clear that traumatized residual limbs represent a very conducive milieu for this process. Although, as will be discussed, the timing of various putative causative factors and prophylactic measures varies, the nucleus of this metabolic cascade lies at the point of injury. Indeed, clinically evident HO can develop very rapidly following injury (Figures 9-1 and 9-2), and ectopic bone due to any cause is reliably present and detectable in some quantity within 2 months of the instigating stimulus onset, although further growth and maturation may continue thereafter.[19,20]

At least 36% of all combat-related amputees from the current conflicts have radiographically proven HO in their residual limbs. The prevalence jumps to an astounding 63% when only limbs with adequate radiographic follow-up are assessed.[10] Although this latter figure likely represents a degree of selection bias, because patients with palpable or symptomatic lesions are more likely to have follow-up radiographs performed, the actual prevalence likely approaches or exceeds 50%. The scope of the clinical problem is therefore vast and not merely a topic of academic discussion.

Proven and statistically significant risk factors for HO formation in residual limbs of traumatic and combat-related amputees include a final amputation within, rather than above, the initial zone of injury (ZOI) and a blast (vs blunt, sharp, or even high-velocity gunshot) mechanism of injury (MOI). However, HO may also develop due to other, non-blast MOIs (Figure 9-3). Final amputation level within the initial ZOI also appears to be predictive of HO magnitude and severity.[10] In addition to these proven risk factors, a number of other potential causative or confounding factors for

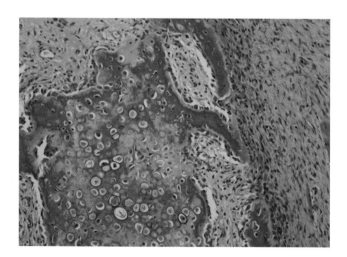

Figure 9-1. Photomicrograph (hematoxylin-eosin stain; original magnification × 20) of a specimen resected from the brachialis muscle of a transhumeral amputation at the time of definitive revision and closure just 15 days after injury. Abundant enchondral heterotopic ossification formation is evident immediately adjacent to normal skeletal muscle.

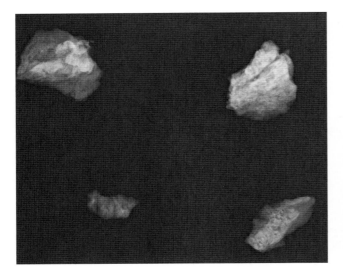

Figure 9-2. Radiograph of resected heterotopic ossification specimens from the soleus muscle belly of a transtibial amputee at the time of definitive amputation and closure 20 days after injury. Although wound vacuum-assisted closure and pulse lavage exposure have been theoretically implicated as potential causes of the apparently increasing prevalence of heterotopic ossification in modern combat-related amputees, the deep superficial compartment of this patient's leg was protected from direct exposure to these devices. The patient underwent elective transtibial amputation for an unreconstructable soft tissue defect associated with a type-IIIB/C tibia fracture after free tissue transfer failed.

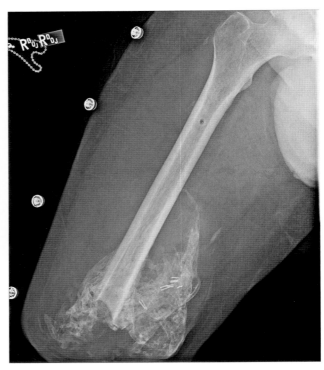

Figure 9-3. Anteroposterior radiograph of a right transfemoral amputation with severe, symptomatic heterotopic ossification following a crush injury sustained in a motor vehicle accident. The patient underwent excision of extensive heterotopic ossification with surgical revision of his residual limb with an excellent clinical result.

the high recent prevalence of HO in residual limbs have been proposed or anecdotally reported. Chief among these is the potentially greater survival of otherwise grievously injured combatants afforded by modern body armor, rapid evacuation and treatment, and medical advances as compared to historical conflicts.

Other potential risk factors for ectopic bone growth within residual limbs include subatmospheric pressure dressings, moderate- to high-pressure pulsatile lavage irrigation systems, occult traumatic brain injury, chronic low-grade local infection, preinjury nutritional supplement use by allied combatants, and other as yet undetermined geographic environmental factors. With the data currently available, none of these has been definitively shown to increase the risk of HO formation in residual limbs.[10] However, such confounding variables, most notably the severity of initial injury to the limb and other body systems, are difficult to adequately control for in statistical data analysis. Further study of these factors is warranted and ongoing.

A wide variety of suppositional prophylactic agents and modalities to prevent HO have been studied, with varied levels of clinical and laboratory evidence of ef-

ficacy, in other patient populations with or at risk for HO. The only modalities definitively proven to prevent HO occurrence are nonsteroidal antiinflammatory drugs (NSAIDs) and local external beam radiation therapy.[20–23] Local radiation therapy within the requisite time frame (24–72 hours of injury) is logistically infeasible in a combat environment, irrespective of concerns about irradiating open wounds and resulting local immunosuppression and inhibition of wound healing, as well as initial uncertainty about the final level of amputation. NSAIDs also have undesirable effects on platelet function, fracture healing, and the renal and gastrointestinal systems. However, in patients with essentially isolated amputations who are putatively able to systemically tolerate this modality, early prophylaxis is reasonable and should be continued for at least 2 and as long as 6 weeks postinjury.

Other proposed prophylactic modalities include vitamin K antagonists, corticosteroids, colchicine, and calcitonin.[24–27] Independent of concerns about coagulopathy, immunosuppression, and other untoward side effects, however, currently available evidence does not support the routine use of any of these agents in the combat-injured amputee. The only agent that has been evaluated for late prophylaxis is the older bisphosphonate etidronate sodium.[28] Enthusiasm for this agent is tempered by frequent symptomatic esophagitis, inhibition of concomitant long-bone fracture healing, and the potential for late "recurrence" of HO after discontinuation of therapy due to delayed mineralization of transiently inhibited ectopic bone. Some long-term benefit may be gained with this modality, however. If bisphosphonate therapy is pursued, etidronate should be used. Newer agents have not been evaluated in relation to HO treatment, and would likely be less efficacious due to greater selectivity and inhibition of osteoclasts, as opposed to the osteoblast suppression desired in HO prophylaxis.

After HO is established within a residual limb, asymptomatic lesions do not require treatment. Particularly in asymptomatic patients in whom the radiographic HO is not palpable, repeated reassurance should be given that the lesion is not a true tumor, no treatment is required, and that asymptomatic HO seldom causes discomfort associated with prosthetic fitting. In dedicated rehabilitation centers where many amputees have HO and some of these have undergone excision, such discussions are critical to avoiding unnecessary and potentially complicated surgery.

The initial treatment of all symptomatic amputees with HO is conservative. The authors have found HO excision with or without amputation revision to be fraught with wound-related and infectious complications. Because of these complications, an exhaustive attempt at nonoperative treatment is indicated prior to excision. This consists of brief periods of rest and activity modification concurrent with adjustments to pain medications, evaluation for alternate causes of residual limb pain (as discussed in the preceding section), and serial prosthetic alignment, socket, suspension, and liner modifications. Using this approach, most patients with symptomatic lesions can be treated conservatively. Of recent combat-related amputees with known HO, nearly 85% were asymptomatic or had been successfully treated conservatively, with only about 7% of all amputees requiring surgical excision of HO.[10]

Once conservative measures have been exhausted and surgery is planned, however, further new socket fitting and prosthesis component changes should be delayed until after the procedure; virtually all patients undergoing HO excision require entirely new sockets postoperatively. Indications for operative intervention include exposed bone, continued skin and soft tissue breakdown, and localizable pain, all of which should be proven refractory to local wound care and/

or repeated prosthetic modifications preoperatively. Patients contemplating an excisional procedure should be counseled that the incidence of wound-related and infection complications requiring additional surgery may approach 25%.

Radiographically, HO may be graded in severity as mild, moderate, or severe based on whether the ectopic bone occupies less than 25%, 25% to 50%, or over 50%, respectively, of the cross-sectional area of the terminal residual limb on plain radiographs.[10] Severe HO is more difficult to excise, requires more extensive surgery for complete excision (including frequent formal myodesis and amputation revision), and is more likely to demand creative soft tissue reconstruction to achieve adequate coverage of the residual limb. However, the shape and depth of heterotopic lesions may be a more critical factor in determining which lesions become symptomatic and require excision (Figures 9-4 and 9-5).

The timing of HO excision has previously been a matter of substantial debate, with many advocates for delayed excision of HO to prevent unacceptable local recurrence rates.[29] The authors have found assessment of historical markers of HO maturity such as bone scan activity and serum alkaline phosphatase to be unhelpful and unnecessary. Plain radiographic evidence of maturity is somewhat helpful (stable, mature cortical rind and no change in appearance on radiographs taken at least 1 month apart), but principally because mature, mineralized bone is technically easier to marginally but completely excise than its softer, cartilaginous precursor. With frequent utilization of adjunctive secondary recurrence prophylaxis (ie, radiotherapy and/or NSAIDs), good results have been obtained, with no clinical recurrences to date, in operations performed as early as 3 months postinjury. The authors therefore advocate excision as soon as required in patients with HO symptoms refractory to conservative measures, which generally take 3 to 4 months to exhaust. At a maximum, 6 months appears to be a more than adequate observation interval from injury to excision for surgeons desiring a more conservative approach.

Preoperative planning and detailed patient counseling are critical to ensuring optimal outcomes following HO excision from residual limbs. In addition to the potential for wound complications, any primary or contingency plans for myodesis takedown, residual limb shortening, or formal revision of the amputation concurrent with the excisional procedure should be discussed with patients preoperatively. All of these factors may affect both subsequent patient function and the postoperative rehabilitation schedule. Although direct data to support secondary HO recur-

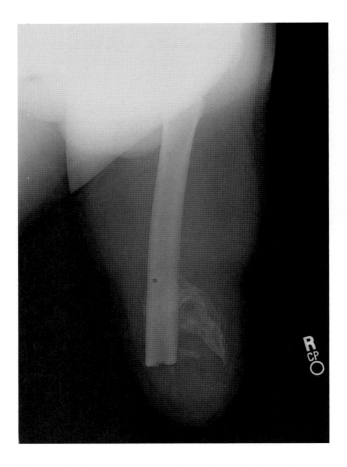

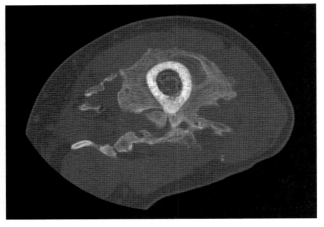

Figure 9-5. Axial computed tomography scan of a left trans-femoral amputee with diffuse heterotopic ossification about his terminal residual limb. Although the patient's preoperative symptoms were greatest laterally, he desired compete excision of the heterotopic ossification. This required complete myodesis takedown and revision amputation concurrent with the heterotopic ossification excision.

Figure 9-4. Anteroposterior radiograph of a left transfemoral amputation demonstrating moderate heterotopic ossification with a prominent, symptomatic distal-lateral spike of ectopic bone. The patient's symptoms were refractory to repeated prosthesis modifications, and he subsequently underwent heterotopic ossification excision through a direct lateral approach without myodesis takedown.

rence prophylaxis are lacking due to a nearly absent control group, the authors advocate routine use of radiotherapy and/or NSAIDs postoperatively based on the potential residual limb compromise that may occur if repeat excision is required. This portion of the postoperative plan should also be discussed with the amputee preoperatively, emphasizing the importance of compliance with, and reporting of side effects related to, postoperative NSAID use.

For relatively uncomplicated cases, orthogonal radiographs of the residual limb are all that is required. For larger, serpentine ectopic bone lesions and those that approach or envelope critical neurovascular structures, preoperative computed tomography scans with coronal, sagittal, and (ideally) three-dimensional reconstructions can be helpful for both preoperative planning and intraoperative reference (Figure 9-6).

Overlying split-thickness skin grafts should be excised concurrently with the HO excisional procedure when practicable. However, soft tissue coverage is often difficult after extensive HO resection, and the majority of any concurrent soft tissue resection should be performed after the HO has been removed. In patients with focal, localizable symptoms or for whom complete excision would require revision with extensive limb shortening or loss of a functional joint level, partial excision of only the most symptomatic HO is a reasonable approach. No evidence indicates that partial excision of HO predisposes the patient to recurrence of the excised portion. A plan for the exact sequence of events during the excisional procedure, including soft tissue coverage and closure as well as the potential need to shorten the residual limb, is helpful in avoiding unsuspected problems.

The authors attribute the relatively high incidence of postoperative infections and wound-related complications to compromised soft tissue envelopes, potentially latent chronic infections, and the frequent culture-positive nature of excised HO specimens. Given the high incidence of postoperative infection and wound-related complications, relatively short-term (~2 weeks) postoperative empiric and subsequently culture-specific antibiotics should be administered, in addition to routine empiric preoperative prophylaxis. Tissue from each resected HO specimen should be sent to microbiology for culture analysis. To further minimize complications, wounds should be irrigated thoroughly following excision, meticulous hemostasis achieved, and layered closure performed over a surgical drain.

Postoperatively, drains should be removed at the bedside generally within 72 hours as indicated by drainage output. Dressings should be changed daily starting on postoperative day 2, and patients should be transitioned back to compressive shrinker stockings as soon as feasible. Sutures should be removed at 2 to 3 weeks postoperatively. For patients with focal excisions and limited dissection, prosthetic fitting and wear may recommence as soon as wound status and comfort allow, in some cases even prior to suture removal. When formal myodesis and amputation revision has been performed, prosthetic rehabilitation should follow a standard protocol and progression similar to, but slightly accelerated from, that utilized for new amputees. New radiographs of the residual limb should be obtained immediately postoperatively, again at 2 to 3 months to assess for possible HO recurrence or myodesis failure, and as clinically indicated thereafter.

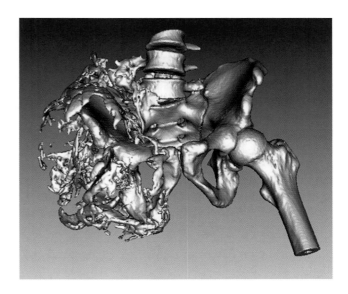

Figure 9-6. Three-dimensional computed tomography scan reconstruction of an amputee with a blast-related right hip disarticulation through the initial zone of injury complicated by severe, diffuse heterotopic ossification.

NEUROMA

Neuroma formation in amputation surgery is inevitable—all transected nerves form neuromas. Currently no technique has been convincingly proven to prevent or ameliorate this process. However, not all neuromas are symptomatic. Persistent symptoms associated with neuromas have been reported in approximately 20% to 30% of amputations,[30,31] and the majority of these can be managed without revision surgery. A discreet area of pain in the vicinity of a palpable nodule and the presence of Tinel's phenomenon are clear indicators of the presence of a symptomatic neuroma. Evaluation of the residual limb with routine radiographs may provide useful information if HO or retained metallic fragments are near the neuroma, but computed tomography or ultrasound rarely provide any information that cannot be determined by a good history, examination, and standard radiographs. Careful evaluation of fine cut MRI scans can occasionally be helpful in identifying neuromas that are otherwise difficult to localize.[14] Prosthetic socket modification is usually sufficient to relieve pressure causing persistent pain from a symptomatic neuroma. However, in recalcitrant cases a diagnostic injection of a local anesthetic at the point of maximal tenderness may help verify the diagnosis as well as provide some prognosis for improvement if surgical excision becomes necessary.

A neuroma that is diagnosed and found to be resistant to all nonoperative measures is best treated with early resection to avoid the development of a "pain generator" and changes in the central neural axis that may result in chronic, refractory pain.[32] The first surgical intervention to remove a painful neuroma is usually the most effective. Tupper and Booth[33] found that in the treatment of 232 neuromas, 65% of patients improved following the first surgery, while only 13% showed improvement following a second operative procedure. Many of the principles outlined in the preceding chapter's section on managing nerves during amputation surgery apply to neuroma surgery. A clean, sharp transection of the nerve proximal to the neuroma, with moderate tension applied, will allow the nerve to retract into the proximal soft tissues. If the surgeon decides to implant the freshly cut nerve end into a local muscle, it is imperative to avoid any tension on the nerve and place the implant in an area free from scar and socket pressure.

Nerves that traverse a relatively superficial anatomic course deserve specific mention. Superficial radial nerve neuromas should be resected so that the remaining nerve end is well beneath the brachioradialis muscle.[34] For neuromas of the peroneal nerve, the surgeon should consider a higher level of resection in the thigh to better insure that the nerve end is beneath the hamstring muscles, while the sural nerve should be allowed to retract deep to the gastrocnemius or into the distal popliteal fossa. When excising a symptomatic neuroma of the sciatic nerve in transfemoral amputees, it is important to remember not to excessively shorten the nerve, which may lead to pain with sitting and is often recalcitrant to repeated attempts at surgical revision. As mentioned previously, pulsatile, throbbing pain, particularly at rest, usually indicates a neuroma in proximity to a blood vessel. Revision surgery for this problem involves separation of the nerve and

blood vessel, repeat ligation of the vessel, and a well-performed traction neurectomy insuring that the nerve is no longer in proximity to the pulsing blood vessel. Adherence to these principles, both conservative and operative, will ensure acceptable relief for the vast majority of amputees with symptomatic neuromas.

MYODESIS FAILURE AND LACK OF SOFT TISSUE PADDING

In response to an increasingly active amputee population, modern amputation techniques emphasize appropriate and durable bone covering as well as anatomic muscle and soft tissue stabilization. In addition to proper socket fit and training, the success and longevity of residual limbs, especially in a young, active population who place supraphysiologic demands on their residual limbs, depend heavily upon the adequacy of this muscular and soft tissue stabilization. Myodesis failure and loss of soft tissue padding are two potential complications facing modern amputees and may contribute significantly to long-term healthcare costs.[35] Thus, it is critical that the treating physician be familiar with the signs and symptoms associated with failure of one or both of these important physiologic constructs.

The approach to the painful or ill-functioning prosthetic limb is multidisciplinary. Close consultation among the patient, orthopaedist, physiatrist, and prosthetist is required to help determine which conditions may respond to socket modifications and which may require further evaluation and surgical treatment (as described in the first section of this chapter). To address failure of myodesis, failure of myoplasty, or loss of soft tissue padding, history and physical examination, weight-bearing radiographs (in and out of the socket), and gait analysis are often successful at identifying the problem.

Myodesis Failure in Transfemoral Amputation

Myodesis of the adductor magnus to the residual femur is critical to restoring proper mechanical alignment and control of the lower extremity.[36,37] Failure to achieve adequate myodesis or catastrophic subsequent rupture of the construct results in a 70% decrease in adduction strength due to a shortened effective movement arm of the weaker adductors longus and brevis (Figure 9-7).[38] The femur, pulled into abduction by the relatively unopposed abductors, can no longer be held in anatomic alignment, even with aggressive socket modifications (Figure 9-8).[37,39–41] The resulting problems, often debilitating, include residual limb pain and ulceration as well as a less-efficient gait cycle, leading to increased energy expenditure during ambulation.[42]

Patients may complain of anterolateral residual limb pain or ulceration despite socket modifications. Subjective weakness in the residual limb, or a decrease in gait velocity, with or without fatigue, often accompanies the discomfort. In highly functional amputees, history may reveal a previously well-functioning limb and well-fitting prosthesis prior to an uncontrolled fall or hyperabduction injury. This may indicate a catastrophic failure of the myodesis. An exaggerated side lurch or a circumduction gait is noticeable as the patient compensates for an inadequate adductor mechanism.

Physical examination may reveal a flexed and abducted residual limb, as well as a bony prominence anterolaterally. An "adductor roll" may be present above the socket line medially, caused, in part, by the retracted adductor musculature. Strength and isometric testing would reveal weak adduction and extension, without a palpable contraction of the adductor longus or hamstring muscle bellies. Radiographic evaluation including weight-bearing anteroposterior and lateral radiographs of the residual limb would reveal an excessively flexed and abducted femur within the soft tissue envelope of the residual limb.

Once the diagnosis of myodesis failure or insufficiency has been made, it is important to assess the amputee's level of functioning before committing to an elective surgical revision. Sedentary or otherwise low-demand patients without ulceration may respond to socket modifications and continue to function adequately despite an insufficient adductor mechanism.[39,40] Most patients, however, may not respond adequately to socket modifications and may desire to achieve (or return to) a higher level of functioning. These amputees require a timely revision procedure to restore proper anatomic alignment to the residual femur.

In these situations, revision or reconstruction of the adductor mechanism should be performed as soon after diagnosis as possible. Scarring and retraction of the adductors and hamstrings can make delayed repair more difficult. Also, some evidence suggests that within a residual limb, retracted muscles atrophy over time, losing up to 60% of their cross-sectional area (and thus the majority of their contractile strength), compared to muscles in which the length-tension relationship

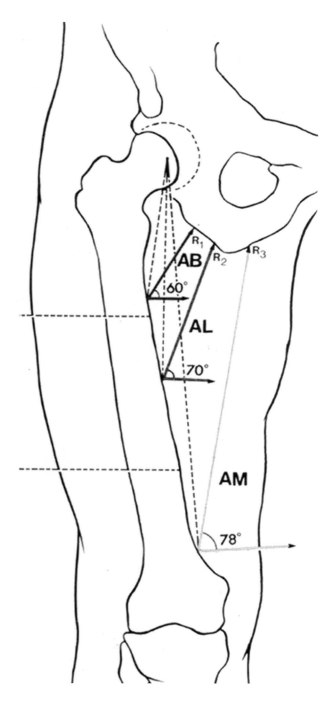

was preserved.[43–45] Early rather than delayed repair of the adductor mechanism is therefore preferred to maximize potential restoration of the residual femur to anatomic alignment, as well as to minimize the difficulty of the reconstruction.

Repair of the insufficient adductor mechanism is technically demanding and consists of meticulous identification of the adductor magnus and hamstring tendons. Previous incisions should be used, and the development of flaps minimized. If adequate tendon length is present, the myodesis is performed in much the same way as a primary transfemoral amputation. The authors recommend the technique described by Gottschalk[38] as outlined in greater detail in the previous chapter. If the adductor and medial hamstring tendons are insufficient for this task, femoral shortening may be required and the patient should be counseled accordingly. In severe or unique cases, reconstruction of the adductor mechanism using soft tissue autograft, allograft, or xenograft may be necessary. Metal vascular clips may be attached to the adductor mechanism near its new insertion in an effort to provide a radiographic indicator of myodesis integrity.

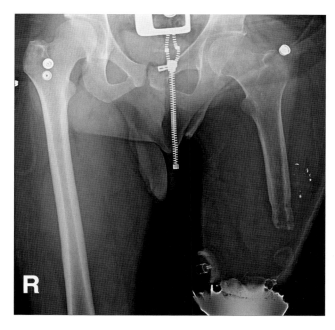

Figure 9-7. Diagram of the resultant forces of the adductor muscles. The relative insertion sites of the adductors are indicated. Progressive shortening of the residual femur results in increasing weakness in adduction as a result of progressive loss of adductor function.
AB: adductor brevis
AL: adductor longus
AM: adductor magnus
Reproduced with permission from: Pinzur MS, Gottschalk FA, Pinto MAG, Smith DG. Controversies in lower-extremity amputation. *J Bone Joint Surg Am.* 2007;89:1118–1127, Figure 7.

Figure 9-8. Standing anterior-posterior radiograph of a transfemoral amputee in his prosthesis demonstrating failure of the adductor magnus myodesis. Due to the resulting deficiency in adductor strength, the residual femur is pulled into progressive abduction, altering the alignment of the residual femur versus the normal mechanical axis in the contralateral sound limb femur, producing a less efficient gait, and causing a focal pressure point against the distal lateral socket, which was a source of the patient's discomfort.

Prolonged adductor pain is common in patients who have undergone revision myodesis. Adequate early pain control with judicious use of muscle relaxants and abduction precautions to protect the myodesis repair is important. Likewise, close consultation with a physical therapist in addition to the prosthetist is critical. After adequate early healing of the wound and myodesis, early rehabilitation should focus on active adduction and extension exercises before a return to prosthetic fitting and rehabilitation.

Inadequate myoplasty or soft tissue padding in the transfemoral amputation is rare, but can be a source of pain and disability. Although most cases result from an inadequate adductor myodesis as discussed above, some can be caused by failure of the quadriceps myoplasty itself. This can often be appreciated clinically via new anterior distal prominence of the residual femur as well as hypermobility of the anterior residual limb skin with active quadriceps contraction. Additionally, traumatic and combat-related amputees may have a paucity of healthy and robust residual limb soft tissue due to appropriate early efforts to maintain maximal residual limb length in the setting of a broad ZOI. Short of revision with substantial shortening of the residual limb or free tissue transfer, both operative options of last resort, reconstructive alternatives may be quite limited in this setting. Fortunately, socket modifications can succeed in improving symptoms in the majority of cases, and it is thus important to maximize the benefits of nonoperative therapy prior to surgery. Revision of the quadriceps myoplasty is unlikely to be successful, especially in a high-demand patient, if the adductor myodesis is inadequate. Therefore, it is important to assess these two structures thoroughly and concurrently.

Myodesis and Myoplasty Failure in Transtibial Amputation

Myodesis and/or myoplasty within the transtibial amputation provides the residual limb with a durable end-bearing muscle mass. Standard posterior (Burgess-type) flaps are perhaps the most durable and employ a myodesis technique.[46,47] Sagittal, skew, and free flaps provide end-bearing bulk by myoplasty alone, or a combination of myoplasty and myodesis.[48–51] The so-called "fishmouth" flap is used in rare cases to salvage bone length when the posterior musculature is inadequate. It is formed by two equal anterior and posterior fasciocutaneous flaps that provide little or no muscular coverage over the distal tibia suitable for end-bearing. For this reason it is not routinely used, but reserved for salvage cases only.

Loss of durable end-bearing musculature in the transtibial amputation causes pressure-related pain with prosthetic wear. Patients may complain of anterior residual limb pain or present with skin breakdown and ulceration. History may reveal a previously well-functioning limb and well-fitting prosthesis prior to a fall onto the residual limb, which may indicate an acute failure of the myodesis or myoplasty.

Physical examination will reveal a prominent anterior and distal tibia. Depending on the type of flap used, retraction of the posterior musculature or a rent in the skew flap myodesis will be palpable. As with any amputation revision, nonoperative management including socket modifications may result in a functional and painless limb and should be exhausted preoperatively. For the same reasons listed above, however, most young, active amputees may not respond adequately to socket modifications and may desire a higher level of function and residual limb durability. This subset of patients requires a timely revision procedure to restore durable end-bearing muscle to the distal tibia. For overt myodesis failure presenting acutely, particularly if occurring relatively early in the soldier's initial rehabilitation, immediate operative repair without a trial of nonoperative treatment is reasonable.

Revision of the transtibial myodesis or myoplasty is challenging. In the acute setting, a simple myodesis or myoplasty repair may be possible; however, retracted posterior compartment muscles are often scarred and difficult to mobilize. Shortening of the residual tibia and fibula is almost always necessary to ensure an adequate, durable myodesis. Care must be taken, however, to avoid overtightening the myofascia of the posterior compartment, which may cause a knee flexion contracture and predispose the patient to early failure of the (revision) myodesis. The anterior bevel of the tibia should also be revised, if needed, and the myodesis performed with stout nonabsorbable sutures. It is important to note that the lateral gastrocnemius undergoes far less atrophy than its medial counterpart, and may contribute a more robust construct to the repair.[52,53] Myoplasty repair, if indicated, may be performed with long-lasting absorbable suture, and consideration should be given to augment the repair with a myodesis technique to prevent recurrence.

As in most amputation revision surgery, previous incisions should be utilized and the development of flaps minimized. Although the development of a knee flexion contracture is undesirable, residual limb rest with the knee in slight flexion for a few days postoperatively is reasonable to permit the muscles to adapt to their new resting length and minimize tension on the myodesis. Early rehabilitation should then focus on gentle passive knee extension and active-assisted knee range-of-motion exercises.

Myoplasty Failure in Transhumeral Amputation

In contrast to lower extremity amputations in which the myodesis and myoplasty form a durable end-bearing pad, myoplasty techniques of the arm serve to stabilize the musculature and contain the residual humerus within the soft tissue envelope. Additionally, for high-demand amputees utilizing myoelectric prostheses, stable myodesis may be required for optimal residual limb and terminal device control.

Failure of the myoplasty is often characterized by the insidious onset of symptoms; catastrophic (or acute) failure is rare. Patients may complain of a painful snapping sensation with range of motion or pressure-related pain with prosthesis wear. Physical examination may reveal a painful bursa overlying an area of inadequate myodesis; however, palpating a defect (rent) in the myoplasty is the key to diagnosis.

As with any amputation revision, nonoperative management must be exhaustive, including socket modifications, local wound care (if necessary), and prosthesis rest. Those amputees who do not improve with nonoperative management require surgical repair. In the authors' experience, higher demand amputees are more likely to fail conservative management for these issues, which should be a consideration when selecting patients for surgery as well as timing the surgery.

Repair of the myoplasty should be performed as soon as possible to minimize the effect of muscular contraction and scarring. The myofascia should be repaired with a mild amount of tension to restore the muscle bellies to resting length and tension. This ensures a maximum myoelectric signal generation for applicable prostheses.[54] Shortening of the humerus is occasionally required, depending on the timing of the repair and general condition of the remaining soft tissues. As with other amputation revisions, previous incisions should be used, and the development of flaps minimized. Postoperative care and rehabilitation are similar to those in primary transhumeral amputations.

Myodesis and Myoplasty Failure in Transradial Amputation

Myodesis in the transradial amputation serves a similar purpose to that performed in a transhumeral amputation. Anterior and posterior muscle flaps are used to contain the residual radius and ulna within a durable, stable myofascial construct. Failure of the myoplasty is rare at this level but is characterized by a prominent distal radius or ulna. As in the transhumeral level, patients may also complain of a painful snapping within their residual limb as well as pressure-related pain with prosthesis wear. Physical examination will indicate an area of inadequate myoplasty and may reveal an overlying painful bursa. Once again, identifying a palpable rent in the myoplasty or new focal area of prominent bone is the key to diagnosis.

Nonoperative management, including socket modifications, local wound care (if necessary), and prosthesis rest will likely provide symptomatic relief and should be exhausted prior to surgery. Those amputees who do not improve with nonoperative management require surgical repair. Again, as with all cases of suspected myodesis or myoplasty failure, conservative options should be pursued expeditiously to minimize muscle retraction and scarring in those cases requiring revision surgery. The myofascia or tendons should be repaired while keeping the muscle bellies at resting length and tension to maximize distal bone stability, residual limb control, and myoelectric signal generation.[54] Shortening of the radius and ulna is sometimes required because more muscle mass is available proximally; however, progressive loss of residual forearm length directly correlates to a decrease in forearm rotation.[55] This must be kept in mind when planning to shorten a transradial amputation, and the patient must be counseled accordingly. For more distal transradial amputations, retracted tendons can often be mobilized sufficiently via proximal dissection so that shortening is not required. Neuromata, if present, may also be addressed during the revision surgery. As with other amputation revisions, previous incisions should be used, and the development of flaps minimized. Postoperative care and rehabilitation are similar to those in primary transradial amputations.

OSTEOMYOPLASTIC TRANSTIBIAL AMPUTATION: THE ERTL PROCEDURE

In 1939 Janos Ertl[56] published a technique for transtibial amputation revision for problematic residual limbs, which he developed treating World War I amputees in Hungary. In 1949 he published his experience treating 6,000 amputees following World War II.[57] His original technique calls for raising periosteum from the

medial aspect of fibula with attached cortical chips and suturing it to the lateral tibial periosteum. A similar flap of periosteum is raised from the anteromedial tibia. The distal tibia and fibula are then cut at the same level, taking care to carefully bevel the tibial crest and round off all cortical edges. The tibial periosteum is then sutured to lateral fibular periosteum. Anteriorly and posteriorly, the edges of the two periosteal flaps are sutured together, forming a tube of periosteum with opposed "cambrial" surfaces and viable bone chips. With time, a synostosis forms between the two bones, with a broad, smooth surface (Figure 9-9). Ertl felt this allowed end bearing in the socket, reducing pain and improving function. He also proposed that, by sealing the medullary canal, "normal bone physiology" was restored.

The procedure continues to have proponents in Europe.[58] In the United States, two generations of Ertl descendants have been proponents of the elder Dr Ertl's techniques.[59] During the Vietnam War, the technique was utilized at Valley Forge General Hospital, the Army's amputee center at the time, for revision of problematic transtibial amputations.[60] Deffer, Moll, and LaNoue[60] reported a case series of 155 patients, giving their opinion that the technique allowed more reliably successful total-contact fitting in their young, active, patient population. In cases of short residual limb length, they successfully utilized free autograft, iliac crest, and rib to form the bone bridge. Pinto and Harris[61] advocated the use of a fibular segment to form the distal tibiofibular synostosis, noting that approximately 7 cm of tibia must be resected to harvest an adequate amount of tibial periosteum. They advocate leaving the adjacent viable lateral compartment muscle attached, performing a closing wedge osteotomy to swing the fibular segment into a slot in the lateral tibial cortex, so the healing will more closely approach fracture healing.

Although the Ertl procedure has many proponents, most of the published literature on the subject consists of case series. A recent review of that literature found a single controlled outcome study.[62] Pinzur and associates[62] reported on 32 consecutive patients with modified Ertl transtibial amputations for a variety of diagnoses, compared to a historical "control" group of 17 transtibial amputees who had been treated by the classic Burgess technique and who were considered to be highly functional. A validated outcome instrument, the prosthetics evaluation questionnaire, measuring "quality of life and functional demands in patients with lower extremity amputations," was administered to the Ertl group at an average of 16.3 months and to the Burgess group and an average of 14.7 years. The Ertl group scored better in ambulation ($P = 0.037$) and frustration ($P < 0.001$) and lower in appearance ($P = 0.025$). The results in the other six domains were similar between the two groups. The authors conclude that bone-bridging "may enhance patient-perceived functional outcomes." No randomized or blinded studies

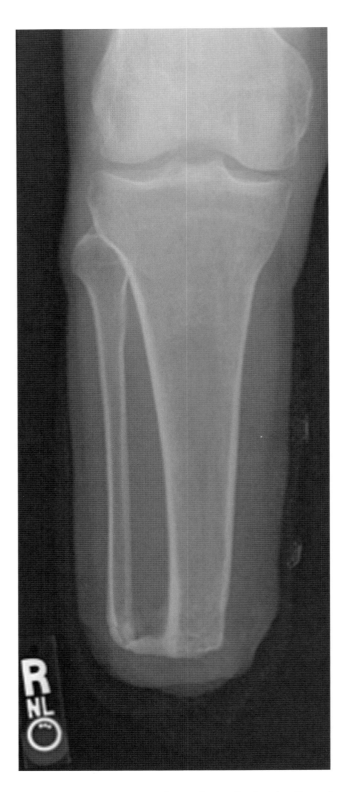

Figure 9-9. Anterior-posterior radiograph after healing of a classic osteomyoplastic transtibial amputation utilizing the classic Ertl technique with strips of tibial and fibular periosteum.

have been performed assessing function or outcomes.

The osteoplastic transtibial amputation technique has been performed on a limited number of amputees from the current wars in Iraq and Afghanistan. Because the current practice is to perform length-preserving amputations in the ZOI, fibular instability due to rupture of the interosseous membrane is not uncommon. There is a general consensus among military orthopaedic surgeons that synostosis is strongly indicated in this clinical situation. A variety of techniques have been used, with roughly an even split between the closing wedge technique and the use of a free segment of autograft fibula. In the latter case, the segment should be relatively short, because a narrower distal tibiofibular distance and osteoplasty length is thought to maximize osseous stability and be less likely to cause a symptomatic osseous prominence. The graft can be stabilized via one of several techniques. Often,

a single 3.5-mm cortical screw is placed through the lateral fibular cortex, through the medullary canal of the graft segment, and through one or two cortices of the tibia (Figure 9-10). The graft can also be secured via intraosseous sutures utilizing devices designed for anterior cruciate ligament graft or syndesmotic stabilization (Figure 9-11). Alternatively, drill holes can be made in both the distal tibia and fibula and the graft secured with heavy, nonabsorbable suture in a fashion resembling a myodesis (Figure 9-12).

If available, the periosteum of the anteromedial tibia, which is invariably thick and easily raised, is then

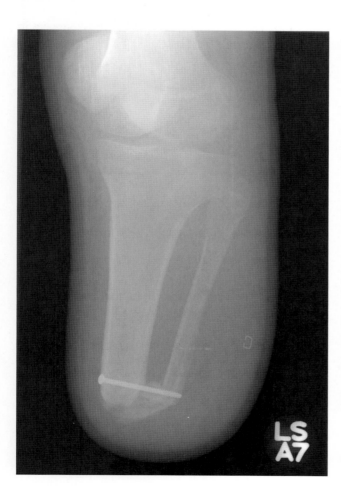

Figure 9-10. Postoperative anterior-posterior radiograph demonstrating a distal tibiofibular synostosis in a transtibial amputation secured with a 3.5-mm cortical screw.

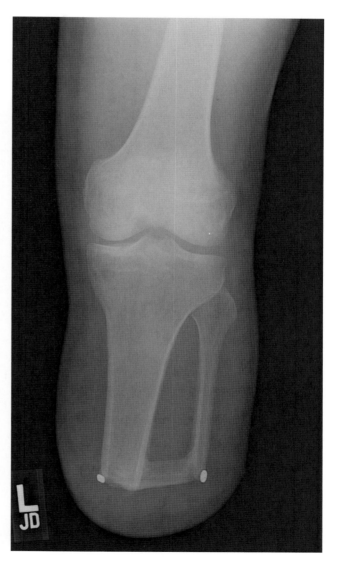

Figure 9-11. Anterior-posterior radiograph demonstrating a healed distal tibiofibular synostosis in a transtibial amputation secured with an intraosseous suture technique.

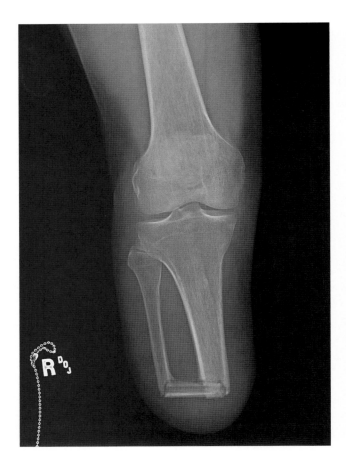

Figure 9-12. Anterior-posterior radiograph demonstrating a distal tibiofibular synostosis in a transtibial amputation utilizing fibular autograft and tibial periosteum and secured with tranosseous heavy, nonabsorbable sutures at both graft junctions. Early postoperative remodeling and healing is evident in this image obtained 8 weeks postoperatively.

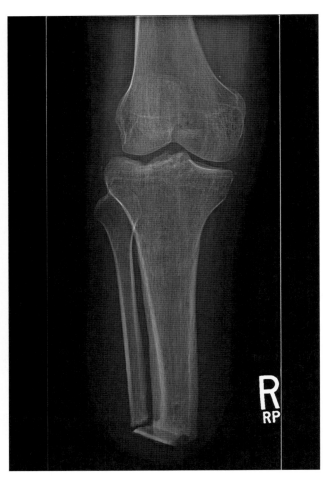

Figure 9-13. Anterior-posterior radiograph demonstrating a nonunion of a distal tibiofibular synostosis at nearly 1 year postoperatively.

sutured over the cut end of the tibia and to the lateral fibular periosteum. This speeds graft incorporation, and extensive remodeling of the synostosis has been noted over time, with its distal profile becoming gradually rounded off in both the anteroposterior and lateral planes. The authors have not noted any frequent problems with graft incorporation when viable periosteum was unavailable, as is the case in most revision cases; although nonunions do occasionally develop (Figure 9-13), they are infrequently symptomatic. Occasionally percutaneous screw removal had to be performed when the screw head became prominent due to osseous remodeling. In revision cases without evidence of latent infection and in which both fibular autograft and tibial periosteum are unavailable without excessive residual limb shortening, use of tricortical iliac crest autograft or fibular allograft may be considered. Finally, as an alternative source of local autograft, the

surgeon may perform a partial tibial osteotomy, hinged distally and utilizing a segment of lateral tibial cortex as graft, while maintaining the overall length of both the tibia and fibula.

The use of the Ertl technique in other clinical situations remains controversial. Because of the risk of infection, many surgeons are reluctant to leave a devascularized fibular segment or a metal implant at the time of delayed primary closure of an amputation through the ZOI. Concern for infection is less in revision surgery above the ZOI, such as transtibial amputation following failed salvage of severe hindfoot injury. The patient with a painful residual limb, who on physical examination has pain with manipulation of the fibula or progressive splaying of the fibula on serial radiographs, may also benefit from synostosis. That said, the surgeon must exercise care to identify and address other causes of lateral residual limb pain, such as peroneal neuroma, or run the risk of a failed outcome and persistent symptoms despite the achievement of radiographic synostosis. Because of the lack of a convincing body of evidence for the superiority of the Ertl over the Burgess technique, synostosis is performed on the basis of surgeon preference and training. Studies are currently in progress that will examine both subjective and objective results comparing the two techniques using outcome instruments such as the SF-36, gait analysis, and videofluorscopy of the residual limb-prosthesis interface, which may provide an evidence-based choice of operative technique.

Much anecdotal advocacy for the Ertl appears on the Internet and in the prosthetic business community.[63] Several patients have requested that highly functional Burgess amputations be revised to Ertls based on this promotional material, including patients successfully running long distances and playing cutting sports. The authors feel these requests are based on limited information, and strongly discourage them. Nonetheless, some patients have found civilian surgeons willing to revise their residual limbs following retirement from active duty.

In summary, the osteomyoplastic transtibial amputation offers the theoretical benefit of allowing distal end bearing, and is definitely indicated acutely in cases where the interosseous membrane has torn and the fibula is unstable. As a revision procedure, it is also useful in cases where fibular hypermobility can be identified as a pain generator. No strong evidence in the literature, however, shows a significant improvement in outcome over amputation without synostosis in patients with a stable fibula. Studies are underway that may further clarify this controversy.

MANAGEMENT OF BURNS AND SKIN GRAFTS

Burn-Related Amputations

Burn injuries may occur due to chemical, electrical, or flash fire-type mechanisms.[64] Burns sustained in combat-related injuries, with or without associated amputation, typically result from fires or thermal injuries secondary to conventional or improvised ordinance and thus fall into the latter category. Burns from volatile compounds such as white phosphorus or actual chemical weapons fortunately remain absent from the present battlefield environment.

In the present conflicts, approximately 5% of all major injuries requiring evacuation from theater have been amputations.[65] A similar proportion of amputees have had concomitant burn injuries, with burns involving the residual limb in nearly 75% of cases. Roughly 6% of patients requiring burn center treatment were amputees, and the proportion of burn patients with multiple limb amputations has not been significantly different from that of amputees without burns. The average burn size has been 40% of total-body surface area (TBSA) involved in the burn amputee group, as compared to 16% TBSA in the entire burn cohort.

In contrast to most combat-related amputations, which often occur as a direct result of the inciting trauma or during early surgical management, nearly 45% of burn-related amputations are ultimately performed at the definitive treatment facility due to early (15%) or late (30%) burn-related complications. Amputees with burn injuries have demonstrated a greater mortality rate (24%) than their nonamputee burn patient counterparts (6%). Thus, burns in the combat-injured amputee complicate treatment and rehabilitation and are associated with higher mortality. Half of the amputations were complete in theater, while 6% had unreconstructable fractures, and 9% required amputation due to progressive ischemia from required vasopressor support. In the delayed amputation group, 21% required amputation due solely to the severity of the burn. The remaining 9% had complications of infection or nonunion. These rates are in direct contradistinction to the available civilian literature on burn-related amputations: the rate of amputations among burn unit patients at civilian centers is 1% to 2%, with the vast majority of these amputations being performed in delayed fashion[66] and burns being more likely to result in multiple limb amputations.[67] Multiple studies have demonstrated a survival benefit to amputation in the management of severe burn patients.[68,69]

Initial in-theater management of the combat-related burn patient with or without amputation follows basic advanced trauma life support and burn protocols. Appropriate early and subsequent attention must be paid to hypothermia, volume resuscitation, electrolyte imbalances, coagulopathy, infection, associated inhalational injuries, and tissue necrosis that may result in sepsis or renal failure.

Surgical principles followed for burn amputees are similar to those recommended for all combat-related amputations, with initial open management and length preservation. In the absence of ongoing sepsis and/or hypotension requiring vasopressors, which may result in additional tissue necrosis and ischemia, tissue viability is generally clinically evident within 4 to 7 days following injury.[64] This time frame coincides with the average arrival time at definitive treatment facilities in the present conflicts. Thus, advanced techniques of tissue viability assessment, such as nuclear medicine scans, have not been routinely required in the authors' experience. Amputees with burn injuries require, in general, a substantially greater number of operative procedures during their initial hospitalization than their counterparts without burns.

Myodesis at the time of definitive treatment is typically performed. One particularly useful technique is to utilize extra-long muscle and/or skin flaps to cover bone and other structures, preserving length and even amputation levels. Even when the entire medial face of the tibia was exposed, a carefully designed very long posterior flap extending down to the plantar foot can preserve a transtibial level (Figure 9-14). Heroic attempts to salvage residual limb length or functional joint levels are indicated in some instances, particularly in multiple limb burn amputees who otherwise would be less likely to achieve independent function

and ambulation.[66] The results of such procedures can be extremely gratifying.[70] However, flap coverage is best performed late, after tissue viability, physiologic status, and residual limb wounds have stabilized; flap failure has been significantly associated with early coverage in burn patients.[71] Eventual skin grafting of residual limbs is routinely required in most patients with burns, and in most cases resulted in a functional residual limb[72] (Figure 9-15).

Most of the civilian medical literature discussing amputations secondary to or associated with burn injuries is limited to case reports or small case series, many of which address electrical injuries. There is general agreement that amputee rehabilitation and prosthetic fitting is complex and frequently delayed secondary to additional surgeries, concomitant medical problems, open wounds and wound instability, edema,

a
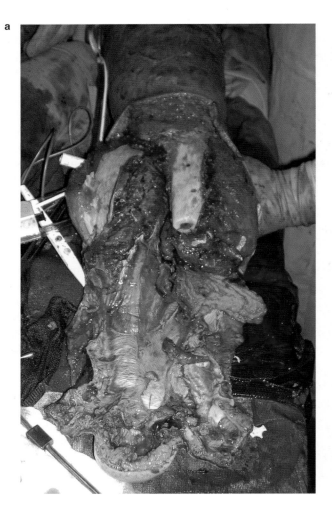

b
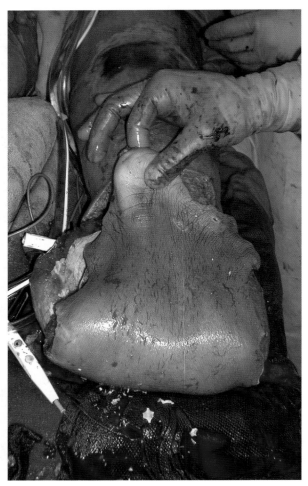

Figure 9-14. Intraoperative photographs of a transtibial amputation with burns of the residual limb. An extra long posterior flap was utilized to compensate for inadequate anterior soft tissue coverage, avoiding the need for a skin graft and salvaging an extremely functional final residual limb length.

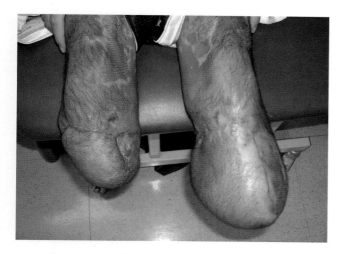

Figure 9-15. Clinical photograph of a healed bilateral transtibial amputee who presented with extensive burns of his residual limbs. Relatively long posterior flaps were utilized, minimizing the need for split-thickness skin grafting. The required skin grafts, which healed uneventfully and functioned well, were not placed over osseous prominences near the terminal residual limb, areas of relatively greater direct pressure and shear forces.

the need for skin graft maturation, hypertrophic and often painful scarring on the residual limb, and joint contractures.[66,68,72,73] The average time to prosthetic fitting of burn amputees in the authors' experience has been over 110 days, or nearly two to three times that of most nonburn amputees. Additionally, burn amputees who had larger burn surface injuries (> 40% TBSA) had a slightly higher average time to prosthetic fitting than burn amputees with less involvement. Due to lower shear forces placed on the residual limb at the skin-prosthesis interface, upper extremity burn amputees without rate-limiting concomitant injuries may be candidates for accelerated prosthetic fitting, training, and rehabilitation.[74]

Skin Grafts

When practicable, skin grafting of residual limbs is best avoided. Although satisfactory results can be achieved in most cases with the techniques described, concerns about chronic and recurrent complications ranging from minor patient discomfort to skin breakdown and ulceration or frank graft failure remain. Split-thickness skin grafts (STSGs) placed over terminal residual limbs or directly over bony prominences are particularly problematic. Current silicone liners, however, have decreased the rate of complications associated with skin grafting of the residual limb. In patients with adequate residual limb length, modest

shortening to achieve adequate native myofasciocutaneous coverage is warranted. However, in many cases, the need for skin grafting cannot be avoided without substantial residual limb shortening or functional joint levels. Furthermore, most combat-related amputees have soft tissue and/or osseous injuries proximal to their residual limb, making shortening or revision to a more proximal level an even less appealing alternative.

When necessary, the authors advocate slightly thicker than typical STSGs (12–16 thousands of an inch) to maximize final residual limb soft tissue durability. With adequate wound bed preparation, including the absence of active infection or nonviable tissue and evidence of early healing granulation tissue formation, failure of these grafts has not been a problem in our experience. However, thicker STSGs may not be possible in burn patients with large TBSA involvement, in whom repeat donor site harvest is sometimes necessary.

Full-thickness pinch grafts can be useful to cover small areas, particularly over the terminal residual limb, but are more prone to early graft necrosis and failure than split-thickness grafts; when utilized, full-thickness grafts should be liberally perforated with a no. 15 blade in order to prevent seroma or hematoma accumulation and subsequent graft separation and failure. In patients undergoing skin grafting at the time of definitive amputation, skin that would otherwise be discarded can sometimes be harvested from the terminal limb or revised viable skin flaps.

Every effort should be made to place grafts over viable underlying muscle, both to ensure graft survival and maximize ultimate function via adequate soft tissue padding. Grafts placed directly on fascia or periosteum, even when "successful," are frequently problematic in the long term. The utilization of creative, atypical myofascial flaps and, occasionally, free flaps, is critical to avoid these problems. When such flaps are not possible, bioartificial dermal substitutes can be useful in restoring soft tissue contour or substituting for the absent native dermis.[75,76] Placed in areas of exposed tendon or bone or otherwise inadequate soft tissue coverage, the grafts should be allowed to incorporate and mature with regular dressing changes for a period of 10 to 21 days, followed by planned, delayed STSG. Grafts can also be layered at 10- to 14-day intervals in an effort to restore normal surface contour to particularly cavitary defects.[76] Treatment with this method is time consuming and can be costly, but the authors have had generally favorable results in a few amputees and a number of nonamputee combat-injured service members.

Myriad conventional graft bolstering techniques have been described in civilian settings. However, when feasible, the authors advocate placement of subatmospheric pressure dressings (VAC; KCI, San Antonio, Tex) to cover STSGs for the first 4 to 5 days postoperatively. Although military medical treatment allows managing these dressings in an inpatient setting in most cases, due to associated injuries, ongoing inpatient rehabilitation, or social concerns not often present in civilian trauma (as well as the general absence of third-party pressure to accelerate discharge), portable units are now available for outpatient use. Numerous series have demonstrated increased graft survival with VAC use compared to conventional techniques.[77–79]

After initial graft healing, careful transition to conventional shrinker compression stocking use can be initiated at 2 to 3 weeks postoperatively. A supplemental dressing beneath the shrinker is generally used initially to protect the graft and cover peripheral areas of ongoing granulation and healing by secondary intention. Prosthetic fitting and, in particular, use are delayed until more definitive graft maturation has occurred. Utilizing this and similar techniques, most amputees requiring skin grafting of their residual limbs can ultimately be fit with and operate a functional prosthesis.[72]

Late wound problems after skin grafting are best managed early and aggressively (albeit nonoperatively) via local wound care, transient activity modification, and prosthetic modification. Problematic grafts can often be treated with late excision and primary closure with adjacent fasciocutaneous advancement after early soft tissue healing and swelling subsidence, or concurrently with excision of symptomatic HO and salvage of redundant native skin. In other cases, catastrophic graft failures following multiple grafting attempts or as a result of prosthesis wear, in addition to patients chronically dissatisfied with their residual limb function or discomfort, may require discussion of more aggressive alternatives including tissue expanders, free tissue transfer, or residual limb shortening or revision to a more proximal level.

JOINT CONTRACTURES

Lower Extremity Contracture

Contracture is a potential complication of any amputation including the lower extremity. Although very uncommon in traumatic amputees, severe contractures may be seen in amputees with neurological injury or vascular disease. Significant contracture can challenge prosthetic fitting and limit functional return. Contractures may also be associated with decubitus ulcers and complicate seating and patient positioning. For these reasons, prevention and aggressive management of contracture are very important in the rehabilitation of war-related amputee care.

Contractures in amputees are caused by many factors. The resulting change in limb length sometimes allows one muscle group to dominate, due to injured, inefficient, or absent antagonist muscle groups, leading to contracture formation. Such a situation is observed in midfoot and hindfoot amputations, when a fixed equinus deformity develops because of unopposed pull of the gastrocsoleus complex, or in a transtibial amputee who develops a knee flexion contracture because of excessive pull of the hamstrings. Contractures are often also exacerbated by delayed prosthetic fitting and mobility training. In addition, pain can often inhibit range of motion of joints and contribute to contracture formation. In the hip, problems are often encountered with prolonged seating or semirecumbent positioning, with shorter residual limbs being at greater risk for contracture development.

The presence of injury proximal to the level of amputation may also be a cause of contracture. In the transtibial amputee, injury to the knee or the distal femur may cause quadriceps scarring, HO, and limited motion in flexion, leading to an extension contracture. Standing is not impaired, but the limitation of flexion makes sitting more difficult in a vehicle and limits high-level function such as running. In these situations, a quick connecting coupler to the prosthetic limb can be a simple solution to facilitate sitting.

The treatment of contracture should be initiated at the time of surgical amputation. It is recommended that midfoot and hindfoot amputation undergo lengthening or tenotomy of the Achilles along with preservation or tenodesis of the tibialis anterior and the peroneal musculature.[80] Similarly, in transfemoral amputees, the myodesis of the adductor and hamstring in adduction and extension reduces the risk of a hip flexion and abduction contracture.[81]

Following surgery, dressings and patient positioning assist in preventing contracture. Hindfoot amputations should be splinted in maximal dorsiflexion. Transtibial amputees should be instructed to initiate active knee extension and range of motion exercises and avoid placing pillows under the knee, producing a flexed resting posture. The transfemoral amputee should be instructed on periodic prone lying, and active hip adduction and extension exercises. For patients unable to tolerate or participate in these activities, periodically lying completely flat in bed and placing a light sandbag on the residual limb to facilitate passive hip extension is an effective preventative measure for supine patients.

Rigid dressings for transtibial amputation have been advocated not only for maintenance of extension but also for edema and pain control.[82,83] The use of rigid dressings was fairly standard in the treatment of war amputees in the Vietnam era. However, in the authors' experience, soft dressings have been very effective in the postoperative management of combat-related amputations and permit regular wound monitoring. In compliant traumatic amputees with appropriate therapy, it has been our experience that amputees have not developed flexion contractures of the hip or knee. Dynamic splinting may be effective in transtibial flexion contracture if the tibial segment is long enough to allow such a device. Another option is to adapt the prosthetic socket in flexion to accommodate the contracture and facilitate mobility and progression with rehabilitation.[64,84]

Generally, surgery is not required in the management of contracture following amputation surgery. Appropriate surgical technique at the time of amputation surgery followed by diligent therapy and patient instruction will generally prevent this complication. In a hindfoot amputation equinus contracture, revision to a transtibial level can be an effective solution. Additionally, consideration can be given to converting a transtibial amputation to a through-knee or transfemoral level when other means of knee contracture treatment have failed.[84,85] However, every effort should be made to save the knee, which has a significant impact on functional recovery. The authors' experience with knee arthrofibrosis release and quadricepsplasty has been generally satisfactory in a few young, motivated amputees. Gas-sterilized custom sockets with attached shafts can be useful

intraoperatively to assist in knee manipulation under anesthesia after contracture release (Figure 9-16). In the hip, contracture up to 25° can be accommodated by the socket. In the hip, as in the knee, a surgical release is difficult, requiring extensive dissection. In these instances, consideration may be given to a femoral corrective osteotomy to improve prosthetic function.

Burn amputees with extensive burns on their limbs represent a separate category of patients with distinct complications.[86] When a skin graft is required, contracture develops slowly, often despite appropriate therapy and positioning.[66,73,87] These contractures may respond to plastic procedures to release the scarred skin but may also require release of contracted muscle-tendon units. When other factors such as very delicate skin grafts make prosthetic wear unlikely, such methods should be avoided.

All patients with contractures should undergo exhaustive conservative attempts to increase motion and function prior to considering operative intervention. Postoperatively, amputees undergoing any contracture release require early mobilization and aggressive physical therapy to maintain and maximize operative gains. Toward this end, indwelling regional anesthesia catheters, continuous passive motion machines, and static and dynamic splinting can be particularly useful. When combined with an appropriately motivated patient, satisfactory results can be achieved in most cases through nonoperative and, in carefully selected patients, operative treatment of contractures. However, it cannot be overemphasized that the primary and most important contracture treatment in combat-related amputees is prevention.

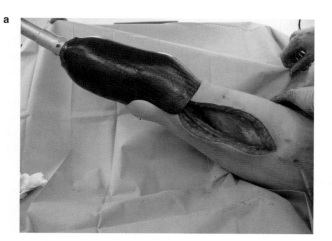 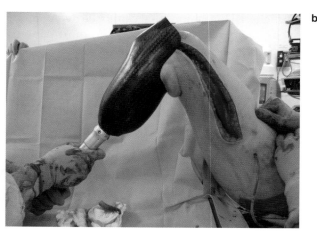

Figure 9-16. Intraoperative photographs of manipulation under anesthesia of a transtibial amputee following knee extension contracture release and quadricepsplasty utilizing a sterilized custom socket. Satisfactory motion was achieved and maintained postoperatively through aggressive rehabilitation.

Upper Extremity Contracture

Among combat-injured personnel with upper extremity amputations, symptomatic contractures are rare. In the absence of additional risk factors, no amputees from the current conflicts have required surgical management or significant modification of prosthetic devices, to the authors' knowledge. Exceptions to this include burn patients, whose injuries may lead to contractures of the elbows and shoulders, patients with concomitant ipsilateral intraarticular elbow fractures, and patients developing HO about the elbow adjacent to short transradial amputations.

In the evaluation and treatment of upper extremity amputees with contractures, decision-making is determined by the condition and function of the terminal limb, the involved joint, and the individual patient's associated injuries as well as his or her real and perceived functional limitations. Consideration for contracture release in burn patients with contracted amputations should be based on the experience gained in the treatment of burn patients without amputations. This may involve capsular release, excision of HO, plastic management of contracted skin (Z-plasty, expanders, and tissue transfer).[88–90] Wound-healing complications are common and often only modest improvements in function are observed.

When HO is limiting functional motion around the elbow, with or without associated fracture, surgical excision and release can be undertaken after conservative measures have been exhausted. A waiting period of 3 to 6 months is recommended to permit initial HO and wound maturation, but longer waiting periods are not necessary.[10,91–93] Typically, at least this much time will transpire while conservative modalities are pursued, patients adapt to their new lives as amputees, functional limitations that cannot be overcome or compensated for become evident, and most patients would even contemplate an additional, elective surgical procedure. The authors advocate standard techniques of scar revision/excision and circumferential capsular release with simultaneous HO excision, followed by postoperative radiotherapy and/or NSAIDs, with aggressive physical therapy.[91–93] Some evidence shows that results of elbow contracture release may be superior in patients with HO compared to those with non-HO posttraumatic fibrosis.[94]

Symptomatic functional loss of shoulder range of motion has not been a frequent problem in the authors' experience, particularly for amputations distal to the elbow. Some patients with short transhumeral amputations likely have markedly decreased shoulder range of motion secondary to a protracted time course of restricted mobility because of multiple surgeries or adjacent soft tissue injury. However, this is seldom if ever bothersome to the amputee; most transhumeral amputees who use functional prostheses seldom use them for overhead activities. For amputees with symptomatic loss of shoulder motion, we recommend standard arthroscopic releases followed by manipulation under anesthesia, soft tissue envelope permitting.[95] Patients in whom the shoulder girdle tissues are too compromised to permit arthroscopy would ostensibly be at dramatically increased risk of wound complications if an open procedure were attempted. Open release should therefore be reserved for patients with a reasonably intact shoulder soft tissue envelope and who fail an attempt at arthroscopic release and manipulation, due to extraarticular causes (eg, subscapularis contracture).

As with most complications, primary treatment of amputation-associated upper extremity contractures is prevention via early motion and therapy as soon after injury as soft tissue and osseous injuries permit. Unique considerations in upper extremity amputation contractures include compromised soft tissue envelopes, which may limit soft tissue healing and durability after operative treatment; shortened lever arms, which may make early passive and active-assisted therapy more difficult; and the patient's desire to return to early prosthetic fitting and use after surgery. Postoperatively, aggressive physical therapy and early return to regular prosthetic use is necessary to maintain operative gains and maximize ultimate patient function. Modalities such as indwelling postoperative nerve catheters, continuous passive motion, and static or dynamic splinting remain relatively unproven with regard to efficacy but can serve as useful adjunctive rehabilitation measures, particularly for patients in whom postoperative pain is too great or motivation too little.

MARQUARDT HUMERAL OSTEOTOMY

Successful prosthesis use by the unilateral transhumeral amputee is by no means guaranteed, despite the availability of the most advanced prosthetic technology and occupational therapy services. Many patients find single-limb strategies for activities of daily living preferable to using a transhumeral prosthesis, be it body-powered, hybrid, or myoelectric. Additionally, many transhumeral amputees who are regular prosthesis users utilize their prostheses only for very specific tasks, and may wear their limbs only for an hour or two per day, a couple of days per week. Among the common reasons cited by patients for low prosthetic use are prosthetic weight and limited functional range of motion. Many suspension systems utilize shoulder caps that are hot and uncomfortable and can chafe and restrict motion. Likewise, suction suspensions on cylindrical residual limbs have limited resistance to torque in the axial plane.

In 1972 Marquardt[96] published a case report of a pediatric patient utilizing a new technique in which a distal angulation osteotomy was performed. He noted improved suspension with unrestricted shoulder motion and improved rotational control in flexion and abduction, giving a much larger functional range for prosthetic use. In 1974 Marquardt and Neff[97] published a case series of adults and children who had undergone the procedure, noting that, in addition to improved motion and control, the incidence of terminal overgrowth in pediatric patients was reduced by the procedure. With the angulation osteotomy, therefore, transhumeral amputation acquired most of the beneficial attributes of elbow disarticulation—without the limitations of external-hinge elbow units needed to keep relative arm and forearm length normal in the disarticulation patient.

The authors have used this technique in selected combat-related amputees. The ideal candidate is a successful prosthetic user who is dissatisfied with a shoulder cap suspension, or who needs greater range of motion or improved rotational control for specific desired bimanual tasks. Most of these transhumeral patients have undergone "length-preserving" amputations closed with nontraditional flaps, and an appropriate portion of the initial closure is utilized. The procedure is performed as a revision only. The risk of placing fixation hardware in these initially highly contaminated wounds is considered too high to be justified until the wound has declared itself and a rehabilitation problem has been identified. Utilizing a portion of the wound closure scar, a 5-cm portion of the distal humerus is exposed. Concomitant revision procedures such as neuroma or HO excision are performed as appropriate. A 70° wedge is then cut anteriorly, with the posterior periosteum preserved as a hinge, if possible. The osteotomy is then closed and fixed with a single 3.5-mm cortical screw placed in compression from distal to proximal (Figure 9-17). (This represents a deviation from Marquardt's original technique, which was performed through a separate posterolateral incision and fixed from proximal to distal.)

Postoperative management includes edema prevention, initially with figure-of-eight elastic wraps, and progressing to a stump shrinker as soon as the patient tolerates application. The patient is transitioned to a Silastic (Dow Corning Corporation, Midland, Mich) liner at about 2 weeks postoperatively. Prosthetic wear is resumed after 3 weeks to allow for early osteotomy healing. The authors have not encountered any problems with nonunion or loss of fixation by resuming

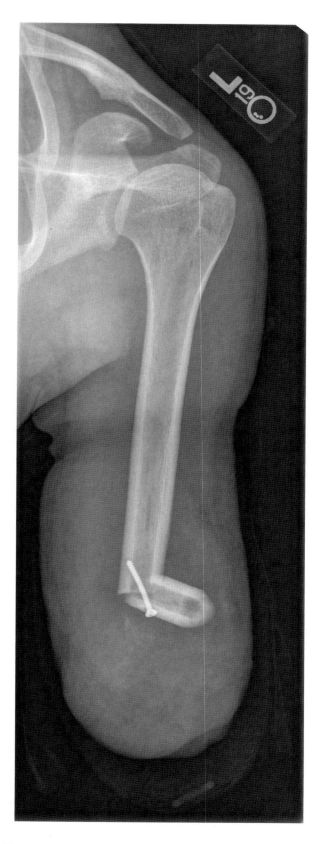

Figure 9-17. Anterior-posterior radiograph of a transhumeral amputee with a healed Marquardt angulation osteotomy.

a

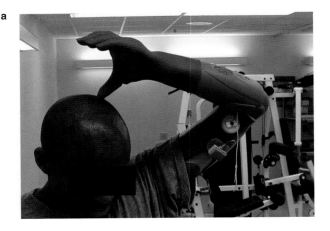

Figure 9-18. Clinical photographs of a transhumeral amputee demonstrating prosthetic use with improved range of motion and prosthesis suspension following a Marquardt angulation osteotomy.

b

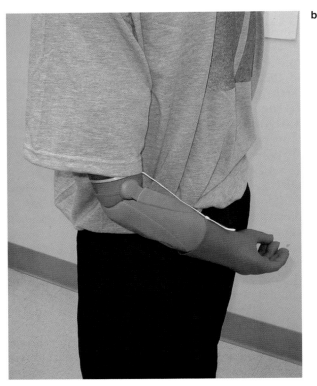

prosthetic wear early and, in spite of some stress at the osteotomy site caused by the prosthesis suspension, the prosthetic socket provides some external, brace-like support. An unexpected benefit is that patients universally perceive a decrease in the weight of their prosthesis (Figure 9-18). We attribute this to the decrease in shear forces on the residual limb soft tissues. The weight of the prosthesis appears to be transferred to the bone, which is better able to tolerate it than the patient's often compromised soft tissues and skin.

Although the best suspension solution for the trans-humeral amputee may be direct skeletal attachment (osseointegration), the Marquardt angulation osteotomy is a useful technique for certain patients until the difficulties of the prosthesis/skin interface and loosening associated with osseointegration are resolved.

KNEE INSTABILITY

The open, length-preserving amputation technique advocated in this textbook, with amputation frequently carried out through the ZOI, is sometimes associated with ligamentous injury to adjacent joints. Two recurrent clinical situations have presented in high-demand transtibial amputees that require ligament reconstruction or repair: (1) anterior cruciate ligament (ACL) deficiency and (2) the short residual limb with an unstable fibula. Although both can be successfully treated with standard surgical techniques, making the correct diagnosis can be challenging. In ACL deficiency, symptoms of "giving way" may be masked by problems with prosthetic fit, weakness, or gait training. The length of the residual limb may make it difficult to perform a Lachman maneuver, and make a classic pivot shift test nearly impossible to perform. Retained ferrous fragments may preclude or obstruct MRI. The symptomatic unstable fibula can be confused with other causes of lateral residual limb pain, such as peroneal

neuroma. Careful physical examination, evidence of fibular splaying on plain radiograph, and peroneal nerve block in the thigh will assist in the diagnosis.

In the authors' experience, high-demand transtibial patients with ACL-deficient knees have not been satisfied with prosthesis modification, incorporating polyaxial hinges in the socket similar to current sports braces used to treat ACL-deficient athletes nonoperatively. Single-bundle ACL reconstruction, however, has had good results. Allograft bone-tendon-bone, Achilles, or tibialis posterior tendons are preferable in reconstructing the ACL-deficient knee in the transtibial amputee, rather than using autograft bone-tendon-bone or semitendinosis/gracilis from the ipsilateral or contralateral knee. Both lower extremities have frequently been severely injured, and the slight delay in incorporation of allograft outweighs the additional insult of autograft harvest. These patients are fitted with hinged, double-upright socket extensions fabricated by prosthetists to protect the reconstruction for 12 weeks postoperatively, allowing early return to prosthetic use. Full weight bearing without ambulatory aides is allowed at 12 weeks, and running and cutting activities are permitted when the quadriceps and hamstrings are within 85% of the contralateral side by Biodex (Biodex Medical Systems, Shirley, NY) testing, usually at about 5 to 6 months.

Patients with extremely short transtibial amputations have achieved high-level functioning: many with amputations 2 or 3 cm distal to the tibial tubercle are runners, and several patients with these short transtibial amputations who have a contralateral transfemoral amputation are able to run and play cutting sports. The function achieved by these young men and women defies conventional wisdom, and speaks volumes about their courage and tenacity.

Some patients with short transtibial amputations, however, have painful, unstable residual fibulas. Frequently, this can be elucidated on physical examination or on plain radiographs. A residual fibula shorter than 5 cm should raise the suspicion that insufficient interosseous membrane remains for fibular stability. Patients with longer residual limbs who have fibular instability can be treated with revision to an Ertl-style amputation with a synostosis between the distal tibia and fibula, but this technique is not easily done in patients with short residual limbs. These patients respond well to fibular excision with repair of the posterolateral corner. In this procedure, the lateral collateral ligament (LCL) and biceps femoris tendon insertion are elevated as a sleeve and fixed to the lateral tibia with a screw and washer at the tibial facet of the proximal tibial-fibular joint, after excision of the articular cartilage. The repair is protected for 6 weeks with a custom clamshell brace before range of motion and active strengthening against resistance are resumed.

If fibulectomy of a very short residual fibula is performed early in a patient's postinjury treatment to facilitate soft tissue closure and prosthetic fitting, the authors advocate securing the released biceps tendon and LCL to the isometric point on the residual tibia with periosteal sutures, suture anchors, or drill holes through bone. However, several early patients in whom this was not performed have not experienced symptomatic instability as a result. For amputees presenting with late LCL/posterolateral corner instability after early fibulectomy, allograft reconstruction using conventional techniques, securing the graft to the residual tibia via a biotendodesis screw, is a reasonable approach.

Elbow or shoulder instability above transradial or transhumeral amputations has not been a common problem in upper extremity amputees. Stiffness of these joints is a more common complaint, due to adjacent fractures, frequent proximate soft tissue injury, and the difficulty of performing early range of motion exercises above an often open or otherwise compromised residual limb. However, in the event that these issues are encountered, standard open and arthroscopic-assisted reconstructive techniques would be indicated.

INFECTION

Despite aggressive medical and surgical care (including serial debridements, judicious use of antibiotics, and local wound adjuvant therapies), as many as 20% to 40% of combat-injured amputees may develop deep infection requiring inpatient care or surgery following attempted definitive revision and closure.[10,98,99] Specific recommendations on point-of-injury care, antibiotic therapy, serial debridements, and the timing and technique of definitive closure for infection prevention are discussed in Chapter 8, General Surgical Principles for the Combat Casualty With Limb Loss. Additionally, combat casualties frequently become malnourished in the postinjury setting because of limited oral intake and high metabolic demands. Nutrition has been repeatedly demonstrated to play a critical role in the wound-healing potential and immunocompetence of diabetic and dysvascular amputees,[100] and the importance of adequate and supplemental nutrition cannot be overemphasized in the care of combat-injured personnel as well.

Given the demonstrated high incidence of early and/or late infectious complications in combat-related and traumatic amputations, appropriate counseling on patient expectations is critical. The probability and likelihood of infection requiring further antibiotic and/or operative treatment should be discussed with patients and families *before* an infection develops so that the psychological and physical setback of an infection, should one develop, is preemptively tempered. Similar to the portrayal of the amputation itself as a reconstructive procedure (rather than an ablative procedure or necessarily a failure of salvage treatment), viewing infection in this setting as an unfortunate but frequently necessary step in the rehabilitative process can prevent both patient and clinician from becoming unnecessarily discouraged.

Once an infection develops, important treatment information can be inferred from both the timing and apparent chronicity of the process. Infections in residual limbs should thus be classified as early (< 6 weeks from closure) or late, and further classified as acute or chronic. The latter distinction is influenced by the duration and type of symptoms or a history of prior infection with the same organism, and frequently this determination cannot be made until after the initial operative debridement permits direct inspection of deep tissues and operative cultures. Acute infections typically present with more fulminant collections of purulence and wound drainage, whereas chronic infections are generally less virulent and may involve well-formed abscesses or slow, gradual destruction of deep tissues or bone. Early infections typically result from bacteria already present and active within the residual limb at the time of definitive closure. Late infections may result from reactivation of a latent process dormant in the deep tissues for long periods, hematogenous seeding of persistent or new fluid collections, or extension of cutaneous infections aggravated by prosthetic wear (eg, cellulitis or folliculitis). Most early infections are acute and most chronic infections are late, but this is not always the case. The timing and chronicity of the infection, as well as the virulence and antibiotic susceptibility of the organism or organisms, are important in determining the need for operative irrigation and debridement, as well as the duration and type of antibiotic therapy. All types of residual limb infections may require one or more operative debridements, but relatively shorter durations of antibiotic therapy are typically required for early, acute infections.

The history and physical examination of a patient with an infected residual limb should include reassessment of mechanism and ZOI, history of prior infections, chronologic relationship with wound closure and prosthetic use, and systemic symptoms, as well as recent exposures, procedures, and antibiotic use. In the authors' experience, most patients with early or acute infections present with a febrile history, but (as is the case in chronic osteomyelitis)[101] fever is less reliably present in late, chronic infections. Patients with focal pain and swelling and symptoms associated with a recent change in activity or prosthesis should have bursitis included in their differential diagnosis. This distinction is important because the treatment of bursitis, particularly aseptic bursitis (discussed in greater detail in the following section), differs substantially from that for abscesses and deep wound infections.

When infection is present, most patients present with an erythematous, swollen, and painful residual limb, with difficulty or inability to tolerate prosthesis wear. The presence or history of a draining sinus should be noted and is strongly suggestive of chronic deep infection (Figure 9-19). Likewise, the presence, quantity, and quality of recent incisional wound drain-

age should be assessed and noted (Figure 9-20). Any palpable fluid collections should be assessed for size, location, tenderness, transillumination, and fluctuance. Routine culture of sinus tracts or draining incisions is not advocated because the results of these cultures are frequently polymicrobial and unreliably indicative of the actual infecting organism.[101,102] If complete evaluation (including laboratory values and imaging studies) is strongly suggestive of infection versus bursitis, bedside aspiration of small palpable fluid collections under sterile conditions is reasonable in the rare instance that this may obviate the need for operative intervention; however, in most cases abscesses should be treated surgically, and multiple operative tissue cultures are preferred to bedside aspirates even under optimal circumstances.

All patients should undergo laboratory evaluation consisting, at a minimum, of blood cultures, complete blood count with manual cell differential, and inflammatory parameter (Westergren erythrocyte sedimentation rate and C-reactive protein level) assessment. Orthogonal radiographs of the residual limb should be obtained with particular attention to soft tissue swelling, osseous changes or new interval bone destruction, and HO. Although the relationship

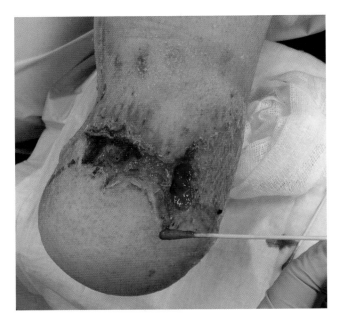

Figure 9-19. Clinical photograph of a transtibial amputation complicated by superficial skin necrosis, eschar formation, and a large draining sinus that probed to bone. The limb was salvaged with serial irrigation, debridements, and vacuum-assisted closure dressing changes followed by delayed split-thickness skin grafting after the excised sinus tract had granulated appropriately.

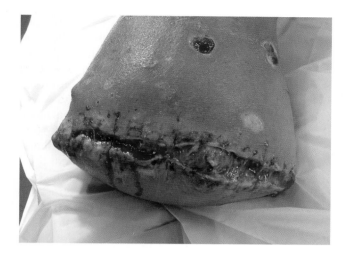

Figure 9-20. Intraoperative photograph of a bilateral transtibial amputee with a deep infection of the right residual limb. Abundant purulence and necrotic tissue is present along the incision line, which dehisced following intraoperative suture removal. The infection was eradicated with two irrigation and debridement procedures with concomitant antibiotic-bead and vacuum-assisted closure dressing use followed by closure over a drain and 2 weeks of parenteral antibiotic therapy.

with infection remains unclear, a high percentage of resected HO specimens from combat-related amputations are culture-positive.[10,102] Advanced imaging modalities are not frequently required, but in patients with equivocal findings, MRI, ultrasound, and indium-111 tagged white blood cell scans can provide useful information.[13,103–105] Isolated technetium-99 three-phase bone scans can remain positive for a prolonged period following revision and closure and may never return to normal in residual limbs due to osseous stress reactions from prosthesis wear,[103] and therefore are generally less helpful in the absence of a paired indium scan.[104,105]

Most residual limb infections should be initially managed with hospital admission. For patients without abscess, fluid collection, or overt wound drainage or draining sinuses, initial treatment should consist of parenteral antibiotics, elevation, adjacent joint and complete prosthetic rest, and continued use of compressive shrinker stockings. Operative intervention should be withheld pending failure to appropriately respond to these conservative measures. Toward this end, patients should be kept non per os (NPO) after midnight for the first 1 or 2 days of admission pending treatment response. This can assist in expediting operative treatment when required, and patients responding appropriately can resume a normal diet without missing any meals following reassessment on early morning rounds.

Patients with active drainage or fluid collections generally require early operative exploration with formal tissue cultures and thorough irrigation and debridement. In these instances, to maximize culture accuracy and yield, empiric antibiotic therapy should be withheld until operative tissue cultures are obtained. When possible, prior surgical incisions and scars should be utilized, but draining sinuses should be excised and some superficial abscesses distant from other incisions are best managed with a direct longitudinal approach, local anatomy permitting. All purulent material and nonviable tissue should be removed and the wound should be thoroughly irrigated. Mixed data regarding the efficacy of gravity, bulb syringe, and pulsatile lavage irrigation preclude a recommendation of a specific irrigation technique,[106–108] which remains a matter of surgeon preference.

Although some patients can be adequately treated with a single irrigation and debridement, closure over a surgical drain, and subsequent systemic antibiotic therapy, the authors prefer a staged approach for most patients. Wounds should be managed in a provisional closure or open fashion, and a return to the operating room for a second look planned. This is performed 2 or 3 days following the initial procedure and permits reassessment of compromised tissue and overall wound status after operative culture speciation and antibiotic susceptibilities have been completed, permitting appropriately tailored subsequent antibiotic therapy. Consultation with an infectious disease specialist is helpful in deciding which antibiotic to use, as well as in determining duration of therapy and monitoring for side effects of antibiotic treatment. Patients who are systemically ill or have locally aggressive infections may require early return to the operating suite within 24 hours. Likewise, patients with ongoing tissue destruction on repeat irrigation and debridement may require further serial irrigation and debridement procedures until the infection is controlled.

In addition to narrowing the antibiotic spectrum while avoiding undertreatment of resistant organisms, a staged approach to infection management may also allow for judiciously less aggressive initial debridement in patients with marginal soft tissue coverage or preexisting suboptimal residual limb length. As a general rule, patients and limbs are best served with eradication of infection via aggressive debridement. In rare instances substantial shortening of the residual limb or even revision to a higher level may be required to both control infection and permit reconstruction of an adequate soft tissue envelope to allow high-demand prosthetic use. Issues of possible limb shortening should be carefully discussed with the patient preoperatively.

A number of local wound adjuncts are available to assist in the staged management of infected residual limbs. Developed in World War I, Dakin moist-to-dry dressing changes are useful for provisional wound management in patients with superficial wounds and others able to tolerate frequent bedside dressing changes. The solution has strong antimicrobial properties without excessive untoward effects on healthy patient tissues, and has been used to good effect in both recent and historical combat-related wounds.[109,110] In some cases of small, superficial abscesses, healing by secondary intention with serial Dakin dressing changes is a reasonable course of action. Subatmospheric pressure VAC dressings encourage vascular ingrowth and granulation tissue formation while removing excess fluid from the wound, reducing soft tissue edema, and preventing excessive soft tissue retraction. These devices also obviate the need for frequent dressing changes and have been utilized with good temporizing and, in some cases, definitive wound management results in both the authors' experience and in the recent open fracture literature.[111–113]

Antibiotic-impregnated polymethylmethacrylate beads achieve supratherapeutic bacteriocidal local antibiotic concentrations with minimal systemic effects and have been utilized with good success in both arthroplasty and fracture-related infections.[114–116] The beads may be placed deep to VAC dressings, in open wounds under an occlusive dressing, or inside provisionally closed residual limbs. A relatively large number of heat-stable antibiotics have been utilized successfully with bone cement, allowing microbe-specific local therapy. Finally, silver-impregnated antimicrobial dressings may be utilized alone or in combination with the aforementioned techniques. These dressings have been repeatedly demonstrated to have good local antimicrobial properties,[117,118] but reports of their use are lacking in the orthopaedic literature. In the authors' experience, antibiotic-bead–associated exudate and silver residue may need to be irrigated from the wound at the time of the repeat procedure

prior to wound assessment. Each of these modalities, used appropriately, may putatively assist in the local control of infection in residual limbs. Although useful in infection control, they should not be viewed as a substitute for adequate debridement, voluminous irrigation, and systemic antimicrobial therapy.

Regardless of the adjuvant wound treatments used, it is prudent to provisionally tag critical structures (eg, released myodesis tendons, skin, and muscle flaps) with monofilament suture and secure them near their intended final locations between staged infection control procedures. This prevents excessive retraction, fibrosis, and scarring, which may make definitive revision and closure of the infected residual limb difficult or impossible days or weeks later. Maintaining as much residual limb length as practical following infection treatment is desirable, but when necessary, freshening the terminal bone end with an oscillating saw and redrilling myodesis holes is useful in achieving satisfactory coverage and closure. Skin closure of previously infected wounds should be performed with nonabsorbable monofilament suture over a closed suction drain and a compressive dressing applied. Drains should be left in place for 1 to 3 days depending on quantity and quality of output and then removed at the bedside. Dressings should be changed daily starting on postoperative day 2, and wound status closely monitored for evidence of recurrent infection. Patients should be transitioned back to compressive shrinker stockings as soon as wound drainage, patient comfort, and edema permit. Sutures should be removed at 2 to 3 weeks postoperatively, after adequate initial wound healing has been achieved and infection-related swelling has subsided. Patients can then be allowed to gradually resume prosthetic fitting, wear, and rehabilitation. Close clinical follow-up is required for several weeks up to and after the completion of systemic antibiotic therapy to monitor for recurrence of infection. As noted, the duration, type, and route of long-term antibiotic therapy are best determined in consultation with an infectious disease specialist.

BURSITIS

Bursitis is a common and likely underreported problem in the residual limbs of amputees with functional pain, especially that which waxes with prolonged prosthetic use and wanes with subsequent rest.[13,119] It can be a disabling and recalcitrant problem in residual limbs, and its treatment can be a matter of great frustration for patient, prosthetist, and physician alike. By definition, synovial (or true) bursae are formed in utero over tendinous or osseous areas of friction or dissimilar motion. In contrast, adventitious bursae

develop postnatally within superficial connective tissues in response to chronic pressure, irritation, and friction. This latter group accounts for the majority of bursae within residual limbs. When these bursae are serially exposed to external stresses that exceed the physiologic tolerance of the involved tissues, they may become inflamed and bursitis results. In the residual limbs of amputees, the majority of symptomatic lesions develop in the subcutaneous tissues, but deep bursitis can develop between a patient's myodesis and the adjacent terminal bone end as well.

Fluid collections are exceedingly common in the early postoperative period following elective amputation or definitive revision and closure of open residual limbs.[120] The majority of these collections undergo biologic resorption and resolve spontaneously. Prior to initiation of regular prosthetic training and rehabilitation, these perioperative collections are unlikely to represent bursae and should be considered hematomas, seromas, or abscesses until proven otherwise. After initial prosthetic fitting and rehabilitation have commenced, a bursa may develop under any area of increased friction or pressure within or near the edge of the prosthetic socket.

Treatment of bursitis begins with prevention. Amputation and wound closure techniques are discussed elsewhere and are therefore beyond the scope of this section. However, bursitis may develop due to either inadequate or redundant mobile soft tissue coverage of a terminal residual limb or bony prominence. Hence, both should be avoided. Likewise, problems with prosthetic alignment, fitting, padding, or suspension may incite or aggravate bursitis and require due diligence on the part of both patient and prosthetist to avoid inadequate prosthetic modifications. Once formed, asymptomatic bursae should be considered part of a normal adaptive physiologic response and do not necessarily require treatment, but socket and liner modifications may be considered to reduce friction in these areas and decrease the potential for bursitis to subsequently develop.

Potential conundrums in bursitis management begin with the frequently difficult diagnosis. The chief differential diagnoses in symptomatic patients include aseptic bursitis, septic bursitis, abscess, and cellulitis. Aseptic bursitis is thus notoriously difficult to distinguish from infection.[121–123] The medical history should include focused questioning about recent changes in activity or wear of the prosthesis or to the prosthesis or liner itself. The duration of symptoms, presence of any constitutional symptoms or fever, and relationship of these to prosthetic wear should be elucidated.

On physical examination, the degree of tenderness, fluctuance, erythema, transillumination, and relative cutaneous warmth[122] of the affected site can be helpful in distinguishing aseptic, mechanical bursitis from septic bursitis or abscesses. A complete blood count with manual cell differential and inflammatory parameters may provide reassurance on the diagnosis of aseptic bursitis or, conversely, guide more aggressive diagnostic and therapeutic modalities for a probable infectious process. Orthogonal radiographs of the residual limb should be obtained, with attention to cystic degeneration of bone, bone spurs, or HO deep

to the symptomatic bursa. Advanced imaging modalities (including ultrasound, MRI, and technetium-99 bone scans) have been advocated.[13,119] However, the appreciation of a fluid collection with adjacent edema is expected, and reciprocal osseous changes may occur in the absence of a septic process; therefore, the utility of these studies in cases of suspected bursitis is limited in the absence of a florid deep infection or overt osteomyelitis.

Diagnostic or therapeutic aspiration should be performed only if sufficient clinical suspicion of septic bursitis or abscess persists following the initial evaluation. There is little evidence that aseptic bursitis outcomes are improved with aspiration alone, and the potential exists for cutaneous fistula formation or bacterial contamination and creation of iatrogenic septic bursitis. Aspiration should therefore not precede more conservative measures in aseptic bursitis patients. At minimum, Gram stain, bacterial cultures, and cell count with differential should be sent from any aspirate.[123,124] If adequate fluid is obtained, additional studies worthy of consideration include aspirate protein, glucose, and lactate dehydrogenase, with corresponding serum levels. Confirmed cases of septic bursitis or abscess should be managed with empiric and subsequently culture-specific antibiotics. The determination of initial intravenous versus oral treatment is predicated upon the severity of the infection and the patient's clinical status. However, when in doubt, initial intravenous therapy with conversion to oral treatment following a positive clinical response is reasonable. The decision to proceed to the operating suite for formal irrigation and debridement of septic bursitis depends on the adequacy of the aspiration and the initial response to antibiotic treatment. Frank abscesses generally require operative intervention for adequate treatment and evacuation.

For cases of suspected aseptic bursitis, initial treatment is conservative and should generally not include antibiotic therapy. Although complete resolution of inflammation and symptoms may require a prolonged period, failure to see tangible early and stepwise improvement within a few days should alert the clinician to a possible underlying infectious process and prompt further evaluation. Conservative treatment should consist of complete prosthetic rest and the required activity modifications, continued compression stocking wear, elevation, ice, and nonsteroidal antiinflammatory medication. Concurrently, investigation should continue in an effort to identify and modify any prosthesis- or activity-related inciting factors. Failure to do so will result in probable and predictable future recurrence of bursitis. Toward this end, particular attention should be paid to relieving pressure and friction over the involved area and prevention of limb pistoning. As symptoms become quiescent, prosthetic wear may gradually be resumed.

For patients with recurrent or refractory aseptic bursitis, further treatment is required. Invasive treatment should be considered only after repeated and exhaustive efforts at prosthetic modification have been completed. Although the results of injection or operative treatment of bursitis are frequently gratifying, the potential complications can be disastrous.[121,123–126] The success of aspiration in aseptic bursitis has been demonstrated only when utilized concurrently with other conservative measures,[123] and only anecdotally noted in amputees.[119] Conversely, corticosteroid injection, while found effective in a small randomized trial of olecranon bursitis patients,[125] may result in atrophy of overlying fat and soft tissue, which is particularly undesirable in amputees with suboptimal soft tissue coverage. Steroid injection is therefore advocated only in patients with a robust soft tissue envelope, and simple aspiration should be the initial invasive treatment of others. Complications of aspiration and injection include tissue atrophy, iatrogenic infection, needle track fistulas, and recurrence of bursitis.

Operative treatment of aseptic bursitis is even more contentious. The difficulties in treating nonamputees with more typical olecranon and prepatellar bursitis have been well documented. Amputees must eventually resume prosthetic wear and, in spite of the benefit of prosthetic modifications, place direct pressure and/or shear on their previously symptomatic sites. This complicates treatment further and may predispose amputees to recurrences in spite of initially successful treatment. Therefore, the authors do not advocate surgical bursectomy for aseptic bursitis in the absence of concurrently modifiable external (eg, prosthesis or activity) or internal (eg, bone spur or HO excision) factors. Regardless of operative technique, completeness of excision, and avoidance of complications, failure to identify and address these factors will reliably lead to early symptomatic recurrence.[121]

Once operative drainage and bursectomy are considered, a preoperative plan should be formulated accounting for the location of the bursitis, the patient's soft tissue envelope, and preexisting surgical incisions, scars, and skin grafts. In contrast to abscess drainage, incisions directly over the involved bursa are ill-advised. Such incisions violate already compromised soft tissue in an area of known chronic irritation and stress, and may be more prone to chronic drainage as well. Therefore, the patient's prior incisions should be utilized when practicable, avoiding skin grafts and flaps if possible. If the local anatomy renders this approach infeasible, a longitudinal incision adjacent to, but not immediately overlying, the involved bursa is recommended. A complete bursectomy should be performed without causing undue damage to uninvolved tissue, and the use of a surgical drain strongly considered. Using these techniques in nonamputees, most authors report favorable results in over 90% of patients,[123,124,126] but wound drainage problems and recurrences in up to 27% and 22% of patients, respectively, have been reported.[121] Endoscopic bursectomy has been reported with limited favorable results but cannot be advocated for routine use in amputees on the basis of the available evidence.[127]

SKIN PROBLEMS

The traumatic amputee who becomes a successful prosthesis user is likely to face lifelong challenges at the skin-prosthesis interface. The skin is subject to many stresses and factors unique to an enclosed and superficial environment. Modern socket liners and suspension have made tremendous progress toward eliminating many of these challenges. However, the surgeon is occasionally called to address issues ranging from wound healing to infections, and even flap failure early in the rehabilitation process. Late sequelae can also occur, such as verrucous hyperplasia, epidermoid cysts or suture abscesses, contact dermatitis, chronic drainage, and even the unlikely development of squamous cell carcinoma after many years of draining sinus tracts or chronic irritation from the prosthetic socket.[128] Most of these conditions, and even more transient problems like hyperhidrosis, terminal limb edema, callus formation, folliculitis, hidradenitis, and fungal infections, can be successfully managed nonsurgically by a skilled team including the therapist, prosthetist, physiatrist, dermatologist, and surgeon.

When the combat amputee eventually undergoes definitive wound closure, it is nearly universal to experience terminal edema. While routine management includes carefully applied dressings and subsequent shrinker appliances, this edema generally resolves once the patient begins socket wear. Whenever a socket is removed for prolonged periods of time edema can return and must be managed accordingly. Over the first several months edema generally stabilizes to a steady state and rarely requires treatment. Similarly with socket wear, issues like hyperhidrosis and maceration improve with hygiene, stump sock use, and, infrequently, topical application of drying materials. The treating physician should regularly monitor for fungal infections or contact dermatitis associated with chronic maceration or reaction to chemicals associated with socket manufacture.

Another condition often associated with prosthetic fit, underlying vascular injury, or chronic bacterial infection is verrucous hyperplasia (Figure 9-21). Verrucous hyperplasia, in keeping with its nomenclature, has a wart-like appearance, often in areas of limited socket contact. While the condition poses superficial hygienic challenges, and pain when associated with skin breakdown, it is best managed with shrinker socks, or socket modification that equalizes the contact pressures throughout the limb.

Chronic conditions that often require surgical intervention are not common. One such condition is an epidermoid cyst, a pocket or invagination of keratin-producing cells, either as a result of overgrowth at the margin of the original amputation incision, or from the original wound closure. These cysts present as localized masses, intermittently draining or painful, and should be excised when recurrent.

Another condition, related to chronic recurring draining fistulae or sinus tracts but reported in amputees with recurrent skin breakdown, is squamous cell carcinoma or Marjolin's ulcer. This condition typically presents years or decades after the original trauma, and is always heralded by a new-onset painful, often malodorous, ulceration at the site of a recurrent sinus tract.

Finally, many combat amputees lack adequate soft tissue coverage to permit closure of native myofascial layers and skin over their terminal residual limbs. Techniques to avoid this problem, including length-preserving initial amputation, subatmospheric pressure dressing use, skin traction, and creative skin flap creation, were discussed earlier. Nonetheless, some patients require split-thickness skin grafting to achieve definitive closure and coverage. Particularly in the lower limb, these grafts may not physiologically withstand high-demand prosthesis use (Figure 9-22). For this reason, somewhat thicker than typical split-thickness skin grafts are advocated. Although the treatment process is lengthened by this intervention and the authors have only anecdotal experience in amputees, in cases of profoundly deficient subcutaneous tissue, dermal substitutes, commonly utilized in burn patients, can be a useful means to achieving an increased thickness of collagenous tissue between prosthesis liner, skin, and bone.[75] Patients experiencing recurrent breakdown of necessary skin grafts are best managed with a truly exhaustive series of conservative measures, including activity, liner, and prosthesis modification. In rare instances, edema subsidence or underlying HO excision may permit delayed skin graft excision and closure with native skin. Some patients, particularly transfemoral amputees with relatively

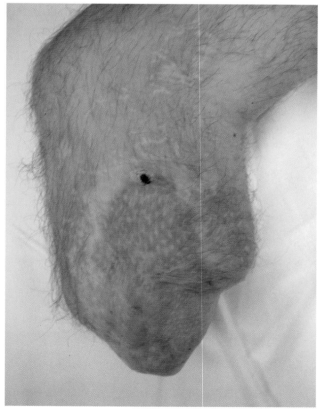

Figure 9-22. Clinical photograph of a transtibial amputee with recurrent skin breakdown of a terminal split-thickness skin graft complicated by underlying heterotopic ossification.

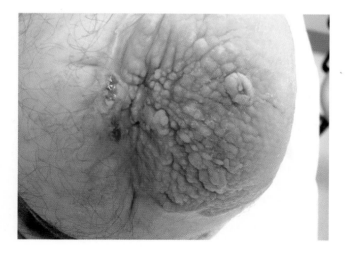

Figure 9-21. Verrucous hyperplasia in a 22-year-old soldier, 18 months after definitive prosthesis. Note the maceration and fissuring within the invaginations.

more adjacent soft tissue, may benefit from plastic surgery consultation and tissue expander use. However, most cases requiring operative treatment will ultimately require free tissue transfer, residual limb shortening, or even revision to a higher level.

Skin conditions are common and require awareness and management with a multidisciplinary approach. Although the majority of these conditions can be successfully managed without surgery, the surgeon may encounter them in the normal postoperative phase and must be prepared to recognize them to direct appropriate management.

CONCLUSION

The surgical management of the combat-related amputee, and amputations in general, remains an elusive and constantly evolving art and science. This chapter and the previous one represent a summary of both the best available published evidence on specific techniques and the sum of the authors' combined clinical experiences in managing hundreds of amputees from the current conflicts in the global war on terrorism. Although specific techniques, such as osseointegration and target nerve transfer or reinnervation, as well as the development of newer and better modern prosthetics, may alter the art of amputation management in future years and conflicts, the general principles described are intended to guide the treating surgeon in making the best operative (and nonoperative) treatment decisions possible for each uniquely complex case and patient. Adherence to these often timeless and proven techniques and principles, coupled with creative thinking, a current knowledge of the available literature, and frequent consultation with experienced peers, will help to ensure the optimal results for both surgeon and patient.

Acknowledgment

The authors gratefully acknowledge Donald A. Gajewski, MD, LTC, for his contributions to this chapter.

REFERENCES

1. Smith DG, Horn P, Malchow D, Boone DA, Reiber GE, Hansen ST Jr. Prosthetic history, prosthetic charges, and functional outcome of the isolated, traumatic below-knee amputee. *J Trauma*. 1995;38(1):44–47.

2. Gunawardena NS, Seneviratne Rde A, Athauda T. Functional outcomes of unilateral lower limb amputee soldiers in two districts of Sri Lanka. *Mil Med*. 2006;171(4):283–287.

3. Fergason J, Smith DG. Socket considerations for the patient with a transtibial amputation. *Clin Orthop Relat Res*. 1999 Apr;(361):76–84.

4. Richardson C, Glenn S, Nurmikko T, Horgan M. Incidence of phantom phenomena including phantom limb pain 6 months after major lower limb amputation in patients with peripheral vascular disease. *Clin J Pain*. 2006;22(4):353–358.

5. Danshaw CB. An anesthetic approach to amputation and pain syndromes. *Phys Med Rehabil Clin N Am*. 2000;11(3):553–557.

6. Hirai M, Tokuhiro A, Takechi H. Stump problems in traumatic amputation. *Acta Med Okayama*. 1993;47(6):407–412.

7. Hoaglund FT, Jergesen HE, Wilson L, Lamoreux LW, Roberts R. Evaluation of problems and needs of veteran lower-limb amputees in the San Francisco Bay Area during the period 1977–1980. *J Rehabil Res Dev*. 1983;20(1):57–71.

8. Denton JR, McClelland SJ. Stump fractures in lower extremity amputees. *J Trauma*. 1985;25(11):1074–1078.

9. Bowker JH, Rills BM, Ledbetter CA, Hunter GA, Holliday P. Fractures in lower limbs with prior amputation. A study of ninety cases. *J Bone Joint Surg Am*. 1981;63(6):915–920.

10. Potter BK, Burns TC, Lacap AP, Granville RR, Gajewski DA. Heterotopic ossification following traumatic and combat-related amputations. Prevalence, risk factors, and preliminary results of excision. *J Bone Joint Surg Am*. 2007;89(3):476–486.

11. Jing BS, Villanueva R, Dodd GD. A new radiological technique in evaluation of prosthetic fitting. *Radiology.* 1977;122(2):534–535.

12. Bocobo CR, Castellote JM, MacKinnon D, Gabrielle-Bergman A. Videofluoroscopic evaluation of prosthetic fit and residual limbs following transtibial amputation. *J Rehabil Res Dev.* 1998;35(1):6–13.

13. Foisneau-Lottin A, Martinet N, Henrot P, Paysant J, Blum A, André JM. Bursitis, adventitious bursa, localized soft-tissue inflammation, and bone marrow edema in tibial stumps: the contribution of magnetic resonance imaging to the diagnosis and management of mechanical stress complications. *Arch Phys Med Rehabil.* 2003;84(5):770–777

14. Henrot P, Stines J, Walter F, Martinet N, Paysant J, Blum A. Imaging of the painful lower limb stump. *Radiographics.* 2000;20 Spec No:S219–235.

15. Brackett EG. Care of the amputated in the United States. In: Ireland MW, ed. *Surgery.* Vol 11. In: *The Medical Department of the United States Army in the World War.* Washington, DC: Department of the Army, Medical Department, Office of The Surgeon General; 1927: 713–748.

16. Otis GA, Huntington DL. Wounds and complications. In: Barnes JK, ed. *The Medical and Surgical History of the War of the Rebellion.* Vol II, Pt III. Washington, DC: Office of The Surgeon General; 1883: 880.

17. Chalmers J, Gray DH, Rush J. Observations on the induction of bone in soft tissue. *J Bone Joint Surg Br.* 1975;57:36–45.

18. Buring K. On the origin of cells in heterotopic bone formation. *Clin Orthop Relat Res.* 1975;110:293–301.

19. Burd TA, Lowry KJ, Anglen JO. Indomethacin compared with localized irradiation for the prevention of heterotopic ossification following surgical treatment of acetabular fractures. *J Bone Joint Surg Am.* 2001;83:1783–1788.

20. Moore KD, Goss K, Anglen JO. Indomethacin versus radiation therapy for prophylaxis against heterotopic ossification in acetabular fractures: a randomized, prospective study. *J Bone Joint Surg Br.* 1998;80:259–263.

21. Potter BK, Burns TC, Lacap AP, Granville RR, Gajewski DA. Heterotopic ossification in the residual limbs of traumatic and combat-related amputees. *J Am Acad Orthop Surg.* 2006;14:S191–S197.

22. Fransen M, Neal B. Non-steroidal anti-inflammatory drugs for preventing heterotopic bone formation after hip arthroplasty. *Cochrane Database Systematic Rev.* 2004;3:CD001160.

23. Pakos EE, Ioannidis JP. Radiotherapy vs. nonsteroidal anti-inflammatory drugs for the prevention of heterotopic ossification after major hip procedures: a meta-analysis of randomized trials. *Int J Rad Onc Bio Phy.* 2004;60:888–895.

24. Gunal I, Hazer B, Seber S, Gokturk E, Turgut A, Kose N. Prevention of heterotopic ossification after total hip replacement: a prospective comparison of indomethacin and salmon calcitonin in 60 patients. *Acta Orthop Scand.* 2001;72:467–469.

25. Guillemin F, Mainard D, Rolland H, Delagoutte JP. Antivitamin K prevents heterotopic ossification after hip arthroplasty in diffuse idiopathic skeletal hyperostosis: a retrospective study in 67 patients. *Acta Orthop Scand.* 1995;66:123–166.

26. Salai M, Langevitz P, Blankstein A, et al. Total hip replacement in familial Mediterranean fever. *Bull Hosp Jt Dis.* 1993;53:25–28.

27. Ahrengart L, Lindgren U, Reinholt FP. Comparative study of the effects of radiation, indomethacin, prednisolone, and ethane-1-hydroxy-1, 1-diphosphonate (EHDP) in the prevention of ectopic bone formation. *Clin Orthop.* 1988;229:265–273.

28. Haran M, Bhuta T, Lee B. Pharmacological interventions for treating acute heterotopic ossification. *Cochrane Database Syst Rev.* 2005;4:CD003321.

29. Garland DE, Orwin JF. Resection of heterotopic ossification in patients with spinal cord injuries. *Clin Orthop.* 1989;242:169–176.

30. Nashold BS, Golder JL, Mullen JB, Bright DS. Long term pain control by direct nerve stimulation. *J Bone Joint Surg.* 1982;62:1–10.

31. Nelson AW. The painful neuroma: the regenerating axon versus the epineural sheath. *J Surg Res.* 1977;23:215–221.

32. Nolan WB, Eaton RG. Painful neuromas of the upper extremity and postneurectomy pain. In: Omer GE, Spinner M, Van Beek AL, eds. *Management of Peripheral Nerve Problems.* Philadelphia, Pa: WB Saunders; 1998:146–149.

33. Tupper JW, Booth DM. Treatment of painful neuromas of sensory nerves in the hand; a comparison of traditional and newer methods. *J Hand Surg.* 1976;1:144–151.

34. Mackinnon SE, Dellon AL. Results of treatment of recurrent dorsoradial wrist neuromas. *Ann Plast Surg.* 1987;19:54–61.

35. MacKenzie EJ, Jones AS, Bosse MJ, et al. Health-care costs associated with amputation or reconstruction of a limb-threatening injury. *J Bone Joint Surg Am.* 2007;89:1685–1692.

36. Gottschalk FA, Stills M. The biomechanics of trans-femoral amputation. *Prosthet Orthot Int.* 1994;18:12–17.

37. Burgess E. Knee disarticulation and above-knee amputation. In: Moore W, Malone MJ, eds. *Lower Extremity Amputation.* Philadelphia, Pa: WB Saunders; 1989:132–146.

38. Gottschalk F. Transfemoral amputation. Biomechanics and surgery. *Clinical Orthop Relat Res.* 1999;361:15–22.

39. Long I. Normal shape-normal alignment (NSNA) above-knee prosthesis. *Clin Prosthet Orthot.* 1985;9:9–14.

40. Sabolich J. Contoured adducted trochanteric-controlled alignment method (CAT-CAM): introduction and basic principles. *Clin Prosthet Orthot.* 1985;9:15–26.

41. Gottschalk FK, Kourosh S, Stills M, McClennan B, Roberts J. Does socket configuration influence the position of the femur in above-knee amputation? *J Prosthet Orthot.* 1989;2:94–102.

42. Waters RL, Perry J, Antonelli D, Hislop H. Energy cost of walking of amputees: the influence of level of amputation. *J Bone Joint Surg Am.* 1976;58:42–46.

43. Jaegers SM, Arendzen JH, de Jongh HJ. Changes in hip muscles after above-knee amputation. *Clin Orthop Relat Res.* 1995;319:276–284.

44. James U. Maximal isometric muscle strength in healthy active male unilateral above-knee amputees, with special regard to the hip joint. *Scand J Rehabil Med.* 1973;5:55–66.

45. Thiele B, James U, Stalberg E. Neurophysiological studies on muscle function in the stump of above-knee amputees. *Scand J Rehabil Med.* 1973;5:67–70.

46. Burgess EM, Romano RL, Zettl JH, Schrock RD Jr. Amputations of the leg for peripheral vascular insufficiency. *J Bone Joint Surg Am.* 1971;53:874–890.

47. Pedersen HE, Lamont RL, Ramsey RH. Below-knee amputation for gangrene. *South Med J.* 1964;57:820–825.

48. Hsieh CH, Huang KF, Liliang PC, Tsai HH, Pong YP, Jeng SF. Below-knee amputation using a medial saphenous artery-based skin flap. *J Trauma.* 2006;61:353–357.

49. Robinson KP, Hoile R, Coddington T. Skew flap myoplastic below-knee amputation: a preliminary report. *Br J Surg.* 1982;69:554–557.

50. Ruckley CV, Stonebridge PA, Prescott RJ. Skewflap versus long posterior flap in below-knee amputations: multicenter trial. *J Vasc Surg.* 1991;13:423–427.

51. Gallico GG 3rd, Ehrlichman RJ, Jupiter J, May JW Jr. Free flaps to preserve below-knee amputation stumps: long-term evaluation. *Plast Reconstr Surg.* 1987;79:871–878.

52. Lilja M, Hoffmann P, Oberg T. Morphological changes during early trans-tibial prosthetic fitting. *Prosthet Orthot Int.* 1998;22:115–122.

53. Golbranson FL, Wirta RW, Kuncir EJ, Lieber RL, Oishi C. Volume changes occurring in postoperative below-knee residual limbs. *J Rehab Res Dev.* 1988;25:11–18.

54. McAuliffe J. Elbow disarticulation and transhumeral amputation/shoulder disarticulartion and forequarter amputations. In: Bowker JM, Michael JW, eds. *Atlas of Limb Prosthetics: Surgical, Prosthetic, and Rehabilitation Principles.* 2nd ed. St Louis, Mo: Mosby-Year Book; 1992: 22.

55. Louis D. Amputations. In: Green D, ed. *Operative Hand Surgery.* 2nd ed. New York, NY: Churchill Livingston Inc; 1988: 61–119.

56. Ertl JV. *Regeneration; ihre Anwendung in der Chirugie, mit einem Anhang, Operationslehre, von Johann v. Ertl.* [Regeneration: The use of the surgical procedure of Johann V Ertl.] Leipzig, Germany: Barth, 1939.

57. Ertl JV. Uber Amputationionsstympfe. [Special amputation synostosis.] *Der Chirurg.* 1949;20:218–224.

58. Murdoch G. Below-knee amputations and prosthetics. In: Murdock G, ed. *Prosthetic and Orthotic Practice.* London, England: Edward Arnold; 1969.

59. Ertl JW, Ertl JP, Ertl WJ, Stokosa J. The Ertl osteomyloplastic transtibial amputation reconstruction: description of technique and long term results. Paper presented at: American Academy of Orthopaedic Surgery Annual Meeting; February 13–17, 1997; San Francisco, Calif.

60. Deffer PA, Moll JH, LaNoue AM. The Ertl osteoplastic below-knee amputation. Paper presented at: American Academy of Orthopaedic Surgery Annual Meeting; January 18–23, 1969; New York, NY.

61. Pinto MA, Harris WW. Fibular segment bone bridging in trans-tibial amputation. *Prosthet Orthot Int.* 2004;28:220–224.

62. Pinzur MS, Pinto MA, Saltzman M, Batista F, Gottschalk F, Juknelis D. Health-related quality of life in patients with transtibial amputation and reconstruction with bone bridging of the distal tibia and fibula. *Foot Ankle Int.* 2006;27(11):907–912.

63. What's past is prologue: Ertl procedure. *O&P Business News.* May 1, 2000.

64. Murnaghan JJ, Bowker JH. Musculoskeletal complications. In: Smith DG, Michael JW, Bowker JH, eds. *Atlas of Amputations and Limb Deficiencies: Surgical, Prosthetic, and Rehabilitation Principles.* 3rd ed. Rosemont, Il: American Academy of Orthopaedic Surgeons; 2004: 683–700.

65. Stansbury LG, Lalliss SJ, Branstetter JG, Bagg MR, Holcomb JB. Amputations in U.S. military personnel in the current conflicts in Afghanistan and Iraq. *J Orthop Trauma.* 2008;22(1):43–46.

66. Kennedy PJ, Young WM, Deva AK, Haertsch PA. Burns and amputations: a 24-year experience. *J Burn Care Res.* 2006;27(2):183–188.

67. Kim YC, Park CI, Kim DY, Kim TS, Shin JC. Statistical analysis of amputations and trends in Korea. *Prosth Orthot Int.* 1996;20(2):88–95.

68. Viscardi PJ, Polk HC Jr. Outcome of amputations in patients with major burns. *Burns.* 1995;21:526–529.

69. Winkley JH, Gaspard DJ, Smith LL. Amputation as a life-saving measure in the burn patient. *J Trauma.* 1965;5:782–791.

70. Acikel C, Peker F, Akmaz I, Ulkur E. Muscle transposition and skin grafting for salvage of below-knee amputation level after bilateral lower extremity thermal injury. *Burns.* 2001;27(8):849–852.

71. Sauerbier M, Ofer N, Germann G, Baumeister S. Microvascular reconstruction in burn and electrical burn injuries of the severely traumatized upper extremity. *Plast Reconstr Surg.* 2007;119:605–615.

72. Ward RS, Hayes-Lundy C, Schnebly WA, Saffle JR. Prosthetic use in patients with burns and associated limb amputations. *J Burn Care Rehabil.* 1990;11:361–364.

73. Ward RS, Hayes-Lundy C, Schnebly WA, Reddy WA, Saffle JR. Rehabilitation of burn patients with concomitant limb amputation: case reports. *Burns.* 1990;16(5):390–392.

74. Fletchall S, Hickerson WL. Early upper-extremity prosthetic fit in patients with burns. *J Burn Care Rehabil.* 1991;12:234–236.

75. Helgeson MD, Potter BK, Evans KN, Shawen SB. Bioartificial dermal substitute use for management of complex combat-related soft tissue wounds. *J Orthop Trauma.* 2007;21:394–399.

76. Jeng JC, Fidler PE, Sokolich JC, et al. Seven years' experience with Integra as a reconstructive tool. *J Burn Care Res.* 2007;28:120–126.

77. Blackburn JH, Boemi L, Hall WW, et al. Negative-pressure dressings as a bolster for skin grafts. *Ann Plast Surg.* 1998;40:453–457.

78. Schneider AM, Morykwas MJ, Argenta LC. A new and reliable method of securing skin grafts to the difficult recipient bed. *Plast Reconstr Surg.* 1998;102:1195–1198.

79. Scherer LA, Shiver S, Chang M, et al. The vacuum assisted closure device: a method of securing skin grafts and improving graft survival. *Arch Surg.* 2002;137:930–934.

80. Bowker JH. Amputations and disarticulations within the foot: surgical management. In: Smith DG, Michael JW, Bowker JH, eds. *Atlas of Amputations and Limb Deficiencies: Surgical, Prosthetic, and Rehabilitation Principles.* 3rd ed. Rosemont, Il: American Academy of Orthopaedic Surgeons; 2004: 29–48.

81. Gottschalk F. Transfemoral amputation: Surgical management. In: Smith DG, Michael JW, Bowker JH, eds. *Atlas of Amputations and Limb Deficiencies: Surgical, Prosthetic, and Rehabilitation Principles.* 3rd ed. Rosemont, Il: American Academy of Orthopaedic Surgeons; 2004: 533–540.

82. Smith DG, McFarland LV, Sangeorzan BJ, Reiber GE, Czerniecki JM. Postoperative dressing and management strategies for transtibial amputations: a critical review. *J Rehab Res Dev.* 2003;40(3):213–224.

83. Harrington IJ, Lexier R, Woods JM, McPolin MF, James GF. A plaster-pylon technique for below-knee amputation. *J Bone Joint Surg Br.* 1991;73-B(1):76–78.

84. Hays RD, Leimkuehler JP, Miknevich MA, Troyer D. An alternative bent knee prosthesis. *Arch Phys Med Rehab.* 1992;73(11):1118–1121.

85. Pinzur MS, Smith DG, Daluga DJ, Osterman H. Selection of patients for through-the-knee amputation. *J Bone Joint Surg Am.* 1988;70(5):746–750.

86. Esselman PC, Thombs BD, Magyar-Russell G, Fauerbach JA. Burn rehabilitation: state of the science. *Am J Phys Med Rehab.* 2006;85(4):383–413.

87. Parrett BM, Pomahac B, Demling RH, Orgill DP. Fourth-degree burns to the lower extremity with exposed tendon and bone: a ten-year experience. *J Burn Care Res.* 2006;27(1):34–39.

88. El-Khatib HA, Mahboub TA, Ali TA. Use of an adipofascial flap based on the proximal perforators of the ulnar artery to correct contracture of elbow burn scars: an anatomic and clinical approach. *Plast Reconstr Surg.* 2002;109:130–136.

89. Aslan G, Tuncali D, Cigsar B, Barutcu AY, Terzioglu A. The propeller flap for postburn elbow contractures. *Burns.* 2006;32:112–115.

90. Tsionos I, Leclercq C. Rochet JM. Heterotopic ossification of the elbow in patients with burns. Results after early ex-cisision. *J Bone Joint Surg Br*. 2004;86:396–403.

91. McAuliffe JA, Wolfson AH. Early excision of heterotopic ossification about the elbow followed by radiation therapy. *J Bone Joint Surg Am*. 1997;79:749–755.

92. Viola RW, Hanel DP. Early "simple" release of posttraumatic elbow contracture associated with heterotopic ossifica-tion. *J Hand Surg Am*. 1999;24:370–380.

93. Moritomo H, Tada K, Yoshida Y. Early, wide excision of heterotopic ossification in the medial elbow. *J Shoulder Elbow Surg*. 2001;10:164–168.

94. Lindenhovius AL, Linzel DS, Doornberg JN, Ring DC, Jupiter JB. Comparison of elbow contracture release in elbows with and without heterotopic ossification restricting motion. *J Shoulder Elbow Surg*. 2007;16:621–625.

95. Warner JJ. Frozen shoulder: diagnosis and management. *J Am Acad Orthop Surg*. 1997;5:130–140.

96. Marquardt E. [Improved effectiveness of upper-arm prostheses through angulation osteotomy]. *Rehabilitation (Stutg)*. 1972;11:244–248.

97. Marquardt E, Neff G. The angulation osteotomy of above-elbow stumps. *Clin Orthop Relat Res*. 1974;104:232–238.

98. Johnson EN, Burns TC, Hayda RA, Hospenthal DR, Murray CK. Infectious complications of open type III tibial frac-tures among combat casualties. *Clin Infec Dis*. 2007;45(4):409–415.

99. Lin DL, Kirk KL, Murphy KP, McHale KA, Doukas WC. Evaluation of orthopaedic injuries in Operation Enduring Freedom. *J Orthop Trauma*. 2004;18(5):300–305.

100. Dickhaut SC, DeLee JC, Page CP. Nutritional status: importance in predicting wound-healing after amputation. *J Bone Joint Surg Am*. 1984;66(1):71–75.

101. Patzakis MJ, Zalavras CG. Chronic posttraumatic osteomyelitis and infected nonunion of the tibia: current manage-ment concepts. *J Am Acad Orthop Surg*. 2005;13(6):417–427.

102. Perry CR, Pearson RL, Miller GA. Accuracy of cultures of material from swabbing of the superficial aspect of the wound and needle biopsy in the preoperative assessment of osteomyelitis. *J Bone Joint Surg Am*. 1994;73:745–749.

103. Goerres GW, Albrecht S, Allaoua M, Slosman DO. Radionuclide imaging in patients with amputations of the lower leg: typical imaging patterns in five cases. *Clin Nuc Med*. 2000;25(10):804–811.

104. Merkel KD, Brown ML, Dewanjee MK, Fitzgerald RH Jr. Comparison of indium-labeled-leukocyte imaging with sequential technetium-gallium scanning in the diagnosis of low-grade musculoskeletal sepsis: a prospective study. *J Bone Joint Surg Am*. 1985;67:465–476.

105. Nepola JV, Seabold JE, Marsh JL, Kirchner PT, el-Khoury GY. Diagnosis of infection in ununited fractures: combined imaging with indium-111-labeled leukocytes and technetium-99m methylene diphosphonate. *J Bone Joint Surg Am*. 1993;75:1816–1822.

106. Boyd JI 3rd, Wongworawat MD. High-pressure pulsatile lavage causes soft tissue damage. *Clin Orthop Relat Res*. 2004;427:13–17.

107. Brown LL, Shelton HT, Bornside GH, et al. Evaluation of wound irrigation by pulsatile jet and conventional methods. *Ann Surg*. 1978;187:170–173.

108. Svoboda SJ, Bice RG, Gooden HA, Brooks DE, Thomas DB, Wenke JC. Comparison of bulb syringe and pulsed lavage irrigation with use of a bioluminescent musculoskeletal wound model. *J Bone Joint Surg Am*. 2006;88(10):2167–2174.

109. Lerner A, Fodor L, Soudry M. Is staged external fixation a valuable strategy for war injuries to the limbs? *Clin Orthop Relat Res*. 2006;448:217–224.

110. McDonnell KJ, Sculco TP. Dakin's solution revisited. *Am J Orthop*. 1997;26(7):471–473.

111. Dedmond BT, Kortesis B, Punger K, et al. Subatmospheric pressure dressings in the temporary treatment of soft tissue injuries associated with type III open tibial shaft fractures in children. *J Ped Orthop*. 2006;26(6):728–732.

112. Dedmond BT, Kortesis B, Punger K, et al. The use of negative-pressure wound therapy (NPWT) in the temporary treatment of soft-tissue injuries associated with high-energy open tibial shaft fractures. *J Orthop Trauma*. 2007;21(1):11–17.

113. DeFranzo AJ, Argenta LC, Marks MW, et al. The use of vacuum-assisted closure therapy for the treatment of lower-extremity wounds with exposed bone. *Plast Reconstr Surg*. 2001;108(5):1184–1191.

114. Calhoun JH, Henry SL, Anger DM, Cobos JA, Mader JT. The treatment of infected nonunions with gentamicin-polymethylmethacrylate antibiotic beads. *Clin Orthop Relat Res*. 1993;295:23–27.

115. Diefenbeck M, Muckley T, Hoffman GO. Prophylaxis and treatment of implant-related infections by local application of antibiotics. *Injury*. 2006;37(Suppl2):S95–S104.

116. Klemm K. The use of antibiotic-containing bead chains in the treatment of chronic bone infections. *Clin Microbiol Infect*. 2001;7:28–31.

117. Burrell RE, Heggers JP, Davis GJ, Wright JB. Effect of silver coated dressings on animal survival in rodent burn sepsis model. *Wounds*. 1999;11(4):64.

118. Thomas S, McCubbin P. A comparison of the antimicrobial effects of four silver-containing dressings on three organisms. *J Wound Care*. 2003;12:101–107.

119. Ahmed A, Bayol MG, Ha SB. Adventitious bursae in below knee amputees: case reports and a review of the literature. *Am J Phys Med Rehabil*. 1994;73(2):124–129.

120. Singh R, Hunter J, Philip A. Fluid collections in amputee stumps: a common phenomenon. *Arch Phys Med Rehabil*. 2007;88(5):661–663.

121. Degreef I, De Smet L. Complications following resection of the olecranon bursa. *Acta Orthop Belg*. 2006;72(4):400–403.

122. Smith DL, McAfee JH, Lucas LM, Kumar KL, Romney DM. Septic and non-septic olecranon bursitis—utility of the surface temperature probe in early differentiation of septic and non-septic cases. *Arch Intern Med*. 1989;149(7):1581–1585.

123. Stell IM. Management of acute bursitis: outcome study of a structured approach. *J R Soc Med*. 1999;92:516–521.

124. Thompson GR, Manshady BM, Weiss JJ. Septic bursitis. *JAMA*. 1978;240(21):2280–2281.

125. Smith DL, McAfee JH, Lucas LM, Kumar KL, Romney DM. Treatment of nonseptic olecranon bursitis. A controlled, blinded prospective trial. *Arch Intern Med*. 1989;149(11):2527–2530.

126. Stewart NJ, Manzanares JB, Morrey BF. Surgical treatment of aseptic olecranon bursitis. *J Shoulder Elbow Surg*. 1997;6(1):49–54.

127. Kerr DR. Prepatellar and olecranon arthroscopic bursectomy. *Clin Sports Med*. 1993;12(1):137–142.

128. Dudek NL, Marks MB, Marshall SC. Skin problems in an amputee clinic. *Am J Phys Med Rehab*. 2006;85(5):424–429.

Chapter 10

MEDICAL ISSUES IN THE CARE OF THE COMBAT AMPUTEE

BRANDON J. GOFF, DO[*]; THANE D. McCANN, MD[†]; RUPAL M. MODY, MD[‡]; JOSHUA D. HARTZELL, MD[§]; PAIGE E. WATERMAN, MD[¥]; LUIS J. MARTINEZ, MD[¶]; ROBERT N. WOOD-MORRIS, MD[**]; CHARLOTTE CARNEIRO, RN, MS, COHN-S, CIC[††]; RICHARD F. TROTTA, MD[‡‡]; JULIE A. AKE, MD, MSC[§§]; AENEAS JANZE, MD[¥¥]; ALLISON FRANKLIN, DO[¶¶]; SHANE McNAMEE, MD[***]; GARTH T. GREENWELL, DO[†††]; VINCENT T. CODISPOTI, MD[‡‡‡]; KEVIN F. FITZPATRICK, MD[§§§]; MICHAEL DEMARCO, DO[¥¥¥]; AND PAUL F. PASQUINA, MD[¶¶¶]

Major, Medical Corps, US Army; Assistant Chief, Amputee Service, Integrated Department of Orthopaedics and Rehabilitation, National Naval Medical Center, 8901 Rockville Pike, Bethesda, MD 20889 and Walter Reed Army Medical Center, 6900 Georgia Avenue, NW, Washington, DC 20307; formerly, Director of Inpatient Rehabilitation, Walter Reed Army Medical Center, 6900 Georgia Avenue NW, Washington, DC

†*Major, Medical Corps, US Army; Staff Physiatrist, Department of Orthopaedics and Rehabilitation, Brooke Army Medical Center, Center for the Intrepid, 3851 Roger Brooke Drive, Fort Sam Houston, Texas 78234; formerly, Resident Physician, Department of Orthopaedics and Rehabilitation, Walter Reed Army Medical Center, 6900 Georgia Avenue, NW, Washington, DC*

‡*Captain, Medical Corps, US Army; Physician, Department of Infectious Diseases, Walter Reed Army Medical Center, 6900 Georgia Avenue, NW, Washington, DC 20307*

§*Captain, Medical Corps, US Army; Infectious Diseases Fellow, Department of Medicine, Walter Reed Army Medical Center, 6900 Georgia Avenue, NW, Washington, DC 20307; formerly, Chief of Medical Residents, Department of Medicine, Walter Reed Army Medical Center, 6900 Georgia Avenue ,NW, Washington, DC*

¥*Major, Medical Corps, US Army; Infectious Diseases Fellow, Department of Medicine, Walter Reed Army Medical Center, 6900 Georgia Avenue, NW, Washington, DC 20307*

¶*Major, Medical Corps, US Army; Infectious Diseases Fellow, Infectious Diseases Clinic, Walter Reed Army Medical Center, 6900 Georgia Avenue, NW, Washington, DC 20307*

**Major, Medical Corps, US Army; Infectious Diseases Fellow, Department of Infectious Diseases, Walter Reed Army Medical Center, 6900 Georgia Avenue, NW, Washington, DC 20307; formerly, Chief of Medicine, Wurzburg Medical Center, Wurzburg, Germany*

††*Infection Control Nurse Specialist, Department of Infection Control and Epidemiology, Walter Reed Army Medical Center, 6900 Georgia Avenue, NW, Washington, DC 20307; formerly, Nurse Manager, Occupational Health, Marriott Wardman Park Hotel, 2660 Woodley Road NW, Washington, DC*

‡‡*Colonel, Medical Corps, US Army; Assistant Chief, Infectious Disease Service, Department of Internal Medicine, Walter Reed Army Medical Center, 6900 Georgia Avenue, NW, Washington, DC 20307*

§§*Captain, Medical Corps, US Army; Infectious Diseases Fellow, Walter Reed Army Medical Center, 6900 Georgia Avenue, NW, Washington, DC 20307; formerly, Chief of Medical Residents, Department of Medicine, Madigan Army Medical Center, Tacoma, Washington*

¥¥*Captain, Medical Corps, US Army; Resident Physician, Department of Physical Medicine and Rehabilitation, Walter Reed Army Medical Center, 6900 Georgia Avenue, NW, Washington, DC 20307*

¶¶*Captain, Medical Corps, US Army; Director of Inpatient Rehabilitation, Department of Orthopaedics and Rehabilitation, Walter Reed Army Medical Center, 6900 Georgia Avenue, NW, Washington, DC 20307; formerly, Resident, Department of Physical Medicine and Rehabilitation, Walter Reed Army Medical Center, 6900 Georgia Avenue, NW, Washington, DC*

***Medical Director, Polytrauma, Assistant Professor, Department of Physical Medicine and Rehabilitation, Virginia Commonwealth University, 1201 Broadrock Boulevard, Richmond, Virginia 23249*

†††*Captain, Medical Corps, US Army; Staff Physiatrist, Department of Physical Medicine and Rehabilitation Services, MCHK-PT, Tripler Army Medical Center, One Jarrett White Road, Tripler Army Medical Center, Hawaii 96859; formerly, Resident, Department of Physical Medicine, Walter Reed Army Medical Center, 6900 Georgia Avenue, NW, Washington, DC*

‡‡‡*Captain, Medical Corps, US Army; Resident Physician, Department of Physical Medicine and Rehabilitation, Walter Reed Army Medical Center, 6900 Georgia Avenue, NW, Washington, DC 20307*

§§§*Captain, Medical Corps, US Army; Staff Physiatrist, Department of Orthopaedics and Rehabilitation, Walter Reed Army Medical Center, 6900 Georgia Avenue, NW, Washington, DC 20307*

¥¥¥*Major, Medical Corps, US Army; Director of Electrodiagnostic Medicine, Department of Orthopaedics and Rehabilitation, Walter Reed Army Medical Center, 6900 Georgia Avenue, NW, Washington, DC 20307*

¶¶¶*Colonel, Medical Corps, US Army; Chair, Integrated Department of Orthopedics and Rehabilitation, Walter Reed Army Medical Center and National Naval Medical Center, Section 3J, 6900 Georgia Avenue, NW, Washington, DC 20307*

ISSUES IN INFECTIOUS DISEASES

Management of Infectious Issues in the Combat Amputee/Extremity Trauma Patient

Prophylactic Antibiotics for the Combat Amputee/Extremity Trauma Patient

Throughout the history of warfare, open extremity fractures have been associated with significant morbidity and mortality. Field surgeons used therapeutic amputations as a last line of defense against sepsis and exsanguination with poor results. During the Franco–Prussian War, management of these injuries accounted for 13,173 amputations with 10,006 reported deaths.[1] During the American Civil War, the mortality rate for lower extremity fractures ranged from 14% to 32%, despite approximately 29,980 amputations reported. Early in World War I an open femoral fracture carried a mortality risk of 80%; however, mortality was reduced to 16% with the advent of the Thomas traction splint.[2] Further advancement in fracture reduction, splinting, surgical debridement, and subsequent healing by secondary intention contributed to even better outcomes. The importance of debridement in decreasing septic mortality from wounds was demonstrated in both the Spanish Civil War and World War I.[2] The often-cited surgeon's creed "cut to cure" should not be dismissed or maligned because this philosophy led to markedly improved survival rates during the preantibiotic era and continues to play a significant part of battlefield injury management in the modern age of broad-spectrum antibiotics and multidrug-resistant organisms (MDROs).

With the discovery of penicillin and subsequently streptomycin and the sulfonamides, physicians anticipated that patient outcomes would improve. Yet, it became evident that even with antibiotics, closure of an infected wound was still prone to failure. Delayed primary closure of an infected wound has evolved into common practice of battlefield medicine. Although it is universally accepted to use antibiotics to treat an infected wound, its use to prevent wound infection is not as clearly defined and may contribute to antibiotic-resistant bacteria.

For 50 years, various prophylactic regimens have been used with varied success. A majority of the data comes from civilian literature and may not always apply to the combat injured. In 1974 Patzakis et al reported the first prospective randomized data demonstrating the effectiveness of prophylaxis in wound infections.[3] Since this report several studies and guidelines have addressed it. In this chapter these data will be reviewed and a framework for the prevention of wound sepsis will be presented.

Initially, the wound should be grossly decontaminated without compromising hemostasis. The wound is then protected with a sterile or clean dressing and orthosis depending on the wound location (ie, wrist hand orthosis on an open distal ulnar fracture). The patient is triaged and transitions through higher levels of care with further wound management to include incision and drainage/debridement and definitive surgical treatment. Tetanus prophylaxis should be provided and documented if not up-to-date or unknown. Although it is mandatory for US service members to have up-to-date tetanus immunization before deployment, this may not be the case for allied soldiers or injured noncombatants.

Characteristics of a fracture determine the risk of infection. The commonly used Gustilo classification scheme for open fractures provides a useful tool for standardizing care, predicting potential complications, and comparing similar injuries in published reports.[4]

There is little value to culturing wounds early in the clinical course. In a series of 1,104 open fractures that were swabbed for aerobic/anaerobic culture before administration of antibiotics, 7% of the positive surveillance wound cultures developed infection with the same bacterium.[5] Another series of 89 consecutive open fractures demonstrated 83% initial surveillance culture growth, but after debridement, 60% of repeat cultures were negative or grew nonpathogenic bacteria.[6] Most wounds at presentation (before debridement/therapeutic irrigation) are colonized or contaminated, but rarely develop true infection. The authors recommend only obtaining wound cultures and initiating antibiotic treatment when clinical symptoms/findings indicate a true infection, such as fever, elevated white blood cell count, change in vital signs, purulent discharge, etc.

Pre- and perioperative antibiotic prophylaxis has repeatedly demonstrated reduced postoperative infectious complications.[7] Significant variation persists in antibiotic selection, timing, and duration of administration. The Surgical Infection Prevention Project guidelines address this topic[8]:

1. *Timing of the first dose of antimicrobial therapy.* The first dose should begin within 60 minutes of the incision. If a fluoroquinolone or vancomycin is used, infusion should begin within 120 minutes of incision to reduce antibiotic-associated reactions. If a proximal tourniquet is used, administering the full antibiotic dose before tourniquet application is desirable.

2. *Duration of antimicrobial prophylaxis.* No compelling evidence indicates that the use of antibiotics until all catheters and drains are removed will lower infection. Prophylactic antimicrobials should be discontinued within 24 hours postoperatively.

Orthopaedic surgical prophylaxis regimens typically involve first or second generation cephalosporins (excellent coverage for anticipated community-based skin flora). Suggested regimens for total joint (hip and knee) arthroplasty are cefazolin 1 to 2 grams intravenous (IV) or cefuroxime 1.5 gram IV. These also would be appropriate for amputation prophylaxis. Vancomycin 1 gram IV may be used if a beta-lactam allergy/intolerance exists. These recommendations should be considered with each hospital's antibiogram (local sensitivities and resistance patterns) because the presence of MDROs may influence the appropriate choice. Consultation with departments of infectious disease, infection control, and surgical services is recommended.

Management of Infectious Issues in Combat Amputee/Extremity Trauma Patients at a Military Tertiary Care Center

War Wound Infections and Appropriate Antibiotic Therapy

The bacteriology of war wounds has changed significantly over the past 100 years. During World War I, *Streptococcus spp* and *Clostridium spp* predominated. Wound infections in World War II showed anaerobic organisms and skin flora such as *Streptococcus spp* and *Staphylococcus aureus*. With the advent of antibiotics and improved wound debridement techniques, there has gradually been a shift to gram-negative wound infections during the Vietnam and Korean wars. Organisms such as *Enterobacter spp, Escherichia spp, Klebsiella spp, Pseudomonas spp,* and present-day *Acinetobacter baumannii-calcoaceticus* complex (ABC) have begun to emerge as predominant pathogens of battle wounds.[9,10]

More than 18,000 service members were injured from 2001 to 2006 while serving in Afghanistan and Iraq. The prevalence of extremity wounds with concomitant infection has been high.[9,10] Murray et al examined wound culture isolates from soldiers admitted to a combat support hospital in Baghdad, Iraq, at the time of initial injury.[11] Of 61 soldiers, 30 (49%) had positive wound cultures, predominantly composed of less pathogenic gram-positive skin commensals (2 cases of which were methicillin-resistant *Staphylococcus*

aureus [MRSA]). Of the three gram-negative organisms isolated, all were drug sensitive. The lack of drug resistance and decreased pathogenicity supported the curtailment of the use of broad-spectrum prophylactic antibiotics in theater.[11]

In contrast to Murray's findings within the theater, wound and blood cultures taken at tertiary care facilities showed increasing gram-negative bacteria, particularly MDROs.[9,10] A report to the Centers for Disease Control and Prevention (CDC) in 2004 demonstrated increasing rates of drug-resistant ABC as a cause of bloodstream infections in 102 soldiers injured in Iraq, Kuwait, and Afghanistan that were treated at military medical tertiary care facilities.[12] Petersen et al identified major pathogens isolated from war trauma-associated infections in 56 soldiers on the USS Comfort from March through May 2003.[10] Of wound cultures obtained, 47% were polymicrobial with ABC the predominant organism (33%), followed by *Escherichia coli* (18%), and *Pseudomonas spp* (17%). Overall, 81% of organisms in wound cultures were gram-negative bacteria, whereas 19% were gram-positive bacteria. Aronson et al reported similar data from Walter Reed Army Medical Center (WRAMC) with ABC, *Pseudomonas aeruginosa, E coli,* and *Klebsiella spp* accounting for a majority of war wound infections.[9] Recent evidence suggests that the outbreak of multidrug-resistant ABC infection in the US military healthcare system likely results from environmental contamination of field hospitals coupled with broad-spectrum antibiotic use and transmission within healthcare facilities.[13]

According to the CDC/Healthcare Infection Control Practices Advisory Committee 2006 guidelines, MDROs are defined as resistant to one or more classes of antibiotics.[14] MDROs such as MRSA, ABC, and extended-spectrum beta-lactamase (ESBL) producing organisms are being isolated from wound infections and other sterile body sites and fluids in soldiers.[9,10,12] The incidence of multidrug-resistant ABC in all culture sites at WRAMC increased from 0.087 cases per 1,000 admissions in 2002 to 0.3 cases per 1,000 admissions in 2005.

Treatment of war wound infections primarily involves surgical debridement of devitalized tissue with adjunctive antibiotics. Antibiotic susceptibility testing must guide treatment for MDROs. Currently, ABC susceptibility testing has increased utilization of polymyxins, carbapenems, and aminoglycosides for treatment.[9,10,12] Severely ill or immunocompromised patients with multidrug-resistant ABC infection have been treated with combination therapy based on in-vitro and some in-vivo reports of synergy with combinations of polymyxins with rifampin and/or carbapenems; however, the clinical relevance of these data remains uncertain.[15,16] A carbapenem is typically the preferred drug for treating ESBL organisms.[17,18] Multiple drugs are available to treat MRSA infections such as vancomycin, linezolid, and trimethoprim-sulfamethoxazole.

The decision to treat war wound cultures and the duration of treatment are challenging. These decisions are dependent on the clinical suspicion for infection and type of infection present (ie, superficial vs deep infection). When MDROs are isolated from sterile sites, an infectious disease specialist should be consulted for further treatment recommendations.

Management and Follow-Up of Surgical Infections for Combat Amputee/Extremity Trauma Patients

Colonization

In postsurgical patients, differentiating between colonization and true infection is critical. Colonization is defined as the isolation of microorganisms in culture without accompanying clinical signs and symptoms of infection. The presence of the organism is not pathogenic and treatment is usually not required because of the lack of active infection, although antimicrobial measures are sometimes undertaken to decolonize a patient for infection control purposes (discussed below). To avoid unnecessary antibiotic use, the authors recommend against culturing wounds and surgical sites without clinical signs or symptoms of infection.

Surgical Site Infections. Surgical site infections (SSIs) are the most common complication of hospitalized surgical patients.[19] Risk for the development of SSIs is related to both patient and operation characteristics. Contaminated and high-risk surgeries are associated with higher frequency of SSI development, with amputations among the highest risk procedures.[20] Organisms commonly causing orthopaedic procedure-associated SSIs include *S aureus*, coagulase-negative staphylococcal species, and gram-negative bacilli. Surveillance data demonstrate that the epidemiology of SSIs in critically ill patients has been changing: the percentage of SSIs associated with gram-negative bacilli decreased from 56.5% in 1986 to 33.8% in 2003. The distribution of gram-negative pathogens also has changed, with decreasing numbers of *E coli* and *Enterobacter* isolates and an increase in the frequency of *Acinetobacter*-associated SSIs.[21] *Acinetobacter spp* and ESBL-producing organisms have presented a particularly difficult clinical challenge to US military hospitals because of high levels of antimicrobial resistance among those pathogens.

SSIs are categorized as follows:

- superficial incisional SSI,
- deep incisional SSI, and
- organ/space SSI.[22]

As defined for surveillance purposes, superficial incisional SSIs occur within 30 days of the operation, involve only the skin or subcutaneous tissue of the incision, and feature at least one of the following: (1) purulent drainage; (2) organisms isolated from culture of fluid or tissue from the incision; (3) local signs or symptoms to include pain or tenderness, swelling, erythema, and warmth; and (4) diagnosis by the surgeon or attending physician.

Deep incisional SSIs occur within 30 days of the operation (within 1 year if an implant is in place); involve the deep soft tissues (muscle and fascial layers) of the incision; feature at least one of the four characteristics listed in the previous paragraph; and involve the patient with a fever greater than 38° Celsius or evidence of abscess or other infection on examination, histopathology, or radiologic examination.

Organ/space SSIs occur within 30 days after the operation if no implant is in place or within 1 year if an implant is in place and involve part of the anatomy that was opened or manipulated. In patients undergoing amputations, the organ/space SSI includes joint or bursa infections and osteomyelitis. Organ/space SSIs are usually treated as infections related to the relevant organ and space, whereas the superficial and deep incisional SSIs are treated as skin and soft tissue infections.

The diagnosis of an SSI is made with emphasis on examination of the incision. Signs of infection include tenderness, swelling, erythema, and purulent drainage. Clinical manifestations of SSIs typically occur 5 days postoperatively. Fever within the first 48 hours postoperatively is only rarely attributable to SSI.[23] Exceptions include SSIs resulting from streptococci and clostridial organisms, which can be diagnosed by the Gram stain of incisional drainage, and staphylococcal toxic shock syndrome, which is accompanied by the early findings of fever, hypotension, elevated liver-associated enzymes, and diarrhea.[24] In the presence of early postoperative fever, the incision should be examined thoroughly and any drainage should be sampled, and a thorough evaluation of all potential causes of common nosocomial infections should be conducted.

The Infectious Diseases Society of America has published guidelines for SSI treatment.[25] The most important aspect of treating SSIs is to open the wound, remove infected material, and perform dressing changes until the wound heals by secondary intention. Following drainage of the wound, antibiotic administration is not recommended without evidence of invasive infection or systemic illness. However, in patients with fever (> 38.5° Celsius) or tachycardia, a short course of antibiotics may be indicated (24–48 hours). The choice of therapy is often empiric, but should be guided by Gram stain or culture results when available. *S aureus* and streptococcal species are the most common infecting pathogens in SSIs following clean procedures (those procedures not entering the gastrointestinal or genital tracts). Consequently, agents with gram-positive coverage such as cefazolin, oxacillin, and clindamycin are recommended. Surgical procedures involving the gastrointestinal and genitourinary tracts as well as incisions involving the axilla or perineum have a higher incidence of gram-negative organisms and anaerobic pathogen infections. In these circumstances, effective choices include cefotetan, ampicillin/sulbactam, or a fluoroquinolone plus clindamycin. In all cases in which the rate of MRSA infection is high, vancomycin or linezolid should be considered while awaiting results of culture and susceptibility testing. In the authors' experience with patients returning from Operation Iraqi Freedom/Operation Enduring Freedom (OIF/OEF), limited-spectra antibiotics have been less useful because of the prevalence of MDROs. Antimicrobials with broader spectra have been required for these wound infections and should be considered as empiric therapy in clinically severe infections.[26]

Implant Infections. SSIs may affect surgical implants. Implant-associated infections occur perioperatively by bacterial contamination during surgery, by hematogenous spread of pathogens through blood from a distant infectious focus, or contiguously from an adjacent infectious focus.[27] Definitive diagnosis of implant-associated infection involves the presence of clinical manifestations, intraoperative signs of infection adjacent to the implant, and the growth of pathogens in cultures of surgical specimens.[28] A full discussion of device-related infections is beyond the scope of this chapter but an overview is provided below.

For infections related to an implanted orthopaedic device, the surgical treatment has traditionally involved resection arthroplasty or removal of the fixation device. The surgical management of infected joint prostheses varies from debridement with prosthesis retention to two-stage replacement, which involves hardware removal, followed by the placement of an antimicrobial-containing spacer. The patient undergoes a prolonged course of systemic antibiotics—typically 6 weeks—and subsequent implantation of a new prosthesis. The two-stage replacement approach is preferred over the one-stage approach because of improved cure rates and superior functional outcomes.[29]

Infections of fracture-fixation devices that involve bone, including pin-site infections, are treated as osteomyelitis with a 6-week course of systemic antibiotics. Superficial infections of these devices can be adequately treated with 10 to 14 days of antibiotic therapy once the possibility of deeper infection has been excluded. Surgical intervention depends on the type of device, the presence of bone union, and the clinical stability of the patient. Infection of intramedullary nails usually requires removal of the infected nail, use of external-fixation pins, and potentially subsequent insertion of a replacement nail. Surgical intervention of infected external-fixation pins[28] involves removing infected pins and, if bone union has not occurred, inserting new pins at a distant site or fusion of the bones.

In the authors' experience, a large number of patients with orthopaedic implant infections have not been able to undergo immediate device removal because of the extent of their injuries. In these patients, the authors recommend infectious disease consultation to determine the optimal antimicrobial regimen often involving an initial parenteral course of antibiotics followed by a long-term oral regimen. Cure rates in trials involving retention of the implant generally have been disappointing. A recent randomized controlled trial of rifampin in implant salvage among a selected group of patients with joint prosthesis or fracture-fixation device staphylococcal infections yielded promising results.[30] Ongoing studies in OIF/OEF patients will hopefully provide valuable data on how to best manage these complex cases.

Protocol for Management of Infections for Amputee/Extremity Trauma Patients

An axiom for the treatment of soft tissue or hardware infections is debridement of infected or devitalized tissues and removal of implanted hardware. Antibiotics serve a secondary role that is effective only with adequate debridement. Without sufficiently removing the infected source, most antibiotic regimens fail regardless of duration of treatment regimen. Recommendations for optimal duration of therapy vary and no standard consensus guidelines exist.

Treatment of osteomyelitis poses several clinical difficulties. No studies have addressed prospective randomized clinical trials assessing the length of antimicrobial therapy in these patients. In the setting of traumatic injury, osteomyelitis has a heterogeneous disease course and the optimal duration of antimicrobial therapy is unknown. In experimental models, 4 weeks of therapy were more effective in sterilizing the bone than 2 weeks of therapy. Surgical debridement was not part of these models; therefore, shorter courses of therapy may be as effective when paired with extensive surgical debridement.[31] Although it typically takes approximately 6 weeks for vascularized soft tissue to cover the debrided bone and anecdotal experiences suggest a higher relapse rate with shorter durations of therapy, most experts recommend 4 to 6 weeks of parenteral antimicrobial therapy.[32]

A similar problem exists for skin and soft tissue infections. The duration of antibiotics for infections involving only the skin and soft tissue has not been definitively proven. Most experts recommend 7 to 14 days of therapy or until resolution of clinical signs and symptoms. Therefore, each patient should be followed closely to ensure adequate treatment and to prevent the spread of the infection to deeper tissues.

Principles of Management. It is difficult to compare the available literature because no standard case definitions, treatments, or patient populations exist, resulting in large discrepancies among outcomes that may not be based exclusively on treatment methods. In addition, small sample sizes in many studies preclude the ability to make definitive conclusions and the sample populations vary (civilian trauma vs combat injury).

The inoculating event is important in determining management. Posttraumatic osteomyelitis may occur as a direct result of bony injury following trauma or arise from nosocomial infection. Ideally, antibiotic selections are guided by wound culture and sensitivity results. Empiric antibiotic regimens should be chosen based on the medical center's antibiogram (local sensitivities and resistance patterns).

Patients with amputations/extremity trauma often have serial debridements ("washouts") prior to wound closure. Interval surgical exams are important in monitoring for resolution of infection. Findings of new purulence, fluid collections, or necrotic tissue should be cultured because it may represent a new infection or an emerging resistant organism. Cultures should not be taken during serial washouts if no evidence of infection exists because positive culture results may represent colonization.

Quantitative operative cultures may be used as a marker of decreased or resolving bacterial burden. Quantitative culture requires weighing and careful preparation of the specimen for serial dilutions to determine whether the colony count is greater than 10^5 colony-forming units per gram of tissue. Colony counts of this magnitude are correlated with a greater likelihood of infection associated with wound closure. Direct Gram smears of known quantities of specimen can be used to give an immediate assessment of organism load. Because quantitative cultures are time consuming and labor intensive, not all laboratories

have procedures for performing these assays. The authors therefore recommend against performing such cultures.[33]

Different inflammatory markers can be used to monitor infection, but none have been studied in the authors' particular patient population. These markers include C-reactive protein, erythrocyte sedimentation rate, and pro-calcitonin level. Unfortunately, these markers differ based on the specific patient's inflammatory response to the initial trauma, surgical trauma, and underlying comorbidities. The most important concept in monitoring these parameters is the observance of trends. A significant increase in any of these serum studies may prompt further radiologic or surgical exploration for unresolved infection.

Orthopaedic consultants often obtain serial plain radiographs. Although plain films are insensitive for monitoring osteomyelitis, findings of osteopenia and thinning of cortical bone or sequestra should prompt closer monitoring or cross-sectional imaging studies. Serial cross-sectional imaging studies (computed tomography [CT], magnetic resonance imaging, etc) may be used, but they are significantly more expensive and patient transport may present challenges. To further complicate imaging study of osteomyelitis, noninfectious postoperative scarring or edema in traumatized bone can persist for up to 1 year.[34] Heterotopic ossification (HO) has also been commonly seen in the OIF/OEF population; however, it does not appear to pose an increased risk of infection.[35]

Infection Control and Surveillance in Returning Warriors

The emergence of MDROs is a worldwide dilemma and adds to the complexity of care for wounded and ill service members returning from theater. The predominant and troublesome MDRO that military personnel face returning from OIF/OEF is ABC.[9,10,12,13] Several reports have focused on the ABC outbreak that appears to be related to contamination in field hospitals.[13] *Acinetobacter* has been appreciated since the Vietnam War and it continues to be a significant problem for personnel returning from OIF/OEF.[36]

Other MDROs of concern in major military hospitals and in civilian hospitals are gram-negative organisms, *Klebsiella pneumoniae*, *P aeruginosa*, vancomycin-resistant enterococcus, and ESBL-producing organisms. These MDROs have a predilection for transmission in healthcare facilities and persist unless diligent control and containment measures are undertaken. Wounded service members, particularly those with open non-healing wounds or burns, are at risk for bacterial colonization and/or infection. Treating these infections with broad-spectrum antimicrobials leads to depletion of normal gut flora, increasing the risk for *Clostridium difficile*-associated disease.

Measures for successful control of MDROs, which have been documented in the United States and abroad, consist of a variety of combined interventions.[14] These interventions include hand hygiene by all healthcare providers, the use of active surveillance cultures for MDRO colonization, contact precautions, infectious control education, enhanced environmental cleaning, and improvements in communication between healthcare providers/facilities about patients with MDRO infections. Each of these measures should be customized for application within each healthcare facility and the local community under the guidance of an active and informed infection control committee of specialists in infectious disease, occupational health, preventative medicine, pharmacy, and clinical laboratory services. However, it is the responsibility of individual healthcare providers to play an active role in the successful elimination of MDROs in their patients, their hospital, and their community.

Initiation and Surveillance of Contact Precautions

Active surveillance of MDROs, particularly with MRSA, is being widely conducted in the United States. In 2003 major military medical treatment facilities began surveillance cultures of groin and axillae for ABC and nares for MRSA on all soldiers directly admitted from theater. Population and need determines targeted surveillance. Contact precautions are used as a containment measure before MDRO isolation from culture when there is a high suspicion for infection (eg, on hospital admission and/or in patients with open draining wounds not contained in a dressing). Methods for determining colonization are not standardized among institutions. CDC guidelines should be used as a reference when making decisions regarding colonization surveillance methods.[14] Any healthcare provider can initiate contact precautions, but they should be removed in conjunction with infection control practitioners and hospital policy.

CDC defines contact precautions as the wearing of gown and gloves when in contact with the patient or anything that has touched the patient.[14] Although visitors who touch the patient do not always need to comply with these measures, the rationale for healthcare providers to wear protective gear is to prevent the transmission of bacteria from one patient to another. In some circumstances it is not feasible for each patient to have a private room. In these cases pa-

tients with the same MDROs can be located together. At WRAMC family members are required to wear a gown and gloves only if they will come into contact with blood or body fluids. Other institutions require family members to wear a gown, gloves, and masks (when concern for airborne transmission exists) at all times. The efficacy of any of these strategies requires strict adherence.

Discontinuing Contact Precautions

Few data support standardized criteria for removing contact precautions for patients colonized or infected with MDROs. The clearing protocol shown in Table 10-1 is used in two major military medical treatment facilities to clear patients and to reduce their social isolation.[37] Providers should know their patients' status and be involved in a clearing protocol as soon as antibiotic therapy has ceased for 72 hours and wounds are healed.

Environmental Cleaning

The environment plays an increasingly significant role in the transmission of nosocomial MDROs. ABC and MRSA can live for weeks on surfaces, especially "high-touch" surfaces.[38] Daily housecleaning of such surfaces, particularly IV poles and bedrails, is critical. Hospital-grade disinfectants with high kill while drying should be used in patient rooms, especially during patient turnover. Assiduous environmental cleaning by hospital housekeeping staff has been shown to reduce the frequency of vancomycin-resistant enterococcus cross contamination.[39]

Once the colonized patient is discharged and returns for rehabilitation in outpatient clinics, the risk for transmission is decreased but not eliminated. Patients with amputations and other combat-related injuries often require multiple readmissions and clinic visits for rehabilitation. They are continually at risk for acquiring a new infection or spreading their colonized microbes. In WRAMC's outpatient clinics patients with open wounds or undergoing dressing changes must be treated in designated areas. In therapy gyms the healthcare provider monitors and cleans mats and other equipment used by patients with the appropriate germicide.

Hand Hygiene

Hand hygiene remains the cornerstone of infection prevention and control in healthcare and community settings; therefore, hospital administrators should give it the highest level of attention.[40] Soap and water may be as effective as antimicrobial soap. Alcohol hand gels with moisturizer have been shown to be effective against all organisms except *C difficile* and spores. Hand hygiene for healthcare workers is required before and after any patient care and after removing gloves. Routine surveillance of handwashing is recommended to enforce its importance and identify areas for intervention within an institution.

Communication and Education

Providers communicating to bed control managers, discharge planners, and others have been very successful in alerting others of a patient's MDRO status. Healthcare providers have a critical role in educating patients of the significance of MDRO colonization or infection. To prevent feelings of isolation and anxiety, simple language should be

TABLE 10-1

CLEARING PROTOCOL SUMMARY CHART

To Clear For	When	Obtain These Cultures	Order as	Repeat	Clear
Acinetobacter	Off antibiotics 72 hours, clinically improved, hardware sites clean and dry	Groin, axillae, nasal swabs Original site if sputum, urine, or open/draining wound	Rule out *Acinetobacter* (ACI), choose site from pick list (groin, axilla, nares, wound, sputum, other)	Same cultures two more times, each 72 hours apart	If all cultures are negative and approved by ICES
MRSA	Off antibiotics 72 hours, clinically improved, hardware sites clean and dry	Nares Original site if sputum, urine, or open/draining wound	Rule out MRSA, select nasal swab and other sites from pick list	Same cultures two more times, each 72 hours apart	If all cultures are negative and approved by ICES
VRE	Off antibiotics 72 hours, clinically improved, hardware sites clean and dry	Stool cultures or rectal swab Original site if sputum, urine, or open/draining wound	Rule out VRE, choose sites from pick list	Same cultures two more times, each 72 hours apart	If all cultures are negative and approved by ICES
MDRO/ESBL Gram negs (*Klebsiella, Pseudomonas*)	Off antibiotics 72 hours, clinically improved, hardware sites clean and dry	Urine or peri-anal/rectal swab Original site if sputum, urine, or open/draining wound	Rule out MDRO choose sites from pick list	Same cultures two more times, each 72 hours apart	If all cultures are negative and approved by ICES
Clostridium difficile	Completed 72 hours of treatment	No cultures necessary	NA	NA	If clinically improved and no diarrhea for 24 hours

ESBL: extended spectrum beta-lactamase
ICES: Infection Control and Epidemiology Service
MDRO: multidrug-resistant organism
MRSA: methicillin-resistant *Staphylococcus aureus*
VRE: vancomycin-resistant enterococcus
Initiate clearance cultures when off effective* antibiotics for 72 hours, wounds are healing, hardware is clean, and patient is clinically healing. For long-term patients readmitted, initiate clearance cultures prior to restart of antibiotics.
Do not culture blood, cerebrospinal fluid, or scabbed/healed wounds if these were originally positive.
*Effective antibiotic = one to which the organism is proven susceptible

used to convey the type and significance of infection/colonization to each patient placed on contact precautions.

Fever in the Returning Service Member

Fever in the returning service member should be recognized for its similarities to routine travelers and for its uniqueness related to the combat environment.[9] Rates of disease and nonbattle injury casualties historically exceed battle injuries in most conflicts. Rates have remained high for conflicts within the past decade, although preventive medicine interventions have dramatically reduced the nonpsychiatric and nonbattle injuries. Nevertheless, certain infections should remain high on the physician's differential when treating a returning service member.

Systemic illness, followed closely by diarrheal and respiratory illnesses, constitutes the majority of syndromes in all travelers when studied across six continents.[41] Diarrheal illness is common in deployed personnel with up to 66% of troops reporting diarrhea, but it is an unlikely cause of fever the longer a patient has been back from theater.[9] Physicians should consider more common etiologies of diarrhea and fever (*C difficile*) for patients who have been out of theater for more than 1 week.

Malaria remains a consideration with travel to endemic areas outside the United States. Malaria is a common etiology of fever in the returning traveler, yet it has attack rates of only 10% in most areas of Afghanistan. Malaria from Iraq is rare with few cases directly attributable to travel there.[42] Most of the malaria cases have been caused by *Plasmodium vivax* (80% to 90% in Afghanistan and 95% in Iraq) with the remainder caused by the more life-threatening strain, *Plasmodium falciparum*.[43] Fever secondary to *P vivax* infection, which can occur months after exposure, should be considered as a potential etiology in at-risk patients for up to 1 year after return from deployment.

Q fever, caused by *Coxiella burnetii*, has been diagnosed in returning service members, with more than 30 cases diagnosed during OIF/OEF.[9,44,45] Classically, patients have been exposed to animals, such as cows and sheep, but several of the cases from OIF/OEF did not have known direct exposure. Q fever, which has a variable clinical course, often presents as a nonspe-

cific febrile flu-like illness with pneumonia and/or hepatitis. Chronic infection most commonly involves the heart, and specific recommendations have been developed to monitor for chronic disease.[46]

Leishmaniasis, spread by the sand fly, represents another potential cause of fever in the returning service member. More than 1,200 cases of cutaneous leishmaniasis and four confirmed cases of visceral leishmaniasis have occurred.[47] Cutaneous leishmaniasis is characterized by a nonhealing skin ulcer, without systemic symptoms. Visceral leishmaniasis is a systemic illness that manifests as a syndrome of fever, fatigue, night sweats, weight loss, gastrointestinal upset, hepatosplenomegaly, impaired liver function tests, and pancytopenia. Patient travel to endemic areas will increase one's suspicion of leishmaniasis, and diagnosis can be made with a serologic assay.[9]

Apart from wound-specific infections, service members are at risk for infections transmitted via blood transfusion. Many service members receive massive transfusions (greater than 10 units of blood products). Although screening of the prepared blood supply is adequate, wartime often necessitates the use of field-expedient donors that may not have had recent screening for potentially newly acquired diseases such as human immunodeficiency virus and viral hepatitis. Unlike hepatitis A, which is rarely acquired via transfusion, hepatitis B and hepatitis C are associated with blood transfusions. One study from 1996 estimated nonwar-related transmission rates of 1 per 64,000 units transfused for hepatitis B virus. Hepatitis C virus was estimated to have transmission rates of 1 per 103,000 per donor exposure in the United States. Human immunodeficiency virus transmission rates have been reported at 1 per 493,000 units transfused in the United States.[48] Although rates are not yet known for deployed service members, new infections have been identified in returning OEF/OIF service members.

Providers caring for hospitalized service members who have sustained injuries during a deployment should be aware of all potential causes of infections. Although it is the tendency to focus on the areas of trauma, potential travel-related infections must also be considered. Using the methods discussed in this section and reviewing the infections that are endemic to a deployed area will help the provider make an expedient diagnosis and decrease morbidity.

WOUND CARE MANAGEMENT

Introduction

Wound care management is a critical component of military medicine, especially in the traumatic amputee's

care. Combat injuries often require complex wound care at multiple sites throughout the body. Because of the advances in body armor, fewer wounds are being seen to the chest and abdomen than had been reported in prior wars. Furthermore, given the combination of immobilization, peripheral nerve injuries, and sedating effects of multiple medications, these patients are at even greater risk of developing problems such as pressure ulcers or compressive neuropathies. Therefore, proper positioning of the patient at all times throughout the echelons of care will likely reduce the risk of iatrogenic injuries. Judicious application of a standardized algorithm may reduce morbidity and mortality associated with wound management as well as economic burden.

Although it would seem reasonable that the amount of training a medical professional receives in wound care management would be commensurate with its degree of overall medical significance, this is not the case. Wound care tends to be an area of healthcare where outdated dogma often supersedes current medical knowledge. In addition, it is often mistakenly judged to be a subject, rather than a required dedicated field of medicine within itself.

A provider cannot make competent decisions regarding the "how" of treatment when there is an incomplete understanding of the "why." In this section a focused discussion of the essential principles of wound care will be presented. Unfortunately, a detailed analysis of wound types, their corresponding nomenclature, and specific treatment algorithms is beyond the scope of this section. Therefore, the following review will address normal wound healing, factors that negatively affect outcomes, and general principles to optimize wound healing.

The Phases of Wound Healing

The four stages of wound healing are

1. hemostasis,
2. inflammation,
3. proliferation, and
4. remodeling.

Hemostasis

The hemostatic phase starts when the skin is first broken and stops when blood loss is controlled. The most immediate reaction to vascular injury occurs at the level of the vessel itself that reflexively vasoconstricts when damaged. The two primary means of hemostasis, however, involve initiation of the coagulation cascade and the formation of a platelet plug. These events are elegantly triggered when normally extraluminal materials such as collagen, thrombin, and tissue factor are exposed to the intraluminal milieu. The time required depends on the wound size and intrinsic factors associated with the patient's health.

Inflammation

The inflammatory phase, under normal circumstances, lasts 3 to 5 days and is defined by the presence of neutrophils. The role of the neutrophils in a wound bed is context dependent and under certain conditions it can be disadvantageous. As a member of the body's innate immune response, neutrophils are critical but their actions are nonspecific. Neutrophils act by releasing cytokines and chemokines within the wound bed, leading to free radical production and creating an unfriendly environment for both pathogens, as well as often the body's own tissue-healing cells. Neutrophils also release the enzymes collagenase and elastase into the wound bed to break down the remaining extracellular matrix in preparation for subsequent wound-healing stages. By preventing pathogens from establishing foci and removing the detritus of an injured wound bed (extracellular matrix, dead pathogens, and native cells), an accessible route of entry for the body's incoming regenerative cells is created.

Neutrophils will generally persist until most of the bacteria and necrotic tissue are removed. Neutrophils are vital acutely following injury, but they become a deficit in subsequent healing stages. Wound debridement at this later stage is therefore vital. The transition to the proliferative phase of wound healing is facilitated by manually cleaning a wound bed of bacteria and necrotic tissue. The success of wound debridement depends on proper technique. Excessive force may lead to renewed involvement of the neutrophils and only reinitiate the wound-healing cascade.

Proliferation

Just as the inflammatory phase was defined by the neutrophil, the proliferative phase is defined by the macrophage. Macrophages consume bacteria and nonviable material, and release enzymes to break down the existing extracellular matrix. However, macrophages, which are more sophisticated and multidimensional than neutrophils in their overall function, can be considered the orchestrators of wound healing. The release of growth factors and cytokines leads to the migration of keratinocytes and fibroblasts into the wound bed to initiate reepithelialization and granulation tissue formation, respectively.

Three steps in the proliferative phase include

1. reepithelialization,
2. granulation tissue formation, and
3. wound contraction.

Reepithelialization. The first step in the proliferative phase, reepithelialization begins as early as
24 hours postinjury. When an area of skin is broken,
the loss of contact inhibition that occurs between
epidermal cells stimulates replication and migration
into the wound bed. This migration is coordinated by
macrophages.

Granulation Tissue Formation. The second step,
the granulation tissue formation, can begin as early
as 3 days postinjury and is visually the hallmark of
the proliferative phase. The wound bed begins to take
on a shiny, reddish-pink, cobblestone appearance.
Macroscopically, each red cobblestone represents a
burgeoning new capillary, and the shiny texture is
imparted by the loose extracellular matrix, which is
produced by fibroblasts. When the intricate processes
of reepithelialization and granulation tissue formation
are not coordinated, they can work in opposition. For
example, a wound will stop granulating once it is
epithelialized, even if the wound has not yet filled in.
Similarly, if epithelialization never occurs, granulation may continue unabated until a heaping mound
of granulating tissue towers over the surrounding
periwound skin. The etiology and treatment of these
conditions will be discussed later in this chapter.

Wound Contraction. The third step in the proliferative phase is wound contraction. When a wound is
mature enough, fibroblasts are signaled to alter their
gene expression, the synthesis of actin filaments is
upregulated, and the fibroblast transforms into a myo-
fibroblast. Myofibroblasts link up across the wound
bed and over time pull the wound closed.

Remodeling

The remodeling phase, the final and longest wound-
healing phase, frequently lasts more than 2 years. It is
largely mediated by fibroblasts and consists primarily
of collagen deposition along the lines of stress. Remodeling is a dynamic process and increases the tensile
strength of the wound where it needs it most.

Abnormal Wound Healing

Abnormal wound healing occurs when a chronic
wound fails to proceed through the aforementioned
phases, resulting in a wound that is deficient in its
anatomic and/or functional integrity. Wound healing
is simplified and described in phases; however, it is a
continuum involving countless cells, cytokines, and
yet to be identified factors. A wound can be further
complicated by extrinsic factors, such as infection, or
intrinsic factors specific to the patient such as malnutrition or defined genetic-dependent characteristics.

The wound-healing mechanisms are overwhelmed,
and intervention is required to facilitate recovery.
The differential diagnosis for a nonhealing wound is
relatively narrow and for the vast majority of cases will
be related to at least one of the following intrinsic or
extrinsic factors. Intrinsic factors may include chronic
inflammation, excessive granulation or insufficient
epithelialization, excessive fluid (maceration) within
the wound bed, poor nutritional status, etc. Extrinsic
factors may include insufficient or excessive debridement and/or inadequate infection management.

Chronic Inflammation

Chronic inflammation in the presence of infection,
for example, is an appropriate and necessary bodily
response. The appropriate clinical action in this situation would clearly be to treat the infection and not
the inflammation. Conversely, if a wound appears
persistently inflamed yet not infected, other etiologies
must be sought.

Insufficient versus Excessive Debridement

Aside from infection, the most likely causes for
persistent inflammation within the wound come from
repeated trauma or necrotic tissue. As discussed previously, fixing one issue can often exacerbate the other.
To clear a wound of its necrotic tissue, for example,
the wound must be debrided. An aggressive debriding
schedule, such as wet-to-dry dressing changes every
4 hours, may cause excessive trauma and a situation
of diminishing returns. Likewise, in an exudative or
otherwise wet wound, applied dressings are unable
to dry and therefore debridement would not be accomplished with subsequent removal. Wounds with
substantial eschar may require sharp debridement,
whereas wounds with less eschar may respond to autolytic or enzymatic debridement. The clinician should
choose the most appropriate means of debridement
depending on the wound characteristics.

Granulation versus Epithelialization

Complications associated with granulation are often compounded with problems of epithelialization.
Specifically, a hypogranulating wound often localizes
the problem to the wound bed. Conversely, a hypergranulating wound often indicates a problem with
epithelialization (ie, the periwound skin).

Consider the following: A wound bed is chronically inflamed from necrotic tissue. The surrounding
skin, however, is supple and healthy. Because of the
persistent inflammation, the wound bed granulates at

a very slow pace, but the surrounding skin continues to migrate in at a normal pace. As a result, the edges of the wound margins are opposed over an insufficient wound bed.

Consider a wound that has a very healthy wound base, but has persistently macerated wound edges. The wound will granulate at a normal pace but the wound margins will fail to oppose secondary to insufficient epithelialization. The granulating tissue, with no signal to stop, will therefore grow unabated, rising above the level of the surrounding skin. This would be referred to as a hypergranulating wound, although a more accurate characterization would be a "hypo-epithelializing" wound.

A wound may fail to epithelialize properly for several reasons. One reason is the rolled edge or epiboly. Under normal circumstances, periwound skin divides and migrates down into the wound bed. Occasionally, however, these cells can become misdirected and like the crest of a breaking wave curl up underneath themselves. Because of contact inhibition, the cells stop dividing and epithelialization fails. A close inspection of the wound can identify this phenomenon. Sharp debridement is usually the quickest and most effective solution. The remaining reasons for insufficient epithelialization are simply related to unhealthy periwound skin, the most common etiologies being a macerated wound edge, unrelieved pressure, persistent inflammation, or infection.

A slowly granulating wound—more often than not—indicates an unhealthy wound base. Desiccation, persistent inflammation, infection, a cold wound bed, and tightly packed gauze are all common causes. Whatever the etiology, it is critical to remember that if epithelialization has already occurred, the wound bed will not granulate even if the underlying problem is corrected. It is therefore occasionally necessary to cauterize the surrounding wound edges with silver nitrate to prevent epithelialization while the wound bed recovers.

Desiccation versus Maceration

The task of balancing optimal moisture levels between wound and skin is often the most challenging aspect of wound care. Depending on age, sex, and body fat, the amount of water in human bodies ranges from 50% to 70%. Moisture is essential for wound healing. Without moisture, migrating cells and chemical signals have no medium in which to travel, and the viability of enzymes and growth factors cannot be maintained.

Although humans need water, they are unable to live in it. The keratinized stratum corneum of human epidermis keeps excess moisture from penetrating to deeper levels; however, this attribute is negated with an open wound. Once upper stratum corneum and basilar layers are interrupted, epidermal cells become exposed to a hypotonic solution and will gradually swell and burst. The desmosomes that anchor the epidermal cells to the dermis and to each other will eventually become disrupted, and the wound will become larger.

A skilled wound care specialist will consider the periwound skin as part of the wound environment because it is from this healthy rim of tissue that most of the regenerative epithelial cells originate. Management of the periwound fluid balance is critical. Through the judicious use of dressings, emollients, and barriers, the wound bed may be kept moist without causing maceration of the wound margin. Likewise, the wound must be kept dry enough without causing desiccation of the wound bed.

Infection versus Antibiotics

By definition a wound is infected when the bacterial load exceeds 100,000 organisms per gram. A clinical diagnosis may be made based on signs and symptoms of infection to include purulence, erythema, or evidence of advancing cellulites. As discussed in the previous section, determination of colonization versus active infection is critical in determining appropriateness of antibiotic management. Additional signs and symptoms of infection include

- induration,
- pain,
- fever,
- changes in color,
- persistently foul odor,
- increased drainage,
- friable granulation tissue that easily bleeds, and
- delayed healing.

The indiscriminate use of topical antibiotics has led to bacterial resistance and the alteration of normal skin flora. In addition, the nonselective nature of these antibiotics also causes damage to native cells. Some bactericidal agents such as hydrogen peroxide and iodine are more toxic to human cells than to bacteria. These characteristics warrant judicious use of topical agents in wound management.

Impaired Healing Response

Thus far, the discussion of abnormal wound healing has revolved around direct extrinsic factors, but an equally important aspect is the health of the wound-healing machinery itself. If a patient's system is already stressed from sepsis, for example, the body simply cannot allocate the resources necessary for wound healing. Broadly speaking (and with some overlap) there are five main categories of problems that can cause an impaired healing response:

1. a diseased state,
2. an impaired immune system,
3. malnutrition,
4. toxins, and
5. medications.

In the inpatient setting special attention should be paid to the patient's nutritional status and medication profile. Immunosuppressants such as corticosteroids and nonsteroidal antiinflammatory medications (NSAIDs) are frequent culprits. Cytotoxic topical agents as discussed above can also slow things down considerably. For a patient whose nutritional status is compromised, weekly prealbumin levels are indicated and a certified nutritionist should be involved as early as possible. Tobacco use also can seriously retard wound healing. Patients must be educated about this and offered a tobacco cessation program. This is an especially important point among traumatic amputees whose wounds have a tenuous blood supply and associated tissue viability; the success of limb preservation depends on optimizing the wound environment.

Wound Treatment

Thousands of wound care products are available and likely an equal number of institution-specific treatment algorithms. To the uninitiated, this abundance of choice can spuriously equate with degree of complexity. Developing expertise in wound care takes years of hands-on experience. Basic proficiency depends on pattern recognition and determining the why, when, and how of the main interventions.

Debridement

Debridement attempts to remove all unwanted elements from a wound such as eschar, slough, fibrin, pus, and bacteria. Because of their common yellow color slough, fibrin and pus are occasionally confused. Slough is loosely adherent, partially solubilized dead tissue that can be stringy or soupy in its texture and usually lacks a persistent foul odor. Fibrin is a very adherent, almost rubbery substance that is formed as a result of fibrinogen leaking into the inflamed wound bed. Pus, which has a milky texture, is usually ac-

companied by other signs of infection and ominously indicates the presence of purulent organisms.

So why debride? The most direct answer is that by not debriding a patient is at increased risk for infection, impaired wound healing, and potentially further surgical revisions. For an amputee this may have a significant impact on his or her functional capabilities if this revision leads to a shorter residual limb. An undebrided wound cannot be properly visualized and therefore cannot be properly assessed. What may initially look like a partial thickness wound, for example, could be deep enough to involve both muscle and bone and could be obscuring a deep infection. In addition, nonviable tissue takes up space and acts as a barrier against further cell entry. In this way, regenerative cells are thwarted from repopulating the wound bed and immune cells are denied access to the growing number of bacteria in the eschar and slough. Chronic inflammation results when nonviable tissue causes persistent neutrophil accumulation that may prohibit cellular progression to granulation and reepithelialization. Debridement is a necessary and powerful tool that can rapidly effect change in a relatively short period.

There are four main techniques to debride a wound:

1. sharp,
2. autolytic,
3. enzymatic, and
4. mechanical.

Sharp Debridement. Sharp debridement involves the use of a cutting instrument, such as a scalpel or scissors, and can be performed at the bedside by qualified personnel. It is the most rapid—and often the most effective—method of debridement. Large wounds that are completely covered in adherent fibrin or eschar are prime candidates for sharp debridement, and depending on patient tolerance may occasionally require more than one session to complete the bulk of the debriding process. The ultimate goal is to expose a healthy pink tissue base, remove all barriers to granulation, and ensure accurate staging and assessment.

Autolytic and Enzymatic Debridement. If a wound contains more than a mild to moderate amount of debris, sharp debridement is usually a necessary initial intervention. After the bulk of necrotic tissue is removed, however, the need for continued debridement must be weighed against the tradeoffs of excessive tissue handling, trauma, and risk of contamination. Under these circumstances and when the wound is otherwise healthy and uninfected, autolytic debridement (with or without exogenous enzymatic debridement) becomes ideal.

Autolytic debridement relies on the body's endogenous enzymes and phagocytes. Toward this end, an occlusive dressing is used that is usually changed no sooner than 72 hours. The occlusive dressing provides a warm, moist, and unperturbed environment that is ideal for wound healing. Because the dressing is not changed multiple times per day, the body's enzymes accumulate in the wound and break down nonviable tissue. To augment this process, exogenous enzymes, such as collagenase, papain, and urea, are occasionally applied to the wound bed. When the dressing is finally changed, much of the debris has become loosened and is easily removed with limited patient discomfort.

Because this method of debridement relies on occlusion, however, presence of active infection is a contraindication to use of this technique. In addition, those that change the dressing should be aware that it is not uncommon for occlusive dressings to have a strong odor. In contrast to infected wounds, however, the odor will not persist once the wound is cleaned.

Mechanical Debridement. Although inferior to sharp debridement at removing recalcitrant fibrin or eschar, mechanical debridement can be a very effective and appropriate means of removing less adherent necrotic tissue from a wound. In addition, most forms of mechanical debridement can be performed with relatively little training. Examples include simple manual scrubbing with gauze, irrigation with pulsatile lavage, and wet-to-dry dressings. The drawback of mechanical debridement is that it nonselectively removes both viable and necrotic tissue from a wound bed. Judicious use of this technique is required.

Wet-to-dry dressing is often a first-line treatment in wound management. However, it may not be appropriate in every clinical situation. In light of the biomechanics of wound healing, this technique may be deleterious to wound healing. The recurrent trauma to the wound bed beyond that necessary for adequate debridement of nonviable tissue may further complicate wound management.

The technique necessary for successful use of wet-to-dry dressings depends on the dressing changes every 12 hours. This frequent inspection of the wound leads to significantly more wound exposure than when using an occlusive dressing, causing inflammation and increasing the risk for contamination. In addition, regular cotton gauze sheds particulate matter when allowed to dry into a wound bed, which can be another source of irritation and inflammation. Wet-to-dry management of wounds is one of the more painful and (additively) time-intensive debridement methods. One benefit of using wet-to-dry dressings is the ability to perform frequent wound inspections particularly between surgical washouts. The disadvantage is the increased risk of excessive moisture leading to maceration of the surrounding skin, with inadequate drying thereby losing the debridement function. Debriding occurs as the adherent gauze is removed from the wound; if the gauze is unable to dry (or, alternatively, if it is remoistened before removal), no debriding occurs.

Another critical point (and this applies to all dressings) is that wounds should not be "packed," but instead they should be "filled." Gauze should be trimmed to an appropriate size, and the wound should be gently filled with the material. Tightly pushing an oversize dressing into the wound or "packing" leads to impaired wound healing. A tightly packed wound creates a pressure gradient that impedes the migration of regenerative cells and prevents adequate perfusion of the wound bed. Furthermore, untrimmed gauze may protrude from the wound bed and macerate the surrounding skin.

When Not To Debride

Although a discussion of specific wound types and their management is beyond the scope of this section, there are a few contraindications to debridement.

- Dry Gangrene: Dry gangrene occurs as a consequence of arterial insufficiency and the wound is poorly perfused. The necrotic tissue under these circumstances is actually protecting the wound underneath from infection. Once this barrier is broken, bacteria can more freely penetrate into the wound bed and cause resistant infection.
- Stable Heel Ulcers: Stable heel ulcers do not need to be debrided and should be left alone.
- Pyoderma Gangrenosum: The pathophysiology of pyoderma gangrenosum is linked to immune system dysregulation, although its specific mechanism remains incompletely understood. An apparently small ulceration can become significantly more problematic following debridement.

Restoring Moisture Balance

The majority of dressings and products fall into one of two major categories: (1) those that wet and (2) those that dry. Moisture balance of the wound bed and surrounding margin is critical and often the greatest challenge when treating a wound.

A wound can be thought of as two populations of cells living side by side, each requiring an environment that is toxic to its neighbor. As previously noted, erring too much on the side of moisture for the sake of the wound bed causes the surrounding skin to become macerated and the wound to ultimately grow. Erring too much on the side of dryness for the sake of the surrounding skin causes the wound bed to become desiccated and prematurely arrests the healing process.

The strategy used to obtain balance depends on the character of the wound. A venous stasis ulcer, for example, is notoriously weepy, such that all efforts are aimed at controlling drainage. Because of the failure of venous return, the wound bed of a venous stasis ulcer is essentially supplied with its own "ground water" making it virtually impossible to dry out. Although wound bed desiccation is unlikely, periwound maceration is a major concern. Barrier creams applied to the periwound skin can help protect against maceration but drainage control is critical. If conventional moisture wicking products such as alginates and hydrofibers fail to be effective, tampons are sometimes used with good results. If all wicking measures fail, the frequency of dressing changes must be increased until the periwound skin is adequately protected.

In contrast to venous ulcers, ulcers caused by arterial insufficiency require the opposite approach. Under these circumstances, venous outflow is not the underlying problem, but rather arterial inflow. Without a healthy blood supply to the skin, the wound bed is easily desiccated and needs to be moistened with products such as hydrogels or impregnated gauze. Barring overzealous hydration, periwound maceration is rarely an issue in this situation.

Similar strategies are used for wounds in between these extremes but to a more graded and balanced degree. For a wound that is producing a modest amount of exudate, for example, highly absorbent materials such as tampons or supersponges should be avoided because they excessively dry out the wound bed. Regardless of the initial strategy, the key is frequent inspection with each dressing change and modifications as the wound matures.

DEEP VENOUS THROMBOSIS AND PULMONARY EMBOLISM

Introduction

Despite advancements in prophylaxis and treatment, deep venous thrombosis (DVT) remains a serious complication in combat casualties with polytrauma and amputation. Consequences of DVT include prolonged hospital stay, delay in rehabilitation, secondary thrombophlebitis, or death from secondary pulmonary embolism. The incidence of DVT in trauma patients without prophylaxis has been estimated at 10% to 65%.[49–52] This variability of incidence rates is likely related to the variety of injury patterns seen in polytrauma and combat amputees. Previous reports have demonstrated that patients with spinal cord injuries (SCIs) have the highest rate of DVT among trauma patients.[53]

Although, in general, prophylaxis greatly reduces the risk of DVT, the choice and method of prophylaxis remain complex, especially in polytrauma and combat amputees.[54–58] Current methods of prophylaxis include adjusted doses of oral warfarin, fixed doses of low molecular weight heparin, subcutaneous heparin, aspirin, TED hose (Tyco Healthcare/Kendall Products, Mansfield, Mass), and sequential compressive devices (SCDs). Each of these methods except TED hose/SCDs carries an increased bleeding risk that presents a particular problem to trauma patients, especially those who require frequent returns to the operating room.[59] The use of TED hose and SCDs in trauma patients—especially those with orthopaedic injuries and amputations—is limited when fractures or wounds involve the extremities. Prevention is the best treatment because the medical therapies to treat venous thromboembolic events are controversial and may have associated risk and complications. DVT/pulmonary embolisms are a severe and life-threatening complication of injury.

Risk factors for DVT include

- immobilization,
- trauma,
- malignancy,
- abnormal coagulation factors,
- obesity,
- estrogen therapy,
- advanced age, and
- prior history of DVT.[60–63]

Given the nature of combat injuries and the (often) lengthy evacuation process required to transport these injured service members through increasing echelons of care, it would appear that this patient population would be at even greater risk for developing venous thromboembolic events.

Incidence and Diagnosis from the Walter Reed Experience

Experience in caring for returning combat amputees from OEF/OIF at WRAMC have shown thrombosis diagnosed in about 30%, with about 60% being DVTs and 40% being pulmonary embolisms. Twenty percent of DVTs were in the arms and 40% were in the leg. The location of the amputation has not been shown to correlate with the location of thromboembolism. The number of days of missed anticoagulation medications did not correlate with clot formation. The number of trips to the operating room correlated highly with clot formation, with more trips to the operating room correlating to a higher incidence of clots. Patients who had a planned trip to the operating room would have medical prophylaxis held the night before and the morning of surgery. In a population of patients undergoing surgery every other day or every third day, the number of days off medical prophylaxis quickly increases. In combination with other accepted prothrombotic factors, including venous stasis, hypercoagulability, and injury to the vascular endothelium, these patients are at increased risk of thrombosis development. Combat amputees with concomitant fracture are more likely to develop a venous thromboembolism (VTE). Comorbid traumatic brain injury (TBI) doubled the likelihood of being diagnosed with a VTE.

For the diagnosis of VTE, computed tomography (CT) was the best screening method for pulmonary embolisms with 100% sensitivity and specificity. The next best screening method was ultrasound, followed by angiography. However, for DVTs, CT scan had 100% sensitivity and 80% specificity, whereas ultrasound demonstrated 100% sensitivity and 91% specificity and angiography was the least sensitive for DVTs. In this young, relatively healthy patient population, physical symptoms of DVT are often vague and rarely readily apparent. Therefore, medical vigilance is critical and providers should have a low threshold for routine screening.

Physical Prophylaxis

Polytrauma and combat amputees are often unable to wear TED hose and SCDs because of their extremity injuries. From the authors' experience at WRAMC, patients able to wear TEDs were less likely to develop a thrombus. A larger number of patients used SCDs, but this higher number may be deceiving. Although the treating physicians order many devices, in practice,

patients do not tolerate them or wear them for much of the day and at night. This magnifies the importance of medical prophylaxis.

Medical Prophylaxis

Medical prophylaxis in this population remains debatable. Lovenox (Sanofi-aventis US, Bridgewater, NJ), a low molecular-weight heparin, tends to be the preferred agent within this population because of the ease in stopping and restarting for procedures. It is also simple to convert from prophylactic dosing to therapeutic dosing. Within the monitored setting of the intensive care units, heparin is often used, in part because of the reversibility of its action with protamine.

Minimizing Immobilization

The air evacuation process also must be considered. Antecedent trauma or surgery followed by prolonged air evacuation may be related to the development of VTE in more than half of those service members evacuated from deployments to the Middle East. Any injured patient who must travel via air evacuation faces several flights lasting approximately 6 hours each and additional ground transport time and other transport time to the evacuation sites. This long period of transportation immobilization should lead the provider to evaluate the need for earlier initiation of medical prophylaxis, although risk of bleeding complications must also be considered. The recognition of complications associated with severe polytrauma and combat wound-related amputations requires careful consideration before initiating anticoagulation and should be made on a case-by-case basis. Upon arrival to a tertiary care hospital (level 4 or 5 echelon), every effort should be given to facilitate early patient mobilization. This may include simple passive range of motion of the extremities for the patient restricted to bed or early transfers and ambulation, whether by wheelchair or other assistive device. Although no clear evidence indicates when medical prophylaxis should be discontinued, it is generally considered necessary to continue it until significant independent mobility is achieved.

WEIGHT-BEARING PROGRESSION

Amputations sustained from high-energy combat trauma generally produce significant comorbidity.[64] Femoral and pelvic fractures with coexisting lower extremity amputation present a significant rehabilitation challenge. These complex fractures must be given an appropriate amount of time protected from large distracted forces to allow proper healing. Operationally this is accomplished by implementing various

degrees of weight-bearing restrictions that must be balanced with the well-known negative physical and psychological consequences of bed rest and inactivity.[65–68] Unfortunately, little standardized information exists to guide the temporal parameters and advancement of weight-bearing restrictions.

Because of advances in military medicine, timely and thorough evaluations of the musculoskeletal system are standard. This generally includes aggressive orthopaedic surgical reduction and fixation as part of fracture management. After initial surgical management, fractures progress through a standard sequence of healing that includes inflammation, repair, and remodeling.[69,70] Initial injury characteristics greatly affect the process. In particular, damage to the blood supply and soft tissue is common and lengthens the course of healing.

Generally the orthopaedic surgeon establishes a guide to the rehabilitation team on a patient's weight-bearing status. Therefore, an individual's weight-bearing status should not be advanced without the surgeon's direct consultation. The determination of weight-bearing tolerance and internal fracture stability, which is multifactorial, includes fracture location, type, apposition of fracture fragments, method of fracture fixation, severity of soft tissue damage, blood supply integrity, nutritional status, and associated injuries. Given the numerous patient-specific variables, no standard guidelines are available for return to full weight bearing.

Existing evidence indicates that fracture healing is optimized through loading of the repair tissue and decreased loading negatively impacts healing time.[71,72] Furthermore, evidence exists that even immediate controlled loading may promote healing.[71,73-78] In the rehabilitation setting, controlled loading is accomplished through the use of tilt tables, parallel bars, and aquatic therapy.[79] Care must be taken to prevent excessive, distracting motion and development of pseudoarthroses or nonunion. Serial radiography to assess evidence of healing (and evidence of nonunion) is recommended. Frequent reassessment of patient symptomatology should be undertaken with particular emphasis on the quality of pain. Changes in quality should prompt further evaluation. The interdisciplinary team of rehabilitation professionals and an orthopedist is critical to ensure successful functional return.

Energy requirements are highest during the first two phases of bone healing, where the need for aggressive early nutritional support is critical.[80-82] Caloric, protein, vitamin C, and vitamin D supplementation are required to meet the anabolic demand of wound healing.[82] The presence of electronegativity at fracture sites has lead to the use of bone stimulators to expedite healing.[83-85] Numerous case reports support their implementation in cases complicated by delayed bone union and nonhealing.[83,86-89] Similarly, ultrasound offers a safe, noninvasive modality that may promote fracture healing.[90-93] Yet, rigid research evidence is still lacking to determine the treatment characteristics of bone stimulation.

During the healing process, the sequelae of combat trauma must be actively managed to promote healing and early functional return. This includes decreasing the metabolic demand of infections and open wounds. TBI, which has a high prevalence in the polytrauma patient, presents numerous barriers including its association with HO development.[94-96] The standard treatments for HO rely on the use of bisphosphonates and NSAIDs. These two pharmacological classes should be avoided with concomitant fractures because of their negative impact on healing. Similarly, nicotine intake should be actively discouraged given its inhibition of fracture healing.[97,98]

In the rehabilitation of the combat-acquired amputation novel plans and individualized recovery trajectories are required. Coexisting lower extremity fractures should be closely followed for appropriate healing and management of potential negative sequelae. The return of full weight bearing and ambulatory function depends on a series of patient-specific variables and ultimately it is decided by collective clinical judgment. Rapid advancement of stable fractures and close multidisciplinary monitoring are preferred in contrast to long periods of inactivity.

HETEROTOPIC OSSIFICATION

Introduction

Among recent military amputees returning from combat in Iraq and Afghanistan, a high rate of HO has been seen in amputated residual limbs.[99] HO is the abnormal formation of bone in soft tissues (Figure 10-1). HO develops when pluripotent mesenchymal cells are inappropriately transformed into osteoblasts that contribute to bone production.[100] The precise cause for this transformation in pluripotent cells is unknown.[100] HO is commonly seen and has been well documented in the setting of SCIs, TBIs, burns, after total joint replacements (especially hips), and with severe soft tissue damage. Before the current military conflict there were few HO reports in amputees' residual limbs.

Bone formation in amputees' residual limbs presents numerous rehabilitation challenges. Bone formed in soft tissues of a weight-bearing limb can result in high-pressure areas, creating a risk for skin breakdown. Skin breakdown can have devastating effects on rehabilitation because it often requires prolonged periods of nonweight bearing and presents a risk for infection. In addition, HO in residual limbs can result in complex residual limb shapes and multiple pressure-sensitive areas that can make prosthesis fitting difficult or impossible. Increased pain, limitations in range of motion, and limitations in ambulation are also complications from HO in residual limbs.

Current diagnosis methods are acceptable. Patients often report changes in pain characteristics, range of motion restrictions, warmth, and socket fitting in their residual limbs. HO is diagnosed by plain radiograph, CT, magnetic resonance imaging, and/or triple phase bone scan. Blood studies such as alkaline phosphatase may also be followed throughout HO development and correlated to bone formation, maturity, and ultimately quiescence.

Current HO treatment methods are less than optimal. Prophylactic measures, which have shown some efficacy, include NSAIDs, bisphosphonates, and/or radiation therapy.[101–105] Once mature, however, treatment of symptomatic HO is limited to surgical resection.

Historical Perspective on Heterotopic Ossification in the Combat Amputee

A thorough literature review reveals few studies describing HO in combat-related traumatic amputees. Those studies are single case reports that demonstrate HO occurring in the amputees' residual limb.[106,107] Prior reports of combat casualties from the Civil War and World War I do not suggest a significant association with HO formation and traumatic amputation.[108–110] A report by Colonel (Retired) Paul Brown, looking at 88 residual limbs in Vietnam combat amputees, reported only 4 limbs (0.5%) as having "bone spur formation" that required surgical excision.[111] Furthermore, Lieutenant General (Retired) Alcide LaNoue, who was chief of orthopaedics at Valley Forge General Hospital in Pennsylvania, reported seeing only a "few cases of ectopic bone in residual limbs" in more than 410 amputations that were treated under his command during Vietnam.[112]

Heterotopic Ossification from the Walter Reed Experience

WRAMC saw a greater than 50% incidence of HO formation in combat amputees returning from OEF/OIF. This is consistent with an estimated 62% incidence noted by Potter et al in a 2006 observational review of a similar patient population.[113]

It is, therefore, important to determine how the identified risk factors from this patient population might differ from those of prior conflicts. Service members with traumatic amputation from the Vietnam War had injuries complicated by retained metal fragments, other fractures, wound infections, and skin grafts.[111] Some factors that do appear to differ from past populations are

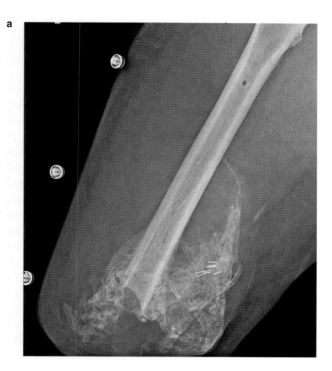

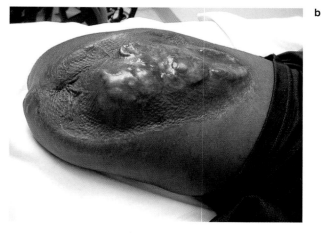

Figure 10-1. (a) Plain radiograph showing heterotopic ossification in a transfemoral amputee and **(b)** photo showing heterotopic ossification manifesting superficially in the limb of an above-knee amputee.

- causative pathogens of wound infections,
- overall increased severity of secondary injuries,
- increased incidence of brain injuries,
- increased numbers, and
- types of surgical procedures/debridements.

One major differentiating factor is modern technology and training of initial responders (ie, the combat medic). Advances in forward care and prompt aeromedical evacuation with better technology in combat personal protective gear have allowed service members to survive injuries that would have been fatal in the past. This has intensified the incidence, type, and severity of secondary injuries and complications. Wound care in the highly advanced surgical arena has changed significantly over the past 40 years. The majority of Vietnam amputees received at Valley Forge General Hospital had open residual limbs, which were debrided with wet-to-dry dressings and rarely required more than one revision.[111] In the current conflict with its emphasis on limb preservation and rapid movement of injured personnel through ascending echelons of care, service members are presenting to continental US tertiary care centers with increased severity of wounds, secondary injuries, and antibiotic-resistant wound infections that necessitate an increased number and complexity of surgical interventions.

Surgical advances such as pulsed lavage debridement and vacuum-assisted wound closure have revolutionized soft tissue injury management and allowed a higher percentage of successful limb preservation attempts. However, the emphasis on limb preservation, which starts at wound triage, leads to tissue preservation with micro- and macro-trauma. This traumatized tissue, which most likely would have been removed in a similarly injured Vietnam War service member, may contribute to the triggering mechanism of cellular differentiation and HO formation.

Another contributing factor is the type and severity of wound infections. Modern weaponry coupled with nontraditional projectiles such as the types of material used in improvised explosive devices appear to cause more contaminated and fragmented wounds. This has contributed to the increased quantity of wound infections and the increased virulence of microorganisms. Approximately 75% of amputee patients with HO at WRAMC had a wound infection. *Acinetobacter baumanni* was the responsible microorganism in half of those infected. Before OIF/OEF *A baumanni* was primarily a hospital-acquired infection and not a common cause of wound infection. Prior studies have also shown *A baumanni* to be more difficult to treat because of increased antimicrobial resistance.[114] The authors'

experience in treating this microorganism is consistent with these findings. Patient infection secondary to this pathogen often required multiple weeks of intravenous antibiotics and multiple wound debridements. Wounds infected with *A baumanni* significantly increased the risk of HO development; however, the mechanism is unclear. HO development may be attributed to factors associated with the bacteria, but the etiology of HO is most likely multifactorial and includes factors intrinsic to the patient. HO development warrants further study.

A comorbidity of TBI was found to have the greatest correlation with HO development. Nearly 40% of the WRAMC OEF/OIF patient population had some degree of brain injury. This incidence is markedly increased compared to the 12% to 14% reported from the Vietnam War.[111] The increased incidence attributed to decreased mortality from brain injury is secondary to technological advances and acute management. Mortality from brain injuries among US combatants in Vietnam was reported at 75% or greater.[115] Studies show that brain injury alone can cause HO in 15% to 40% of patients.[116] Studies also suggest that having a brain injury in combination with structural trauma has an additive effect on HO frequency.[116]

The decisions to use prophylactic medications by the primary medical teams were determined largely by extrapolating evidence from other disorders. An abundance of evidence supports the efficacy of multiple types of NSAIDs to prevent HO, especially involving traumatic injuries.[117] Banovac et al[118] showed treatment with the cyclooxygenase (COX)-2 inhibitor, Rofecoxib, to be clinically significant in preventing HO in patients with SCI. The advantage of a COX-2 inhibitor versus a traditional NSAID is based on the gastrointestinal protective properties of the COX-2 inhibitors. It is believed that these medications inhibit prostaglandin synthesis and thus reduce the inflammation and proliferation of mesenchymal cells.[119] Etidronate is in the class of medications known as bisphosphonates. Numerous studies show its efficacy in preventing HO in SCIs and TBIs.[120,121] However, some studies have demonstrated HO recurrence with treatment cessation.[122] Etidronate is thought to decrease HO formation by inhibiting the conversion of amorphous calcium phosphate compounds into hydroxyapatite crystals, which is one of the final steps in bone formation.[123]

Radionuclide bone imaging roentgenographic studies have shown that the onset of HO—regardless of etiology—ranges from 3 to 12 weeks postinjury. It peaks at about 2 months and then evolves for an average of about 6 months. Then it reaches maturity and metabolic activity ceases.[124] The authors' patients treated with either Etidronate within 3 weeks or Rofecoxib at any time were less likely to develop HO compared to those who took no prophylactic medication. The standard dose of Etidronate was 20 mg/kg per day for 2 weeks followed by 10 mg/kg per day for 10 weeks based on the original dosing scheme used by Stover et al[120] in their study on prophylaxis after SCI. Standard doses of Rofecoxib, Valdecoxib, and Celecoxib were 25 mg/20 mg/200 mg per day, respectively, for 8 to 12 weeks.

HO incidence appears to be markedly increased in OIF/OEF compared to prior military conflicts. Additionally, risk factors for HO development have been elucidated from the WRAMC population. Five of the risk factors are associated with increased structural trauma to soft tissue and bone. The sixth risk factor (brain injury) is neurogenic in nature and appears to have an additive effect on HO incidence when combined with structural trauma. Prophylactic medical treatment with Etidronate and Rofecoxib (no longer available) appears to decrease the probability of developing HO if started within 3 weeks of injury. To better determine a risk-benefit analysis, randomized controlled studies are needed to further determine the long-term effectiveness of both Etidronate and Celecoxib (the only COX-2 available) and identify complicating side effects, optimal dosage, and duration. However, if a decision is made to use any class of medication based on data from the Stover et al study and historical knowledge of HO's natural evolution, the authors recommend starting the medication as soon as is feasible, preferably within 3 weeks of injury.

In the authors' experience, most HO manifestations can be treated conservatively with treatments such as range-of-motion exercises and appropriate prosthetic prescription to include liner and socket modifications. However, the definitive treatment for mature HO that fails conservative therapy is surgical removal.

Heterotopic Ossification and Three-Dimensional Modeling

Because of the number and severity of the complications associated with HO, surgical excision of the abnormal bone may become necessary. Excision is an accepted treatment for symptomatic HO when conservative treatment measures fail.[116,125–127] Excision is frequently a difficult procedure because of the often intimate relationship of ectopic bone with native muscles, blood vessels, and nerves (Figure 10-2), and complications resulting from excision are common.[128] Excision of HO requires careful planning to ensure that all ectopic bone is identified and excised, to minimize

the resection of muscle and soft tissue surrounding the ectopic bone, and to prevent injuries to nearby nerves and blood vessels.

Currently accepted imaging techniques, such as CT and magnetic resonance imaging, do not adequately provide a useful representation of the ectopic bone for planning and performing HO excision and for designing and fabricating prosthetic sockets. The emergence of technology that allows for the construction of three-dimensional models to display a patient's anatomy based on CT scans can now be used to plan for HO excisions and socket design.

The process that makes the construction of these models possible combines high-resolution CT, software rendering technology, and three-dimensional modeling. When construction of a model is indicated to facilitate prosthetic socket construction or surgical excision of HO, a CT scan of the residual limb is obtained using 1.5-mm slices throughout the area to be modeled. The digital data from CT images are imported to software that allows for the selection of tissues to be modeled based on pixel density (Hounsfield values). The resulting images are delivered to the 3D Systems Inc. SLA-7000, which constructs a three-dimensional

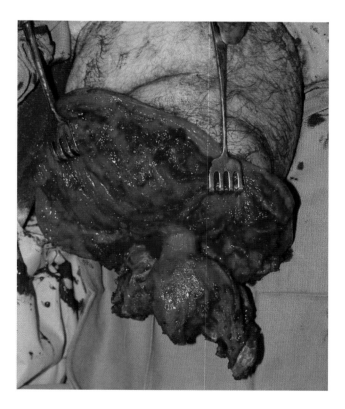

Figure 10-2. Intraoperative view of heterotopic ossification excision.

resin model of the patient's anatomy (Figure 10-3).

Several benefits and advantages result from using CT-based three-dimensional models for prosthetic socket design and surgical HO excision planning. When used for prosthetic socket design, the models improve the anatomical contouring of the socket and assist in identifying anatomic anomalies for avoidance of stress to those areas.[129] When used for planning surgical HO excision, the models helped allow for limited surgical incisions by preventing the need for complete takedown and revision of the amputation. In addition, they permitted preoperative planning of skin incisions and soft tissue revision, thereby allowing for complete HO excision while preserving enough soft tissue to adequately close the wound. The models provided a three-dimensional understanding of the ectopic bone's anatomy and, therefore, the relationship of the HO to the patient's native anatomy, which helped prevent damage to nearby nerves and blood vessels. Patients can use these models to localize pain areas in the residual limb that is attributed to specific spicules of the ectopic bone. The models also allowed for three-dimensional documentation of the extent of the HO to permit excision of all troublesome ectopic bone.[130]

In addition to being a tool for planning surgical HO excision, CT-based three-dimensional models have other uses in managing amputees and the combat wounded. Amputees returning from combat in Iraq and Afghanistan often have other traumatic injuries, many of which can hinder their progress more than the amputation. Comminuted fractures of the long bones of the extremities and pelvic fractures are common comorbid injuries. Because of the complexity of pelvic and acetabular fractures, the anatomical details and full extent of the damage are not easily demonstrated by routine radiographs. It is vital to assess the integrity of the anterior and posterior columns, hip joint spaces for debris, and the medial walls of the acetabula.[33] This assessment can often be achieved with routine CT (Figure 10-4). However, CT in conjunction with three-dimensional imaging can provide information regarding the extent of the fractures, help determine the spatial arrangement of fracture fragments, and assist the radiologist and physician understand complex fracture patterns (Figure 10-5).[131,132]

Damage to the bony structure of the pelvis often can be extensive as a result of gunshot wounds or shrapnel, forcing the patient to remain on bed rest until the fracture heals. Management consists mainly of reestablishing a joint congruence to allow for adequate weight bearing and to prevent early coxarthrosis.[133] CT-based three-dimensional models can greatly assist with assessing fracture healing because they can help monitor bony deficits in the pelvic ring until adequate continuity is established. These models, which provide accurate information on callus formation and potential areas of poor healing, can also help the patient to visualize the nature and extent of his or her injuries (Figure 10-6).

Although patients with extensive pelvic fractures remain on bed rest, it is essential for them to receive

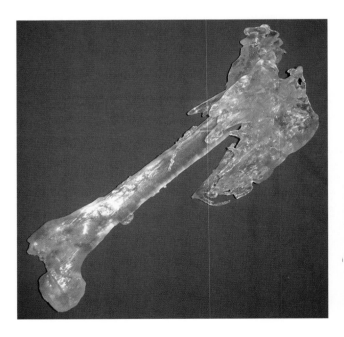

Figure 10-3. Three-dimensional resin model of heterotopic ossification in a combat amputee.

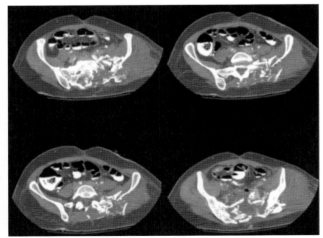

Figure 10-4. Computed tomography axial images of comminuted L5 and sacrum fractures 2 weeks postinjury.

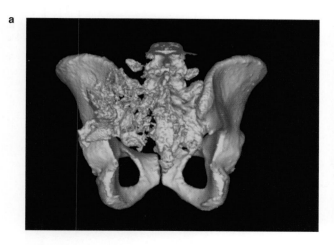
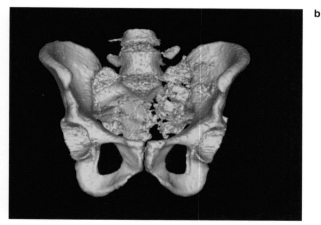

Figure 10-5. Graphic representation of three-dimensional model of the pelvis 2 weeks postinjury. (**a**) anterior view (**b**) posterior view.

bedside physical and occupational therapy to maintain upper extremity strength, lower extremity range of motion, and bed mobility. In addition, they should receive proper bowel and bladder management and their medical needs should be closely managed. Once callus formation is sufficient as indicated on CT imaging and three-dimensional models, the patient can advance to weight bearing. Training is initiated using a tilt table for improved orthostasis and the patient can ultimately progress to full weight bearing and ambulation.[134] In lower extremity amputees, fitting and casting for an initial prosthetic limb can begin while they are on bed rest. They can begin bearing weight on the prosthetic limb once improved orthostasis is achieved and they can bear weight on the intact or residual limbs.

ELECTRODIAGNOSTIC EVALUATION OF PERIPHERAL NERVE INJURIES IN COMBAT AMPUTEES/EXTREMITY TRAUMA

Patient Identification

Peripheral nerve injuries are not always apparent at the time of injury. The primary and secondary surveys are focused on life and limb preservation. Severely injured patients will be obtunded on arrival and may remain so for days to weeks. Some neurologic deficits are subtle and the diagnosis is not entertained until the patient fails to meet therapy goals or has unexplained limb pain.

All patients should have a complete neurologic exam at regular intervals for several reasons:

- It increases the likelihood that the nerve injuries will be diagnosed, especially the more subtle injuries, in the individuals who are regaining consciousness.
- It provides several data points to track the patient's recovery or failure to recover.
- These data points provide temporal context in the patient with a prolonged hospital course exposed to numerous complications.

Patients with peripheral nerve injuries can present with symptoms of pain, numbness, paresthesias, or weakness in a region or extremity. Any losses of muscle strength, sensation, or reflexes are signs of nerve injury. Swelling, increased warmth, deepened color, or lack of sweating in the distal extremity may indicate autonomic signs of nerve injury. These findings do not necessarily localize the injury to the peripheral nervous system. Central nervous system injuries can mimic or coexist with peripheral nervous system injuries.

Clinical Evaluation

The goals of the clinical evaluation are to (*a*) define the distribution of nerve(s) injured, (*b*) determine the severity of injury, and (*c*) localize the presumed site of injury. Nerve injuries can cause deficits in the distribution of nerve roots, multiple peripheral nerves, or individual peripheral nerves. In brachial plexus lesions, trunk injuries will appear as deficits in multiple dermatomes and myotomes, whereas cord injuries present as multiple peripheral nerve injuries.

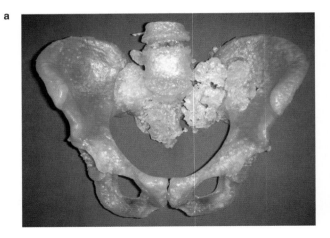 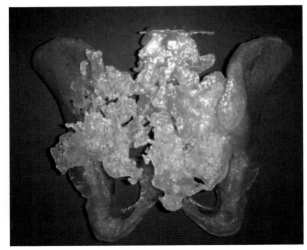

Figure 10-6. Three-dimensional model of the pelvis from Figure 10-5, 2 weeks postinjury. (**a**) anterior view, (**b**) posterior view.

For example, an upper trunk injury will present with shoulder abduction and elbow flexion weakness, and impaired sensation in the lateral forearm and thumb. A posterior cord lesion will appear as coexistent radial and axillary nerve injuries.

Different clinical and electrophysiologic severity scales exist. The initial clinical evaluation should define complete versus incomplete motor and sensory loss in a particular nerve because operative intervention is rarely required for initially incomplete injuries. When intact motor function exists in the most distal muscles innervated by a particular nerve, the injury is considered "incomplete." Key muscles in the upper extremity include the flexor digitis indicis, abductor pollicis brevis, and extensor indicis proprius for the ulnar, median, and radial nerves, respectively. In the lower extremity, the extensor hallucis longus is easily demonstrated with great toe extension for deep peroneal nerve function and palpating the adductor hallucis during great toe abduction or flexion demonstrates tibial nerve function. It is helpful to palpate the muscle being tested because substitution can sometimes create the same movement.

All patients should receive a detailed sensory exam of autonomous zones. This information can be used to support or refine the diagnosis and to help formulate an electrodiagnostic further work-up. A bedside sensory examination is very subjective and considerable anatomic variation may exist. Furthermore, after an injury adjacent nerves can expand to previously anesthetic areas. For example, if there is no motor function in median-innervated muscles but sensation is present in the palmar thumb, the injury should not

be immediately categorized as incomplete.

Inspection of the trunk and extremities can provide a presumed injury site. All entry and exit wounds and surgical scars should be documented. Sometimes extensive soft tissue damage and scars exist in the distal extremity with only a single entry wound more proximal. Both must be entertained as potential injury sites. Fasciotomy scars, which are also very common in combat casualties, are usually done at the time of injury prophylactically because of vascular disruption. If the fasciotomy was performed to decompress an acute compartment syndrome, there may have been nerve injury from the compartment syndrome. Atrophy is also important because disuse atrophy is mild and more generalized, whereas denervation atrophy is profound and focal. Documentation of limb circumferences, while not validated, is a reasonable objective measurement. In the fully recovered patient with significant axonal disruption, atrophy may persist despite symmetric clinical strength. The exact location of a Tinel's sign should be documented. Distal progression of the Tinel's sign supports spontaneous recovery before return of muscle function.

A detailed history should uncover the mechanism of injury and a timeline of when nerve deficits appeared. Sometimes patients can recall immediate loss of motor function on the battlefield. Surgical reports might comment on the continuity of nerves encountered during exploration. If the nerve is found not in continuity, the ends may have been tagged and fixed to adjacent structures for future reattachment. This level of detail is often difficult to find in the medical records during medical evacuation. Patients occasionally report to the surgeon that the "nerve is bruised" or that it is a "neuropraxia." The conclusions drawn from these particular historical reports generally mean that nerve continuity is intact.

Electrodiagnostic Evaluation

The goals of any electrodiagnostic examination are to (*a*) determine the presence or absence of nerve injury, (*b*) rule out confounding diagnoses, (*c*) localize the lesion, (*d*) characterize the nerve lesion and determine severity, and (*e*) establish prognosis.

Goals of the Electrodiagnostic Examination

1. **Determine the presence or absence of nerve injury**. Usually, the first sentence of the conclusion of an electrodiagnostic consultation is whether the study is normal or abnormal. Many individual abnormalities exist in the exam components: abnormal spontaneous potentials, abnormal motor unit morphology or recruitment, low amplitude compound muscle action potentials or sensory nerve action potentials, and conduction slowing. There are two major themes when determining an abnormal examination: (1) having multiple internally consistent abnormalities and (2) surrounding abnormalities with normality. These principles help prevent both false positive and false negative studies. False positive studies arise when conclusions are drawn on limited data. There are usually abnormalities of motor unit morphology or recruitment used to support a presumed diagnosis, ie, the self-fulfilling prophecy. False negatives arise when insufficient adjacent nerves and muscles are tested, eg, a diagnosed ulnar neuropathy that is really a lower trunk plexopathy.

2. **Rule out confounding diagnoses**. Similar to excluding a cervical radiculopathy in a patient with carpal tunnel syndrome, care must be taken to exclude more proximal or more systemic nerve lesions in patients with peripheral nerve trauma. The concept of a "double crush" nerve injury is important here. The assumption is that a nerve injury in one location has a causal relationship with a nerve injury elsewhere along a common pathway, perhaps resulting from impaired axoplasmic flow. Despite this, it is important to exclude entrapment neuropathies along an injured peripheral nerve. These represent eas-

ily treatable conditions that would otherwise interfere with recovery.

3. **Localize the lesion**. There are two ways to localize an injury on the electrodiagnostic examination. The first is to demonstrate conduction slowing or conduction block across a lesion. The second is the evaluation of the distribution of needle electromyography abnormalities. Using the second technique, there is always the possibility that "selective fasicular vulnerability" of a more proximal lesion explains the distribution of findings, eg, a sciatic injury involving only the fibers destined for the deep peroneal nerve. The electrodiagnostic localization also should be correlated with the mechanisms of injury. Both open penetrating wounds and closed blunt force injuries should be considered. This presumed site of injury is important in determining the progress.

4. **Characterize the lesion and determine severity**. The first characterization is whether the nerve injury is complete or incomplete. "Complete" does not imply nerve transection; it simply connotes that all axons are involved. However, demonstrating intact voluntary motor units in the most distal muscles of the injured nerve confirms incompleteness and at least partial nerve continuity. It is mandatory that those motor units have a rise time of less than 500 microseconds to ensure one is not looking at volume conducted motor units from nearby intact muscles. When the needle electrode exam shows positive sharp waves and fibrillations, with no voluntary recruitment of motor units, one is tempted to assume a complete injury. Performing motor and sensory nerve conductions on that nerve, distal to the presumed site of injury, allows one to demonstrate conduction block if present. A recordable response will appear if the conduction-blocked nerve is stimulated below the lesion. The partial axonal disruption explains the abnormal spontaneous potentials, and the conduction block of the remaining axons explains the inability to voluntarily recruit any motor units. The net effect is a muscle that will not activate. This demonstration of conduction block is important because it improves the patient's prognosis. The conduction block should resolve fully within 3 months.

    If the lesion is incomplete, an attempt should be made to approximate the degree of axon loss with primarily motor amplitude measurement.

Preinjury motor amplitudes would be most reliable, but are rarely available. Total body electrodiagnostic exams are not yet part of the predeployment examinations. Comparisons can be made to the contralateral limb. Although an up to 50% side-to-side motor amplitude variation exists in nonamputees, they should be considered equivalent in a patient with clear nerve injury for estimation of axon loss. This technique will underestimate the degree of axon loss after 2 to 3 months because of collateral sprouting. Unfortunately, most combat casualties do not have a true "sound side" for comparison. The contralateral limb is frequently injured or frankly absent. In those cases, amplitude comparisons with normal values with standard deviations provide a rough estimate. The utility of percentage amplitude preservation in prognosticating eventual outcome is unclear. One assumes the lower the percentage the worse the prognosis, but the real question is at what percentage is treatment altered? The answer to this typically lies with the peripheral nerve surgeon's threshold for nerve exploration. At one of the authors' institution, most incomplete injuries, regardless of percentage axon disruption, are treated conservatively.

Another characterization is the presence of ongoing reinnervation. This can be a powerful conclusion to report to the referring physician. Documenting "reinnervation" implies an improved prognosis, even if not necessarily proven. "Reinnervation" is usually documented based on the presence of polyphasic motor unit potentials. Polyphasia, however, is a normal finding in all muscles, up to a certain percentage. Quantitative techniques may add objectivity and likely improve specificity. Polyphasic motor unit potentials should also be assessed for stability. An immature polyphasic potential, either from a collateral sprout or a regenerating axon, will show instability on conventional needle electromyography. Triggering on the potentials and then superimposing them will demonstrate the stability. "Instability" is the manifestation of increased jitter and blocking seen on single fiber electromyography. When looking for stability, it may be helpful to use the "apparent single fiber" technique. Distant motor unit activity is excluded when using a concentric needle electrode and a low frequency filter of 500 Hertz.

5. **Establish prognosis**. No studies provide Class I evidence of electrodiagnostic findings and eventual outcomes. Generally, the purely neuropraxic lesions usually do well, whereas more severe nerve injuries rarely spontaneously recover. Electrodiagnostics cannot distinguish between a moderate and severe nerve injury. The diagnosis of a higher grade lesion can be based on one of four things:
   a. Direct visualization of a nerve transection.
   b. Direct visualization of a nerve lesion in continuity, but failure to conduct an action potential across the lesion site and entirely below the lesion site.
   c. Imaging, using either magnetic resonance neurography or ultrasound. Both are promising, but not readily available, and unvalidated.
   d. Failure to progress (most common). Identify the most proximal muscle that has no voluntary motor units. If axons regenerate 1 to 5 mm per day, then the maximum recovery time is 1 inch per month. One can then predict, in months, when the most proximal nonfunctioning muscle should begin working based on its distance from the presumed site of injury. Assume a median nerve injury in the distal brachium with no voluntary units in the pronator teres. If no voluntary motor units are seen in the pronator by 3 months (3 inches), then the injury is unlikely to recovery spontaneously. Assume a sciatic nerve injury in the proximal thigh. The peroneal division is complete and the tibial division demonstrates incompleteness in all muscles including the foot intrinsics. One would predict the short head of the biceps femoris would begin functioning by 12 months. The tibial division injury is incomplete from outset and will likely be followed clinically.

Mechanisms of Recovery

A nerve injury that is incomplete recovers by several mechanisms:

- resolution of conduction block (typically 0–3 months);
- collateral sprouting from the nerve terminals to innervate nearby muscle fibers that have lost their axons; and
- regeneration of the axons from the injury site.

The complete nerve injury can only recover by axonal regeneration. Once the target muscle is reached, then collateral sprouting also occurs. Muscles with some innervations may undergo muscle hypertrophy to increase strength. All patients also improve using adaptive techniques. This manifests as improvements on scales such as the functional independence measure.

Surgical Intervention

There are several types of surgical procedures to repair peripheral nerve injuries. An external neurolysis involves removal of necrotic and scar tissue from the outside of a neuroma. An internal neurolysis includes splitting the fascicles and resecting necrotic fascicles and those that cannot conduct an action potential. Those resected fibers can then be reapproximated or grafted. If no recordable action potential exists, then the entire neuroma can be resected and the nerve can be reapproximated or grafted. Neurotization involves taking fascicles from an intact nerve and performing an end-to-end or end-to-side anatamosis into the distal nonfunctioning nerve, eg, taking fascicles from the anterior interosseous nerve distal to the flexor pollicis longus and anastamosing it to the ulnar nerve near the wrist.

Nerve repairs can be immediate, early, delayed, or late. Immediate repair is done within the first hours to days for sharp, complete, but otherwise uncomplicated transections. The ends are mobilized and reapproximated. An early repair is performed several weeks after a complete injury to allow time for demarcation of the necrotic tissue to be removed. A graft may be required to achieve a tension-free repair. A delayed repair is performed between 3 and 6 months. These patients have complete deficits, but the initial Sunderland grade is unclear. They do not show recovery in the most proximal muscles as predicted by the 1 inch per month estimation. A late repair is a salvage procedure or performed for pain control. Tendon transfers are also a viable option for patients with forearm and lower leg injuries, and they are usually performed late.

Once a nerve repair—with or without graft—is performed, it must recover by axonal regeneration. Sufficient time must be given to reach the target muscles. In denervated muscle, the motor end plate degenerates sometime between 12 and 24 months. Using 18 months as a time frame will help dictate the latest a delayed repair can be performed.

Rehabilitation Intervention

The initial rehabilitation intervention is to ensure the appropriate diagnosis has been made. Repeat testing and second opinions are sometimes necessary. Patient and family education about the treatment plan and goals is important to express that progress is measured in weeks and months rather than days. Providing symptomatic treatment for neuropathic pain is covered elsewhere in this textbook (see Chapter 11, Pain Management Among Soldiers With Amputations). Interval examinations will help detect the development of complex regional pain syndrome as early as possible.

Emphasizing the importance of maintenance of range of motion is imperative. Nerve regrowth to a contracted hand is of little use. If patients are unable to demonstrate their home exercise program, then they require closer supervision. Physical and occupational therapy can assist with modalities before range-of-motion exercises, pain control, adaptive mobility, and activity of daily living strategies.

LONG-TERM EFFECTS OF LIMB AMPUTATION

The connection between health and disease is a dynamic process of salutogenesis and pathogenesis, with the individual's health dependent on the delicate balance of homeostasis.[135] The trauma associated with the combat amputee can be seen as a powerful disturbance of homeostasis because effects are experienced long after the initial injury. Longitudinal studies of traumatic amputees suggest that this population ages differently than age-matched uninjured individuals. These differences not only may be attributed directly to the amputation (altered anatomy and physiology), but also may be related to disturbance of homeostatic mechanisms. Throughout OIF/OEF, military amputee clinics have continued to focus on short-term and intermediate goals for its service members that focus on rapid function recovery and reducing impairment through adaptive techniques or assistive equipment. The main focus of the acute interventions is wound healing, pain control, prosthesis optimization, and return to high-level activities. The long-term goals of amputee rehabilitation are either return to duty or transition to the civilian community with reintegration. Regardless of initial disposition, the eventual separation of the service member from the military requires that special attention be given to the aging combat amputees and their associated greater vulnerability to certain medical complications.

Musculoskeletal Topics of Concern

Osteoarthritis has occurred in the unilateral lower extremity amputees with higher incidence than predicted based on age alone, with osteoarthritic changes found in both the ipsilateral and contralateral hips. This incidence is increased threefold in the individual with a transfemoral as compared to transtibial amputation.[135] The prevalence of symptomatic osteoarthritis of the knees has been found to be greater in amputees compared to age-matched, uninjured individuals. Factor analysis of the amputees suggests that biomechanical changes and body weight alone do not account for increased osteoarthritis incidence. In the unilateral lower extremity amputee, forces transmitted through the intact limb can be three to five times greater than total body weight (transfemoral greater than transtibial).[136] In an age-matched comparison of healthy athletic amputees and nonamputees, the incidence of contralateral knee osteoarthritis and pain was 65% greater in the amputee population.[137]

Back pain has also been shown to be a chronic and significant issue in amputees, much more than in the nonamputee population. It has been referred to as a secondary disability because 57% of amputees claimed it to be persistent and bothersome, with pain ratings of greater than 5 of 10 on the Visual Analogue Scale.[138] Functional limitations were found to be more significant in the lower extremity amputee with low back pain.[139] Bone density testing in amputees shows significant early and sustained loss over time in amputees. This is important because some studies indicate scores commonly in the range of osteopenia and often osteoporosis. The bone loss is throughout the whole body but much worse in the amputated limb.[140,141] A study by Leclercq et al correlated the loss of bone mass etiology of amputation (traumatic vs dysvascular), level of amputation (more severe bone loss when above-knee amputation), and prosthesis fit and use.[142]

Osteoarthritis and decreased levels of bone density in amputees are multifactorial. However, steps may be taken to reduce functional limitations, such as socket fit, prosthetic fit and suspension, and prescription of components, for the appropriate associated activity (eg, a multiaxial energy-storing foot for ambulating on uneven terrain). It is also vital to evaluate gait through both clinical observation and formal gait laboratory analysis. An improved understanding of the kinetics and kinematics will help the clinician and rehabilitation team provide an appropriate prescription for both prosthetic and assistive equipment and associated therapies. When feasible, eligible amputees should be referred for a formal gait and motion analysis.

Cardiovascular and Metabolic Topics of Concern

The aging amputee population has significantly worse cardiovascular and metabolic issues that appear to be directly related to their traumatic amputation and not accounted for by obesity, sedentary lifestyle, or tobacco use.[142–144] Reports demonstrate a positive correlation between a rise in norepinephrine and mean arterial blood pressure after walking in a prosthesis, a phenomenon attributed to mechanical irritation of the residual limb.[145] Studies of traumatic amputees compared to a cohort sample of the general population identify increased hypertension, ischemic heart disease, and diabetes mellitus. The traumatic amputee has a 65% greater risk of death from coronary and peripheral vascular diseases.[146,147] Rose et al hypothesized that insulin may be a causative factor in maturity-onset obesity-hypertension in his study of Vietnam War veterans who had undergone bilateral traumatic leg amputation.[148] In this study, the differences that were observed in insulin response between obese and lean bilateral above-knee amputees could not be attributed to lean body mass or physical fitness, inferring that these differences may be related to factors such as insulin-induced renal salt retention, increased sympathetic nervous stimulation, or increased cardiac inotropy.

Evidence also suggests that lower extremity amputees should be monitored for aortic aneurysms; occurring at a reported rate of 6% versus 1% in the nonamputee population. It is postulated that the asymmetric blood flow changes in the lower limb amputee lead to an unbalanced mechanical stress on the aortic wall with eventual asymmetric degeneration of the aortic wall elastic elements, resulting in an aneurysm.[149] Additionally, the metabolic costs of ambulation are substantially higher compared to the nonamputee, with much greater energy required for dysvascular amputees as compared to traumatic amputees. With aging and the aforementioned increased risk of cardiovascular disease and peripheral vascular disease in amputees, many of these demonstrate the metabolic derangements typically described in the dysvascular amputee.

The issues above underlie the importance of comprehensive nutritional, exercise, and wellness counseling for amputees. Wellness promotion and preventive measures should be part of one's lifestyle. Vigilant medical monitoring for cardiovascular diseases, including aortic aneurysms, should be routine in amputee clinics.

Endocrine Topics of Concern

The blast injuries sustained by service members in Iraq and Afghanistan are best described as polytrauma because all organ systems are affected. Comorbidities in this patient population often include TBIs, visceral organ damage, large soft tissue defects, concomitant fractures, and peripheral nerve injuries. Service members with multisystem injury are often managed acutely in the intensive care unit and require prolonged hospitalization for multiple surgical and medical issues. Previous studies in the critical care literature have elucidated the posttraumatic inflammatory response and the negative systemic effects of critical illness and polytrauma on hypothalamic-pituitary function.[150,151] Studies in patients with isolated SCI and TBI have identified associated chronic endocrinologic deficiencies, most notably hypogonadism. Total serum testosterone levels are significantly reduced in those with SCIs or TBIs.[152–155] The specific etiology of these hormonal deficiencies is multifactorial, but the question for the clinician is: once a deficiency is identified, should it be addressed through supplementation? Androgen supplementation has been beneficial in maintaining skeletal muscle following SCI[155] and has been used to augment wound healing in severe burns.[156] Deficiency of testosterone and growth hormone in the individual with TBI has been theorized to result in the observed visual-spatial impairment memory and neurovegetative symptoms such as depression. Studies evaluating the utility of hormone supplementation in TBI are pending.

The issue of sexual function and fertility in the polytrauma patient—specifically the traumatic amputee—requires evaluation. The long-term effect of endocrine derangements on reproductive health in the male and female traumatic amputee has not been described in the literature. Impaired fertility has been documented in SCI,[157] and recent animal models of SCI demonstrate that sperm integrity and genetic structure are altered following injury with an associated fertility reduction.[158] From these findings about SCIs, service members with traumatic amputations should be screened early in their periprosthetic rehabilitation to identify hormonal deficiencies and consider appropriate supplementation. In those service members considering procreation, the consultation of a fertility specialist may be appropriate in those couples having difficulty with conception.

SUMMARY

This chapter has shown that there are a number of important medical issues that must be considered in the trauma care and eventual rehabilitation of the combat amputee. Following lifesaving surgical stabilization, these issues rise in their importance and cannot be ignored. In addition to the orthopaedic and vascular surgeons, these medical issues require teamwork among a host of nonsurgical specialists from infectious diseases, physical medicine and rehabilitation, neurology, internal medicine, and hematology. In summary, whether reading for initial knowledge or review, this chapter provides an overview of basic approaches to some of the more prominent medical issues encountered in the care of the combat amputee.

REFERENCES

1. Border J. Death from severe trauma: open fractures to multiple organ dysfunction syndrome. *J Trauma*. 1995;39:12–22.

2. Luchette F, Bone L, Born C, et al. East Practice Management Guidelines Work Group: Practice management guidelines for prophylactic antibiotic use in open fractures. 2000. Available at: www.east.org/tpg/openfrac.pdf. Accessed July 24, 2007.

3. Patzakis MJ, Harvey JP Jr, Ivler D. The role of antibiotics in the management of open fractures. *J Bone Joint Surg Am*. 1974;56:532–541.

4. DeCoster T. Open fractures and osteomyelitis. In: Fry D, ed. *Surgical Infections*. Boston, Mass: Little, Brown; 1995:399–405.

5. Patzakis MJ, Wilkins J. Factors influencing infection rate in open fracture wounds. *Clin Orthop Relat Res*. 1989;243:36–40.

6. Robinson D, On E, Haddas N, Halperin N, Hofman S, Boldur I. Microbiologic flora contaminating open fractures: its significance in the choice of primary antibiotic agents and the likelihood of deep wound infection. *J Orthop Trauma*. 1989;3:283–286.

7. Classen DC, Evans RS, Pestotnik SL, Horn SD, Menlove RL, Burke JP. The timing of prophylactic administration of antibiotics and the risk of surgical-wound infection. *N Engl J Med.* 1992;326:281–286.

8. Bratzler D, Houck P. Antimicrobial prophylaxis for surgery: an advisory statement from the National Surgical Infection Prevention Project. *Clin Infect Dis.* 2004;38;1706–1715.

9. Aronson NE, Sanders JW, Moran KA. In harm's way: infections in deployed American military forces. *Clin Infect Dis.* 2006;43:1045–1051.

10. Petersen K, Riddle MS, Danko JR, et al. Trauma-related infections in battlefield casualties from Iraq. *Ann Surg.* 2007;245:803–811.

11. Murray CK, Roop SA, Hospenthal DR, et al. Bacteriology of war wounds at the time of injury. *Mil Med.* 2006;171:826–829.

12. Centers for Disease Control and Prevention. *Acinetobacter baumanni* among patients at military medical facilities treating injured U.S. members, 2002-2004. *MMWR Morb Mortal Wkly Rep.* 2004;53:1063–1066.

13. Scott P, Deye G, Srinivasan A, et al. An outbreak of multidrug-resistant *Acinetobacter baumannii-calcoaceticus* complex infection in the US military health care system associated with military operations in Iraq. *Clin Infect Dis.* 2007;44:1577–1584.

14. Siegel JD, Rhinehart E, Jackson M, Chiarello L; Healthcare Infection Control Practices Advisory Committee. Management of multi-drug resistant organisms in health care settings, 2006. Available at: http://www.cdc.gov/ncidod/dhqp/pdf/ar/mdroGuideline2006.pdf. Accessed July 6, 2007.

15. Timurkaynak F, Can F, Azap OK, Demirbilek M, Arslan H, Karaman SO. In vitro activities of non-traditional antimicrobials alone or in combination against multidrug-resistant strains of *Pseudomonas aeruginosa* and *Acinetobacter baumannii* isolated from intensive care units. *Int J Antimicrob Agents.* 2006;27:224–228.

16. Motaouakkil S, Charra B, Hachimi A, et al. Colistin and rifampicin in the treatment of nosocomial infections from multiresistant *Acinetobacter baumannii. J Infect.* 2006;53:274–278.

17. Jacoby GA, Munoz-Price LS. The new beta-lactamases. *N Engl J Med.* 2005;352:380–391.

18. Ramphal R, Ambrose PG. Extended-spectrum beta-lactamases and clinical outcomes: current data. *Clin Infect Dis.* 2006;42(Suppl 4):S164–S172.

19. Brennan TA, Leape LL, Laird NM, et al. Incidence of adverse events and negligence in hospitalized patients: results of the Harvard Medical Practice study I. *N Engl J Med.* 1991;324:370–376.

20. Gaynes RP, Culver DH, Horan TC, Edwards JR, Richards C, Tolson JS. Surgical site infection (SSI) rates in the United States, 1992–1998: the National Nosocomial Infections Surveillance System basic SSI risk index. *Clin Infect Dis.* 2001;33(Suppl 2):S69–S77.

21. Gaynes R, Edwards JR; National Nosocomial Infections Surveillance System. Overview of nosocomial infections caused by gram-negative bacilli. *Clin Infect Dis.* 2005;41:848–854.

22. Mangram AJ, Horan TC, Pearson ML, Silver LC, Jarvis WR. Guideline for prevention of surgical site infection, 1999: Hospital Infection Control Practices Advisory Committee. *Infect Control Hosp Epidemiol.* 1999;20:250–278.

23. Dellinger EP. Approach to the patient with postoperative fever. In: Gorbach SL, Bartlett JG, Blacklow NR, eds. *Infectious Diseases.* Philadelphia, Pa: WB Saunders; 1998:903–909.

24. Bartlett P, Reingold AL, Graham DR, et al. Toxic shock syndrome associated with surgical wound infections. *JAMA.* 1982;247:1448–1450.

25. Stevens DL, Bisno AL, Chambers HF, et al. Practice guidelines for the diagnosis and management of skin and soft-tissue infections. *Clin Infect Dis.* 2005;41:1373–1406.

26. Murray CK, Hospenthal DR. Treatment of multidrug resistant *Acinetobacter*. *Curr Opin Infect Dis*. 2005;18:502–506.

27. Trampuz A, Widmer AF. Infections associated with orthopedic implants. *Curr Opin Infect Dis*. 2006;19:349–356.

28. Darouiche RO. Treatment of infections associated with surgical implants. *N Engl J Med*. 2004;350:1422–1429.

29. Grimer RJ, Belthur M, Chandrasekar C, Carter SR, Tillman RM. Two-stage revision for infected endoprostheses used in tumor surgery. *Clin Orthop Relat Res*. 2002;395:193–203.

30. Zimmerli W, Widmer AF, Blatter M, Frei R, Ochsner PE. Role of rifampin for treatment of orthopedic implant-related staphylococcal infections: a randomized controlled trial. Foreign-Body Infection (FBI) Study Group. *JAMA*. 1998;279:1537–1541.

31. Lew DP, Waldvogel FA. Ostemoyelitis. *Lancet*. 2004;364:369–379.

32. Calhoun JH, Manring MM. Adult osteomyelitis. *Infect Dis Clin North Am*. 2005;19:765–786.

33. Gill VJ, Fedorko DP, Witebsky FG. The clinician and the microbiology laboratory. In: Mandell GL, Bennett JE, Dolin R, eds. *Mandell, Douglas and Bennett's Principles and Practice of Infectious Diseases*. 6th ed. New York, NY: Elsevier Churchill Livingstone; 2005:2060–2085.

34. Ledermann HP, Kaim A, Bongartz G, Steinbrich W. Pitfalls and limitations of magnetic resonance imaging in chronic posttraumatic osteomyelitis. *Eur Radiol*. 2000;10:1815–1823.

35. Potter BK, Burns TC, Lacap AP, Granville RR, Gajewski DA. Heterotopic ossification following traumatic and combat-related amputations. Prevalence, risk factors, and preliminary results of excision. *J Bone Joint Surg Am*. 2007;89:476–486.

36. Murray CK, Yun HC, Griffith ME, Hospenthal DR, Tong MJ. Acinetobacter infection: what was the true impact during the Vietnam conflict? *Clin Infect Dis*. 2006;43:383–384.

37. Harris AD, McGregor JC, Furuno JP. What infection control interventions should be undertaken to control multidrug-resistant gram-negative bacteria? *Clin Infect Dis*. 2006;43(Suppl 2):S57–S61.

38. Jawad A, Seifert H, Snelling AM, Heritage J, Hawkey PM. Survival of *Acinetobacter baumannii* on dry surfaces: comparison of outbreak and sporadic isolates. *J Clin Microbiol*. 1998;36:1938–1941.

39. Hayden MK, Bonten MJ, Blom DW, Lyle EA, van de Vijver DA, Weinstein RA. Reduction in acquisition of vancomycin-resistant enterococcus after enforcement of routine environmental cleaning measures. *Clin Infect Dis*. 2006;42:1552–1560.

40. Roup B, Kelley PW. Principles of infection control and prevention during military deployment. In: Kelley PW, ed. *Military Preventive Medicine: Mobilization and Deployment Volume 2*. In: Lounsbury DE, Bellamy RF, eds. *Textbooks of Military Medicine*. Washington, DC: Department of the Army, Office of The Surgeon General, Borden Institute; 2005:1249–1266.

41. Wilson ME, Weld LH, Boggild A, et al. Fever in returned travelers: results from the GeoSentinel Surveillance Network. *Clin Infect Dis*. 2007;44:1560–1568.

42. Ciminera P, Brundage J. Malaria in U.S. military forces: a description of deployment exposures from 2003 through 2005. *Am J Trop Med Hyg*. 2007;76:275–279.

43. Kotwal RS, Wenzel RB, Sterling RA, Porter WD, Jordan NN, Petruccelli BP. An outbreak of malaria in US Army Rangers returning from Afghanistan. *JAMA*. 2005;293:212–216.

44. Hartzell JD, Peng SW, Wood-Morris RN, et al. Atypical Q fever in US soldiers. *Emerg Infect Dis*. 2007;13:1247–1249.

45. Leung-Shea C, Danaher PJ. Q fever in members of the United States armed forces returning from Iraq. *Clin Infect Dis*. 2006;43:e77–e82.

46. Landais C, Fenollar F, Thuny F, Raoult D. From acute Q fever to endocarditis: serological follow-up strategy. *Clin Infect Dis*. 2007;44:1337–1340.

47. Aliaga P. Leishmaniasis in relation to service in Iraq/Afghanistan, U.S. Armed Forces, 2001-2006. In: *Medical Surveillance Monthly Report*. Vol 14. Silver Spring, Md: US Army Center for Health Promotion and Preventive Medicine; April 2007:2–5.

48. Kaur P, Basu S. Transfusion-transmitted infections: existing and emerging pathogens. *J Postgrad Med*. 2005;51:146–151.

49. Sevitt S, Gallagher N. Venous thrombosis and pulmonary embolism: a clinico-pathological study in injured and burned patients. *Br J Surg*. 1961;48:475–489.

50. Freeark RJ, Boswick J, Fardin R. Posttraumatic venous thrombosis. *Arch Surg*. 1967;95:567–575.

51. Kudsk KA, Fabian TC, Baum S, Gold RE, Mangiante E, Voeller G. Silent deep vein thromboses in immobilized multiple trauma patients. *Am J Surg*. 1989;158:515–519.

52. Geerts WH, Code KI, Jay RM, Chen E, Szalai JP. A prospective study of venous thromboembolism after major trauma. *N Engl J Med*. 1994;331:1601–1606.

53. Weingarden SI. Deep venous thrombosis in spinal cord injury: overview of the problem. *Chest*. 1992;102:636S–639S.

54. Collins R, Scrimgeour A, Yusuf S, Peto R. Reduction in fatal pulmonary embolism and venous thrombosis by perioperative administration of subcutaneous heparin: overview of results of randomized trials in general, orthopedic, and urologic surgery. *N Engl J Med*. 1988;318:1162–1173.

55. Clagett GP, Reisch JS. Prevention of venous thromboembolism in general surgical patients: results of meta-analysis. *Ann Surg*. 1988;208:227–240.

56. Raskob GE, Hirsh J. Controversies in timing of the first dose of anticoagulant prophylaxis against venous thromboembolism after major orthopedic surgery. *Chest*. 2003;1249(6 Suppl):379S–385S.

57. Geerts W, Selby R. Prevention of venous thromboembolism in the ICU. *Chest*. 2003;124(6 Suppl):357S–363S.

58. Kearon C. Duration of venous thromboembolism prophylaxis after surgery. *Chest*. 2003;124(6 Suppl):386S–392S.

59. Cushner FD. Bleeding associated with thromboprophylaxis: a multifactorial issue. *Orthopedics*. 2003;26(2 Suppl):s251–s254.

60. Eriksson BI, Wille-Jorgensen P, Kalebo P, et al. A comparison of recombinant hirudin with a low-molecular-weight heparin to prevent thromboembolic complications after total hip replacement. *N Engl J Med*. 1997;337:1329–1335.

61. Kearon C. Natural history of venous thromboembolism. *Semin Vasc Med*. 2001;1:27–37.

62. White RH, Gettner S, Newman JM, Trauner KB, Romano PS. Predictors of rehospitalization for symptomatic venous thromboembolism after total hip arthroplasty. *N Engl J Med*. 2000;343:1758–1764.

63. Grady D, Wenger NK, Herrington D, et al. Postmenopausal hormone therapy increases risk for venous thromboembolic disease. The Heart and Estrogen/progestin Replacement Study. *Ann Intern Med*. 2000;132:689–696.

64. Scott SG, Belanger HG, Vanderploeg RD, Massengale J, Scholten J. Mechanism-of-injury approach to evaluating patients with blast-related polytrauma. *J Am Osteopath Assoc*. 2006;106:265–270.

65. Buschbacker R, Porter CD. Deconditioning, conditioning and benefits of exercise. In: Braddom RL, ed. *Physical Medicine and Rehabilitation*. 2nd ed. Philadelphia, Pa: WB Saunders; 2000: 702–723.

66. Li XJ, Jee WS, Chow SY, Woodbury DM. Adaptation of cancellous bone to aging and immobilization in the rat: a single photo absorptiometry and histomorphometry study. *Anat Rec*. 1990;227:12–24.

67. Muller EA. Influence of training and of inactivity on muscle strength. *Arch Phys Med Rehabil.* 1970;51:449–462.

68. Uhtoff HK, Jaworski ZF. Bone loss in response to long-term immobilization. *J Bone Joint Surg Br.* 1978;60:420–429.

69. Buckwalter JA, Einhorn TA, Bolander ME, Cruess RL. Healing of the musculoskeletal tissues. In: Rockwood CA, Green DP, Bucholz RW, Heckman JD, eds. *Fractures in Adults.* Philadelphia, Pa: Lippincott-Raven; 1996:261–304.

70. Einhorn TA. The cell and molecular biology of fracture healing. *Clin Orthop Relat Res.* 1998;(355 Suppl):S7–S21.

71. Buckwalter JA, Woo S-Y. Effects of repetitive loading and motion on musculoskeletal tissues. In: DeLee JC, Drez D, eds. *Orthopaedic Sports Medicine: Principles and Practice.* Vol 3. Philadelphia, Pa: WB Saunders; 1994:60–72.

72. O'Sullivan ME, Bronk JT, Chao EY, Kelly PJ. Experimental study of the effect of weight bearing on fracture healing in the canine tibia. *Clin Orthop Relat Res.* 1994;302:273–283.

73. Buckwalter JA. Activity vs. rest in the treatment of bone, soft tissue and joint injuries. *Iowa Orthop J.* 1995;15:29–42.

74. Goodship AE, Kenwright J. The influence of induced micromovement upon the healing of experimental tibial fractures. *J Bone Joint Surg Br.* 1985;67:650–655.

75. Kenwright J, Goodship AE. Controlled mechanical stimulation in the treatment of tibial fractures. *Clin Orthop Relat Res.* 1989;241:36–47.

76. Kenwright J, Richardson JB, Cunningham JL, et al. Axial movement and tibial fractures: a controlled randomized trial of treatment. *J Bone Joint Surg Br.* 1991;73:654–659.

77. Kenwright J, Richardson JB, Goodship AE. Effect of controlled axial micromovement on healing of tibial fractures. *Lancet.* 1986;2:1185–1187.

78. Kershaw CJ, Cunningham JL, Kenwright J. Tibial external fixation, weight bearing and fracture movement. *Clin Orthop Relat Res.* 1993;293:28–36.

79. Becker B, Cole AJ. Aquatic rehabilitation. In: Delisa J, Gans G, eds. *Textbook of Physical Medicine and Rehabilitation.* 4th ed. Philadelphia, Pa: Lippincott Williams and Wilkins; 2005:484–485.

80. Leung KS, Sher AH, Lam TS, Leung PL. Energy metabolism in fracture healing. Measurement of adenosine triphosphate in callus to monitor progress. *J Bone Joint Surg Br.* 1989;71:657–660.

81. Michelsen CB, Askanazi J. The metabolic response to injury: mechanisms and clinical implications. *J Bone Joint Surg Am.* 1986:68:782–787.

82. Taylor SJ, Fettes SB, Jewkes C, Nelson RJ. Prospective, randomized, controlled trial to determine the effect of early enhanced enteral nutrition on clinical outcome in mechanically ventilated patients suffering head injury. *Crit Care Med.* 1999; 27:2525–2531.

83. Brighton CT, Hozack WJ, Brager MD, et al. Fracture healing in the rabbit fibula when subjected to various capacitively coupled electrical fields. *J Orthop Res.* 1985;3:331–340.

84. Lavine LS, Grodzinsky AJ. Electrical stimulation of repair of bone. *J Bone Joint Surg Am.* 1987;69:626–630.

85. Lavine LS, Shamos MH. Electrical enhancement of bone healing. *Science.* 1972;175:1118–1121.

86. Brighton CT. The semi-invasive method of treating nonunion with direct current. *Orthop Clin North Am.* 1984;15:33–45.

87. Brighton CT, Pollack SR. Treatment of recalcitrant non-union with a capacitively coupled electrical field; a preliminary report. *J Bone Joint Surg Am.* 1985;67:577–585.

88. Scott G, King JB. A prospective, double-blind trial of electrical capacitive coupling in the treatment on non-union of long bones. *J Bone Joint Surg Am.* 1994;76:820–826.

89. Sharrard WJ. A double blind trial of pulsed electromagnetic fields of delayed union of tibial fractures. *J Bone Joint Surg Br.* 1990;72:347–355.

90. Hadjiargyrou M, Halsey MF, Ahrens W, Rightmire EP, McLeod KJ, Rubin CT. Enhancement of fracture healing by low intensity ultrasound. *Clin Orthop Relat Res.* 1998;355(Suppl):S216–S229.

91. Heckman JD, Ryaby JP, McCabe J, Frey JJ, Kilcoyne RF. Acceleration of tibial fracture healing by non-invasive, low-intensity pulsed ultrasound. *J Bone Joint Surg Am.* 1994;76:26–34.

92. Klug W, Franke WG, Knoch HG. Scintigraphic control of bone-fracture healing under ultrasonic stimulation: an animal experimental study. *Eur J Nucl Med.* 1986;11:494–497.

93. Pilla AA, Mont MA, Nasser PR. Non-invasive low-intensity pulsed ultrasound accelerates bone healing in the rabbit. *J Orthop Trauma.* 1990;4:246–253.

94. Burnett DM, Watanabe TK, Greenwald BD. Congenital and acquired brain injury. 2. Brain injury rehabilitation: medical management. *Arch Phys Med Rehabil.* 2003;84(3 Suppl 1):S8–S11.

95. Flin C, Curalucci H, Duvocelle A, Viton JM. Heterotopic ossification and brain injury. *Ann Readapt Med Phys.* 2002;45:517–520.

96. Garland DE, Blum CE, Waters RL. Periarticular heterotopic ossification in head-injured adults. Incidence and location. *J Bone Joint Surg Am.* 1980;62:1143–1146.

97. Raikin SM, Landsman JC, Alexander VA, Froimson MI, Plaxton NA. Effect of nicotine on the rate and strength of long bone fracture healing. *Clin Orthop Relat Res.* 1998;353:231–237.

98. Riebel GD, Boden SD, Whitesides TE, Hutton WC. The effect of nicotine on incorporation of cancellous bone graft in an animal model. *Spine.* 1995;20:2198–2202.

99. Potter BK, Burns TC, Lacap AP, Granville RR, Gajewski DA. Heterotopic ossification following traumatic and combat-related amputations. Prevalence, risk factors, and preliminary results of excision. *J Bone Joint Surg Am.* 2007;89:476–486.

100. Balboni TA, Gobezie R, Mamon HJ. Heterotopic ossification: pathophysiology, clinical features, and the role of radiotherapy for prophylaxis. *Int J Radiat Oncol Biol Phys.* 2006;65:1289–1299.

101. Ellerin BE, Helfet D, Parikh S, et al. Current therapy in the management of heterotopic ossification of the elbow: a review with case studies. *Am J Phys Med Rehabil.* 1999;78:259–271.

102. Stein DA, Patel R, Egol KA, Kaplan FT, Tejwani NC, Koval KJ. Prevention of heterotopic ossification at the elbow following trauma using radiation therapy. *Bull Hosp Jt Dis.* 2003;61:151–154.

103. Banovac K, Sherman AL, Estores IM, Banovac F. Prevention and treatment of heterotopic ossification after spinal cord injury. *J Spinal Cord Med.* 2004;27:376–382.

104. Pakos EE, Ioannidis JP. Radiotherapy vs. nonsteroidal anti-inflammatory drugs for the prevention of heterotopic ossification after major hip procedures: a meta-analysis of randomized trials. *Int J Radiat Oncol Biol Phys.* 2004;60:888–895.

105. Banovac K, Gonzalez F, Wade N, Bowker JJ. Intravenous disodium etidronate therapy in spinal cord injury patients with heterotopic ossification. *Paraplegia.* 1993;31:660–666.

106. Dudek NL, DeHaan MN, Marks MB. Bone overgrowth in the adult traumatic amputee. *Am J Phys Med Rehabil.* 2003;82:897–900.

107. Warmoth JE, Riegel B, McFall TL, et al. Case report forum: heterotopic ossification associated with traumatic amputa-

tion. *J Prosthet Orthot.* 1997;9:33–37.

108. Brackett EG. Care of the amputated in the United States. In: Ireland MW, ed. *The Medical Department of the United States Army in the World War.* Washington, DC: Government Printing Office; 1927:11(pt 1):713–748.

109. Otis GA, Huntington DL. Wounds and complications. In: Barnes JK, ed. *The Medical and Surgical History of the Civil War.* Washington, DC: Government Printing Office; 1883:2(pt 3):880.

110. Dougherty PJ. Wartime amputations. *Mil Med.* 1993;158:755–763.

111. Brown PW. Rehabilitation of bilateral lower-extremity amputees. *J Bone Joint Surg Am.* 1970;52:687–700.

112. LaNoue AM. Lieutenant General, US Army (Ret). Personal communication, 2007.

113. Potter BK, Burns TC, Lecap AP, Granville RR, Gajewski D. Heterotopic ossification in the residual limbs of traumatic and combat-related amputees. *J Am Acad Orthop Surg.* 2006;14(10 Suppl):S191–S197.

114. Fournier PE, Richet H. The epidemiology and control of *Acinetobacter baumannii* in health care facilities. *Clin Infect Dis.* 2006;42:692–699.

115. Okie S. Traumatic brain injury in the war zone. *N Engl J Med.* 2005;352:2043–2047.

116. Melamed E, Robinson D, Halperin N, Wallach N, Keren O, Groswassen Z. Brain injury-related heterotopic bone formation: treatment strategy and results. *Am J Phys Med Rehabil.* 2002;81:670–674.

117. Fijn R, Koorevaar RT, Brouwers JR. Prevention of heterotopic ossification after total hip replacement with NSAIDs. *Pharm World Sci.* 2003;25:138–145.

118. Banovac K, Williams JM, Patrick LD, Levi A. Prevention of heterotopic ossification after spinal cord injury with COX-2 selective inhibitor (rofecoxib). *Spinal Cord.* 2004;42:707–710.

119. Nilsson OS, Bauer HC, Brosjo O, Tornkvist H. Influence of indomethacin on induced heterotopic bone formation in rats. Importance of length of treatment and age. *Clin Orthop Relat Res.* 1986;207:239–245.

120. Stover SL, Niemann KM, Miller JM III. Disodium etidronate in the prevention of postoperative recurrence of heterotopic ossification in spinal-cord injury patients. *J Bone Joint Surg Am.* 1976;58:683–688.

121. Spielman G, Gennarelli TA, Rogers CR. Disodium etidronate: its role in preventing heterotopic ossification in severe head injury. *Arch Phys Med Rehabil.* 1983;64:539–542.

122. Banovac K. The effect of etidronate on late development of heterotopic ossification after spinal cord injury. *J Spinal Cord Med.* 2000;23:40–44.

123. Fleisch H. Diphosphonates: history and mechanisms of action. *Metab Bone Dis Relat Res.* 1981;3:279–287.

124. Orzel JA, Rudd TG. Heterotopic bone formation: clinical, laboratory, and imaging correlation. *J Nucl Med.* 1985;26:125–132.

125. Hunt JL, Arnoldo BD, Kowalske K, Helm P, Purdue GF. Heterotopic ossification revisited: a 21-year surgical experience. *J Burn Care Res.* 2006;27:535–540.

126. Fuller DA, Mark A, Keenan MA. Excision of heterotopic ossification from the knee: a functional outcome study. *Clin Orthop Relat Res.* 2005;438:197–203.

127. Anderson MC, Lais RL. Excision of heterotopic ossification of the popliteal space following traumatic brain injury. *J Orthop Trauma.* 2004;18:190–192.

128. Garland DE, Orwin JF. Resection of heterotopic ossification in patients with spinal cord injuries. *Clin Orthop Relat Res.*

1989;242:169–176.

129. Fitzpatrick KF, et al. The use of CT-based 3-D model construction to aid in the fitting of upper extremity prosthetic sockets in patients with heterotopic ossification: a case series. Poster presented at: Association of Academic Physiatrists Annual Conference; February 2005; Tucson, AZ.

130. Fitzpatrick KF, et al. The use of CT-based 3-D model construction to aid in resection of heterotopic ossification after traumatic transfemoral amputation: a case series. Oral presentation at: 2006 Medicine Meets Virtual Reality Meeting 15; January 2006; Long Beach, CA.

131. Howie JL. Computed tomography of the bony pelvis: a protocol for multiplanar imaging. Part II: Trauma. *J Can Assoc Radiol*. 1985;36:287–295.

132. Falchi M, Rollandi GA. CT of pelvic fractures. *Eur J Radiol*. 2004;50:96–105.

133. Theumann NH, Verdon JP, Mouhsine E, Denys A, Schnyder P, Portier F. Traumatic injuries: imaging of pelvic fractures. *Eur Radiol*. 2002;12:1312–1330.

134. Codispoti VT, et al. Three-dimensional CT modeling as a tool for rehabilitation of a patient with a comminuted pelvic fracture: a case report. Poster presented at: American Academy of Physical Medicine and Rehabilitation Conference; September 2007; Boston, MA.

135. Davies P. Between health and illness. *Perspect Biol Med*. 2007;50:444–452.

136. Kulkarni J, Adams J, Thomas E, Silman A. Association between amputation, arthritis, and osteopenia in British male war veterans with major lower limb amputation. *Clin Rehabil*. 1998;12:348–353.

137. Norvell DC, Czerniecki JM, Reiber GE, Maynard C, Pecoraro JA, Weiss NS. The prevalence of knee pain and symptomatic knee osteoarthritic among veteran traumatic amputees and nonamputees. *Arch Phys Med Rehabil*. 2005;86:487–493.

138. Melzer I, Yekutiel M, Sukenik S. Comparative study of osteoarthritis of the contralateral knee joint of male amputees who do and do not play volleyball. *J Rheumatol*. 2001;28:169–172.

139. Friel K, Domholdt E, Smith DG. Physical and functional measures related to low back pain in individuals with lower-limb amputation: an exploratory pilot study. *J Rehabil Res Dev*. 2005;2:155–166.

140. Ehde DM, Smith DG, Czerniecki JM, Campbell KM, Malchow DM, Robinson LR. Back pain as a secondary disability in persons with lower limb amputations. *Arch Phys Med Rehabil*. 2001;82:731–734.

141. Rush PJ, Wong JS, Kirsh J, Devlin M. Osteopenia in patients with above knee amputation. *Arch Phys Med Rehabil*. 1994;75:112–115.

142. Leclercq MM, Bonidan O, Haaby E, Pierrejean C, Sengler J. Study of bone mass with dual energy x-ray absorptiometry in a population of 99 lower limb amputees. *Ann Readapt Med Phys*. 2003;46:24–30.

143. Stocker D, Stack A, Goff B, Pasquina P, Marin R. Patients experience rapid, substantial bone loss following a trauma-related amputation: the Walter Reed experience. *J Nucl Med*. 2007;48(Suppl 2):286P.

144. Rose HG, Schweitzer P, Charoenkul V, Schwartz E. Cardiovascular disease risk factors in combat veterans after traumatic leg amputations. *Arch Phys Med Rehabil*. 1987;68:20–23.

145. Peles E, Akselrod S, Goldstein DS, et al. Insulin resistance and autonomic function in traumatic lower limb amputees. *Clin Auton Res*. 1995;5:279–288.

146. Modan M, Peles E, Halkin H, et al. Increased cardiovascular disease mortality rates in traumatic lower limb amputees. *Am J Cardiol*. 1998;82:1242–1247.

147. Grubeck-Loebenstein B, Korn A, Waldhausl W. The role of adrenergic mechanisms in the blood pressure regulation

of leg-amputees. *Basic Res Cardiol.* 1981;76:267–275.

148. Rose HG, Yalow RS, Schweitzer P, Schwartz E. Insulin as a potential factor influencing blood pressure in amputees. *Hypertension.* 1986;8:793–800.

149. Yekutiel M, Brooks ME, Ohry A, Yarom J, Carel R. The prevalence of hypertension, ischaemic heart disease and diabetes in traumatic spinal cord injured patients and amputees. *Paraplegia.* 1989;27:58–62.

150. Aller MA, Arias JL, Nava MP, Arias J. Posttraumatic inflammation is a complex response based on the pathological expression of the nervous, immune, and endocrine functional systems. *Exp Biol Med.* 2004;229:170–181.

151. Kohl B, Deutschman C. The inflammatory response to surgery and trauma. *Curr Opin Crit Care.* 2006;12:325–332.

152. Schopp LH, Clark M, Mazurek MO, et al. Testosterone levels among men with spinal cord injury admitted to inpatient rehabilitation. *Am J Phys Med Rehabil.* 2006;85:678–684.

153. Naderi AR, Safarinejad MR. Endocrine profiles and semen quality in spinal cord injured men. *Clin Endocrinol.* 2003;59:177–184.

154. Woolf PD, Hamill RW, McDonald JV, Lee LA, Kelly M. Transient hypogonadotrophic hypogonadism after head trauma: effects on steroid precursors and correlation with sympathetic nervous system activity. *Clin Endocrinol.* 1986;25:265–274.

155. Gregory CM, Vandenborne K, Huang H, Ottenweller JE, Dudley GA. Effects of testosterone replacement therapy on skeletal muscle after spinal cord injury. *Spinal Cord.* 2003;41:23–28.

156. Jeschke MG, Finnerty CC, Suman OE, Kulp G, Mlcak RP, Herndon DN. The effect of oxandrolone on the endocrinologic, inflammatory, and hypermetabolic responses during the acute phase postburn. *Ann Surg.* 2007;246:351–362.

157. Brown DJ, Hill ST, Baker H. Male fertility and sexual function after spinal cord injury. *Prog Brain Res.* 2006;152:427–439.

158. Talebi A, Khalili M, Hossaini A. Assessment of nuclear DNA integrity of epididymal spermatozoa following experimental chronic spinal cord injury in the rat. *Int J Androl.* 2007;30:163–169.

Chapter 11

PAIN MANAGEMENT AMONG SOLDIERS WITH AMPUTATIONS

RANDALL J. MALCHOW, MD*; KEVIN K. KING, DO[†]; BRENDA L. CHAN[‡]; SHARON R. WEEKS[§]; AND JACK W. TSAO, MD, DPHIL[¥]

*Colonel, Medical Corps, US Army; Chief, Regional Anesthesia and Acute Pain Management, Department of Anesthesia and Operative Services, Brooke Army Medical Center, 3851 Roger Brooke Drive, Fort Sam Houston, Texas 78234; formerly, Chief of Anesthesia, Brooke Army Medical Center, 3851 Roger Brooke Drive, Fort Sam Houston, Texas, and Program Director, Anesthesiology, Brooke Army Medical Center-Wilford Hall Medical Center, Fort Sam Houston, Texas
[†] Major, Medical Corps, US Army; Resident Anesthesiologist, Department of Anesthesiology, Brooke Army Medical Center, 3851 Roger Brooke Drive, Fort Sam Houston, Texas 78234
[‡] Research Analyst, CompTIA, 1815 South Meyers Road, Suite 300, Villa Park, Illinois 60181; Formerly, Research Assistant, Department of Physical Medicine and Rehabilitation, Walter Reed Army Medical Center, 6900 Georgia Avenue, NW, Washington, DC 20307
[§] Research Assistant, Physical Medicine and Rehabilitation, Walter Reed Army Medical Center, 6900 Georgia Avenue, NW, Washington, DC 20307
[¥] Commander, Medical Corps, US Navy; Associate Professor, Department of Neurology, Uniformed Services University of the Health Sciences, 4301 Jones Bridge Road, Room A1036, Bethesda, Maryland 20814; Traumatic Brain Injury Consultant, US Navy Bureau of Medicine and Surgery, 2300 E Street, NW, Washington, DC

INTRODUCTION

Pain management is increasingly recognized as a critical aspect of the care of the polytrauma patient. Aggressive analgesia not only decreases pain but also produces myriad benefits such as improving sleep–wake cycles; decreasing anxiety, stress, and depression; improving pulmonary mechanics; decreasing ileus; reducing hospital stay; decreasing cost; and improving overall outcome. Additionally, aggressive acute pain control leads to a reduction in chronic pain, which remains a persistent challenge: chronic pain rates are over 50% following many surgeries and trauma conditions.[1–6]

HISTORY

Various methods to reduce pain were tried before the development of specific analgesics. In the 17th century, the Italian surgeon Marco Aurelio Severino applied ice to injured areas to reduce pain, but the technique was limited by resultant frostbite, slow onset of relief, painful administration, and limited depth of analgesia. In the 18th century, various compression devices used to reduce pain in extremities were somewhat effective yet limited by their associated ischemic pain and the direct discomfort of the device. The mid-19th century brought several pivotal developments in acute pain management.[7–11] First, Friedrich Serturner extracted morphine from the opium plant in 1803, naming it "morphia" after the Greek god of dreams. Local anesthesia for analgesia became possible through the inventions of the syringe by Charles Gabriel Pravaz of France, the hollow needle by Alexander Wood of Scotland, and the extraction of cocaine from the coca leaf by Albert Niemann of Germany. Carl Koller demonstrated the effectiveness of topical cocaine at the Congress of Ophthalmology in Germany.

Regional anesthesia quickly followed when American William Stewart Halsted performed various peripheral nerve blocks (PNBs), usually via cut-down techniques, in the late 1880s. James Leonard Corning injected cocaine in the lower thoracic "dorsal vertebrae," with numbness occurring 20 minutes later, probably due to epidural blockade. In 1897 George Washington Crile, surgeon and founder of the Cleveland Clinic, performed one of the first leg blocks for a traumatic amputation and introduced the term "block" to describe the effect of blocking afferent input from the periphery to the brain. The desire for safer local anesthetics led Heinrich Braun of Germany to develop procaine (Novocain; Hospira, Inc, Lake Forest, Ill) at the turn of the century as well as the addition of epinephrine to prolong the duration of blockade. Harvey Williams Cushing furthered the use of "cocainization of nerve trunks" prior to amputation as a means to block neural fibers, which were felt to cause shock and hemorrhage in the early 1900s.

Brachial plexus blockade techniques expanded at the outbreak of the First World War when three German physicians, G Hirshel, D Kulenkampff, and M Kappis, demonstrated the first axillary block, supraclavicular block, and interscalene block, respectively. In 1939 meperidine became the first synthetic opioid available, and fentanyl followed 20 years later. Building on the continuous spinal anesthesia techniques of William Lemmon and EB Touhys, F Paul Ansbro introduced continuous supraclavicular techniques in 1946, followed by Manuel Martinez Curbelo's 1949 continuous epidural technique.[12–14] Early nerve localization techniques relied on paresthesias; later anesthesiologists pursued nerve stimulation in the 1960s and 1970s and most recently began using portable high-resolution ultrasound machines.[15–21] Finally, Susan Steele and Ottmar Kick introduced continuous peripheral nerve blocks (CPNBs) in 1998 and 1999.[22,23]

Phantom limb pain (PLP) has been recognized as a significant problem in the amputee patient for centuries; as 16th century French surgeon Ambroise Paré noted, "Truly, it is a thing wondrous, strange, and prodigious which will scarce be credited, unless by such as have seen with their own eyes and heard with their own ears, the patients who many months after cutting away the leg, grievously complained that they yet felt exceeding great pain of that leg so cut off." Silar Weir Mitchell, a surgeon during the US Civil War, is credited with the term "phantom limb pain" to describe this phenomenon.[24]

NEUROPHYSIOLOGY AND MECHANISMS OF PAIN

Neurophysiology

Understanding the normal nociceptive pathway, including the four processes in the sensory pathway of pain perception (transduction, transmission, perception, and modulation), is critical to understanding the specific types of neuropathic pain that many amputees experience. In addition, knowledge of the nociceptive pathway lays the foundation for an understanding of how regional analgesia at various points in the pathway may be beneficial, and demonstrates that regional analgesia is pathophysiologically a crucial part of the multimodal regimen, which is most effective in the treatment of pain.[25,26]

Transduction

Peripheral nociceptors such as free nerve endings and mechanoceptors convert noxious stimuli into neural impulses that travel along A-δ (fast, myelinated) fibers and C (slow, unmyelinated) fibers, which transmit first (sharp, injurious) pain and second (dull, visceral) pain, respectively. Peripheral sensitization, or lowering of the pain transduction threshold, occurs in severe tissue injury and is maintained by a cycle of mediators, including prostaglandins, leukotrienes, kinins, histamines, substance P, and serotonin, causing more tissue damage. These products of the arachidonic acid pathway are major mediators of hyperalgesia, so inhibitors of this pathway are likely key to any analgesic regimen for pain secondary to severe limb injury.[25]

Transmission

Nociceptive impulses including first (sharp, injurious) pain and second (dull, visceral) pain are transmitted via A-δ (fast, myelinated) fibers and C (slow, unmyelinated) fibers, respectively, which synapse with second order neurons within laminas I, II, and IV of the dorsal horn of the spinal cord using substance P and excitatory aminoacids (aspartate, glutamate). The contralateral spinothalamic tract comprises the majority of second order neurons and ascends to the thalamus; third order neurons transmit pain from the thalamus to the sensory cerebral cortex, the cingulate cortex, the amygdala, and the insulate gyrus.

Perception

The third order neurons, including lateral thalamic projections to the cerebral cortex and medial thalamic projections to the reticular formation (emotional aspect), contribute to the perception of pain. Many medications including opioids, anticonvulsants, antidepressants, and α_2-agonists affect the perception of pain in these areas.

Modulation

The efferent descending inhibitory fibers from the corticospinal tract, hypothalamus, and periaqueductal gray areas modulate afferent input at laminas I and V (primarily) of the dorsal horn by decreasing neurotransmitter release. Serotonin, norepinephrine, and opioid-like encephalins (especially within lamina II at the substantia gelatinosa) are known neurotransmitters in the descending pathways. Modulation is augmented by intrathecal spinal opioids and intrathecal α-agonists.

Mechanism of Phantom Sensations and Phantom Limb Pain

A phantom limb experience is defined as the continued perception of a missing limb, the simple tactile awareness of the missing limb, and the perceived ability to move the missing limb, most likely due to a persisting central nervous system representation of the limb.[26] Between 90% and 98% of all patients who have undergone limb amputation experience a vivid phantom, with even higher incidences following traumatic limb loss or following a preexisting painful condition in the limb. Phantom limb sensations, including tingling, itching, burning, movement, temperature changes, pressure, and pain occur as soon as an anesthetic wears off in 75% of cases, but development of these sensations may be delayed up to several weeks.[27–30] PLP and phantom sensations tend to be brief and last from days to weeks for most amputees, but can become chronic. Sherman et al[31] found in a study of several thousand amputees that over 70% continue to experience PLP as long as 25 years following a limb amputation. A recent epidemiologic study by Richardson and Turo[32] was performed to investigate all postamputation phenomena in a homogenous group of amputees (all with peripheral vascular disease). Sixty amputees were recruited, but only 52 survived until a 6-month postoperative interview. Phantom sensations (kinetic, kinesthetic, exteroceptive) were universal (100%). "Telescoping," the sensation of the distal end of the phantom limb becoming progressively closer to the residual limb, was the most common kinesthetic aspect reported in 67.3% of cases, PLP occurred in 78.8% of cases, and residual limb pain occurred in 51.2% of cases.[32]

The phantom limb tends to occupy a fixed or "habitual" posture. For example, following upper limb amputation, many patients report experiencing the limb as partially flexed at the elbow, with the forearm pronated. However, the phantom limb sometimes occupies a painful or awkward posture (ie, a tightly clenched fist).[28] A soldier who was holding a grenade that exploded in his hand reportedly experienced a phantom hand clenched in a painful posture,[33] and the authors have heard similar experiences from Operation Enduring Freedom and Operation Iraqi Freedom patients treated at Walter Reed Army Medical Center. Thus, the phantom limb may sometimes be experienced as a reactivation of preamputation memories of the limb. Telescoping occurs in two-thirds of limb amputees.

Many theories have been proposed for the etiology of PLP.[34] The development of neuromas was once thought to cause phantom sensations and pain. Neuromas are bundles of severed nerve fibers that can send ectopic pain impulses through the spinal cord and the thalamus to the somatosensory cortex. However, removal of neuromas does not relieve phantom limb sensation or phantom pain.[35] Modifications of spinal neurons that were dependent on the neurons that subserved the formerly innervated limb may be another explanation for phantom limb sensations. Excessive spontaneous firing of spinal neurons that have lost their proper sensory input from the deafferented limb may be interpreted as PLP or phantom sensations when these abnormal impulses reach the brain.[36–38] However, studies of individuals who were born without limbs but still exhibit phantom limb sensations show no excessive firing of spinal neurons because peripheral nerves connected to these neurons have never developed, suggesting that this theory is probably incorrect.[27]

Most likely, a central representation of the limb persists and is responsible for meaningful experiences of the limb, as proposed by Melzack's "neuromatrix theory."[39] According to this theory, a central representation of the limb is formed and modified within a neuromatrix, a neural network that subserves body sensation; contains the somatic, visual, and limbic systems; and produces characteristic nerve-impulse patterns.[39] This network of neurons is present throughout the brain and has synaptic links that are genetically determined but later sculpted by sensory inputs. The repeated cyclical processing and synthesis of nerve impulses creates a characteristic pattern called the neurosignature. The phantom limb experience is produced by the same neuromatrix that underlies the intact bodily experience. Phantom pain may thus result from the deprivation of modulating inputs from the limbs to the neuromatrix, which can then cause an abnormal neurosignature to be produced.[39]

Therefore, PLP is most likely the result of cortical reorganization within the somatosensory and motor cortices. The brain contains several complete somatotopic maps (homunculi) of the body surface.[40] The primary motor area, lateral premotor area, supplementary motor area, parietal cortex, and basal ganglia all contain complete somatotopic representations of the body.[41,42] It was once believed that these maps were fixed following critical periods during infancy.[43] However, many studies suggest that sensory maps can undergo remodeling in the adult brain.

Experimental evidence demonstrates that the amount of cortical reorganization is associated with the severity of PLP and likely plays a prominent role

in its emergence.[44] Studies using noninvasive imaging techniques, such as functional magnetic resonance imaging, have demonstrated changes within the somatosensory and motor cortices in amputees.[45,46] Ramachandran and Hirstein[28] found that sensory maps reorganize in such a way that specific points along the neighboring sensory area evoke modality-specific referred sensations such as warmth and pain. However, if there is a slight error in cortical reorganization such that some of the touch input is accidentally connected to pain areas, it is theorized that amputees may experience pain when these regions are touched.[28] Finally, a sympathetic mechanism that increases sympathetic activity may maintain pain by noradrenergic stimulation of the neuromas or nerve endings in a residual limb.[37]

Residual Limb Pain

Residual limb pain, previously referred to as stump pain, can be a painful and frustrating postamputation phenomena. Residual limb pain is common in early postoperative and rehabilitation phases but regresses to a greater extent than any other of the postamputation phenomena. After 2 years postamputation, prevalence may be as low as 20%.[37] Typically, residual limb pain should subside with healing, but if it persists more than a few months, poor prosthetic fit or overuse and overtraining is often the cause. Residual limb pain is more likely if chronic pain was a problem before surgery and will likely persist longer if postoperative analgesia is inadequate. A survey of veteran amputees in the early 1980s revealed that the severity and duration of residual limb pain correlated well with presence and persistence of phantom pain.[31,47] Multiple other reasons may explain why residual limb pain can persist beyond the normal healing period.

The treatment of residual limb pain is typically the domain of the physiatrist or physical therapist; however, anesthesiologists and surgeons can also be helpful in the early postoperative period by screening for anatomic residual limb pathology that may be causative. Anatomic causes include ulcers or inflammation secondary to improper prosthesis fit; bony abnormalities (ischemia, spurs, heterotopic ossification, and osteomyelitis); neuroma formation; and, rarely, malignancies or tumors, many of which may be amenable to surgical correction such as neuroma excision and repositioning of the nerve within bone or muscle.[37] Nonsurgical treatments include botulinum toxin injection; nerve blocks; transcutaneous electrical nerve stimulation (TENS); acupuncture; Farabloc (Farabloc, Coquitlam, British Columbia, Canada) steel fiber sheet sheaths or socks; and oral medications, such as nonsteroidal antiinflammatory drugs (NSAIDs), cyclooxygenase (COX)-2 inhibitors, and acetaminophen for somatic pain, and tricyclic antidepressants and anticonvulsants (eg, gabapentin, pregabalin) for neuropathic pain.[48] Mexiletine and clonidine have also been used successfully for PLP, and are likely effective for residual limb pain as well.[49] A recent case report by Nikolajsen et al[50] proposes that low-dose ketamine is effective in treating residual limb pain when conventional tricyclic antidepressants and opioid therapy have failed. Ketamine decreases the hyperactivity of *N*-methyl-ᴅ-aspartate (NMDA) receptors and thus decreases neuronal excitability. Ketamine reduced allodynia and wind-up response, and increased the pressure-pain threshold. Amputee soldiers and veterans may benefit from ketamine therapy to allow reductions in residual limb pain caused by neuromas, which may allow more function with prostheses.[50] Other medications such as mirtazapine, a serotonin-norepinephrine reuptake inhibitor antidepressant, may be more cost-effective than newer generation anticonvulsants and are probably more efficacious than older tricyclic antidepressants.[35] Each component of this multimodal approach is described more extensively below.

MULTIMODAL PAIN MANAGEMENT IN AMPUTEE CARE

Rationale

Capitalizing on synergy among various medications and modalities, multimodal therapy affects the nociceptive pathway at multiple points (Figure 11-1). Synergy among medications should allow the provider

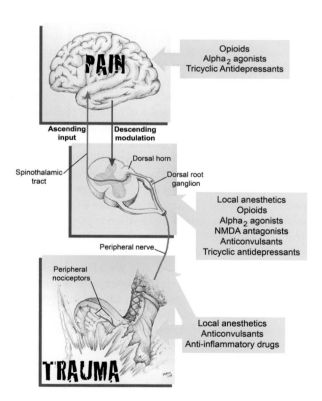

Figure 11-1. Multiple sites of action with multimodal therapy.
NMDA: *N*-methyl-ᴅ-aspartate
Reproduced with permission from: Buckenmaier C, Bleckner L. *Military Advanced Regional Anesthesia and Analgesia Handbook*. Washington, DC: Borden Institute; 2009: Figure 27-1.

to use less of each medication, thereby reducing side effects and the potential risks of each medication. Treating pain at various points of the nociceptive pathway allows multimodal therapy to be more effective than simply increasing the treatment at one point in the pathway. "Practice Guidelines for Acute Management in the Perioperative Setting"[51] recommends that all patients receive an around-the-clock regimen of NSAIDs, selective COX-2 inhibitory blockers, and/or acetaminophen unless contraindicated,[51] because all of these medications reduce inflammatory mediators (which increase after tissue injury), thereby decreasing the transduction aspect of the pain pathway. Regional anesthesia, however, blocks the transmission process in the pain pathway. PNBs and epidurals use local anesthetics to decrease or halt transmission at large peripheral nerves and the dorsal root, respectively. Epidural local anesthetics also diffuse into the intrathecal space and spinal cord to a lesser degree and thus have an effect at the dorsal horn. Intuitively, if pain cannot be transmitted, it will not be perceived or modulated. Adjunctive medications, such as anticonvulsants, antidepressants, and α₂-agonists affect primarily spinal and supraspinal sites. Finally, intrathecal opioids, ketamine, and α-agonists modulate the pain pathway at the dorsal horn.[52]

The basis for multimodal therapy is achieving optimal acute and subacute pain management to optimize the polytrauma patient's overall recovery and rehabilitation. Excellent postoperative analgesia aids postoperative healing by increasing oxygenation and mobility and also reduces anxiety, stress, and depression. Multimodal therapy reduces the potential for opioid-related physical dependence, addiction, and the recently recognized phenomenon of opioid-induced hyperalgesia (OIH)[53,54] resulting from opioid-centered analgesia. Of course, postoperative respiratory depression is a continual threat with opioid-centered postoperative pain plans such as intermittent dosing and patient-controlled analgesia (PCA).[55] The practice guidelines[51] state that acute perioperative pain management helps maintain the patient's functional abilities and psychological well-being, enhances the quality of life, and prevents the results of undertreatment of perioperative pain. The adverse outcomes of undertreatment include thromboembolic and pulmonary complications, increased intensive care or hospital time, needless suffering, and possibly the development of chronic pain. The guidelines continue by stating that interdisciplinary perioperative analgesia programs with dedicated acute pain service and 24-hour anesthesiologist availability enhance patient comfort and prevent analgesic gaps. Multimodal techniques are specifically recommended.[51]

Treatment Modalities

Regional Anesthesia and Analgesia

Although perioperative regional anesthesia and analgesia (PRAA) has strong support,[51,56,57] the literature on its success in reducing chronic postamputation pain has been inconclusive.[58] However, the weight of evidence suggests a long-term benefit. Studies have demonstrated an association between acute and chronic pain as well as between preamputation pain and chronic pain[4,59]; therefore, postamputation phantom pain may be reduced by inducing local anaesthesia in the limb prior to a planned surgical amputation.[60]

Benefits. Significant benefits to the use of PRAA, including epidural analgesia or PNBs, in the polytrauma patient have been established. Intraoperatively, PRAA provides a stable hemodynamic profile, minimal pulmonary concerns, avoidance of side effects from general anesthesia if used as a sole technique, improved operating room efficiency, and decreased blood loss. Postoperatively, recovery in the postanesthesia care unit improves, postoperative analgesia improves, overall hospital costs diminish, overall outcome improves, and both patient and surgeon satisfaction scores are high.

Intraoperative Hemodynamic Stability. Following the Vietnam War, San Diego Naval Medical Center (California) treated a large number of patients, but the patient demand exceeded the supply of operating room time. Therefore, a system was designed whereby patients underwent surgical procedures in the orthopaedic clinic after a regional anesthetic was placed by the anesthesia department. Over 15,000 patients were safely given regional anesthesia over a 30-year period. In 1997 Waters et al[61] reported findings in a 1-year prospective study of 677 patients. Upper and lower extremity blocks were placed without sedation, after which patients were transported to the clinic for their procedures accompanied only by a corpsman, with

minimal monitors. The incidence of complications was low (0.3%) with no postoperative sequelae, attesting to the overall hemodynamic and respiratory safety of peripheral blocks.

In centroneuroaxis blockade, PRAA generally has fewer hemodynamic perturbations than single-shot spinal anesthesia. Auroy and colleagues[62] reported provocative findings in a 1997 French prospective study of over 103,000 regional anesthetics, including over 40,000 spinal blocks, over 30,000 epidural blocks, over 20,000 PNBs, and over 11,000 intravenous (IV) regional anesthetics. The study surveyed 736 anesthesiologists, half in private practice and half in academic settings, with an average of 12 years of experience. The risk of cardiac arrest was 1 per 1,500 for spinal anesthesia, 1 per 10,000 for epidural anesthesia, and 1 per 7,000 for PNB, suggesting a higher cardiac arrest rate for spinal anesthesia compared to other regional anesthetics. Although the authors acknowledged the possibility of selection bias because sicker patients received spinal anesthesia, other studies also report a relatively high rate of cardiac arrest during spinal anesthesia, ranging from 1 per 500 to 1 per 4,000.[63-66] Caplan et al[67] reviewed 14 cases of cardiac arrest in a closed claims analysis, all of which involved healthy patients for minor surgery who suffered cardiac arrest after decreasing blood pressure and pulse. All but one patient had a poor outcome. de Visme and colleagues[68] reported in 2000 "more prolonged hemodynamic effect" in isobaric spinal anesthesia compared to PNBs for hip fractures in 29 elderly patients. Finally, spinal anesthesia often results in significant hypotension and severe bradycardia (33% and 13% incidence, respectively).[69]

Likewise, PNBs may have a greater safety profile than centroneuroaxis blockade. In a 1996 French prospective study by Giaufre et al,[70] over 24,000 regional anesthetics were studied in a pediatric population. The group included 89% receiving a combined anesthetic and general anesthesia, 61% with a centroneuroaxis block, 17% with a PNB, and 22% with local infiltration. Only the centroneuroaxis group reported complications, including dural puncture, cardiac arrhythmias, IV injections, and paresthesias.

Avoiding General Anesthesia Side Effects. If used as a sole anesthetic, regional anesthesia minimizes the risk of central nervous system complications such as postoperative delirium and excessive drowsiness. The likelihood of airway complications including sore throat, traumatized airway, aspiration, and potential for loss of airway in a difficult airway are minimized. Both elevated rate-pressure products during laryngoscopy and intubation as well as potentially low perfusion states during patient positioning and preparation are avoided. Finally, PRAA minimizes the risk of postoperative nausea and vomiting.[71]

Improving Operating Room Efficiency. Surgeons are often concerned about the additional time required for the placement of regional anesthesia; however, use of central and peripheral blocks can actually decrease "anesthesia-controlled time" if managed by a separate "block team" prior to surgery. In 2000 Williams and colleagues[72] studied 369 patients for anterior cruciate ligament repair in a retrospective review using the same surgeon for all the operations. Total time, including intraoperative anesthesia-controlled time plus turnover time, was 31 minutes for PNBs, 36 minutes for PNB combined with general anesthesia, and 41 minutes for general anesthesia.[72] Additionally, regional anesthesia can significantly reduce or eliminate phase I recovery and expedite phase II recovery.[73,74]

Decreasing Blood Loss. Central neuroaxis blockade can decrease perioperative blood loss by 37% to 46%, as demonstrated in many studies,[75,76] but PNBs may also accomplish this benefit. Lumbar plexus blocks have been demonstrated to decrease total blood loss by 49% in total hip arthroplasty.[77,78] Mechanisms by which regional anesthesia decreases blood loss include shunting of blood from the operative site, decreased venous pressure by blockade of sympathetic tone, and the lack of positive-pressure ventilation.

Improving Early Recovery Period. Regional anesthesia potentially improves the recovery period. Ford and colleagues[71] reported a retrospective review of 801 patients comparing general anesthesia to PNBs and a combined general and regional anesthetic. Regional anesthesia patients had less nausea and vomiting (6% vs 20%), less supplemental oxygen requirement (12% vs 81%), and quicker discharge times (51 min vs 104 min). Along with less nausea and vomiting, regional anesthesia patients have less postoperative ileus due to decreased opioid use and decreased sympathetic tone with epidural analgesia.

Decreasing Deep Vein Thrombosis. Regional anesthesia, especially when extended into the postoperative period, has been shown to decrease the rate of deep vein thrombosis in many studies[79–81]; this finding is particularly evident when no further pharmacologic prophylaxis is prescribed. Modig et al[79] examined 60 patients undergoing total hip arthroplasty who received either epidural analgesia or systemic narcotics. Only 13% experienced a deep vein thrombosis, and 10% had a pulmonary embolism in the epidural group compared to 67% and 30%, respectively, in the systemic narcotic group.[79] In 1991 Tuman and colleagues[82] showed a decrease in the alpha angle and maximum amplitude value on postoperative thromboelastogram in 80 major vascular patients, as well as fewer arterial occlusions in the epidural group compared to the systemic narcotic group. Finally, in 1993 Christopherson et al[83] examined the effect of epidural analgesia with lower extremity vascular surgery and found a decreased need for revascularization in the epidural group.

Decreasing Hospital Costs. In addition, regional anesthesia can save hospitals significant costs. In 2004 Williams and colleagues[84] reviewed 948 anterior cruciate ligament repairs, comparing the overall hospital costs between patients with and without PNBs. Of those who received blocks, 82% were able to bypass phase I recovery and only 4% required unplanned admissions, compared with an admission rate of 17% for those who did not receive blocks. Based on an average of 3,000 outpatient orthopaedic cases annually, hospital savings could reach $1.8 million annually through the use of regional anesthesia. Other studies also support fewer costs associated with regional anesthesia.[85–87]

Improved Postoperative Analgesia. Many studies report improved postoperative analgesia utilizing regional analgesia with fewer side effects.[76,87–89] Regional analgesia minimizes the risk of central nervous system side effects such as delirium and drowsiness compared to systemic opioids. Grass[76] reported less sedation with sufentanil patient-controlled epidural analgesia compared to IV morphine PCA and intramuscular (IM) opioids, while Guinard et al[87] demonstrated greater sedation with IV fentanyl compared to epidural fentanyl. Salomaki and colleagues[90] showed decreased nausea and vomiting with epidural fentanyl (20%) compared to IV fentanyl (65%). Regional analgesia patients have less nausea and vomiting, less supplemental oxygen requirement, and less postoperative ileus resulting from fewer opioids and the resultant sympathectomy with epidural analgesia.[71] Horlocker et al[91] eliminated the need for any opioids through the use of multimodal analgesia with a continuous lumbar plexus catheter in addition to acetaminophen and ketoroloc for a total knee replacement, and Mulroy et al[92] demonstrated extended relief with up to 24 hours of analgesia using single shot femoral nerve blocks following anterior cruciate ligament reconstruction. PNBs may also decrease pruritis, urinary retention, hypotension, difficulty with ambulation, and respiratory depression.[76] Because of improved analgesia with fewer side effects and fewer opioids used, nursing requirements are significantly diminished.

Improving Patient Outcome. Several studies have shown improved patient outcome with PRAA,[93,94] including decreased intensive care unit stay,[82,86] decreased hospital stay,[86,89] decreased cardiac morbidity,[82,86,95,96] decreased pulmonary dysfunction,[82,87–89,90] earlier return of bowel function,[89,93] decreased neuroendocrine stress,[86,97] fewer infections,[86] decreased mortality,[86,98] and improved rehabilitation. Yeager et al[86] examined 53 patients after abdominal, thoracic, and vascular surgery in 1987, and Tuman et al[82] examined 80 major vascular patients in 1991. Both studies reported decreased intensive care unit stays with epidural analgesia versus systemic narcotics. In addition, Yeager's epidural group had a 14% incidence of cardiac morbidity (myocardial infarction, congestive heart failure, angina, or arrhythmia) compared to 52% in the systemic narcotic group; Tuman also demonstrated a significant difference (10% vs 27%) in cardiac events. Blomberg and others[95,96] in a series of studies demonstrated a favorable myocardial oxygen supply versus demand balance with a decrease in heart rate, contractility, preload, and afterload, yet an increased coronary blood flow to the endocardium during thoracic epidural blockade. Furthermore, coronary perfusion pressure was maintained, and stenotic but not nonstenotic coronary vessels became dilated.[96,99–104] Studies[88,89] demonstrated fewer pulmonary complications including atelectasis, infiltrates, and cough in an epidural group compared to a systemic narcotic group, and Boylan and colleagues[88] demonstrated earlier tracheal extubation in the epidural group.

Liu et al[105] examined various analgesic techniques on recovery of bowel function and found a local anesthetic plus opioid combination to provide the optimal result, especially compared to systemic opioids. Epidural opioids have been shown to decrease the stress response, specifically free cortisol levels, compared to systemic opioids.[97] Yeager[86] showed a 7% incidence of major infections (pneumonia, sepsis) in the epidural analgesia group, compared to 40% in the systemic narcotic group. In addition, Yeager's epidural group had no deaths while the systemic narcotic group had a 16% mortality rate.[86] Wu and colleagues[98] reported an analysis of the Medicare claims database in 2004 over a 4-year period and showed significantly lower odds of death at 7 and 30 days postoperatively for those patients who had postoperative epidural analgesia. Finally, PRAA has been shown to decrease pain scores, increase range of motion, decrease hospital stay, and decrease rehabilitation time compared to IV PCA, although CPNBs had fewer side effects compared to epidural analgesia.[106,107]

Improving Patient Satisfaction. In 2001 Wu and colleagues[108] reviewed 18 trials that examined patient satisfaction with PRAA and reported that over 70% of these studies demonstrated greater patient satisfaction with regional anesthesia and analgesia compared to general anesthesia with IV PCA. Specifically, Vloka et al[109] demonstrated greater patient satisfaction with PNBs compared to spinal anesthesia for varicose vein surgery, and Borgeat et al[110] demonstrated greater patient satisfaction with postoperative interscalene analgesia compared to IV PCA for shoulder anesthesia. Although patient satisfaction is a complex issue, critical determinants are judicious sedation during the

regional procedure as well as optimal postoperative analgesia.[108,111–113]

Risks of Perioperative Regional Anesthesia and Analgesia. Although PRAA has many significant benefits, its use also introduces potential risks, which must be considered for each individual patient. This section will focus first on the "big three" risks, as termed by Finucane,[114,115] namely, local anesthetic toxicity, pneumothorax, and nerve injury. Additionally, the provider should consider other miscellaneous risks before employing PRAA.

Local Anesthesia Toxicity. Local anesthetic toxicity resulting in seizures, cardiac arrest, or both can be a devastating complication that all anesthesia providers must consider. With PNBs, the incidence of seizures is roughly 1 per 1,000, whereas the incidence with epidural anesthesia is roughly 1 per 8,000.[62,116] Brown et al[116] completed a retrospective review of over 25,000 patients with caudal, epidural, and brachial plexus blocks and found the highest rate of local anesthetic toxicity with caudal anesthesia, followed by PNBs, followed by epidural anesthesia. Most cases of seizures occurred after bolusing local anesthesia through needles or catheters, as opposed to perioperative infusions, and did not necessarily result in cardiac arrest even with bupivacaine in this series of patients. The incidence of cardiac arrest, resulting from several different mechanisms, appeared to be similar between epidural anesthesia and PNBs, approximately 1 per 10,000 and 1 per 7,000, respectively.[116] Both epidurals and PNBs may elicit the vasovagal reaction, which is usually self-limiting, as well as cardiac arrest due to local anesthetic toxicity.[117] In addition, accidental intrathecal (spinal) injection and the Bezold-Jarisch reflex may cause cardiac arrest during epidural anesthesia.

Because local anesthetic toxicity can be life-threatening, efforts to decrease this event have largely focused on prevention, including using the lowest effective dose, frequent aspiration with intermittent boluses, the use of a vascular marker such as epinephrine, and avoiding agents with a low therapeutic index (eg, bupivacaine) in highly vascular areas. However, determining meaningful maximum dosages for local anesthetics has been elusive, since the maximum dose depends primarily on where the local anesthetic is given; a standard maximum dose of a particular local anesthetic is not helpful unless location is specified. For example, a greater dose is allowed moving within a continuum from IV, to intercostals, to caudal, to epidural, to PNBs, and finally to subcutaneous administration.[118–120] On the one hand, although 5 to 7 mg/kg of lidocaine is frequently quoted as a maximum dose, twice that dose could be used for PNBs and subcutaneous administration.[114,121–130] On the other hand, even 5 mg/kg lidocaine intravenously could have disastrous consequences. Therefore, rather than relying on set maximum dosages, the provider must be sure not to inject within a vessel, to use the lowest effective local anesthetic dose possible, and to have Intralipid (KabiVitrum Inc, Alameda, Calif) readily available.

Unfortunately, detection of an intravascular injection can be difficult; merely aspirating for heme prior to injection does not preclude the possibility of an intravascular injection. Therefore, a test dose is critical, which most commonly is epinephrine 15 μg (6 mL of 1:400,000 solution). If the heart rate increases more than 10 points, the practitioner should withdraw the needle and either abandon the procedure or reattempt it if the patient is stable. Additionally, extreme vigilance is required during the bolus injection, especially when using an immobile needle with fractionated 5-mL doses; mobile or multiple injection techniques may decrease the rate of local anesthestic toxicity by spreading local anesthesia in multiple locations.

Choice of the local anesthetic is a critical aspect of decreasing patient risk, because local anesthetics can have varying effects on different organ systems. Lidocaine, for example, can cause seizures and eventually cardiac shock at high concentrations.[131] In addition, according to numerous studies, lidocaine is less cardiotoxic than ropivacaine, which is less cardiotoxic than bupivacaine.[132-136] Providers must be aware of the potential for cardiac complications with the use of local anesthetics, and early treatment of cardiac complications is essential (decreasing mortality from 83% to 33% for bupivacaine and 17% to 0% for ropivacaine in one study).[137,138] The cardiotoxicity of these anesthetics results from both depressed left ventricular function as well as arrhythmogenicity. Animal studies have shown significantly less cardiovascular depression and arrhythmias, greater rate of successful resuscitations, and less mortality after cardiac arrest with ropivacaine compared to bupivacaine. For constant infusions, maximum epidural bupivacaine rates should not exceed 0.5 mg/kg/hr (0.25 mg/kg/hr in infants),[139-143] and this rate should be decreased in the elderly, pregnant women, and those with uremia or liver failure.

Finally, treatment of local anesthesia toxicity should focus on airway management, possible administration of induction agents and/or benzodiazepines to control seizure activity, and control of arrhythmias with amiodarone, vasopressin, epinephrine, Intralipid therapy, and/or defibrillation. Perhaps the most remarkable recent discovery about local anesthesia toxicity is the ability for Intralipid to act as an antidote: the free plasma local anesthetic binds to Intralipid, thereby dramatically decreasing circulating local anesthesia levels.[144-147] In 2003 Weinberg et al[145] reported a study in which 12 dogs were given lethal doses of IV bupivacaine, and the group treated with Intralipid all survived while the control group all died. The currently recommended dosing is 1 mL/kg over 1 minute, followed by 3 mL/kg over 10 minutes, followed by an infusion of 0.25 mL/kg/min after establishment of normal sinus rhythm until hemodynamics have been stabilized. Maintaining an immediately available supply of Intralipid, which is inexpensive and stable at room temperature for long periods, while blocks are performed has become the standard of care.

Pneumothorax. Pneumothorax, the second of the "big three" risks of PRAA, is primarily a risk with supraclavicular brachial plexus block and thoracic paravertebral block, but has been seen with other blocks as well.[148] The risk of pneumothorax during supraclavicular blockade has been reported as high as 5%,[107] but other studies indicate this risk is much less in experienced hands; Franco and Vieira[149] reported no pneumothorax in 1,001 supraclavicular blocks. Incidence of pneumothorax with thoracic paravertebral block is roughly 1 per 300, but it is highly dependent on patient factors such as the presence of scoliosis, as well as provider experience.[150] During block placement, cough, chest pain, or aspiration of air are signs of possible pleural puncture. To reduce the risk of pneumothorax after block placement, nitrous oxide and positive pressure ventilation should be avoided, and a chest film should be considered, particularly if the patient is symptomatic. Outpatients undergoing supraclavicular or thoracic paravertebral blocks should be instructed to report immediately to the emergency room for dyspnea or chest pain. Treatment includes a chest tube if pneumothorax is greater than 25% or symptomatology is severe. Again, prevention is critical and requires adequate training, education, and experience as well as the use of ultrasound imaging techniques.

Nerve Injury. Nerve injury is the third major risk associated with PRAA. Due to an inconsistent definition (various etiologies, sensory versus motor deficits, duration of persistent block, severity, etc), the incidence of nerve injury varies widely among studies, ranging from 0.2% to 2%.[151] Auroy et al[62] reported an incidence of 1 in 5,000 for both epidural and PNBs, compared to 1 in 1,670 for spinal anesthesia. Although the number of patients with persistent neural deficits was small, all patients in the epidural and PNB groups had either paresthesias during block placement or pain on injection.[62] Nerve injury may be more common after general anesthesia than regional anesthesia: the American Society of Anesthesiologists closed-claims analysis found that 61% of the total number of nerve injuries occurred during general anesthesia, and 39% during regional anesthesia, although 90% of lower extremity claims involved regional anesthesia, especially spinal anesthesia.[152] The incidence of nerve injury appears to decrease with time, as Borgeat et al[148] demonstrated in a prospective study examining interscalene blockade and shoulder surgery, finding that 14% of the patients had persistent sensory deficits on the 10th postoperative day, but the number had decreased to 4% at 3 months and 0.2% at 9 months. Bergman and colleagues[153] showed that using continuous techniques in over 400 axillary catheter placements did not increase the risk of neural injury compared to using single injections. Still, many surgeons perceive that PNBs are associated with a relatively high rate of neural deficits; 21% of hand surgeons reported having seen a "major nerve injury" following axillary blockade.[154]

Sources of nerve injury include trauma, toxicity, ischemia, or more frequently a combination of thesemechanisms.[114] Neural trauma could result from the needle, intraneural injection, compression, or stretch. Whether the choice of technique (paresthesia or nerve stimulation) or the use of short bevel needles affects neural trauma is controversial.[155,156] Toxicity from local anesthetic correlates with potency (2-chloroprocaine < lidocaine < etidocaine), although 4% lidocaine or greater causes the greatest injury. High concentrations of local anesthetics can be neurotoxic, but concentrations used at clinical concentrations are considered safe. Clearly, any substance injected within the epineurium can result in neural injury as a result of all three mechanisms. Intraneural or extraneural compression, edema, and vasoconstriction could result in neural ischemia. Partridge[157] examined the use of epinephrine and found that lidocaine with 1:200,000 epinephrine decreased neural blood flow, but so did plain lidocaine, also probably as a result of the coupling of neural activity with oxygen requirements and blood flow. No evidence exists that 1:400,000 epinephrine significantly decreases neural blood flow, and this concentration appears to be an acceptable balance between maintaining a reliable intravascular marker and avoiding neural ischemia.[157]

Prevention of neural injury involves adequate informed consent and effective communication with the patient preoperatively, minimizing sedation to obtain feedback during a 1-mL test dose to help rule out pain on injection that could be associated with intraneural injection, avoiding high concentrations of local anesthesia, avoiding 1:200,000 epinephrine, and possibly implementing the use of ultrasound, which allows visualization of neural tissue, the needle, and local anesthesia spread. Treatment of a possible neural injury begins with a comprehensive yet focused history and physical examination of the complaint with consideration of a wide range of possible etiologies, including preexisting nerve injury, prolonged use or high pressure of the tourniquet, surgical trauma, local edema and swelling, patient position, tight splints or casts, and regional anesthesia. Workup may include imaging studies to evaluate for hematoma, which could be evacuated with return of function, and possibly electromyogram/nerve conduction velocity studies to record baseline function, because changes in these studies lag weeks behind neural injury.[158] Treatment should focus on reversible causes (hematoma, casts), multimodal therapy to treat possible neuropathic pain, and reassurance that most neural injuries improve with time.

Other Risks. Other risks associated with PRAA include epinephrine toxicity, phrenic blockade, bronchospasm, failure of the technique, inadvertent epidural or spinal spread, hematoma, and infection. Epinephrine toxicity may occur with a small, inadvertent IV dose in a susceptible patient or from slow systemic uptake if epinephrine is mixed in the local anesthesia solution, especially if total epinephrine dose exceeds 250 μg, including the surgeon's possible use of epinephrine-containing solutions. Phrenic blockade occurs with virtually all interscalene blocks and deep cervical plexus blocks, although it is well tolerated in patients who don't have significant pulmonary disease. Roughly 40% of supraclavicular blocks result in phrenic blockade. Bronchospasm has also been reported after interscalene block[159] but is not typically seen after other regional anesthetics. Failure of the technique comprises 5% to 15% of regional anesthetics that required a backup plan for all patients; higher failure rates occur with poor patient selection, insufficient time allowed for local anesthesia onset, surgery outside the area of blockade, surgery outlasting the duration of the regional block, and minimal experience or training in regional techniques.

Inadvertent epidural spread occurs frequently with paravertebral blockade,[160] occasionally with lumbar plexus blockade (up to 10% of the time), and rarely with interscalene and deep cervical plexus block. Inadvertent spinal anesthesia possibly resulting in total spinal anesthesia can occur during lumbar plexus block, paravertebral block, interscalene block, and epidural anesthesia via inadvertent dural puncture. Hematoma formation is a well-known complication of epidural/spinal anesthesia, with an incidence between 1 per 5,000 and 1 per 150,000, depending the presence of anticoagulation and needle size.[161,162] The American Society of Regional Anesthesia has specific guidelines on its Web site (www.asra.com) that pertain to central neuroaxis blockade in the presence of anticoagulants. Particularly concerning is the recent relatively high rate of epidural hematoma formation especially with high-risk dosing of low-molecular-weight heparin. Hematoma has also been associated with PNBs, namely lumbar plexus block with Lovenox[163] (Sanofi Aventis, Bridgewater, NJ) as well as axillary catheters.[153]

Finally, infection can result particularly from catheter techniques, varying from 1 case in 10,000 with epidural catheters to up to 1% of cases with CPNB catheters.[153] As many as 30% of catheters become colonized with skin flora, and a small percentage of patients develop either superficial or deep infections. Risk factors associated with catheter infections include diabetes, traumatic placement, longer duration of catheter, frequent unnecessary dressing changes, and lack of systemic antibiotics. Additionally, type and concentration of local anesthesia may affect the risk of infection. In a series of deep CPNB catheter infections treated at Brooke Army Medical Center, patients noted primarily pain deep to the catheter site in the absence of erythema, induration, or drainage.[164]

Evidence-Based Medicine for Regional Analgesia in the Prevention of Phantom Limb Pain. This section reviews both positive and negative epidural and PNB studies that focus on the potential benefits of preemptively administering regional anesthesia to decrease the incidence of PLP. PRAA plays a pivotal role as part of a multimodal plan. Therapies for chronic PLP should address the above hypothesized mechanisms of pain. Regional analgesia addresses two of the putative sites of PLP: the peripheral nerves and the dorsal horn of the spinal cord. Additionally, preemptive analgesia may affect all four components of the nociceptive pathway. As Birbaumer et al[165] revealed, regional anesthesia may prevent cortical reorganization, which may decrease pain perception. Ong and colleagues[58] reported that intraoperative spinal anesthesia alone benefited the amputee with less postoperative pain during the first week, compared to those who did not receive neuraxial anesthesia. Presumably, a mechanism related to spinal modulation and preemptive analgesia accounts for the analgesia lasting long after the sensory blockade has subsided. Preemptive analgesia is also supported by better postoperative analgesia in patients who received regional anesthesia interventions prior to surgical stimulus.[25,34] Regional analgesia with continuous epidural infusion or CPNBs is beneficial because of the ability to provide preoperative, intraoperative, and postoperative analgesia during much of the inflammatory period.[107] First, studies demonstrating a reduction of PLP with PRAA will be discussed, followed by studies that fail to demonstrate a specific benefit.

Epidural studies demonstrating benefit:

1. In 1988 Bach et al[166] published an often referenced article, "Phantom Limb Pain in Amputees During the First 12 Months Following Limb Amputation, After Preoperative Lumbar Epidural Blockade," a prospective, randomized, controlled trial of 25 geriatric vascular patients. The epidural group of 11 patients received analgesia for 3 days preoperatively to alleviate preoperative limb pain, and the control group of 14 patients received perioperative opioids. Both groups had either epidural or spinal anesthesia for their amputation surgery and postoperative meperidine and acetaminophen for analgesia. At 6 and 12 months postamputation, none of the epidural patients reported PLP, while the control group reported incidences of 38% and 27%, respectively. However, the study was small and six patients died before follow-up was complete (see Table 11-1). The relatively low incidence of PLP even in the control group could possibly be attributed to the intraoperative use of preemptive regional anesthesia.[166]

2. Jahangiri and colleagues[167] reported in 1994 that perioperative epidural infusion of diamorphine, clonidine, and bupivicaine 0.125% is safe and effective in reducing the incidence of phantom pain after amputation. Thirteen epidural study patients were compared to 11 control patients who received on-demand opioids. The epidural solution was infused at 1 to 4 mL/hr for 1 to 2 days preoperatively and at least 3 days postoperatively, and both groups received general anesthesia intraoperatively. The study group reported significantly less PLP at 7 days, 6 months, and 1 year, with 8% incidence in the epidural group compared to 73% in the control group at 1 year.[167]

3. In 1996 Katsuly-Liapis[168] reported that preemptive epidural analgesia reduces the incidence of phantom pain in lower limb amputees. This prospective study divided 45 patients for lower-limb amputation into three

TABLE 11-1

INCIDENCE OF PHANTOM LIMB PAIN IN BACH'S STUDY

Study Group	Time Since Operation		
	7 day	6 mo	12 mo
Epidural	27%	0%	0%
Control	64%	38%	27%

Data source: Bach S, Noreng MF, Tjellden NU. Phantom limb pain in amputees during the first 12 months following limb amputation, after preoperative lumbar epidural blockade. *Pain*. 1988;33:297–301.

groups. Group A received 3 days of preoperative and 3 days of postoperative epidural analgesia with 0.25% bupivacaine and morphine. Group B received opioids and NSAIDs for preoperative pain followed by epidural analgesia for postoperative pain. Group C received no epidural analgesia. At 6 months and 1 year, the patients in group A reported no phantom pain, while a significant portion of groups B and C did experience phantom pain. The authors concluded that preemptive epidural analgesia reduced the incidence of phantom pain in lower limb amputees during the first year following amputation.[168]

Epidural studies demonstrating no benefit:

1. Nikolajsen et al published a relatively large study in 1997 titled "Randomised Trial of Epidural Bupivicaine and Morphine in Prevention of Stump and Phantom Pain in Lower-Limb Amputation."[169] The 29 patients in the epidural group received bupivacaine 0.25% at 4 to 7 mL/hr with epidural morphine at 0.16 to 28 mg/hr preoperatively, bupivacaine 0.5% intraoperatively (with general anesthesia), and 0.25% bupivacaine at 4 to 7 mL/hr with epidural morphine in 2- to 8-mg boluses as needed postoperatively for an average of 6.9 days. The control group's 31 patients received epidural saline intraoperatively and postoperatively. All patients received postoperative parental opioids as needed as well. Although Nikolajsen found no reduction in PLP at 1 week, 3 months, 6 months, or 12 months postamputation (Table 11-2), the results are questionable because half the patients were lost to follow-up due to death,

TABLE 11-2

INCIDENCE OF PHANTOM LIMB PAIN IN NIKOLAJSEN'S STUDY

Study Group	Time Since Operation			
	1 wk	3 mo	6 mo	12 mo
Epidural	52%	82%	81%	75%
Control	56%	50%	55%	69%

Data source: Nikolajsen L, Ilkjaer S, Christensen JK, Kroner K, Jensen TS. Randomised trial of epidural bupivacaine and morphine in prevention of stump and phantom pain in lower-limb amputation. *Lancet*. 1997;350:1353-1357.

reamputation, or inability to contact them. In addition, the infusion rate was somewhat low for lumbar epidural, which may have resulted in inadequate spread.[169]

2. In 2001 Lambert[170] reported on a study designed to compare the effect of two different regional techniques, perioperative epidural analgesia and postoperative sciatic catheter analgesia, on PLP. The 14 patients in the epidural analgesia group received bupivacaine 0.166% with morphine at 0.2 to 0.8 mg/h for 24 hours preoperatively, intraoperatively, and continued for 3 days postoperatively. In the sciatic analgesia group, 16 patients had a perineural sciatic catheter placed intraoperatively, which was infused postoperatively with bupivacaine 0.25% at 10 mL/hr for 3 days. Epidural analgesia was shown to provide greater relief of residual limb pain during the first 3 days, yet there was no significant difference in the incidence and severity of PLP at 6 and 12 months. Like Nikolajsen's study, this unblinded study lost 40% of patients to follow-up due to death, and had low epidural infusion rates. Additionally, it was hampered by the lack of a control group (without regional analgesia).[170]

Continuous peripheral nerve block studies demonstrating benefits:

1. In 1991 Fisher and Meller[171] reported on a small, prospective study of 11 vascular patients in whom sciatic catheters were placed intraoperatively and infused postoperatively with bupivacaine 0.125% at 10 mL/h for 72 hours, concluding that perineural catheters may have a role in diminishing PLP. These patients demonstrated a 50% decrease in morphine administration within the first 3 days and, more importantly, no PLP at 12 months after above-knee or below-knee amputation; however, the study used retrospective controls and studied a limited number of patients.[171]

2. In 1997 Birbaumer et al published a study titled "Effects of Regional Anesthesia on Phantom Limb Pain Are Mirrored in Changes in Cortical Reorganization"[165] that supports a benefit of PRAA in treating established PLP and possibly in preventing PLP in amputees. As noted above, studies have revealed that substantial reorganization of the primary somatosensory cortex occurs subsequent to amputation and that such cortical reorgani-

zation is positively correlated with PLP. The Birbaumer study hypothesized that pain reduction induced by regional anesthesia leads to less cortical reorganization and thus less phantom pain. Six males with trauma-induced unilateral arm amputations with established PLP were investigated and controlled against four arm amputees without PLP. After the patients were given brachial plexus anesthesia to influence their PLP, researchers performed neuroelectric source imaging while stimulating the fingers and the mouth of each subject, as cortical reorganization was assessed as a dependent variable. The blockade abolished all aspects of cortical reorganization seen by neuroelectric source imaging and simultaneously eliminated the current experience of PLP. Birbaumer concluded that cortical reorganization likely contributes to PLP but probably does not maintain PLP by itself.[165]

3. In 1998 Lierz and colleagues[172] published a case report that demonstrated successful elimination of PLP with regional analgesia after unsuccessful extensive pharmacologic therapy. A 39-year-old male with 39% total-body surface area burns requiring bilateral upper extremity amputations developed severe phantom pain by postoperation day 18, which was treated with NSAIDs, calcitonin, amitriptyline, and carbamazepine, as well as TENS therapy. Due to unrelenting PLP, the patient had bilateral brachial plexus catheters placed on postoperation day 39 (left interscalene and right axillary perineural catheters), which were infused with ropivicaine 0.2% at 4 to 6 mL/hr for 6 days. The regional analgesia resulted in complete pain relief through the 7 months of follow-up.[172]

Continuous peripheral nerve block studies demonstrating no benefit:

1. Elizaga et al[173] reported a retrospective, unblinded study of 19 lower extremity amputees in which study patients received a sciatic catheter placed intraoperatively and maintained postoperatively for an average of 4 days. Patients in the treatment group received 10 mL of bupivacaine 0.5% bolused intraoperatively, then 2 to 6 mL/hr of bupivacaine 0.5% infused intraoperatively and postoperatively; patients in both the treatment and control group received an IV PCA. No differences were found in opioid use or

PLP between the two groups, although 70% of patients were lost to follow-up and the intraoperative anesthetic technique was not controlled.[173]

2. Pinzur and colleagues[174] published a prospective, randomized study for the prevention of PLP in 1996. Twenty-one vascular patients scheduled for lower extremity amputations for peripheral vascular disease were given spinal anesthesia intraoperatively as well as perineural sciatic nerve catheters, which were infused with either bupivacaine 0.5% at 1 mL/hr or saline for 72 hours. Residual limb and PLP were assessed for the first 72 hours as well as at 3 and 6 months. While patients who received bupivacaine via the sciatic catheters reported lower pain scores and decreased opioid use for the first 48 hours, there was no difference in the incidence of PLP. Weaknesses of the study included lack of any attempt at preemptive analgesia, and very low infusion rate, resulting in probable inadequate blockade.[174]

Considering the quality of the studies that examined the benefit of epidural and CPNB analgesia in reducing chronic postamputation pain, a greater weight of evidence favors PRAA having some degree of prevention of the development and successful treatment of established PLP. Therefore, regional analgesia may be central to a successful multimodal approach to preventing and treating chronic postamputation pain.

Techniques of Regional Analgesia. This section reviews the placement of epidural and continuous peripheral nerve catheters, localization of nerves, and administration of solutions used during continuous infusions. Because many seriously injured patients present with multiple injuries, ongoing, adequate analgesia naturally remains a paramount patient concern as well as a significant provider challenge. Examining the timing and duration of regional analgesia, Kissin[175] reviewed the need for continuous regional anesthesia techniques when attempting to provide preemptive analgesia by preventing central hypersensitivity. Ideally, regional anesthesia techniques should cover the entire "initiation phase"—the initial inflammatory response, which lasts days or sometimes weeks in the case of polytrauma—which may require sequential catheters to provide optimal long-lasting analgesia.[25,34,175,176] In the current military conflict, these continuous regional analgesia techniques have been successfully placed in the combat theater or at the earliest opportunity in Europe with pumps that accompany the service member back to the United States.

Epidural Catheters. Epidural analgesia has been the mainstay of perioperative regional analgesia for several decades. Using a dilute solution of local anesthesia often combined with an opioid, the anesthesia provider can effectively block transmission of afferent nociception and achieve profound analgesia. Epidural catheters should be placed at the "epicenter" of the incision to optimize segmental analgesia, thereby targeting only those nerve roots requiring blockade. For example, a standard thoracotomy incision at T6 should have a T6 epidural catheter, whereas a standard exploratory laparotomy should have a low thoracic epidural placed for optimal analgesia. Standard technique incorporates a sterile preparation and drape, skin localization, advancement of an epidural needle either with a midline or paramedian approach, confirmation of epidural needle placement by a "loss of resistance" technique, and threading a 20-gauge multiorifice catheter 3 to 5 cm within the epidural space. Typical local anesthetic and opioid concentrations, boluses, and rates are listed in Table 11-3. In addition to the above risks and benefits, epidural analgesia can result in hypotension in up to 30% of cases, particularly with larger boluses of high-concentration local anesthesia in hypovolemic patients. However, establishment of blockade after volume resuscitation in a stable patient with dilute solutions can provide excellent analgesia while maintaining stable hemodynamics.

Peripheral Nerve Blocks. PNBs, which may reduce the risk of hypotension, respiratory depression, urinary retention, and difficulty with ambulation, offer an attractive alternative to epidural analgesia. PNBs include upper and lower extremity blocks, head and neck blocks, and paravertebral blocks. Upper extremity blocks include interscalene, supraclavicular, infraclavicular, and axillary approaches to the brachial plexus; lower extremity approaches include lumbar plexus, sciatic, femoral, popliteal, and ankle blocks. The approach to the brachial plexus (Figure 11-2) is based primarily on the location of the injury or surgery: the interscalene approach is used for shoulder analgesia and the axillary approach for forearm and hand surgery. Similarly, proximal lower extremity blocks can provide analgesia to a neural plexus; for example, the lumbar plexus block results in femoral, obturator, and lateral femoral cutaneous nerve blockade with a single injection. Paravertebral blockade can be performed in the thoracic or lumbar region, resulting in excellent unilateral blockade of nerve roots with minimal risk for hypotension, bradycardia, or respiratory depression.

TABLE 11-3

ROUTINE VOLUMES AND RATES FOR REGIONAL ANESTHESIA TECHNIQUES IN ADULTS

Approach	Single Injection (using 0.5% ropivacaine)*	Continuous Infusion (using 0.2% ropivacaine)*	Patient-Controlled Bolus (total rate should be < 20 mL/hr)
Interscalene	30–50 mL	6–10 mL/hr	2–5 mL bolus q 20–60 min
Supraclavicular	30–40 mL	6–10 mL/hr	2–5 mL bolus q 20–60 min
Infraclavicular	30–40 mL	6–10 mL/hr	2–5 mL bolus q 20–60 min
Axillary	30–50 mL	6–10 mL/hr	2–5 mL bolus q 20–60 min
Paravertebral	3–5 mL each level	6–10 mL/hr	2–4 mL bolus q 20–30 min
Lumbar plexus	30 mL	6–10 mL/hr	2–4 mL bolus q 20–30 min
Femoral	30 mL	6–10 mL/hr	2–5 mL bolus q 20–60 min
Sciatic	20–30 mL	6–10 mL/hr	2–5 mL bolus q 20–60 min
Popliteal	30–40 mL	6–10 mL/hr	2–5 mL bolus q 20–60 min
Epidural-thoracic	6–10 mL	6–10 mL/hr w/ opioid	2–3 mL bolus q 20–30 min
Epidural-lumbar	10–20 mL	10–20 mL/hr w/ opioid	3–4 mL bolus q 20–30 min
Epidural-morphine	3–5 mg	40 μg/mL at 0.4–0.8 mg/hr	NA
Epidural-fentanyl	50–100 μg	2–5 μg/mL at 0.3–1.0 μg/kg/hr	NA

*Ropivacaine percentages not applicable to morphine or fentanyl epidural.
NA: not applicable

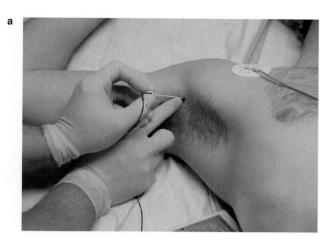
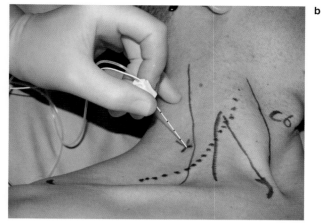

Figure 11-2. Peripheral nerve block of the brachial plexus. **(a)** Axillary approach. **(b)** Interscalene approach.
Reproduced with permission from: Buckenmaier C, Bleckner L. *Military Advanced Regional Anesthesia and Analgesia Handbook.*
Washington, DC: Borden Institute; 2009: Figures 10-5 (a) and 7-5 (b).

Localization techniques:

- **Nerve stimulation**, which originated in the 1960s, is now used for most PNBs. This technique provides a quantifiable endpoint for needle placement without causing a potentially uncomfortable paresthesia.[18,19,177] However, little evidence exists that the widespread use of nerve stimulation has increased the safety of neural blockade.[178] Typically, the needle is advanced close to the nerve as the nerve stimulator is dialed to a final stimulation between 0.2 and 0.5 mA.[179] After negative aspiration, a 1-mL test dose ("Raj test") is injected to rule out a possible intraneural injection (marked by pain or high pressure on injection) and to confirm proper needle position, followed by an intravascular test dose using local anesthesia with 15 μg of epinephrine (6 mL with a 1:400,000 solution); an increase of greater than 10 beats/minute or greater than 15 points on the systolic blood pressure over the resting values indicates intravascular position of the needle, requiring its withdrawal. After negative test doses, the total local anesthesia dose (see Table 11-3) is given in 5-mL aliquots with frequent aspiration.
- **Ultrasound technology** specifically for regional anesthesia has revolutionized regional anesthesia within the past 5 years. Nerve blocks using ultrasound may be performed with either ultrasound alone or in combination with nerve stimulation. The potential benefits of ultrasound-guided regional

anesthesia are numerous. Higher success rates and decreased onset times have been demonstrated in several studies, because the anesthesiologist can optimize needle placement during injection to ensure appropriate spread.[21,180,181] Because vascular and neural structures, as well as others such as pleura, can be well-visualized, fewer complications from needle penetration or vascular injection occur. In the case of trauma, the sole use of ultrasound technique should also decrease pain compared to nerve stimulation, which causes extremity movement. In the case of amputation, ultrasound allows for block placement when the loss of a limb precludes the ability to observe motor stimulation from a nerve stimulator. The risks of the application of ultrasound are minimal; however, indirect challenges do exist, including potential breaks in sterile technique with extra equipment or inability to see the actual needle tip on ultrasound, resulting in inadvertent needle advancement.

Continuous Peripheral Nerve Blocks. CPNBs offer improved analgesia over single shot nerve blocks by virtue of longer duration with minimal motor block. Many combat-wounded service members present with multiple-extremity injury, and ongoing, adequate analgesia remains a paramount concern. Occasionally, dual catheters may be required in a single patient to achieve adequate analgesia in multiple areas. Ganesh and Cucchiaro[182] reported on a study in which adolescents were discharged 24 hours following extremity surgery with dual CPNBs with good to excellent analgesia. This practice will likely become more common because it potentially reduces hospital stay, economic impact, opioid use, and opioid side effects. Ropivacaine may be preferred for its greater safety margin in cases when multiple infusions are employed, and until more data is available, total infusion rates should be less than 0.5 mg/kg/hr.[139]

Catheters and Pumps. Peripheral catheters are either stimulating or nonstimulating devices, most commonly a "catheter through needle" technique. The stimulating system (eg, Arrow StimuCath, Teleflex Medical, Research Triangle Park, NC) employs an insulated needle as well as a stimulating, single-orifice catheter that is advanced 3 to 5 cm through the needle; once proper stimulation is achieved, incremental boluses are administered through the catheter. The nonstimulating catheter system utilizes an insulated needle with a side port for aspiration and injection; after proper needle placement, injection of local anesthesia is made through the needle, followed by advancement of the multiorifice catheter an additional 3 to 5 cm through the needle.

Electronic pumps, such as Stryker (Stryker Instruments, Kalamazoo, Mich) and AmbIT (Sorenson Medical Inc, West Jordan, Utah; Figure 11-3), as well as elastomeric pumps, such as Accufuser (McKinley Medical, Wheat Ridge, Colo) and On-Q (I–Flow Corporation, Lake Forest, Calif; Figure 11-4), are commercially available. Electronic pumps are very reliable and programmable for various settings, including patient-control settings. Both the Stryker and the Sorenson pumps are approved for flight within the Department of Defense. Elastomeric pumps are simple devices that

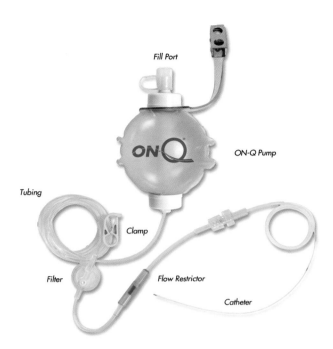

Figure 11-4. On-Q pump (I–Flow Corporation, Lake Forest, Calif; used with permission).

allow dependable infusion rates and do not require batteries. Both types are small, portable, and disposable, although the Sorenson pump may be reused by replacing a disposable cassette.

Solutions. When utilizing epidural analgesia, the combination of local anesthesia and opioids appears to afford the greatest advantage, resulting in synergistic analgesia.[105,183–186] Opioid choices include morphine, a hydrophyllic, and fentanyl and sufentanyl, which are lipophyllic. Morphine can be used in lesser amounts: its epidural/IV dose ratio is 0.25, compared to 1.0 for fentanyl and over 1.0 for sufentanyl; however, some studies suggest that fentanyl and sufentanyl have fewer side effects.[187] Epidural hydromorphone has steadily gained in popularity over the past decade, with one study showing that it causes less pruritis.[188] Typically, either 0.0625% to 0.125% bupivacaine or 0.1% to 0.2% ropivacaine is used in conjunction with an opioid at 10 to 20 mL/hr (6–10 mL/hr for thoracic and 2–3 mL every 20–30 min for lumbar epidural analgesia).[183,189,190] As noted above, maximum epidural bupivacaine rates should not exceed 0.5 mg/kg/hr (0.25 mg/kg/hr in infants),[139–143] and the rate should be decreased for pregnant or elderly patients or those with uremia or liver failure. Morphine rates should be infused at 0.4 to 0.8 mg/hr, and fentanyl typically ranges from 0.25 to 1.0 µg/kg/hr. Higher opioid rates should prompt increased monitoring within the intensive care unit.

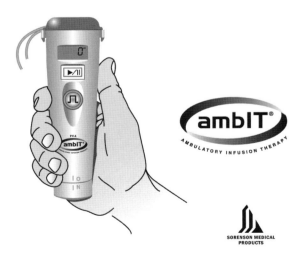

Figure 11-3. AmbIT (Sorenson Medical Inc, West Jordan, Utah) portable electronic pump (used with permission).

Medications

The treatment of PLP has been a difficult process, with a variety of treatments attempted but few providing consistent long-term relief. Drug therapies are the most commonly used treatment modalities for PLP. Drug therapies used to treat PLP include opioids, anticonvulsants, lidocaine/mexiletene, clonidine, ketamine, amitriptyline, NSAIDs, and calcitonin. These drugs have been shown to reduce PLP severity and have an analgesic effect on pain in some cases, but few have demonstrated long-term PLP relief.[191]

Opioids

Traditionally, opioids form the cornerstone of acute pain management; however, they are often overused, and recent studies have revealed more problems with an opioid-based regimen. Still, as a component of multimodal therapy, opioids complement both oral analgesics and regional analgesia. Opioids notably bind with opioid receptors peripherally and centrally, providing analgesia without loss of touch, proprioception, or consciousness. Peripherally, they reduce neurotransmitter release and nociceptor sensitization, particularly in inflammatory tissue; centrally, they modulate afferent input in the substantia gelatinosa of the dorsal horn lamina where C fibers terminate, as well as in cortical areas to blunt perception of pain. Acute pain specialists currently are armed with a wide range of opiate choices including (in increasing potency) meperidine, morphine, methadone, hydromorphone, and fentanyl, with various route of administration such as IV (including PCA), intramuscular, oral, transmucosal, transdermal, subcutaneous, epidural, intrathecal, and intraarticular. Providers should remember that morphine-6-glucuronide can accumulate in the presence of renal insufficiency.[191] Methadone is unique in acting through NMDA receptor antagonism and serotonin reuptake inhibition, yet can be challenging to manipulate because of its long half-life.[192] Transdermal fentanyl (Duragesic, Ortho-McNeil-Janssen Pharmaceuticals, Inc, Raritan, NJ) is approved for chronic pain management but not for acute pain management, in which its use has resulted in several negative outcomes.

PCAs offer a significant advantage over opioids administered by nurses, empowering the patient to self-administer analgesia as needed, thereby decreasing analgesia gaps and decreasing excess opioid dosing that could result in excess sedation and respiratory depression. Expanding the PCA arsenal to include various agents (eg, morphine, hydromorphone, fentanyl) at equianalgesic doses allows the opioid to be easily changed if it is ineffective or causes side effects. A novel, transdermal fentanyl PCA, IONSYS (Janssen-Cilag International, Beerse, Belgium) is currently available that could dramatically reduce some of the drawbacks of the PCA modality. IONSYS uses an iontopheretic transdermal system in which a small current is applied to a reservoir of fentanyl, allowing a 40-µg dose to move effectively across the dermis and be readily absorbed via cutaneous capillaries. The system significantly reduces both nursing and pharmacy workload. It has a built-in 10-minute lockout and requires replacement after 80 doses or 24 hours, whichever occurs first.[193,194] Table 11-4 lists various PCA options.

Oral opioid choices include short-acting agents such as Percocet (Endo Pharmaceuticals, Chadds Ford, Pa), a combination of oxycodone and acetaminophen; Vicodin (Abbott Laboratories, Abbott Park, Ill), made of hydrocodone and acetaminophen; and hydromorphone; as well as long-acting agents including methadone, sustained-release morphine, and sustained-release oxycodone (OxyContin, Purdue Frederick Co, Stamford, Conn). When changing either the opiate or the route of administration, the

TABLE 11-4

PATIENT-CONTROLLED ANALGESIA MODALITIES

Drug	Equianalgesic Dose (mg/mL)	Basal (mg/hr)	PCA Dose (mg)	Lockout (min)	Load (mg)
Morphine	1	0, 1	1, 2, 3	6–12	5–10
Meperidine	10	0, 10	10, 20, 30	6–10	50–100
Hydromorphone	0.2	0, 0.2	0.2, 0.4, 0.6	6–10	1–2
Fentanyl (µg)	25	0, 25	20, 25, 30	6–10	100–200

PCA: patient-controlled analgesia

TABLE 11-5

NARCOTIC CONVERSION CHART

Narcotic	IV Dose (mg)	PO Dose (mg)
Morphine	10	30–60
Hydromorphone	2	10
Methadone	10	20
OxyContin (Purdue Frederick Co, Stamford, Conn)	15	30

IV: intravenous
PO: orally

provider must use great care in converting the dose (Table 11-5). Once a new 24-hour dose is calculated based on a different medication or route, half the calculated dose should be given in divided doses in an appropriate frequency to allow for varying pharmacodynamics and pharmacokinetics. In addition, multimodal therapy with adjunctive agents requires reduced dosing as well.

In spite of their popularity, opioids cause both short- and long-term sequelae that are particularly problematic in the trauma patient.[56] Besides the side effects of sedation and the potential for respiratory depression, as well as their ineffectiveness in dynamic and neuropathic pain, opioids frequently are associated with nausea, vomiting, constipation, ileus, urinary retention, and pruritis. Long-term consequences include possible immunosuppression of B and T cell function, opioid tolerance, OIH, and the potential for opioid addiction in susceptible patients. OIH can occur even after short-term administration and results in a paradoxical decrease in a patient's pain threshold such that they are more sensitive to pain. The mechanism of OIH appears to include enhanced NMDA activity, increased levels of the pronociceptive spinal dynorphin, and increased excitatory pathways from the rostral ventromedial medulla to the dorsal horn. "Rekindling" of OIH may occur with a subsequent administration of a small dose of opioid after the apparent resolution of OIH.[53,56,195]

In the acute treatment of amputation pain in 31 patients, Wu et al[196] compared an IV bolus and infusion of morphine and lidocaine administration with a diphenhydramine control group in a cross-over study. They found that morphine relieved 45% of residual limb pain and 48% of PLP, while IV lidocaine relieved only 33% of residual limb pain and only 25% of PLP.[196] In another cross-over study, Huse et al[197] reported the efficacy of oral morphine for chronic PLP. They admin-

istered long-acting, oral morphine (70–300 mg daily) to 12 patients in a cross-over method, half receiving morphine for 12 weeks and the other half receiving placebo, followed by 6- and 12-month follow-ups. Although 42% of patients had greater than 50% reduction in pain, 50% of patients reported no pain relief. In three patients who responded to morphine, somatosensory evoke potential evaluations demonstrated decreased cortical reorganization.[197] Loeser[6] may offer the best advice on opioid use with amputees: as long as the patients' activities of daily living increase, a cautious trial of opioids is reasonable; however, if their activities of daily living decrease while their opioid dose increases, then the provider should wean them off of opioids.

Anticonvulsants

Anticonvulsants have long played a role in the treatment of neuropathic pain conditions, including peripheral diabetic neuropathy, postherpetic neuralgia, causalgia, and reflex sympathetic dystrophy (now called chronic regional pain syndrome). With the advent of newer and safer anticonvulsants, researchers have demonstrated a significant benefit with their use in acute pain management. Gabapentin and pregabalin, which are structural analogs of γ-aminobutyric acid, reduce calcium influx at the calcium channel and activate spinal noradrenergic activity, thereby reducing spinal cord excitatory amino acids, glutamate, and aspartate.[198] Pregabalin is the newest agent and although more expensive, it has a more favorable pharmacokinetic profile, allowing more rapid titration as well as twice daily dosing. Most commonly, gabapentin is dosed at 300 mg three times daily, then increased by 300 mg per dose every 3 days to a maximum daily dose of 3,600 mg. The most frequent side effects of these drugs are dizziness and drowsiness in roughly 10% of patients, yet both drugs seem to be well-tolerated in most patients. In several studies, including a look at the use of gabapentin in the treatment of PLP, their benefits include improved analgesia with an average use of 50% less opioids, decreased opioid-induced hyperalgesia and tolerance, decreased anxiety, possibly decreased chronic pain, and increased patient satisfaction.[199–202]

Carbamazepine reduces intense, brief, lancinating PLP, but has not been demonstrated to be effective for other types of phantom pain.[24,203] Gabapentin had little immediate effect on PLP but was shown to reduce pain intensity and visual analog scale scores after a 5-week treatment period in one study,[201] but this pain reduction was not replicated in subsequent studies,[204,205] although gabapentin was shown to be opioid-sparing.

Lidocaine/Mexiletene

The local anesthetic lidocaine and the oral analog mexiletene, class Ib antiarrhythmics, provide analgesia separate from their direct local anesthetic properties. Administered systemically, local anesthetics can decrease pain and opioid requirements, possibly through decreasing ectopic afferent neural activity at the NMDA receptor within the dorsal horn. IV lidocaine continuous infusion (1–2 mg/min) and topical lidocaine have been shown to decrease pain in the burn patient.[206] Mexiletene (with an initial dose of 150 mg twice daily) can be administered empirically or following a positive IV lidocaine test, after documenting the absence of conduction abnormalities on a 12-lead electrocardiogram. Mexiletene can be increased by 150 mg every 3 days to a maximum of 900 mg daily, although nausea and vomiting may limit dose escalation.

The combination of clonidine and mexiletene appears particularly beneficial in difficult, central-mediated pain syndromes such as PLP, as reported by Davis[49] and in one author's (RJM) personal experience in treating Brooke Army Medical Center patients from 2003 to 2007. As indicated above, Wu et al[196] demonstrated minimal benefit from the acute administration of IV lidocaine in PLP, and Davis[49] reported good to excellent relief from oral mexiletene alone in 58% of patients and good relief with a combination of mexiletene and clonidine in an additional 35% of patients, for a total 83% response rate for mexiletene when used in conjunction with clonidine.

Clonidine

Clonidine is an α_2-agonist acting at the locus caeruleus and in the dorsal horn of the spinal cord at α_2 antinociceptive receptors, causing analgesia, sedation, and anxiolysis from a supraspinal, spinal, and peripheral site of action. Whether given by an oral, IV, intrathecal, epidural, transdermal, or perineural route, it has been shown to decrease pain scores, decrease opioid requirements, decrease opioid-induced hyperalgesia, and prolong nerve blocks in a synergistic manner with other analgesics. In a hemodynamically stable patient, clonidine should be initiated at 0.1 mg by mouth twice daily, increasing to a maximum of 0.3 mg twice daily, observing for hypotension. While Davis[49] reported success with transdermal clonidine for outpatients, especially combined with mexiletene, providers at Brooke Army Medical Center found oral clonidine effective and easier to titrate for inpatients.

Ketamine

Historically, ketamine has played a central role in anesthesia for the trauma patient due to the profound analgesia and hemodynamic stability it provides. However, ketamine has increasingly been used for postoperative analgesia and acute pain management in the trauma patient; in fact, its use throughout the inflammatory period of injury may result in decreased central hypersensitivity resulting from the continual C fiber wind-up phenomenon in the polytrauma patient. Ketamine binds noncompetitively to the phencyclidine site of the NMDA receptor as well as to the σ-opioid receptor, resulting in intense analgesia; other benefits include prevention of opioid-induced hyperalgesia, decreased opioid tolerance, decreased opioid requirements, increased sense of well-being and patient satisfaction, decreased nausea and vomiting, decreased risk of respiratory depression, and decreased chronic pain. Although anesthetic doses may be associated with secretions as well as agitation and hallucinations, subanesthetic doses, with the addition of a benzodiazepine if necessary, are tolerated extremely well. The combination of ketamine and morphine in low PCA doses (1 mg morphine and 1 mg ketamine) has been shown to be particularly beneficial, with few side effects when ketamine doses are below 150 μg/kg/hr (2.5 μg/kg/min).[207–209]

Studies on ketamine have shown that it does not reduce the occurrence of PLP, but may temporarily reduce the severity of pain. A prospective observational study of 14 limb amputees showed that following administration of ketamine, 72% of subjects continued to experience PLP. However, only 9% of subjects given ketamine reported severe PLP, compared to 71% of controls.[210] Nikolajsen et al[211] reported profound acute reduction of both residual limb pain and PLP after a 0.1-mg/kg bolus followed by a 7-μg/kg/min infusion for 45 minutes. Nikolajsen[50] also reported on the efficacy of oral ketamine on chronic residual limb pain over a 3-month period. Another NMDA antagonist, dextromethorphan, was given daily (120–180 mg/day) to three amputation patients with PLP for 3 months, resulting in a significant reduction in PLP without side effects.[212] However, a further follow-up study randomizing 53 subjects to either epidural ketamine plus bupivacaine or epidural saline plus bupivacaine failed to demonstrate increased efficacy of epidural ketamine in treating PLP.[213]

Antidepressants

Tertiary amines, most notably amitriptyline, as well as secondary amines such as nortriptyline and desipramine, are effective in neuropathic and central hypersensitivity conditions primarily by blocking norepinephrine and serotonin reuptake in the dorsal horn. Their limitations result from a broad side-effect profile including antihistamine, anticholinergic, and antiadrenergic effects that together frequently cause sedation, dry mouth, constipation, and possible tachycardia and orthostasis. Although amitriptyline has been most studied, the secondary amines may be equally effective and have fewer side effects. After ruling out significant cardiac contraindications by history, physical, and electrocardiogram, amitriptyline can be started at 10 to 25 mg every evening, increasing to 50 mg after 1 week of therapy, although its analgesic properties may take 3 to 4 weeks to take effect.

Amitriptyline has not been shown to be a consistently effective treatment for PLP. A randomized, placebo-controlled study of amitriptyline showed that it did not significantly reduce chronic PLP over a 6-week period.[214] Panerai et al,[215] however, demonstrated efficacy of both chlorimipramine and nortriptyline in central pain syndromes such as PLP in a randomized, controlled trial. Finally, mirtazapine, a newer antidepressant that modulates both serotonin and norepinephrine with fewer side effects than the tricyclic antidepressants, demonstrated efficacy in reducing PLP in one case series.[35]

Acetaminophen

Atlhough acetaminophen is a relatively weak analgesic, it is attractive as part of a multimodal pain regimen because it does not cause platelet dysfunction, gastritis, significant renal toxicity, bone-healing concerns, or associated nausea and vomiting. The mechanism of action is reported to function at a central COX-3 receptor, producing analgesia. Numerous studies have demonstrated synergy with other analgesics with at least 20% opioid sparing,[216,217] as well as decreased nausea, vomiting, and sedation using up to 4,000 mg daily in divided doses.

Nonsteroidal Antiinflammatory Drugs

NSAIDs also play a potentially critical role in multimodal therapy although with notable limitations. Traditional NSAIDs inhibit both COX-1 and COX-2 receptors, thereby decreasing the production of prostaglandins and thromboxane, and also decreasing nociception, respectively. Traditional NSAIDs bind receptors only peripherally, whereas the newer COX-2 agents work both peripherally and centrally, decreasing both peripheral and central sensitivity.[3] Their use is associated with many benefits including decreased opioid requirements, decreased pain scores, decreased nausea and vomiting, decreased constipation, decreased sedation, and finally decreased heterotopic ossification, a complication frequently associated with

the polytrauma patient. Traditional NSAIDs are limited by potential adverse effects such as platelet dysfunction, gastritis, renal impairment, and impaired bone healing, most of which is dose-dependent. Oral COX-2 agents, currently only celecoxib, may be an attractive alternative because they do not cause platelet dysfunction and have decreased gastritis risk, although their risk of renal impairment and bone-healing problems is similar to traditional NSAIDs. Unfortunately, the COX-2 inhibitors have been associated with increased thromboembolic events including myocardial infarction, as well as higher rates of congestive heart failure and hypertension. Recently, some of the traditional NSAIDs have also been associated with an increased thromboembolic risk.[218,219] However, in some patients, traditional NSAIDs, including ketorolac (for up to 5 days) and COX-2 inhibitors can be helpful in achieving greater analgesia, particularly for dynamic pain and as part of a multimodal regimen.[220–222]

Calcitonin

Salmon calcitonin has been noted to have analgesic properties in the treatment of Paget disease, possibly related to binding with serotonin receptors within the hypothalamus and limbic system. Calcitonin has been shown to provide analgesic effects for PLP.[170,223] Jaeger and Maier[223] reported a prospective, double-blinded, cross-over trial with calcitonin 200 units over 30 minutes. Each of the calcitonin groups showed a significant reduction in pain scores compared to placebo.

Nontraditional Therapies

TENS, acupuncture, and virtual reality mirror treatments have also shown some success in reducing PLP or delaying the onset of chronic phantom pain.[192,224,225]

Transcutaneous Electrical Nerve Stimulation, Spinal Cord Stimulation, and Deep Brain Stimulation

TENS has shown some success in relieving PLP, but again, study results have been varied. Spinal cord stimulation and deep brain stimulation of the ventral caudal thalamic nucleus are techniques that have led to short-term relief of PLP in several studies.[226–230] A series of studies showed that the stimulation of the posterior columns of the spinal cord led to 65% of patients having a 25% reduction in pain levels immediately after surgery, but only 33% showing long-term reduction in pain levels.[231,232] Other reports have shown little or no reduction in PLP following dorsal column stimulation.[233,234]

Sympathetic Blocks for Postamputation Pain

An infrequent intervention for amputation pain is sympathetic blocks, specifically lumbar sympathetic block and stellate ganglion block. A practitioner must first recognize the signs of sympathetically mediated pain, which include allodynia, decreased range of motion, edema, and possible skin changes such as a cold and clammy or sweaty extremity with possible hair changes. Pain may become worse during physical or emotional stress due to catecholamine release, which may activate nerve terminals and neuromas. Classically, local anesthetics are injected near the sympathetic ganglia, which relieves pain and sympathetic symptoms within minutes, making the extremity warm with improved blood flow and color. Pain physicians have documented the effective use of stellate ganglion blocks to prevent reactivation and worsening of pain in patients with a history of chronic regional pain syndrome who are undergoing upper extremity surgery. In addition, there are case reports of stellate ganglion block to treat acute postoperative pain in patients without chronic regional pain syndrome.[235] A stellate ganglion block with fentanyl alone has also been reported to be effective.[236] Temperature increase in the extremity without motor or sensory blockade is indicative of effective stellate ganglion or lumbar sympathetic block; stellate ganglion blocks may be accompanied by a possible Horner syndrome (ptosis, miosis, and anhydrosis). However, pain relief following sympathetic blocks may result from undetected somatic block from local anesthetic spread to the epidural space or lumbar nerve roots.[237]

Acupuncture

Some amputees have gained relief from PLP by rubbing their intact limb and stimulating normal afferent input at the peripheral, spinal, and cortical levels. Based on this concept, acupuncture in the intact limb has been used as a means to stimulate normal afferent input to the nervous system and elicit an analgesic effect that reduces the intensity of PLP and phantom sensations.[238,239] Bradbrook[239] found that acupuncture was an effective treatment in two patients who had had nontraumatic limb amputation (following congenital talipes and myeloma of the pelvis). These two patients reported immediate and significant reduction in severity of PLP as measured with a visual analog scale following several sessions of acupuncture in regions of the intact limb anatomy in relation to the subjects' PLP and phantom sensations.[239] However, in another single case of a patient who had undergone traumatic limb amputation following a motor vehicle accident, acupuncture was not effective in reducing the severity of PLP and phantom sensations. It remains unclear through what specific mechanism acupuncture alleviates PLP, and as with many other therapies, accupuncture has not been shown to consistently relieve PLP in patients who have undergone traumatic limb amputations.

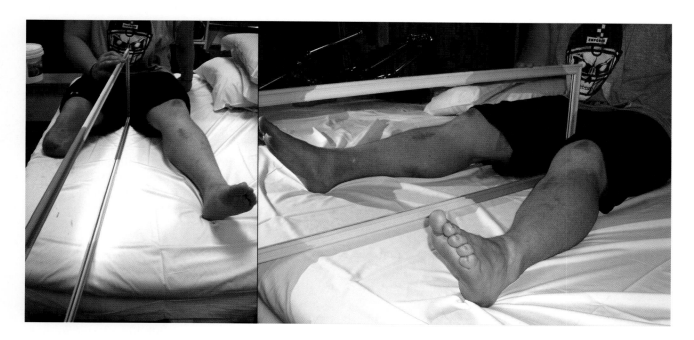

Figure 11-5. Right lower extremity amputee participating in mirror therapy as treatment for phantom limb pain.

Mirror Therapy

Another proposed treatment is based on the concept that the perception and experience of PLP may emerge due to conflicts within the brain between visual and proprioceptive feedback mechanisms.[224] Based on this visual-proprioceptive dissociative feedback postulate, Ramachandran and colleagues[224] proposed that using the reflected image of the intact limb in a mirror to create the visual illusion of the missing limb might reduce the conflict between visual and proprioceptive inputs and, consequently, reduce PLP. They used this technique in upper extremity amputees and found that approximately 60% of subjects in one case series of 15 amputees reported an improvement in their PLP.[224] This technique required the amputee to view the reflected image of the intact hand performing specific movements, while performing the same movements with the amputated, or "phantom," hand. While performing these movements with the intact hand, many subjects reported feeling the phantom hand moving simultaneously, accompanied by pain relief.

Two of the authors (BLC and JWT) were part of a recently concluded randomized, sham-controlled study of unilateral lower extremity amputees using mirror therapy (Figure 11-5) compared to cover mirror and mental visualization therapies, finding a strong benefit of mirror therapy (Figure 11-6).[225] This study showed that all six amputees (100%) who were randomized to mirror therapy had pain relief and eight of nine subjects (89%) who crossed over to mirror therapy after being randomized initially to either covered mirror or mental visualization therapies had benefit from mirror therapy, so that a total of fourteen of fifteen subjects (93%) using mirror therapy had pain relief.

Although the results of these studies appear to provide further support for the postulate that a mismatch between visual and proprioceptive inputs contributes to the generation of PLP, it is not clear why a mismatch would cause pain. Head first posited the existence of two major somatesthetic sensory systems, one he termed epicritic and the other protopathic.[240] The epicritic system is rapid and is transmitted to the brain by lemniscal afferent pathways. In contrast the protopathic system is slow and is carried to the brain by a chain of neurons. Head suggested that the epicritic

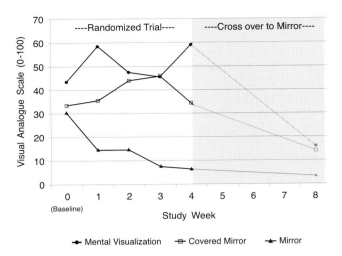

Figure 11-6. Results of controlled trial of mirror therapy. Change in phantom limb pain measured using the VAS. Group medians are depicted for each time point.
Reproduced with permission from: Chan BL, Witt R, Charrow AP, et al. Mirror therapy for phantom limb pain. *N Engl J Med.* 2007;357:2206–2207. Copyright 2007 Massachusetts Medical Society. All rights reserved.

system gates the protopathic system and that loss of the epicritic system can induce pain because the protopathic system is uninhibited.[240] Melzack and Wall[27] subsequently put forth a similar gating hypothesis.

Rossi et al[241] postulated and provided evidence to demonstrate that imagery of movements or actual movements reduces the amplitude of the somatosensory evoked potentials (ie, a gating effect), suggesting that this gating may help reduce phantom pain. The mirror therapy paradigm has been more successful than imagery alone because it led to the activation of mirror neurons, neurons that fire both when a person performs an action and when observing the same action performed, in the cortex contralateral to the amputated limb. Since the activation of these mirror neurons modulates somatosensory inputs, their activation may have blocked protopathic pain perception in the phantom limb.[241] Mirror therapy has now been adopted as part of the routine treatment for PLP offered by several military medical centers, including Walter Reed Army Medical Center.

LOW BACK PAIN

Low back pain (LBP) is reported as a significant impairment in approximately 71% of patients with lower limb amputations.[242] Patients with transfemoral amputations tend to have a greater incidence and severity of LBP than those with transtibial amputations.[243] Leg

length discrepancy, excessive lumbar lordosis, and excessive trunk motion may be related to LBP in transfemoral patients. Friel et al[244] found that patients with transfemoral amputations exhibited greater strength but less endurance in their back extensor muscle than those with transtibial amputation. Friberg[245] found that amputees with LBP tended to have greater leg length discrepancies than those without pain. Back pain tends to decrease following leg length discrepancy correction. In some studies, lumbar lordosis has been correlated with increased LBP, particularly in circumstances with poor prosthetic fit.[245] Leg length discrepancy, lumbar lordosis, and excessive motion of the lumbar spine may lead to abnormal spinal loads, which produce abnormal stress distributions in the tissues. No specific evidence is available to guide treatment of LBP in patients with lower extremity amputations. However, the high prevalence of LBP among patients with lower extremity amputations may have as strong an impact on disability, function, and rehabilitation as residual limb pain and phantom sensations.

FUTURE RESEARCH

Research into methods for preventing and treating postoperative residual limb pain and PLP have demonstrated several therapeutic options. It is likely that a combination of therapies may be needed to effectively treat pain through acute, subacute, and chronic pain conditions following limb amputation. Areas that require additional research are more effective analgesics to be deployed in the battlefield setting, pain immediately following amputation, and treatments for chronic pain (eg, headaches, osteoarthritis, PLP, and LBP). The appropriate timing and duration of regional anesthesia in the acute and subacute period to decrease both acute and chronic pain needs further evaluation. Understanding the mechanism for the development of pain sensation will lead to improved pharmacologic as well as nontraditional methods for controlling and regulating the pain response. Also, further understanding of the cognitive response to pain, especially phantom pain, will help in the development of more effective treatments for PLP and possibly a means for tracking the response to therapies.

SUMMARY

In summary, PLP and pain in the residual limb are significant medical problems after amputation. Many different therapies have been tried with few successes, although multimodal therapy appears to be most effective. Multimodal therapy including appropriate continuous regional analgesia, multiple medications aimed at various locations along the nociceptive pathway, and nontraditional therapies such as mirror therapy, is a promising method of treatment that may bring desperately needed pain relief to service members with limb loss.

REFERENCES

1. Clark ME. Post-deployment pain: a need for rapid detection and intervention. *Pain Med*. 2004;5:333–334.

2. ClarkME, Blair MJ, Buckenmaier CC III, Gironda RJ, Walker RL. Pain and combat injuries in soldiers returning from Operations Enduring Freedom and Iraqi Freedom: implications for research and practice. *J Rehabil Res Dev*. 2007;44: 179–194.

3. Eisenach JC. Preventing chronic pain after surgery: who, how, and when? *Reg Anes Pain Med*. 2006;31:1–3.

4. Iohom G, Abdalla H, O'Brien J, et al. The associations between severity of early postoperative pain, chronic postsurgical pain and plasma concentration of stable nitric oxide products after breast surgery. *Anes Analg*. 2006;103:995–1000.

5. Perkins FM, Kehlet H. Chronic pain as an outcome of surgery. A review of predictive factors. *Anesthesiology*. 2000;93:1123–1133.

6. Loeser JD. Pain after amputation: phantom limb and stump pain. In: Loeser JD, Bonica J, eds. *Bonica's Management of Pain*. 3rd ed. Philiadelphia, Pa: Lippincott Williams and Wilkins; 2001: Chap 26.

7. Bacon D. Regional anesthesia and analgesia. In: Brown D, ed. *Regional Anesthesia and Chronic Pain Treatment: A History*. New York, NY: WB Saunders Co; 1996: Chap 2.

8. Davison M. *Evolution of Anaesthesia*. Baltimore, Md: Williams and Wilkins Co; 1965.

9. Faulconer A, Keys TE. *Foundations of Anesthesiology.* Vol II. Springfield, Ill: Charles C Thomas Publisher; 1965.

10. Keys TE. *The History of Surgical Anesthesia.* New York, NY: Schuman's; 1945.

11. Cole F. *Milestones in Anesthesia: Readings in the Development of Surgical Anesthesia, 1665–1940.* Lincoln, Nebr: University of Nebraska Press; 1965.

12. Winnie A, Hakansson L, Buckhoj P. *Plexus Anesthesia.* Vol I. New York, NY: WB Saunders Co; 1983.

13. Touhy E. Continuous spinal anesthesia: its usefulness and technic involved. *Anesthesiology.* 1944;5:142–148.

14. Ansbro F. A method of continous brachial plexus block. *Am J Surg.* 1946;71:716–722.

15. Greenblatt G, Denson J. Needle nerve stimulator locator: nerve blocks with a new instrument for locating nerves. *Anesth Analg.* 1962;41:599–602.

16. Koons RA. The use of the block-aid monitor and plastic intravenous cannulas for nerve blocks. *Anesthesiology.* 1969;31:290–291.

17. Raj P. Use of the nerve stimulator for peripheral blocks. *Reg Anesth.* 1980;5:14–21.

18. Ford DJ, Pither C, Raj PP. Comparison of insulated and uninsulated needles for locating peripheral nerves with a peripheral nerve stimulator. *Anesth Analg.* 1984;63:925–928.

19. Pither C, Raj PP, Ford D. The use of peripheral nerve stimulators for regional anesthesia; a review of experimental characteristics, technique, and clinical applications. *Reg Anesth.* 1985;10: 49–58.

20. LaGrange P, Foster PA, Pretorius LK. Application of the Doppler ultrasound blood flow detector in supraclavicular brachial plexus block. *Br J Anaesth.* 1978;50:965–967.

21. Marhofer P, Schrögendorfer K, Koinig H, Kapral S, Weinstabl C, Mayer N. Ultrasonographic guidance improves sensory block and onset time of 3-in-1 blocks. *Anesth Analg.* 1997;85:854–857.

22. Steele SM, Klein SM, D'Ercole FJ, Greengrass RA, Gleason D. A new continuous catheter delivery system. *Anesth Analg.* 1998;87:228.

23. Kick O, Blanche E, Pham-Dang C, Pinaud M, Estebe JP. A new stimulating stylet for immediate control of catheter tip position in continuous peripheral nerve blocks. *Anesth Analg.* 1999;89:533–534.

24. Patterson JF. Carbamazepine in the treatment of phantom limb pain. *South Med J.* 1988;81:1100-1102.

25. Kelly DJ, Ahmad M. Preemptive analgesia I: physiological pathways and pharmacological modalities. *Can J Anesth.* 2001;48:1000–1010.

26. Downs TH. *Movement and Motor Imagery of Phantom Limbs: A Study in Cortical Reorganization* [dissertation]. Waco, Tex: Baylor University; 1992.

27. Melzack R, Wall PD. *The Challenge of Pain.* 2nd ed. London, England: Penguin Books; 1988.

28. Ramachandran VS, Hirstein W. The perception of phantom limbs. The D.O. 1998 Hebb lecture. *Brain.* 1999; 121:1603–1630.

29. Haber W. Effects of loss of limb on sensory functions. *J Psychol.* 1995;40:115–123.

30. Moser H. Schmerzzustande nach amputation [Pain management after amputation]. *Arztl Mh.* 1948;11:977.

31. Sherman RA, Sherman CJ, Parker L. Phantom and stump pain among American veterans: results of a survey. *Pain.* 1984;18:83–95.

32. Richardson C, Turo N. Incidence of phantom phenomena including phantom limb pain 6 months after major lower limb amputation in patients with peripheral vascular disease. *Clin J Pain*. 2006;22:353–358.

33. Browder EJ, Gallagher JP. Dorsal cordotomy for painful phantom limb. *Ann Surg*. 1948;128:456–469.

34. Kelly DJ, Ahmad M. Preemptive analgesia II: recent advances and current trends. *Can J Anesth*. 2001; 48:1091–1101.

35. Kuiken T, Schechtman L, Harden RN. Phantom limb pain treatment with mirtazapine: a case series. *Pain Pract*. 2005;5:356–360.

36. Livingston K. The phantom limb syndromes: a discussion of the role of major peripheral nerve neuromas. *J Neurosurg*. 1945;3:251–255.

37. Raja S, Benzon H. Phantom pain. In: Benzon HT, ed. *Essentials of Pain Medicine and Regional Anesthesia*. 2nd ed. Philadelphia, Pa: Elsevier Churchill Livingstone; 2005: Chap 49.

38. Wall JT. Variable organization in cortical maps of the skin as an indication of the lifelong adaptive capacities of circuits in the mammalian brain. *Trends Neurosci*. 1988;11:549–557.

39. Melzack R. Phantom limbs and the concept of a neuromatrix. *Trends Neurosci*. 1990;13:88–92.

40. Penfield W, Rasmussen T. *The Cerebral Cortex of Man*. New York, NY: Macmillan; 1950.

41. Adrian ED, Zotterman Y. The impulses produced by sensory nerve endings, part 2. *J Physiol Lond*. 1926;61:157–171.

42. Garraghty PE, Kaas JH. Functional reorganization in adult monkey thalamus after peripheral nerve injury. *Neuroreport*. 1991;2:747–750.

43. Wiesel TN, Hubel DH. Single-cell responses in striate cortex of kittens deprived of vision in one eye. *J Neurophysiol*. 1963; 6:1003–1017.

44. Ramachandran VS. Behavioral and magnetoencephalographic correlates of plasticity in the adult human brain. *Proc Natl Acad Sci USA*. 1993;90:10413–10420.

45. Lotze M, Grodd W, Birbaumer N, et al. Does use of a myoelectric prosthesis prevent cortical reorganization and phantom limb pain? *Nat Neurosci*. 1999;2:501–502.

46. Lotze M, Montoya P, Erb M, et al. Activation of cortical and cerebellar motor areas during executed and imagined hand movements: an fMRI study. *J Cogn Neurosci*. 1999;1:491–501.

47. Sherman RA, Sherman CJ. Prevalence and characteristics of chronic phantom limb pain among American veterans. Results of a trial survey. *Am J Phys Med*. 1983;62:227–238.

48. Kern U, Martin C, Scheicher S, Muller H. Effects of botulinum toxin type B on stump pain and involuntary movements of the stump. *Am J Phys Med Rehabil*. 2004;83:396–399.

49. Davis RW. Successful treatment for phantom pain. *Orthopedics*. 1993;16:691–695.

50. Nikolajsen L, Hansen PO, Jensen TS. Oral ketamine therapy in the treatment of postamputation stump pain. *Acta Anaesthesiol Scand*. 1997;41:427–429.

51. American Society of Anesthesiologists Task Force on Acute Pain Management. Practice guidelines for acute pain management in the perioperative setting: an updated report by the American Society of Anesthesiologists Task Force on Acute Pain Management. *Anesthesiology*. 2004;100:1573–1581.

52. Shorten G, Carr D, Harmon D, Puig M, Browne J, eds. *Postoperative Pain Management: An Evidence-Based Guide to Practice*. Philadelphia, Pa: Saunders Elsevier; 2006.

53. Celerier E, Rivat C, Jun Y, et al. Long-lasting hyperalgesia induced by fentanyl in rats—preventive effect of ketamine. *Anesthesiology*. 2000;92:465–472.

54. Angst MS, Clark JD. Opioid-induced hyperalgesia. *Anesthesiology*. 2006;104:570–587.

55. Weinger M. Dangers of postoperative opioids. *Anesthesia Patient Safety Foundation Newsletter*. 2006;21:61–68.

56. Kehlet H, Dahl J. The value of "multimodal" or "balanced analgesia" in postoperative pain treatment. *Anesth Analg*. 1993;77:1048–1056.

57. Richman JM, Liu SS, Courpas G, et al. Does continuous peripheral nerve block provide superior pain control to opioids? A meta-analysis. *Anesth Analg*. 2006;102:248–257.

58. Ong BY, Arnega A, Ong EW. Effects of anesthesia on pain after lower-limb amputation. *J Clin Anesth*. 2006;18:600–604.

59. Hanley MA, Jensen MP, Smith DG, Ehde DM, Edwards WT, Robinson LR. Preamputation pain and acute pain predict chronic pain after lower extremity amputation. *J Pain*. 2007;8:102–109.

60. Schug SA, Burrell R, Payne J, Tester P. Pre-emptive epidural analgesia may prevent phantom limb pain. *Reg Anesth*. 1995;20:256.

61. Waters JH, Leivers D, Maher D, Scanlon T, DeGuzman GM. Patient and surgeon satisfaction with extremity blockade for surgery in remote locations. *Anesth Analg*. 1997;84:773–776.

62. Auroy Y, Narchi P, Messiah A, Litt L, Rouvier B, Samii K. Serious complications related to regional anesthesia: results of a prospective survey in France. *Anesthesiology*. 1997;87:479–486.

63. Olsson GL, Hallen B. Cardiac arrest during anaesthesia: a computer-aided study in 250,543 anaesthetics. *Acta Anaesthesiol Scand*. 1988;32:653–664.

64. Geffin B, Shapiro L. Sinus bradycardia and asystole during spinal and epidural anesthesia: a report of 13 cases. *J Clin Anesth*. 1998;10:278–285.

65. Mackey DC, Carpenter RL, Thomspon GE, Brown DL, Bodily MN. Bradycardia and asystole during spinal anesthesia: a report of three cases without morbidity. *Anesthesiology*. 1989;70:866–868.

66. TarkkilaPJ, Kaukinen S. Complications during spinal anesthesia: a prospective study. *Reg Anesth*. 1991;16:101–106.

67. Caplan R, Ward RJ, Posner K, Cheney FW. Unexpected cardiac arrest during spinal anesthesia: a closed claims analysis of predisposing factors. *Anesthesiology*. 1988;68:5–11.

68. de Visme V, Picart F, LeJouan R, Legrand A, Savry C, Morin V. Combined lumbar plexus and sacral plexus blockade compared with plain bupivacaine spinal anesthesia for hip fractures in the elderly. *Reg Anesth Pain Med*. 2000;25:158-162.

69. Carpenter RL, Caplan RA, Brown DL, Stephenson C, Wu R. Incidence and risk factors for side effects of spinal anesthesia. *Anesthesiology*. 1992;76:906–916.

70. Giaufre E, Dalens B, Gombert A. Epidemiology and morbidity of regional anesthesia in children: a one-year prospective survey of the French-Language Society of Pediatric Anesthesiologists. *Anesth Analg*. 1996;83:904–912.

71. Ford RP, Gerancher JC, Rich R, et al. An evaluation of immediate recovery after regional and general anesthesia: a two year review of 801 ambulatory patients undergoing hand surgery. *Reg Anesth Pain Med*. 2001;26(suppl):41.

72. Williams BA, Kentor ML, Williams JP, et al. Process analysis in outpatient knee surgery: effects of regional and general anesthesia on anesthesia-controlled time. *Anesthesiology*. 2000;93:529–538.

73. Maurer P, Greek R, Torjman M, et al. Is regional anesthesia more time efficient than general anesthesia for shoulder surgery. *Anesthesiology*. 1993;79:A897.

74. Chan V. A comparative study of general anesthesia, IV regional anesthesia, and axillary block for outpatient hand surgery: clinical outcome and cost analysis. *Anesth Analg*. 2001;93:1181–1184.

75. Modig J. Beneficial effects on intraoperative and postoperative blood loss in total hip replacement when performed under lumbar epidural anesthesia. An explanatory study. *Acta Chir Scand Suppl*. 1989;550:95–103.

76. Grass J. Surgical outcome: regional anesthesia and analgesia versus general anesthesia. *Anes Rev*. 1993;20:117–125.

77. Twyman R, Kirwan T, Fennelly M. Blood loss reduced during hip arthroplasty by lumbar plexus block. *J Bone Joint Surg*. 1990;72-B:770–771.

78. Stevens RD, Van Gessel E, Flory N, Fournier R, Gamulin Z. Lumbar plexus block reduces pain and blood loss associated with total hip arthroplasty. *Anesthesiology*. 2000;93:115–121.

79. Modig J, Borg T, Karlstrom G, Maripuu E, Sahlstedt B. Thromboembolism after total hip arthroplasty: role of epidural and general anesthesia. *Anesth Analg*. 1983;62:74–80.

80. Benzon HT, Wong CA, Wong HY, Brooke C, Wade L. The effect of low-dose bupivacaine on postoperative epidural fentanyl analgesia and thromboelastography. *Anesth Analg*. 1994;79:911–917.

81. Rosenfeld BA, Beattie C, Christopherson R, et al. The effects of different anesthetic regimens on fibrinolysis and the development of postoperative arterial thrombosis. *Anesthesiology*. 1993;79:435–443.

82. Tuman KJ, McCarthy RJ, March RJ, et al. Effects of epidural anesthesia and analgesia on coagulation and outcome after major vascular surgery. *Anesth Analg*. 1991;73:696–704.

83. Christopherson R, Beattie C, Frank SM, et al. Perioperative morbidity in patients randomized to epidural or general anesthesia for lower extremity vascular surgery. *Anesthesiology*. 1993;79:422–434.

84. Williams BA, Kentor ML, Vogt MT, et al. Economics of nerve block pain management after anterior cruciate ligament reconstruction: potential hospital cost savings via associated postanesthesia care unit bypass and same-day discharge. *Anesthesiology*. 2004;100:697–706.

85. D'Alessio JG, Rosenblum M, Shea KP, Freitas DG. A retrospective comparison of interscalene block and general anesthesia for ambulatory surgery shoulder arthroscopy. *Reg Anesth*. 1995;20:62-68.

86. Yeager MP, Glass DD, Neff RK, Brinck-Johnsen T. Epidural anesthesia and analgesia in high risk surgical patients. *Anesthesiology*. 1987;66:729-736.

87. Guinard JP, Mavrocordatos P, Chioloer R, Carpenter RL. A randomized comparison of intravenous versus lumbar versus thoracic epidural fentanyl for analgesia after thoracotomy. *Anesthesiology*. 1992;77:1108–1115.

88. Boylan JF, Katz J, Kavanagh BP, et al. Epidural bupivacaine-morphine analgesia versus patient-controlled analgesia following abdominal aortic surgery: analgesic, respiratory, and myocardial effects. *Anesthesiology*. 1998;89:585–593.

89. Rawal N, , Sjöstrand U, Christoffersson E, Dahlström B, Arvill A, Rydman H. Comparison of intramuscular and epidural morphine for postoperative analgesia in the grossly obese. *Anesth Analg*. 1984;63:583–592.

90. Salomaki TE, Laitinen JO, Nuutinen LS. A randomized double-blind comparison of epidural versus intravenous fentanyl infusion for analgesia after thoracotomy. *Anesthesiology*. 1991;75:790–795.

91. Horlocker TT, Hebl JR, Kinney MA, Cabanela ME. Opioid-free analgesia following total knee arthroplasty—a multimodal approach using continuous lumbar plexus (psoas compartment) block, acetominophen, and ketorolac. *Reg Anesth Pain Med*. 2002;27:105–108.

92. Mulroy M, Larkin KL, Batra MS, Hodgson PS, Owens BD. Femoral nerve block with 0.25% or 0.5% bupivacaine improves postoperative analgesia following outpatient arthroscopic anterior cruciate ligament repair. *Reg Anesth Pain Med*. 2001;26:24–29.

93. Liu S, Carpenter RL, Neal JM. Epidural anesthesia and analgesia. Their role in postoperative outcome. *Anesthesiology*. 1995;82:1474–1506.

94. de Leon-Casasola OA. Thoracic epidural anesthesia and analgesia for thoracic surgery in high risk surgical patients: a physiological appraisal of pulmonary and cardiac function and its influence on patient outcome. *Techniques Reg Anesth Pain Manage*. 1998;2:35–40.

95. Blomberg S, Emanuelsson H, Ricksten SE. Thoracic epidural anesthesia and central hemodynamics in patients with unstable angina pectoris. *Anesth Analg*. 1989;69:558–562.

96. Blomberg S, Emanuelsson H, Kvist H, et al. Effects of epidural anesthesia on coronary arteries and arterioles in patients with coronary artery disease. *Anesthesiology*. 1990;73:840–847.

97. Norris EJ, Parker S, Breslow MJ, et al. The endocrine response to surgical stress: a comparison of epidural anesthesia/ analgesia vs general anesthesia/patient controlled analgesia. *Anesthesiology*. 1991;75:A696.

98. Wu CL, Hurley RW, Anderson GF, Herbert R, Rowlingson AJ, Fleisher LA. Effect of postoperative epidural analgesia on morbidity and mortality following surgery in Medicare patients. *Reg Anesth Pain Med*. 2004;29:525–533.

99. Gramling-Babb P, Miller MJ, Reeves ST, Roy RC, Zile MR. Treatment of medically and surgically refractory angina pectoris with high thoracic epidural analgesia: initial clinical experience. *Am Heart J*. 1997;133:648–655.

100. Davis RF, DeBoer LW, Maroko PR. Thoracic epidural anesthesia reduces myocardial infarct size after coronary artery occlusion in dogs. *Anesth Analg*. 1986;65:711v717.

101. Kock M, Blomberg S, Emanuelsson H, Lomsky M, Stromblad SO, Ricksten SE. Thoracic epidural anesthesia improves global and regional left ventricular function during stress-induced myocardial ischemia in patients with coronary artery disease. *Anesth Analg*. 1990;71:625–630.

102. Meissner A, Rolf N, Van Aken H. Thoracic epidural anesthesia and the patient with heart disease: benefits, risks, and controversies. Review Article. *Anesth Analg*. 1997;85:517–528.

103. Rolf N. Thoracic epidural anesthesia in cardiac risk patients. In: Chaney M, ed. *Regional Anesthesia for Cardiothoracic Surgery*. Philadelphia, Pa: Lippincott Williams and Wilkins; 2002: 21-38. Society of Cardiovascular Anesthesiologists Monograph.

104. Scott NB, Turfrey DJ, Ray DA, et al. A prospective randomized study of the potential benefits of thoracic epidural anesthesia and analgesia in patients undergoing coronary artery bypass grafting. *Anesth Analg*. 2001;93:528–535.

105. Liu SS, Carpenter RL, Mackey DC, et al. Effects of perioperative analgesic technique on rate of recovery after colon surgery. *Anesthesiology*. 1995;83:757–765.

106. Capdevila X, Barthelet Y, Biboulet P, Ryckwaert Y, Rubenovitch J, d'Athis F. Effects of perioperative analgesia technique on the surgical outcome and duration of rehabiliation after major knee surgery. *Anesthesiology*. 1999;91:8–15.

107. Singelyn FJ, Devaert M, Joris D, Pendeville E, Gouverneur JM. Effects of intravenous patient-controlled analgesia with morphine, continuous epidural analgesia and continuous three-in-one block after postoperative pain and knee rehabilitation after unilateral total knee arthroplasty. *Anesth Analg*. 1998;87:88–92.

108. Wu CL, Nagibuddin M, Fleisher LA. Measurement of patient satisfaction as an outcome of regional anesthesia & analgesia: a systematic review. *Reg Anesth Pain Med*. 2001;26:196–208.

109. Vloka JD, Hadzić A, Mulcare R, Lesser JB, Kitain E, Thys DM. Femoral and genitofemoral nerve blocks versus spinal anesthesia for outpatients undergoing long saphenous vein stripping surgery. *Anesth Analg*. 1997;84:749–752.

110. Borgeat A, Perschak H, Bird P, Hodler J, Gerber C. Patient-controlled interscalene analgesia with ropivacaine 0.2% versus patient-controlled intravenous analgesia after major shoulder surgery: effects on diaphragmatic and respiratory function. *Anesthesiology*. 2000;92:102–108.

111. Allen HW, Liu SS, Ware PD, Nairn CS, Owens BD. Peripheral nerve blocks improve analgesia after total knee replacement surgery. *Anesth Analg*. 1998;87:93–97.

112. Logas WG, el-Baz N, el-Ganzouri A, et al. Continuous thoracic epidural analgesia for postoperative pain relief following thoracotomy: a randomized prospective study. *Anesthesiology*. 1987;67:787–791.

113. Cooper K, Kelley H, Carrithers J. Perceptions of side effects following axillary block used for outpatient surgery. *Reg Anesth*. 1995;20:212–216.

114. Finucane BT. *Complications of Regional Anesthesia*. New York, NY: Churchill Livingstone; 1999.

115. Cheney FW. The American Society of Anesthesiologists Closed Claims Project: what have we learned, how has it affected practice, and how will it affect practice in the future? *Anesthesiology*. 1999;91:552–556.

116. Brown DL, Ransom DM, Hall JA, Leicht CH, Schroeder DR, Offord KP. Regional anesthesia and local anesthetic-induced systemic toxicity: seizure frequency and accompanying cardiovascular changes. *Anesth Analg*. 1995;81:321–328.

117. D'Alessio JG, Weller RS, Rosenblum M. Activation of the Bezold-Jarisch reflex in the sitting position for shoulder arthroscopy using interscalene block. *Anesth Analg*. 1995;80:1158–1162.

118. Pihlajamaki KK. Inverse correlation between the peak venous serum concentration of bupivacaine and the weight of the patient during interscalene brachial plexus block. *Br J Anaesth*. 1991;67:621–632.

119. Palve H, Kirvela O, Olin H, Syvalahti E, Kanto J. Maximum recommended doses of lignocaine are not toxic. *Br J Anaesth*. 1995;74:704–705.

120. Reynolds F. Maximum recommended doses of local anesthetics: a constant cause of confusion. *Reg Anesth Pain Med*. 2005;30:314–316.

121. Vanderpool S, Steele SM, Nielsen KC, Tucker M, Klein SM. Combined lumbar plexus and sciatic nerve blocks: an analysis of plasma ropivacaine concentrations. *Reg Anesth Pain Med*. 2006;31:417–421.

122. Urmey WF, Stanton J, Sharrock NE. Interscalene block: effects of dose, volume, and mepivacaine concentration on anesthesia and plasma levels. *Reg Anesth*. 1994;19:34.

123. Scott DB. "Maximum recommended doses" of local anaesthetic drugs. *Br J Anaesth*. 1989;63:373–374.

124. Robinson C, Ray DC, McKeown DW, Buchan AS. Effect of adrenaline on plasma concentrations of bupivacaine following lower limb nerve block. *Br J Anaesth*. 1991;66:228–231.

125. Moore DC, Mather LE, Bridenbaugh LD, Balfour RI, Lysons DF, Horton WG. Arterial and venous plasma levels of bupivacaine following peripheral nerve blocks. *Anesth Analg*. 1976;55:763–768.

126. Hahn MB, McQuillan PM, Sheplock GJ, eds. *Regional Anesthesia: An Atlas of Anatomy and Techniques*. St Louis, Mo: Mosby; 1996.

127. Cousins MJ, Bridenbaugh PO, eds. *Neural Blockade in Clinical Anesthesia and Management of Pain*. 2nd ed. Philadelphia, Pa: Lippincott; 1988.

128. Raj PP. *Practical Management of Pain*. 2nd ed. St Louis, Mo: Mosby Year Book; 1992.

129. Misra U, Pridie AK, McClymont C, Bower S. Plasma concentrations of bupivacaine following combined sciatic and femoral 3 in 1 nerve blocks in open knee surgery. *Br J Anaesth*. 1991;66:310–313.

130. Dentz S, D'Ercole F, Edgar R, et al. Safety and efficacy of supplementing interscalene blocks. *Reg Anesth*. 1996;21(suppl 2):22.

131. Munson ES, Gutnick MJ, Wagman IH. Local anesthetic drug-induced seizures in rhesus monkeys. *Anes Analg*. 1970;49(6):986–994.

132. Pitkanen M, Feldman HS, Arthur GR, Covino BG. Chronotropic and inotropic effects of ropivacaine, bupivacaine, and lidocaine in the spontaneously beating and electrically paced isolated, perfused rabbit heart. *Reg Anesth*. 1992;17:183––192.

133. Scott DB, Lee A, Fagan D, Bowler GM, Bloomfield P, Lundh R. Acute toxicity of ropivacaine compared with that of bupivacaine. *Anesth Analg*. 1989;69:563–569.

134. Ruetsch YA, Fattinger KE, Borgeat A. Ropivacaine-induced convulsions and severe cardiac dysrhythmia after sciatic block. *Anesthesiology*. 1999;90:1784–1786.

135. Korman B, Riley RH. Convulsions induced by ropivacaine during interscalene brachial plexus block. *Anesth Analg*. 1997;85:1128–1129.

136. Feldman HS, Arthur GR, Covino BG. Comparative systemic toxicity of convulsant and supraconvulsant doses of intravenous ropivacaine, bupivacaine, and lidocaine in the conscious dog. *Anesth Analg*. 1989;69:794–801.

137. Groban L, Deal DD, Vernon JC, James RL, Butterworth J. Cardiac resuscitation after incremental overdosage with lidocaine, bupivacaine, levobupivacaine, and ropivacaine in anesthetized dogs. *Anesth Analg*. 2001;92:37–43.

138. Feldman HS, Arthur GR, Pitkanen M, Hurley R, Doucette AM, Covino BG. Treatment of acute systemic toxicity after the rapid intravenous injection of ropivacaine and bupivacaine in the conscious dog. *Anesth Analg*. 1991;73:373–384.

139. Berde CB. Toxicity of local anesthetics in children. *J Pediatr*. 1993;122:S14–20.

140. Scott DA, Emanuelsson BM, Mooney PH, Cook RJ, Junestrand C. Pharmacokinetics of long-term ropivacaine infusion for postoperative analgesia. *Anesth Analg*. 1997;85:1322–1330.

141. Wulf H, Winckler K, Maier C, Heinzow B. Pharmacokinetics and protein binding in postoperative epidural analgesia. *Acta Anaesthesiol Scand*. 1988;32:530–534.

142. Ecoffey C, Dubousset AM, Samii K. Epidural bupivacaine in children. *Anesthesiology*. 1986;65:87–90.

143. Berde C. Epidural infusion in children. *Can J Anesth*. 1994;41:555–560.

144. Weinberg GL, Ripper R, Murphy P, et al. Lipid infusion accelerates removal of bupivacaine and recovery from bupivacaine toxicity in the isolated rat heart. *Reg Anesth Pain Med*. 2006;31:296–303.

145. Weinberg G, Ripper R, Feinstein DL, Hoffman W. Lipid emulsion infusion rescues dogs from bupivacaine induced cardiac toxicity. *Reg Anesth Pain Med*. 2003;28:198-202.

146. Weinberg G. Lipid infusion resuscitation for local-anesthetic toxicity. *Anesthesiology*. 2006;105:7–8.

147. Rosenblatt MA, Abel M, Fischer GW, Itzkovich CJ, Eisenkraft JB. Successful use of a 20% lipid-emulsion to resuscitate a patient after a presumed bupivacaine-related cardiac arrest. *Anesthesiology*. 2006;105:217–218.

148. Borgeat A, Ekatodramis G, Kalberer F, Benz C. Acute and nonacute complications associated with interscalene block and shoulder surgery: a prospective study. *Anesthesiology*. 2001;95:875–880.

149. Franco CD, Vieira ZE. 1,001 subclavian perivascular brachial plexus blocks: success with a nerve stimulator. *Reg Anesth Pain Med*. 2000;25:41–46.

150. Lonnqvist PA, MacKenzie J, Soni AK, Conacher ID. Paravertebral blockade-failure rate and complications. *Anaesthesia.* 1995;50:813–815.

151. Stan TC, Krantz MA, Solomon DL, Poulos JG, Chaouki K. The incidence of neurovascular complications following axillary brachial plexus block using a transarterial approach. *Reg Anesth.* 1995; 20:486–492.

152. Cheney FW, Domino KB, Caplan RA, Posner KL. Nerve injury associated with anesthesia: a closed claims analysis. *Anesthesiology.* 1999;90:1062–1069.

153. Bergman BD, Hebl JR, Kent J, Horlocker TT. Neurologic complications of 405 consecutive continuous axillary catheters. *Anesth Analg.* 2003;96:247–252.

154. Stark RH. Neurologic injury from axillary block anesthesia. *J Hand Surg.* 1996;21:391–396.

155. Selander D. Peripheral nerve injury caused by injection needles. *Br J Anaesth.* 1993;71:323–325.

156. Selander D, Edshage S, Wolff T. Paresthesiae or no paresthesiae? Nerve lesions after axillary blocks. *Acta Anaesth Scand.* 1979;23:27–33.

157. Partridge BL. The effects of local anesthetics and epinephrine on rat sciatic nerve blood flow. *Anesthesiology.* 1991;75:243–250.

158. Robaux S, Bouaziz H, Boisseau N, et al. Persistent phrenic nerve paralysis following interscalene brachial plexus block. *Anesthesiology.* 2001;95:1519–1521.

159. Thiagarajah S, Lear E, Azar I, Salzer J, Zeiligsohn E. Bronchospasm following interscalene brachial plexus block. *Anesthesiology.* 1984;61:759–761.

160. Malchow R, Aikele S. Spread of single and multiple injections in the paravertebral space. *Eur J Anesth.* 2007;24(suppl 39):90.

161. Horlocker T. Regional anesthesia and anticoagulation: are the benefits worth the risks? In: Chaney M, ed. *Regional Anesthesia for Cardiothoracic Surgery.* Philadelphia, Pa: Lippincott Williams and Wilkins; 2002: 139–162. Society of Cardiovascular Anesthesiologists Monograph.

162. Rao TL, El-Etr AA. Anticoagulation following placement of epidural and subarachnoid catheters: an evaluation of neurologic sequelae. *Anesthesiology.* 1981;55:618–620.

163. Klein SM, D'Ercole F, Greengrass RA, Warner DS. Enoxaparin associated with psoas hematoma and lumbar plexopathy after lumbar plexus block. *Anesthesiology.* 1997;87:1576–1579.

164. Malchow R, Chief, Regional Anesthesia and Acute Pain Management, Brooke Army Medical Center; Kaderbek E, Air Force Anesthesiology Resident, Brooke Army Medical Center; Tristan L, Air Force Anesthesiology Resident, Brooke Army Medical Center. Unpublished data from Acute Pain Service, Brooke Army Medical Center, Fort Sam Houston, Texas. 2005.

165. Birbaumer N, Lutzenberger W, Montoya P, et al. Effects of regional anesthesia on phantom limb pain are mirrored in changes in cortical reorganization. *J Neurosci.* 1997;17:5503–5508.

166. Bach S, Noreng MF, Tjellden NU. Phantom limb pain in amputees during the first 12 months following limb amputation, after preoperative lumbar epidural blockade. *Pain.* 1988;33:297–301.

167. Jahangiri M, Jayatunga AP, Bradley JW, Dark CH. Prevention of phantom pain after major lower limb amputation by epidural infusion of diamorphine, clonidine and bupivicaine. *Ann R Coll Surg Engl.* 1994;76:324–326.

168. Katsuly-Liapis I. Pre-emptive extradural analgesia reduces the incidence of phantom pain in lower limb amputees. *Br J Anaesth.* 1996;76(suppl 2):A401.

Care of the Combat Amputee

169.   Nikolajsen L, Ilkjaer S, Christensen JK, Kroner K, Jensen TS. Randomised trial of epidural bupivicaine and morphine in prevention of stump and phantom pain in lower-limb amputation. *Lancet*. 1997;350:1353–1357.

170.   Lambert AW. Randomized prospective study comparing preoperative epidural and intraoperative perineural analgesia for the prevention of postoperative stump and phantom limb pain following major amputation. *Reg Anesth Pain Med*. 2001;26:316–321.

171.   Fisher A, Meller Y. Continuous postoperative regional analgesia by nerve sheath block for amputation surgery—a pilot study. *Anesth Analg*. 1991;72:300–303.

172.   Lierz P, Schroegendorfer K, Choi S, Felleiter P, Kress HG. Continuous blockade of both brachial plexus with ropivicaine in phantom pain: a case report. *Pain*. 1998;78:135–137.

173.   Elizaga AM, Smith DG, Sharar SR, Edwards WT, Hansen ST Jr. Continuous regional analgesia by intraneural block: effect on postoperative opioid requirements and phantom limb pain following amputation. *J Rehabil Res Dev*. 1994;31:179–187.

174.   Pinzur MS, Garla PG, Pluth T, Vrbos L. Continuous postoperative infusion of a regional anesthetic after an amputation of the lower extremity. *J Bone Joint Surg*. 1996;8A:1501–1505.

175.   Kissin I. Preemptive analgesia. *Anesthesiology*. 2000;93:1138–1143.

176.   Kissin I, Lee SS, Bradley EL Jr. Effect of prolonged nerve block on inflammatory hyperalgesia in rats. *Anesthesiology*. 1998;88:224–232.

177.   Sia S, Lepri A, Ponzecchi P. Axillary brachial plexus using peripheral nerve stimulator: a comparison between double- and triple-injection techniques. *Reg Anesth Pain Med*. 2001;26:499–503.

178.   Choyce A, Chan VW, Middleton WJ, Knight PR, Peng P, McCartney CJ. What is the relationship between paresthesia and nerve stimulation for axillary brachial plexus block? *Reg Anesth Pain Med*. 2001;26:100–104.

179.   De Andres J, Sala-Blanch X. Peripheral nerve stimulation in the practice of brachial plexus anesthesia: a review. *Reg Anesth Pain Med*. 2001;26:478–483.

180.   Perlas A, Niazi A, McCartney C, Chan V, Xu D, Abbas S. The sensitivity of motor response to nerve stimulation and paresthesia for nerve localization as evaluated by ultrasound. *Reg Anesth Pain Med*. 2006;31:445–450.

181.   Perlas A, Chan VW, Simons M. Brachial plexus examination and localization using ultrasound and electrical stimulation: a volunteer study. *Anesthesiology*. 2003;99:429–435.

182.   Ganesh A, Cucchiaro G. Multiple simultaneous perineural infusions for postoperative analgesia in adolescents in an outpatient setting. *Br J Anaesth*. 2007;98:687–689.

183.   Laveaux MM, Hasenbos MA, Harbers JB, Liem T. Thoracic epidural bupivacaine plus sufentanil: high concentration/low volume versus low concentration/high volume. *Reg Anesth*. 1993;18:39–43.

184.   de Leon-Casasola OA, Parker B, Lema MJ, Harrison P, Massey J. Postoperative epidural bupivacaine and morphine therapy experience with 4,227 surgical cancer patients. *Anesthesia*. 1994;81:368–375.

185.   Kaneko M, Saito Y, Kirihara Y, Collins JG, Kosaka Y. Synergistic antinociceptive interaction after epidural coadministration of morphine and lidocaine in rats. *Anesthesiology*. 1994;80:137–150.

186.   Mourisse J, Hasenbos MA, Gielen MJ, et al. Epidural bupivacaine, sufentanil, or the combination for post-thoracotomy pain. *Acta Anaesthesiol Scand*. 1992;36:700–704.

187.   Eisenach JC. Epidural and spinal opioids. In: Barash PG, ed. *ASA Refresher Courses in Anesthesiology*. Philadelphia, Pa: JB Lippincott Company; 1993: 65–79.

260

188. Chaplan, SR, Duncan, SR, Brodsky JB, Brose WG. Morphine and hydromorphone epidural analgesia: a prospective, randomized comparison. *Anesthesiology.* 1992;77:1090–1094.

189. Badner NH, Bhandari R, Komar WE. 0.125% bupivacaine is the optimal concentration for continuous postoperative epidural fentanyl analgesia. *Reg Anesth.* 1993;18(2 suppl):27.

190. Snijdelaar DG, Hasenbos MA, van Egmond J, Wolff AP, Liem TH. High thoracic epidural with bupivacaine: continuous infusion of high volume versus low volume. *Anesth Analg.* 1994;78:490–494.

191. McQuay H. Opioids in pain management. *Lancet.* 1999;353:2229–2232.

192. Manchikanti L, Singh V. Managing phantom pain. *Pain Physician.* 2004;7:365–375.

193. Hartrick CT, Bourne MH, Gargiulo K, Damaraju CV, Vallow S, Hewitt DJ. Fentanyl iontophoretic transdermal system for acute pain management after orthopedic surgery: a comparative study with morphine intravenous patient controlled analgesia. *Reg Anesth Pain Med.* 2006;31:546–554.

194. Minkowitz H. Fentanyl iontophoretic transdermal system: a review. *Tech Reg Anesth Pain Mgmt.* 2007;11:3–8.

195. Koppert W, Schmelz M. The impact of opioid-induced hyperalgesia for postoperative pain. *Best Pract Res Clin Anaesthesiol.* 2007;21:65–83.

196. Wu CL, Tella P, Staats PS, et al. Analgesic effects of intravenous lidocaine and morphine on postamputation pain: a randomized double-blind, active placebo-controlled, crossover trial. *Anesthesiology.* 2002;96:841–848.

197. Huse E, Larbig W, Flor H, Birbaumer N. The effects of opioids on phantom limb pain and cortical reorganization. *Pain.* 2001;90:47–55.

198. Hayashida K, Degoes S, Curry R, Eisenach JC. Gabapentin activates spinal noradrenergic activity in rats and humans and reduces hypersensitivity after surgery. *Anesthesiology.* 2007;106:557–562.

199. Dirks J, Fredensborg BB, Christensen D, Fomsgaard JS, Flyger H, Dahl JB. A randomized study of the effects of single-dose gabapentin versus placebo on postoperative pain and morphine consumption after mastectomy. *Anesthesiology.* 2002;97:560–564.

200. Hurley RW, Cohen SP, Williams KA, Rowlingson AJ, Wu CL. The analgesic effects of perioperative gabapentin on postoperative pain: a meta-analysis. *Reg Anesth Pain Med.* 2006;31:237–247.

201. Rowbotham DJ. Gabapentin: a new drug for postoperative pain? *Br J Anaesth.* 2006;96:152–155.

202. Bone M, Critchley P, Buggy DJ. Gabapentin in postamputation phantom limb pain: a randomized, double-blind, placebo-controlled, cross-over study. *Reg Anesth Pain Med.* 2002;27:481–486.

203. Elliott F, Little A, Milbrandt W. Carbamazephine for phantom limb phenomena. *N Engl J Med.* 1976;295:678.

204. Smith DG, Ehde DM, Hanley MA, et al. Efficacy of gabapentin in treating chronic phantom limb and residual limb pain. *J Rehabil Res Dev.* 2005;42:645–654.

205. Nikolajsen L, Finnerup NB, Kramp S, Vimtrup AS, Keller J, Jensen TS. A randomized study of the effects of gabapentin on postamputation pain. *Anesthesiology.* 2006;105:1008–1015.

206. Cohen SP, Christo PJ, Moroz L. Pain management in trauma patients. *Am J Phys Med Rehabil.* 2004;83:142–160.

207. Himmelseher S, Durieux M. Ketamine for perioperative pain management. *Anesthesiology.* 2005;102:211–220.

208. Sveticic G, Gentilini A, Eichenberger U, Luginbuhl M, Curatolo M. Combinations of morphine with ketamine for patient-controlled analgesia. *Anesthesiology.* 2003;98:1195–1205.

209. Bell RF, Dahl JB, Moore RA, Kalso E. Perioperative ketamine for acute postoperative pain. *Cochrane Database Syst Rev.* 2006;1:CD004603.

210. Dertwinkel R, Heinrichs C, Senne I, et al. Prevention of severe phantom limb pain by perioperative administration of ketamine—an observational study. *Acute Pain.* 2002;4:9–13.

211. Nikolajsen L, Hansen CL, Nielsen J, Keller J, Arendt-Nielsen L, Jensen TS. The effect of ketamine on phantom pain: a central neuropathic disorder maintained by peripheral input. *Pain.* 1996;67:69–77.

212. Ben Abraham R, Marouani N, Kollender Y, Meller I, Weinbroum AA. Dextromethorphan for phantom limb pain attenuation in cancer amputees: a double-blind crossover trial involving three patients. *Clin J Pain.* 2002;18:282–285.

213. Wilson JA, Nimmo AF, Fleetwood-Walker SM, Colvin LA. A randomised double blind trial of the effect of pre-emptive epidural ketamine on persistent pain after lower limb amputation. *Pain.* 2008; 135:108–118.

214. Robinson LR, Czerniecki JM, Ehde DM, et al. Trial of amitriptyline for relief of pain in amputees: results of a randomized, controlled study. *Arch Phys Med Rehabil.* 2004;85:1–6.

215. Panerai AE, Monza G, Movilia P, Bianchi M, Francucci BM, Tiengo M. A randomized, within-patient, crossover, placebo-controlled trial on the efficacy and tolerability of the tricyclic antidepressants chlorimipramine and nortriptyline in central pain. *Acta Neurol Scand.* 1990;82:34–38.

216. Remy C, Marrett E, Bonnet F. Effects of acetaminophen on morphine side-effects and consumption after major surgery: meta-analysis of randomized controlled trials. *Br J Anaesth.* 2005;94:505–513.

217. Elia N, Lysakowski C, Tramer MR. Does multimodal analgesia with acetaminophen, nonsteroidal antiinflammatory drugs, or selective cyclooxygenase-2 inhibitors and patient-controlled analgesia morphine offer advantages over morphine alone? Meta-analyses of randomized trials. *Anesthesiology.* 2005;103:1296–1304.

218. Bombardier C, Laine L, Reicin A, et al. Comparison of upper gastrointestinal toxicity of rofecoxib and naproxen in patients with rheumatoid arthritis. VIGOR Study Group. *N Engl J Med.* 2000;343:1520–1528.

219. Levesque LE, Brophy JM, Zhang B. The risk for myocardial infarction with cyclooxygenase-2 inhibitors: a population study of elderly adults. *Ann Int Med.* 2005;142:481–489.

220. Thompson JP, Sharpe P, Kiani S, Owen-Smith O. Effect of meloxicam on postoperative pain after abdominal hysterectomy. *Br J Anaesth.* 2000;84:151–154.

221. Joshi GP. Multimodal analgesia techniques and postoperative rehabilitation. *Anesth Clin North America.* 2005;23:185–202.

222. Reuben SS, Buvanendran A. Preventing the development of chronic pain after orthopaedic surgery with preventive multimodal analgesic therapy. *J Bone Joint Surg Am.* 2007;89:1343–1358.

223. Jaeger H, Maier C. Calcitonin in phantom limb pain: a double-blind study. *Pain.* 1992;48:21–27.

224. Ramachandran VS, Rogers-Ramachandran D. Synaesthesia in phantom limbs induced with mirrors. *Proc Biol Sci.* 1996;263:377–386.

225. Chan BL, Witt R, Charrow A, et al. Mirror therapy for phantom limb pain. *N Engl J Med.* 2007;357:2206–2207.

226. Long DM. Cutaneous afferent stimulation for relief of chronic pain. *Clin Neurosurg.* 1974;21:257–268.

227. Melzack R. Prolonged relief of pain by brief, intense transcutaneous somatic stimulation. *Pain.* 1975;1:357–373.

228. Shealy CN. Transcutaneous electrical stimulation for control of pain. *Clin Neurosurg.* 1974;21:269–277.

229. Winnem MF, Amundsen T. Treatment of phantom limb pain with TENS. *Pain.* 1982;12:299–300.

230. Carabelli RA, Kellerman WC. Phantom limb pain: relief by application of TENS to contralateral extremity. *Arch Phys Med Rehabil.* 1985;66:466–467.

231. Krainick JU, Thoden U, Riechert T. Pain reduction in amputees by long-term spinal cord stimulation: long-term follow-up study over 5 years. *J Neurosurg.* 1980;52:346–350.

232. Krainick JU, Thoden U, Riechert T. Spinal cord stimulation in post-amputation pain. *Surg Neurol.* 1975;4:167–170.

233. Nielson KD, Adams JE, Hosobuchi Y. Phantom limb pain: treatment with dorsal column stimulator. *J Neurosurg.* 1975;42:301–307.

234. Wester K. Dorsal column stimulation in pain treatment. *Acta Neurol Scand.* 1987;75:151–155.

235. Kakazu CZ, Julka I. Stellate ganglion blockade for acute postoperative upper extremity pain. *Anesthesiology.* 2005;102:1288–1289.

236. Wassef MR. Phantom pain with probable reflex sympathetic dystrophy: efficacy of fentanyl infiltration of the stellate ganglion. *Reg Anesth.* 1997;22:287–290.

237. Molloy RE. Diagnostic nerve blocks. In: Benzon HT, Raja SN, Molloy RE, Liu S, Fishman SM, eds. *Essentials of Pain Medicine and Regional Anesthesia.* London, England: Churchill Livingstone; 2005: Chapter 19.

238. Xing G. Acupuncture treatment of phantom limb pain—a report of 9 cases. *J Trad Chin Med.* 1998;18:199–201.

239. Bradbrook D. Acupuncture treatment of phantom limb pain and phantom limb sensation in amputees. *Acupunct Med.* 1997;22:93–97.

240. Henson RA. Henry Head: his influence on the development of ideas on sensation. *Br Med Bull.* 1977;33:91–96.

241. Rossi S, Tecchio F, Pasqualetti P, et al. Somatosensory processing during movement observation in humans. *Clin Neurophysiol.* 2002;113:16–24.

242. Ehde DM, Czerniecki JM, Smith DG, et al. Chronic phantom sensations, phantom pain, residual limb pain, and other regional pain after lower limb amputation. *Arch Phys Med Rehabil.* 2000;81:1039–1044.

243. Smith DG, Ehde DM, Legro MW, Reiber GE, del Aguila M, Boone DA. Phantom limb, residual limb, and back pain after lower extremity amputations. *Clin Orthop Relat Res.* 1999;361:29–38.

244. Friel K, Domholdt E, Smith DG. Physical and functional measures related to low back pain in individuals with lower-limb amputation: an exploratory pilot study. *J Rehabil Res Dev.* 2005;42:155–166.

245. Friberg O. Leg length inequality and low back pain. *Lancet.* 1984;2:1039.

Chapter 12

PSYCHIATRIC INTERVENTION WITH THE ORTHOPAEDICALLY INJURED

HAROLD J. WAIN, PhD[*]; ANDREE BOUTERIE, MD[†]; MARVIN OLESHANSKY, MD[‡]; AND JOHN C. BRADLEY, MD[§]

[*]Chief, Psychiatry Consultation Liaison Service, Department of Psychiatry, Walter Reed Army Medical Center, 6900 Georgia Avenue, NW, Building 2, Room 6238, Washington, DC 20307
[†]Staff Psychiatrist, Psychiatry Consultation Liaison Service, Department of Psychiatry, Walter Reed Army Medical Center, 6900 Georgia Avenue, NW, Building 2, Room 6237, Washington, DC 20307
[‡]Staff Psychiatrist, Department of Psychiatry, Tripler Army Medical Center, 1 Jarrett Hite Road, Honolulu, Hawaii 96859
[§]Colonel, Medical Corps, US Army; Chief, Department of Psychiatry, Walter Reed Army Medical Center, 6900 Georgia Avenue, NW, Building 2, Room 6237, Washington, DC 20307

INTRODUCTION

Injuries that result from disasters, whether natural or human made, have a deleterious impact not only on the injured, but also on their families and caregivers. The psychological trauma of combat may be overwhelming, especially when combined with physical injuries. Freud suggested that trauma is an extraordinary stimulus that disrupts homeostasis and can be too powerful to be worked through in a normal way. Variables contributing to this disruption include the physical injuries, recovery from and long-term adjustment to the injuries, and associated losses and psychiatric sequelae. This is most obvious in the polytrauma patient, who may have orthopaedic injuries combined with other injuries, such as burns; traumatic brain injury (TBI); spinal cord, peripheral nerve, and genital injuries; internal organ damage; poor wound healing; blindness; deafness; or facial disfigurement.

TRAUMA AS A RISK FACTOR FOR PSYCHIATRIC DISORDERS

Morgan et al stated that nearly all survivors exposed to traumatic events briefly exhibit one or more stress-related symptoms.[1] In many instances, these symptoms dissipate within a reasonable period of time. However, O'Donnell et al reported that 20% to 40% of patients followed 1 year after trauma had a psychiatric disorder.[2] Hoge et al reported that 18% to 20% of soldiers met screening criteria for psychiatric diagnoses 3 to 4 months after duty in Iraq, where combat exposure was deemed high.[3] Injury appears to increase the risk of developing psychiatric disorders above that of exposure to combat alone. Koren et al suggested that in the combat-injured, rates of posttraumatic stress disorder (PTSD) are more than 5-fold higher (16.7% vs 2.5%) than in similarly combat-exposed soldiers 15 months following injury.[4] A study by Grieger et al shows that injured soldiers at Walter Reed Army Medical Center (WRAMC) had posttraumatic rates of psychiatric disorders equivalent to rates found in the combat-exposed soldiers in Hoge's study, suggesting that early interventions during the acute medical–surgical care of combat casualties as WRAMC reduces the impact of injury as a risk factor for developing psychiatric sequelae.[3,5]

Although most survivors of trauma will not manifest severe psychiatric disturbances, some appear more susceptible than others. Research demonstrates that low intelligence, low education level, poor vocational endeavors or achievement, absence of social support following the event, and female gender are risk factors for psychiatric sequelae to occur subsequent to trauma.[6] Severity of the traumatic event, prior traumatic exposure, and additional life stressors may also contribute to psychiatric morbidity. Premorbid psychiatric disorders and personality disorders are thought to predispose individuals to posttraumatic psychiatric disorders. Smells, heat, light, sand, the backfiring of a car, and holiday fireworks are just some of the environmental stimuli that can trigger thoughts of past trauma and psychiatric symptomatology.

TRADITIONAL RESPONSES TO COMBAT AND INJURY

Service members have traditional fears as they engage in battle. Psychological responses to combat include the normal fear of injury or death, constant threats of being attacked, and existential worries about life. While in theater, sleep deprivation is an almost universal problem, as is the need for alertness in case of attack and a sense of vulnerability. These behaviors are all components of what is frequently described as the "battle-mind mentality," which may prevail for a long period of time even after a soldier returns home. Upon being injured, a soldier may initially exhibit disbelief (denial), begin prayer (taking a bargaining approach with religion), show anger or rage, and eventually express grief or depression. Emotional reactions resulting from physical injuries may persist even after evacuation to safety. Negative reactions may complicate recovery and rehabilitation and may lead to poor interactions with family members and staff.

Unit cohesion reportedly helps decrease the incidence of PTSD. It is therefore important to consider the impact of removing injured soldiers from their units and understand the importance of finding a strong environmental support structure for them.

Separation anxiety and "survivor guilt" may also play a significant role in a service member's psychological adjustment after an injury. The service member may experience overwhelming guilt for surviving a wartime experience that led to the death of a battle buddy. Survivor guilt may also extend beyond the injured soldier, adversely affecting many of the members within the unit. This may play a role in the subsequent interactions between injured service members and their units and may impact the support they receive. Although most patients deal with feelings of survivor guilt effectively, professional intervention is sometimes necessary to help reframe a patient's perceptions in an appropriate manner. Surviving service members often feel their fallen comrades' families expect to hear comforting words about their loved ones' last moments. Whenever possible, service members are encouraged to attend their colleagues' funerals or military unit reunions because these events are often helpful during the recovery process. Most wounded warriors want to rejoin their former units when they are redeployed and every effort should be made to advocate for this reunion. Service members should be encouraged to let go of grief to maximize their own life potentials and thereby honor the fallen and their sacrifices.

Trauma victims employ various psychological defenses in an attempt to maintain homeostasis. Some of the more common defense mechanisms include dissociation, regression, intellectualization, rationalization, and denial. Dissociation may occur during or subsequent to trauma and is an attempt to delay the impact of the trauma. Regression occurs when a person temporarily reverts to an earlier stage of psychological development. For example, an adult who is hospitalized may become more dependent and act several years younger. In the early stages of hospitalization, dependency can be helpful. It can become pathological, however, if it lasts too long or is too extreme. Intellectualization is a mental mechanism in which the person engages in excessive abstract thinking or extreme reasoning to avoid confronting conflicts or disturbing feelings. Rationalization is a similar defense mechanism in which patients develop elaborate explanations for their behavior that appear logical only to themselves, allowing them to escape anxiety about their actions and continue with the behavior. Denial can also be a healthy defense because it allows patients to distance themselves from the impact of the injury and perhaps decrease the immediate likelihood of being overwhelmed. However, it too can become a hindrance if prolonged.

When psychological defenses are overwhelmed, normal coping mechanisms may become dysfunctional. Generally, psychiatric disorders that emerge soon after injury are best characterized as adjustment disorders or acute stress disorders. More prolonged reactions include various anxiety and depressive disorders, such as generalized anxiety disorder, panic disorder, social phobia, agoraphobia, major depressive disorder, and other mood disorders, which may also be associated with more chronic forms of PTSD. Somatoform disorders and volitional symptoms are also observed in some service members returning from combat. Psychotic disorders are rarely observed in injured service members. Cognitive disorders may result from a comorbid TBI or from postconcussive sequelae.

CONCERNS OF THE SERVICE MEMBER WITH POLYTRAUMA AND LIMB LOSS

Service members who have sustained traumatic injuries, including amputation, present with myriad issues. In addition to physical limitations, they may fear failure, rejection, loss of military careers, and future under-employability. Orthopaedically and neurologically injured service members must also deal with pain and loss of body integrity and function. Psychological responses to this state include the classic symptoms of acute and chronic PTSD, such as emotional numbing, flashbacks, avoidance of reminders of the experience, and hyperarousal. They may express resentment, frustration, helplessness, hopelessness, and self-pity. Body image concerns may also be prominent (eg, one of the earliest concerns of many service members is fear they have sustained physical injury to or loss of their genitals). As recovery progresses, many service members wonder if they are going to be the same men or women that they were before they were injured. Those who are single may focus negatively on the future prospects of dating; all may question whether they will be able to play with children or partake in physical activities, such as athletics, recreational events, hobbies, and, in particular, sexual activities. The latter concern may be exacerbated by the lack of opportunity to test out sexual functioning in the earlier stages of rehabilitation. Later, medication-related problems may decrease libido and impair performance, further increasing these concerns.

Service members who have lost one or more limbs or other body parts experience a host of additional concerns. They often struggle with a severely altered body image, and low self-esteem may ensue. They frequently worry about the impact of further surgical revisions, which may come to be seen as cutting them down in size. They may particularly fear rejection by loved ones and social stigma. Rybarczyk et al showed that a negative body image is correlated with an increase in adjustment problems following amputation.[7] Phantom pain, though troublesome, may later exacerbate psychological sequelae by delaying focus on the emotional trauma.[8,9] Others suggest that phantom pain may have nothing to do with psychological concerns, emphasizing that each individual's needs must be addressed independently.[10]

The loss of a body part is similar to the loss of a loved one and may be associated with a prolonged grieving process. The reintegration of self for the amputee has been described as occurring in three phases. The first phase involves shock, with feelings of cold and numbness; being dazed and confused; and feeling empty.[11] This manifests as the service member feeling overwhelmed and immobilized by daily tasks. The second phase is the period of mourning, in which internal focus leaves little energy for others. In this phase, the service member's internal body image awareness comes in line with external awareness, but the patient still does not give up the past.[12] A prolonged period of mourning may hamper eventual adjustment. Following the mourning phase, an adjustment phase ensues.[13] As the patient deals with the demands of life, present resources and abilities are reorganized. Through a gradual increase in satisfying experiences and newfound competencies, the patient finally emerges with a new sense of self and worth.[14]

FACTORS INTERFERING WITH RECOVERY

There are many factors that interfere with physical and psychological recovery after injury. Lack of support from family, caregivers, and even the general public can be detrimental and can impede recovery. The Department of Defense provides travel and housing allowances to nonmedical attendants who stay with service members during recovery. The nonmedical attendants, who are often family members, can help with activities of daily living, dressing changes, and medication administration. Nonmedical attendants also provide companionship and often serve as advocates for the service member.

Feelings of low self-esteem, loss of wholeness, and fear of the future are common early in the recovery phase for combat-related trauma. Frierson and Lippmann describe social isolation as a common occurrence after amputation that needs to be addressed.[15] Similarly, social discomfort and body image anxiety must be addressed and overcome with appropriate support and therapy.[16] Some amputees may exhibit initial discomfort with their prostheses, which may represent rejection of themselves and their ongoing mourning. It is not uncommon for severely injured service members to believe that their injuries have left them less than human. Additionally, grief and sorrow over their personal loss may be complicated by grief over the loss of combat buddies injured in the same incident. Survivor guilt can contribute to depressive symptoms. Grief and sorrow are often expressed as anger, which may threaten relationships with spouses and families. Anger may eventually lead to emotional withdrawal.

A significant stressor in the orthopaedically injured service member is the need for frequent washouts of the affected limbs. Service members are often apprehensive of these procedures, which usually require general anesthesia and may be associated with significant pain. Service members also fear additional surgeries that may result from poor healing of the affected tissues. A significant number of service members without initial limb loss may ultimately require amputation. Some service members fear losing a limb and plead for its preservation, while others seek elective amputation to minimize pain and shorten recovery and rehabilitation time. Before elective amputation, however, a thorough psychological evaluation is performed to assess capacity, ascertain secondary gain, and address underlying issues. Some injured service members who are hesitant to return to the community or who fear limited access to healthcare upon discharge may seek to prolong their hospital stays. A small number of service members may be motivated to extend their hospital stays because they believe (incorrectly) that will enhance their disability benefits.

It is important that professionals caring for injured service members believe in a positive outcome for their patients because their expectations will be reflected in their interactions and resultant care. However, this may be problematic in situations where the service member is not likely to return to full physical function. Providers must be aware that their verbal and nonverbal interactions are keenly observed by their patients and their patients' families. Providers often feel the need to correct their patients' overly negative and overly positive appraisals for recovery; however, hope and determination are important motivators for recovery and need to be encouraged. Providers should keep in mind that during the initial inpatient hospitalization, it is often too early to understand the full extent of even the most severe injuries and the impact they will have on the service member.

A PSYCHIATRIC APPROACH TO SERVICE MEMBERS WHO HAVE SUSTAINED TRAUMA OR COMBAT-RELATED INJURIES

A major concern in providing mental health care to service members is their reluctance to seek treatment because of a fear of stigmatization.[3] To address this issue at WRAMC, the psychiatric consultation-liaison service developed a preventive medical psychiatry (PMP) service.[9] This service performs, without formal consult, routine initial screening evaluations of every service member admitted to the hospital for medical or surgical sequelae of the global war on terror. The goal of the PMP service is to foster acceptance of mental

---

EXHIBIT 12-1

CASE STUDY 1: AN EXPERIENCE OF THE PREVENTIVE MEDICAL PSYCHIATRY SERVICE

A 36-year-old soldier with a soft tissue injury to right eye, left femur and tibia fractures, and a right below-the-knee amputation responded in a sullen manner to his orthopaedic and physical therapy teams. Upon the initial visit, he denied any psychiatric problems had resulted from the improvised explosive device blast that had resulted in his injuries. He claimed he did not need psychiatric intervention and was concerned that the team referred him. The team reported poor compliance with treatment and disrupted sleep. When the soldier became aware that the psychiatric approach was routine and preventive, he began describing his concerns about his decision-making process while in theater that may have led to his unit receiving the blast it sustained. The preventive medical psychiatry service worked to reframe his experiences while advocating for him. As he accepted the routine of the approach, the soldier began to respond more favorably, appeared to assimilate the intervention, and cooperated more fully with his rehabilitation.

---

health issues and decrease stigmatization, thereby preventing or decreasing chronic disabling psychiatric disorders following trauma.

The approach to psychiatric intervention with injured service members has evolved over the years. The contemporary model of intervention has been developed based on lessons learned from past conflicts and events.[17] For example, after the Pentagon attack on September 11, 2001, WRAMC staff were deployed to local hospitals to meet with injured survivors where, instead of using classic debriefing techniques that had not proven effective in the past, caregivers practiced empathic exposure (see below) and provided ongoing follow-up. Anecdotally, this technique was well perceived by those who were contacted, so the practice was continued with the casualties returning to WRAMC from Iraq and Afghanistan. While it has been reported that prolonged exposure may be a more efficacious treatment than cognitive restructuring for patients with acute stress disorder,[18] the experience of the WRAMC staff has shown that injured service members may not be able to tolerate the stress of more aggressive psychotherapies while dealing with physical loss, pain, and profound life change. Following injury, all means must be taken to help the patient overcome losses and facilitate recovery. Initially, patients must believe the staff is there to protect them from further harm. Care providers should work

to facilitate sleep and rest and reduce physiological arousal and pain. This may be accomplished through medical and surgical means or through pharmacological interventions, hypnotic techniques, and psychological support. Care providers and family members of injured service members must strive to reduce unnecessary stressors.

It is important for caregivers to connect with their patients so patients can see providers as a healthy adjunct to their recovery. At times, patients may only need basic information as to what services or treatment options are available; other times, they may need guidance toward more direct coping strategies, such as distracting themselves and reframing conflicts. Negative appraisals by patients or their families must also be corrected; however, providers must take care to remind patients that although they will not be returned to their premorbid states, they can still achieve their goals and have satisfying lives. As patients join in a therapeutic alliance with their caregivers, they become more open to discussing complex issues, fears, and concerns about the future. This is facilitated with a flexible evaluation and treatment approach. Patient assets and strengths should be recognized and reinforced. The PMP service acts as a patient advocate and serves as a liaison between families and medical and support staff (Exhibit 12-1).

THERAPEUTIC INTERVENTION FOR PREVENTING PSYCHIATRIC STRESS DISORDERS

At WRAMC, the PMP service employs an approach known as the "Therapeutic Intervention for the Prevention of Psychiatric Stress Disorders." This program was developed to address the psychological needs of trauma victims, provide support to the individuals and their families, assess psychiatric status,

provide early intervention (when needed) without stigmatization, and support the medical and surgical staff. The major components of the approach include making mental health a routine part of trauma care, using a biopsychosocial approach to care, developing a strong therapeutic alliance with the patient

EXHIBIT 12-2

CASE STUDY 2: USING REFRAMING AND AFFIRMING TECHNIQUES

Following the blast from an improvised explosive device, the right ankle of a 22-year-old male was severed such that he could not stand to run. He described seeing his driver bleeding from a gunshot wound and he crawled to the driver's side, applied a tourniquet to his fellow soldier, and pulled him to safety. The caregiver focused positively on the soldier's actions, asking how he had the strength to assist the driver and help save his life.

EXHIBIT 12-3

CASE STUDY 3: USE OF EMPATHIC EXPOSURE

Following the blast from an improvised explosive device, a 41-year-old service member with a soft tissue injury to the left eye and bilateral lower extremity fractures was hospitalized with an external fixator on his leg. The patient began having episodic tremors and seizure-like behavior without any explanation (his electroencephalography result was normal). A thorough psychological evaluation also appeared to be normal. After the development of a therapeutic alliance and applying techniques such as hypnosis and pharmacological management of sleep, it was discovered that the noise that was being generated multiple times a day from the patient's external fixator was similar to that created by the blast that had caused his injury; the sound was contributing to his symptom manifestation. As he was empathically exposed to his trauma, his symptoms dissipated.

and family, normalizing the patient's experience and psychological response to the trauma, providing education, using pharmacology and hypnosis when appropriate, providing empathic exposure therapy (see below), treating identified psychiatric symptoms, reinforcing resiliency, and promoting positive coping behaviors. Traditional psychotherapeutic and psychodynamic perspectives are also employed to help conceptualize specific patient problems and find solutions.[19]

Intervention timing is particularly important to the success of the approach. Following trauma, victims are less likely to attend to internal psychological distress until they are medically stabilized. Maslow described a hierarchy of needs, with a specific time and place for all interventions.[20] He suggested that patients' physiological needs have to be met first, followed by their needs for safety, belongingness, esteem, and self-actualization. Ultimately, therapy for resilience is ineffective while the patient is struggling for life or feels unsafe.

Horvath and Symonds found that the therapeutic alliance is meaningfully correlated with treatment outcomes,[21] and Crits-Christoph et al found the therapeutic alliance is important in developing interactions that repair problematic ones.[22] Marmar et al reported that addressing feelings leads to positive outcomes only after the therapeutic alliance has been established.[23]

Therapeutic alliances with injured service members are used to help the injured process their ordeals through empathic exposure therapy. During this therapy, service members are usually seen for 15 to 20 minutes several times per week. They are asked to reflect on their traumatic experiences, with the suggestion that talking about them at the present will be helpful in the future. Empathic exposure allows patients to normalize their experiences and consolidate them in their memory, and may help them integrate the past trauma into a normal stream of consciousness. Providers are trained to offer rapid empathic responses to the patient's recall of the trauma and injury. Caregivers avoid confrontational approaches and instead employ nonthreatening techniques, responding in ways that emphasize patients' positive assets, such as, "How did you know to do that?" and "Where did you learn that?" Clinicians are encouraged to display acceptance, respect, empathy, warmth, advice, praise, affirmation, and a sense of hope while working with these patients. It is critical that providers are viewed as genuine in their concern and support of the patient while encouraging patients to elaborate on reactions relevant to the trauma and offering empathic validation (Exhibits 12-2 and 12-3).

PHARMACOLOGY AND OTHER TREATMENT INTERVENTIONS FOR ANXIETY, DEPRESSION, AND PAIN

In addition to the psychotherapeutic interventions discussed above, medications can be used to address patient needs and psychiatric symptoms. Although it is beyond the scope of this chapter to present a detailed medication or other treatment approach to combat-trauma–injured patients, an overview of symptoms and disorders most frequently encountered and general treatment approaches are discussed below.

In order to address the combat-injured patient's most urgent needs and to provide comfort (barring frank delirium), the primary focus should be on encouraging sleep, controlling pain, and alleviating anxiety symptoms, which most prominently present in the form of nightmares, hyperarousal, intrusive thoughts, and flashbacks. Before recommending medication, it is important to consider the patient's underlying medical condition, current medications, and allergies. Potential interactions should be reviewed because most psychoactive medications have the propensity to interact with other medications and antibiotics. Sleeping agents are recommended as needed, according to the patient's preference and medical situation. Hypnotic agents, such as zolpidem, may be helpful for problems with sleep initiation, but may not be as efficacious for problems with sleep maintenance, early morning wakefulness, or nightmares. Sedating antidepressants, such as trazodone and mirtazapine (both of which are fairly well tolerated, have few medication interactions, and may help address comorbid anxiety or depressive symptoms), are frequently used. Atypical antipsychotics have also been successfully employed to treat sleep disturbances with nightmares, and may be indicated in the presence of flashbacks or disorientation and emotional dysregulation due to multiple or high doses of pain medications or other medical issues. Quetiapine is used in low doses (25–75 mg) to capitalize on its sedative properties in this dose range and to minimize potential, although rare, adverse side effects. In this dose range, quetiapine appears to work largely by blocking histamine receptors, an action that has been associated with a decrease in the rapid eye movement stage of sleep. Prazosin has also proven effective for reducing nightmares in outpatients with PTSD,[24] but has not been studied in the inpatient polytrauma setting, in part because of concern over its cardiovascular effects.

Pain control is an important consideration for patients in all stages of recovery, but is particularly important in the earlier stages of treatment because proper management can set the stage for future adequate responses. Conversely, poor pain control may heighten a patient's anticipatory anxiety for all procedures, interfere with sleep, and may eventually lead to problems with chronic pain. The psychiatric consultation-liaison service at WRAMC works closely with the medical, surgical, and pain services to achieve maximum patient comfort. Hypnotic techniques are frequently employed to help in this area.

More specific treatments for anxiety and depression depend on the associated disorder (if present), the severity of symptoms, and the patient's stage of medical recovery. Early during the course of medical treatment, anxiety may be associated with delirium because of the underlying medical condition, in which case a neuroleptic medication may be used to address anxiety, agitation, and disorientation. As the patient stabilizes, anxiety symptoms tend to ameliorate or consolidate into more recognizable disorders. As the service member physically heals and develops more cognitive reserve, more standardized treatment strategies may be used for the particular disorder identified (eg, more formalized cognitive behavioral therapy for anxiety or depression). Service members may then participate in supportive group or psychodynamic therapy, particularly if more developmental and interpersonal concerns appear to be impacting the current condition.

Selective serotonin reuptake inhibitors remain the medications of first choice to treat PTSD[25] and depression. Of these, sertraline and citalopram are generally preferred because of their tolerability and relatively decreased potential for drug-to-drug interactions. Benzodiazepines are generally avoided where possible, particularly in PTSD, because data that supports their use is lacking and they may result in addiction and worsen PTSD in the long term.[1] However, benzodiazepines are occasionally used to temporarily relieve severe anxiety and panic attacks. Patients are frequently already prescribed benzodiazepines for conditions such as muscle spasms or phantom limb pain. In this case, patients should be educated on the impact benzodiazepines have on anxiety, and the effects should be monitored. Treatment for persistent conditions may ultimately extend beyond the period of hospitalization.

HYPNOSIS

Absorption, focused attention, decreased vigilance, suggestion, dissociation, trance logic, rapid data assimilation, and time distortion are all components of hypnosis.[26] Patients often tend to be self-absorbed and focused on their somatic complaints in the presence of medical or surgical illness, and many psychologically healthy individuals may have a hypnotic gift.[27] These individuals can constructively employ dissociation to distract themselves from physical and emotional trauma. When appropriate, they can weave dissociative elements into a normal stream of consciousness. By capitalizing on the rapid assimilation of data, they can also learn new techniques at a faster pace. Hypnotic techniques that guide constructive thought processes help individuals cope with pain, insomnia, and injuries by allowing them to distance themselves from their treatment, feel safe, rapidly learn new coping techniques, and become productively engaged in the healing process.[28–30] Experience at WRAMC has shown that service members can use hypnosis to control pain from surgery, wounds, washouts, burns, and phantom sensations, as well as to assist with medication augmentation. Hypnosis can provide a safe place for patients to work through or restructure their emotional conflicts (Exhibit 12-4).

EXHIBIT 12-4

CASE STUDY 4: USE OF HYPNOSIS IN TREATING PHANTOM LIMB PAIN

A 28-year-old male with a left below-the-knee amputation complained of phantom limb pain, which was described as the painful curling of his missing toes. He was taught to envision relaxing his foot and uncurling his toes. Using this hypnotic technique, he was able to reduce pain from an 8 to a 0 on a 10-point pain scale.

TRAUMATIC BRAIN INJURY ASSOCIATED WITH POLYTRAUMA AND AMPUTATION

Approximately one third of the service members injured in Iraq who require medical evacuation to WRAMC have been found to have TBI. Of these, about 50% are classified as having mild TBI, with the remaining half having moderate or severe TBI. Most TBIs occur with polytrauma and are common in service members with traumatic amputations. All service members with an injury history that may be associated with TBI (eg, blast exposures, motor vehicle accidents, falls, etc) are screened during the initial phase of their hospitalization by a specialized team from the Defense Veterans Brain Injury Center (this screen is in addition to the routine screening performed by the PMP service). A multidisciplinary team from the departments of neurology, neuropsychology, physical medicine and rehabilitation, psychiatry, physical therapy, occupational therapy, and speech language pathology provides ongoing assessment and treatment of these patients.

The PMP service provides clinical assessment of TBI and treats associated behavioral sequelae. This begins in the intensive care unit (ICU) for more severely injured service members, who generally arrive at WRAMC on ventilator support. In addition to the common problems of disorientation and frank delirium seen in patients with polytrauma as they are weaned from sedation, patients with TBI take considerably longer to become alert, are often agitated and disorganized, and are generally less able to participate in their own care. Families of service members with TBI are provided support and made aware that the prognosis for moderate to severe TBI is hard to predict and may be frightening and upsetting. In addition, staff members treating patients with more severe TBI can be nihilistic—a disposition that needs to be addressed by the consultation-liaison psychiatrist. Treatment of delirium and agitation often involves modifying the intravenous pain regimen, minimizing external stimulation, adding neuroleptic medication,

and, when other modalities fail, restraining the patient. Symptoms of hyperarousal, such as sleep disturbances, nightmares, and flashbacks, are common in service members in the ICU, and they can be worse with existing TBI. Preemptive treatment of hyperarousal with low-dose, atypical neuroleptics has proven to be especially effective in improving sleep and decreasing nightmares and flashbacks.

TBI in amputees often complicates rehabilitation. Significant deficits in cognition, memory, and awareness may preclude prosthetic fitting and training. Additionally, patients with TBI may manifest problems with impulse control. Their disinhibition and impulsivity may interfere with their care as well as disrupt others in treatment. Similarly, problems with mood and emotional regulation can manifest as anxiety, depression, and emotional liability and can complicate recovery. Behavioral problems, including apathy, lack of motivation, dependency, and passive childlike behavior, are also commonly seen in this patient population. Somatic symptoms, such as sleep disturbances, fatigue, slowness, dizziness, headaches, and noise sensitivity, are likely to be magnified in patients with TBI.

Because of the magnitude of complications associated with TBI and their disruption of amputee rehabilitation, service members with significant cognitive, emotional, or behavioral problems related to TBI are best managed in a TBI center of excellence, such as those that have been established in the Veterans Affairs polytrauma centers. For this reason, nearly all service members with severe TBI are rapidly transferred from the military healthcare system to a Veterans Affairs polytrauma center. Once brain injury has recovered to the point where the patient can begin learning new tasks and attend therapy training, those with amputation are typically returned to one of the Department of Defense amputee centers of excellence for amputee-specific rehabilitation.

TREATING THE TRAUMA PATIENT'S FAMILY

Initially, it is important that the families of injured service members have access to food, clothing, and shelter. Many spouses of injured service members communicate a sense of hopelessness and helplessness in the face of their loved one's injuries. They worry about lack of information, support, and control in the injured service member's care and rehabilitation. This experience may be very traumatic.[31–34] It is also often difficult for families to absorb the amount of information presented to them from the multiple healthcare providers treating their loved one. Uncertainty within the healthcare team adds to the family members' feelings of anxiety and helplessness.[35] Conflicts between family members may cause some members to be unwilling to share information with others, exacerbating the challenges of information exchange. It is difficult to predict how family members will react to the injuries sustained by the service member or to the "trauma" with which they themselves are faced. Helping these families cope with the traumatic event may lessen their chances of developing secondary PTSD.[33] Family members are often better than the medical staff at providing emotional support and reassurance to trauma patients.[32]

Preexisting conflicts between family members or between the injured service member and the family may be exaggerated with the added stress of the injury. At times, having a severely injured family member may exacerbate family malfunctioning,[35] and the family's built-in support system may need to be augmented with professional help.[33] Effective therapeutic family interventions may not only help family members cope with the traumatic events, but may help the patient as well. Support group therapy sessions can help the families of trauma victims address their needs and feelings.[36] Harvey at al found that families were more willing to attend group therapy sessions when the focus was on education and families sharing their stories with one another.[36] Families attending these support groups realized that they were not alone and were able to offer support to each other. They were able to share their

---

EXHIBIT 12-5

CASE STUDY 5: FAMILY INTERVENTION

A 28-year-old male with a right above-the-knee amputation and left below-the-knee amputation was injured in Afghanistan. The patient was flown to Germany, where his wife and mother met him. His wife began having difficulty adjusting to his injury. Problems with her and her in-laws were prominent. The patient's wife and mother frequently argued about what care was appropriate for the patient, causing more stress for the family, service member, and medical staff. The service member's mother was particularly angry that her daughter-in-law of 1 year was taking charge of her son, whom she had raised by herself since he was 5 years old. Upon arrival at Walter Reed Army Medical Center, the family and patient were assessed by the preventive medical psychiatry team and interventions were initiated. The problems were eventually resolved and continued therapy was established upon hospital discharge.

---

feelings, reduce their anxiety, garner hope, and gain a better understanding of their family member's injuries, medical treatments, and hospital procedures. Many support groups are run by social workers and allow for empathetic sharing and support. Session topics may include issues such as fear, frustration, the need to protect the injured patient, depression, anger, education, coping with disabled spouses, and feelings of alienation and disappointment. The purpose of family intervention is to build up the family's coping skills and resolve symptoms associated with psychological trauma. Further activities, such as sharing meals with other families of trauma patients, may provide the family with additional support.[33] Brief supportive counseling has also proven effective at reducing anxiety in individual family members of trauma victims (Exhibit 12-5).[37]

FOLLOW-UP

The PMP service continues to support those who need help and attempts to reach out to those screened as inpatients. At discharge, each patient is given a contact number and is encouraged to call the PMP service office if concerns develop. The PMP service at WRAMC calls patients at 30, 90, and 180 days following discharge. If crises occur, patients appear more willing to accept referral recommendations from behavioral health providers they have known previously or whom they perceive as allies. Additionally, they may find it easier to receive and respond to psychiatric interventions once they have returned home. In general, patients who need treatment upon leaving WRAMC are referred to resources within the military, Veterans Health System, or civilian community.

SUMMARY

The impact of a traumatic event resulting in physical injuries frequently extends beyond the bodily disruptions sustained by the victim to encompass the psychological realm. Although medical trauma teams are designed to respond to physical injuries, equal emphasis needs to be placed on the mental health interventions necessary to assist these victims and their families. The WRAMC PMP service is the first mental health service to see every hospitalized, traumatically injured patient without a formal consult. This approach appears to have reduced the need for emergent psychiatric services in this population.

REFERENCES

1. Morgan CA, Krystal JH, Southwick SM. Toward early pharmacological posttraumatic stress intervention. *Biol Psychiatry*. 2003;53(9):834–843.

2. O'Donnell ML, Creamer M, Pattison P, Atkin C. Psychiatric morbidity following injury. *Am J Psychiatry*. 2004;161:507–514.

3. Hoge CW, Castro CA, Messer SC, McGurk D, Cotting DI, Koffman RL. Combat duty in Iraq and Afghanistan, mental health problems, and barriers to care. *N Engl J Med*. 2004;351:13–21.

4. Koren D, Norman D, Cohen A, Berman J, Klein EM. Increased PTSD risk with combat-related injury: a matched comparison study of injured and uninjured soldiers experiencing the same combat events. *Am J Psychiatry*. 2005;162(2):276–282.

5. Grieger TA, Cozza SJ, Ursano RJ, et al. Posttraumatic stress disorder and depression in battle-injured soldiers. *Am J Psychiatry*. 2006;163:1777–1783.

6. Brewin CR, Andrews B, Valentine JD. Meta-analysis of risk factors for posttraumatic stress disorder in trauma-exposed adults. *J Consult Clin Psychol*. 2000;68(5):748–766.

7. Rybarczyk B, Nyenhuis DL, Nicholas JJ, Cash SM, Kaiser J. Body image, perceived social stigma, and the prediction of psychosocial adjustment to leg amputation. *Rehabil Psychol*. 1995;40(2):95–110.

8. Lundberg SG, Guggenheim FG. Sequelae of limb amputation. *Adv Psychosom Med*. 1986;15:199–210.

9. Wain HJ, Grammer G, Stasinos J. Psychiatric intervention for medical and surgical patients following traumatic injuries. In: Ritchie EC, Watson PJ, Friedman MJ, eds. *Interventions Following Mass Violence and Natural Disasters: Strategies for Mental Health Practice*. New York, NY: The Guilford Press; 2007: 278–298.

10. Katz J. Reality of phantom limbs. *Motiv Emot*. 1993;17:147–179.

11. Shontz FC, Fink S. A method for evaluating psychosocial adjustment of the chronically ill. *Am J Phys Med*. 1961;40:63–69.

12. Parkes CM. *Bereavement: Studies of Grief in Adult Life*. New York, NY: International Universities Press; 1972.

13. Lazarus RS. *Psychological Stress and Coping Process*. New York, NY: McGraw-Hill; 1966.

14. Katz S, Florian V. A comprehensive theoretical model of psychological reaction to loss. *Int J Psychiatry Med*. 1986–1987;16(4):325–345.

15. Frierson RL, Lippman SR. *The Psychological Rehabilitation of the Amputee*. Chicago, Ill: Charles Thomas; 1978.

16. Horgan O, MacLachlan M. Psychosocial adjustment to lower-limb amputation: a review. *Disabil Rehabil*. 2004;26:837–850.

17. Wain HJ, Grammer GG, Stasinos JJ, Miller CM. Meeting the patients where they are: consultation-liaison response to trauma victims of the Pentagon attack. *Mil Med*. 2002;167(Suppl 9):19–21.

18. Bryant RA, Mastrodomenico J, Felmingham KL, et al. Treatment of acute stress disorder: a randomized controlled trial. *Arch Gen Psychiatry*. 2008;65(6):659–667.

19. Wain HJ, Gabriel G. Psychodynamic concepts inherent in a biopsychosocial model of care of traumatic injuries. *J Am Acad Psychoanal Dyn Psychiatry.* 2007;35(4):555–573.

20. Maslow AH. *Toward a Psychology of Being.* 2nd ed. Princeton, NJ: Van Nostrand; 1968.

21. Horvath A, Symonds V. Relation between working alliance and outcome in psychotherapy: the meta-analysis. *J Couns Psychol.* 1991;38:139–149.

22. Crits-Christoph P, Barber J, Kurcias J. The accuracy of therapists' interpretations and the development of the therapeutic alliance. *Psychother Res.* 1993;3:25–35.

23. Marmar CR, Weiss DS, Gaston L. Toward the validation of the California Therapeutic Alliance Rating System. *Psychol Assess.* 1989;1:46–52.

24. Raskind MA, Peskind ER, Kanter ED, et al. Reduction of nightmares and other PTSD symptoms in combat veterans by prazosin: a placebo-controlled study. *Am J Psychiatry.* 2003;160:371–373.

25. Davidson JR, Rothbaum BO, van der Kolk BA, Sikes CR, Farfel GM. Multicenter, double-blind comparison of sertraline and placebo in the treatment of posttraumatic stress disorder. *Arch Gen Psychiatry.* 2001;58:485–492.

26. Wain HJ. Medical hypnosis in medical psychiatric practice. In: Stoudemire A, Fogel BS, eds. *Medical Psychiatric Practice.* Vol 2. Washington, DC: American Psychiatric Press; 1993; 39–66.

27. Wain HJ. Hypnosis on a consultation-liaison service. *Psychosomatics.* 1979;20:678–689.

28. Beshai JA. Toward a phenomenology of trance logic in posttraumatic stress disorder. *Psychol Rep.* 2004;94:649–654.

29. Patterson DR, Jensen MP. Hypnosis and clinical pain. *Psychol Bull.* 2003;129(4):495–521.

30. Spiegel D, Spiegel H. Hypnosis in psychosomatic medicine. *Psychosomatics.* 1980;21:35–41.

31. Solursh DS. The family of the trauma victim. *Nurs Clin North Am.* 1990;25:155–162.

32. Brown V. The family as victim in trauma. *Hawaii Med J.* 1991;50(4):153–154.

33. Flannery RB Jr. Treating family survivors of mass casualties: a CISM family crisis intervention approach. *Int J Emerg Ment Health.* 1999;1:243–250.

34. Alexander DA. The psychiatric consequences of trauma. *Hosp Med.* 2002;63:12–15.

35. Landsman IS, Baum CG, Arnkoff DB, et al. The psychosocial consequences of traumatic injury. *J Behav Med.* 1990;13(6):561–581.

36. Harvey C, Dixon M, Padberg N. Support group for families of trauma patients: a unique approach. *Crit Care Nurse.* 1995;15(4):59–63.

37. Lenehan GP. Emotional impact of trauma. *Nurs Clin North Am.* 1986;21(4):729–740.

Chapter 13

REHABILITATION OF BURN CASUALTIES

TRAVIS L. HEDMAN, PT[*]; CHARLES D. QUICK, OTR/L[†]; REGINALD L. RICHARD, MS, PT[‡]; EVAN M. RENZ, MD[§]; STEVEN V. FISHER, MD[¥]; ELIZABETH A. RIVERS, OTR, RN[¶]; JAMES C. CASEY, MOT, OTR/L[**]; KEVIN K. CHUNG, MD[††]; PETER A. DESOCIO, DO[‡‡]; WILLIAM S. DEWEY, PT, CHT, OCS[§§]; JAIME L. DROOK, OTR/L[¥¥]; NICOLE J. LEHNERZ, OTR/L[¶¶]; CHRISTOPHER V. MAANI, MD[***]; ALFREDO E. MONTALVO, MSN, BSN, APN[†††]; BETH A. SHIELDS, RD, LD, CNSD, MS[‡‡‡]; MELISSA Z. SMITH, MOT, OTR/L[§§§]; CHARLES K. THOMPSON, PA-C[¥¥¥]; ALICIA F. WHITE, PT, DPT[¶¶¶]; JAMES F. WILLIAMS, PA-C, MPAS[****]; AND ALAN W. YOUNG, DO[††††]

Captain, US Army, Medical Corps; Chief, Burn Rehabilitation Department, US Army Burn Center, US Army Institute of Surgical Research, 3400 Rawley E. Chambers Avenue, Fort Sam Houston, Texas 78234

†*Major, US Army, Medical Corps; Chief, Occupational Therapy Service, Burn Rehabilitation Department, US Army Burn Center, US Army Institute of Surgical Research, 3400 Rawley E. Chambers Avenue, Fort Sam Houston, Texas 78234*

‡*Clinical Research Coordinator, Burn Rehabilitation Department, US Army Burn Center, US Army Institute of Surgical Research, 3400 Rawley E. Chambers Avenue, Fort Sam Houston, Texas 78234*

§*Lieutenant Colonel, US Army, Medical Corps; Director, US Army Burn Center, US Army Institute of Surgical Research, 3400 Rawley E. Chambers Avenue, Fort Sam Houston, Texas 78234*

¥*Chief, Department of Physical Medicine and Rehabilitation, Hennepin County Medical Center, Minneapolis, MN 55415; Associate Professor, Department of Physical Medicine and Rehabilitation, University of Minnesota Medical School*

¶*Burn Rehabilitation Specialist (Retired), Burn Center, Regions Hospital, formerly known as St. Paul Ramsey Medical Center, 640 Jackson Street, St. Paul, Minnesota 55101*

**Occupational Therapist, Burn Rehabilitation Department, US Army Burn Center, US Army Institute of Surgical Research, 3400 Rawley E. Chambers Avenue, Fort Sam Houston, Texas 78234*

††*Major, US Army, Medical Corps; Medical Intensivist, US Army Burn Center, US Army Institute of Surgical Research, 3400 Rawley E. Chambers Avenue, Fort Sam Houston, Texas 78234*

‡‡*Captain, US Army, Medical Corps; Anesthesiologist, US Army Burn Center, US Army Institute of Surgical Research, 3400 Rawley E. Chambers Avenue, Fort Sam Houston, Texas 78234*

§§*Occupational Therapist, Burn Rehabilitation Department, US Army Burn Center, US Army Institute of Surgical Research, 3400 Rawley E. Chambers Avenue, Fort Sam Houston, Texas 78234*

¥¥*Occupational Therapist, Burn Rehabilitation Department, US Army Burn Center, US Army Institute of Surgical Research, 3400 Rawley E. Chambers Avenue, Fort Sam Houston, Texas 78234*

¶¶*Occupational Therapist, Burn Rehabilitation Department, US Army Burn Center, US Army Institute of Surgical Research, 3400 Rawley E. Chambers Avenue, Fort Sam Houston, Texas 78234*

***Major, US Army, Medical Corps; Chief, Anesthesiology, US Army Burn Center, US Army Institute of Surgical Research, 3400 Rawley E. Chambers Avenue, Fort Sam Houston, Texas 78234*

†††*Lieutenant Colonel, US Army, Medical Corps; Psychiatric Clinical Nurse Specialist, US Army Burn Center, US Army Institute of Surgical Research, 3400 Rawley E. Chambers Avenue, Fort Sam Houston, Texas 78234*

‡‡‡*Dietitian, US Army Burn Center, US Army Institute of Surgical Research, 3400 Rawley East Chambers Avenue, Fort Sam Houston, Texas 78234*

§§§*Occupational Therapist, Burn Rehabilitation Department, US Army Burn Center, US Army Institute of Surgical Research, 3400 Rawley E. Chambers Avenue, Fort Sam Houston, Texas 78234*

¥¥¥*Physician Assistant, US Army Burn Center, US Army Institute of Surgical Research, 3400 Rawley E. Chambers Avenue, Fort Sam Houston, Texas 78234*

¶¶¶*Physical Therapist, Burn Rehabilitation Department, US Army Burn Center, US Army Institute of Surgical Research, 3400 Rawley E. Chambers Avenue, Fort Sam Houston, Texas 78234*

****Physician Assistant, US Army Burn Center, US Army Institute of Surgical Research, 3400 Rawley E. Chambers Avenue, Fort Sam Houston, Texas 78234*

††††*Physiatrist, Burn Rehabilitation Department, US Army Burn Center, US Army Institute of Surgical Research, 3400 Rawley E. Chambers Avenue, Fort Sam Houston, Texas 78234*

INTRODUCTION

Rehabilitation is critical to the long-term survival of the burn casualty.[1] For the most favorable outcomes to occur, endurance, active range of motion (AROM), fine motor dexterity, coordination, and psychosocial and community reintegration must be achieved, and strength must be integrated into purposeful activity. After a major burn injury, casualties depend on a comprehensive, interdisciplinary rehabilitation treatment plan designed to expeditiously recover their premorbid level of independence, the end goal being return to duty and other activities with maximum functional independence.[1] Additional rehabilitative interventions implemented along the continuum of care help minimize edema and infection, promoting durable, soft, supple, flat, properly colored, and pain-free wound coverage.

Following stabilization from an acute burn injury, battlefield casualties are rapidly evacuated from the theater of operations to the burn center at the US Army's Institute of Surgical Research (USAISR) at Fort Sam Houston, Texas. The establishment of comprehensive burn centers and advancements in treatment have resulted in a significant decline in burn injury mortality.[2] The LD_{50}, or total-body surface area (TBSA) burned that is lethal to 50% of casualties, has improved dramatically, from 65% in 1984 to over 81% in the early 1990s (Figure 13-1).[3] This improvement in survival, combined with efforts to improve long-term

function, is the clinical focus of burn centers.[4]

The healing process is impeded by battlefield and regional conditions (eg, extremes of climate and contaminated environments), dehydration, inadequate nutrition, psychological and physiological stressors, and burn pain. Managing and recovering from a burn is a demanding material and human resource endeavor. Casualties with serious burns stress the assets available to deployed combat support hospitals in a theater of operations.[5]

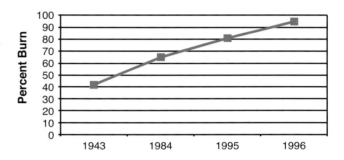

Figure 13-1. Graph of burn patient mortality.
Data source: Saffle JR, Davis B, Williams P. Recent outcomes in the treatment of burn injury in the United States: A report from the American Burn Association Patient Registry. *J Burn Care Rehabil.* 1995;16(3 pt 1):219–232.

PATHOPHYSIOLOGY OF BURNS

Inflammatory Response and Burn Shock

Thermal insult results in physiological changes affecting both injured and noninjured tissue.[6] Burn shock begins at the cellular level, decreasing cellular transmembrane potential.[7] Inflammatory and vasoactive mediator release, activated by thermal injury, results in increased capillary micropermeability and hypovolemia, leading to cellular edema.[7,8] Over the 48 hours following injury, fluid continues to be lost through the wound and edema continues to form.

As the burn wound exceeds 20% to 25% TBSA, capillary permeability and intravascular volume deficits can exceed the body's compensatory mechanisms and result in circulatory compromise.[7] If distance and time of transport are lengthy, casualties may suffer burn shock by the time they arrive at a treatment facility, and self-aid or buddy aid will be ineffective. During evacuation, casualties must receive emergency medical treatment by providers trained in burn management.

Burn Resuscitation

A fluid resuscitation program is designed to overcome the acute period of massive fluid shifts, electrolyte derangements, acid–base imbalance, edema formation (see further discussion below), and fluid and protein losses. Replenishing circulatory volume using one of several formulas restores and maintains organ perfusion and function (Table 13-1).

A key component in most resuscitation fluids is the sodium ion; the fluid (free water) is the vehicle that delivers the sodium. Depending on the choice of formula, fluid volumes range from 2 to 5 mL/kg/% TBSA. Burn resuscitation formulas are similar in the milliequivalents of sodium they provide.[9] Some formulas use only crystalloid fluids and omit colloid, while others vary the amount and timing of colloid administration. The role of crystalloid or colloid resuscitation remains an ongoing debate. However, a prescribed formula is a guideline to help resuscitate a burn casualty. The individual response to a prescribed formula may be unpredictable and variable, requiring continual corrective adjustments. None of these formulas reflects evolving trends that add a sophisticated medical resuscitation component to the already existing fluid protocol. Several components are currently being used or investigated to improve resuscitation and decrease edema and the inflammatory response in the early phase, including:

- low molecular weight dextran,
- fresh frozen plasma,
- pentastoid,
- mannitol,
- ibuprofen,
- cimetidine,
- vitamin C, and
- vitamin E.[9–18]

The current approach to fluid therapy has led to reduced mortality rates.[7] Not long ago, approximately 50% of deaths occurred within the first 10 days following burn injury because of multiple organ failure syndrome and devastating sepsis. A principal cause, particularly of multiple organ failure syndrome, is inadequate fluid resuscitation and maintenance. Because burn shock is both hypovolemic and cellular in etiology, fluid management following successful resuscitation

TABLE 13-1

FLUID RESUSCITATION FORMULAS

Formula	Fluid Composition	Calculation
Brooke	Ringers lactate; Na 130, Cl 130, Lactate 28, K 4, Ca 3	2–4 cc/kg/% TBSA
Parkland	Ringers lactate; D5W + 0.5–2.0 L	4 cc/kg/% TBSA
Hypertonic saline	Na 200–300 mEq/L, Cl 100 mEq/L, HCO3 150 mEq/L	2 cc/kg/% TBSA

D5W: dextrose 5% in water
TBSA: total-body surface area

is as important as that performed during the initial revival process.[19] Multiple organ dysfunction resulting from inadequate resuscitation has become less common with the use of weight- and injury-size based formulas.[7] However, increased fluid regimens, known as "fluid creep," are also associated with adverse outcomes, including edema formation, increased compartment pressures, acute respiratory distress syndrome, and multiple organ dysfunction.[7] The goal of proper fluid resuscitation is to prevent burn shock.[7]

CLASSIFYING AND ASSESSING BURNS

Burn casualties typically comprise between 5% and 20% of service members wounded during conventional warfare.[19–22] Burn injury occurs in a young population, with a high incidence of inhalation injury and Injury Severity Score (an anatomical trauma severity measure that can be used to predict mortality).[23] Military burn injuries have a broad impact, affecting everything from the individual to the overall status of military operations.[24]

Burns are classified by mechanism of causation (ie, thermal, chemical, electrical, or radiation), as well as size, depth, and location of the burn and other associated trauma. Regardless of mechanism or severity, rehabilitation goals for burn casualties are the same.

Thermal Injuries

Thermal injury accounts for approximately 95% of military burn casualties, with chemical and electrical making up the most of the remainder.[20,24] Burns resulting from flash fire and flame are the most common in wartime.[20,24] The detonation of explosive devices, such as landmines, artillery munitions, mortar rounds, and improvised explosives, has been a significant source

of combat burns.[20,24,25] The most common causes of noncombat burns in service members are related to burning waste materials, inappropriately handling ammunition and pyrotechnics, and misusing fuels. Efforts to prevent noncombat injuries continue to reduce their impact on military operations.[20,24] Other causes of military burn injury include exposure to hot liquids or superheated steam, typically from ship or submarine boilers, resulting in scald burns. Inhalation injury is frequently associated with superheated steam burns.

Chemical Injuries

Chemical burns appear to be uncommon in military casualties,[26] with reported incidences ranging from 0.9% to 6.5% (Figure 13-2).[20,27–29] However, the widespread use of chemicals and their ready availability creates the potential for a large number of this type of casualty. Chemical burns are caused by acids, alkalis, or organic compounds.[26] Except for white phosphorus,[26,27] most chemical burns should be immediately treated with copious water lavage. Wounds caused by white phosphorus, which ignites on contact with air, should be covered

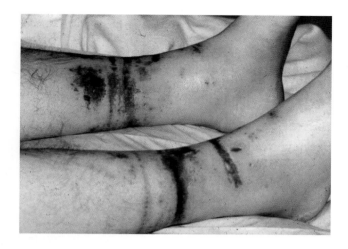

Figure 13-2. Chemical burn to the lower extremities of a burn casualty.

with water or saline until the wound can be debrided of all chemical.[26] Powdered chemical should be brushed away prior to water lavage to decrease the quantity of exposure. The process of neutralization generates heat, which can add thermal injury to the chemical insult. The duration of irrigation is variable depending on the agent. In general, alkalis require a much longer period of irrigation than acids. At a minimum, 30 minutes of continuous irrigation are required for all burns, and at least 1 hour of irrigation is necessary for alkali burns.[28] A period of up to 6 hours of irrigation has been recommended for acid burns, and one of up to 48 hours has been suggested for ocular alkali burns. A good rule of thumb is to irrigate at least until there has been a significant decrease in pain.[29]

Chemical agents produce direct tissue damage by a variety of reactions. Acid burns tend to be superficial in depth, whereas alkali burns tend to burrow into the tissues and cause more significant destruction. Acids cause coagulation necrosis, whereas alkaline materials cause liquefaction necrosis. Hydrofluoric acid requires copious water lavage, followed by topical calcium gluconate, which, when injected into the area, may decrease the severity of the injury. Using intraarterial calcium gluconate on wounds of the hands and feet is beneficial. Mustard agent, a chemical previously used in warfare, is rapidly absorbed by the skin, conjunctiva, and mucous membranes, and within minutes irreversibly combines with tissue proteins, damaging the lungs, eyes, and skin.[30] Over time, the exposed tissues blister and ulcerate.[31] Ophthalmic injuries are best treated with copious water irrigation. Skin should be decontaminated with 0.5% hypochlorite. In general, skin burns from mustard are superficial and heal without difficulties; injuries to the mucosal linings are much more serious and disabling.

Electrical Injuries

Electrical injuries result from the conduction of electrical energy through tissue or from heat that is released as the current arcs through the air (Figure 13-3). Current arcs may generate temperatures as high as 3,000°C. As they arc, they ignite clothing, which results in a combination electrical and thermal injury. Injuries caused by low voltage current (< 1,000 V) are occasionally fatal because of immediate ventricular fibrillation. Survivors rarely have significant tissue damage. High voltage (> 1,000 V) current can damage tissue anywhere along its route.

Electrical injuries are heat related. Electrical energy is converted to heat energy as expressed by Joule's law: power or heat equals amperage squared times resistance ($P=I^2 \bullet R$). As voltage or amperage increases, so does the heat produced. Measurement of tissue temperature experimentally reveals that it is highest directly underneath and adjacent to the contact site of the wounds. Deep tissue destruction is always greatest in areas of the body with small volume, such as the fingers, toes, wrists, or ankles. The farther away the tissue is from the contact point, the lower the current density, and the less heat is generated. Various tissues have different resistance to current flow; for example, nerves and blood vessels have low resistance, while cartilage and bone have high resistance. Because bone is highly resistant, current tends to flow at its surface, making temperature greatest at the periosteum. Thus, muscle damage is often extensive adjacent to the bone,

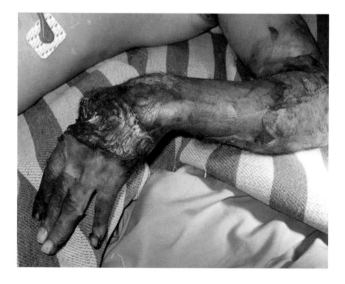

Figure 13-3. Electrical burn to the upper extremity of a burn casualty. Note the extent of injury indicated by the presence of exposed subcutaneous structures on the dorsum of the hand.

and many times the periosteum and portions of the outer cortex of the bone may not be viable. For these reasons, the extent of electrical injury is often not well reflected in the cutaneous burn size.[20] An electrical injury may be deceiving and not initially appear severe, with only small areas visible superficially, but the casualty may have severe limb injury that will ultimately lead to amputation.[32]

A sensitive indicator of total muscle damage following electrical injuries is serum creatine kinase (CK). Ahrenholz et al[33] found that casualties with a total CK concentration of under 400 international units (IU) had no significant tissue loss; a few casualties with total CK concentration ranging between 400 IU and 2,500 IU required digit amputations or skin grafts. Casualties with a CK total greater than 2,500 IU had a high risk of major amputation, and those with a CK total greater than 10,000 IU had an 84% risk of major amputation or permanent neurologic deficit. More recently, Cancio et al reported age, myoglobinuria, and fasciotomy are independent predictors of amputation following high voltage electrical injuries.[20]

SEVERITY OF BURNS

The overall severity of a burn is related to the casualty's age, TBSA affected, burn depth, associated injuries, and, to a lesser extent, associated illnesses.[34]

Age

The very young and the very old do not tolerate illness and trauma (particularly burn trauma) as well as those between 10 and 50 years of age. Military burn casualties typically range from 18 to 48 years of age.[5,24,25,35] Individuals at the extremes of age are generally more physiologically fragile and poorly tolerate the massive fluid shifts and infectious complications associated with burn and its treatment. These factors should be considered during triage when the number of casualties exceeds available resources.

Burn Size

Evaluating and treating a burn requires an accurate assessment of the injury's size. The three most commonly used methods of determining burn size include using the casualty's palm as a reference, the rule of nines, and the Lund and Browder chart. The area of the palm, excluding the digits, represents approximately 0.5% of the body surface over a wide range of ages.[36] Using a casualty's palm to determine burn size is particularly useful for spotty burns in multiple areas. The rule of nines is a convenient way of estimating adult TBSA (Figure 13-4). Developed in the 1940s by Pulaski and Tennison, it is easily remembered because it divides the body surface into areas of 9% or multiples of 9%. The head and neck equal 9%, each upper extremity is 9%, the anterior and posterior trunk are 18% each, each lower extremity is 18%, and the perineum is 1%. The rule of nines is easily applied in field situations, but is relatively inaccurate.[37] The Lund and Browder chart, developed over 50 years ago, more accurately defines burn size and is commonly used in most burn centers (Figure 13-5). This chart assigns a percent of surface area to body segments,[38] taking into account the disproportionate growth of the trunk, head, and lower extremities based on the age of the casualty. However, the chart is not always readily available and is too complex to commit to memory.

Recent reports show that the average burn size for both combat and noncombat injuries is between 7% and 15%.[20,23–25] Despite the low average burn size for military casualties, the use of unconventional incendiary devices has resulted in casualties with large burns exceeding 95% TBSA.[24]

Burn Depth

Historically, burns have been classified into degree categories (ie, first, second, third, and fourth).[39] More recently, however, burns have been classified by depth in relation to the tissues involved (epidermal, superficial partial-thickness, deep partial-thickness, full-thickness, or subdermal; Table 13-2). For example, a sunburn is a standard epidermal burn, and typically heals in 3 to 6 days without long-term sequelae (Figure 13-6).[40] Superficial partial-thickness burns are deeper than epidermal burns (Figure 13-7). They are best treated with daily dressing changes and heal without surgical intervention. A superficial partial-thickness burn may heal with minor color and texture changes, but it does not develop hypertrophic scarring.[41] In contrast, a deep partial-thickness burn results in fragile skin, requires increased time to heal, and may create severe scarring (Figure 13-8). This type of burn is best treated with early excision and grafting.[39] A full-thickness burn larger than 3 cm in diameter is best treated with early excision and grafting to prevent significant scarring (Figure 13-9).[39] Subdermal burns should be treated by debriding devitalized tissues, ensuring exposed bone and tendons are covered by soft tissue, and expeditiously grafting skin to prevent significant scarring (Figure 13-10).[39] Extensive soft tissue reconstruction may be required to cover these wounds.

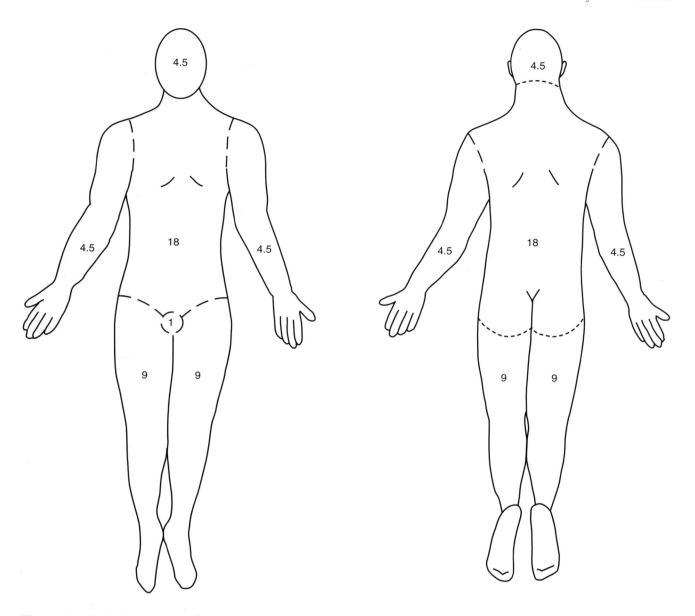

Figure 13-4. Rule of nines body chart for estimating burn size.
Reproduced from Pulaski EJ, Tennison CW. Exposure (open) treatment of burns. *U S Armed Forces Med J*. 1951:2;769.

In the case of a hand burn, knowledge of wound depth and location is imperative to determine an appropriate treatment plan. In particular, the presence of a deep palmar burn should be noted and taken into consideration when designing a splinting program. The location of eschar should also be noted prior to burn excision. If tendon involvement is suspected with a full-thickness burn, precautions should be made as if tendon involvement is confirmed.[42]

The dorsal hand is one of the most common sites for tendon exposure, especially over the proximal interphalangeal (PIP) joint. Hunt and Sato found that damage to the extensor tissue over the PIP joint resulted in the worst functional outcomes.[43] Damage to the central slip of the extensor mechanism can lead to a boutonnière deformity. If tendon exposure is suspected or confirmed, care must be taken to protect the integrity of the tendon; exposed tendons can desiccate rapidly.[44] A moist environment must be maintained with antibiotic ointments and petroleum-based gauze to prevent drying.

Reports from current military operations indicate the average TBSA full-thickness burn is between 4% and 8%.[23,24] The impact of combat versus noncombat injuries on burn depth has been shown to be insignificant.[24]

CHART FOR ESTIMATING SEVERITY OF BURN WOUND

NAME _____ WARD _____ NUMBER ____ DATE _____
AGE _____ ADMISSION WEIGHT _____

LUND AND BROWDER CHARTS

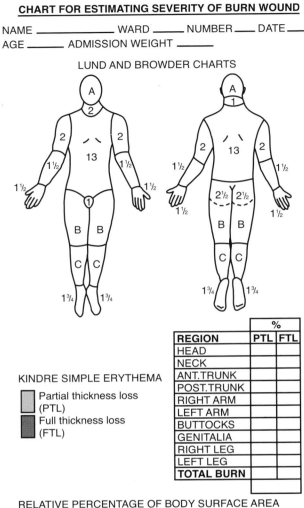

KINDRE SIMPLE ERYTHEMA

▢ Partial thickness loss (PTL)
▣ Full thickness loss (FTL)

REGION	%	
	PTL	FTL
HEAD		
NECK		
ANT. TRUNK		
POST. TRUNK		
RIGHT ARM		
LEFT ARM		
BUTTOCKS		
GENITALIA		
RIGHT LEG		
LEFT LEG		
TOTAL BURN		

RELATIVE PERCENTAGE OF BODY SURFACE AREA AFFECTED BY GROWTH

AREA	AGE 0	1	5	10	15	ADULT
A = ½ OF HEAD	9½	8½	6½	5½	4½	3½
B = ½ OF ONE THIGH	2¾	4¼	4	4½	4½	4¾
C = ½ OF ONE LEG	2½	2½	2¾	3	3¼	3½

Figure 13-5. Lund and Browder chart for estimating burn size.
Adapted from Cioffi WG Jr, Rue LW III, Buescher TM, Pruitt BA. A brief history and the pathophysiology of burns. In: Bellamy RF, Zajtchuk R, eds. *Conventional Warfare: Ballistic, Blast, and Burn Injuries*. Part 1, Vol 5. In: *Textbooks of Military Medicine*. Washington, DC: Office of The Surgeon General, Department of the Army, and Borden Institute; 1991: 341.

Location

The anatomical location of burns is important in determining burn severity.[45] Burns, even of similar size, to various areas of the body have differing and significant impacts on survival, functional outcome, and cosmesis, especially when depth of injury is factored in (Figure 13-11). Additional considerations for critical care, wound care, and rehabilitation management must be made for specialized anatomical areas, such as the face, hands, feet, and genitalia.[41] Burns that cross skin creases require special rehabilitation to prevent contracture and minimize hypertrophic scarring.[46]

For military casualties, the most frequently burned anatomical areas include the head, face, and hands.[23–25,47] Injuries to these areas are due to several factors, including the need for unimpeded accessibility for vision, breathing, and communications, as well as for activities requiring maximal hand dexterity. Other anatomical locations frequently burned include the upper arm, forearm, thigh, and lower leg.[23–25] New advances in body armor and flame-resistant protective clothing are being examined and fielded to decrease the incidence of burns to these areas.[47] There is no noticeable difference in burn distribution between combat- and noncombat-related burn injuries, except that the face is more likely to be burned in combat operations.[24]

The burn location on the hand is important when determining an appropriate treatment plan. Range-of-motion (ROM) exercises, splinting, or serial casting should be implemented in the direction of tissue tension to provide optimal tissue realignment. For example, a dorsal hand burn needs to be placed in the safe resting position to put mild tension on the involved structures. Exercises should emphasize regaining a composite flexion of the digits. A palmar burn will contract into thumb flexion, thumb adduction, and finger flexion. Splints or casts used for palmar burns should hold the hand in the position of thumb radial abduction and finger metacarpophalangeal (MCP), PIP, and distal interphalangeal (DIP) extension. Caution should be taken to avoid MCP hyperextension of the thumb when positioning into radial abduction. Exercises should emphasize finger extension and radial abduction. Flexion exercises can be performed to prevent joint capsule tightness of the MCP and interphalangeal (IP) joints; however, caution should be taken to avoid digital extension losses.

Associated Illnesses and Injuries

Most military casualties are healthy adults. However, 37% to 52% of combat burn casualties sustain associated injuries (Table 13-3).[23,24,48] Additionally, combat burn casualties are significantly more likely to sustain associated trauma than noncombat burn casualties.[24] Acute injuries, whether due to penetrating or blunt trauma, are given first priority. Inhalation injury affects about 16% of combat and 6% of noncombat burn casualties.[24] An associated injury may complicate care, interfere with surgical treatment, and impede normal rehabilitation.

TABLE 13-2

BURN TERMINOLOGY

Old Classification	New Classification	Description
First degree	Epidermal burn	Involves only the epidermis, is erythematous or deeply tanned in appearance, does not blister
Second degree	Superficial partial thickness burn	Involves both the epidermis and dermis, blisters, is moist and erythematous, reepithelializes in less than 3 weeks
	Deep partial thickness burn	Cream colored or white beneath blisters, takes longer than 3 weeks to heal
Third degree	Full thickness burn	Involves the entire depth of the skin, destroys both the epidermis and dermis, must heal from the wound margins
Fourth degree	Subdermal burn	Occurs when damage is deep to the skin and involves muscle, bone, and other deeper tissues

Data sources: (1) Richard R. Assessment and diagnosis of burn wounds. *Adv Wound Care*. 1999;12(9):468–471. (2) Devgan L, Bhat S, Aylward S, Spence RJ. Modalities for the assessment of burn wound depth. *J Burns Wounds*. 2006;5;e2. (3) Peitzman AB. Burns/inhalation injury. In: Peitzman AB, ed. *The Trauma Manual: Trauma and Acute Care Surgery*. 3rd ed. Philadelphia, PA: Wolters Kluwer Lippincott Williams & Wilkins; 2008: Chapter 45. (4) Johnson RM, Richard R. Partial-thickness burns: identification and management. *Adv Skin Wound Care*. 2003;16(4):178–189.

Clinical Relevance

The severity of a burn has an impact on casualty survival, as well as on nutritional and surgical considerations. Additionally, severity largely influences rehabilitation outcomes.[49] The physical manifestations of burn scar contracture, hypertrophic scarring, and overall long-term functioning are often directly attributable to how severely a casualty is burned.

The development and number of burn scar contractures have been directly related to the extent of TBSA burned (Figure 13-12).[50] If less than 20% TBSA

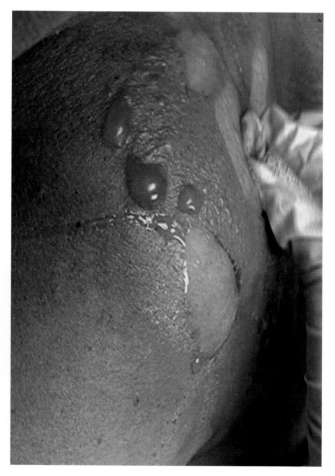

Figure 13-7. Superficial partial-thickness burn with intact blisters.

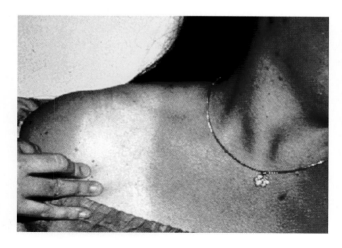

Figure 13-6. Typical appearance of an epidermal burn.

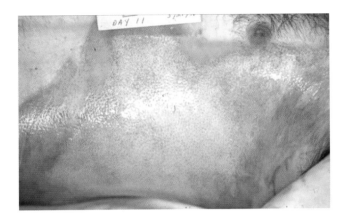

Figure 13-8. Deep partial-thickness burn demonstrating mottled appearance.

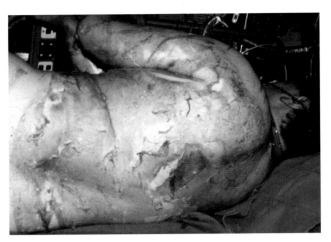

Figure 13-9. Full-thickness burn showing eschar on flank.

is burned, a casualty is expected to do well, unless the hands are heavily involved, in which case the potential for impaired functional outcomes is considerable.[45] If more than 20% TBSA is burned, casualties begin to manifest burn scar contractures during the intermediate and long-term phases of burn rehabilitation. Recently, the incidence of burn scar contracture has been identified to be as high as 50%.[51] Additionally, burn depth has long been implicated in the appear-

ance of burn scar contractures, based on healing either by secondary intent or skin grafting and burn wound location relative to anatomic functional sites.[50,52,53] In recent combat operations, TBSA burned, inhalation injury, associated trauma, and length of hospitalization were found to be the most influential parameters determining whether or not an injured service member would return to duty.[54]

CRITICAL CARE OF BURN CASUALTIES

Skin, the largest organ of the body, is vital for survival. Aside from protecting the body from losing temperature, fluid, electrolytes, and other solutes, skin provides the first line of protection from a hostile microbial world. Severely burned casualties experience a cascade of metabolic and physiologic consequences, including recurrent infections, organ failure, and, in

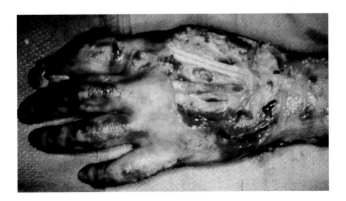

Figure 13-10. Subdermal burn displaying exposed tendon and bone on the dorsum of the hand.

the worst cases, death. Until every open wound can be closed with functional skin, a burn casualty remains at risk for infection and organ failure. Open wounds must be closed with autograft and healing conditions must be optimized before organ failure and death can ensue. Organ support, nutrition, and early rehabilitation should optimize the conditions for successful graft take.

Burns involving critical locations must be identified immediately to be managed appropriately. The head, face, hands, feet, genitalia, perineum, and major joints are considered critical areas by the American Burn Association and must be managed at a burn center.

Early Life Support Evaluation and Management

In most cases, especially during military conflict, it is crucial to remember that burn injury is a traumatic event, often associated with other possibly life-threatening injuries. Isolated burns are rarely immediately life threatening; however, burn casualties must be viewed within the context of a multisystem injury that could reveal varying degrees of life-threatening conditions. Other conditions that may result in immediate

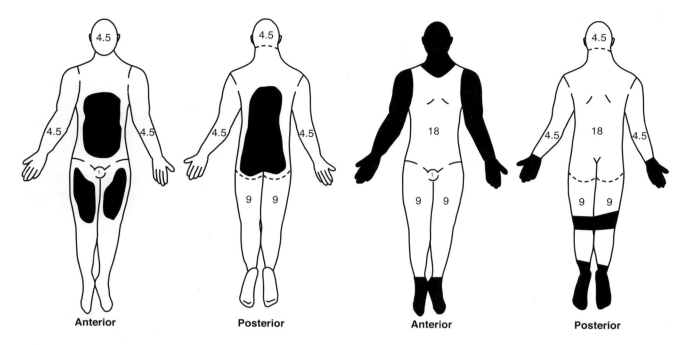

Figure 13-11. Body diagrams of equal size burn depicting the difference that location of burn has on functional areas.

death include a compromised airway and uncontrolled hemorrhage, and should be identified and treated first. A thorough and rapid assessment of the casualty helps prioritize care during the initial critical phase. Primary and secondary surveys are designed to help rescuers identify and treat the most life-threatening conditions.

Service members often initially manage and treat burn casualties. This treatment should follow the three basics of first aid: (1) stop the burning process, (2) evaluate and secure the airway, and (3) treat other life-threatening injuries. If the airway is compromised,

ventilation should be maintained by mask and oxygen, or intubation if possible (see "Respiratory Considerations" below). When facial or neck edema is anticipated from fluid administration and prolonged transport times (ie, > 4 hours), intubation is usually necessary prior to transfer. The burn wound should be covered with a clean sheet or simple dry dressing to minimize further contamination and to help conserve body heat. The basics of trauma emergency care apply to initial burn treatment.

Vascular venous access is established peripherally for immediate use, or centrally for when necessary or

TABLE 13-3

INCIDENCE OF ASSOCIATED TRAUMA IN BURN CASUALTIES

Type of Injury	Incidence
Eye injury	8.5%
Skull fracture	7.5%
Neck/Torso fracture	3.5%
Upper limb fracture	10.0%
Lower limb fracture	16.6%
Intracranial injury	2.0%
Internal torso injury	4.2%
Fragment wounds	38.4%
Traumatic amputation	2.3%

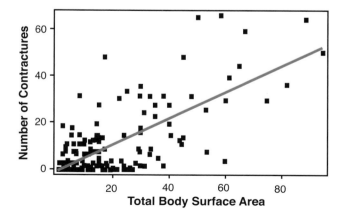

Figure 13-12. Graph displaying the relationship between total body surface area burned and the incidence of burn scar contractures.

when multiple ports are required. Obtaining central venous access is not without risks; however, central venous lines provide a means of monitoring central venous pressure and ease serum sampling. Casualties with cardiovascular instability or inhalation injuries often benefit from arterial lines, which provide hemodynamic values and allow blood to be drawn without repeated arterial punctures.

The secure maintenance of intravascular devices warrants special care as well. Loss of these devices places a casualty at unnecessary risk of additional invasive procedures. Intravascular devices should be securely sutured or stapled in place at multiple anchor points, with care and attention given to these sites during rehabilitation activities.

Fluid Resuscitation

Severe burn injury results in massive fluid shifts from the intravascular space into the interstitium and intracellular space of both burned and unburned tissues.[55] This fluid shift results in intravascular volume depletion and hemoconcentration, with blood hematocrit elevated in the first 24 hours after burn.[56] Several formulas exist to calculate the required amount and rate of volume repletion for burn casualties,[57] such as the modified Brooke formula,[58] in which volume is replenished by providing crystalloids (Ringers lactate, 2 mL/kg/% burn) over the first 24 hours post burn. No colloids are given during the first 24 hours. Over the next 24 hours, colloids are provided in the amount of 0.3 to 0.5 mL/kg/% burn. No crystalloids are given during the second 24 hours. Glucose in water is also provided over the second 24 hours and titrated to maintain good urinary output.

The Starling equation indicates that two forces, capillary hydrostatic pressure and interstitial colloid osmotic pressure, push fluid out of the vasculature into the interstitium (Exhibit 13-1).[6] The remaining two forces, capillary colloid osmotic pressure and interstitial hydrostatic pressure, work to counterbalance this shift by holding fluid in the vasculature. These forces are balanced in a healthy organism.[6] Based on this principle, fluid resuscitation is managed to maintain organ perfusion with minimal physiological cost.[7]

Delayed or inadequate replacement of intravascular volume results in suboptimal tissue perfusion and can lead to end-organ failure and death. The goal of fluid resuscitation after severe burn is to replace lost intravascular volume with intravenous (IV) crystalloid, maintaining adequate tissue perfusion throughout the 48-hour period of increased capillary leak and relative hypovolemia at the lowest physiologic cost.[59]

Casualties with severe burns, extensive soft tissue trauma, inhalation injury, or electrical injury require increased amounts of fluid to prevent burn shock. In certain casualties, burn shock and resuscitation failure occur, despite optimal resuscitation by experienced personnel, because of factors associated with limits in cardiovascular reserve and adverse host responses.[60]

Under resuscitation, which contributes to shock, and acute renal failure must be avoided. On the other hand, the consequences of over resuscitation have been termed "resuscitation morbidity" and have severe, long-ranging effects. Resuscitation morbidity includes complications such as extremity eschar and compartment syndromes and abdominal compartment syndrome (ACS).[61] Extremity eschar and compartment syndromes resulting from over resuscitation have immediate and long-term rehabilitation consequences. Eschar syndrome is characterized by a leathery, noncompressible, circumferential burn that prevents skin expansion as tissues become edematous. This leads to compromised tissue perfusion. Early mobility may be restricted when edema impairs joint motion (Figure 13-13). In addition to

---

EXHIBIT 13-1

STARLING EQUATION

$$J_v = K_f\,([P_c - P_i] - \sigma\,[\pi_c - \pi_i])$$

K_f: filtration coefficient
π_c: capillary oncotic pressure
π_i: interstitial oncotic pressure
P_c: capillary hydrostatic pressure
P_i: interstitial hydrostatic pressure
σ: reflection coefficient

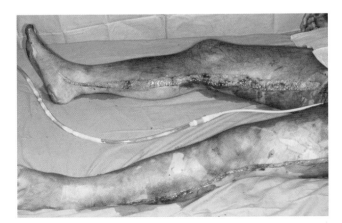

Figure 13-13. Example of an escharotomy of the lower extremities.

early escharotomy, early extremity elevation and range-of-motion exercises are encouraged to decrease gravity-dependent edema.

Extremity compartment syndrome differs from eschar syndrome in that it is characterized by tissue expansion occurring specifically within a fascial compartment, resulting in decreased tissue perfusion and cell death. The mainstay of management is early recognition through monitoring of compartment pressures, and release of the involved compartment via fasciotomy if compartment pressures are elevated (Figure 13-14).

Delaying escharotomy or fasciotomy can result in myonecrosis. Acutely, myonecrosis can lead to acute renal failure and lung injury secondary to the systemic release of intracellular contents into the circulation. The long-term consequences of myonecrosis are linked to the muscle groups involved. From a rehabilitation standpoint, loss of significant muscle groups can severely impact a casualty's functional outcome in various ways, ranging from the loss of independence with ambulation or transfers acutely to increased risk for overuse and degenerative processes due to muscle imbalances over the long term.

ACS results in decreased renal blood flow and subsequent renal failure, intestinal ischemia, respiratory failure, and death if not recognized and treated early.[62] A resuscitation volume greater than 237 mL/kg over 12 hours (or 16 liters over a 12-hour period in a 70 kg male) appears to be the threshold for the development of ACS.[63] Treating ACS by placing a drain and performing an abdominal escharotomy (or a decompressive laparotomy as a last resort) may improve survival but is associated with dramatic increases in morbidity. The mortality rate after decompressive laparotomy for ACS in burn casualties is documented to be 60% to 100%.[64] For those few survivors, the added catabolic load of an open abdomen (and all the potential subsequent complications thereof) can significantly increase wound healing times, muscle catabolism, and functional recovery time.

Respiratory Considerations

Intubation entails passing an endotracheal tube from either the nose or the mouth through the pharynx into the trachea. This tube is then connected to a mechanical ventilator to cause inspiration and passive exhalation through the lungs. General indications for intubation in burn casualties are to improve oxygenation and ventilation, or to maintain gas exchange during respiratory distress or clinical conditions expected to compromise the airway. Indications include:

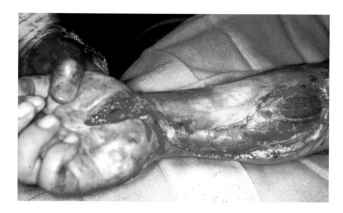

Figure 13-14. Example of a fasciotomy (carpal tunnel release) of the upper extremity.

- tachypnea,
- hypoxia,
- impending need for airway maintenance,
- initial management of smoke inhalation injury, and
- expected massive edema.

The importance of securing an airway device cannot be overemphasized. During rehabilitation activities, caution must be exercised and all efforts should be made to prevent the loss of the airway. The inadvertent displacement or removal of an endotracheal tube is often fraught with difficulties and can (rarely) result in death. Commercially available, function-specific devices are not ideal for burn casualties, especially those with burns of the face and neck. Tape does not adhere to burned tissue, and the edema associated with resuscitation is often marked.

To ensure security of an endotracheal tube, a cotton umbilical tape is tied securely around the tube, then around the head. As facial edema increases and decreases, adjustments in the ties should be made to prevent skin breakdown. Alternatively, stainless steel wire may be routed around a molar tooth and the wire subsequently attached to the endotracheal tube. This technique is sturdy and eliminates the need for constricting materials across the face. The challenge of this technique is routing the wire. Wire cutters should be readily accessible for removing the securing wire if necessary.

Endotracheal intubation and respiratory support treat burn casualties in two general groups: those who need a definitive airway for airway protection, and those who need mechanical ventilation. Casualties needing airway protection may include those whose airways have been compromised by upper airway inhalation injury, airway edema from massive resuscitation, or loss of consciousness from carbon monoxide poisoning. Casualties needing ventilatory support include those with severe smoke inhalation injury, acute lung injury, acute respiratory distress syndrome, or those who require deep sedation for extensive burns.

Endotracheal tubes can be placed either via the nasotracheal or orotracheal route. If orotracheal intubation is used, a bite block should be placed between the teeth to prevent the casualty from biting the tube and obstructing it. The nasotracheal route is preferred because the tube can be better secured, and oral care and rehabilitation can be performed that intubation via the orotracheal route would not allow. The disadvantages of using the nasotracheal route include inability to pass the tube, discomfort, and the potential for sinus infection. Occasionally, severe burns involving the face and neck preclude traditional nasotracheal or orotracheal intubation, and performance of a cricothyroidotomy may be required. The cricothyroidotomy is generally followed by a formal tracheostomy when appropriate surgical support is available.

A tracheostomy may be necessary for some casualties, either acutely due to the inability to access the airway via the orotracheal or nasotracheal route, or long term because of a prolonged need for mechanical ventilation. Tracheostomies often offer the advantage of better comfort, improved oral care, and improved ability to clear pulmonary secretions. However, the risks and benefits of the tracheostomy must be weighed because complications, although uncommon, can be fatal.

The tracheotomy tract usually matures in 5 to 10 days. If the tube is unintentionally pulled out before the stoma and if the tract has matured, replacing the tube can be difficult. It is therefore crucial that careful attention is given to the tracheotomy site during all rehabilitation activities or whenever there is a significant position change. It is recommended that a respiratory therapist be present at all times during any major casualty movement when an endotracheal tube or a fresh tracheotomy is present.

There are various modes of ventilatory support, including:

- **Controlled mechanical ventilation.** The casualty receives a breath from the ventilator at predetermined rates, whether or not the casualty attempts to breathe. This mode is rarely used in the intensive care unit.
- **Assist control (volume or pressure).** The casualty receives a ventilator breath, either volume- or pressure-targeted, whenever an attempt to breathe is made; a minimal rate is provided if no attempt to breathe is made.

- **Synchronized intermittent mandatory ventilation.** Regular predetermined breaths are delivered and casualties are allowed to breathe first at their own tidal volume, later between ventilated breaths. This mode is frequently used for weaning.
- **Pressure support.** The casualty initiates every breath, which is supported with a set amount of pressure.
- **Continuous positive airway pressure.** Continuous positive airway pressure restores the glottic mechanism of intrapulmonary pressure maintenance, which has been eliminated by intubation. This allows the casualty to take full spontaneous negative-pressure breaths. It is the setting most used during spontaneous breathing trials.
- **Other modes.** High-frequency oscillatory ventilation, high-frequency percussive ventilation, airway pressure release ventilation, and bilevel continuous positive airway pressure are alternative modes of ventilation that can be used for ventilatory support.

Ventilation and oxygenation must be monitored in casualties on mechanical ventilation. Adequate ventilation is assessed via arterial carbon dioxide tension. A casualty's minute ventilation (the amount of carbon dioxide exchanged in 60 sec) is the product of the volume of each breath (tidal volume) and respiratory rate over a minute. A minute ventilation requirement can be affected by a variety of conditions, including exercise. Thus, it is possible that simple ROM exercises in a severely burned casualty, already pushed to the limit in terms of catabolic workload at baseline, can result in carbon dioxide accumulation. An acute rise in carbon dioxide (hypercapnea) can result in respiratory acidosis, leading to a variety of systemic effects (eg, coagulopathy, hemodynamic compromise, and mental status changes). A casualty's ventilatory status must be closely monitored during rehabilitative sessions. Arterial carbon dioxide is typically measured via blood gas analysis. After assessing the partial pressure of carbon dioxide, ventilatory settings can be made to adjust minute ventilation.

Oxygenation is determined using the partial pressure of oxygen in arterial blood. In general, 60 mmHg of oxygen has been considered sufficient oxygenation. Another frequently used monitor is pulse oximetry, which is an optical measurement of oxygenated hemoglobin in pulsatile vessels. The percentage of oxygenated hemoglobin in the arteries can be calculated using differences in absorption of red and infrared light. Because of the shape of the oxyhemoglobin dissociation curve, when the saturation of oxygen exceeds 90% and the partial pressure of oxygen in arterial blood is greater than 60 mmHg, the curve is flat, and the latter can change considerably with little change in the former. Regardless, it is assumed that an oxygen saturation value greater than 90% is indicative of adequate oxygenation. Like minute ventilation, the impact of exercise on oxygenation can be significant. This is particularly important in casualties who have a high oxygen requirement (ie, needing > 50% fraction of inspired oxygen [FiO$_2$]). It may be necessary to closely monitor oxygen saturation to determine the limits of an activity. In general, activity should be curtailed or stopped when oxygen saturation is less than 90%.

Ventilator-associated pneumonia is a common complication in intubated and ventilated casualties and is associated with high morbidity and mortality. Hospital-acquired pneumonia can occur in nonintubated casualties with an equally morbid impact. In burn casualties, especially those with smoke inhalation injury, both ventilator-associated pneumonia and hospital-acquired pneumonia occur at a much higher frequency, and all efforts must be made to minimize this nosocomial complication. Simple interventions, such as frequent handwashing, daily oral care with chlorhexidine oral rinse, and head-of-bed elevation above 30° can decrease the incidence of hospital-acquired pneumonia and ventilator-associated pneumonia.[65]

Early mobilization out of bed to an upright position, either chair or standing frame, can optimize pulmonary function in spontaneously breathing casualties. Compared to the supine position, the upright position allows for easier diaphragmatic excursion with each breath, bibasilar recruitment of atelectatic alveoli, and improved aeration. In casualties with abdominal distension, a standing position may be preferred over a sitting position to allow optimum excursion. In addition to optimal positioning, burn casualties use secretion-clearing devices for aggressive pulmonary toilet.

In general, those casualties who require only airway protection may be good candidates for early mobilization out of bed. Casualties who are cooperative, minimally sedated, and have minimal lung pathology, may even be able to ambulate, with assistance of frequent bagging. Aggressive mobilization out of bed for rehabilitation activities, such as tilting and transfers to sitting position, can be safely performed with—and is recommended for—intubated casualties. Respiratory parameters during mobilization of intubated casualties out of bed include a peak inspiratory pressure equal to or less than 30 cm H$_2$O and a FiO$_2$ equal to or less than 40%.

Once airway edema has subsided and it is determined that casualties are able to protect their own airways, extubation may be considered. Typically, those who are placed on a ventilator for pulmonary problems remain on mechanical ventilation until the underlying reason for needing the support has resolved. These casualties are placed on a spontaneous breathing trial when the provider feels they no longer require as much or any ventilator support. Breathing trials can last anywhere from 30 minutes to 2 hours, during which it is important that casualties are not overly stimulated or anxious.

A significant amount of interdisciplinary coordination is necessary in order to perform spontaneous breathing trials around daily wound care and rehabilitation. In some cases, casualties no longer need a ventilator, but may continue to require airway protection. The use of continuous positive airway pressure or a minimal spontaneous mode of ventilation may be appropriate.

Once the casualty is liberated from a ventilator, aggressive pulmonary hygiene is crucial to maintain the airway. Proper casualty care includes frequent deep breathing, coughing, position changes, use of incentive spirometer, nebulizer treatment, and provision of humidified oxygen. Suctioning may be required if a casualty is not able to adequately clear secretions. Continued monitoring of arterial blood gasses or oximetry and serial chest radiographs are required.[66]

Gastrointestinal Considerations

The gastrointestinal response to burn is highlighted by mucosal atrophy, changes in digestive absorption, and increased intestinal permeability.[67] Atrophy of the small bowel mucosa occurs within 12 hours of injury in proportion to the burn size. Given the changes in the gut, it is common to see evidence of gut dysfunction after burn manifested by feeding intolerance and mucosal ulceration and bleeding, particularly in the stomach and duodenum. Enteral feeding is one of the most important means of providing nutrition to burn casualties and has led to a decrease in mortality, but at times the gut will not cooperate.[68] Reduced motility and ileus are common, at times requiring parenteral nutrition to meet caloric needs. At the present time, there is no specific treatment for burn-induced ileus, but it seems that early enteral feeding will prevent some of these potential complications. Gastric distention can be avoided by nasogastric tube decompression of the stomach, accompanied by enteral feeding through a tube placed beyond the ligament of Treitz. Failure to decompress the stomach can result in respiratory complications that need to be considered when deciding optimal positioning of the casualty. Furthermore, the risk of aspiration must be considered, and the head of the bed elevated to greater than 30° as often as possible.

Curling's ulcer, with erosion of the stomach and duodenal mucosa, results in upper gastrointestinal bleeding or perforation. However, its incidence has been largely eliminated by the use of histamine-2 blockers, proton-pump inhibitors, early enteral feeding, and antacids. Burn casualties with significant anemia and resultant hemodynamic instability should be evaluated for stress-induced gastrointestinal bleed.

Occasionally, severe burns involving the face and neck preclude traditional nasotracheal or orotracheal intubation, and performance of a cricothyroidotomy may be required. The cricothyroidotomy is generally followed by a formal tracheostomy when appropriate surgical support is available.

Metabolic Considerations

Over the course of hospitalization, catabolic derangement in burn injury results in a tremendous loss of lean body mass. This occurs over the entire first year after injury, and the impact on the rehabilitative course can be significant, ranging from isolated strength impairments to decreased independence with activities of daily living (ADLs). Time to full functional recovery may also increase.

One of the responses to severe burn is a dramatic increase in catecholamine production. This has been linked to a number of metabolic abnormalities, including increased resting energy expenditure (REE), muscle catabolism, and altered thermoregulation.[69] The effects of this sustained catecholamine surge on the cardiac system are to increase heart rate and, therefore, myocardial work. Propranolol, a nonspecific β-blocker, has been used to decrease heart rate and myocardial work in casualties with severe burns. Propranolol can be given intravenously and orally to equal effect on heart rate and myocardial work without detrimental effect on cardiac output or response to stress. Propranolol administration also decreases peripheral lipolysis and muscle catabolism, which are additional beneficial effects.[70]

Oxandrolone, an anabolic agent that helps decrease lean mass catabolism and improves wound healing, was recently shown to significantly decrease length of hospital stay.[71] Oxandrolone should be considered in all casualties with a burn size greater than 20% TBSA. Liver function tests should be monitored for the potential for hepatotoxicity and stopped if significant elevations in enzymes are detected.

Renal Considerations

Acute renal failure, usually in the form of acute tubular necrosis, is characterized by deterioration of renal function over a period of hours to days, resulting in the failure of the kidney to excrete nitrogenous waste prod-ucts and to maintain fluid and electrolyte homeostasis.[72] In burn casualties, the causes can generally be narrowed to renal hypoperfusion from volume depletion or sepsis, or nephrotoxic iatrogenic insults (eg, aminoglycosides or IV contrast agents). Acute renal failure may be isolated or may occur in conjunction with other organs (ie, multiple organ dysfunction syndrome).

Generally, a conservative approach is applied in managing acute renal failure. Supportive care, optimization of hemodynamics, and prevention of further insults will result in resolution. In severe cases, renal replacement therapy or extracorporeal renal support is needed to eliminate toxins. Various modalities can be used, including intermittent hemodialysis and continuous renal replacement therapies.[73] To date, trials have not shown any differences in outcomes between continuous modes of renal replacement and traditional intermittent dialysis.[74]

The rehabilitative implications of renal replacement therapy depend on the modality. In hemodynamically stable casualties with renal failure, intermittent hemodialysis is generally well tolerated and, because casualties are off dialysis the majority of the day and are allowed to participate in rehabilitation sessions, it does not hinder rehabilitation. Casualties who are hemodynamically unstable and need vasopressor support are often unable to tolerate intermittent hemodialysis. For these casualties, treatment with continuous renal replacement therapy may be effective. While a casualty receives treatment, rehabilitation is limited to therapeutic bed exercises and positioning because working vascular access must be maintained without bending or kinking the catheter. Casualties typically remain in bed for the duration of treatment.

Cardiac Considerations

Early rehabilitative care in severely burned casualties requires an understanding of cardiovascular physiology in the acute period. There is a direct link between cardiac performance and casualty function. Several factors, including ventricular preload, myocardial contractility, ventricular afterload, and heart rate and rhythm, determine cardiac function, and thus tissue perfusion of blood, at the whole body level. Understanding the effects of each of these components on heart function, as well as the effects of added activity, is necessary for the optimal rehabilitative care of the casualty.

Ventricular Preload

The force that stretches the cardiac muscle prior to contraction is known as "preload." Severe burns reduce preload to the heart through volume loss into the burned and nonburned tissues. Therefore, volumes predicted by resuscitation formulas must be used to maintain blood pressure and hemodynamics. The Frank-Starling relationship describes the increase in cardiac performance via preload augmentation by volume resuscitation.[75] Preload is measured clinically by either central venous pressure or by pulmonary capillary wedge pressure (PCWP) obtained with a pulmonary artery catheter. Of these, the PCWP is the best estimate because it assesses the left side of the heart.

Myocardial Contractility

The force with which the heart contracts is referred to as "cardiac contractility." Severe burns can induce myocardial depression early (characterized by abnormalities in contraction and relaxation),[76] reducing cardiac output. This is followed by a hyperdynamic phase of increased cardiac output that generally persists throughout hospitalization.

Ventricular Afterload

Afterload is the force that impedes or opposes ventricular contraction. Elevated afterload is most evident early in the course of injury; however, shortly thereafter, it is decreased primarily through vasodilation and an increase in heart rate.

Heart Rate and Rhythm

For the heart to function properly, the electrical conduction system must be intact and provide regular contractions sufficient to propel blood through the circulatory system. If heart rate exceeds 160 beats per minute, the heart may not have time to fill completely, thus decreasing myocardial fiber stretch and heart function. The same effect is seen with frequent premature ventricular or irregular beats. Heart rate and rhythm are continuously monitored in critically ill casualties.

Hemodynamic Therapy: Preload Augmentation and Use of Vasopressors

When a patient exhibits hypotension or other signs of inadequate cardiac function (eg, decreased urine output), the usual response is to augment preload by increasing intravascular volume. This sound physiologic approach is based on the Frank-Starling principle, and should be the first therapy for a casualty in shock. Intravascular volume can be increased with either crystalloid or colloid to increase the central venous pressure and PCWP to a value between 10 and 20 mmHg. The effects of this therapy can be monitored

by the restoration of arterial blood pressure, a decrease in tachycardia, and a urine output greater than 0.5 mL/kg/h.

If volume replacement is insufficient to improve hemodynamics in burn casualties in shock, vasopressor support may be required. Agents with primary effects on the α-adrenergic receptor can be used to induce vasoconstriction and increase blood pressure. These agents consist of norepinephrine and phenylephrine, and can be used effectively during septic shock or neurogenic shock to increase vascular tone. In burn casualties, it is believed that these agents cause vasoconstriction of the skin and splanchnic circulation to preserve blood flow to major organs, such as the heart and brain. This redistribution in blood flow can convert partial-thickness skin injuries to full-thickness injuries and result in ischemic injury to the gut. The benefits of specific vasoconstrictors must be weighed against these effects. Alternative agents include vasopressin, dopamine, dobutamine, and epinephrine. Vasopressin acts primarily by augmenting the effects of existing catecholamines. Dopamine has a dose-related response at different receptors. Dobutamine, which is considered an inotrope, acts primarily on β-receptors and increases contractility (and thus stroke volume). Epinephrine has both β and α properties.

The cardiac implications of physical activity during rehabilitation are extremely important. Casualties who have inadequate preload, as determined by central venous pressure or PCWP, are likely to exhibit orthostatic symptoms when going from the supine position to an upright chair or standing position. Inadequate preload, when further decreased by gravity via venous pooling in the lower extremities, can lead to tachycardia and hypotension because the casualty cannot maintain or augment sufficient cardiac output. In these instances, intravascular volume loading (with crystalloid, colloid, or blood products) may allow the casualty to tolerate positioning changes more readily.

Contractility and afterload varies in the post-burn period. Early on, physical activity may not be tolerated due to depressed myocardial function. Later, profound tachycardia may prohibit activity and limit rehabilitation potential. A casualty may also be hemodynamically unstable, requiring vasopressor support, and unable to tolerate rehabilitation. Physical activity is not necessarily prohibited when a vasopressor is required. Constant communication between the rehabilitation team and the critical care team is vital to determine a casualty's threshold for any type of activity. An understanding of cardiovascular physiology and its impact in the post-burn period is important in order to optimize rehabilitation and promotion to functional recovery.

Hematological Considerations

Severely burned casualties develop a variety of hematologic conditions that may impact the rehabilitative process.

Anemia

Over the last 10 years, restrictive transfusion practices have led to clinicians being more tolerant of lower hemoglobin and hematocrit levels; studies demonstrated improved outcomes for casualties who tolerated anemia with hemoglobin levels as low as 7 g/dL.[77] Unless anemia is acute, lower hemoglobin levels are not only well tolerated, limiting unnecessary, potentially harmful blood transfusions, but can save lives. Severely burned casualties are generally not transfused blood products unless they are symptomatic from anemia; it has become more common to transfuse blood only when hemoglobin levels fall below 7 g/dL, unless there is active bleeding, shock, or evidence of myocardial ischemia. Thus, rehabilitation occurs routinely in casualties with stable anemia and is, in most cases, well tolerated.

Thromboembolic complications

Thromboembolic complications were thought to be rare in the burn population; however, recent reports have suggested an incidence at an estimated 2.9%.[78] This is much lower than the general trauma population, but remains clinically significant. As a result, on admission, burn casualties are placed on chemoprophylaxis with either low-molecular–weight heparin or unfractionated heparin. Those who are at highest risk (eg, those who are morbidly obese or have sustained spinal cord trauma) may be considered for inferior vena cava filter placement. Development of deep venous thrombosis is not a contraindication for early mobilization out of bed. Generally, after a deep venous clot has been identified, the casualty is fully anticoagulated with IV heparin. Casualties may be as physically active as they can tolerate; there is no evidence that early activity increases risk of clot dislodgement and pulmonary embolism. However, anticoagulation is recommended for at least 24 hours prior to any activity.

Nutritional Considerations

Severe burn injury results in a hypermetabolic and catabolic state. For burn casualties, adequate nutrition is vital for wound management and rehabilitation. Without it, wounds, grafts, and donor sites will not heal, and the casualty will become more susceptible to infection. Additionally, weight loss can be associated with impaired immune function, decreased wound healing, functional impairments, and morbidity.[79] All the members of the interdisciplinary burn team must be familiar with the importance of providing nutrition to burn casualties. Providing adequate nutrition is a difficult task, considering that resting energy can be as high as double normal levels. The needs of casualties with less than 20% TBSA burns can usually be met with a high-calorie, high-protein diet and supplemental multivitamins. Casualties with greater than 20% to 30% TBSA burned often require nutritional support via feeding tubes. Many complications and treatments can inhibit feeding, and careful monitoring is essential. The goals of nutrition support are to avoid malnutrition without overfeeding, to promote wound healing and graft retention, to preserve immune function and gut integrity, and to maximally support functional rehabilitation.

After burn injury, the body goes through ebb and flow phases. The ebb phase is characterized by decreased cardiac output, oxygen consumption, body temperature, blood volume, and insulin levels. The flow phase is characterized by increased cardiac output, oxygen consumption, body temperature, insulin levels, and gluconeogenesis.[80] In 1979 Long et al discussed the ebb and flow phases in subjects with major burns, describing the loss of nitrogen through the urine and the REE by indirect calorimetry.[81] Burn casualties have been shown to have a prolonged flow phase. Pereira et al found that the initial increase in REE can be as high as double, 150% at full healing, 140% at 6 months, 120% at 9 months, and as high as 110% after 12 months.[82] The magnitude and duration of the flow phase can be minimized by placing casualties in a warm environment, providing adequate pain relief, completing early wound closure, applying occlusive wound dressings, and preventing sepsis.

Burn injury results in major changes in metabolism that are believed to be largely hormone-mediated. These changes are likely due to increased catecholamines, glucocorticoids, and glucagon-to-insulin ratios, and they include increased gluconeogenesis, proteolysis, and ureagenesis, and decreased lipolysis and ketone utilization. In addition, skin barrier destruction results in physiologic losses of heat, water, and water-soluble nutrients. These changes result in increased energy expenditure, increased nitrogen losses, and changes in nutrient metabolism. The body's available kilocalorie stores are quickly consumed after a burn injury, and gluconeogenesis must occur to further fuel the body (Table 13-4). This results in the expense of lean body mass.

Nutritional support for burn casualties should be

TABLE 13-4

AVAILABLE ENERGY STORES

Source	Type	Available Kilocalories
Liver	Glucose	300
Muscle	Glucose	600
Liver	Triglyceride	500

initiated early. Studies have shown early feeding after burn injury increases gut size in animals,[83] promotes better nitrogen balance in humans,[84] and can be safely initiated.[83,85] Nutritional support should be monitored closely to ensure that nutritional needs are being met that promote wound healing. Underfeeding can affect wound healing and immunocompetence.[86] Overfeeding can result in hyperglycemia, elevated carbon dioxide, and fatty liver, leading to delayed ventilator weaning and liver dysfunction.

Energy needs can be estimated using equations that are based on factors such as body size, age, activity level, and percentage of burn. A casualty's preburn weight should be used in figuring energy needs because weight is affected by massive edema, as well as bulky dressings and external fixations. Many other factors affect a burn casualty's metabolic rate, such as body composition, body temperature, circadian rhythm, ambient temperature,[87] chemical paralysis,[88] the energy costs of protein synthesis and respiratory

stress, evaporative heat loss from wounds, infection,[89] other trauma, pain, the thermogenic effect of food, and surgery. No metabolic rate equation can incorporate this vast range of variables.

The most well-known equation for calculating burn energy needs was developed by Curreri et al, and uses weight and burn size to determine needs.[90] Later studies show that it is likely that this formula overestimates the calorie needs.[91,92] USAISR also developed an equation for determining calorie needs (Exhibit 13-2).[93] Carlson et al noted a linear relationship between burn size and REE,[93] and Milner et al validated this formula during the first month following burn injury.[94] Initial feeding based on the USAISR equation is an appropriate approach until a metabolic cart study can be completed.

Because of the many factors affecting a burn casualty's metabolic rate, the most precise method of measuring energy requirements is by taking serial measurements of REE by indirect calorimetry. Indirect calorimetry uses a portable metabolic cart at the casualty's bedside that can be attached to the ventilator or to a canopy if the casualty is not on a ventilator. The cart measures respiratory gas exchange and calculates REE from this data. This measured energy expenditure includes increased needs because of the injury, but not the energy needed for activity because it is performed when the casualty is at rest. Total calorie needs can be estimated by adding 10% to 40% to the measured expenditure to account for activity.

With the USAISR formula, Carlson et al used an

EXHIBIT 13-2

US ARMY INSTITUTE OF SURGICAL RESEARCH EQUATION FOR DETERMINING CALORIE NEEDS*

$$EER = [BMR^\dagger \times (0.89142 + \{.01335 \times TBSA^\ddagger\})] \times BSA \times 24 \times AF^\S$$
Male BMR $= 54.337821 - (1.19961 \times Age) + (0.02548 \times Age^2) - (0.00018 \times Age^3)$
Female BMR $= 54.74942 - (1.54884 \times Age) + (0.03580 \times Age^2) - (0.00026 \times Age^3)$
BSA (m^2) = square root of:

$$\frac{Ht(cm) \times Wt\ (kg)}{3600} \quad or \quad \frac{Ht\ (in.) \times Wt\ (lb)}{3131}$$

*This applies to burns ≥ 20% total body surface area; for burns < 20% total body surface area, use 30–35 kcal/kg.
†This is determined using the Fleisch equation.
‡For example, for 30% TBSA burn, use "30."
§Use 1.25 or a value appropriate for the specific patient.
AF: activity factor
BMR: basal metabolic rate
BSA: body surface area
EER: estimated energy requirement
Ht: height
TBSA: total-body surface area burn (eg, for 30% TBSA, use "30")
Wt: weight

estimated activity factor of 1.25.[93] Wall-Alonso et al used the doubly labeled water technique, along with resting metabolic rate, and determined an activity factor of 1.05 to 1.15.[95] Hart et al found that an activity factor of 1.4 can lead to weight maintenance but results in an increase in body fat, while an activity factor of 1.2 can maximize lean body mass retention.[89]

If tube feeds are a patient's only source of calories, a goal rate derived from the REE times 1.4 is appropriate. At least the REE times 1.2 must be provided. Many sources of calories need to be considered in tube-fed patients, including food and beverages taken orally and IV fluids (eg, a solution of 5% dextrose in water contains 170 cal/L; albumin contains 200 cal/L in a 5% solution, 1,000 cal/L in a 25% solution; and propofol contains 1,100 cal/L).

Burn injury results in profound changes in protein metabolism, increasing liver synthesis of acute phase proteins. Energy needs are met by muscle proteolysis. In addition, significant amounts of protein are lost through urine, feces, and open wounds. Losses can lead to as much as 2 to 3 lb of muscle in a day. The protein needs of burn casualties are difficult to determine with available data. It is currently recommended that 20% to 25% of a burn casualty's calories come from protein.[96–98] Protein intake should be adjusted serially, based on nitrogen balance. The Waxman formula is used to determine nitrogen loss from open burn wounds.[99] Total body nitrogen losses are determined by urinary urea nitrogen, insensible losses, and wound losses. The surface area of open wounds is entered into the Waxman formula for the appropriate post-burn day to determine nitrogen lost through the wound. The urinary, wound, and estimated insensible losses are added to determine the current rate of nitrogen loss. The goal is to provide more nitrogen to the casualty than what is being lost, promoting overall anabolism. Increased nutritional protein does not stop catabolism; rather, it serves in anabolism to replace lost tissue.

Recent studies have focused on the role of specific amino acids in nutritional support of the burn casualty. In the past, arginine supplementation was shown to improve cell-mediated immunity and wound healing and decrease morbidity and mortality.[100–102] However, its safety has been called into question, especially in septic casualties. Use of another amino acid, glutamine, is now advocated because it is the primary fuel for enterocytes and immune cells. Its use purportedly preserves gut integrity and decreases translocation and infections.[103] Branched-chain amino acids, leucine, isoleucine, and valine, although once believed to spare endogenous muscle catabolism, have not been proven to improve outcomes in burn casualties.[104–108] More research is needed to determine the utility and proper use of amino acids and to examine safety and efficacy.

Carbohydrate metabolism is altered during the acute post-burn phase. For example, glucose is produced from gluconeogenesis. Carbohydrates are the primary energy substrate during this period, and a high carbohydrate diet (3% fat) may decrease muscle protein degradation.[109] Although this may be convincing evidence to provide high-carbohydrate, low-fat nutritional support, excess carbohydrate use is also likely to lead to increased carbon dioxide production.

The optimal amount and type of lipid to use in nutritional support of the burn casualty is controversial and currently the subject of extensive research. During the acute post-burn phase, lipolysis decreases because protein is the preferred fuel source, and serum free fatty acids and triglycerides increase. Lipids are a concentrated source of calories for burn casualties, but high levels of lipid intake may impair immune function. Because adequate essential fatty acids aid in wound healing (among other things), it is necessary to prevent their deficiency in burn casualties.[96,110,111]

Specific vitamin and mineral requirements for burn casualties have not been established, although it is believed there are increased needs for at least those nutrients involved in wound healing and tissue synthesis (zinc and vitamins C and A). Providing a vitamin-mineral supplement equal to the recommended dietary allowances is commonly recommended. Additional daily supplements of 1 g ascorbic acid and 250 mg zinc sulfate are also recommended.[112–114]

The levels of the trace elements copper, iron, selenium, and zinc are of interest because they decrease plasma levels in the acute phase after thermal injury.[115] A deficiency in iron, which is involved in adenosine triphosphate production, can lead to decreased performance and decreased immunity.[116] Copper is involved in wound healing and collagen production.[117,118] A copper deficiency can lead to decreased synthesis,[117] decreased immune function,[119] heart and lung dysfunction, and bone demineralization.[120] The loss of copper in the first week after thermal injury is as high as 20% to 40% of the body's stores.[121] Selenium is involved in immunity, lipid peroxidation,[122] tissue oxygenation,[123] and the phagocytic activity of neutrophils.[124] Selenium deficiency can cause cardiomyopathy,[125] myalgia,[126] and decreased immunity.[127–129] A deficiency in zinc, which is involved in the function of metalloenzymes[130] and bone metabolism,[118] can lead to decreased wound healing and impaired immunity.[130]

Developing a nutritional care plan involves selecting the appropriate route of nutritional support and the specific formula, diet, or supplement to be used. Early enteral support (within the first 24 hours) is preferred.[131] Nutritional support for burn casualties may include an oral diet, oral supplements, enteral nutrition, or parenteral nutrition.

PAIN MANAGEMENT

Pain is a negative sensory or emotional response to a stimulus that may or may not be associated with actual tissue damage.[132,133] Nociceptive pain results from stimulation of nocioreceptors within the body, neuropathic pain is due to nerve damage, and central pain is associated with central nervous system (CNS) lesions.[134] Purely psychogenic pain, which is secondary to mental illness, is very rare in burn casualties.[135]

Pain impacts interpersonal relationships, as well as a casualty's ability to carry out ADLs and participate in rehabilitation. Poor pain control is associated with increased incidence of posttraumatic stress disorder (PTSD), anxiety, conditioning, and development of avoidance behaviors,[136] as well as a decreased willingness to remain actively engaged in the rehabilitation plan.[137] Casualties frequently cite inadequate pain control as the reason for noncompliance with their medical treatment plans.[138] Pain management can rely on both a multimodal pharmacological approach and an interdisciplinary approach.

The pharmacological management of pain is heavily dependent on opioids.[139] Moderate- to long-acting medications, such as continuous release morphine and methadone, are generally used on a scheduled basis for background pain. Methadone is especially useful for prolonged treatment when casualties become intolerant to morphine.[140] Rescue medications intended for breakthrough pain include short-acting agents, such as oxycodone and acetaminophen/oxycodone. Fentanyl transmucosal lozenges work in minutes and last longer than IV doses because they are absorbed through the stomach and the oral mucosa.[141]

Anxiolytics, such as benzodiazepines, alleviate anxiety in burn casualties.[142] A casualty's level of sedation must be closely monitored because of the synergism anxiolytics have with other drugs. Ketamine, commonly used with midazolam,[143] is often used for burn dressing changes because it provides analgesia with minimal respiratory depression[144]; however, it may cause prolonged sedation, dysphoric reactions, and delusional hallucinations.

Several other classes of drugs also improve pain control and decrease narcotic use. Anticonvulsants, such as gabapentin, pregabalin, and carbamazepine, are especially useful as neuronal membrane stabilizers whenever there is a component of neuropathic pain.[145] Local anesthetics, which act to block sodium channel conductance of the pain signal, can be used as topical analgesics and in regional anesthesia,[146] which will be addressed later in this chapter.

Antidepressants, such as tricyclics, are another class of drugs commonly used to manage chronic pain. Nonsteroidal antiinflammatory drugs (NSAIDs) and acetaminophen relieve minor pain; however, NSAIDs are less commonly prescribed because of concerns over their antiplatelet and nephrotoxic effects. Other medications used or soon to be available may include topical sprays, salves, and creams or iontophoretic and lozenge-based fentanyl. Intranasal applications of ketamine, butorphanol, morphine, and hydromorphone are also being developed.

In addition to a pharmacological approach to pain management, an interdisciplinary approach has also been successful. Clinics with pain management specialists are a staple, but alternative and complementary medicine techniques, including acupressure, music therapy, and massage therapy, are also being welcomed.[141] Additionally, virtual reality and hypnosis are being investigated as pain management techniques.[147] Pain populations that were difficult to manage in the past, including those with phantom limb pain or sensation, have achieved some success with pain psychology professionals.[148] Group therapy and counseling, support groups, psychotherapy, and behavioral modification, such as breathing and relaxation techniques, have all been used to deal with severe and life-altering pain.[149]

Burn pain is unique in many ways. Most pain decreases with time from the original insult and throughout the recovery period; however, burn pain may increase with time, increase with recovery (full-thickness burns are insensate initially) and are more likely to result in chronic pain (>6 months' duration).[150] Predictors of burn pain include depth and location of burn. Extent, age, gender, ethnicity, educational history, occupation, history of drug or alcohol abuse, and other psychiatric illness do not predict the severity of burn pain.[133] Although many people have lasting impressions of burn injury related to momentarily touching hot stoves or scalding water, few can actually understand the pain associated with a major burn. For example, with superficial partial-thickness burns, even air currents moving over the affected tissue may result in excruciating pain.

Chronic pain—an intense, prolonged pain—is common in burn casualties and is aggravated by the need for frequent wound care, dressing changes, and rehabilitation activities. The repetitive and extensive nature of dressing changes cause anxiety and depression, which can further decrease pain thresholds.[151] The sequelae of poor pain control can affect the psyche, including self-image, motivation, and will to live.[152] Burn injuries cause significant pain during the entire recovery period, and although complete elimination may not be possible without a general anesthetic, thorough assessment and planning can make pain more tolerable.

During the acute phase, burn pain is managed through emergency care. The American Burn Association recommends the use of morphine during this phase, but many other opioids could be titrated to be effective.[153] Burn casualties experience intense pain and usually require large doses of opioids to remain comfortable, even in the absence of movement or surgical procedures. Because airway compromise is an ever-present concern, ketamine may also be considered to decrease opioid requirements.[143] When possible, subcutaneous and intramuscular administration should be avoided in favor of IV delivery because the former result in unpredictable absorption. When IV access is unobtainable, intraosseous placement may be considered by skilled personnel in urgent need of temporary venous access.[23]

Inhalational agents, such as volatile anesthetic gases and IV agents, form the main portion of an intraoperative anesthetic regimen.[154] Casualties may develop opioid tolerance. Regional anesthesia may also be indicated, either alone or combined with general anesthesia, but is often limited to casualties with small burns and for analgesia of donor sites.

Operative intervention often leads to a change in pain focus because donor sites are commonly more painful than excision sites, which may be insensate.[137] Neuraxial techniques, such as epidural or spinal anesthetics, may help with postoperative analgesia in affected areas, especially when more caudad. For example, femoral or iliac fascia compartment nerve block may be used to provide analgesia for the anterior flank donor site. Blood loss may be increased from the resultant sympathectomy after neuraxial techniques, and percutaneous technique risks infection.

Severe burn injuries often present significant perioperative challenges to providers and therapists secondary to reported inadequate pain management.[155] A characteristic hospital course for burn casualties includes frequent operative visits, long hospital stays, and extended rehabilitation, during which casualties are placed on chronic opioid therapy to manage pain.[156] Burn rehabilitation is unique because it is repetitive, painful, and prolonged, increasing the difficulty of achieving goals.

In addition to use of systemic pain medications during potentially painful acute and intermediate rehabilitation sessions, regional anesthesia (in the form of peripheral nerve block) can be added to a multimodal pain management regimen. Historically, regional anesthesia has been used in the form of CNS block or neuraxial techniques to control intraoperative pain and labor-induced pain (eg, epidural and spinal anesthesia). However, advancements in peripheral nerve block techniques, with targeted placement of local anesthetic medications via peripheral nerve stimulation and ultrasound guidance, has created new interest in peripheral nerve blocks to control intraoperative, acute postoperative pain, and chronic pain syndromes during the recovery phase following burn.

In addition to opioids, regional anesthesia of the extremities and of the trunk is useful for burn casualty rehabilitation. Intramuscular, oral, and IV opioid medications have a long history of use as part of acute and chronic pain control regimens. However, based on the known side effects of sedation, respiratory depression, and inadequate pain control, exclusive use of opioids for analgesia has been replaced by multimodal approaches, including regional anesthesia for the extremities. Benefits of regional anesthesia include reducing pain during rehabilitation, avoiding side effects of respiratory depression caused by opioid and sedative medication use, and minimizing limits imposed on therapists secondary to casualties' intolerance to pain, allowing the advancement of rehabilitation goals.

In the extremities, regional anesthesia is given using a needle attached to a low-current electrical impulse generator, which stimulates motor fibers and identifies the targeted nerves.[157] Once the nerve fibers are identified, large volumes (20–40 mL) of local anesthetic are injected to produce nerve block. An alternative technique uses an ultrasound probe to identify targeted nerve bundles and uses direct visualization of the needle during local anesthetic injection.

Peripheral nerve block can be performed by a single injection or continuous catheter technique. Single injection techniques are limited in duration, based on the local anesthetic medication used, but can be extremely useful in immediate rehabilitation.[157] The most commonly used local anesthetic medications for peripheral nerve block can be classified as either amide or ester local anesthetics. The local anesthetic drug class affects onset of action, duration of drug effects, rate of systemic absorption versus elimination, and distribution throughout the body. Commonly used local anesthetics for peripheral nerve block include lidocaine (short duration, 1–2 hrs), mepivacaine (intermediate duration, 2–4 hrs), ropivacaine (long duration, 5–8 hrs), and bupivacaine (long duration, 4–12 hrs).[157]

Continuous catheter techniques can extend the duration of analgesia to the desired length of time. Continuous peripheral nerve catheters have commonly been reserved for the inpatient population, secondary to provider concerns over potential systemic toxicity, potential nerve toxicity, infection at the catheter site, and risk of accidental limb injury as outpatient. In an ambulatory setting, casualty selection is critical. Only casualties who are capable of accepting the additional responsibility of the catheter and infusion pump should be selected. Ambulatory use of continuous nerve block is contraindicated when a casualty is cognitively impaired and without a home caregiver, unable to attend scheduled follow-up catheter care, or is at high risk for systemic toxicity (ie, hepatic or renal insufficiency).[158]

During regional anesthesia procedures, casualties frequently require minimal to moderate sedation to tolerate the pain from placing the peripheral nerve block. Preoperative fasting practices have been established to reduce the risk of pulmonary aspiration from gastric contents during elective procedures, based on American Society of Anesthesiologists Task Force on Preoperative Fasting guidelines.[159] These guidelines do not apply to casualties who undergo procedures without anesthesia or with only local anesthesia, when upper airway protective reflexes are unimpaired, and when there is no apparent risk of pulmonary aspiration. An anesthesiologist should be consulted before discontinuing oral intake for peripheral nerve block.[159] In addition, care must be taken to ensure the daily anticoagulation dose is discontinued prior to regional technique.[160] Therapists, anesthesiologists, and primary team physicians should consult one another before performing regional block and discontinuing scheduled medication.

Complications of peripheral nerve block, although rare, must be considered when weighing the risks and benefits of the procedure. When complications arise, it is imperative that the provider and therapist be aware of the symptoms and take appropriate action. Systemic drug toxicity is caused by excessive absorption or accidental injection of greater-than-recommended blood concentrations of local anesthetic. Signs of generalized CNS toxicity are dependent on plasma concentration. Lower plasma concentrations may cause CNS depression (eg, lightheadedness, tinnitus, numbness of tongue), whereas higher plasma concentrations of local anesthetic may result in CNS excitation (eg, seizures, unconsciousness, coma, respiratory arrest,

cardiovascular depression).[157] Additional procedure complications include the following:

- nerve injury during needle placement,
- bleeding from vascular puncture,
- intravascular injection of local anesthetic,
- allergic reaction to local anesthetic,
- lung injury during peripheral nerve block placement in the upper extremities or trunk,
- temporary phrenic nerve paralysis during upper-extremity blocks, and
- high local anesthetic cerebral spinal fluid level, causing respiratory depression.

During the long term, burn pain management relies on controlling both baseline (often chronic) and breakthrough pain. "Pain soup" refers to a group of pain medications that target different receptors to attempt synergistic pain management while minimizing adverse effects related to overuse of any one class of drugs. Chronic use often escalates the requirement for opioids, secondary to the development of drug tolerance. A multireceptor approach helps reduce drowsiness, nausea, vomiting, constipation and addiction potential seen with narcotics by interfacing with receptors other than just the μ-opioid receptor.[150]

Peripheral nerve block techniques can also be effective over the long term. When developing therapeutic plans, anesthesiologists or interventional pain specialists should be consulted. Outpatient follow-up at a pain clinic is often an ideal solution to best tailor a pain management plan for each burn casualty.[161] Nonpharmacological pain control modalities to consider include behavior modification (conditioning),[148] transcutaneous electrical nerve stimulation, acupressure (to the external ear), massage or music therapy, virtual reality,[147] and counseling and group therapy. Enlisting the assistance of professionals, such as psychiatric nurses, psychotherapists, and fellow burn survivors, is also often advantageous.[2]

REHABILITATION OF THE BURN CASUALTY

Rehabilitative interventions are paramount to a casualty's total functional outcome and are required through all phases (acute, intermediate, and long term) of the recovery process (Figure 13-15).[162] On a daily basis, burn therapists treat burn casualties with the goal of achieving maximum physical and functional recovery.[163] Occupational therapy and physical therapy evaluations performed throughout the rehabilitation community initially resemble typical burn rehabilitation evaluations. They include acquiring a baseline of neurocognitive function, ROM, strength, sensation,

activity tolerance, and intervention response. These components of the evaluation are performed following an appropriate chart review to understand the expected physiological, psychological, and emotional involvement from the described injury or insult.

Burn Edema

Massive tissue edema develops following thermal injury (Figure 13-16).[6] Current evidence indicates biochemical mediators, released in response to thermal

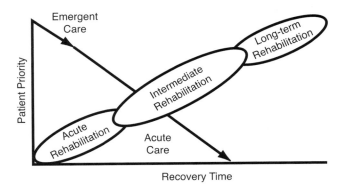

Figure 13-15. Interaction between medical care and rehabilitation of burn casualties.

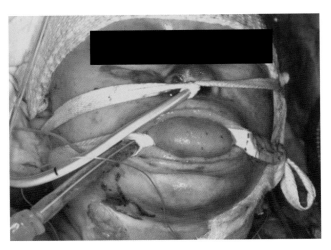

Figure 13-16. Burn casualty displaying massive facial edema.

injury, play a significant role in edema development.[6] The pathogenesis of tissue edema following thermal injury involves changes in the physical forces controlling fluid flux across the capillary, as well as fluid accumulation in the interstitium.[6] Edema forms at the expense of the vascular and extracellular compartments. Electrolyte concentrations can vary considerably, due in part to large potassium intracellular losses, urinary excretion, and large sodium intracellular and extracellular gains.[164]

Although edema is common to most significant burn injuries, no modalities have proven completely effective at managing it in severe burn casualties.[6] To better understand edema formation, one must appreciate the basis of fluid management and its role in resuscitation, both positive and negative (see "Fluid Resuscitation" above).

Edema Evaluation

Measuring edema is an important aspect of a burn casualty's physical examination. Edema can impair joint ROM, slow wound healing, and compromise circulation.[165] All areas of the body can be affected by edema that results from a burn. Hands are commonly affected and are particularly troublesome to rehabilitate.

Typically, edema is first assessed on a subjective scale by a therapist and is rated as minimal, moderate, or severe. If edema persists or progresses, therapists use objective measurement to more accurately assess the quantity of edema and the effectiveness of treatment measures and to document progress.[166] Although traditional methods of objectively assessing edema, especially in burns, are difficult to perform clinically or have limited validity, recent literature demonstrates an objective edema measurement that provides a more

valid assessment and can be performed just as expeditiously as a subjective measure.[167]

The most commonly used methods of objective edema assessment include circumferential measurement, water volumetry, and the figure-of-eight measurement. Circumferential measurements give therapists a value to quantify edema at a specified site along an extremity. The therapist identifies a site along an edematous area to be evaluated, and the site is either marked or measured at a set distance from an anatomical landmark, allowing for future reference or measurement. A circumferential measurement is then taken at the designated point to quantify the edema.[168] Circumferential measurements are practical for all body areas, but provide only a point estimate of volume for an area. Depending on the site chosen to measure, the results can be significantly different. This method is best reserved for use on areas of isolated edema, such as the fingers, or where other measurement techniques are not available, such as the trunk. Although they are clinically expedient and more useful for monitoring the effectiveness of treatment and progress than a subjective assessment, the limited reliability and validity of circumferential measurements limits their usefulness.[168]

Volumetry, a measurement based on the principle of water displacement as a measure of volume, is considered the "gold standard" for measuring edema.[169] The volumeter is a standardized tool that allows a therapist to measure edema, most commonly of the hand and foot.[166] Reliability and validity of volumetric measurements is well established[169,170]; however, volumetry has several limitations.[171] For example, it is time consuming, requires expensive specialized equipment, and great care must be taken to ensure a consistent position for each measurement.[168–170,172] Also, whenever possible, open wounds and immature skin grafts should not be immersed in water.

The figure-of-eight technique offers an alternative that is reliable, valid, and clinically expedient (Figure 13-17).[167,173–175] It uses a tape measure and defined anatomical landmarks to quantify edema. Although the reliability and validity of this technique are superior or equal to other forms of objective measurement, its applicability to areas of the body other than the ankle and hand are limited.

Edema Management

Excessive edema can have severe, long-lasting consequences. The complications resulting from severe edema include tissue hypoxia and massive loss of intravascular fluid (which results in hypovolemia). Tissue hypoxia may develop as a result of increased tissue pressures from an impending compartment syndrome, and over-aggressive fluid therapy, often used to correct suspected hypovolemia, catalyzes the edema process.[6] Organ systems, such as the brain, lungs, and heart, do not function well under the stress of severe edema. Circulation to an edematous extremity can also be compromised. Early escharotomy is indicated when massive edema is anticipated or observed to compromise tissue.

Severe edema that does not require escharotomy may also have a profound effect on a burn casualty. Loss of dexterity in edematous hands and digits can further compound a casualty's feelings of helplessness following injury, leading to a cycle of decreased use, joint stiffness, contracture, tendon shortening, and long-term disability (Figure 13-18). It is imperative to provide adequate resuscitation to burn casualties while making every effort to minimize edema formation.

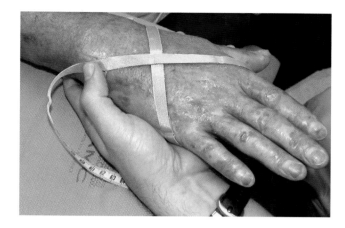

Figure 13-17. Figure-of-eight technique for measuring hand edema.

Acute Phase. Generally, edema peaks within 48 hours following burn.[165] Ongoing burn resuscitation can compound and prolong edema. If left untreated, edema can progress to critical levels, leading to eschar and compartment syndromes that require escharotomy or fasciotomy.[165] During the acute phase, the burn team must regularly examine the casualty for signs of vascular compromise.

Initially, edema is managed by elevating the affected areas. To facilitate edema reduction, the upper and lower extremities should be positioned such that the hand or foot is above the elbow or knee, which is above or at the level of the heart (Figure 13-19). ROM exercises are also an effective edema reduction tool in the acute phase. Passive range-of-motion (PROM) and AROM exercises have been shown to be effective, depending on the responsiveness of the casualty.[176,177] ROM exercise activates the muscle pump and

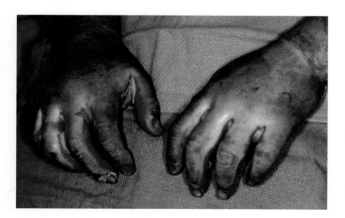

Figure 13-18. Burn casualty with edematous hands resulting in decreased dexterity.

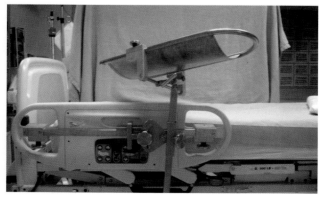

Figure 13-19. Positioning device used to elevate the upper extremity to facilitate edema reduction.

promotes edema reduction through enhanced venous and lymphatic flow.[178] Hand edema should be measured using the figure-of-eight technique.[167] The optimal position to control hand edema is placing the hand above the elbow and elbow above the heart.[168,179,180] AROM exercise of the digits can also help control edema; however, muscle contraction must be sufficient enough to act as a pumping mechanism and help venous and lymph return.[181]

Compression with elastic wraps can reduce edema when combined with elevated positioning and ROM exercises. The wrap should be applied uniformly to prevent a tourniquet effect and must have a greater perpendicular pressure distal to proximal. Elastic wraps are typically applied in a figure eight (Figure 13-20). For compression to be effective, the wrap must remain in place for prolonged periods of time. Generally, wraps are applied daily after completing wound care, and remain in place until wound care is performed the following day. Caution should be exercised when using compression in the acute phase because elastic wraps can contribute to increased compartment pressures or graft loss if applied too early or incorrectly. Therapists should frequently monitor vascular status distally on all areas being compressed. Burn casualties should be positioned with joints opposite the tendency for contracture. The individual's medical history and potential comorbidities should be considered at this stage of developing a positioning plan. Previous arthritis, strokes, brain injury, or residual functional motion deficit may require a modification to the positioning plan. A thorough history, physical examination, and sensory evaluation will reveal accompanying injuries that must be considered when developing plans for prolonged positioning. After sustaining a burn, a casualty's inflammatory response initiates a process by which any position maintained for more than 8 hours without active motion may cause early contracture formation.

During the acute phase, appropriate positioning decreases the potential to develop contractures; assists venous return, minimizing edema and the risk for compartment syndromes; protects the neurovascular bundles from further trauma; assists proper respiratory function; and protects the healing wound. The typical anticontracture bed positioning method during this phase should hold the neck in extension, with the shoulders abducted to 110° and forward flexed 15° or in the position of scaption.[182] Elbows should be extended and in supination, wrists and hands in functional position, hips extended and abducted 20° without external rotation, knees in extension, and ankles neutral. Although described as the anticontracture position, there is no single position that

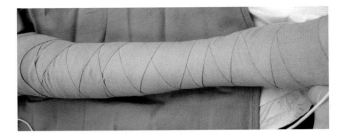

Figure 13-20. Figure-of-eight application of elastic wraps to the lower extremity.

completely ameliorates contractures. For those at risk for ACS, preventive measures incorporate the reverse Trendelenburg's position used to elevate the head of the bed while keeping the rest of the body straight, reducing intraabdominal pressure.[183]

As the initial, acute resuscitation process resides, the risk of compartment syndrome reduces; however, acute protective position techniques continue to assure optimal effectiveness for combating burn scar contracture, which will be addressed daily until the newly formed tissue matures. The incidence of joint contracture is high in this population and it is indicated that joint contracture has a significant detrimental impact on a burn casualty's quality of life.[51]

Each burned part of the body must be considered independently and in conjunction with other parts when planning positioning. Independent considerations include the various positioning and splinting devices available or required to achieve maximum benefit from the intervention (Table 13-5 and Figure 13-21). The concept of positioning must be well understood for optimal effectiveness in edema management and contracture prevention as well as to avoid adverse affects throughout the course of therapeutic interventions. Casualties with burn injuries are at high risk to develop pressure sores due to the nature of the injury and specifically identified risk factors related to the development of pressure sores. Although the cause of pressure sores is multifactorial, several of the factors listed include shear, friction, and unrelieved pressure.[184] All opportunities must be taken to get casualties out of bed to the highest level of functional position and activity possible.

Requisite repositioning is essential in preventing tissue contracture. Repositioning is recommended, at a minimum, every 2 hours to alleviate pressure from susceptible areas, such as the sacrum, coccyx, and heels. Heels are extremely vulnerable to pressure sores and require additional protection beyond specialty beds.[185] Other areas susceptible to pressure sores are the ankles, buttocks, and occipital area.

TABLE 13-5

POSITIONING AND SPLINTING DEVICES USED TO MANAGE EDEMA

Position	Device/Technique	Indications
Bed Position, Supine		
Head	Gel donut	Alternate flat to round every 2 hrs to avoid pressure sores to occipital region
	Foam pad	Used for custom requirements to maintain neutral alignment and avoid ear pressure
Face	Wide tie tapes	Used to distribute pressure over a larger area
Ears	Pillows are removed	Alleviates pressure and reduces edema
	Gel or foam donut	Used to prevent ear contact with the bed; irritation of ears increases the risk of chondritis
	Ear glock (see Figure 13-21a)	Used to prevent contact to the ear if the risk of chondritis is high
Nose	Foam or gel face support	If the prone position is required, a foam face support with a cutout is used to prevent pressure on the nose; a gel horseshoe pad can also be used
	Wide tie tapes	Used to distribute pressure under the nose for implementation of nasal airway, feeding, or gastrostomy tubes
Mouth	Bite block	Used to position the jaw and oral opening
	Microstomia	Used to extend the oral commissures; uses an expansion screw
Neck	Pillows are removed	Allows for improved neck extension
	Foam wedge	Used if additional neck extension is required
Shoulder	Arm slings	Used to position the shoulder in a supported posture to achieve between 90° and 120° of abduction and 15° forward flexion, or scaption[1]
Elbow	Positioned in extension with the forearm in supination on the sled of the shoulder sling	Supination and scaption remove undue tension from the neurovascular and muscular structures and elevate the upper extremity to improve vascular return
Wrist	Volar-based functional position hand splint	Wrist placed in functional position extended 20° to 25° and without ulnar or radial deviation
Hand	Volar-based functional position hand splint (see Figure 13-21b)	Places the thumb in palmar abduction with the MCP and IP joints in extension; the MCP joints of the index through small fingers is flexed to 70° and all IP joints are extended
Torso	Body wedges or tumble forms	Used to adjust the torso to relieve pressure from side to side and directly from the back
Hip	Positioned in full extension with 20° abduction and no external rotation	Alleviates pressure and reduces edema
	Abduction wedge	Maintains full extension position when the casualty is unable to maintain the position due to concomitant injury
	Elevation of lower extremity	Assists with fluid return, reducing the risk of compartment syndromes; protects the neurovascular bundles from further trauma; protects the healing wound
Knee	Extension	Alleviates pressure and reduces edema

(**Table 13-5** *continues*)

Table 13-5 *continued*

Position	Device/Technique	Indications
Feet, ankles, and legs	Inflatable booties	Used to keep the ankle at 90° and the toes extended; removes pressure from the heel of the foot
	L'nard boot	Used if the foot begins to develop an equines deformity
	Leg net	Made with copper tubing and fittings with surgical netting stretched over the frame (see Figures 13-21c and 13-21d); used to elevate the leg to reduce the risk of compartment syndrome acutely; used to prevent pressure sores from developing on the heels, typically alternated with the inflatable bootie and positioned so that there is a bootie on the contra-lateral lower extremity; reduces the degree of direct pressure on the sacrum, therefore reducing the risk of pressure sores; helps dry donor sites postoperatively, and prevent maceration and further tissue damage[2]
Seated Position		
Head, face, ears, nose, mouth, neck, shoulder, elbow, wrist, and hand	See above	See above
Torso	Body wedges, tumble forms	Used to assure posture is maintained in a midline posture
Hip	Positioned in flexion between 60° and 90° through chair recline; hip abduction is maintained at 20° and external rotation is avoided	Alleviates pressure and reduces edema
Knee	Full extension while seated (can alternate between flexion and extension if not contraindicated)	Alleviates pressure and reduces edema
Feet and ankles	Ankles are maintained at 90° and the toes extended	Alleviates pressure and reduces edema
Miscellaneous	Total lift chair	Used for its versatility in casualty transfer and positioning adaptability
	Roho cushion	Used to protect against pressure sores in the seated posture
	Slings, sandbags, foam blocks, and sponge positioning devices	Used to reduce edema and protect the healing wound

IP: interphalangeal
MCP: metacarpophalangeal
(1) Chapman TT, Hedman TL, Quick CD, Dewey WS, Wolf SE, Holcomb JB. Airplane sling with seven degrees of freedom used to position the burned upper extremity. Poster presented at: Southern Region Burn Conference; November, 2006; Durham, NC. (2) Hedman TL, Chapman TT, Dewey WS, Quick CD, Wolf SE, Holcomb JB. Two simple leg net devices designed to protect lower-extremity skin grafts and donor sites and prevent decubitus ulcer. *J Burn Care Res.* 2007;28(1):115–119.

Techniques used in repositioning for pressure relief include various forms of ROM exercise. AROM, active assisted range-of-motion (AAROM), and PROM exercises allow for changes in body position to remove direct pressure from a susceptible area, therefore reducing the risk of pressure sores. Positioning order sets or turning schedules can be placed on a casualty's order profile so nursing staff will know to reposition the casualty every 2 hours when active intervention is not occurring (eg, at night during a sleep pattern).

Mobility training and activity progression help manage pressure relief as well.

Postoperatively, casualties are placed in splinting and positioning devices to prevent disruption of new grafts. Positional splints and devices are used to assist in graft protection, pressure relief, and donor site healing. Most significantly noted are for the torso, elbow, and legs (Table 13-6 and Figure 13-22). Normal therapeutic ROM, mobility, and ADL activities are continued to the areas unaffected by surgery.

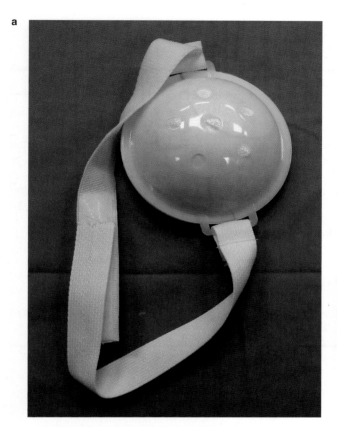

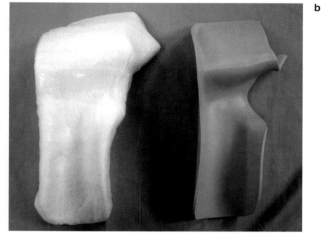

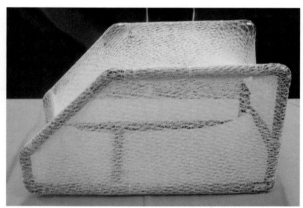

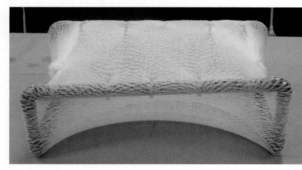

Figure 13-21. (**a**) Ear glock for protection of ear burns and grafts. (**b**) The Safe Position Burn Splint (Northcoast Medical, Morgan Hill, Calif) is a functional position hand splint that properly positions hands following burn. The (**c**) high profile leg net device and (**d**) low profile leg net device are used to position lower extremities.
Photograph (**b**): Courtesy of North Coast Medical Inc., Morgan Hill, California.

Intermediate Phase. The majority of edema resolves during the acute phase as the initial physiological response to burn injury, fluid resuscitation, and wound closure are completed. However, residual, chronic edema and the episodes of acute edema associated with ongoing surgical procedures pose the same limitations for casualties in the intermediate phase as they did in the acute phase.

As in the acute phase, during the intermediate phase edema is managed through a combination of elevation, ROM exercises, and compression. A casualty's responsiveness is typically improved and wounds are healed or nearly healed during this phase, allowing for more vigorous AROM and increased compression to mobilize edema. Compression wraps commonly used in this phase include elastic wraps and Isotoner (totesIsotoner Corporation, Cincinnati, Ohio) edema gloves. Dependent positioning of the affected areas must be avoided at night, and elevation at night is recommended to sustain the edema-reducing benefits of activity throughout the day.

Retrograde massage may be beneficial for persistent edema during this phase. During the acute phase, the casualty's wound status, pain tolerance, and risk for skin breakdown do not typically permit the use of retrograde massage. Therapists can use retrograde massage to mobilize persistent, chronic edema that has proven recalcitrant to more conservative edema management strategies.

Long-Term Phase. As casualties progress into the

TABLE 13-6

POSTOPERATIVE SPLINTING AND POSITIONING

Body Area	Device/Position	Indications
Torso	Back net (see Figure 13-22)	Used to air the donor site on the back; alternated on and off every 4 hrs[1]
Elbow	Hyalite low-temperature thermoplastic material is modeled to the elbow	Used to maintain the extended position following initial excision and grafting
Knee, feet, and ankles	Leg splints	Used to maintain the knee in extension, the ankle at 90°, and extend the toes; a heel dropout prevents pressure sores from developing
Miscellaneous	KinAir (Kinetic Concepts Inc, San Antonio, Tex) bed	Minimizes contractures
	The grafted sites are immobilized	Minimizes contractures
	Splints and other positioning devices	Keeps casualty immobile
	Bed rest	Used only when immobility of the graft cannot be achieved through splinting and positioning devices

(1) Salinas RD, Hedman TL, Quick CD, Wolf SE, Holcomb JB. Ventilation back ramp designed to prevent suppurative donor sites and accelerate healing time. *J Burn Care Res.* 2007;28:S109.

long-term rehabilitation phase, the focus of edema management shifts substantially. The persistent, chronic edema associated with this phase generally does not respond to passive elevation. Vigorous ROM exercises and retrograde massage, in conjunction with a comprehensive compression regimen, are the most effective ways to treat chronic edema.

Casualties generally receive custom compression garments during this phase. Casualties should wear compression garments 23 hours a day, removing them only for daily hygiene activities. A strict compression regimen and daily therapeutic activities effectively reduce edema.

Wound and Skin Care

Proper wound assessment and adequate wound care strategies are paramount during all phases of wound healing. Appropriate, timely, and effective wound care techniques can make the difference between successful healing and prolonged, problematic rehabilitation. Rehabilitation providers must be vigilant and aware of how wounds progress in order to recognize adverse changes and avoid setbacks in rehabilitation.

Acute Phase

During the acute phase, strategies are developed to manipulate the wound healing process, minimize

wound progression, and avoid involvement of deeper tissue.[186] Goals of therapeutic intervention in this phase focus on reducing the chance or rate of further burn damage to the involved tissue; positioning and splinting devices, in conjunction with fluid mobilization techniques, improve tissue viability.[187] Common rehabilitation goals during the acute phase include:

- educating casualties about the rehabilitation processes and expectations,
- reducing edema,
- facilitating wound healing,
- preventing skin breakdown,
- protecting skin graft and donor sites,
- preserving ROM,
- maximizing ADLs,
- accomplishing mobilization, and
- managing psychological coping and adjustment.

The acute phase of wound healing includes the initial injury assessment and evaluation. Loose tissue must be removed and the injury thoroughly cleansed to properly evaluate the extent of the burns and depth of the injury. IV narcotic medications are usually required to facilitate the initial wound cleansing. Small wounds can initially be cleaned in bed or in the shower. Additional space is often required to inspect larger wounds; shower carts and hand-held showerheads are

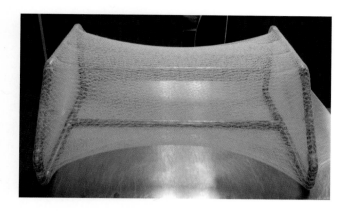

Figure 13-22. Back net device used to provide protection and ventilation for skin grafts and donor sites on the back.

used to adequately cleanse larger areas. Larger carts facilitate quick draining of water spray and provide an area that can be accessed by multiple caregivers. A shower cart basin can be covered in propylene drapes to guard against cross contamination. The use of Hubbard tanks (large full-body immersion tanks) has been largely abandoned due to the risk of cross contamination, space requirements, and difficulty in transferring casualties to and from beds.

Infection related to skin loss can be life threatening for a burn casualty, making meticulous wound care crucial. All areas of the body should be exposed and inspected to determine the extent and depth of the injury on an interval basis. During wound care, plastic aprons, gloves, hats, masks, and protective eye wear should be used. Plastic aprons prevent scrubs from becoming contaminated with body fluids and also prevent cross contamination to other casualties.

Wounds are gently cleaned using a mild cleanser and loose damaged skin is removed and blisters debrided to prevent infection. Thick blisters of the palms or soles of feet may be aspirated instead of unroofed to reduce pain.[188] Shaving body hair adjacent to the wound is beneficial in exposing the burn for evaluation and makes it easier to apply topical agents and dressings. Shaving is repeated as necessary until the wound is closed. Wound touch plate cultures are done on initial wound cleansing and thereafter for bacterial surveillance. Progression of wound healing is documented using the Lund and Browder chart.

After evaluating a burn, a wound dressing is chosen based on the operative plan, if indicated. If a casualty has areas of all partial-thickness burns that have been recently debrided and may be lightly weeping serous fluid, a synthetic skin substitute may be considered (Figure 13-23). After applying the synthetic skin, the wound is wrapped first with dry gauze, then with an elastic bandage to ensure conformity and adherence

of the contact dressing. After 24 to 48 hours, the outer dressing is removed and the synthetic skin is exposed to air. Keeping the skin substitute dry appears to aid in its adherence and overall performance. A synthetic skin substitute will spontaneously separate from the reepithelialized wound in 10 to 14 days.

A contact dressing that uses a combination of silver fibers incorporated into nylon can be left in place for an extended period of time. Silver-nylon dressings may be useful when treating burns that are deeper partial-thickness burns that exude large amounts of serous fluid or are dry. Silver-nylon dressings are easy to apply, conform effectively, and, because silver ion is an antimicrobial agent, they can be left in place for up to 72 hours, making them very effective during long-range transport. All of these dressing materials are available in varying sizes, including glove-shaped designs for easier application over burned hands.

Deeper partial-thickness, marginal full-thickness, and full-thickness burns that may require surgery can be treated with dressings that will facilitate daily wound care and evaluation. Most bacteria are found in the burn eschar, so dressings that guard against infection are preferred and topical, rather than systemic, antibiotics are effective.[189] Gauze dressings soaked with antimicrobial agents (eg, mafenide acetate in a 5% solution) and placed in contact with the burn are known as "bolsters." Bolster dressings provide the necessary wound protection and moist environment to improve wound outcome and aid in wound-bed preparation for future excision. Other solutions commonly used include dilute sodium hypochlorite (0.25% Dakin's solution) or silver nitrate. Topical burn ointments and creams are also used for antimicrobial protection include mafenide acetate cream, 1% silver sulfadiazine, polymixin, and bacitracin. Mycostatin can be added to provide additional antifungal protection if indicated.

Burn Wound Excision. Full-thickness burn wounds require excision and subsequent application of donor autograft, or temporary application of homograft (cadaver skin), a bilaminar dermal substitute, or xenograft

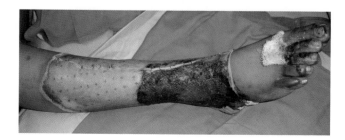

Figure 13-23. A synthetic skin substitute applied to partial-thickness burn of the lower extremity.

if the casualty does not have adequate donor skin. Prompt application of split-thickness skin grafts expedites wound closure and decreases risk of infection, scarring, contracture, loss of function, and the time needed for dressing changes (see "Plastic and Reconstructive Surgery" below). A principle goal of burn care is to debride nonviable tissue and provide early and functional wound coverage. Estimation of wound depth determines whether the burn can be managed conservatively or will require surgical intervention. Superficial and full-thickness burns are generally readily determined, and appropriate management can be immediately initiated. Partial-thickness burns are more difficult to evaluate and often require a serial assessment of the burn over several days to determine the actual depth of injury and initiate the appropriate intervention. A partial-thickness burn may also vary in depth within a small area, thus, healing may be patchy or delayed. A burn that fails to heal by 21 days after injury typically requires skin grafting.

For burns that require surgical intervention, expedited wound closure minimizes inflammation, wound contraction, and scar formation. Early excision and grafting are the modern standard of care for full-thickness burns. Early excision is based on the principles of general surgical wound management and has been clinically proven effective in diminishing morbidity in the burn casualty.[190–194]

The estimated depth of the burn wound often determines the choice of excision technique (tangential, sequential tangential, or fascial). Partial-thickness burns are generally excised with either tangential or sequential tangential methods until viable tissue is exposed. Hydrosurgery can provide an alternative to sharp excision. Full-thickness burns deep into subcutaneous fat are excised in segments to the fascia.

Tangential Excision. Dermal burns are excised with either a single pass (tangential) or multiple passes (sequential tangential) with the debridement instrument until viable tissue is reached (Figure 13-24). This method of debridement allows maximum preservation of viable dermis, which ultimately leads to better long-term results in the quality of the healed grafted skin.

There are a number of manual and mechanical instruments available for wound debridement. Debridement involves excising tissue in the range of 0.008 to 0.012 inches for partial-thickness burns, and up to 0.030 inches for full-thickness burns. Areas requiring intricate or delicate work, such as digit web spaces and the dorsum of the hand and fingers, are best approached using small instrumentation with shallow settings in multiple passes.

Areas that have been adequately debrided show brisk punctate bleeding in healthy white dermis (Figure 13-25). Poor bleeding in grayish dermis indicates inadequate debridement and a need for further excision. As debridement progresses deeper into and through the dermis, more fat appears and capillary bleeding gives way to brisker flow from arterioles and veins.

Hemostasis of the debrided wound bed is accomplished using one or more proven methods, including directed electrocautery on larger vessels and dilute, epinephrine-soaked lap pads on the diffuse capillary bleeding bed. Local pressure and temporary elastic wraps can reduce bleeding. Topical epinephrine solutions in concentrations ranging from 1:10,000 to 1:100,000 can be safely used with few systemic effects in acutely burned casualties. Topical thrombin spray has also been used for this purpose.

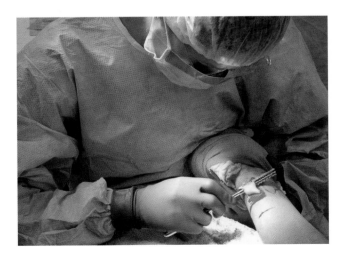

Figure 13-24. Tangential excision of a burn injury.

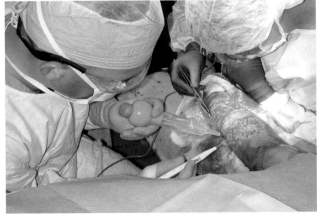

Figure 13-25. Punctate bleeding of healthy dermis following adequate burn excision.

It is important for a surgeon to consider a casualty's overall status, the available resources, and the capabilities of the team when formulating the operative plan. Blood loss from a debrided wound bed can be significant and require serial monitoring of hemoglobin and hematocrit levels, platelet counts, levels of coagulation factors, body temperature, blood pressure, and urine output. With adequate planning and preparation, it is safe and practical for an experienced surgical team to rapidly excise and cover very large TBSA burns in a single operation.

Excision to Fascia. Subdermal burns extending well into the subcutaneous tissue are often excised to the fascial plane using a combination of sharp dissection and electrocautery (Figure 13-26). Excision at this level can generally proceed rapidly with minimal to moderate blood loss. On extremity burns, blood loss can be minimized by tourniquets. To use a tourniquet, a surgeon must be confident of the level of injury because punctuate bleeding cannot be used to determine tissue viability until the tourniquet is released and perfusion restored.

Engraftment on fascia is often more effective than placing autograft onto subcutaneous fat. However, this improved graft take can result in inferior cosmetic appearance, increased edema in distal extremities, decreased sensation, and inferior function, especially without early and progressive rehabilitation.

Skin Grafts.

Split-Thickness Skin Grafts. A split-thickness skin graft is usually harvested in a range from 0.007 to 0.012 inches (Figure 13-27). Donor sites for split-thickness skin grafts heal in 7 to 10 days, may be reharvested once healed, and heal with little or no scar formation. Split-thickness skin grafts may be placed as either a sheet or meshed graft.

The typical healing time for a split-thickness skin graft is 3 to 5 days for adherence to the wound bed and up to 7 days for durable engraftment. Rehabilitation of areas that have been grafted should be implemented during the first 3 days after grafting. Mobilization activities, such as ROM exercise and transfers, can be performed during this time if the area of grafting can be protected from shear forces. As the split-thickness skin graft matures, rehabilitation activities may progress, but consideration must be given to the healing graft until approximately 7 days after grafting. Excellent functional outcomes with split-thickness skin graft coverage can be achieved with early and progressive rehabilitation and through the comprehensive development of a safe and effective rehabilitation plan.

Sheet Grafts. Faster wound closure and cosmetic uniformity (without the appearance of a pattern) are some advantages of sheet grafting. Unlike meshed grafts, sheet grafts do not have perforations or incisions and are not expanded. Examples of areas best served by sheet grafting include the hands, face, and neck. The use of sheet grafts is often limited by the availability of adequate donor tissue.

When blood or serum collects under sheet grafts, the grafts may separate from the vascularized bed, resulting in graft loss. Hemostasis is critical to the success of a sheet graft. Large fluid collection can threaten the entire graft and may result in local drainage or aspiration to rescue the graft.

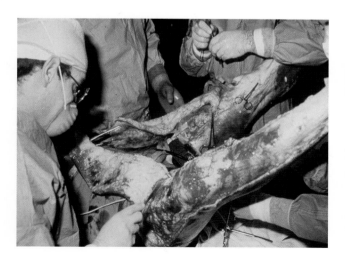

Figure 13-26. Fascial excision of subdermal burns to the lower extremities.

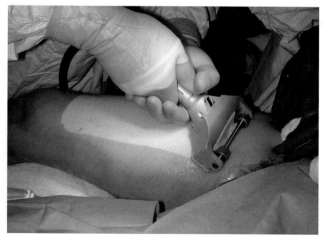

Figure 13-27. Harvesting of a split-thickness skin graft using a dermatome.

Meshed Skin Grafts. The instrumentation to accurately and reproducibly mesh skin (Figure 13-28) revolutionized burn care by providing a method of skin coverage for massively burned casualties. Skin expansion allows for greater graft coverage from limited donor sites. The surgeon has a choice of multiple expansion ratios, ranging from 1:5 to 9:1. One-to-one meshing is essentially uniform perforation without expansion. As the expansion ratio increases, the quality and cosmesis of the skin decreases, and healing time increases for the graft interstices or the perforations made in the skin graft because of the meshing and expansion process (Figure 13-29). As a general rule, most coverage is accomplished with a mesh ratio of 3:1 or less.

Full-Thickness Skin Grafts. The depth of harvest for a full-thickness skin graft depends on the skin thickness of the designated donor site. The technique involves excising slightly into the subcutaneous layer, then preparing the full-thickness skin graft by removing as much of the subcutaneous tissue as possible from the bottom side of the dermis. A full-thickness skin graft provides appropriate wound coverage for small full-thickness and subdermal burns, especially over anatomical areas requiring durability, extensibility, or cosmesis, such as the hands and face (Figure 13-30). Full-thickness skin grafts are associated with less wound contraction and scar formation than split-thickness skin grafts and are placed on the burn wound as a sheet graft only. Donor sites for full-thickness skin grafts may require grafting with a split-thickness skin graft for improved healing, minimizing wound contraction and scar formation.

The typical healing time for a full-thickness skin graft is 10 to 14 days. Rehabilitation of areas with full-thickness skin grafts during this time should focus on

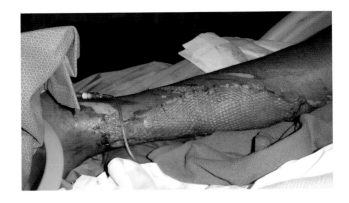

Figure 13-28. Meshed split-thickness skin graft applied to the lower extremity.

graft protection through splinting and positioning. Mobilization activities, such as transfers and ambulation, can be performed during this time, depending on the location of the full-thickness skin graft and if the area of grafting can be safely protected. As the full-thickness skin graft matures, rehabilitation activities may progress, but consideration must be given to the healing graft until day 14 following operation. As with split-thickness skin grafts, functional outcomes are best achieved with early and progressive rehabilitation and through a safe and effective rehabilitation plan.

Skin Graft Adherence. Skin graft adherence is a two-part process. The first phase, known as plasmatic imbibition, lasts for 24 to 48 hours. During this phase, the graft is held in place with fibrin bonding and nourished by direct diffusion. The second phase, inosculation, follows plasmatic imbibition and is marked by neovascularization.[195]

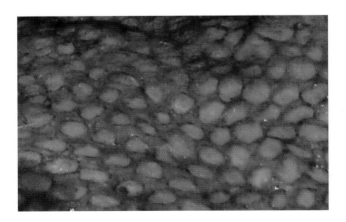

Figure 13-29. Interstices (perforations) in a meshed skin graft.

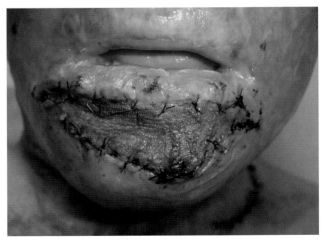

Figure 13-30. Full-thickness skin graft to the face of a burn casualty.

Proper management during the immediate postoperative period can significantly affect the final outcome of a scar graft. Graft movement or shear is generally the first cause of graft failure; infection is the second. Securing the graft to the wound bed is important to avoid shear. Grafts are often secured with staples or sutures. Sutures are typically used in sensitive areas, such as the eyelid. Biological glue is occasionally used to supplement adherence, such as in areas with irregular contours. Splints incorporated into the final dressing help maintain the desired position and prevent graft loss due to motion, especially over joints. Negative-pressure wound dressings, such as vacuum-assisted closure devices, can also prevent shear and have been shown to significantly increase skin graft take when used over freshly grafted wounds (Figure 13-31).[196]

Techniques used to cover fresh skin grafts are wide ranging and often depend on surgeon preference. Skin grafts may be treated in either an open or closed fashion, which corresponds to the degree to which the graft is covered. Regardless of the exact type of dressing used, most fresh grafts are protected to prevent desiccation. This necessitates maintaining a moist environment while avoiding a wet wound bed.

Generally, autografts can be left uncovered by the fifth day following grafting, and can be protected with an antimicrobial emollient, such as petrolatum impregnated gauze, to retain moisture in the recently grafted tissue and protect reepithelialization at the grafted site. Grafts can usually withstand gentle cleansing in a shower by day seven.

In contrast to the highly vascular peritendineum, exposed tendons have poor vascular supply and autograft will not "take" over an exposed tendon.[44,197] Granulation tissue is needed to cover exposed tendon

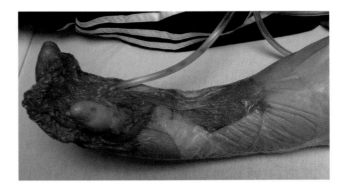

Figure 13-31. Application of a negative-pressure wound dressing following skin grafting to the hand.

and allow the wound to be closed with skin grafting. Negative-pressure wound dressings can be used to promote wound bed granulation. Therapists should pay particular attention to exposed tendons over the PIP joint. If tendon exposure is noted, the PIP joint should be immobilized continuously in full extension to prevent stress on the central slip caused by PIP flexion.

Flap Grafts. Deep subdermal wounds that injure muscle and bone can be covered by flaps. A pedicle flap involves rotating tissue (typically a flexor surface) from an unburned area into the defect (Figure 13-32). When suitable donor tissue is not available directly adjacent to the defect, free tissue transfer may be required. This technique, requiring a surgical microscope, is commonly employed for complex injuries (Figure 13-33). Free flaps are also occasionally needed to cover areas prone to contracture, such as the neck. Some common flaps include the parascapular flap, anterolateral thigh flap, and groin flap.[198]

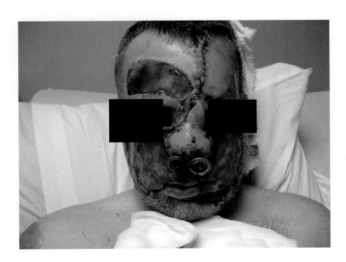

Figure 13-32. Pedicle flap to the nose of a burn casualty.

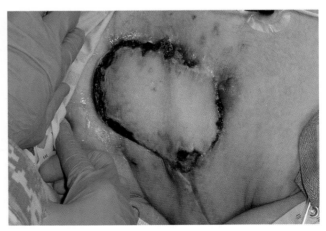

Figure 13-33. Free tissue transfer (free flap) on the torso of a burn casualty.

Cultured Autologous Keratinocyte (Epidermal) Grafts. Human epithelial cells can now be grown in cultures with techniques developed by Rheinwald and Green[199] and modified by Pittelkow and Scott.[200] The multistep process starts with the harvesting of a small piece of thin skin from an unburned site. Epithelial cells are enzymatically cleaved and separated, then placed in a serum-free culture medium where, under ideal conditions, they grow rapidly. Thin, fragile keratinocyte sheets are approximately 7 to 10 cell layers thick and have the consistency of wet tissue paper (Figure 13-34).

Before grafting with cultured grafts, the wound bed must be carefully prepared. Most grafts adhere by fibrin adhesion. Casualties grafted with cultured epithelium do not develop hair, sweat or oil glands, or normal sensation in the grafted area. The epidermis remains relatively fragile and requires extra protection from exposure to sun, chemicals, and trauma. Rehabilitation is challenging because the epithelium does not tolerate exercise, splinting, or external supports. Casualties may have the cultured graft replaced with autograft as donor sites become healed enough for reharvesting.

Artificial Dermal Replacement. Another approach to providing more rapid coverage is through the use of an artificial dermis (Figure 13-35). One type of artificial dermis is composed of bovine collagen fibers bonded to chondroitin-6-sulfate, a component of shark cartilage.[201] Thin split-thickness skin grafts are later placed on the neodermis, resulting in a closed wound. A multicenter controlled study of this dermal replacement system showed favorable results, concluding that the

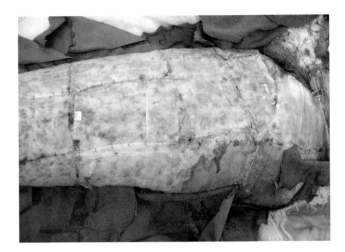

Figure 13-34. Multiple keratinocyte sheets applied to the lower extremity of a burn casualty.

healed artificial dermis covered with thin epidermal graft is essentially equivalent to standard skin grafts but with faster healing at the donor sites.[201]

Biological Dressings. The ideal biological dressing would function as natural skin and come prepackaged off the shelf, ready to apply and perform as a complete skin replacement on a permanent basis. Synthetic dressings are laboratory designed to mimic their biological counterpart, skin. Because these act as biological dressings, for the purpose of this discussion, they will be reviewed along with true biologic dressings. Satisfactory biological dressings undergo the same bonding process as skin grafts. Most importantly, when they

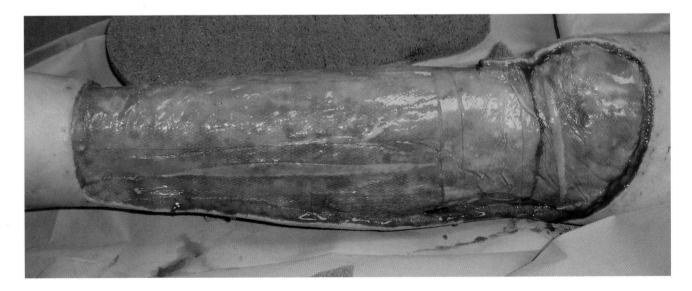

Figure 13-35. Artificial dermis applied to the lower extremity following excision.

adhere, the wound gains resistance to infection.

Biological dressings are designed to function in a similar manner as their more expensive natural counterpart, cadaver skin. There are many biological dressings available, but none is a true skin replacement. Biological dressings provide temporary coverage and time for adequate donor sites to become available for repeated graft harvest. This coverage is important in the overall physiological well being of a burn casualty because it provides better wound and pain management, helps decrease metabolic rate, reduces fluid losses through the wound, and suppresses the growth of granulation tissue.

Homograft or Allograft. Human cadaver skin is commonly used for grafting and is the standard against which other biological and synthetic dressings are measured. Banked frozen human skin is becoming more widely available, but is inferior to its fresh counterpart. Improved salvage of major burn casualties is based on early aggressive burn excision and coverage with homograft, followed by sequential replacement with autologous skin.

Fresh homograft adherence and capillary ingrowth is similar to that seen with autografts. Burn casualties with greater than 50% TBSA injury are autoimmunosuppressed. This state of immunosuppression can result in slowing of the natural rejection process, especially when the homograft skin is ABO compatible. Aside from providing excised wound coverage, homografts can also be used as overlay grafts to protect thin, widely expanded autografts or cultured keratinocytes, providing protection to the underlying grafts.

Homograft rejection occurs anywhere from 14 to more than 60 days after grafting, depending on the casualty's immune status. Replacement homografts tend to reject at a faster rate than original grafts, and the rejection process affects the wound bed and may negatively influence further grafting. The wound bed should be completely excised prior to grafting with autograft.

Availability, cost, and the potential risk of viral transmission are the major drawbacks of fresh homograft. Procurement, preparation, and storage costs are relatively high. Despite testing, there remains the possibility of viral transmission, including hepatitis, cytomegalovirus, and human immunodeficiency virus (HIV). There is at least one known case of HIV transmission involving autograft from England in 1987.[202,203] Amnion is used for temporary coverage in underdeveloped countries but not in the United States, and carries the same infectious risks.[204,205]

Because cadaver graft take is expected to be prolonged, the area is protected postoperatively in a method similar to that used with autografts. Rehabilitation of cadaver-grafted areas can commence in 3 to 7 days.

Heterograft and Synthetic Dressings. Porcine skin heterograft (xenograft) is occasionally used in the United States. However, it has limited value for short-term, temporary wound coverage. It has no advantage over homograft, but does have numerous disadvantages. Most importantly, xenograft does not incorporate into the wound, and therefore does not stimulate neovascularization.[206] If used, rehabilitation activities should mirror those following grafting with homograft.

Numerous synthetic dressings are currently available, and many more are expected to be developed in the future. Some dressings have been designed for a specific purpose (eg, use in a combat zone), while others are adapted to a wide variety of clinical applications. The choice of a particular dressing is usually based on a mixture of tradition, art, and science.

Synthetic dressings range from simple transparent polyurethane or polyurethane membranes to a more complicated bilaminate membrane. The former often work well to relieve pain and protect skin donor sites, as well as to decrease pain, protect, and decrease fluid loss in small, isolated, minor burns treated in an outpatient burn clinic. There is no restriction in ROM exercises with these products. A bilaminate membrane dressing is composed of collagen peptides bound to a silicone nylon mesh. To function properly, it must be bound to the tissue by ingrowth into the collagen network. Bilaminate membrane dressings have proven effective on partial-thickness burns and excised wound beds,[207] but they are contraindicated for use over full-thickness burns. To allow for adequate adhesion, ROM exercises are temporarily restricted for 24 hours following application of a bilaminate membrane dressing.

Donor Sites. As burn size increases, the donor site takes on added importance (Figure 13-36). The donor site can be considered analogous to a partial-thickness burn, which heals in the same way. Essentially, donor-site healing involves epithelial regeneration via migration of replicating epithelial cells, which originate from remaining hair follicle shafts and adnexal structures left in the dermis.[208] It is imperative that donor sites heal quickly because numerous repeat harvestings are required to close massive burns. The scalp is an ideal donor site because it heals rapidly and has few associated complications. A scalp donor site covered with an appropriate dressing can be expected to heal in 5 to 7 days for a graft harvested at 0.0008 to 0.010 inches. As a general rule, the further the donor site is from the heart, the longer it will take to heal.

Donor sites are dressed to decrease pain and promote rapid healing. Donor site dressings can consist

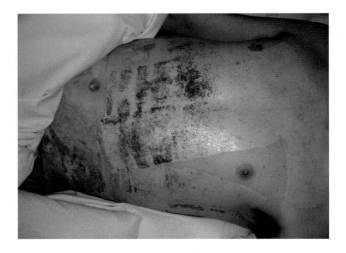

Figure 13-36. Donor site on the chest and abdomen of a burn casualty.

of fine mesh gauze with or without antibiotics or ointments (Figure 13-37). An open-to-air technique may also be used, but is not typically tolerated as well by casualties. Donor site dressing should be applied so that it overlaps by several centimeters onto the normal skin surrounding the site. If a donor site exceeds the size of the largest dressing, multiple dressings can be patched together to achieve complete coverage. Elastic or tubular support bandages may be applied over donor site dressings to provide external compression to the site microvasculature, especially in the case of the lower extremities. This technique decreases pain and the potential for tattooing of the donor site when rehabilitation activities force the extremity into various dependent positions.

The donor site dressing becomes problematic when the site is adjacent to or between burns, as it often is in massive burn casualties. If this donor site is covered with a traditional dressing, it may rapidly become infected, so it is preferable to treat the donor site with a nonadherent dressing and a topical antimicrobial, similar to the way the adjacent burned or grafted areas are treated.

Donor sites can also cause problems when the harvested grafts increase in depth, such as in the case of a full-thickness skin graft. The donor site may become as deep as the original burn and often heals slowly, and hypertrophy of the donor site can occur, resulting in a cosmetic appearance that is less favorable than that at the grafted sites. To avoid problems with slow or nonhealing donor sites, a thin split-thickness skin graft can be harvested, expanded at a ratio of 3:1, and regrafted to the donor sites.[209]

Healed donor sites can have problems with blisters

and pigmentation changes. To minimize splotchy pigmentation, sun exposure should be avoided for a year or more. Educating casualties on donor site care mitigates these occurrences.

Intermediate Phase

The intermediate phase of rehabilitation, which begins after grafting, can be a trying time for the casualty, family, and staff. Casualties may see it as a setback if they are unable to continue exercising areas that were grafted. Grafting and the period of immobilization should be thoroughly explained to casualties and their families to prepare them emotionally for the postoperative period. Postoperative positioning and splinting should be discussed with the physician, therapist, and nursing staff preoperatively. Whenever possible during preoperative teaching, the nurse should assist the casualty into the position that will be assumed postoperatively; this will help alleviate discomfort issues in advance. Preoperatively, a low-air–loss bed or air-fluidized bed should be considered, not only for comfort reasons, but also for pressure reduction on healed, unhealed, old, or new graft sites, as well as donor sites.

During the intermediate phase, rehabilitation efforts continue to focus on wound healing, managing edema, and restoring ROM; however, increased emphasis is now directed towards strength, endurance, independence with ADLs and mobility, psychological adjustment and initiation of scar management. Common goals during this phase include:

- progressing toward independence with ADLs and mobility;
- preserving and restoring ROM;
- initiating strengthening;

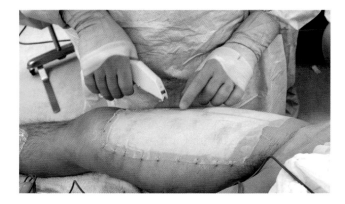

Figure 13-37. Application of petrolatum gauze dressing to a donor site on the anterior thigh.

- developing self-management skills;
- facilitating wound closure with graft adherence;
- modifying edema;
- preventing complications, such as skin breakdown;
- maintaining joint and skin mobility;
- educating the casualty and family about the expected results;
- conducting behavioral interventions; and
- counseling to focus on the positive final outcome, rather than on loss of independence, pain, or inactivity.

During this phase, wounds in nonsurgical areas need to be cared for at least daily. Surgical areas should be observed for signs of increased bleeding and infection, or because of complaints of pain from splints or dressings throughout the period of immobilization.

Negative pressure wound dressings enable casualties to resume limited mobility earlier during the immediate period following grafting. The negative pressure effect of the dressing splints the graft into the wound bed and prevents disturbing the engraftment process. A nonadherent overlay dressing is applied directly over new grafts. Immediately after grafting, a nonadherent dressing can be soaked with bacitracin and used to protect and hold the graft in place. After applying the interface dressing over the graft, an open-cell sponge can be placed to fit slightly larger than the graft. The open-cell sponge must be applied with a nonadherent interface dressing. A thin, adhesive-backed occlusive film is applied over the sponge and adjacent wound area to form an airtight seal. The entire dressing is then negatively pressurized to 125 mmHg. This dressing decreases risk for maceration, improves engraftment, and provides an effective splint. It is usually placed on the casualty in the operating room and is removed after 3 to 5 days at the direction of the physician.[210] Secondary dressings also applied in the operating room include agent-soaked bolsters, tie-down bolsters, or negative pressure wound dressings.

The first postoperative dressing change can be done at the bedside or in the shower area. Thoroughly soaking the gauze outer dressings with water or saline facilitates their removal without disrupting the underlying grafts or overlay dressings that may be used to secure and protect grafts. The contact dressing is usually left in place for 24 hours after the first dressing change. Bending the dressing back 180° as it is pulled away from the wound, rather than lifting it at 90°, is less disruptive to the graft. After this time, graft dressings can be changed daily. If the contact layer adheres to the graft, applying an antibiotic ointment or white petrolatum 1 hour prior to removal decreases sticking and bleeding. Acute pain management with IV narcotics and anesthesia may be necessary for larger, more extensive, or painful dressing changes that require removal of numerous staples, negative pressure dressings, or further debridement. Subsequent dressings are placed considering the location of the graft, facilitation of rehabilitation, and casualty tolerance. In general, moist bolsters are continued until interstices are closed or nearly closed, at which time a topical moisturizer and dry protective dressings may be applied. Splinting, compression, and mobilization facilitate the quickest time to mobility and function.

Postoperative rehabilitation of a hand that has been grafted consists of an immediate protective phase of full-time immobilization. The hand can be immobilized with a splint or a negative-pressure wound dressing, and must be immobilized for 3 to 5 days for split-thickness skin grafts. If the dorsal hand is grafted, it should be immobilized in the resting position full time. A palmar split-thickness or full-thickness skin graft must be immobilized in finger extension and thumb radial abduction. Full-thickness grafts are usually immobilized continuously for 5 to 7 days following operation.

AROM and gentle PROM exercises usually begin 3 to 5 days after operation for split-thickness skin grafts, and 5 to 7 days after full-thickness skin grafting. Dorsal hand ROM exercises following split-thickness skin grafts should emphasize composite flexion of the digits (concurrent MCP, PIP, and DIP flexion), thumb opposition, and thumb palmar abduction. Splinting should be discontinued after the protective phase if the casualty is able to perform adequate ROM. Continued splinting should be considered for nighttime and as needed during the day if adequate ROM is not obtained with ROM exercises and ADLs.

Once the graft is well adhered, interim compression can be applied to the involved areas. Interim compression can be provided using self-adhesive elastic wrap and is usually initiated 7 to 10 days following split-thickness skin grafting. A nonadherent dressing can be used underneath the elastic wrap to prevent adherence of the compression dressing to the skin graft. ROM exercises should be performed as prescribed while wearing the interim compression.

Topical Treatment. Burns are cleansed once or twice daily, followed by application of a topical agent. A soothing ointment can be applied to small wounds (less than 10% TBSA), such as bacitracin, which is relatively inexpensive but does not penetrate well and is ineffective against gram-negative bacteria. Mafenide acetate can be used as a solution in bolsters or in cream form. Bolsters soaked in 5% mafenide acetate are often used to improve marginally full-thickness burns.

Alternating mafenide acetate with silver sulfadiazine and a dry protective dressing over deep burns with leathery eschar has proven effective in helping separate eschar from wound beds, and penetrates more effectively than other topical agents alone. Alternating these agents helps with tolerance because silver sulfadiazine is soothing after the irritating mafenide acetate cream. All previously applied agents must be thoroughly removed before applying subsequent topicals. Meticulous wound care between dressing changes is the hallmark of progressive burn healing. Although mafenide acetate has been shown to cause metabolic acidosis when applied over very large areas, it is the preferred treatment when dealing with burns to the outer ear because it penetrates well into cartilaginous tissues and is the most effective antimicrobial agent for preventing chondritis of the outer ear. Burns that are obviously full-thickness or are potentially infected are treated twice daily with mafenide acetate until the burn is healed or nearly healed,[211] at which time transition is made to topical bacitracin ointment or plain white petrolatum. Silver sulfadiazine does not penetrate well, but has a good spectrum of coverage, is easy to apply, and is the least painful agent, but sensitivity and leukopenia are not uncommon. Silver sulfadiazine is avoided in casualties with sulfa drug allergy.

Topical treatments vary depending on location, extent of injury, and surgical excision and grafting. Wounds that do not appear they will heal within 2 to 3 weeks are usually excised and grafted 1 to 5 days following burn.

Wound care and wound management are large parts of the recovery process for injured casualties. Rehabilitation is also vital in returning the injured to normalcy or optimal function. Discharge criteria include particular levels of independence in ambulation, ADLs, hygiene, transfers, and ability to manage wounds. Pain and pain management must also be considered when determining discharge eligibility. Today, there are numerous wound dressings that require little more care than regular follow-up for progress evaluation. Pain medications traditionally given in IV form can now be given orally.

Long-Term Phase

Rehabilitation focus continues to shift in the long-term phase. By this time, edema, ROM, strength, ADLs, and mobility are typically well managed. Rehabilitation efforts are now more specifically targeted toward reintegration, psychological adjustment, return to duty, and continued scar management. However, if impairments persist from the acute or intermediate rehabilitation phases, continued focus for these will be required. Common goals include:

- societal reintegration;
- improving aerobic capacity;
- preventing hypertrophic scarring;
- remediating scar contracture;
- modifying edema;
- increasing joint and skin mobility;
- increasing strength;
- facilitating casualty and family participation in resumption of family roles;
- learning self-care activities;
- mastering compensation techniques for exposure to friction, trauma, ultraviolet light, chemical irritants, and extremes of weather or temperature;
- developing a profile for active-duty training, return to part-time modified duty, or to full-time active duty; and
- continued counseling to deal with life and psychological stresses regarding permanently changed appearance, altered ability levels, and difficulties with PTSD symptoms.

As a casualty transitions into the long-term rehabilitation phase, the healing burn is very fragile, and if not protected, is prone to shearing, pressure, and subsequent breakdown until matured. It is not uncommon to have small blisters form during this time, because the epidermal layer is not firmly attached to the underlying dermis for several months.[212] All wound areas should be gently cleansed and rinsed well with water. Infection is no longer a significant consideration; therefore, antibiotic ointments are generally discontinued. However, multiple topical agents may be used for cleansing, barrier protection, and antimicrobial control, and may lead to complications of contact and irritant dermatitis, further complicating reepithelialization and wound healing.[213] Blistered areas should have a light, nonadherent dressing applied for protection. The intact blister should not be opened or debrided. If the blister is large and spreads when external vascular support is applied, the blister should be drained and the wound protected with the dry skin. If the dry skin peels away, a protective nonadherent dressing can be applied and changed daily.

During the end stages of wound epithelialization, the wound is assessed to determine whether compression by elastic wraps, interim compression garments, or custom compression garments will be most effective. The integument should be continually inspected for changes resulting from increased activity, exercise, or in response to treatment procedures. External vascular support should be applied to the lower extremities prior to dependent positioning or ambulation.[214] Standing in the shower with legs dependent is permitted only after all open areas are closed and purple color exhibited by dependent wounds in this position decreased.

After a burn, the number of sebaceous and apocrine glands are decreased, leaving healed skin dry and flaky. Casualties may be irritated by pruritus, but vigorous rubbing or scratching results in newly opened areas. Moisturizing lotions should be applied to all healed areas after bathing and routinely as needed. The lotion should not be perfumed, have an alcohol base, or be so viscous that it causes blisters during application. Long-acting oral antipruritic medications should be used[215] in conjunction with lotion to relieve the itch. Fingernails should be kept trimmed, smooth, and clean to prevent excoriation of fragile skin. Desensitization exercises and vibration massage may reduce itching.[216] When exercising outside, a casualty's healed burn or donor areas should be protected from sunlight until all the red color has faded.

The long-term phase emphasizes addressing deficits to allow optimal return of function following a hand burn. Finger amputations, poor autograft take, age, full-thickness TBSA burned, and full-thickness hand burn area are all long-term predictors of hand function following a burn.[217] Management during this phase is primarily dependent on scar maturation; mobility of skin, joint, and soft tissue; and neuropathy.

Chronic Nonhealing Wounds. Occasionally, chronic nonhealing wounds will develop. In these instances, it is important to identify the underlying problem causing the healing delay. Pressure, shear forces, infections, and poor nutrition are common factors that delay healing. Interventions such as pressure relief, properly fitting compression garments, and nutritional counseling may be needed to promote healing. Occasionally hypertrophic granulation tissue may keep wound edges from migrating effectively, resulting in a chronically open wound. Silver nitrate as a cauterizing agent, surgical excision, and regrafting have all proven beneficial in managing chronically open wounds.

Biomechanics of Skin and Scar

A severe burn is both a physical injury to the integumentary system and a physiologic insult to several other organ systems. Skin is unique because one piece of tissue encapsulates the entire body while permitting unrestricted flexibility to the extremities and trunk. When naturally pliable skin is replaced by scar tissue or skin grafts, tissue contractures can develop.

The viscoelastic nature of native skin is derived from the interactive combination of a fibrous matrix of collagen and elastic fibers surrounded by an amorphous gel generically referred to as "ground substance."[218] Collagen fibers lend strength to the skin, while elastic fibers give the skin its extensibility and subsequent retraction after deformation. The ground substance lubricates the fibers and partially absorbs energy applied to the skin during movement.

The collagen network of the dermis in undamaged skin is made up of long, undulating fibers that are somewhat randomly oriented under relaxed conditions.[218,219] Elastic fibers are straighter than individual collagen fibers and are interconnected as well as attached to the collagen strands. As traction is applied to the skin, the elastic fibers elongate, pulling on the collagen fibers to orient them in the direction of applied force.[220] During this action, the viscous ground substance is displaced from between the fibrous network.[218]

The interaction of these three biomechanical components of skin can be described on a stress-strain curve (Figure 13-38). Initially, skin can be significantly elongated with minimal force because mostly the highly pliable elastic fibers are being stretched.[221] As additional tension is added to elongate the skin, more collagen fibers reorient themselves in the direction of the applied stress. As collagen fibers accumulate in the direction of the applied force, a greater force is required to overcome the resistance by the aligning collagen fibers to gain further length. Once all the collagen fibers have aligned parallel to one another in the direction of the force, the slope of the curve becomes linear, with little further elongation attainable despite the input of greater force. At the physical terminus of skin elongation, applying additional force causes the skin to rupture. Cessation of an elongating force allows

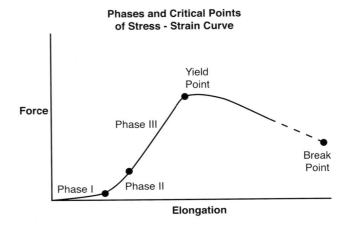

Figure 13-38. Stress-strain curve of tissue.

the fibrous network to revert back to its original resting length by a recoil action of the elastic fiber attached to the straightened collagen fibers (Figure 13-39).[221] Undamaged skin has the capacity to elongate up to 50% to 60% of its original resting length.[222]

The dermis injured by burn is replaced by scar tissue. Scar tissue differs from normal dermis in that elastic fibers do not regenerate,[223] the composition of ground substance changes, and the fibrous portion is only collagen. Morphologically, untreated burn scar develops into a disarray of randomly oriented collagen fibers. Characteristically, nodules form in the extracellular matrix, which may be under the influence of ground substance changes.[224] Biomechanically, burn scar behaves much like tendon, resisting deformation. Immature burn scar is only 16% extensible, which decreases to approximately 4% at maturity.[225]

Acute Phase

Burn scar must be managed while it is being produced. Physical intervention is an imperative part of the early rehabilitation phase. Arem and Madden have shown that stress applied to newly developing scar tissue causes it to orient in the direction of the force.[226] Burn scar begins to form during the proliferative stage of wound healing, which begins approximately 5 to 7 days after injury.

The effect of burn rehabilitation interventions is based on biomechanics principles. Repeated ROM exercise or the use of reciprocal pulleys, for example, harness the principle of successive length induction.[227] With successive length induction, each time the body segment is moved, the tissue further elongates (Figure 13-40). However, tissue length increase from successive length induction is not permanent because as soon as stress is relieved from the tissue, the tissue begins to return to its original resting length. Also, it is important to consistently use ROM measurements from either the beginning of the treatment session or the end to accurately compare improvement between treatment sessions. Improvements in ROM achieved within a given treatment session are misleading because the improved ROM is temporary.

Positioning, static and static-progressive splinting, and serial casting incorporate the biomechanical principle of stress relaxation.[228] With stress relaxation, tissue is elongated to a set point and held at that given length by the selected intervention. The set point should cause slight discomfort for the casualty. As time passes (within an hour), stress on the tissue eases and the tissue relaxes, making the intervention more tolerable (Figure 13-41). Stress relaxation prevents scar tissue from shortening.

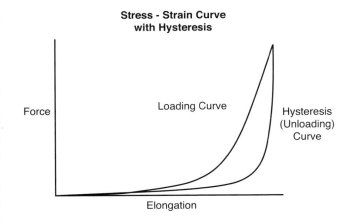

Figure 13-39. Tissue hysteresis.

Another biomechanical principle used in burn rehabilitation is based on tissue creep.[229] When controlled stress is applied to tissue over a prolonged period of time, such as with dynamic splints, the tissue continually undergoes elongation (Figure 13-42).

Strain rate, or how quickly tissue should be elongated, is another biomechanical consideration (Figure 13-43).[230] Tissue responds to stress that is applied either rapidly or over a prolonged period, as long as the force of the stress is at a therapeutic level. However, rapidly elongating tissue causes casualties more pain than if the intervention is performed or applied over a prolonged period of time.

Regardless of the therapeutic approach or biomechanical principle, casualty tolerance of the procedure

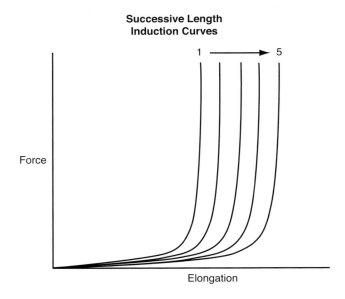

Figure 13-40. Successive length induction.

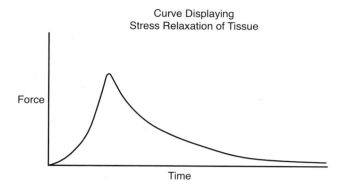

Figure 13-41. Stress relaxation of tissue.

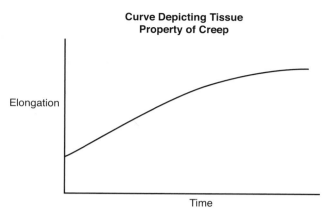

Figure 13-42. Tissue creep.

should guide rehabilitation. Furthermore, a sustained-approach treatment minimizes the chance of damaging tissue.

Intermediate Phase

Positioning during the intermediate phase is based on several factors relevant to tissue recruitment and creep. If a body part has a direct burn injury resulting in grafting or healing of native skin, positioning in the intermediate phase continues in the same fashion as it did acutely, so as to place the body part in anticontracture or a maximum wound length position while at rest or between active therapeutic interventions. If a body part has residual healthy native skin and is involved as recruited tissue due to close proximity to the burn wound, positioning in the intermediate phase continues in the same fashion while at rest or between active therapeutic interventions.

Burn casualties increase their daily activity level in the intermediate phase. The primary function of positioning now becomes more focused on stressing the grafted and healing sites beyond what is accomplished in active therapeutic intervention to create tissue creep and increase native skin recruitment. Success in this phase requires creative interventions beyond the standard positioning and splinting devices. The therapist should always consider various interventions to prevent contracture; aside from positioning and repositioning, ROM exercise, strengthening, and ADLs are implemented to reduce contracture risk.

Additional activity integrates postural awareness and dependant posture demands on wounds. A therapist will instruct a casualty in postural adaptations and explain the need to adjust from dependant to nondependent postures throughout the day, allowing the casualty to avoid undue stress to the wounds and preventing acute swelling.

Long-Term Phase

Many different interventions applying these biomechanical principles have been successfully employed to treat established burn scar contractures. A study investigating approaches to remediating burn scar contracture documented that serial casting and splinting, as well as dynamic splinting, were the most efficacious methods to reverse burn scar contractures.[231] By using one of these three interventions, contracture resolution took approximately half the time than it took using various other methods. These methods were effective on immature scar tissue.

Positioning requirements continue to be a key factor in contracture prevention and burn scar management until the wounds reach maturation. As the casualty

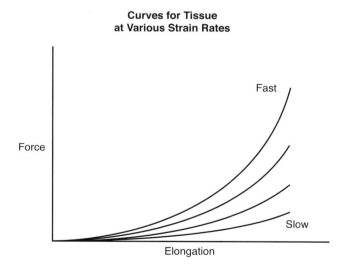

Figure 13-43. Graph displaying the difference in various strain rates of tissue.

reaches the long-term rehabilitation phase, wounds are closed and essentially healed. The casualty then endures the process of wound maturation as the scar tissue gradually slows in formation, flattens, and reestablishes a color presentation more similar to native skin. This process can last as long as 2 to 3 years after injury.

The techniques for positioning during the long-term rehabilitation phase closely resemble those of the intermediate rehabilitation phase. The most significant adjustment in implementing contracture prevention techniques includes increased use of custom splinting and positioning devices. Initially, dependent positioning of the extremities will be painful, which will remind the casualty to elevate the hands or feet. By this time, casualties must take responsibility for varying their own positions while at rest. However, it will still be necessary to apply various splinting devices to critical areas that have lost strength or active motion to produce burn scar contracture.

Splinting

A splint is defined as "an orthopedic device for immobilization, restraint, or support of any part of the body."[232] Splints can also mobilize, position, and protect a joint or specific body part.[233] Different types of splints are used throughout a burn casualty's rehabilitation, depending on the phase the casualty is in.

Acute Phase

There have been 93 splints used for burn rehabilitation described in the English language; *An Atlas and Compendium of Burn Splints*[234] provides a description and summary of each. During the acute phase, the primary goal of splinting is to maintain proper positioning of the burn casualty's extremities in order to reduce edema, prevent soft tissue contracture, and protect skin grafts, all of which minimize burn scar contracture and deformity. Proper positioning is vital because burn casualties may not be alert enough to maintain ROM with active movement. Static splints are used most frequently and may be custom or prefabricated, depending on the burn casualty's specific needs. Splints are generally applied 72 hours after burn. If implemented during the first 72 hours after burn, complications may develop because of the confining nature of splints and the active edema accumulation from fluid resuscitation.

A commonly used, prefabricated hand splint maintains the hand in the intrinsic plus position, also known as "the position of safe immobilization" (Figure 13-44). This position involves 20° to 30° of wrist extension,

maximum flexion of the MCP joints, maximum extension of the IP joints, and palmar abduction of the thumb to avoid contracture of the first web space.[235]

Prefabricated burn splints are clinically expedient and generally meet the needs of burn casualties during this phase. Also, they are oversized and can accommodate bulky dressings. These early burn splints are secured with a gauze wrap; straps are contraindicated at this time because they do not accommodate for changing edema, have the potential to compromise circulation, and do not evenly distribute pressure over the edematous extremity.

When using splints, it is essential to constantly assess the burn casualty's skin integrity. Pressure areas can increase the risk for skin breakdown, nerve compression, or burn wound conversion. The safe position can also be achieved with a custom splint, which may be more appropriate for a burn casualty with fluctuating edema, associated orthopaedic conditions, or digit amputations. Custom splints may also be indicated for the hand in the presence of full-thickness burns of the dorsal hand that result in exposed tendons. During the acute phase, static splinting can be used to maintain proper joint alignment and to help prevent contractures.

Dorsal hand edema encourages wrist flexion, MCP joint hyperextension, and IP flexion.[42] Intrinsic muscle edema encourages PIP joint flexion.[236] Therefore, the resting hand splint is the most common splint used during this phase. The resting position maintains 20° of wrist extension and 60° to 70° of MCP flexion, and keeps the thumb in palmar abduction.[42]

The PIP joint can be immobilized with a gutter splint or with surgical placement of Kirschner wires, and the PIP should be immobilized until the tendon is no longer exposed. MCP and DIP joint motion should be maintained as long as there is no tendon exposure in these areas. If the tendon over the PIP joint is ruptured, immobilizing the PIP joint in extension for 6 weeks

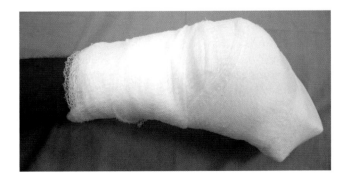

Figure 13-44. Hand splint secured with gauze wrap.

may prevent volar migration of the lateral bands that contributes to a boutonnière deformity. The scar over the PIP joint may form a pseudotendon that assists with PIP extension.[237]

A palmar burn will contract into thumb flexion, thumb adduction, and finger flexion. Splints or casts used for palmar burns should hold the hand in the position of thumb radial abduction and finger MCP, PIP, and DIP extension. Caution should be taken to avoid MCP hyperextension of the thumb when positioning into radial abduction. Exercises should emphasize finger extension and radial abduction. Flexion exercises can be performed to prevent joint capsule tightness of the MCP and IP joints; however, caution should be taken to avoid digital extension losses.

Splints are not usually necessary for superficial partial-thickness burns unless there is minimal active motion of the hand and poor exercise participation because of pain. Resting hand splints are more commonly used for deep partial-thickness or full-thickness burns because of the higher risk of joint or skin contracture. Prefabricated resting splints covered with gauze are primarily used during the acute phase.

Intermediate Phase

Although reducing edema and preventing soft tissue contracture remain priorities, the primary goal of splinting is to protect skin grafts during the intermediate phase of rehabilitation. One of the most important responsibilities of the rehabilitation staff is to promote skin graft adherence. The most common type of splint indicated is a static splint, or a splint that does not allow movement. Newly grafted areas are generally immobilized with static splints for 3 to 5 days following operation for split-thickness skin grafts, and 5 to 7 days for full-thickness skin grafts. Preventing burn scar contracture from forming is also important at this point and can be accomplished concurrently with skin graft protection using the appropriate splint.

Ears. An ear-dressing kit can be used to protect ears before and after grafting. A typical kit includes a hard plastic cup to cover the ear and is lined with gauze for wound protection

Mouth. A microstomia prevention appliance[238] or a mouth spacer can maintain the horizontal component of mouth opening after a burn to the commissural region (Figure 13-45).

Neck. There are several options for immobilizing the neck in the intermediate phase of recovery. A soft neck collar, consisting of foam placed circumferentially around the neck, can serve as a positioning device to promote neutral neck positioning (Figure 13-46).[239] Custom thermoplastic splints may be fabricated to

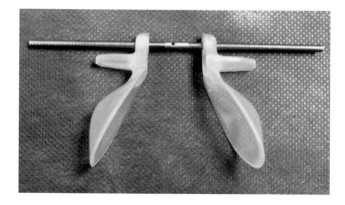

Figure 13-45. Jouglard's mouth spacer (Medical Z, San Antonio, Tex) for the prevention of correction of microstomia. Photograph: Courtesy of Medical Z, San Antonio, Texas.

protect neck grafts or to provide optimal positioning, most commonly in neutral or slight neck extension. An anterior neck splint is conformed along the anterior neck, the upper chest, chin, and lower mandible.[240] The splint can be secured with hook-and-loop fasteners around the posterior of the neck, and can protect the graft and provide optimal positioning to limit the formation of burn scar contracture.

Both the soft collar and the anterior neck splint can provide contact pressure to help minimize scar hypertrophy while providing neutral or slight cervical extension. Both splints can be used past the immobilization phase to provide prolonged neck positioning. Providers must frequently perform skin integrity checks when using these splints, as both can cause

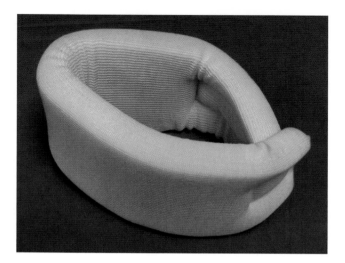

Figure 13-46. A soft neck collar for neutral positioning of the neck.

mechanical shear to skin grafts with any movement or excessive pressure.

A halo neck splint[241] and three-point anterior neck splint[242] are two types of "open" neck splints that can immobilize the neck after grafting (Figure 13-47). These splints do not permit direct wound contact and allow the wounds to ventilate. The halo neck splint consists of a posterior thermoplastic post with a skull cup and a circumferential head strap. These are connected to a thermoplastic base over bilateral anterior and posterior shoulder girdles. The three-point anterior neck splint is similar to the anterior neck splint, but there is an opening over the anterior neck, with three thermoplastic posts connecting the chin and shoulder girdle components.

Axilla. In the event that traditional positioning is not enough to immobilize and protect the axilla area, a thermoplastic splint may be fabricated. An airplane splint with a support rod[243] can be custom fit to the burn casualty in order to keep the axilla positioned in at least 90° of flexion or abduction for optimal positioning after burning or grafting. This splint can also be used to protect lateral trunk grafting.

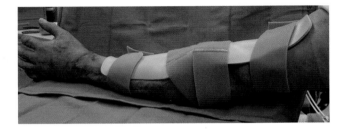

Figure 13-48. Thermoplastic static elbow plank for optimal post-grafting positioning.

Elbow. A static elbow splint, or elbow plank, is commonly used for graft protection or for optimal post-burn positioning (Figure 13-48). This splint can be fabricated out of thermoplastic material and can be placed posterior[244] or anterior.[245] The splint is usually worn until 3 to 5 days after split-thickness skin grafting when used for graft protection.

Wrist and Hand. There are several splints that can immobilize the hand or wrist after skin grafting. A prefabricated splint is the most common type used for protection following grafting (see Figure 13-21b). An advantage of this oversized splint is that it can accommodate the typical bulky postoperative dressings. These splints are usually worn continuously until at least 3 to 5 days after grafting, when ROM exercises are again permitted. A custom resting splint is indicated if a proper fit is not obtained due to anatomical restrictions or dressing limitations.[246] A custom splint is also indicated if specific positioning other than the "safe" position is indicated (Table 13-7 and Figure 13-49). Static or serial static splinting are the primary splint types used during the intermediate rehabilitation phase. Dynamic or static-progressive splints should be implemented if sufficient ROM gains are not achieved with static or serial static splinting. Serial casting is an effective alternative to splinting that provides the low force and long duration positioning needed for optimal tissue elongation.[247] It can protect open wounds, facilitating healing. Antimicrobial wound dressings that remain effective for at least several days should be used underneath the casts on open wounds. ROM gains made in a cast can be maintained with static splinting or improved with static-progressive or dynamic splinting once casting is no longer indicated.

Deep partial and full-thickness burns also require interim compression for scar control during the intermediate rehabilitation phase. Permanent custom compression garments are not appropriate during this phase because of open wounds, edema, and skin fragility. However, interim compression can help with edema control and protect fragile skin from friction.

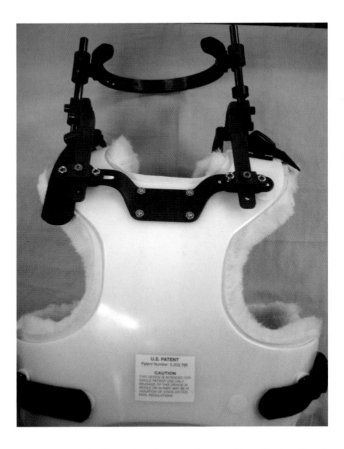

Figure 13-47. Halo neck splint used to position the head and neck after grafting.

TABLE 13-7

CUSTOM HAND AND WRIST SPLINTS

Type	Indication
C-bar	Stretches first web space; places the thumb in palmar abduction for optimal dorsal web space positioning, or in radial abduction for optimal palmar or thenar positioning following burn or skin grafting (see Figure 13-49a)[1,2]
Slot-through	Used when combined wrist and palmar extension is indicated following grafting to the palm or for adequate positioning after a palmar burn with or without volar wrist involvement (see Figure 13-49b); a C-bar component can be added to place the thumb into optimal radial abduction if the thenar eminence is involved (see Figure 13-49c)[3]
Volar wrist extension	May be fabricated with thermoplastic material to immobilize the wrist following skin grafting or volar wrist burn; may also be indicated if wrist support is needed due to a neurological deficit, such as a radial neuropathy[4]
Finger gutter or finger tunnel	Fabricated to hold interphalangeal joints in extension, protect exposed tendons, immobilize after skin grafting, or prevent a boutonniere deformity[5,6]

Data sources: (1) Fess EE, Philips CA. *Hand splinting, Principles and Methods.* 2nd ed. Saint Louis, Mo: Mosby; 1987. (2) Walters CJ. *Splinting the Burn Patient.* Laurel, MD: RAMSCO Publishing Company; 1987. (3) Forsyth-Brown E. The slot-through splint. *Physiotherapy.* 1983;69:43–44. (4) Miller H, Posch JL. Acute burns of the hand. *Am J Surg.* 1950;80(6):784–798. (5) Von Prince KMP, Yeakel MH. *The Splinting of Burn Patients.* Springfield, Ill: Thomas; 1974: 60–70. (6) Salisbury RE, Bevin AG. *Atlas of Reconstructive Burn Surgery.* Philadelphia, PA: WB Saunders; 1981: 164.

a

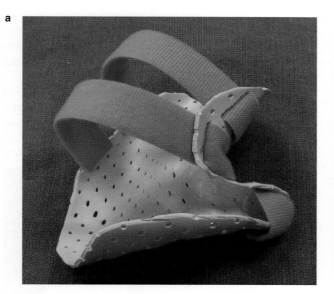

b

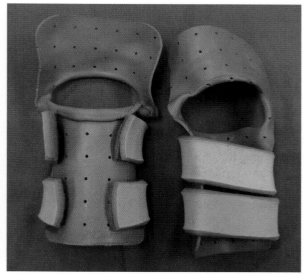

c

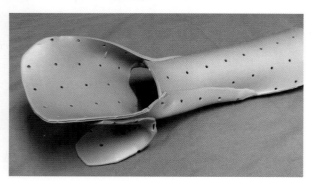

Figure 13-49. (**a**) C-bar splint for preventing and correcting contracture to the first web space (top view).
(**b**) Slot-through splint for combined wrist and palmar extension. (**c**) Slot-through splint with C-bar component for optimal thumb positioning.

Interim compression options for the hands are self-adherent elastic wrap or commercially available nylon gloves. Superficial partial-thickness burns do not require scar compression, but a nylon glove can reduce edema or protect the involved hand from friction.

Knee and Ankle. There are several options available to immobilize the knee and ankle after grafting or for proper positioning. A long leg splint—a static, prefabricated, metal-based splint lined with foam inserts, cast padding, and gauze dressing—may be indicated when it is necessary to simultaneously immobilize the knee and ankle (Figure 13-50). A long leg splint immobilizes the ankle in a neutral position and the knee in full extension. It extends posteriorly from the plantar surface of the foot to the posterior thigh and is typically applied to the burn casualty using gauze. When it is necessary to isolate either the knee or the ankle, a custom thermoplastic splint can be fabricated.[244,246] Ankles can be isolated and immobilized or held in a neutral position with a prefabricated boot (Figure 13-51).

Long-Term Phase

The primary goal of splinting during the long-term rehabilitation phase is to prevent skin or joint contractures. Because collagen fibers are aligned along lines of stress,[189] splinting is an important component of rehabilitation. The three types of splints used during this period are static, dynamic, and static progressive. Static splints are indicated if an achieved position needs to be maintained during the scar maturation phase. Static splints can also be serially fabricated. Serial static splints get remolded progressively at the maximum tolerable end ROM to increase tissue length.[247]

A dynamic splint allows for or provides movement. A dynamic splint can be used correctively or functionally. A corrective splint is indicated to correct burn scar or joint contracture. The movement provided should include a low-load force in the direction of tension.[248] The most common dynamic force used for dynamic splinting is rubber band or elastic tension. If the goal for this splint is to gain motion, a period of 6 to 8 hours of cumulative wear time, with wear intervals lasting at least 30 minutes, is recommended. The key to successful dynamic splinting and tissue elongation is to provide a low-load force for a long duration.[248]

Corrective dynamic splints are most frequently used for the elbow, wrist, and hand, and the involved area must be frequently inspected for skin breakdown. A 90° angle of pull is required to provide optimal dynamic force.[249] Dynamic splints for the elbow, wrist, forearm, hand, knee, and ankle are also commercially available, providing many options depending on the

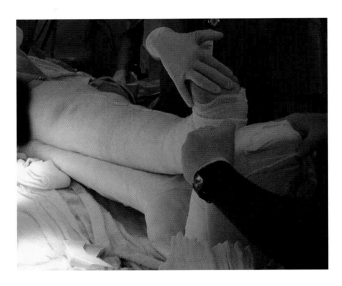

Figure 13-50. A long leg splint used for simultaneous knee extension and ankle dorsiflexion positioning.

targeted movement or joint. However, commercially available splints may not adequately fit a casualty; therefore custom fabricated dynamic splints are sometimes indicated. A dynamic supination splint can be effective for increasing ROM if limited by burn scar or joint contracture.[250] A thermoplastic wrist extension splint has also been used to address burn scar and joint limitations (Figure 13-52).[251]

Dynamic splints are also useful during this phase to substitute for loss of function from concomitant nerve injuries or amputations. The most commonly used

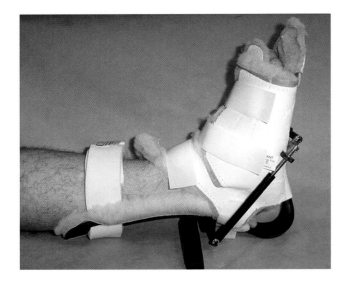

Figure 13-51. Commercial ankle-foot orthosis for ankle positioning.

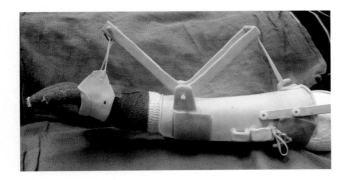

Figure 13-52. Fulcrum wrist extension splint.

adaptive splint for burn casualties is the mobilization splint for radial nerve palsy, originally designed at the Hand Rehabilitation Center in Chapel Hills, North Carolina, in 1978 (Figure 13-53).[252] This mobilization splint reestablishes the tenodesis pattern of the hand[253] and includes a dorsal base splint with a low-profile outrigger that spans from the wrist to each proximal phalanx.[233]

Another type of corrective splint, a static progressive splint, uses inelastic components to apply torque to a joint at end range to increase available ROM.[254] Unlike the dynamic splint, the static progressive splint does not permit active-resisted ROM against the line of pull.[255] Flowers states that static progressive splints are indicated when the targeted tissue is stiff and requires the most aggressive intervention.[256] The principle of a low-load force for long duration should be implemented with static progressive splints. Wearing schedules and precautions are similar to those observed with dynamic splints. A variety of static progressive splints for the upper and lower extremities are also commercially available.

There are several different types of static progres-

sive splints used to correct contractures of the upper extremity. An elbow extension turnbuckle splint or elbow flexion splint may be used when joint or burn scar limitation results in elbow flexion or extension contractures.[257] Wrist and hand splints can also be fabricated to address burn scar or joint limitations, and various other static progressive splints can be fabricated for the upper extremities, depending on the target joint or tissue.[255] A common static progressive splint used to regain hand ROM following burn or skin grafting is a composite flexion splint, which includes combined flexion of the MCP, PIP, and DIP joints (Figure 13-54).

Casting

Serial casting is typically recommended for managing burn scar contracture when the involved structures are resistant to traditional methods of treatment, such as AROM exercises, paraffin baths, massage, progressive resistive exercise, and splinting (**Figure 13-55**).[258,259] Casting can help throughout the various phases of burn recovery.

Acute Phase

In the acute phase, casting can be used for immobilization, edema reduction, and tissue protection.[260] Burn casualties often present with a significant soft tissue defect that leaves underlying structures exposed. Some of the qualities of Plaster of Paris make it the perfect material to intercede, including unparalleled conformity, decreased pressure (which is due to the conforming quality of the material), and reduced shear force compared to alternative materials.[260,261] Plaster of Paris is also porous and retains heat well, which is important for individuals with friable tissue. These qualities decrease the likelihood of maceration

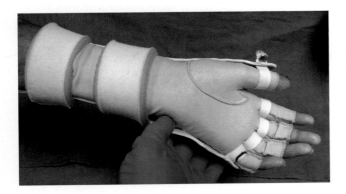

Figure 13-53. Volar view of radial nerve palsy mobilization splint, displaying elastic straps around first phalanx that assist with metacarpophalangeal extension.

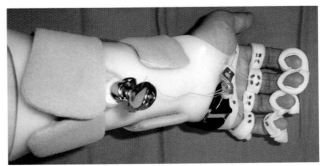

Figure 13-54. Static progressive finger composite flexion splint.

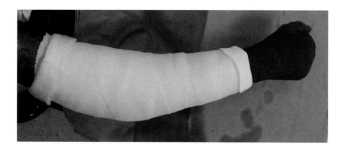

Figure 13-55. Elbow cast used to serially correct burn scar contracture.

and create neutral warmth, required because casualties with large burns have difficulty regulating their temperature.[260]

Intermediate Phase

The clinical focus in the intermediate phase moves from tissue protection toward mobilization while maintaining emphasis on reducing and managing edema. The indication for casting as an intervention during the intermediate phase is based on the same factors as in splinting: tissue recruitment and creep. If a body part has healthy, native skin and is involved as recruited tissue because of close proximity to the burn wound, aggressive total active motion is sought throughout each intervention. All active components of ROM progression, such as AROM, sustained stretch, strengthening exercises, and daily functional activities, should precede casting. Keeping in mind that the chosen modality should help restore ROM, serial or dropout casting may be considered to stimulate tissue creep or native tissue recruitment. Skin and joint tightness suggest serial or dropout casting will be effective.[260] The extended gentle stress of serial casting results in the repose of links between collagen fibers and realignment of collagen into a parallel and lengthened state. The realignment of collagen structures around the affected joint is also protected.[262]

Guidelines to Serial Casting

Serial casting is indicated for the following:

- casualties who have scar contractures for less than 18 months,
- casualties with contractures that are not responding to traditional methods of therapy,
- casualties with exposed tendons,
- casualties who do not comply with traditional therapy,

- casualties willing to comply with inconveniences of wearing a cast,
- casualties with multiple joint involvement,
- casualties with increased muscle tone, and
- when extra contour or compression must be applied for scar management.

Serial casting is contraindicated when a casualty exhibits heterotopic ossification (HO), excessive edema, or agitation, or does not comply with follow-up appointments.

A thorough chart review, followed by a complete physical examination, will help determine if serial casting will be therapeutically beneficial. The assessment must include radiographs to rule out HO in the affected joint. ROM and the functional components of the affected joint should be assessed to acquire joint feel and mobility while using proper alignment. The end range test should be concluded just beyond the point of resistance to achieve an appropriate end feel.[262] Fragile or friable skin, open wounds, an insensate extremity, and cognitive or emotional impairments should be taken into account when considering serial casting. These considerations are weighed against the advantages of a noninvasive procedure. Serial casting allows for continuous intervention with total contact in addition to continuous stretch, which allows for more concentrated intervention on other affected areas.[260,262]

Long-Term Phase

Casting techniques during the long-term rehabilitation phase closely resemble the interventions of the intermediate rehabilitation phase, but with a focus on mobilization and edema management. Casting is key in reducing and preventing contracture until the wounds reach maturation and full active ROM can be achieved and sustained. A variety of casting techniques are available to help burn casualties recover ROM. Any design that can be made with splinting material can also be made with casting material.[260]

Range-of-Motion Exercise

Acute Phase

Burns heal naturally by contraction, and shortened connective tissue responds to the stress imparted by ROM exercise. A thorough history is required to determine the type of ROM exercises that will meet the casualty's, physician's, and therapist's goals. Additionally, service members who sustain battlefront burns often incur accompanying injuries, such as penetrating wounds or fractures, which require consideration when selecting appropriate ROM exercise.

Acutely burned service members must move gently through full ROM each day to improve peripheral circulation, keep joints nourished, and prevent contractures or decubitus ulcers. All areas injured, including the face, neck, bilateral upper extremities, hands, bilateral lower extremities, feet, and trunk, require attention. Contractures of the flexor surfaces of joints are noted most frequently. However, exercise in all planes of motion must take place. Therapists and casualties collaborate to form the ROM exercise plan most appropriate to the individual injury (Exhibit 13-3). The progression of ROM differs based on the casualty and injury characteristics. All types of ROM exercise apply to all casualties at some point in the recovery and rehabilitation process.

Casualties with larger burns (> 30% TBSA burned) are typically intubated, sedated, and admitted to the intensive care unit, rendering AROM impossible. In these cases, PROM is the mainstay of daily ROM treatment. In the case of smaller burns, casualties are capable of beginning with AAROM or AROM in the acute phase. Casualties admitted with acute hand burns should be evaluated by a therapist within 24 hours of admission.

Although PROM may be the least desirable type of ROM exercise, it can be useful when treating a comatose casualty, and it helps maintain joint mobility and integrity.[263] PROM should be performed gently, slowly and cautiously by a therapist, and precautions should be taken to avoid overstretching joint structures.[177] PROM should be performed in the appropriate planes of motion for each joint while stabilizing the joints above and below. Some clinicians believe that PROM may cause tissue damage that leads to increased scarring, but this theory has not been substantiated.[263–265] Scar tissue responds well to passive force when applied in a steady, controlled manner (Exhibit 13-4).[177] Special instances where PROM is called for include after an escharotomy or fasciotomy, or when it is necessary to preserve tendon gliding and the casualty is unable to perform AAROM or AROM exercises.[177,263] Caution should be exercised when tendons are exposed, especially at the PIP joint of the finger. PROM exercise should be restricted to the amount of force required for an observable tendon excursion to occur.[177] Additional force provides no increased benefit and places exposed tendons at risk for rupture, leading to joint deformities. Once hemostasis has been achieved, any type of ROM exercise is permissible to obtain full ROM and preserve joint integrity.[177]

Continuous passive motion (CPM) devices reduce edema[266] and preserve motion. The deleterious effects

---

EXHIBIT 13-3

RANGE-OF-MOTION EXERCISE CATEGORIES

- Passive range of motion (PROM) is movement of the joint through the range of movement, which is produced entirely by an external force.[1] The prime mover muscle for the joint does not voluntarily contract to complete the range of movement. Movement performed without assistance on the part of the casualty is considered passive exercise.
- Active assistive range of motion (AAROM) is movement in which AROM by the casualty is supplemented with assistance by an external force.[1] The prime mover muscle for the joint needs assistance to complete the range of movement. AROM with terminal stretch means the casualty vigorously moves the joint through available motion, then the therapist gently stretches the joint in its proper plane of motion, toward the extremes of full motion.
- Active range of motion (AROM) is movement within the range of movement, which is produced by voluntary active contraction of the muscles crossing that joint by the casualty.[1] The prime mover muscle for the joint voluntarily contracts to complete the range of movement.
- Low-load prolonged stretch is a relatively long-term stretch, applied in a controlled manner at a tolerable load.[2] Typically achieved through positioning, splinting, casting or with the use of equipment, this type of stretch is used for a prolonged time and therefore must be tolerable for the long-term benefit to be realized. As it is characterized by length of time rather than number of repetitions, it is different from all other range-of-motion definitions.

Data sources: (1) Kisner C, Colby LA. *Therapeutic Exercise: Foundations and Techniques.* 3rd ed. Philadelphia, Pa: FA Davis; 1996. (2) Humphrey C, Richard RL, Staley MJ. Soft tissue management and exercise. In: Richard R, Staley MJ, eds. *Burn Care and Rehabilitation: Principles and Practice.* Philadelphia, Pa: FA Davis; 1994: 334.

EXHIBIT 13-4

CONSIDERATIONS FOR USE OF PASSIVE RANGE-OF-MOTION EXERCISE

- Level of consciousness
- Level of medication
- Severity of condition
- Decreased range of motion
- Scar contractures
- Peripheral nerve injury
- Preservation of joint mobility
- Anesthesia
- Area of escharatomy
- Preservation of tendon glide

---

of prolonged immobilization of the synovial joints, demonstrated by numerous orthopaedists,[267] inspired the development of CPM machines. There are two basic CPM designs. One is an anatomical design that moves the joint in an arc of motion as similar to actual anatomical movement as is possible. The other design is free linkage, which moves body parts adjacent to the involved joint. For example, it can move the forearm while allowing the casualty to move an elbow or shoulder if possible.

The anatomical motion machine is probably the more comfortable of the two devices. Most of the machines can be set to pause at the end range and resemble slow, prolonged stretch. Machines may be portable, free-standing, or attached to a bed or chair. Those who are most likely to benefit from use of CPM in addition to customary physical and occupational therapy include individuals who have burns involving multiple joints; comatose casualties; and casualties who refuse to perform active motion because of pain, swelling, or anxiety. The specific protocol of use for CPM machines depends on a casualty's tolerance and limitations.

The hand CPM device restores hand ROM. It does not damage skin grafts or newly healed tissue, and the pain experienced is the same as that with conventional hand stretching and exercise therapy.[266] Adaptations can be made to block MCP or PIP motion, and some splints can be used over the dorsum of the hand to achieve improved composite MCP and IP flexion. AROM exercise of the involved hand joints should be measured daily to assess for skin tightness and to evaluate joint mobility. If the casualty is able, hourly AROM exercise and ADL participation should be encouraged at home to maximize ROM. If the casualty is unable to participate in sufficient AROM exercise,

then PROM exercise should be performed at least three times a day on the involved joints. Dressings should be applied with digits individually wrapped to permit participation in ROM exercises. To maximize tissue elongation, PROM activities should include low-load force with a long duration of hold.[249]

Shoulder CPM machines, which attach to a bed or chair and move the shoulder through 180° of flexion or abduction, help prevent axillary scar bands and nourish shoulder joint cartilage. Additional models move the shoulder in other planes, including a figure-eight pattern. Some models incorporate the elbow, providing ROM for both joints simultaneously.

The elbow CPM can be set for low-load stretching and auto reverse, so there is little risk of overloading the joint or surrounding tissues (Figure 13-56). The degree of elbow flexion, extension, pronation, and supination can be adjusted to the casualty's tolerance. When set for gentle motion, this device provides thorough ROM while minimizing the risk of HO.

Knee CPM machines should be used when the casualty is not participating in active therapy (Figure 13-57). They provide improved motion at the knee and can be set up to address the ankle and hip joints, as well. These CPMs are useful until ambulation is possible, or longer if joints continue to exhibit ROM limitations.

Showering and dressing changes are good opportunities to perform ROM exercises. During these procedures, bandages and wraps that typically inhibit ROM are removed, allowing for more thorough treat-

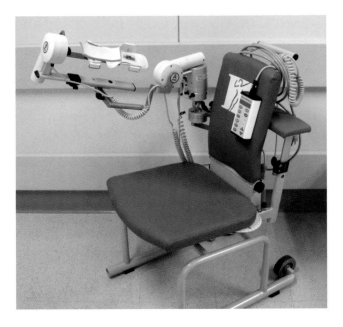

Figure 13-56. Continuous passive motion device for the elbow.

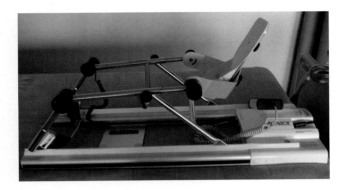

Figure 13-57. Continuous passive motion device for the knee.

ment. Therapists can see the affects of ROM exercise on the tissue and can ensure enough force is being exerted to elongate the tissue. Additionally, because the casualties' pain will already be managed for the wound care procedure, ROM exercises will be better tolerated (however, casualties must not be overloaded with pain from both wound care and ROM exercises).

When casualties are under anesthesia for skin grafting or debridement, ROM exercises can be used to evaluate range and determine the cause of limitations. ROM may be limited because of soft tissue contracture or pain; anesthetizing the casualty can help distinguish the cause. If the primary cause of the limitation is pain, the pain management plan can be adjusted to improve the casualty's tolerance. If the primary cause is determined to be soft tissue contracture, the casualty should be encouraged to increase the frequency and vigor of rehabilitation. A gentle, slow, controlled force in the correct orientation is the key to safe ROM exercise, particularly when the casualty is anesthetized.

Intermediate Phase

Casualties generally regain responsiveness in the intermediate phase, and PROM exercise should be replaced with AAROM exercise if full ROM has not been achieved. AROM exercises should be initiated when the casualty has full ROM. Alert casualties must learn to move past the painful range to the extremes of joint motion; this can be accomplished with gentle terminal stretching. AAROM exercises with terminal stretching teach casualties how to move the affected body part and achieve the extremes of motion that are not used spontaneously during activity (Exhibit 13-5).[177]

For AAROM exercises, healing and healed tissue should be stretched to the point of tissue blanching and maintained until the tissue becomes more pliable or tissue color returns.[177] A casualty's tolerance to the force applied must also be considered. Typically, 1 to

2 lb of force is required to cause blanching.[177] Several preliminary repetitions must be performed to ensure tissue is at its optimal length prior to sustaining the force applied.[177] Best results are achieved when a casualty performs AROM exercises to the limits of pain or tissue restriction, and then the therapist applies the required slow and controlled overpressure to complete the ROM exercise.

Additional AAROM exercises can be performed with various devices, such as pulleys, finger and dowel ladders, and weights. These activities use the casualty's unaffected limbs as the source of overpressure to achieve full ROM at the affected joint. A stationary bike or upper-body ergometer can also be used for AAROM exercise, as can the casualty's body weight. These AAROM techniques allow casualties some control, improving tolerance and promoting compliance and independence.

AROM is the most desirable form of ROM exercise.[265] It tends to be less painful and activates the muscle pump, enhancing venous and lymphatic return and reducing edema.[178] However, AROM should only be used with casualties who can achieve full ROM within a reasonable amount of time (Exhibit 13-6).[177] AROM is also the safest form of ROM exercise and is recommended for joints with exposed tendons or immature skin grafts, or those at risk for HO, where PROM exercise and AAROM exercise must be used sparingly and cautiously. Casualties generally self-limit voluntary muscle contractions because of pain and will not produce the force required to rupture a tendon or disrupt skin grafts.[265] Active motion decreases the risk of HO at the elbow joint.[268,269] Occasionally, casualties need encouragement and relaxation reminders in order to tolerate ROM exercises. If casualties are still unable to tolerate the force required to achieve scar tissue blanching, their pain management plan must

---

EXHIBIT 13-5

CONSIDERATIONS FOR USE OF ACTIVE ASSISTED RANGE-OF-MOTION EXERCISE

- Limited range of motion
- Scar contractures
- Area of escharotomy
- Skin graft adherence
- Increased physiological demands
- Decreased cardiac reserve
- Poor ventilation and respiratory status
- Decreased strength secondary to prolonged hospitalization

> **EXHIBIT 13-6**
>
> **CONSIDERATIONS FOR USE OF ACTIVE RANGE-OF-MOTION EXERCISE**
>
> - Edema reduction from muscle pumping
> - Increased circulation
> - Initiation of exercise first week after skin grafting
> - Conditioning of uninvolved areas
> - Exposed tendons (except the proximal interphalangeal joint)
> - Prevention of soft tissue shortening
> - Prevention of muscle atrophy

be reviewed and modified to improve tolerance of ROM exercise.

Full ROM returns most quickly when inflammation is minimal, wound healing is complete, and a casualty complies with rehabilitation. Applying heat prior to ROM exercises may also be beneficial.[263,265,270–272] Joint mobilization and distraction of joint surfaces, in conjunction with stretching, may decrease pain and muscle spasm and increase the effectiveness of stretching.[273]

Casualties must invest a significant amount of mental concentration and vigorous physical energy for ROM exercises to be effective. Distractions, such as visitors, should be minimized to allow casualties to concentrate on restoring greater function.

A clock that announces time intervals, such as one that rings every 15 minutes, can help a casualty remember to stretch eyelids or other important contractures throughout the day without the verbal cues that may come to seem like nagging from a therapist. A casualty may also be able to relax and benefit more from ROM exercises when the therapist uses another activity, such as conversation, to distract the casualty from the pain at the treatment site. During the latter phases of recovery, casualties wear external vascular supports, which may need to be removed for 10-minute periods for ROM exercises but donned immediately after.

Post-burn management of a superficial partial-thickness burn differs from management of a deep partial-thickness or full-thickness burn. Superficial partial-thickness burns are at minimal risk for contracture.[274] Full ROM is usually restored with AROM exercises performed in a home program, and AROM exercises are initiated as soon as possible. Adequate pain control is imperative to allow participation in a home program. Splinting is only necessary if poor exercise participation is noted over a prolonged period of time and ROM gains are not being made.

Deep partial-thickness and full-thickness burns are at a high risk for contracture.[274] AROM and PROM exercises should be consistently performed throughout the intermediate rehabilitation phase. Home exercises and supervised therapy should include low-load force and long duration PROM exercises and should place the involved tissue at its greatest length. Isolated joints should be stretched, with the involved skin in a shortened position prior to elongation. For example, isolated MCP, PIP, and DIP PROM exercises should precede a composite stretch involving combined MCP, PIP, and DIP flexion stretching. AROM exercises in the same movement pattern should immediately follow passive exercises.

Long-Term Phase

During the long-term rehabilitation phase, as with the early phases, low-load, prolonged stress is recommended for minimizing and preventing burn scar and joint contractures.[275] Gentle, graded, and prolonged ROM stretching, preferably achieved actively by the casualty, will help collagen fiber realign into a longer, less tightly convoluted, mat-like configuration. At this point, if burn scar contractures are present, they are usually so severe that they will not resolve with prolonged ROM stretching alone. Additional interventions, such as positioning, splinting, casting, strengthening exercises, and functional activities will be required. However, the burn therapist must reserve adequate time for prolonged individual joint and composite ROM stretching because casualties will need encouragement, supervision, and hands-on treatment during this phase of rehabilitation.

Low-load, prolonged ROM stretching has the additional benefit of gently, slowly overcoming muscular cocontraction in casualties who fear pain. With prompting, casualties who have had adequate analgesia during the first two phases will put forth maximum effort to move through the extremes of motion, preventing joint motion from becoming painful, nourishing joint cartilage, and elongating surrounding burn scar and soft tissue. Low-load, prolonged ROM stretching may also be combined with work-equivalent activities. All other types of ROM exercise should be applied and incorporated into written home programs during the long-term rehabilitation phase.

Strengthening and Conditioning

Acute Phase

Casualties recovering from burn injuries will require strength training and cardiovascular reconditioning. These treatments can begin as soon as the casualty is admitted to the hospital, and may continue throughout several years. Although each burn casualty is unique, all will experience some form of deconditioning. When designing a rehabilitation program, therapists should consider the casualty's phase of recovery, the percentage of TBSA burned, the etiology of the burn, comorbitities (including inhalation injuries), postsurgical skin grafting precautions, and prior level of function.[276] Depending on the casualty's status, strength and conditioning programs can commence on the same day as admission.

In the sitting position, casualties experience reduced pulmonary congestion, facilitated diaphragmatic expansion and ventilation, and ease of dyspnea. If possible, a casualty can be transferred to a bedside chair, with or without assistance, and remain sitting for as long as tolerated. When a casualty is sedated or otherwise unable to assist with the transfer, a total lift chair may be used (Figure 13-58). A casualty can be transferred laterally from a bed to a chair in a flattened position. From there, a therapist can manipulate the chair into an upright sitting position, where the casualty may remain for as long as tolerated to receive the benefits of upright sitting. Some hospital beds may also have specific settings that move the bed from a supine position to an upright sitting position if the casualty is unable to be laterally transferred to the total lift chair.

When a casualty is medically cleared for lower-extremity weight bearing but is unable to stand without great assistance, a therapist may use a tilt table. With a tilt table, the casualty is secured to the plinth with a series of straps while in the supine position. A therapist can mechanically tilt the table into the upright position and can pause the tilt at any interval to allow a casualty to slowly become acclimatized to the upright standing position. The casualty's response to the activity will dictate the progress of the tilt. Because the straps restrict casualty movement, the motion is generally passive and recruits mainly postural muscles. The primary benefit of a tilt table is its ability to decrease orthostatic hypotension through gradual retraining of the cardiovascular system to the upright position.[277] It also allows gradual weight bearing through the lower extremities.

If a casualty is able to tolerate the standing position of the tilt table but does not have the endurance to stand for any great length of time, the standing frame may be appropriate. The standing frame uses a system of levers to raise a casualty from the sitting position to the standing position with a solid support, allowing the casualty to receive the cardiovascular benefits of an upright position while experiencing weight bearing to increase lower-extremity and trunk strength.

If a casualty is cleared for lower-extremity weight bearing but still unable to stand without great effort, a therapist may use a modified tilt table (Figure 13-59). The modified tilt table has a system of pins and locks that allow the plinth to slide so the casualty may

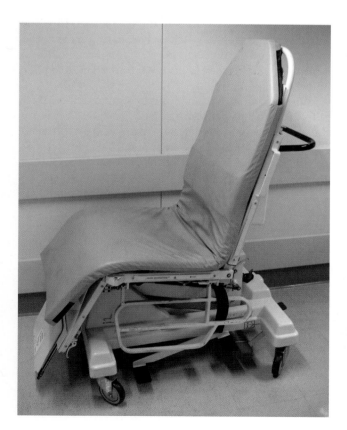

Figure 13-58. Total lift chair used for early out-of-bed transfers.

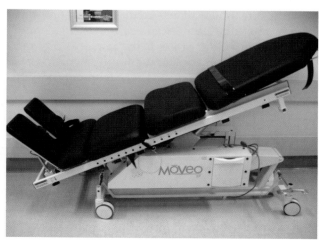

Figure 13-59. Modified tilt table.

perform an inclined squat unilaterally or bilaterally in an environment of decreased gravity resistance. This permits the casualty to increase lower-extremity strength in preparation for ambulation.[277]

Early ambulation is vital to the success of all casualties. Ambulation may begin while a casualty is still intubated if deemed safe. If the casualty is recovering from lower-extremity skin grafting over a joint, ambulation may begin as early as the third day following operation. Casualties that ambulate within this timeframe experience increased ROM, cardiopulmonary function, and muscular strength compared to those that remain immobilized for a longer period of time.[278,279]

ROM exercise also promotes cardiovascular reconditioning. PROM of all extremities requires the casualty to exert 1 metabolic equivalent (MET), AROM exercise of all extremities requires 1 to 1.5 METs, and AROM with moderate resistance requires 1.5 to 2 METs. ROM exercises not only increase joint mobility and integumentary movement, but promote proper cardiovascular reconditioning and increase muscular strength.[280]

Intermediate Phase

When burn casualties have 50% to 100% wound closure, they transition to an outpatient program. Prior to discharge from the hospital, the casualty should be able to transfer and complete ADLs with little to no assistance. Practicing these activities is a functional method of increasing strength and cardiovascular endurance. When casualties are preparing for discharge, strengthening and conditioning therapy sessions should focus on increasing independence with ADLs.

Resisted ROM exercises can be provided by the therapist, resistance bands, or weight-lifting equipment, and should progress in accordance with the casualty's treatment plan. Circuit training programs increase muscular strength and cardiovascular endurance while providing variety in the casualty's program. Pilates exercises, on a mat or with equipment, increase strength, promote proper body alignment, and improve ROM.[281]

Casualties can use gym equipment to increase cardiovascular conditioning and muscle strength. Recumbent bicycles and elliptical machines increase cardiovascular strength without increasing weight bearing. The NuStep machine (NuStep Inc, Ann Arbor, Michigan), a recumbent cross-training machine, promotes lower-extremity strength and ROM without increasing weight bearing in the hip and knee joints. The American College of Sports Medicine recommends that adults exercise at moderate intensity for at least 30 minutes on most, if not all, days of the week.[282] Casualties with burns are no exception to this recommendation. Casualties should begin their reconditioning slowly, with the long-term goal of meeting the American College of Sports Medicine standard.

Long-Term Phase

Once a casualty transitions to the long-term rehabilitation phase, high-level functional activities should be encouraged. In the rehabilitation gym, isokinetic exercises can be used to improve strength and power, in addition to maintaining ROM.[283] When participating in outdoor activities, casualties should be aware of their own limitations concerning thermoregulation. Many areas of healed burn scar or skin grafts are unable to produce sweat to cool the body; therefore, the casualty is at a greater risk for overheating and should take the necessary precautions.[284] Casualties should also keep water close at hand and remain in the shade when possible if outside.

Burn casualties have a higher resting metabolic rate than individuals without burns. Despite having an elevated resting metabolic rate, the stress on the casualty's cardiopulmonary system resulting from activity increases resting metabolic rate proportional to that of an individual without burns.[285] The Karvonen method should be used to determine the appropriate heart rate range because it takes into consideration the casualty's resting heart rate (Exhibit 13-7).[276] Ultimately, proper rehabilitation for burn casualties should consist of a cardiovascular reconditioning and muscle strengthening program that maximizes functional outcome and return to duty.

EXHIBIT 13-7

THE KARVONEN METHOD FOR DETERMINING HEART RATE RANGE

Target heart rate = ([maximum heart rate − resting heart rate] • percent intensity) + resting heart rate

Activities of Daily Living

Acute Phase

Functional activities should be practiced around the clock when possible. Not only should the burn team be aware of what a casualty is capable of doing in areas of self-care, but the casualty's family should know as well. Frequently, the burn team and family perform activities that a casualty is capable of performing independently. This is detrimental because casualties gain self-esteem and self-confidence by being as independent as possible. Families can be directed to participate with casualties in activities such as applying lotion, organizing get-well cards, answering mail, or playing games, rather than assisting with essential tasks, such as feeding, that a casualty must learn to perform independently.

ADLs, such as independent phone use, self-feeding, shaving, brushing teeth, and self-toileting, are beneficial exercises for the upper extremities. Repetitive calisthenics may be boring; however, casualties understand the importance of practicing daily living skills and are often motivated by the desire to regain independence. It is helpful for casualties to be reminded of the goals of regaining maximum independence with the fewest possible scar bands and with the least possible disfigurement while struggling with self-care or uncomfortable exercises.

Participation in functional ADLs is important in the rehabilitation of the burn casualty.[286] The major ADL classifications are:

- Mobility: including movement in bed, wheelchair mobility and transfers, indoor ambulation with special equipment, outdoor ambulation with special equipment, and management of public or private transportation.
- Self-care: including feeding, bathing, toileting, grooming, and dressing.
- Managing environmental hardware and devices: including the ability to use telephones, doors, faucets, light switches, scissors, keys, windows, and street control signals.
- Communication skills: including the ability to write, operate a personal computer, read, type, and use the telephone, a tape recorder, or a special communications device.
- Home management activities: including shopping, meal planning and preparation, cleaning, doing laundry, caring for children, and operating household appliances.[287]

There are numerous benefits gained from independently performing functional tasks and activities. Physical benefits include improving ROM, fine motor dexterity, and overall endurance. The psychological benefits include increased self-reliance, improved self-esteem, and positive feelings about the future. Involving casualties in planning and implementing functional activities early on allows them to more easily resume social roles and decreases posttraumatic disability later. Independent performance of ADLs also hastens hospital discharge to home or a less-supervised setting.

Several factors can influence the overall outcome of a functional activity program, including medical status (percent of TBSA burned, degree, and location of burns); age; degree of cooperation and motivation; premorbid physical, psychological, educational, intellectual, economic, and functional status; and social resources. Additional factors that impact independent living include memory loss from medication, pain or severity of illness, cognitive changes due to anoxia or accompanying head injury, preburn or medication-induced impaired judgment, depression, and pain. Successful programs involve the casualty and family in prioritization, goal setting, and problem solving for accomplishing functional activities.

Functional activity performance can be analyzed in terms of independence, speed of performance, and safety when considering how a casualty accomplishes tasks. Independence in ADLs can be achieved in a number of ways. Burned soldiers need to perform ADLs without adaptive equipment, using repetitions to improve strength and endurance. When adaptive equipment is used in the earliest phase of rehabilitation, it should be discontinued as soon as possible. Occupational therapists can make recommendations concerning adaptive equipment, task alteration, adaptive techniques, and environmental modifications.

Burn casualties are encouraged to self-feed, despite hand burns. Conventional silverware with handles enlarged by elastic rolls and an elevated table are often adequate to encourage self-feeding. Adaptations for self-care are discontinued as soon as possible to avoid dependence and to increase hand and upper-extremity ROM. Adaptive feeding devices include long-handled silverware, utensils with built-up handles, and universal cuffs (Figure 13-60). Universal cuffs with hook-and-loop fasteners or D-ring attachments allow casualties to don them without assistance. Expanded universal cuffs can be fabricated for bulky dressings, casts, or splints. Additional devices, such as bent-angled silverware or bendable, foam-handled spoons, are available if wrist radial deviation is permanently limited (Figure 13-61).

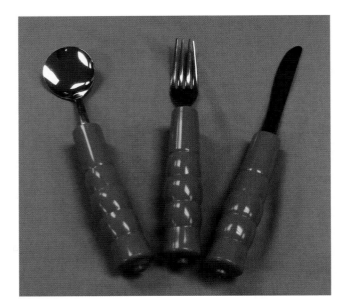

Figure 13-60. Adaptive eating utensils with built-up handles.

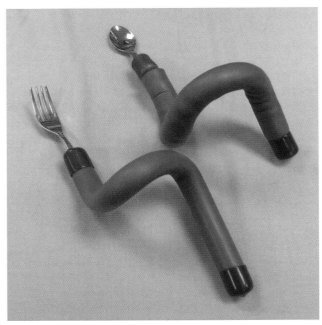

Figure 13-61. Bendable foam-handled eating utensils.

Utensils with extensions can be helpful when there is limited mobility in decreased shoulder or elbow flexion. Utensils with swivel attachments or horizontal handles replace forearm supination. Vertical handles can be used when the forearm is fixed for midposition. Long straws held in place by straw clips, adaptive mugs and glasses, easy-grip mugs with protruding handles, glasses with a cutout area for the nose, and bilateral glass holders can aid in drinking. Sealed mugs are also helpful when a casualty lacks hand control. Weighted mugs can be used when a casualty exhibits a tremor. When inhalation injuries result in swallowing difficulties, vacuum flow suction mugs can prevent choking by controlling the rate at which liquid is released.

There are several types of adaptive equipment that provide stabilization when a casualty has use of only one hand. Nonskid mats can be placed on counters or tabletops to prevent plates and bowls from slipping. Scoop dishes and plate guards provide stability for utensils (**Figure 13-62**). A rocker knife can be used for cutting when a casualty is permanently unable to use one hand. Pan and bowl holders also provide stability. Adaptive cutting boards have a nail to stabilize items for cutting, and built-up corners to hold bread while buttering. Special openers for jars, cans, or bottles are helpful for casualties with only one functional hand or decreased hand strength or control.

Grooming is another self-care activity that can be performed early. Oral care and hair brushing and combing are initiated when bathroom privileges begin. Although rarely needed, a built-up handle

or universal cuff can compensate for the inability to grasp a toothbrush, hairbrush, or comb. A temporary extended handle can make teeth brushing easier while ROM improves. Toothpaste tube squeezers are available if fine motor dexterity is limited. Denture brushes with suction cups are also useful when only one hand is functional. Adding extended handles (straight or bent-angled) to hairbrushes and combs is useful when shoulder flexion, shoulder external rotation, or both are lacking.

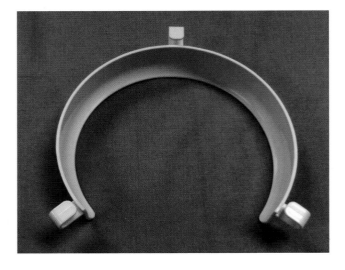

Figure 13-62. Plate guard used to assist with self-feeding.

During the acute phase, toileting skills vary according to the extent of the burn. Casualties with larger TBSA burns may be unable to participate in self-toileting because of sedation, intubation, catherization, and limited upper-extremity use. Less-involved casualties can use a variety of large-handled urinals and spill-proof containers at the bedside, and can transfer to and from the bedside commode for bowel activities (which will help advance mobility as well as toileting skills). As casualties progress, they may be left with some level of deficit requiring use of a toileting aid to manipulate toilet paper, or they need to incorporate assistive technology such as a bidet, autoflush commodes, or a raised commode seat to assist with sit–stand transfers.

Communication is a functional activity that is very important in all phases of rehabilitation. This is a broad category that includes expression, reading, use of environmental controls, writing, and telephone and typewriter or computer use. Large button, programmable phones can be adapted with speakers, allowing early independent telephone use. Because telephones keep burn casualties in touch with their support systems, adaptations are requested early. An adjustable gooseneck phone holder allows a casualty to speak and hear without holding the telephone. The gooseneck holder affords more privacy than the speakerphone. There are also special phone holders for casualties with weak grasps. A phone flipper lever can be added to the base of a telephone to activate the connection button if a casualty cannot press it. A flipper can be operated by hand or by mouth stick. Another type of phone adaptation is a touchtone adapter, which enlarges regular push buttons and can be operated by a very light touch.

Expression is important because it allows casualties to interact with others in the environment and decreases fear and frustration. A casualty with a severe burn may be intubated, ventilator-dependent, and unable to speak. Prolonged exposure to smoke can result in vocal cord injuries, leaving speech unintelligible or contraindicated. Communication boards composed of letters, pictures, body maps, words, or complete sentences are commonly used to convey thoughts if the casualty can point to them. There are also sophisticated communication devices with voice outputs that can be operated by touch or by a light-activated beam. However, because casualties are often medicated or too ill, complicated communication devices are best used in the later stages of recovery.

As a casualty progresses, a number of environmental controls can be adapted for independent use. Environmental controls are available in a wide variety of switching systems with specific mounting devices. The basic plate, light touch plate, air cushion, rocker, foot, wobble, sip-and-puff control, and joystick are common switch options. The same switch and input device method can also be used to operate a communication device, computer, or electric wheelchair in other phases of rehabilitation. Switches can be specially ordered or can be purchased from electronics retail stores.

Reading can be a very important functional exercise when a casualty is confined to bed. There are several types of book and magazine stands that can assist with reading. Bed readers, positioned slightly overhead, are useful when an alert casualty must stay supine. A prone casualty can use a floor stand or music stand with pages stabilized by clothespins. Height- and angle-adjustable bookstands can be clamped to a bedside table or headboard. Bookstands with automatic page turners can be used if a casualty is unable to turn pages independently. A mouthstick can also be used to turn pages. Mouthstick devices have increased friction at the end and can be adapted to fit universal cuffs. Prism glasses allow a casualty to look down at pages to read while the head is positioned forward. In cases of preexisting visual acuity deficits, a variety of magnifiers can be used, in addition to large-print books.

Writing is another important self-care activity that can be performed in early stages of burn rehabilitation. Pen and pencil holders are useful temporary adaptations when a casualty's ability to grasp or pinch is decreased. Built-up foam handles or plastic easy-grip adapters facilitate holding a pen. Special splints or adaptive writing utensils can be fabricated out of thermoplastic materials, or commercially available splints can be obtained to customize writing devices. A clipboard can be used to stabilize paper when the nondominant hand is unable to hold it steady for writing. A writing device can be attached to a mouth stick if neither hand can write.

Intermediate Phase

As a casualty becomes more independent in the hospital, it is important to identify home management responsibilities, including general maneuvering, operating home appliances, cooking, and cleaning. It is important for casualties and their families to identify the tasks that the individual wants or needs to perform. Ideally, a survey of home needs is accomplished with the casualty, family, and a staff member, but it can also be performed by just the casualty and family. A home evaluation focusing on independence and safety can identify functional or environmental limitations, and casualties can use mobility aids and adaptive equipment in the home to determine the level of assistance that will be required after hospital discharge.

It is important to avoid trauma or shearing the skin surface while practicing ADLs during the intermediate phase. Functional activities, such as feeding, grooming, and communication, should be performed, and adaptive equipment can continue to be used. Applying lotion to healed or unburned areas increases sensory input and decreases hallucinations from sensory deprivation.

Casualties usually view hospital discharge as a welcome termination of burn care, exercise, and pain, and they often eagerly anticipate what they believe is a well-deserved rest. Recalcitrant casualties who endure exercise and scar control devices at the hospital may abandon custom-made elastic stockings, traction, total contact splints, and activity once they feel safe at home. Many casualties believe returning home will restore their previous physical and emotional status. However, it quickly becomes obvious that achieving adequate epithelial healing at home is only the beginning of rehabilitation and return to active duty.[288] Work-hardening programs—graded work activities that simulate a casualty's work requirements— are appropriate for severely burned casualties. The activities are adapted to assure success in the simulated activity and are designed to lead to progress in work performance. Acitivities can be sequentially redesigned to require less adaptation until adaptation is minimized. Work hardening also reinforces protective measures for friction, trauma, chemical irritants, and extremes of weather or temperature.

The best outcomes result when the casualty, therapist, and physician formulate an appropriate active-duty limitation outline with each clinic visit. It can be helpful for casualties to return part time to as many active-duty tasks as possible, even if their ability to perform tasks is limited. Jobs done by habit eliminate the need for casualties to constantly think about the discomfort of exercising.

Long-Term Phase

In the long-term rehabilitation phase, casualties continue to actively participate in functional activities that are consistent with life roles and return to active duty. As they become medically stable and burn scars and skin grafts become more durable, casualties can pursue a variety of activities; however, caution is required because maturing burn scars and skin grafts remain fragile in this phase. Casualties must learn proper interventions to compensate for sensory, pigmentation, and circulatory changes while performing ADLs. At this time, casualties must begin to wean off adaptive equipment used in the initial phases of rehabilitation. However, casualties with electrical injuries, amputa-

tions, or burns greater than 70% TBSA may continue to use adaptive equipment if residual impairments exist. For severely impaired casualties, sophisticated orthoses and adaptive equipment should be used to reduce disability.

Adaptive silverware, drinking aids, and stabilization devices are rarely used in the long-term rehabilitation phase. If decreased shoulder ROM and proximal weakness are permanent, suspension slings or mobile arm supports can be used when a casualty is seated. These devices support the entire arm, assist shoulder flexion, and allow the elbow to move in a gravity-eliminated plane. The mobile arm support is available in standard, elevating, and table-mounted models. Battery-powered or electric feeding machines operated by microswitch control are available for casualties in which severe burn has resulted in upper-extremity amputations. The switches can be operated by various body parts that can predictably and consistently control the machine.

Casualties can participate in additional grooming tasks, such as shaving with special holders for electric or regular razors (Figure 13-63). Casualties should regularly care for nails to prevent excoriation of skin during scratching. Mounted nail clippers (Figure 13-64) or files are available to assist with such activities.

At this stage, casualties should begin to assume responsibility for the condition of their skin, burn scars, and skin grafts, inspecting them regularly to identify any areas of concern. Flexible inspection mirrors are available to assist with this task. Casualties can also assume responsibility for wound care and should demonstrate the ability to safely cleanse and apply medication and dressings to any remaining wounds. Casualties should also massage scars and apply moisturizer as indicated.

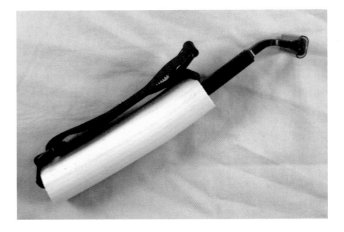

Figure 13-63. Adaptive holding device for a shaving razor.

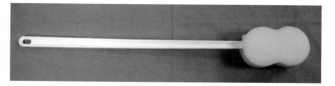

Figure 13-65. Adaptive long-handled sponge for self-bathing.

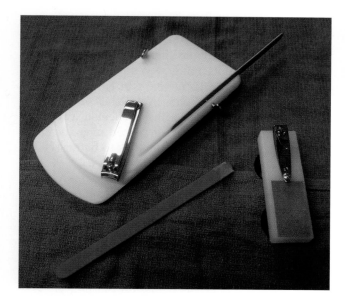

Figure 13-64. Commercially available adaptive mounted nail clippers and file.

or bath mats, can be applied to the bottom of the tub to prevent slipping.

Casualties assume total responsibility for donning external vascular support garments, orthoses, and clothing during the long-term rehabilitation phase. Casualties must be cautioned against pulling too rigorously on garments while donning them, which could injure fragile skin. A nylon stocking contact layer worn over wound dressings secures them and facilitates donning external vascular supports. Casualties must demonstrate donning facemasks, microstomia splints, hand splints, and lower extremity orthoses independently in front of a mirror to ensure proper fit.

There are a number of adaptive aids that assist with donning pressure garments and regular clothing. It is often more effective to use practice time donning items without adaptations when a casualty is expected to achieve enough ROM in a short period of time to make adaptations unnecessary. Long-handled aids are helpful in cases where there is decreased trunk, hip, and knee flexion, and hip external rotation. Many different "reachers" can be used to don pants; they are available in a standard size, extended length, and a self-closing model for decreased hand grasp (Figure 13-66). Long-handled shoehorns and stocking aids help with donning shoes and socks (Figure 13-67). A dressing stick can be used for donning pants and shirts if upper-extremity ROM is limited.

Other adaptive aids are useful if finger dexterity is limited or if a casualty has use of only one hand. Elastic shoelaces and button and zipper aids are available in

As casualties progress, they will want to perform toileting tasks independently. A variety of adaptive equipment is available to ensure safety and independence. Safety rails can be mounted on either side of the toilet to increase transfer stability. Use of a raised toilet seat is usually discouraged, but it can be helpful when a casualty permanently lacks strength or control in the lower extremities and cannot perform transfers with a standard seat. A bedside commode is necessary in the hospital or at home only when ambulation to the bathroom is not possible. Toilet aids are also helpful if a casualty lacks the necessary upper-extremity ROM for hygiene.

A number of adaptive safety aids also allow independent bathing. It is often safer for casualties to bathe in a seated position if endurance is low. Edema can be minimized by keeping burned legs elevated until bathing is finished and external vascular supports are reapplied. Shower seats, with or without backs, provide stability in walk-in showers. Extended tub benches allow casualties to bathe independently on a seat if they are unable to step over the tub safely. Grab bars can be mounted on the tub or wall to further increase stability with transfers. A flexible shower hose permits casualties to bathe independently in a seated position if they are unable to stand for a prolonged period of time. Long-handled sponges compensate for decreased trunk or upper-extremity ROM and allow a casualty to wash feet and back independently (Figure 13-65). A bath mitt can stabilize a bar of soap if the casualty's grasp is weak. Safety features, such as nonskid surfaces

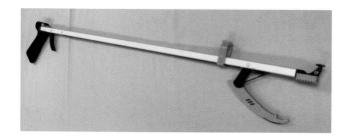

Figure 13-66. Adaptive reaching device used for a variety of self-care activities.

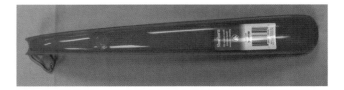

Figure 13-67. Long-handled shoehorn for donning shoes.

standard and easy-grasp varieties (Figures 13-68 and 13-69). Hook-and-loop fasteners can replace buttons and zippers, and large loops can be sewn onto pants to help casualties with donning. In general, some types of clothing are relatively easy to put on, such as large shirts, gym pants, and hook-and-loop closure tennis shoes, and many varieties of easy-to-don clothing are available through special-order catalogues.

A number of home accessibility aids can also facilitate independence. Wheelchair ramps are important modifications for some casualties. Stair glides are often used within a house to allow movement from one floor to another. High-rise furniture leg extenders make independent transfers to chairs and couches easier, and lamp and light switch extensions are helpful if a casualty has decreased finger dexterity or is functioning from a wheelchair. A variety of turning adaptations can help a casualty operate doors, faucets, stoves, and radiators when grasp is limited or weak (Figure 13-70).

As burn casualties continue in the rehabilitation process, they will generally resume kitchen activities. In addition to the adaptive kitchen and feeding tools already mentioned, home kitchen modifications can be made to make cooking safe and efficient. For example,

special devices can be used to safely operate an oven. Push/pull devices can be used to manipulate hot oven racks when a casualty has limited finger dexterity or sensory impairments. Long oven mitts made of flame-retardant fabric protect sensitive skin. Kitchen roll carts can move hot or heavy pans and dishes; if the cart is sturdy, it may also be used like a wheeled walker for stability. A positioning mirror placed over the stove allows wheelchair-bound casualties to better see the stovetop and cook safely.

As with many of the other functional activities, adaptive housekeeping aids compensate for a decreased ability to reach or grasp. Examples include extended dustpans and brushes, long-reach sponge mops, extended dusters, and housekeeping cuffs with hook-and-loop attachments that permit casualties with weak grasps to hold a broom or mop handle.

During the long-term rehabilitation phase, some of the communication devices used in earlier phases are unnecessary, although others will still be required. Casualties who are able to be out of bed in a seated position can practice typing and computer activities. Typing aids that fit over the hand and depress keys are commercially available or can be custom made. These aids are useful when fine motor dexterity is lacking and a casualty is unable to access the keyboard in a traditional way. If a casualty has limited ROM in the shoulders or elbows, a keyboard can be mounted on a special device to allow access. Detachable keyboards are also available for casualties unable to access the keys in the usual location. Key guards that separate keys are useful for casualties who have impaired coordination. One-handed users can use a key lock to simultaneously press multiple keys, and there are a variety of special switches casualties can use to operate environmental controls or activate computers.

Mobility

Acute Phase

Early initiation and aggressive progression of mobility activities are critical during the acute rehabilitation phase. ADLs orient casualties to the upright position,

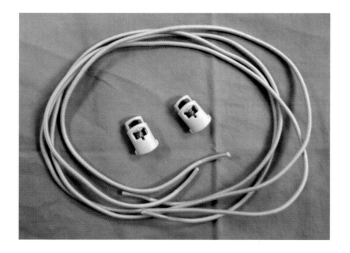

Figure 13-68. Elastic shoelaces.

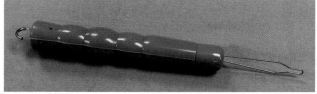

Figure 13-69. Button aid for self-dressing.

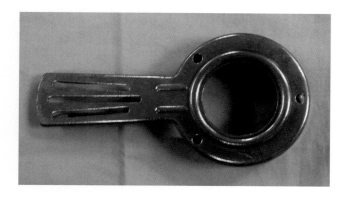

Figure 13-70. Door knob extension.

decreasing risk for pulmonary infection and complications, improving cardiovascular function, preventing orthostatic hypotension, preventing skin breakdown and decubitus ulcers, and restoring strength and independent functional mobility.[289] Exercise has also been shown to increase energy and decrease depression[290] as well as facilitate wound healing and pain reduction by more rapidly decreasing edema and inflammation.[289]

Mobility activities are commonly divided into three categories: (1) bed mobilities, (2) transfers and pregait activities, and (3) gait or ambulation activities. Bed mobilities include rolling, scooting, bridging, bed chair positioning, bed tilts, and supine-to-sitting transfers. Pregait activities include transfers (sit-to-stand, squat pivot, stand pivot, and stand step), and out-of-bed activities, such as sitting upright in a chair and standing frame or tilt table sessions. Trees et al described a novel therapeutic device that allows casualties to be challenged orthostatically while simultaneously performing body-weight–resisted squatting exercises for lower extremity strengthening.[277] This device has recently become commercially available (see Figure 13-59). Gait activities, or ambulation, complete the casualty's progression of mobility activities. Casualties may require assistive devices, such as canes, crutches, or walkers, depending on medical status and associated injuries. Close communication and coordination of the interdisciplinary burn team is critical to developing a mobility plan that safely enhances the casualty's recovery.

During the acute rehabilitation phase, several factors must be taken into consideration when determining the appropriate mobility activities. Factors to consider include the following:

- the casualty's level of alertness and orientation,
- the casualty's ability to follow commands,
- the casualty's baseline vital signs,
- the presence of new (< 1–3 days old) skin grafts that require immobilization or protection,

- the casualty's respiratory status (ie, on a ventilator, undergone a tracheostomy with oxygen support, or spontaneously breathing room air),
- the casualty's mobility activities, which may be precluded by certain treatments or procedures (eg, blood transfusion, dialysis, or respiratory treatments),
- the presence of orthopaedic issues that require accommodations,
- the need for vascular support wraps to the dependant extremities, and
- the physician's expectations for mobility activities.

Generally, some type of mobility activity along the continuum of activities may be safely performed after close coordination with the interdisciplinary burn team (Figure 13-71).

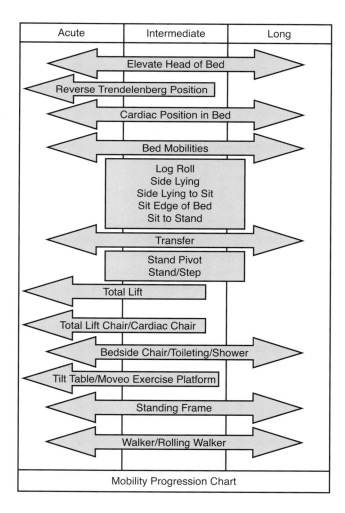

Figure 13-71. Continuum of mobility activities throughout the phases of burn rehabilitation.

Depending on the severity of injury and the casualty's status, a casualty may begin mobility activities anywhere along the continuum and progress as appropriate. For severely injured burn casualties (TBSA burned > 30%), the casualty is usually initially positioned in a bed chair position or bed tilt and alternated every 2 hours, or as indicated by a physician. As the casualty's status improves, bed mobilities and lateral transfers to a chair are implemented. Casualties are encouraged to spend several hours (> 4 hrs) sitting in a chair each day. ROM, strengthening, and other functional activities are performed while in the chair and on the tilt table, and distract casualties enough to improve tolerance of the activity. When a casualty can tolerate 30 minutes of tilting to 70° for 3 consecutive days, more advanced pregait or gait activities can begin.

It is not unusual for a casualty in the acute rehabilitation phase to require several IV lines, chest and feeding tubes, or a Foley catheter. In these cases, it is imperative that all lines and tubes are properly secured before, during, and after mobility activities. Chair positioning, tilting, standing frame activities, and ambulation all require use of gait belts at the torso, waist, buttocks, and thighs for safety. Gait belts may need to be placed in such a way as to protect skin graft sites and prevent shearing.

Intermediate Phase

During the intermediate rehabilitation phase, the emphasis of mobility activities shifts from reorientation and improving tolerance to the upright position to improving endurance and functional independence. In this phase, casualties are typically more medically stable and are capable of tolerating more aggressive mobility activities. However, some mobility activities may carry over from the acute rehabilitation phase and should continue until the casualty demonstrates the strength and endurance to progress to more advanced functional activities.

The primary focus of this phase is independence with transfers, ambulation, and ADL training, such as bathing and toileting. Casualties are introduced to equipment in the rehabilitation gym, such as stationary bikes, upper-body ergometers, treadmills, parallel bars, and stair trainers to improve strength, endurance, and independence. An ADL room is also useful at this point in the casualty's recovery. Casualties must be encouraged and motivated to participate in mobility activities on a daily basis. Maximum participation will result in the expeditious return of function and prepare the casualty for discharge from the burn center and return home.

Long-Term Phase

Advanced mobility activities are the mainstay of the long-term rehabilitation phase. By this time, casualties have already met the functional mobility requirements for discharge from the burn center and are ready to begin mobility activities that will prepare them to return to duty. Advanced mobility activities focus on transitioning back to duty through advanced physical training and simulated work activities. Mobility training, such as jogging, running, swimming, weight lifting, sports, driving, and firearm training simulation, is implemented to improve a casualty's strength, cardiovascular endurance, and capacity to return to duty. At this time, it may be appropriate to refer a casualty to an advanced rehabilitation center, such as the Center for the Intrepid at Brooke Army Medical Center, Fort Sam Houston, Texas.

Psychosocial Aspects

Acute Phase

The psychological characteristics of the acute phase of rehabilitation include dealing with stressors of the intensive care environment, uncertainty about outcome, and the struggle for survival. Tremendous stress affects burn casualties' mental abilities, including their alertness, attention to detail, perception, reasoning, comprehension, memory, motor responses, communication, self-control, and interpersonal relations. Shock, numbness, and detachment, which protect casualties while they collect emotional coping resources, are commonly noted at the time of injury. Reorientation helps increase trust and lower anxiety, and reassurance can help casualties feel optimistic and lower anxiety. Families are encouraged to learn deep breathing relaxation techniques, and humor is often used throughout rehabilitation to lower a casualty's anxiety. Giving the casualty control and choices can also prevent serious psychological issues and can lead to a strong working relationship.

Casualties with minor burns who will return to duty as soon as their wounds heal need to be treated using the principles of proximity, immediacy, and expectancy. The mental health section at the unit level can provide support that focuses on mild and moderate battle fatigue and burns. Keeping casualties as close as possible to their units makes it easier for them to return to normal duty. Expectancy refers to the understanding that casualties will return to normal duty when they are healed. Treatment using the principle of expectancy is appropriate not only for casualties returning to duty within a short recuperation time, but also for casualties who will require extensive rehabilitation.

For casualties with severe enough burns to be evacuated, early psychological intervention and support help with motivation and encourage cooperation with treatment. Burn casualties separated from their units do not have ready access to family or friends for psychological support; therefore, an important role of the treatment team at all echelons is to provide emotional support and reassurance to reduce casualties' anxieties and fears. The evacuation team provides ongoing orientation information, including calling casualties by name. Part of the chaplain's mission is to provide comfort, assurance, and encouragement. Positive affirmations and encouragement, even during initial delirium, reinforce a casualty's motivation.[291]

The speed of physical recovery may be affected by the early emotional adjustment to an acute burn.[292] It is important to continually provide preparatory information before performing procedures and to encourage simple relaxation techniques during treatments. It is also important to frequently repeat instructions, provide orientation, and allow verbalization of fears.

The immediate reaction of a massive burn casualty includes psychological shock. This reaction usually lasts a short time and may involve disorientation delirium, emotional instability and liability, and sleeping problems with nightmares of being burned.[293] Fear and anxiety also accompany the initial part of the acute phase of burn recovery. Casualties should be allowed to express fears regarding death. These fears should be met with a realistic response regarding the chance of survival.[294] Behavioral manifestations, such as increased startle response, difficulty concentrating or following instructions, withdrawal, resistance to treatment, overt hostility, or other inappropriate behavior, are often noted immediately after burn.[295] Burn casualties may perceive a major threat to their survival. Information regarding the seriousness of the burn should be given, if possible, before pain medications cloud awareness.

Following resolution of the initial shock of the burn incident, casualties become more aware of the impact of their injuries. Orientation improves and survival anxiety diminishes. Thoughts are more focused on concerns about self, including the effects of changed appearance and altered function or lifestyle. The casualty's preburn physical, emotional, intellectual, social, and spiritual characteristics provide the basis for initial coping skills. Rehabilitation counselors, psychologists, social workers, and chaplains help casualties focus on regaining as much control as possible and on redefining the meaning of the accident, desensitizing the reminders of the injury, dealing with stress in a positive way,[296] and gradually accepting loss and trauma.

Adequate pain control, correction of sleep disturbances, decreasing the fear of long-term consequences, and cooperation with the burn team are crucial for optimal outcome.[293] Numerous interventions are appropriate and may include providing the casualty with as much physical comfort as possible; providing ongoing orientation information, including calling the casualty by name; mentioning the date and time of day; providing explanations about the procedures that are being used, even if the casualty is comatose; providing relaxation training after orientation is established; providing routine for bathing time, exercise, and meal times to decrease unexpected procedures; encouraging family involvement as soon as possible; and emphasizing individual control over as many situations as possible.

Losses and changes related to the burn injury affect each casualty differently. Casualties grow, find new strengths and coping mechanisms, recover from grief, and develop renewed goals sometime after realizing the impact and disruption they will experience from the injury. When casualties determine that there is potential for survival, their focus may turn to the perceived pain and its alleviation. This focus frequently results in increased reports of pain, as well as requests for analgesia. When adequate pain control is not provided, casualties begin to believe that pain will be associated with each treatment, which may result in poor compliance. The anticipation of pain may be complicated when painful procedures occur at different times, increasing a casualty's anxiety level. Medication dosage for pain, anxiety, and sleep is increased because of the hypermetabolic state of the casualty. When IV lines are in place, patient-controlled analgesia is allowed during the day, interspersed with comfortable rest periods. This improves cooperation with antigravity positioning and elevated exercise that ultimately also results in diminished pain. Relaxation training, counseling, and behavioral management are effective, nonpharmacological ways to deal with pain. However, they cannot replace analgesic, hypnotic, or tranquilizing medications. The goals of pain management are to maximize comfort, minimize disruptive behavior, and increase cooperation and productivity.[293]

When casualties complain of dysesthesias and pain as medications are being tapered, short continuance of narcotics combined with desensitization techniques reduces the problem. Most neuropathies resolve slowly. However, in addition to being taught desensitization and compensation techniques, casualties will appreciate assistance with reintegrating sensory information. Relaxation techniques (eg, Benson's relaxation technique, which involves slow breathing and repetition of a single, meaningless word[296]), practiced daily, can help casualties tune out sensations they would not have been aware of before the accident. For some casualties, dysesthesias from the healed tissue become a central, compelling part of their awareness. Individual counseling and reassurance by the physicians and therapists help casualties accept the return of sensation as a positive sign, even if it is temporarily distorted and therefore painful. Casualties slowly come to realize that the burn emergency has passed and, by using vision and tactile sensation from the burned and unburned parts, sensory information will be more quickly reintegrated.

As orientation improves, additional behavioral methods of relaxation may be implemented. These include Benson's relaxation response, autogenic training, biofeedback, imagery, and distraction. Deep breathing exercises may also be used, though they may alter sensation in a negative way, especially if a casualty hyperventilates when attempting deep breathing. Progressive muscle relaxation is another option, though it can be painful if the overlying skin is burned. Combining familiar techniques with non-pharmacological techniques can provide the casualty with greater control of the situation.

Intermediate Phase

During the intermediate phase, burn casualties are able to communicate with others, including staff members, family, and friends. Behavioral health providers and other medical staff provide support and information related to their specialty. Pain control may remain an issue. Rehabilitation remains aggressive to maximize function. The surgeon and rehabilitation team help casualties see grafting operations positively and allay fears related to loss of control during anesthesia.

Casualties are unable to exercise the grafted area or perform many activities because of potential skin shearing from movement. The resultant lack of movement and sensory deprivation create the potential for confusion and hallucinations, but this is reduced by sensory stimulation, provided by staff or family.[297] Rubbing lotion on closed areas controls itching and provides reassurance through therapeutic touch. Auditory and visual input may be emphasized through the use of television, radio, music, and frequent family and staff interaction.

Explaining procedures before they are performed can reassure casualties. Adequate analgesia and sedation, as well as the use of familiar relaxation exercises, help casualties tolerate discomfort during this phase. Avoiding repeated, unexpected, painful, and frightening treatments reduces the potential for develop-

ing PTSD. Staff should provide casualties as many choices as possible, and casualties should be invited to participate in procedures, such as staple removal, wound cleansing, and antigravity positioning, to reinforce the sense of control and responsibility in the healing process.

During this phase, burn casualties may come to terms with their injuries and prepare to leave the safe environment of the burn unit and reenter society. Reentry may be accomplished in steps, including excursions outside the burn unit, day passes for outings with family or friends, passes to restaurants, or trips home. These outings help casualties adjust to the rude reactions they may receive from the public. It can also help determine what adaptive equipment will be needed at home. At this stage, casualties can benefit from talking to other burn casualties, rehabilitation counselors, psychologists, psychiatrists, and social workers, and from viewing videos about other burn casualties and their families to learn how they coped. Along with physical and emotional recovery, ongoing social support is necessary. Nurses provide psychological support and encouragement to burn casualties as they prepare to leave acute care and return to society. Nurses also refer casualties to appropriate services, such as alcohol and drug treatment facilities (studies have confirmed that burn victims who abused drugs or alcohol before the accident are likely to do so again[298]) or chronic pain programs. Outpatient treatment may be indicated in these situations.

Long-Term Phase

Research on lifelong psychological issues as a result of combat-related burn injuries is limited. The Department of Defense and the Department of Veterans Affairs are taking proactive steps to identify and treat combat-related psychosocial issues stemming from Operation Iraqi Freedom and Operation Enduring Freedom.[299]

Normal responses to a major burn injury often include crying, degrees of fear, depression,[300] grief, loss of hope, and other reactions unfamiliar to the casualty. Discharged casualties report it takes about 6 to 7 months of being at home before they can cope, as they did before the injury, with emotions and activities that require concentration; however, distractibility gradually subsides. Impatience, irritability, and frustration are common. Casualties must learn to accept gradually improving function instead of perfection in activities. Family members can often help sort out the realistic reactions from overreactions.

Casualties at home or in the rehabilitation center

must learn how to safely return to duty and routine life despite their injuries. Physical changes are often bothersome, and physical fitness is now a prolonged, daily struggle. Reconditioning may take place at a much slower pace than before the burn.[301]

Another factor to consider is psychological adjustment when a casualty returns to work in the area where the injury occurred. Few casualties return to the injury site easily. Referring a casualty to a psychologist is appropriate at this time. Return to duty at the earliest possible time provides casualties with the benefits of buddy support as well as routine and work. Strength and coordination improve much sooner from work than from therapy. Ego strength and social interaction are also improved with return to duty. Feelings of anger, fear, loneliness, or helplessness make casualties acutely aware of pain.[302] Casualties benefit from sharing personal experiences of pain relief. Former burned casualties report being helped by participating in trauma survivors' groups. With leadership from social workers and psychologists (or both), trauma survivors' groups are able to deal positively with symptoms, including the following:

- disturbing dreams,
- appetite disturbances,
- difficulty with sleep,
- feelings of estrangement or detachment,
- recurrent intrusive memories of the event,
- memory impairment,
- difficulty concentrating,
- reluctance to accept a changed body image,
- decreased interest in sex,
- sensitivity to loud noises or other cues related to the accident,
- irritability, and
- fear of returning to field duty or other work.

Return to active duty improves the casualty's self-concept. Burn physicians must consider the duty tasks and the progress of the healing burn scars and skin grafts when recommending return to active duty. Food handlers must remain off-duty until open areas are closed and wound cultures reveal no pathogens. Heavy laborers may need job modifications when they first return to duty. Often casualties need a transition period of half-day work, progressing slowly to full-time work. Rehabilitation counselors, nurses, or occupational therapists can help with changes in the work setting when these are encountered. The adaptations are often inexpensive. For example, a footstool may be placed near a bench or counter, and casualties may alternately place their feet on it for half-hour periods. Similarly, items can be arranged so casualties avoid

reaching beyond their center of balance when first returning to duty.

Appraising the extent of burn injury and objectively estimating residuals that affect performance are most accurate when based on objective criteria[303] and experienced prediction. Rating permanent impairment is a physician's function. Disability is related to performance loss, preinjury age, education, economic and social situations, sex, and the burn casualty's attitude toward recovery. The physician has the final responsibility in determining when it is medically safe for casualties to return to active duty.

Community Reintegration

Acute Phase

The ultimate goal of burn casualty rehabilitation is reintegration into casualties' previous roles in their homes, schools, workplaces, and communities. Until recently, the goal for burn casualties was simply survival, with little emphasis focused on the quality of life after a severe burn injury. Advances in the medical care of casualties with major burn injuries have led to increased focus and need for rehabilitation services, as well as the need to improve intervention programs at acute, intermediate, and long-term phases of burn recovery. For a more successful and complete reintegration into society, research has indicated the need for a multidisciplinary team approach to ensure all areas of reintegration are addressed appropriately.

Sheridan describes three things needed for burn casualties to successfully reintegrate into their previous roles: rehabilitation, reconstruction, and reintegration, with the emphasis placed on long-term rehabilitation.[304] Sheridan further divided burn care into four general phases: initial resuscitation; initial excision and grafting; definitive wound closure; and the rehabilitation, reconstruction, and reintegration phase.[304] Rehabilitation and reintegration begins at the acute stages and can continue up to 2 years after the casualty is discharged from inpatient care.

In the acute stage, basic goals for rehabilitation and reintegration include positioning and splinting, reducing edema, and completing ROM exercises. This enables more functional mobility as the burn casualty continues to recover. These rehabilitation goals are important in the acute stage because they address the needs of the burn casualty and maximize the long-term functional outcome of reintegration into society. Educating families on positioning, splinting, and exercises to help maintain a burn casualty's functional mobility is crucial to the casualty's recovery and reintegration into society.

Intermediate Phase

In the intermediate rehabilitation phase, burn casualties begin to further comprehend the extent of their deficits secondary to their injuries and the potential impact on their previous functional roles. During this time, limited reintegration into society is accomplished with day passes and excursions outside the burn unit. Family education is another key element of successful reintegration. Proper training and information of assistance programs has led to family members and burn casualties reporting more successful reintegration into society and higher satisfaction with quality of life.[305] Burn casualties should be put in contact with veterans' service organizations as they reintegrate into their communities and seek to return to work.

Long-Term Phase

Once discharged from the hospital, many burn casualties report feelings of self-consciousness, anxiety, sadness, and anger about their physical appearance as well as in everyday social interactions with other individuals.[305] In the past, burn casualties reported receiving little assistance from burn care professionals beyond discharge from the hospital. Others, however, expressed empowerment from burn casualty organizations, such as the Phoenix Society, that provide support for burn casualties and their families in the challenges they face during reintegration into society.[305] Most research on community reintegration has focused on the "psychological adjustment" versus the physical or social adjustments burn casualties face.

A community reintegration program must be designed to support the needs of burn casualties and their family members as they transition back into society or past performance roles. The purpose of such a program is to assist in the development of appropriate psychosocial skills, peer-to-peer interactions, executive functions, motor planning, and physical components. The program must also provide a real-world environment in which casualties can develop the skills required to handle social interactions and environmental challenges. Casualties should be screened by the interdisciplinary team to ensure that they are ready to participate in community outings and that the outings will be therapeutic. The goal of a community reintegration program is for the burn casualty to achieve complete reintegration into the community. In order for the casualty to complete a community reintegration program, the casualty must meet all short-term and long-term goals. Some common goals include interacting appropriately and independently with peers, the general public, and burn team members.

Casualties have successfully completed a community reintegration program once they have developed effective coping skills or adaptive techniques to interact appropriately with the environment.

Casualties with associated injuries, such as traumatic brain injury or spinal cord injury, may require transfer to a Department of Veterans Affairs rehabilitation center. Casualties being transferred should be medically stable and able to tolerate and benefit from a minimum of 3 hours of therapy a day.

The decision for a burn casualty to transition to an outpatient burn clinic should be made by the interdisciplinary burn team, casualty, and family. However, this may be challenging when the casualty has unrealistic expectations or when there is a lack of family presence or involvement. The success of outpatient treatment involves proper wound care, pain management, and rehabilitation by experienced burn team members. A patient should be followed up with at least weekly for the first 30 days after discharge, then monthly for 3 months, and finally every 3 months until the casualty's outcome has been maximized. Casualties are evaluated and treated by several members of the burn team at each follow-up visit, including a surgeon, physician assistant, nurse, therapist, mental health professional, and case manager.

In addition to a burn clinic, all outpatient casualties requiring continuing rehabilitative services are evaluated and treated by an outpatient rehabilitation service. These casualties must remain engaged in goal-oriented and outcome-based rehabilitation programs supervised by therapists.

Sexuality

Resuming sexual activity and relationships is an important part of recovery after a burn injury.[306] A casualty's partner should to be included in discussions about changes that take place during recovery and the expected final outcome. Most partners appreciate participating in an open discussion prior to resuming sexual activity. Casualties often worry about rejection; counseling to encourage trusting, honest communication can become the basis of a loving, caring, and exciting relationship. Understanding, communication, imagination, and experimentation can expand opportunities for a fulfilling relationship.[306] Potential problems related to sexual activity and birth control should be addressed by the physician. Friction or trauma to healed burns during sexual activity may cause blisters that are slow to heal. As burn scars and skin grafts mature and become more durable, blisters will be less likely to occur. Lubricants may help reduce friction and blister formation.

The areas least affected by the burn can often be used to enhance sexual activity. Because the lips and tongue are rarely burned, patients and their partners should be encouraged to use their mouths as a means of sexual expression. The lips and tongue are also more sensitive to touch and temperature than other body parts. Any part of the body that can be made clean enough for oral contact should be explored. Pregnancy may cause hypertrophy of burn scars and should be avoided until scars are mature. Stretching the tissue away from the direction of contracture and frequent erections assist with burn scar and skin graft maturity. Vigorous exercise and stretching of these areas results in the best outcome. Contracture releases are possible if required to improve function.[307]

COMPLICATIONS ASSOCIATED WITH REHABILITATION

Orthopaedic Complications

Bone and joint changes are common complications of burns, especially following thermal and electrical injuries.[308] Common changes include internal changes in bone, such as osteoporosis; bone necrosis; bone growth disorders in children; and periosteal bone formation. Early mobilization and weight bearing is thought to diminish the risk and severity of osteoporosis. Periarticular changes can include HO and calcific tendonitis. Generally, periarticular ossification is noted in the area of deep burn, although it has been noted in areas distant from the burn, as well.[309]

Joint changes, such as septic arthritis and ankylosis, occur when the injury is deep into the joint or when bacteremia seeds the joint. When a joint is thought to be infected, in addition to appropriate medical management, the joint should be positioned and rested using a static orthotic device in a functional position. If ankylosis does occur secondary to the septic process, the joint will then be at a maximal position of function.

Dislocation can occur from improper positioning of an injured joint or, more commonly, by scar contracture. If a joint is subluxed by a contracture, orthotic management, such as an IP extension serial cast, should be instituted immediately. If the orthosis cannot adequately control the deformity, internal fixation or release of the contracture (or both) should be considered.[310]

Heterotopic Ossification

HO is the ectopic deposition of bone around joints and tendons.[170] Incidence is variable in the literature, and ranges from 4% to 23%.[268,310] When it occurs in muscle body, it is more appropriately termed "myositis ossificans." It most frequently occurs at the elbow, hip, and shoulder, and to a lesser degree at the temporal mandibular joint, wrist, hand, knee, and ankle.[268,310] Usually the amount and location of the extra bone is clinically insignificant, but it can be severe enough to completely lock a joint in place.

Occurrence seems most likely to be related to the extent of the burn, size of open areas, and bed rest.[311] Inflammation may also contribute to HO or fibrosis.[269] The exact etiology has yet to be determined. HO should be suspected if there is a sudden onset of joint pain, swelling, or redness. When the diagnosis is confirmed by plain radiograph or bone scan, rehabilitation consists of AROM exercises without passive stretching and orthotic positioning in the maximal functional position.

There is currently no prophylactic treatment available for HO. Etidronate disodium has been used to prevent HO in the treatment of spinal cord injury.[309,312] However, a recent retrospective review found that it was ineffective in preventing HO in burn casualties.[313] Prospective studies need to be performed. Etidronate disodium has been used after early resection of HO, with significant improvement in functional ROM and without recurrence after periods of 6 months to 2 years. Early resection has been supported in the literature.[314]

Other techniques to prevent recurrence include irradiation and the use of NSAIDs, both of which may have significant complications in the burn population.[310] There is also controversy regarding thermo exercise. Some data suggest that vigorous AROM exercise can cause HO.[315] Splinting, combined with AROM exercise and PROM exercise, is appropriate unless HO occurs, in which case, ROM exercise should be limited to AROM activity only within the casualty's pain-free range.[315,316]

Amputations

Amputation can occur as a separate injury concurrent with a burn, particularly with explosive mechanisms of injury. The use of improvised explosive devices in Operations Enduring Freedom and Iraqi Freedom has resulted in a high rate of amputations associated with burn injury.[23,24]

Amputation can also occur as the direct result of an electrical injury, or as the sequela of a full-thickness or subdermal burn. The rate of occurrence varies with the etiology. Amputations from burn injury usually occur in 2 to 4 weeks and are related to infection.[317,318] Amputations are treated concurrently with the burn.

Electrical burns are associated with a 10% to 50% incidence of amputation.[317,319–323] An electrical current may result in an explosive loss of all or part of a limb. Because the current follows the path of least resistance, damage tends to follow the nerves, arteries, veins, and muscle tissue, with the potential for deep tissue necrosis. Generally, it takes 4 to 5 days for an electrical burn to completely declare itself and for the need for amputation to become apparent. The need for amputation may also arise later in the course of care, such as when neurologic function or sensation does not recover, leaving an extremity that appears healthy without function or sense of temperature, pressure, or pain.

When considering amputation, preserving length is important; however, it should not result in a functional disadvantage or problematic prosthetic care, such as occurs with a knee or elbow disarticulation. Burn injury can often delay fitting and application of a prosthesis because of the healing status of the skin. Grafted and healed areas of burned skin may require a prolonged course of treatment before they are able to tolerate the shear and pressure requirements of prosthetic use. Applying compression to the residual limb with stump shrinkers or elasticized tubular, self-adhesive, or compression bandages is important in preventing complications and may offset the delay in actual prosthetic fitting if done early.

Fitting a prosthesis to an extremity with healed burns is problematic because of various factors, including irregular length and shape, inability to tolerate pressure and shear, inadequate tissue for suspension, and limited ROM and strength to power myoelectric devices. Fitting must be approached with patience and innovation. Skin must be diligently monitored because breakdown can occur even after months of seemingly normal wear.

Another significant problem after amputation is phantom pain. It is normal for amputees to sense that an amputated limb is still attached, and the phantom limb may even seem to be in an odd position. Phantom sensation may last for many years and does not require any treatment other than education. However, if the sensation is painful, it should be aggressively treated using gabapentium or pregabalin and amitriptyline at night.[324] Desensitization techniques, such as rubbing, tapping, and contrasting temperatures and textures, are also helpful. Compression wraps and prostheses may help or exacerbate the pain. Treatment can include a single modality or combinations of the above. Narcotics have not proven beneficial in treating phantom pain.[324]

Neurological Considerations

Neurologic problems result from various etiologies. Although there may not be direct CNS damage from a burn, most burn casualties notice changes in reflexes and their perception of tactile and visual information. It is important to understand the etiologies of these deficits so precautions can be taken for prevention. Peripheral neuropathies may occur, resulting in decreased motor, sensory, and proprioceptive input. Early recognition and treatment may help prevent permanent deformity. The itching and pain sensations associated with burns subside gradually and may benefit tremendously from desensitization techniques.

A desensitization program can enhance the neurological recovery of a burn casualty and allows the casualty to control the level, frequency, duration, and pressure of differing external stimuli applied to a healed wound.[325] As the casualty's tolerance increases, the ability to withstand unexpected stimuli improves. Sensations from the healed wound, such as pain and itching, decrease and return to preinjury sensation. This occurs more rapidly when a desensitization program, including massage, vibration, and exposure to varying textures and temperatures, is practiced regularly.[325]

Texture desensitization involves introducing various textures to the healing tissues. Desensitization through texture contrast is commonly accomplished using cloth-covered wooden dowels to produce differing stimuli over the affected area (Figure 13-72). The repeated use of graded contact increases the sensory

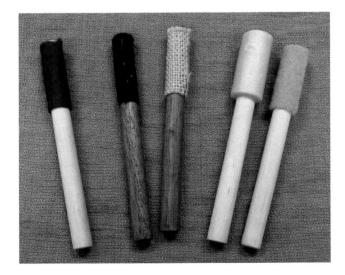

Figure 13-72. Wooden dowels with varying textures used for desensitization.

tolerance of the affected area. A hand or foot may be immersed in a basin that contains various objects, such as cotton, rice, plastic squares, or beans. The use of fluidotherapy may also be beneficial for desensitizing the hands.

Temperature desensitization is performed through controlled exposure to warm and cool water. The affected area is maintained at heart level if possible, and water is allowed to run over the healed wound—first cool water for 20 seconds, then warm water for 5 seconds—repeated for up to 10 minutes. Contrast baths of warm, followed by cool, water may be used for dipping hands or feet.

Peripheral neuropathies are relatively common among burn survivors, yet the diagnosis is often delayed or missed. Clinical weakness or atrophy is attributed to disuse after prolonged hospitalization with periods of forced immobility. The incidence of peripheral neuropathy has been reported to be as high as 30%. There is a greater incidence of peripheral neuropathies as the burn size increases above 20% TBSA. Casualties with electrical burns develop neuropathies at an even higher rate. Predisposing factors, such as alcohol abuse and diabetes, also increase casualties' susceptibility to neuropathies.[15]

The most frequently diagnosed neuromuscular abnormality observed in a burn casualty is generalized peripheral neuropathy, which commonly presents as distal weakness in the upper and lower extremities. The casualty's complaint, however, is usually lack of endurance and easy fatigability, not weakness. When weakness is noted, it occurs in the burned as well as unburned extremity. The cause of generalized neuropathies is not entirely understood but is probably multifactorial, related to toxic, nutritional, management, and metabolic factors.

Local peripheral neuropathies are also concerning because they are probably related to preventable causes, such as compression or stretch injuries of a peripheral nerve or damage from intramuscular injections.[326] The ulnar, radial, and median nerves are the most commonly affected peripheral nerves. However, neuropathies of the peroneal (fibularis) nerve and brachial plexus have also been observed. For example, the ulnar nerve is at risk of compression as it passes through the cubital tunnel at the elbow. When a burn casualty is positioned, for purposes of edema reduction, with the elbow elevated on pillows or arm troughs, flexed at approximately 90° and pronated, the cubital tunnel is narrowed. In this position, the ulnar nerve receives both external and internal compression and can be damaged, resulting in weakness of the ulnar intrinsic muscles of the hand and a claw hand deformity with loss of sensation to the ulnar side

of the hand. Neuropathies are best prevented with frequent position changes and positioning that limits external pressure and avoids positions that impose internal compression. Thorough initial and logitudinal neuromuscular examinations are essential to properly manage burn casualties.

Manual muscle testing should be performed to evaluate for the presence of upper-extremity peripheral neuropathy, especially in the presence of circumferential, full-thickness burns. The resting position of the hand can be indicative of neuropathy. For example, radial nerve involvement should be suspected if the wrist is held in flexion and the casualty is unable to actively extend the wrist, MCP joints of the fingers, and the thumb. Signs of ulnar neuropathy are clawing of the fingers and the inability to adduct the thumb. A median neuropathy should be suspected if the casualty is unable to oppose or abduct the thumb.

Median, ulnar, and radial neuropathy also influence positioning needs. The loss of active palmar thumb abduction associated with a median neuropathy increases the risk for adduction contracture. Splinting should include a resting splint or a C-bar splint, positioning the thumb in palmar abduction.

Emphasis should be placed on avoiding MCP joint extension and IP flexion contractures, which can result from an ulnar neuropathy and manifest with the fingers (especially the ring and small) maintaining a clawing position. When the skin is durable enough, an "anticlaw" splint can place the involved MCP joints into flexion and block hyperextension.

The absence of wrist extension, finger MCP extension, and thumb radial abduction is indicative of a radial neuropathy. Positioning and exercise should prevent wrist flexion contracture or contracture of the flexor compartment in the volar forearm. Splinting should hold the wrist and fingers in extension and thumb in radial abduction. MCP joint extension contractures must be avoided if dorsal hand burns are present; thus splinting the casualty into a resting position of 70° of MCP flexion may be indicated. In this case, the therapist needs to modify the splinting program, which may include alternating each type of splint indicated for day or night use.

Burn casualties often experience symptoms of pruritus.[2] In some cases, these symptoms can be worse than other pain a casualty experiences. Histamine release was previously thought to be the cause of the itching, but this has been proven incorrect. The exact mechanism remains unknown. It may be that pruritus, in some cases, is a manifestation of neuropathic pain. Nevertheless, initial treatment of pruritus is antihistamines, which do clinically benefit the casualty by managing symptoms. Diphenhydramine hydrochloride or hydroxizine, taken alone or in combination, are reasonable choices. Neuropathic pain medication (gabapentium or pregabalin) may be reasonable for resistant cases. Massage and transcutaneous electrical nerve stimulation may also be helpful.[216,327] Pruritus will improve over time, frequently in conjunction with scar maturation.

Psychological Considerations

The psychological effects of being burned in combat are complicated and challenging to identify and treat. While grief, bereavement, and sadness are understandable and natural feelings, when not managed appropriately, combat-related burn injuries can result in more serious reactions and lead to more debilitating mental illness.[328] Significant psychological distress occurs in over a third of casualties. Psychological management must be initiated early on, because evidence shows there is little clinically significant, reliable change in symptom severity when casualties are followed as outpatients.[329] Operations Iraqi Freedom and Enduring Freedom have presented a unique opportunity to study the psychological effects of burns because the number of individuals affected by the same event permit comparison not possible in individual trauma.[330]

The following principles and presented guidelines, consolidated by Faber et al,[331] should be implemented when managing burn casualties:

- **Routine care.** Psychological screening and support should be routine from the start for the casualty and family and continue well into the completion of physical care.
- **Promotion of a casualty- and family-centered approach.** In light of the complexity and cultural considerations, a holistic approach based on the casualty's psychosocial needs should be addressed in conjunction with the requisite medical model.
- **Staff should be sensitive, trained, and fully integrated members of the burn care team.** Psychosocial support is critical to the degree that casualties' long-term psychosocial adaptation is largely dependent on their successful community reintegration.[305]
- **The survivor is assumed to be a "normal" person and is expected to fully recover.** The burn casualty's sense of well-being is contingent on the ease with which they relate with the nonburned community.[305]
- **Difficulties are normal experiences.** It is natural for a casualty to struggle to develop a new life, new body image, and new ways of feeling good. The entire process has been described as achieving a "new normal." The burn center team plays a vital role in this process.
- **The family is critical to success.** Next to the casualty's desire to reintegrate into societal roles, family support is the most important component to healthful recovery.[331]

Appropriate pain management is also important when providing psychological and emotional support. Special attention should be made to address pain, especially as it relates to wound care, patient activity, therapies, and patient expectations. Anxiety often amplifies pain and therefore must also be addressed. Providers should be aware that acute pain may become chronic if not treated early and aggressively. Both background and breakthrough pain need to be aggressively monitored and appropriately managed. In addition to medical interventions, modalities such as hypnosis, acupuncture, deep breathing relaxation exercises, and distractions (eg, music and positive imagery) may ameliorate pain and its deleterious emotional effects.[332]

Agitation is frequently observed in sedated and intubated casualties and must be assessed for cause (eg, pain, anxiety, or sleep deprivation). Sleep deprivation can cause various other conditions, such as stress, pessimism, and anger.[333] Sleep deprivation and restriction diminish vigilance (which can negatively impact performance), alter neuroendocrine control, and negatively impact immune function.[334] This deficit can be the difference between a successful outcome and one that is less than adequate. A sleep hygiene protocol that allows for uninterrupted sleep and reduced environmental stimuli can augment restorative sleep. Relaxing music or a cool dark room may also help a casualty fall asleep.

Nightmares are common in burn casualties,[335] which may explain agitation in sedated and intubated casualties. Atypical antipsychotic medication may prevent nightmares. Antihypertensive medications and β-blockers can block the adrenergic response to nightmares. One way casualties may confront the fears and issues in their nightmares is by recording them in a journal and changing their endings.[335]

Delirium is a common and usually reversible disorder that occurs during a period of illness and must be aggressively assessed and treated.[336] Possible causes of delirium include pain, pain medications, sleep deprivation, and witnessing loss of life, limbs, and horrific trauma. Recognizing these triggers is crucial when assessing work in war-injured casualties. Reorientation, restorative sleep, reassurance, and relaxation techniques can be effective in preventing and minimizing delirium symptoms.[334] Atypical antipsychotic medication can also be extremely effective.[337] Benzodiazepines are not recommended because casualties may have sustained traumatic brain injury, resulting disinhibition and respiratory depression.[336]

Armed conflicts have a long-lasting impact on the mental health of those affected.[338] PTSD, acute stress disorder, and their associated anxiety disorders are common psychological problems secondary to combat-related burns.[338] PTSD is the most common and predictable mental health problem that results from exposure to war and terrorism.[339] Most casualties will have symptoms of PTSD weeks to months following the event. A high incidence of PTSD among burn casualties has been noted from current conflicts.[328]

A burn casualty's response to a recognizable stressor signals PTSD if it evokes distress symptoms. Casualties also often experience vivid, intrusive dreams or recollections of the traumatic incident. Other frequently noted characteristics of PTSD are an exaggerated startle response, impaired memory, concentration problems, avoidance of cues of the accident, and withdrawal from normal social interaction, chores at home, tasks at work, or participation in active duty.[340] Treatment is aimed at giving casualties as many choices as possible during recovery, thereby relieving a sense of helplessness. Stress reduction strategies and goal-directed individual counseling can also be beneficial. Short-term pharmacological intervention may also be appropriate. It is helpful for casualties returning to active duty to know that PTSD may be exacerbated by distant yet significant events, such as the dedication of a war memorial or reunion event.[330] Reading about an individual who sustained a similar burn may also revive PTSD symptoms.

Losing fellow service members during combat is a significant source of distress.[341] Grief and depression are common concurrent with combat-related burns.[341] A number of medical interventions are effective in treating combat-related grief and depression, including antidepressant medications and grief counseling. Combat casualties have experienced numerous losses and changes that may take time to resolve, and they should be allowed to express their feelings and concerns.[341]

It is important to provide behavioral health support to casualties and their families from the earliest phases of hospitalization throughout the hospital course.[342]

The Red Cross may relay information between casualties and their families while separated, and can help families secure quarters near the medical treatment facilities where their loved ones will be treated. Intact and supportive families have been influential in the successful long-term psychosocial adjustment of casualties of severe burn injury.[343] Family members may be interviewed by social workers, nurse specialists, psychologists, psychiatrists, and chaplains to get an accurate history of the casualty's preburn personality, coping styles, and reactions. This facilitates the development of rehabilitation strategies.

It is important to involve casualties' families in support groups and to provide them with educational classes to inform them about burn injuries and treatment. Families' reactions to burn injuries and their ability to support casualties through recovery and reintegration into society is critical to casualties' successful life adjustment.[342] Support groups may help family members deal with the stress and uncertainty of caring for a combat-injured casualty.

Family members are often responsible for immediate communication with loved ones, extended family, colleagues, and community groups or churches. Family and friends at home can provide significant support and focus toward the future by letter writing and maintaining positive contacts with burn casualties. Evidence shows psychosocial adjustment is a function of both coping responses and social resources.[340]

Alcohol and substance abuse or dependence research over the past decade has demonstrated a strong association between PTSD and substance abuse and dependence.[344] The assessment and treatment of alcohol withdrawal is challenging in burn casualties because hyperthermia, tachycardia, and narcotic medications may mask these symptoms. Some of these signs, symptoms, and behaviors may not reveal themselves until long after the casualty is discharged from the service.

Combat casualties who have sustained burns are neither exempt from, nor more prone to report, suicidal or homicidal ideations than other casualties who have experienced severe trauma. Risk assessment should be performed during the course of the behavior health assessment. Concerns for suicidal or homicidal ideations should be assessed and interventions provided by mental health professionals.

SCAR MANAGEMENT

Scar management is an essential component in burn casualty rehabilitation. Appropriately managing burn wounds can minimize the resultant functional limitations. As burn wounds heal, scar tissue, comprised of collagen fibers, forms over all affected areas. The impetus of the healing process is to achieve closure as quickly as possible to achieve tissue contraction.[345] Tissue contracture protects a casualty's survival, but also creates a setting for joint contracture and restrictive scarring that interferes with functional independence.

Tissue Contracture

When considering the rehabilitation of burn casualties, most clinicians think about the deleterious physical effects of burn wound healing in the form of scar tissue contractures that appear after wound closure. However, burn scar contractures develop during the acute rehabilitation phase, making early therapist intervention important. Additionally, it is important to differentiate between burn scar contracture and burn scar hypertrophy. It is likewise important for clinicians to be able to differentiate between burn scar contracture, which occurs early, and contracture from muscle or joint capsule, which occurs following prolonged immobilization.[346]

During the inflammatory phase of wound healing, edema can cause body parts to become malaligned, positioning body segments to develop scar contractures.[6] In the proliferative phase of wound healing, granulation tissue, which contains the elements that can ultimately lead to scar tissue contracture, forms.[347] Simultaneously, wounds naturally undergo contraction, which, by action of myofibroblasts, pulls the edges of the surrounding tissue centripetally, reducing the pliability of the surrounding tissue.[348] All areas of the body do not contract to the same extent. Areas where skin is loose, such as over the abdomen or buttock, can contract further than areas where skin is tighter, such as around the leg. Because of these biological processes, casualties will develop burn scar contractures if proper interventions are not instituted, especially during the intermediate phase of burn rehabilitation.[53]

Because of known poor outcomes associated with the formation of granulation tissue, early excision of burn wound and skin grafting is a common practice.[348] Nonetheless, burn wounds that are skin grafted still undergo contraction. Partial-thickness skin grafts contract more than full-thickness skin grafts.[349] More important than the overall thickness of the skin graft is the makeup of the skin graft. Partial-thickness skin grafts from an area where skin is thin, but that transplant a large portion of the reticular layer of the dermis, contract less than skin grafts taken more superficially. Therefore, even if casualties are skin grafted, they will need rehabilitation beyond the intermediate phase of burn rehabilitation and well into the long term, until the tissue no longer demonstrates a tendency to contract.

Hypertrophic Scarring

Hypertrophic scarring is the most common and debilitating complication of burn injury and occurs when burns extending into the dermis of the skin heal through scar formation (Figure 13-73).[350] Hypertrophic scarring is defined as an overgrowth of dermal elements that remains within the boundaries of the original wound, a distinguishing characteristic from keloid scarring (see below).[350] Hypertrophic scarring frequently occurs in cases of burns extending into the deep layer of the dermis (the reticular layer) or if there is a delay in wound healing longer than 3 weeks.[351,352] It also tends to occur in areas of full-thickness burns or where donor sites have been harvested too deeply, reharvested several times, or in which healing has been delayed because of infection or trauma.[350]

Hypertrophic scarring may be painful, limit range of motion, impair sensation, and result in loss of function. Compression garments, scar massage, dynamic splinting, serial casting, and other conservative therapies may prevent or minimize hypertrophic scarring. Some burn casualties may need to undergo reconstructive surgery to deal with these scars.

Keloid Scarring

Another complication of scar formation in burn healing is keloid scarring. Keloid scarring occurs when an overgrowth of dermal elements extends beyond the boundaries of the original wound.[189,350] According to Linares, keloid scarring is the most severe degree of hypertrophic scarring, with the differentiating factor being quantity.[351]

Keloid scarring is not as commonly observed as

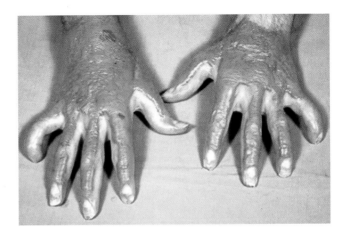

Figure 13-73. Severe hypertrophic scarring of the hands.

hypertrophic scarring, but depending on the location of development it can be, by its progressive and proliferative nature, more debilitating. Keloid scars go beyond limiting function because they are also disfiguring. Intradermal steroid injections, excision, and compression are often used to manage keloids. There is currently no preferred therapeutic modality to treat keloids. Location, size, disfigurement, debilitation, and depth of the scar are all considerations when deciding on a particular therapy.[353]

Hyperpigmentation

As a scar matures, it may become hyperpigmented (Figure 13-74). This occurs because newly formed epithelial cells eventually contain a relatively greater number of melanocytes than surrounding unburned tissue.[354] The amount of color contrast varies from one individual to another. Exposure to sun must be gradual; avoiding sun exposure for about 1 year after injury is the best way to prevent permanent hyperpigmentation, and healed skin will tolerate graded sun exposure 3 to 18 months following injury. Damaged, thinned skin will turn very dark brown with even brief sun exposure. If sunscreen is being used, it is important to prescribe the type appropriate for the casualty's natural skin condition. A commercially available, waterproof sunscreen with a sun protection factor rating of 15 or more should be applied to all burned areas. A wide-brimmed hat can protect the ears and nose during exercise in the sun. It is common for areas underneath custom-fitted, elastic, external vascular support garments to burn in the sun.

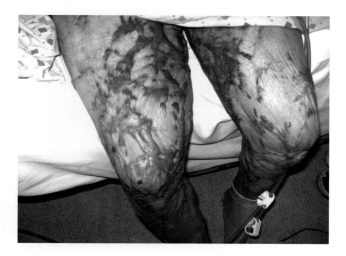

Figure 13-74. Hyperpigmentation of burn scar on the lower extremities.

Once a scar has matured, steps can be taken to modify its appearance. The simplest modification is applying camouflage or makeup. When combined with prosthetic facial components, makeup can significantly change appearance. Skin may be lightened over a period of months with daily topical application of hydroquinone, which can be purchased over the counter in strengths up to 4%, or prescribed in strengths up to 10%. Ruby laser may also lighten the skin. Hydroquinone and ruby laser are most effective in lighter skinned casualties because of the greater contrast between the affected and nonaffected areas.

Burn scar contractures can lead to decreased ROM and decreased mobility, resulting in a functional deficit in ADL performance as well as an altered aesthetic appearance and ending in a dysfunctional outcome. Various modalities can reduce the severity of burn scar contracture and the extent of surgical reconstruction required to preserve function. Appropriate burn scar control can effectively decrease the adverse affects of burn scar contractures and hypertrophic scarring.[345]

From the rehabilitation perspective, burn scar management includes using external vascular support to avoid excessive edema and compartment syndromes, positioning to create an environment for tissue elongation, and AROM and PROM exercises to retain joint motion and functional capacity as the healing tissue initiates typical contraction behavior.[355] As the wound area heals and scar is formed, the immature scar tissue will receive heat treatment and massage to enhance tissue pliability. Rehabilitation will also include additional compression interventions, occlusive dressings for hydration, custom splinting devices for tissue elongation and flattening, more aggressive AROM exercise, and reintroduction of ADLs.

Characteristics of Burn Scars

An increased healing time can result in hypertrophic scarring. In such a case, the wound-healing process begins like it does with normal scarring, but the additional healing time results in a protracted course of repair matrix accumulation, increasing morphologic and biochemical abnormality.[345] According to Burd and Huang, "although the hypertrophic scar follows the same cycle as the normal scar, time to heal is considerably prolonged and the adverse effects of the scar on form and function, particularly caused by contraction, are significantly worse than those of normal scars."[345] Hypertrophic scars also have an increased microcirculation compared to normal skin and mature scar tissue. Clinically, active lesions are firm and erythematous, resulting in maturation related to microvascular regeneration.[345] As scar tissue forms, the early, immature presentation is often described by appearance using the "3 Rs": red, raised, and rigid (see Figure 13-73).

Burn scar management begins at the time of insult. Following a dermal injury, a cascade of events results in the formation of a collagen-rich repair matrix; in normal scar tissue it presents clinically with increased height, firmness, and redness, indicating increased vascularity.[345] At this time the interdisciplinary staff is focused on wound management and closure. Reepithelialization, or wound healing, following a split-thickness skin graft, can take from 2 days to several months; however, most wounds heal within a few weeks.[356] Graft loss, hypergranulation tissue, and malnutrition can all result in lengthy healing of a split-thickness skin graft.[356]

Compression

Pressure therapy helps restore the extracellular matrix organization identified in normal scar.[357] External vascular support, begun early in the acute phase, uses a thin, moist contact layer to prevent the appliance from sticking to the epithelium at the wound edge. The initial purpose of external vascular support is to protect fragile, newly healed skin from blistering; improve venous and lymphatic return; decrease extremity pain; decrease itching; prevent sunburn or frostbite; moisturize the epithelium; modify overly bulky, thick, hard, scars; and elongate maturing contracture bands. Complete baseline descriptions of the healed wound, open areas, and areas of early scar symptoms or contractures are documented. Pressure must be adequate to decrease capillary circulation and must be continued until the scar matures. Pressure adequate to decrease edema and compress scar tissue cannot be applied to the middle of an extremity without impairing lymphatic return. Therefore, the principle of gradient pressure (the greatest support at the distal limb and the least at the proximal limb) must be observed.

For external vascular support of the hand, the fingers can be individually wrapped in a supportive, self-adherent elastic wrap (Figure 13-75). Several compression companies provide elastic digi-sleeves, also called edema sleeves. Isotoner gloves are an economical, off-the-shelf support glove manufactured in three sizes for hands that are not extraordinarily large or small. The most universally used early external vascular support is the elastic bandage wrap applied in a gradient figure eight, distal to proximal. Because early excision and grafting have become the norm, external vascular support is provided in the acute phase of healing primarily for the upper and lower extremities.[358]

Burned legs have generally been supported with figure-eight elastic bandage wraps from the acute phase through discharge from the hospital. This method of support facilitates ambulation and prevents pain and lower extremity edema or hemorrhage.[214] Elastic wraps are applied while the casualty is recumbent to avoid edema and poor venous return when standing. The most distal part of the extremity (ie, the hand or foot) must be properly managed first; then the support can be worked proximally.

Wound exudate may cause elastic wraps or garments to stick, so they should be soaked off during bathing to prevent denuding skin. Unless worn only for protection, the external vascular support appliance must apply continuous pressure in a gradient manner.

Massage and Vibration

Massage may break up bands of scar tissue that can cause contracture and decrease sensitivity and pain in the healed scar.[355] Massage therapy often helps desensitize the skin and scar and assists with venous return. It involves manipulating the soft tissues with the hands

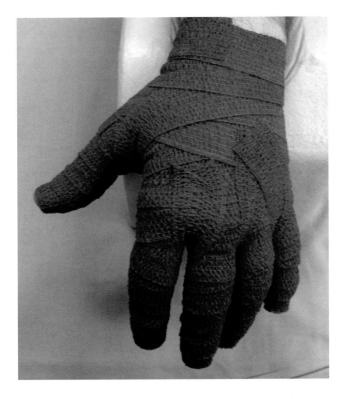

Figure 13-75. Self-adherent elastic wrap of the hand and fingers for vascular support.

to produce effects on the neuromuscular and circulatory systems. The massage should generally work in the direction of the venous and lymphatic circulation. Massage should be a slow, repetitive motion, moving distal to proximal, with the affected area elevated above the heart, if possible. However, applying too much pressure can cause pain or blisters.

Massage with lotion or mineral oil softens and increases the pliability of scar tissue. Nongreasy sunscreen and adequate medication to decrease pruritus help individuals avoid damaging newly healed tissue. In addition to increased pliability, massage with lotion lubricates dry scar tissue and skin grafts, which may prevent dehiscence of the less mature scar tissue.[355] Topical silicone gel is effective in both preventing and managing hypertrophic scar.[358,359] Silicone gel sheeting has been used for decades to effectively manage scars. Silicone therapy's mechanism of action has not been completely determined, but is likely to involve occlusion and hydration of the stratum corneum.[360] Applying self-adhesive silicone gel sheeting to a scar allows for a comfortable, reusable silicone product that implements the occlusion and hydration necessary to manage and prevent hypertrophic scarring. Silicone sheeting is also easy to apply under vascular support garments.

Vibration is a controlled method of massage that stimulates nerve endings and may lessen pain or irritation. An electric or battery-operated vibrator can be used to massage around affected areas. As tolerance increases, the vibrator can be placed directly over the healed wound, first with a stocking covering the skin and then directly against the healed skin. Vibration is used to decrease pruritus associated with healing scar tissue. It is also indicated for flattening scar tissue.[361] Casualties and their families are typically taught vibration therapy in clinic instruction.

Range of Motion

ROM and stretching exercises increase joint movement and lengthen scar tissue to reduce the restrictions of joint ROM. Preparing the tissue with massage allows for less restrictive scar tissue while performing ROM and functional activities. Goal-directed progress in ROM is required daily throughout all phases of recovery to prevent contracture and deformity and to increase function.[355,361]

Splinting and Positioning

Splints and casts are used to manage scar tissue. Compressive forces flatten scars and positional forces create a stretch by imposing a constant tension on the scar.[355,361] These modalities are used from day of admission on all casualties and modified or advanced depending on a casualty's needs.

For casualties who have sustained facial burns, preventing and managing microstomia contracture is essential for maintaining premorbid quality of life. Mouth opening is imperative for speaking, eating, performing dental hygiene, interacting, and restoring psychosocial well-being. Opposing horizontal, vertical, and circumferential forces are necessary for effective scar management.[362]

Heat

Initially heat packs, and later paraffin, are used to increase pliability and tissue flexibility and to prepare the tissue for elongation stresses prior to progressive ROM exercise programs.[355,361] Heat should not be applied to insensate areas.

Compression

Casualties wearing external vascular supports or orthoses for the face and neck must be closely observed for complications such as sleep apnea,[363] changed bone growth,[364] and posterior migration of the teeth. A separate nose orthosis may be fitted under the clear facial orthosis to maintain patent nostril openings. Custom-fitted inserts may be made of soft silicone or hard acrylic. If the ear meatus is scarring closed, it can be maintained with a silicone elastomer or acrylic insert or hard plastic.

It is difficult to properly fit a neck orthosis because there are no bony landmarks on the anterior neck, the larynx must be able to move during speech or swallowing, and the sternocleidomastoid muscles change as they contract and relax for neck movement. However, with practice, a neck orthosis may be fitted that reduces edema and supports the tissue between the sternal notch and the chin at the maximum possible length. Wearing an orthosis should never replace AROM exercises to improve the quality and length of the healing epithelium and underlying connective tissue.

When the extremity is healed, it is usually durable enough for tubular external vascular support on a foot and leg, or Isotoner gloves on a hand. The prefabricated garments are made of a variety of materials, including unidirectional, stretchable rubber; elasticized cotton; elasticized nylon; nylon/spandex; spandex; and rayon.[365] Many casualties tolerate prefabricated cotton and rubber garments well; scars recede and no other support is needed.[366] In addition, fabrics with varying elasticity are available from most custom garment manufacturers. Multiple types of custom-fitted orthoses are available for external vascular support and scar compression. Once wound closure is complete, a wide variety of commercially available support designs are available, as well.[348]

Transparent Facemasks

Casualties with extensive facial burns can use custom-made, silicone-lined, transparent facemasks (Figure 13-76). Facial skin is loosely connected to underlying structures, and permanent distortion of the nose, eyelids, mouth, ears, and neck may result if this connective tissue is allowed to contract around the face or neck. Face-scanning technology, which digitizes the complex surfaces of a burn casualty's face, and rapid prototyping on a computer-controlled milling machine can create a transparent facemask that provides compression.[367]

Body Garments

Weight gain and loss should be stabilized before measuring for custom garments. Custom garments are usually measured circumferentially for the extremities and at the waist, hips, and chest for the trunk. Joints are marked on a circumferences record and measured on a pictorial form. Each garment company has its own forms, tapes, and measuring style. Measurements are usually taken by a company representative. Tape measure designs include longitudinal paper tape with cross-sections taped on an extremity, and lightly adhesive measuring devices placed directly on the body. Knowledge of the casualty's injury and course of recovery helps in planning the proper design and individual op-

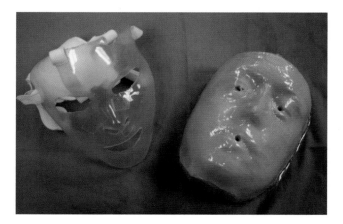

Figure 13-76. Transparent facemask providing compression for scar management.

tions.[368] Climate, employment conditions, physical limitations, and psychological status also influence the garment type. Casualties should be measured as early in the morning as possible, when extremities are the least edematous. Measurements are taken in direct contact with the casualty's skin, not over clothing or dressings. The tape measure should be placed firmly but not tightly. When there are two adjacent garments—for example, a glove and an arm sleeve—measurements should be overlapped so the garments themselves overlap and do not gap or pinch. A tracing should be done with a thin marking pen. The garments are produced and mailed, and the casualty usually tries the garments on in the therapy department of a burn center.

Burn site, casualty age, burn depth, the presence of split-thickness skin grafts, and wound healing time influence garment design. Of primary importance is predicting whether a wound will scar and the location and size of the potential scar area. The garment should completely cover the potential scar area with a 2- to 3-inch overlap at each end so that when the casualty moves, the garment will still be in contact with the area being treated. Because edema and deep vein thrombosis are always concerning, the garment design must include tissue distal to the burn. Fingertips and feet can be either open or closed, depending on the casualty's needs. Liners can be placed around joints with bony prominences.

Garments need firm attachment points so they do not roll, slide down, or ride up. Attachment points could be at the waist, forearm, shoulders, or hips. Ending the garment on the muscle belly should be avoided because the edge may constrict when the muscle is flexed. Ending the garment directly on a joint can decrease circulation.

The initial, custom-measured, full glove with closed or open fingertips is appropriate for the hands. This glove should also have slanted interdigital seams and a thumb design that allows radial and palmar abduction without losing fit over the dorsum of the hand. The initial glove is often made of soft fabric; the density of the fabric is increased to heavy duty when the skin can tolerate it.

For the thorax and limbs, basic designs can be varied to create several options. A thorax garment can be a basic sleeveless vest, or a full suit with long arms and thighs with a crotch that is opened, closed, or has a hook-and-loop fastener, zipper, or snap flap. If the vest rides up and a body brief is not desired, the vest can be made several inches longer, or a heavy-duty snap or hook-and-loop fastener crotch strap can be added. Hook-and-loop fasteners allow for some adjustment in tightness. For females, breast cups are measured and front closures are used in vests. Unburned arms can have short sleeves, which are useful because the open armholes put little pressure on the chest and upper back. Vests with only one arm pull the neck opening away from the open side, take away chest and back pressure, and exaggerate poor posture. Various arm sleeve lengths are feasible. However, if the shoulder requires compression, a vest style is most effective. The axillary area may be made larger if no compression is needed there. Pants can be waist high, and wide clip-on suspenders or elastic bands may keep the waist from rolling down. If a vest is also required, overlapping hook-and-loop fastener tabs or heavy-duty snaps can be used. Garter belts can be used to secure bilateral thigh-high stockings. A garter belt will not work on a unilateral thigh-high stocking. If the skin is durable enough, some skin adhesive or foam tape can be used.

Anklets and knee-length stockings usually stay up well, especially if the skin is well moisturized before donning the stocking. Zippers can be placed on any of the extremities to assist initial donning and doffing when the skin is still fragile; however, zippers decrease the uniform compression of the garment and at times need to be padded, so it is best to avoid them if possible. Other options to add to compression garments are inserts, gussets, pads, and darts.

The initial fitting of a garment should always be done in the clinic to assure an accurate measurement and fit. To be therapeutic, the correct level of compression should slightly blanch the hypertrophic scar areas. There should not be any restrictions in motion, circulation, or skin integrity. Color, motion, and sensation should be checked before the casualty leaves the clinic. Fingers and toes should be observed for swelling, coolness, and dusking, as well as numbness or tingling. Casualties should be instructed to discontinue the garment, reapply elastic wraps, and call the therapist if problems occur at home.

Applying the new garment for the first time is challenging. It should fit tightly, like a wet suit, and should take several minutes to don. The fit can be checked by how the garment feels to the casualty and how the scars feel through the garment. The garment should be tight enough that it is not possible to grab hold of it easily and pull it away from the skin, and should not wrinkle. Shoulders, elbows, and knees should have adequate relief for full AROM without allowing open areas. Often the first garment does not fit correctly and alterations or new measurements may be required. Most commercial companies will replace a problematic garment.

The body garment is worn 23 hours a day throughout the duration of the skin maturation process. The garment must be removed for bathing, and occasionally it is necessary to remove it during vigorous exercise sessions when it causes blisters. It should be washed daily to remove perspiration, body oils, and dirt. Meticulous hygiene is essential for the skin, as well. Garments should be cared for according to the manufacturer's recommendations.

A light dusting with cornstarch or powder may help with garment donning; however, casualties should be reminded to wash the powder away each day to avoid plugging pores. Wearing nylon under the body garment can decrease the shear on skin and increase the ease of donning. Foam pads at the joint creases of the knee and ankle can prevent garments from cutting into underlying skin. A protective hydrocolloid patch on the olecranon, the antecubital area, or both, can prevent scrapes in these vulnerable spots.

Initially, reassessment is best done weekly to ensure wearing tolerance and to watch for complications and changes in weight or muscle mass. If an aggressive therapy program is not required, the scars are becoming soft and light in color, and the casualty is doing well, visits can be decreased to biweekly, monthly, and bimonthly through the maturation process. Generally, prefabricated garments last only 1 to 2 months, depending on the casualty's activity level. A weight change of 10 lb or more may require new measurements be taken. A new garment should be issued at each clinic visit until the casualty has five garments that fit well. Custom garments generally last 2 to 3 months. Some casualties may require more than two sets, depending on their work or leisure situations. It may be necessary to set aside one set of garments for dress and use stained ones for daily activities.

Bothersome open areas should be checked for infection. If they interfere with motion or cause excessive pain, garments can be removed for exercise. It may be necessary to wear elastic bandages for a few days before reapplying the garments.

Skin covered with support garments may develop offensive odors. Daily bathing, washing open areas and body wrinkles thoroughly, drying skin meticulously, and applying a lotion every day improves wound hygiene. Heavy petrolatum or oil-based lotions should be avoided because they liquefy natural sebum, and it is then washed away. Deodorant is appropriate if it does not cause contact dermatitis. If blisters form or open areas increase in size, the casualty should discontinue wearing the support garment, resume elastic wrapping of the extremity, and explore the causes of blistering. If excoriation has resulted from scratching, antihistamine medications can be increased or changed. Ambulation and exercise should be continued.

Inserts

A mature scar will never return to a high degree of organization of normal dermal architecture.[345] However, an insert can accelerate hypertrophic scar maturation process.[369] Inserts that fill in concave areas that a custom-measured garment cannot reach are usually placed between the skin and the compression garment over a thick hypertrophic scar, tight skin, contracture, or a concavity where a bridging area has begun. Some inserts have been used successfully alone, for small areas, without compression. Overlays are placed over the custom-measured garment with an elastic wrap or another garment to press the garment into concavities between bony prominences or anatomical structures that compression garments "tent" over. The overlay or insert fills in the negative spaces for a smooth, total-contact compression from the external vascular support garment. Inserts are also used to help flatten and soften the taut, rope-like contractures that are often noted over joints.

As tissues eventually become longer, blanching decreases when the skin is stretched, and contractures decrease. Inserts add extra pressure over thick, nodular, hyperemic scars. When used in this manner, tapering the edges of the inserts assures total contact by preventing tenting from the elevated ridges. Inserts can be used as padding for protection over bony prominences, under zippers, and at the inner angle of flexor creases, such as the ankles or elbows, to prevent garments from cutting into the skin. Closed-cell inserts may need to be worn with an open-cell, fabric, or disposable gauze, or paper liner to absorb perspiration.

Wounds must be healed before inserts can be used. Inserts can be fabricated prophylactically for areas of anatomical vulnerability, such as the thumb web space, or for concave areas, such as between the breasts. When the skin begins to shrink and before contracture can form, properly placed inserts can prevent more difficult problems later. As dynamic scars change, inserts can be serially made for increasingly larger anatomical spaces. As the scar flattens, impressions can be filled in until the insert is flush with the surface and the scar impression is no longer seen in the insert.

There are a wide variety of materials to use for inserts or overlays to increase pressure over a hard scar. The creativity of both therapists and casualties has resulted in many successful scar modifications. Fabric, open-cell or closed-cell foam, rubber or plastic pieces, and silicones are all appropriate inserts or overlays (Figure 13-77). Silicone can be placed between two Isotoner gloves or between two tubular compression stockings to increase the pressure on the scar and prolong the life of the insert. When the insert causes contact dermatitis, it must be discontinued and, after the area is healed, a different insert material can be tried.

The insert and support must be applied to maintain gradient pressure. As with the vascular support garment, they cannot be applied like a tourniquet in the middle of an extremity, which would impair venous return and cause edema in the distal hand or foot. Even if edema is not severe enough to be seen with the naked eye, the distal circulation will change. Therefore, the insert must be placed under or over a support that is donned from the hand or foot to the shoulder, knee, or hip. Certain prefabricated, commercially available fabrics and foams can be used. Lamb's wool, in coil form, is a very soft, natural fiber that absorbs moisture in interdigital web spaces and protects fragile areas. Fibers adhere and incorporate into open wounds, so wool should be covered if applied where open areas or drainage is present. Cushioned strapping materials made of thin foam work well as finger inserts. They are loose fabric compatible with hook-and-loop fasteners.

Silicones and elastomers can also be useful, such as a protective skin care pad with a solid, gelatinous consistency (described as artificial fat). These pads are lightly adherent and can be cut into any shape to provide cooling comfort. Thicker pads eliminate friction and absorb pressure. Thinner flexible pads are effective on mobile joints, such as the elbow. Both increase compression. The pad's surface is oily, and

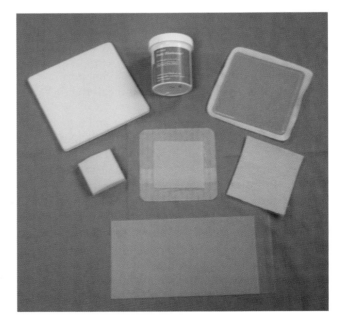

Figure 13-77. Variety of insert materials for scar management.

the scar must be protected or observed for maceration. Using these pads for periods of 8 to 12 hours, then leaving them off for 12 to 16 hours, may relieve skin over-moisturization.

Silicone gel sheeting is another compression insert option. This clear, soft, slightly adherent, semiocclusive, flexible insert is made from medical-grade silicone polymers without fillers (Figure 13-78).[242,370] One version is very tacky and stays in place well, but crumbles fairly easily. Another type has a netted back woven through and is advertised to modify a scar with or without pressure. It is effective when worn a minimum of 12 hours per day (rather than the usual 23 hours).[359,371]

Putty-based, white silicone elastomers can also be used for compression. In this case, the elastomer is mixed with a red tube catalyst, resulting in a firm, pink, rubbery, closed-cell insert. It does not run, sets in 5 minutes, is odorless, and is semirigid but flexible. It is easy to work with in small quantities, and works well for interdigital web spacers and as a shock absorber, decreasing contractures and filling in cavities.

A closed-cell, gray-liquid–based, taffy-like elastomer mixed with a clear catalyst can also be used. It cures to a rubbery texture, and the setting rate depends on the amount of catalyst used. Handling it can be challenging and requires a tongue depressor. It sticks to hair, so a protective layer of lotion or plastic wrap should be used. It stains before the catalyst is added, and it requires refrigeration or storage and has a 1-year shelf life. It picks up very fine detail and works well on large areas. Serial inserts can be made by filling in the scar impression with medical adhesive as it improves. Repetitive fabrications can be made on a revised scar until the insert is flush. On large body areas, a pattern can be made and the insert fabricated on old radiographic material; this works well on flatter surfaces with less mobility, such as the trunk, lateral ankle, or palmar arch. This elastomer can be mixed with prosthetic foam.

Hot and cold gel pads can be used under compression garments. They have a cloth covering on the back that protects the garment from oils. The pads are occlusive, can be used on open wounds, and can be cut to size, but should extend 1 to 2 inches beyond the wound or be 25% larger than the wound. They can be worn over topical medication and made waterproof by applying a film dressing over the top. They can be secured with tape, gauze, or elastic compression.

If both compression and silicone gel sheeting are used, they should only be worn together 12 hours a day. For the other 11 hours that compression garments should be worn, one or the other can be used separately; otherwise, skin irritation may develop and the gel sheet will disintegrate from too much wear.

Although scar tissue usually looks shiny and is lighter in color than surrounding tissue, the optimal final healed wound should appear flat, soft, mobile, durable, supple, of proper color, and have minimal thinning and wrinkling. The wound is mature when the skin texture is soft and the scar is flat and thin. There may be some loose, excess skin folds that appear to be wrinkled, but overall the skin should be more flexible and exhibit some extensibility. Erythema will have faded or lightened from purple to red, then pink, then dark brown or white. The skin will return closer to its normal pigmentation in darker-skinned individuals than in fairer-skinned individuals. Often a graft site that required mesh continues to present the mesh pattern. Even with optimal results, there is usually some change in color tone. External vascular supports decrease the amount of hyperpigmentation deposited in the wounds of casualties with darker skin.

When a scar appears to be mature, external vascular support is discontinued for a trial period lasting at least 1 to 3 days, but not longer than 1 to 2 weeks. If the symptoms or signs of active scar formation do not recur, the ultimate outcome has been achieved.

For burned hands, compression should continue on burned or grafted areas until the scar is mature.[192] Custom compression gloves should be introduced approximately 6 weeks following the burn for deep partial-thickness burns and full-thickness burns or after skin graft. All burn wounds should be closed and there should be minimal or no edema present. ROM exercises should continue during the long-term phase to emphasize tissue elongation. If adequate skin length is not obtained, the risk for joint capsular tightness

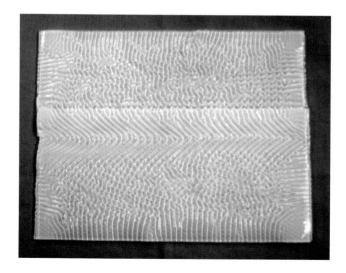

Figure 13-78. Silicone gel sheeting for scar management.

increases. Therapists should continually assess for joint capsular tightness, skin tightness, tendon adherence, or intrinsic muscle tightness. ROM exercises should address the appropriate deficits.

If adequate ROM gains are not achieved with exercise alone, splinting or serial casting should be considered. Dynamic or static-progressive splints are the most common splints used during the long-term rehabilitation phase, when the goal is to increase ROM. Static splints are usually sufficient if the goal is to maintain what was achieved with exercises. Static-progressive or dynamic splints should be worn for at least 6 to 8 hours a day, for intervals of at least 30 minutes, to provide the optimal duration for tissue elongation.

PLASTIC AND RECONSTRUCTIVE SURGERY

Reconstructive surgery and subsequent rehabilitation must be appropriately timed for the casualty to improve functionally, cosmetically, and psychologically. Otherwise, when inaccurately timed, the inverse is probable, resulting in loss of function, wasted valuable donor areas, and failure to benefit from the procedure.

Burn surgery is reconstructive rather than cosmetic. The American Society of Plastic Surgery defines reconstructive surgery as a surgical intervention "performed on abnormal structures of the body, caused by birth defects, developmental abnormalities, trauma or injury, infection, tumors, or disease. It is generally performed to improve function, but may also be done to approximate a normal appearance."[372] In addition to reconstructive surgery, plastic surgeons recommend makeup to enhance appearance and self-confidence for both male and female casualties.

The phases of recovery addressed by plastic surgeons include the acute phase, during which the wounds are closing, and the long-term phase, during which the scars are maturing. The ideal time to undertake reconstructive surgery is after scars have matured; however, there are a few specific situations in which reconstruction must begin earlier. In many cases, casualties want reconstruction early, and they must be made aware of the disadvantages of increased inflammatory scar deposition during the early scar maturation phase. As time progresses and the scars mature, casualties often become more satisfied with the appearance of their scars.[373] Additionally, as casualties become involved in former activities, they are less interested in prolonged interruptions for operations or in-hospital care.

The reconstructive process requires communication between members of the interdisciplinary team, including the surgeon and therapy staff, and the casualty. The process requires clinical evaluation, assessment, and planning to select the most troubling functional deficits or disfiguring scars. Casualties take an active part in the planning process. After considering multiple ways of correcting significant problems, the reconstruction surgeon chooses the optimal method for a particular casualty, as well as a backup procedure in case of postoperative complications or tissue loss.

Surgical teams frequently perform multiple operations under the same anesthetic so procedure time is used efficiently and recovery time is minimal. For instance, a fifth finger flexion contracture is often released the same time a web space contracture is corrected with a Z-plasty (see "Flaps" below) on the same hand. Only one hand is operated on at a time, and early motion cases are not mixed with procedures that require immobilization. In most cases, external vascular support garments are not worn and compression is usually not helpful after reconstructive operations. If hypertrophic scarring becomes difficult after reconstruction, the rehabilitation team uses pressure, gel sheets, or intralesional steroids.

Flaps

Skin flaps are frequently used in burn reconstruction when vital structures need coverage. They may be used in any phase of the reconstruction, and various flaps are used for different purposes. Musculocutaneous flaps, or muscle flaps, are often used acutely to cover bone, vascular grafts, or vital organs exposed by the burn. Musculocutaneous flaps are also used during reconstructive procedures. Muscle provides excellent blood supply, new lymphatics, and thick composite coverage. In some cases, the initial reconstructions are bulky and do not shrink adequately, so volume must be reduced at a later procedure.

Free flaps are used to provide blood supply to large avascular areas, such as the scalp, following electrical injury. These flaps require microvascular anastomosis and a specialized and individualized donor site. For example, a free flap of omentum may be used to cover a complete scalp defect. An overlying skin graft is then required. If abdominal burns or gastrointestinal pathology make this choice unwise, a latissimus dorsi flap may be used.[374,375]

A thin, free flap including skin, such as a dorsalis pedis flap, may be better than a muscle flap reconstruction, which requires an additional overlying skin graft. Free flaps are useful in all phases of burn healing and provide sufficient options for the plastic surgeon.

Axial flaps are long, cutaneous flaps that contain an anatomically recognized artery and vein. The flap is turned, rotated, or moved into position. Axial flaps are usually used for hand procedures, such as a pollicization or island pedicle finger pulp reconstruction.

Random, or local flaps, were the earliest flaps used. They do not contain a recognized artery and are used almost anywhere on the body surface. The skin flap survives on the subdermal plexus of vessels. A delay procedure may be needed to enlarge these flaps. Tissue expansion may expand the size of available tissue.

Z-plasty is a procedure using multiple small flaps to lengthen a contracture. Z-plasties may set multiple flaps around a specific joint or along a contraction line. These flaps are occasionally mixed with small skin grafts.

Timing a reconstruction may depend on the type of burn. Chemical and thermal burns may not need reconstruction because they slowly improve. In contrast, radiation burns tend to be chronic and gradually worsen. These injuries require late debridement and flap coverage years after the initial trauma. Skin grafts in these cases are ineffective; musculocutaneous flap coverage ideally provides a new blood supply.

Electrical burns often require reconstruction during the acute phase of burn rehabilitation because they usually expose vital structures, such as tendons, bones, or viscera. Split-thickness skin grafts rarely provide the quality of coverage needed, and flaps are vital to introducing new blood supply during the first few weeks following injury. Musculocutaneous flaps and free flaps are the most adaptable methods for coverage of electrical wounds.

In the face, reconstruction and function begin to merge. Functionally, facial skin identifies an individual, transmits emotion in communication, protects the corneas, and forms the mouth and nose. Eyelids, vital to the protection of the eye, may require reconstruction at a very early stage in the acute phase of burn recovery. To correct eyelid eversion or contraction, full-thickness donor skin must be obtained in sufficient quantity to replace the eyelid skin. If hair-bearing skin or scarred skin is used, the results may give an unacceptable appearance and rapid reoccurrence of ectropion. Reconstructing aesthetic units of the face during the acute phase provides an optimal appearance that may not be matched by another procedure until the casualty's burn wounds have matured. In the interim, facial orthoses (eg, transparent facemasks) are the primary option for improving the appearance.[376] Facial features are not reconstructed until scar tissue has become inactive, supple, and mature. In many cases spontaneous healing, with the use of a microstomia appliance, produces such favorable results that no further reconstruction is necessary.

Timing of functional hand burn surgery is fairly independent of reconstruction considerations for appearance. After initial wound closure, finger motion is vital and surgery assumes a secondary role until the wound has become mature. Once the skin starts to feel supple, reconstruction can begin. Skin grafts to the hand require immobilization for 10 to 14 days, followed by aggressive remobilization using prolonged stretch and AAROM, AROM, and CPM equipment as necessary. Extensor tenolysis is undertaken only when skin coverage is good. Casualties must start ROM exercises within 24 to 48 hours of extensor tenolysis surgery. Web space reconstruction using Z-plasties is managed like skin grafts, with 10 to 14 days of immobilization and 6 to 8 weeks of spacers at night. It is not unusual to need an unexpected skin graft during a web space release because, as the scars are incised and defects are opened, the need for additional skin coverage becomes obvious. Functional problems with hands, eyelids, mouth, axillae, elbows, and neck are the most important to the well-being of the casualty. Because muscles, tendons, and nerves shorten when the skin over a joint is contracted, reconstruction takes precedence, even if the maturation phase has not been completed.

It is important for all team members to understand the objectives and timing of reconstructive surgical interventions in the burn casualty. Proper postoperative rehabilitation is best directed by communication between the plastic surgeon, who knows the surgical intervention and proper timing to resume therapy, and the rehabilitation team, who understands splinting needs and a casualty's independent activity.

SPECIAL CONSIDERATIONS

Special Senses

Casualties injured from burns and explosives can sustain a variety of trauma and complications. For example, blast trauma can leave a casualty with a ruptured tympanic membrane as well as external injury to the ear, resulting in profound hearing loss. If a casualty is burned during the trauma, there may also be injuries to facial skin affecting the ears, eyes, nose, and throat, impairing the casualty's ability to see, smell, taste, eat, or speak. Other types of exposure or idiopathic injury, such as chemical splashes or toxic epidural necrolysis, may result in a number of conditions (eg, purulent conjunctivitis, corneal abrasions, epithelial defects, and retinal detachments), leaving the casualty with temporary vision loss or a residual deficit. Rehabilitation professionals must be prepared to address these issues because they can affect the casualty's ability to participate in rehabilitation and to recover critical independence with ADLs.

During the acute care phase, all deficits must be defined and addressed in the casualty's care plan. Rehabilitation professionals must be familiar with the many types of equipment a casualty may present with (eg, protective ear coverings, moisture chambers or eye coverings that help protect the exposed cornea from drying injury, eye bolsters, a variety of lubricating and antibacterial creams for the injured eye, and eye patches).

Casualties with reduced sensorium require increased safety measures as a daily part of their care. Clear and concise verbal cues enable casualties to follow commands and directions. Written signage above a casualty's bed and daily rounds reports alert staff and family to the casualty's needs. Casualties with significant speech and hearing loss must have alternative types of communication, including writing or pictures on a board to allow them to point and make their needs known. Manual expressions or demonstration of directions can also be used to perform ROM exercises.

As rehabilitation continues from acute care to intermediate care, the casualty's ability to perform basic mobility tasks may improve, but some deficits will continue to be problematic, such as diminished vision or hearing. Rehabilitation goals must shift to accommodate this and advance a casualty's mobility and ability to perform ADLs despite the continued deficits. Rehabilitation specialists should be proficient in adaptive technologies, techniques for low vision training, and assistive devices that may be introduced to continue towards rehabilitation goals.

In the long-term recovery stage, it is hoped that casualties will have regained many of the lost sensory deficits; however, many casualties continue to have additional procedures that prolong visual and hearing deficits. Technologies for coping with permanent vision and hearing loss, and education to protect extremities with decreased protective sensation remain important throughout the rehabilitation process.

Thermoregulation

Full-thickness burns damage dermal appendages, including sweat glands, leading to a decreased ability to sweat in areas of deep burns.[2] Skin grafting of these wounds does not replace the dermal appendages, and the density of sweat glands decreases in areas used for donor sites.[284] Areas of superficial and partial-thickness burns will regenerate lost glands.

As perspiratory function returns, it is common to see an increase in perspiration and sebum in both burned and nonburned tissue because of the body's continued need for thermoregulation within the environment. The loss of glands in the deeper portion of the burn requires the remaining and regenerating sweat glands to work harder to maintain homeostasis.

Austin et al reported no significant difference in the rise of body temperature of subjects with burns after 1 hour of cycle ergometer exercise in a 35°C environment.[284] These subjects were able to maintain heat tolerance through increased sweat rates in areas of healthy skin, and whole body sweat rates were comparable to those of normal subjects.[284] Other studies, however, have shown thermoregulation problems do exist, especially when exercising in warmer environments.[377–379] These studies demonstrated that subjects with greater than 40% TBSA burned had increased sweat rates but were unable to adequately maintain thermoregulation after exercise in a 40°C environment,[377,379] resulting in a significant increase in core temperature and heart rate.

If a casualty has sustained burns equal to or greater than 40% TBSA, there is potential for hyperthermia during exercise, especially in environments with high ambient temperatures. Prolonged exposure to temperatures above 35°C should be avoided. A fan or air conditioner may be needed to help body cooling by evaporation. Casualties must remove garments and orthoses and must shower and cool down after vigorous exercise or work-related activities. Clinical experience shows that the ability to maintain temperature homeostasis at rest and with minimal to extreme exertion is an individual response. Work and exercise tolerance has to be evaluated on a case-by-case basis and requires careful, supervised therapy to maximize a casualty's potential.

Medical Evaluation Boards

An injured service member may remain on temporary physical profile for up to 1 year. During this time, the rehabilitation team makes every attempt to maximize the casualty's recovery potential. Casualties are referred to the Physical Disability Evaluation System if they are unable to meet medical retention standards after ample time or if they are unable to return to duty.

The US Army Physical Disability Agency, under the operational control of the commander of the Human Resources Command, is responsible for operating the Physical Disability Evaluation System.[380] According to Army Regulation 635-40, Physical Evaluation for Retention, Retirement, or Separation, the system's goals are to:

- maintain an effective and fit military organization with maximum use of available labor,
- provide benefits for eligible soldiers whose military service is terminated because of service-connected disability, and
- provide prompt disability processing while ensuring that the rights and interests of the government and the soldier are protected.[381]

The medical evaluation board process begins when optimal medical recovery has been reached, when the

service member's ability to perform further duties can be determined, when the service member has been on temporary profile exceeding 1 year, or when the service member has been given a permanent profile of a three (3) or a four (4), indicating a permanent functional deficit exists for which functional recovery is unlikely. The medical evaluation board is comprised of at least two physicians whose job is to assess and evaluate the medical history of a soldier and determine how the injury or disease will respond to treatment protocols.[382]

SUMMARY

Treatment of combat-related burn injuries includes recovering optimal function to maximize participation in societal, psychological, and physical roles. Increased rates of survival have led to greater concern for potential morbidity. Surgical and medical technology has improved to such an extent that now, in most cases, burn care providers must assume that burn casualties will survive. Even during the initial or acute phases of care, the burn team must be aware of what will be important to the casualties they treat in the long term. Burn casualties experience a series of traumatic assaults to the body and mind that present extraordinary challenges to their psychological resilience. Contrary to what might be expected, empirical data regarding the long-term sequelae of burn indicate that many burn casualties do achieve a satisfying quality of life and that most are judged to be well-adjusted individuals. Outcomes studies not only report status of burn casualties following treatment, but can also indicate those factors that seem necessary to good outcomes. These studies have also found that the extent of the

injury, the depth of the burn, the area of the body burned, and even amputations are not determining factors of good psychosocial recovery. The two most important factors that have consistently been found to be related to psychological and social adjustment are the quality of family and social support received by the casualty and the willingness of the casualty to take social risks.[383]

Burn casualties must be reassured that confusion, mistrust, anger, guilt, sorrow, and other issues are normal when they consider that their experiences are part of a very abnormal situation. Casualties should be prepared to handle stares and insensitive comments. Casualties must focus on what they can still do and on what functionality they still have, and should be encouraged to keep a sense of humor and nourish their spirits by whatever means possible. Successful reintegration into the community is the ultimate goal for the remainder of their lives. Every individual who interacts with a casualty impacts the psychosocial world of that casualty.

REFERENCES

1. Harden NG, Luster SH. Rehabilitation considerations in the care of the acute burn patient. *Crit Care Nurs Clin North Am.* 1991;3(2):245–253.

2. Esselman PC, Thombs BD, Magyar-Russell G, Fauerbach JA. Burn rehabilitation: state of the science. *Am J Phys Med Rehab.* 2006;85:383–413.

3. Saffle JR, Davis B, Williams P. Recent outcomes in the treatment of burn injury in the United States: A report from the American Burn Association Patient Registry. *J Burn Care Rehabil.* 1995;16(3 pt 1):219–232.

4. Pruitt BA, Goodwin CW, Mason AD. Epidemiological, demographic, and outcome characteristics of burn injury. In: Herndon DN, ed. *Total Burn Care.* 2nd ed. New York, NY: WB Saunders; 2002: 16–30.

5. Cancio L. Burn care in Iraq. *J Trauma Inj Infect Crit Care.* 2007;62(6):S70.

6. Demling RH. The burn edema process: current concepts. *J Burn Care Rehabil.* 2005;26(3):207–227.

7. Pham TN, Cancio LC, Gibran NS. American Burn Association practice guidelines burn shock resuscitation. *J Burn Care Res*. 2008;29(1):257–266.

8. Demling RH, Kramer GC, Harms B. Role of thermal injury-induced hypoproteinemia on edema formation in burned and non-burned tissue. *Surgery*. 1984;95:136–144.

9. Gelin LE, Solvell L, Zederfeldt B. The plasma volume expanding effect of low viscous dextran and Macrodex. *Acta Chir Scand*. 1961;122:309–323.

10. Demling RH, Kramer GC, Gunther R, Nerlich M. Effect of nonprotein colloid on postburn edema formation in soft tissues and lung. *Surgery*. 1984;95:593–602.

11. Du GB, Slater H, Goldfarb IW. Influences of different resuscitation regimens on acute early weight gain in extensively burned patients. *Burns*. 1991;17(2):147–150.

12. Waxman K, Holness R, Tominaga G, Chela P, Grimes J. Hemodynamic and oxygen transport effects of pentastarch in burn resuscitation. *Ann Surg*. 1989;209(3):341–345.

13. Wallace BH, Caldwell FT Jr, Cone JB. Ibuprofen lowers body temperature and metabolic rate of humans with burn injury. *J Trauma*. 1992;32(2):154–157.

14. Demling RH, Zhu D, Lalonde C. Early pulmonary and hemodynamic effects of a chest wall burn (effect of ibuprofen). *Surgery*. 1988;104(1):10–17.

15. Haberal M, Mavi V, Oner G. The stabilizing effect of vitamin E, selenium and zinc on leucocyte membrane permeability: a study in vitro. *Burns Incl Therm Inj*. 1987;13(2):118–122.

16. Matsuda T, Tanaka H, Williams S, Hanumadass M, Abcarian H, Reyes H. Reduced fluid volume requirement for resuscitation of third-degree burns with high-dose vitamin C. *J Burn Care Rehabil*. 1991;12:525–532.

17. Boykin JV Jr, Crute SL, Haynes BW Jr. Cimetidine therapy for burn shock: a quantitative assessment. *J Trauma*. 1985;25:864–870.

18. Boykin JV Jr, Manson NH. Mechanisms of cimetidine protection following thermal injury. *Am J Med*. 1987;83:76–81.

19. Brunicardi FC, Andersen DK, Billiar TR, Dunn DL, Hunter JG, Pollock RE. Basic considerations, fluid management. Part I. In: Schwartz SI, Brunicardi FC, eds. *Schwartz's Principles of Surgery*. 8th ed. New York, NY: McGraw-Hill Medical Publishing Division: 2005.

20. Cancio LC, Horvath EE, Barillo DJ, et al. Burn Support for Operation Iraqi Freedom and related operations, 2003 to 2004. *J Burn Care Rehabil*. 2005;26:151–161.

21. Champion HR, Bellamy RF, Roberts CP, Leppaniemi A. A profile of combat injury. *J Trauma*. 2003;54:S13–S19.

22. Thomas SJ, Kramer GC, Herndon DN. Burns: Military options and tactical solutions. *J Trauma*. 2003;54:S207–S218.

23. Wolf SE, Kauvar DS, Wade CE, et al. Comparison between civilian burns and combat burns from Operation Iraqi Freedom and Operation Enduring Freedom. *Ann Surg*. 2006;243(6):786–795.

24. Kauvar DS, Cancio LC, Wolf SE, Wade CE, Holcomb JB. Comparison of combat and non-combat burns from ongoing U.S. military operations. *J Surg Res*. 2006;132:195–200.

25. Kauvar DS, Wolf SE, Wade CE, Cancio LC, Renz EM, Holcomb JB. Burns sustained in combat explosions in Operations Iraqi and Enduring Freedom (OIF/OEF explosion burns). *Burns*. 2006;32:853–857.

26. Barillo DJ, Cancio LC, Goodwin CW. Treatment of white phosphorus and other chemical burn injuries at one burn center over a 51-year period. *Burns*. 2004;30:448–452.

27. Curreri PW, Asch MJ, Pruitt BA. The treatment of chemical burns: specialized diagnostic, therapeutic, and prognostic considerations. *J Trauma.* 1970;10:634–641.

28. McCarthy JG. Cold, chemical, and irradiation injuries. In: McCarthy JG, May JW, Littler JW, eds. *The Hand.* Part 2. In: McCarthy JG, May JW, Littler JW, eds. *Plastic Surgery.* Vol. 8. Philadelphia, Pa: W.B. Saunders; 1990: 5438.

29. Jurkiewicz MJ, Krizek TJ, Mathes SJ, Ariyan S. *Plastic Surgery, Principles and Practice.* Vol 2. Saint Louis, MO: CV Mosby; 1990: 1399.

30. Khateri S, Ghanei M, Keshavarz S, Soroush M, Haines D. Incidence of lung, eye, and skin lesions as late complications in 34,000 Iranians with wartime exposure to mustard agent. *J Occup Environ Med.* 2003; 45(11):1136–1143.

31. Cox BM. Torald Sollmann's studies of mustard gas. *Mol Interv.* 2007;7:124–128.

32. Hunt JL. Electrical injuries. In: Fisher SV, Helm PA, eds. *Comprehensive Rehabilitation of Burns.* Baltimore, Md: Williams & Wilkins; 1984: 249–266.

33. Ahrenholz DH, Schubert W, Solem LD. Creatine kinase as a prognostic indicator in electrical injury. *Surgery.* 1988;104:741–747.

34. Zawacki BE, Azen SP, Imbus SH, Chang YT. Multifactorial probit analysis of mortality in burned patients. *Ann Surg.* 1979;189:1–5.

35. Wolf S. Modern burn care. *J Trauma Inj Infect Crit Care.* 2007;62(6):S67.

36. Sheridan RL. Evaluating and managing burn wounds. *Dermatol Nurs.* 2000;12(1):17–28.

37. Knaysl GA, Crikelair GF, Cosman B. The role of nines: its history and accuracy. *Plast Reconstr Surg.* 1968;41:560–563.

38. Lund C, Browder N. The estimation of area of burns. *Surg Gynecol Obstet.* 1944;79:352–355.

39. Holmes JH, Heimbach DM. Burns/inhalation injury. In: Peitzman AB, Rhodes M, Schwab CW, Yealy DM, Fabian TC, eds. *The Trauma Manual: Trauma and Acute Care Surgery.* 3rd ed. Philadelphia, Pa: Lippincott Williams & Wilkins; 2007: 387–492.

40. Devgan L, Bhat S, Aylward S, Spence RJ. Modalities for the assessment of burn wound depth. *J Burns Wounds.* 2006;5;e2.

41. Richard R. Assessment and diagnosis of burn wounds. *Adv Wound Care.* 1999;12:468–471.

42. Grigsby deLinde L, Miles WK. Remodeling of scar tissue in the burned hand. In: Hunter JM, Mackin EJ, Callahan AD, eds. *Rehabilitation of the Hand: Surgery and Therapy.* 4th ed. Saint Louis, Mo: Mosby; 1995.

43. Hunt JL, Sato RM. Early excision of full-thickness hand and digit burns: factors affecting morbidity. *J Trauma.* 1982;22(5):414–419.

44. Saffle JR and Schnebly WA. Burn wound care. In: Richard RL, Staley MJ, eds. *Burn Care and Rehabilitation: Principles and Practice.* Philadelphia, Pa: FA Davis; 1994.

45. Anzarut A, Chen M, Shankowsky H, Tredget EE. Quality-of-life and outcome predictors following massive burn injury. *Plast Reconstr Surger.* 2005;116(3):791–797.

46. Richard R, Steinlage R, Staley M, Keck T. Mathematic model to estimate change in burn scar length required for joint range of motion. *J Burn Care Rehabil.* 1996;17(5):436–43.

47. Hedman TL, Renz, EM, Richard RL, et al. Incidence and severity of combat hand burns after All Army Activity message. *J Trauma.* 2008;64(suppl 2):169–173.

48. Cioffi WG, Rue LW, Buescher TM, Pruitt BA. The management of burn injury. *Mil Med*. 1981:349–377.

49. Staley M, Richard R, Warden GD, Miller SF, Shuster DB. Functional outcomes for the patient with burn injuries. *J Burn Care Rehabil*. 1996;7(4):362–368.

50. Kraemer MD, Jones T, Deitch EA. Burn contractures: incidence, predisposing factors, and results of surgical therapy. *J Burn Care Rehabil*. 1988;9(3):261–265.

51. Leblebici B, Adam M, Bagis S, et al. Quality of life after burn injury: the impact of joint contracture. *J Burn Care Res*. 2006;27:864–868.

52. Dobbs ER, Curreri PW. Burns: analysis of results of physical therapy in 681 patients. *J Trauma*. 1972;12:242–248.

53. Richard RL, Hedman TL, Chapman TT, et al. Atlas of burn scar contractures: a patient education tool. *J Burn Care Res*. 2007;28:S152.

54. Chapman TT, Richard RL, Hedman TL, et al. Military return to duty and civilian return to work factors following burns with focus on the hand and literature review. *J Burn Care Res*. 2008;29(5):756–762.

55. Cope O, Moore F. The redistribution of body water and the fluid therapy of the burned patient. *Ann Surg*. 1947;126:1010–1045.

56. Demling RH, Mazess RB, Witt RM, Wolberg WH. The study of burn wound edema using dichromatic absorptiometry. *J Trauma*. 1978;18:124–128.

57. Warden G. Fluid resuscitation and early management. In: Herndon DN, ed. *Total Burn Care*. Philadelphia, Pa: WB Saunders; 1996: 55.

58. Sheridan RL. Comprehensive treatment of burns. *Curr Probl Surg*. 2001;38(9):657–756.

59. Shwartz S. Consensus summary on fluid resuscitation. *J Trauma*. 1979;19:876–877.

60. Pruitt BA Jr. Fluid and electrolyte replacement in the burned patient. *Surg Clin North Am*. 1978;58:1291–1312.

61. Chung KK, Blackbourne LH, Wolf SE, et al. Evolution of burn resuscitation in Operation Iraqi Freedom. *J Burn Care Res*. 2006;27(5):606–611.

62. Sugrue M. Abdominal compartment syndrome. *Curr Opin Crit Care*. 2005;11:333–338.

63. Hobson KG, Young KM, Ciraulo A, Palmieri TL, Greenhalgh DG. Release of abdominal compartment syndrome improves survival in patients with burn injury. *J Trauma*. 2002;53:1129–1133.

64. Sheridan RL, Tompkins RG, McManus WF, Pruitt BA Jr. Intracompartmental sepsis in burn patients. *J Trauma*. 1994;36:301–305.

65. Kollef MH. The prevention of ventilator-associated pneumonia. *N Engl J Med*. 1999;340:627–634.

66. Bayley E. Care of the burn patient with inhalation injury. In: Trofino RB, ed. *Nursing Care of the Burn-Injured Patient*. Philadelphia, Pa: FA Davis; 1991: 325–348.

67. Ryan CM, Yarmush ML, Burke JF, Tompkins RG. Increased gut permeability early after burns correlates with the extent of burn injury. *Crit Care Med*. 1992;20:1508–1512.

68. Herndon DN, Barrow RE, Stein M, et al. Increased mortality with intravenous supplemental feeding in severely burned patients. *J Burn Care Rehabil*. 1989;10:309–313.

69. Wilmore DW, Long JM, Mason AD Jr, Skreen RW, Pruitt BA Jr. Catecholamines: mediator of the hypermetabolic response to thermal injury. *Ann Surg*. 1974;180:653–669.

70. Herndon DN, Hart DW, Wolf SE, Chinkes DL, Wolfe RR. Reversal of catabolism by beta-blockade after severe burns. *N Engl J Med*. 2001;345:1223–1229.

71. Wolf SE, Edelman LS, Kemalyan N, et al. Effects of oxandrolone on outcome measures in the severely burned: a multicenter prospective randomized double-blind trial. *J Burn Care Res*. 2006;27:131–139.

72. Thadhani R, Pascual M, Bonventre JV. Acute renal failure. *N Engl J Med*. 1996;334:1448–1460.

73. John S, Eckardt KU. Renal replacement strategies in the ICU. *Chest*. 2007;132:1379–1388.

74. Vinsonneau C, Camus C, Combes A, et al. Continuous venovenous haemodiafiltration versus intermittent haemodialysis for acute renal failure in patients with multiple-organ dysfunction syndrome: a multicentre randomised trial. *Lancet*. 2006;368:379–385.

75. Suzuki K, Nishina M, Ogino R, Kohama A. Left ventricular contractility and diastolic properties in anesthetized dogs after severe burns. *Am J Physiol*. 1991;260:H1433–H1442.

76. Cioffi WG, DeMeules JE, Gamelli RL. The effects of burn injury and fluid resuscitation on cardiac function in vitro. *J Trauma*. 1986;26:638–642.

77. Hébert PC, Wells G, Blajchman MA, et al. A multicenter, randomized, controlled clinical trial of transfusion requirements in critical care. Transfusion Requirements in Critical Care Investigators, Canadian Critical Care Trials Group. *N Engl J Med*. 1999;340:409–417.

78. Harrington DT, Mozingo DW, Cancio L, Bird P, Jordan B, Goodwin CW. Thermally injured patients are at significant risk for thromboembolic complications. *J Trauma*. 2001;50(3):495–499.

79. Lee JO, Benjamin D, Herndon DN. Nutrition support strategies for severely burned patients. *Nutr Clin Pract*. 2005;20(3):325–330.

80. Mahan LK, Krause MV, Escott-Stump S. *Krause's Food, Nutrition & Diet Therapy*. 9th ed. Philadelphia, Pa: WB Saunders Company; 1996.

81. Long CL, Schaffel N, Geiger JW, Schiller WR, Blakemore WS. Metabolic response to injury and illness: estimation of energy and protein needs from indirect calorimetry and nitrogen balance. *JPEN J Parenter Enteral Nutr*. 1979;3(6):452–456.

82. Pereira CP, Muphy KD, Herdon DN. Altering metabolism. *J Burn Care Rehabil*. 2005;26(3):194–199.

83. McDonald WS, Sharp CW Jr, Deitch EA. Immediate enteral feeding in burn patients is safe and effective. *Ann Surg*. 1991;213(2):177–183.

84. Gottschlich MM, Jenkins ME, Mayes T, Khoury J, Kagan RJ, Warden GD. The 2002 Clinical Research Award. An evaluation of the safety of early vs delayed enteral support and effects on clinical, nutritional, and endocrine outcomes after severe burns. *J Burn Care Rehabil*. 2002;23(6):401–415.

85. Hansbrough WB, Hansbrough JF. Success of immediate intragastric feeding of patients with burns. *J Burn Care Rehabil*. 1993;14:512–516.

86. Cunningham JJ, Hegarty MT, Meara PA, Burke JF. Measured and predicted calorie requirements of adults during recovery from severe burn trauma. *Am J Clin Nutr*. 1989;49(3):404–408.

87. Kelemen JJ 3rd, Cioffi WG Jr, Mason AD Jr, Mozingo DW, McManus WF, Pruitt BA Jr. Effect of ambient temperature on metabolic rate after thermal injury. *Ann Surg*. 1996;223(4):406–412.

88. Barton RG, Craft WB, Mone MC, Saffle JR. Chemical paralysis reduces energy expenditure in patients with burns and severe respiratory failure treated with mechanical ventilation. *J Burn Care Rehabil*. 1997;18(5):461–468.

89.   Hart DW, Wolf SE, Herndon DN, et al. Energy expenditure and caloric balance after burn: increased feeding leads to fat rather than lean mass accretion. *Ann Surg*. 2002;235(1):152–161.

90.   Curreri PW, Richmond D, Marvin J, Baxter CR. Dietary requirements of patients with major burns. *J Am Diet Assoc*. 1974;65(4):415–417.

91.   Saffle JR, Medina E, Raymond J, Westenskow D, Kravitz M, Warden GD. Use of indirect calorimetry in the nutritional management of burn patients. *J Trauma*. 1985;25(1):32–39.

92.   Turner WW Jr, Ireton CS, Hunt JL, Baxter CR. Predicting energy expenditures in burned patients. *J Trauma*. 1985;25(1):11–16.

93.   Carlson DE, Cioffi WG Jr, Mason AD Jr, McManus WF, Pruitt BA Jr. Resting energy expenditure in patients with thermal injuries. *Surg Gynecol Obstet*. 1991;174(4):270–276.

94.   Milner EA, Cioffi WG, Mason AD, McManus WF, Pruitt BA Jr. A longitudinal study of resting energy expenditure in thermally injured patients. *J Trauma*. 1994;37(2):167–70.

95.   Wall-Alonso E, Schoeller DA, Schechter L, and Gottlieb LJ. Measured total energy requirements of adult patients with burns. *J Burn Care Rehabil*. 1999;20(4):329–337.

96.   Gottschlich MM. Nutrition support in burns. In: Shronts EP, ed. *Nutrition Support Dietetics: Core Curriculum*. Silver Spring, Md: American Society of Parenteral and Enteral Nutrition; 1989: 213–219.

97.   Matsuda T, Kagan RJ, Hanumadass M, Jonasson O. The importance of burn wound size in determining the optimal calorie:nitrogen ratio. *Surgery*. 1983;94(4):562–568.

98.   Alexander JW, MacMillan BG, Stinnett JD, et al. Beneficial effects of aggressive protein feeding in severely burned children. *Ann Surg*. 1980;192(4):505–517.

99.   Waxman K, Rebello T, Pinderski L, et al. Protein loss across burn wounds. *J Trauma*. 1987;27(2):136–40.

100.   Saito H, Trocki O, Wang S, Gonce SJ, Joffe SN, Alexander JW. Metabolic and immune effects of dietary arginine supplementation after burn. *Arch Surg*. 1987;122(7):784–789.

101.   Daly JM, Reynolds J, Thom A, et al. Immune and metabolic effects of arginine in the surgical patient. *Ann Surg*. 1988;208(4):512–523.

102.   Gottschlich MM, Jenkins M, Warden GD, et al. Differential effects of three enteral dietary regimens on selected outcome variables in burn patients. *JPEN J Parenteral Enteral Nutr*. 1990;14(3):225–236.

103.   Hammarqvist F, Wernerman J, Ali R, von der Decken A, Vinnars E. Addition of glutamine to total parenteral nutrition after elective abdominal surgery spares free glutamine in muscle, counteracts the fall in muscle protein synthesis, and improves nitrogen balance. *Ann Surg*. 1989;209(4):455–461.

104.   Yu YM, Wagner DA, Walesreswski JC, Burke JF, Young VR. A kinetic study of leucine metabolism in severely burned patients. Comparison between a conventional and branched-chain amino acid-enriched nutritional therapy. *Ann Surg*. 1988;207(4):421–429.

105.   Cerra FB, Mazuski JE, Chute E, et al. Branched chain metabolic support: a prospective, randomized, double-blind trial in surgical stress. *Ann Surg*. 1984;199(3):286–291.

106.   Cerra F, Blackburn G, Hirsch J, Mullen K, Luther W. The effect of stress level, amino acid formula, and nitrogen dose on nitrogen retention in traumatic and septic stress. *Ann Surg*. 1987;205(3):282–287.

107.   Mochizuki H, Trocki O, Dominioni L, Alexander JW. Effect of a diet rich in branched chain amino acids on severely burned guinea pigs. *J Trauma*. 1986;26(12):1077–1085.

108. Yu YM, Wagner DA, Walesreswski J, Burke JF, Young VR. A kinetic study of leucine metabolism in severely burned patients. Comparison between a conventional and branched-chain amino acid-enriched nutritional therapy. *Ann Surg.* 1988;207(4):421–490.

109. Hart DW, Wolf SE, Zhang XJ, et al. Efficacy of a high-carbohydrate diet in catabolic illness. *Crit Care Med.* 2001;29(7):1318–1324.

110. Gottschlich MM, Warden GD, Michel M, et al. Diarrhea in tube-fed burn patients: incidence, etiology, nutritional impact, and prevention. *JPEN J Parenteral Enteral Nutr.* 1988;12(4):338–345.

111. Gottschlich MM, Alexander JW. Fat kinetics and recommended dietary intake in burns. *JPEN J Parenteral Enteral Nutr.* 1987;11(1):80–85.

112. Williamson J. Actual burn nutrition care practices. A national survey (Part II). *J Burn Care Rehabil.* 1989;10(2):185–194.

113. Gottschlich MM, Warden GD. Vitamin supplementation in the patient with burns. *J Burn Care Rehabil.* 1990;11(3):275–279.

114. Boosalis MG, Solem LD, McCall JT, Ahrenholz DH, McClain CJ. Serum zinc response in thermal injury. *J Am Coll Nutr.* 1988;7(1):69–76.

115. Berger MM, Cavadini C, Chiolero R, Guinchard S, Krupp S, Dirren H. Influence of large intakes of trace elements on recovery after major burns. *Nutrition.* 1994;10(4):327–334.

116. American Society for Parenteral and Enteral Nutrition. *The A.S.P.E.N. Nutrition Support Core Curriculum: a Case-Based Approach—the Adult Patient.* Silver Spring, Md: ASPEN; 2007: 145.

117. Voruganti VS, Klein GL, Lu HX, Thomas S, Freeland-Graves JH, Herndon DN. Impaired zinc and copper status in children with burn injuries: need to reassess nutritional requirements. *Burns.* 2005;31(6):711–716.

118. McCord JM. Free radicals and inflammation: protection of synovial fluid by superoxide dismutase. *Science.* 1974;185(150):529–531.

119. Selmanpakoğlu AN, Cetin C, Sayal A, Işimer A. Trace element (Al, Se, Zn, Cu) levels in serum, urine and tissues of burn patients. *Burns.* 1994;20:99–103.

120. Gropper SAS, Groff JL, Smith JL. *Advanced Nutrition and Human Metabolism.* Belmont, Calif: Thomson Wadsworth; 2005.

121. Berger MM, Cavadini C, Bart A, et al. Cutaneous copper and zinc losses in burns. *Burns.* 1992;18(5):373–380.

122. Allen JI, Kay NE, McClain CJ. Severe zinc deficiency in humans: association with reversible T-lymphocyte dysfunction. *Ann Intern Med.* 1981;95(2):154–157.

123. Levander OA. Considerations in the design of selenium bioavailability studies. *Fed Proc.* 1983;42(6):1721–1725.

124. Dimitrov NV, Ullrey DE, Primack S, Meyer C, Ku PK, Miller ER. Selenium as a metabolic modulator of phagocytosis. In: Combs GR Jr, Spallholz JE, Levander OA, Oldfield JE, eds. *Selenium in Biology and Medicine: Proceedings of the Third International Symposium on Selenium in Biology and Medicine, Held May 27–June 1, 1984, Xiangshan (Fragrance Hills) Hotel, Beijing, People's Republic of China.* New York, NY: Van Nostrand Reinhold; 1987: 254–262.

125. Johnson RA, Baker SS, Fallon JT, et al. An occidental case of cardiomyopathy and selenium deficiency. *N Engl J Med.* 1981;304(20):1210–1212.

126. Fleming CR, Lie JT, McCall JT, O'Brien JF, Baillie EE, Thistle JL. Selenium deficiency and fatal cardiomyopathy in a patient on home parenteral nutrition. *Gastroenterology.* 1982;83(3):689–693.

127. Duhr A, Galan P, Hercberg S. Relationship between selenium, immunity and resistance against infection. *Comp Biochem Physiol C.* 1990;96(2):271–280.

128. Porter EK, Karle JA, Shrift A. Uptake of selenium-75 by human lymphocytes in vitro. *J Nutr.* 1979;109(11):1901–1908.

129. Karle JA, Kull FJ, Shrift A. Uptake of selenium-75 by PHA-stimulated lymphocytes: effect on glutathione peroxidase. *Biol Trace Elem Res.* 1983;5:17–24.

130. Gamliel Z, DeBiasse MA, Demling RH. Essential microminerals and their response to burn injury. *J Burn Care Rehabil.* 1996;17(3):264–272.

131. Chiarelli A, Enzi G, Casadei A, et al. Very early nutrition supplementation in burned patients. *Am J Clin Nutr.* 1990;51(6):1035–1039.

132. Walsh EN, Dumitru D, King J C, Ramamurthy S. Management of acute and chronic pain. In: Kottke FJ, Amate EA, eds. *Clinical Advances in Physical Medicine and Rehabilitation.* Washington, DC: Pan American Health Organization, Pan American Sanitary Bureau, Regional Office of the World Health Organization; 1991: 373–401.

133. DeJong RH. Defining pain terms. *JAMA.* 1980;244(2):143–147.

134. Choinière M, Melzack R, Rondeau J, Girard N, Paquin MJ. The pain of burns: characteristics and correlates. *J Trauma.* 1989;29(11):1531–1539.

135. Andreasen NJ, Noyes R Jr, Hartford CE, Brodland G, Proctor S. Management of emotional reactions in seriously burned adults. *N Engl J Med.* 1972;286(2):65–69.

136. Taal LA, Faber AW. Burn injuries, pain and distress: exploring the role of stress symptomatology. *Burns.* 1997;23(4):288–290.

137. Choinière M. The pain of burns In: Wall PD, Melzack R, Bonica JJ, eds. *Textbook of Pain.* 3rd ed. Edinburgh, Scotland: Churchill Livingstone; 1994.

138. Meyer WJ, Marvin JA, Patterson DR, et al. Management of pain and other discomforts in burned patients In: Herndon DN, ed. *Total Burn Care.* Philadelphia, Pa: WB Saunders; 1996.

139. Ulmer JF. Burn pain management: a guideline-based approach. *J Burn Care Rehabil.* 1998;19(2):151–159.

140. Williams PI, Sarginson RE, Ratcliffe JM. Use of methadone in the morphine-tolerant burned paediatric patient. *Br J Anaesth.* 1998;80(1):92–95.

141. Loeser JD, Bonica JJ, Bulter SH, Chapman CR, Turk DC, eds. *Bonica's Management of Pain.* Philadelphia, Pa: Lippincott Williams & Wilkins; 2001.

142. Pal SK, Cortiella J, Herndon D. Adjunctive methods of pain control in burns. *Burns.* 1997;23(5):404–412.

143. Slogoff S, Allen GW, Wessels JV, Cheney DH. Clinical experience with subanesthetic ketamine. *Anesth Analg.* 1974;53(3):354–358.

144. Dickenson AH, Sullivan AF. Evidence for a role of the NMDA receptor in the frequency dependant potentiation of deep rat dorsal horn nociceptive neurones following C fibre stimulation. *Neuropharmacology.* 1987;26:1235–1238.

145. Cuignet O, Pirson J, Soudon O, Zizi M. Effects of gabapentin on morphine consumption and pain in severely burned patients. *Burns.* 2007;33(1):81–86.

146. Wasiak J, Cleland H. Lidocaine for pain relief in burn injured patients. *Cochrane Database Syst Rev.* 2007;3:CD005622.

147. Hoffman HG, Patterson DR, Carrougher GJ. Use of virtual reality for adjunctive treatment of adult burn pain during physical therapy: a controlled study. *Clin J Pain.* 2000;16(3):244–250.

148. Rainville P, Hofbauer RK, Paus T, Duncan GH, Bushnell MC, Price DD. Cerebral mechanisms of hypnotic induction and suggestion. *J Cogn Neurosci.* 1999;11(1):110–125.

149. de Jong AE, Gamel C. Use of a simple relaxation technique in burn care: literature review. *J Adv Nurs*. 2006;54(6):710–721.

150. Choinière M. Burn pain: a unique challenge. *Pain Clin Updates*. 2001;9:1–4.

151. Foertsch CE, O'Hara MW, Stoddard FJ, Kealey GP. Treatment-resistant pain and distress during pediatric burn-dressing changes. *J Burn Care Rehabil*. 1998;19(3):219–224.

152. Schreiber S, Galai-Gat T. Uncontrolled pain following physical injury as the core-trauma in post-traumatic stress disorder. *Pain*. 1993;54(1):107–110.

153. Singer AJ, Brebbia J, Soroff HH. Management of local burn wounds in the ED. *Am J Emerg Med*. 2007;25(6):666–671.

154. MacLennan N, Heimbach DM, Cullen BF. Anesthesia for major thermal injury. *Anesthesiology*. 1998;89(3):749–770

155. Summer GJ, Puntillo KA, Miaskowski C, Green PG, Levine JD. Burn injury pain: the continuing challenge. *J Pain*. 2007;8(7):533–548.

156. Latarjet J, Choinière M. Pain in burn patients. *Burns*. 1995;21(5):344–348.

157. Barash P, Liu S, Joseph R, et al. Peripheral nerve blocks. In: Barash PG, Cullen BF, Stoelting RK, eds. *Clinical Anesthesia*. 5th ed. Philadelphia, Pa: Lippincott Williams & Wilkins; 2006: 453–471.

158. Viscusi E, Jan R, Schechter L, et al. *Organization of an Acute Pain Management Service Incorporating Regional Anesthesia Techniques*. Available at: http://nysora.com/regional_anesthesia/index.1.html. Accessed 2007.

159. Practice guidelines for preoperative fasting and the use of pharmacologic agents to reduce the risk of pulmonary aspiration: application to healthy patients undergoing elective procedures: a report by the American Society of Anesthesiologists Task Force on Preoperative Fasting. *Anesthesiology*. 1999;90(3):896–905.

160. Horlocker T, Wedel DJ, Benzon H, et al. Regional anesthesia in the anticoagulated patient: defining the risk (the second ASRA Consensus Conference on Neuraxial Anesthesia and Anticoagulation). *Reg Anesth Pain Med*. 2003;28(3):172–197.

161. Choinière M. Prescribing practices for analgesia in adults and children with minor burns. Paper presented at: 10th Congress of the International Society for Burn Injuries; November 1998; Jerusalem, Israel.

162. Edgar D, Brereton M. Rehabilitation after burn injury. *BMJ*. 2004;329(7461):343–345.

163. Ferguson SL, Voll KV. Burn pain and anxiety: the use of music relaxation during rehabilitation. *J Burn Care Rehabil*. 2004;25(1):8–14.

164. Baxter CR. Fluid volume and electrolyte changes in the early postburn period. *Clin Plast Surg*. 1974;1(4):693–703.

165. Kramer G, Lund T, Herndon D. Pathophysiology of burn shock and burn edema. In: Herndon DN, ed. *Total Burn Care*. 2nd ed. New York, NY: WB Saunders; 2002.

166. Fess EE. The need for reliability and validity in hand assessment instruments. *J Hand Surg [Am]*. 1986;11(5):621–623.

167. Dewey WS, Hedman TL, Chapman TT, Wolf SE, Holcomb JB. The reliability and concurrent validity of the figure-of-eight method of measuring hand edema in patients with burns. *J Burn Care Res*. 2007;28(1):157–162.

168. Villeco J, Mackin E, Hunter J. Edema: therapist's management. In: Hunter JM, Mackin EJ, Callahan AD, eds. *Rehabilitation of the Hand*. 5th ed. Saint Louis, MO: Mosby; 2002: 186–188.

169. Schultz-Johnson K. *Volumetrics: a Literature Review*. Glenwood Springs, CO: Upper Extremity Technology; 1988: 16–23.

170. Waylett-Rendall J, Seibly D. A study of accuracy of a commercially available volumeter. *J Hand Ther*. 1991;4:10–13.

171. DeVore GL, Hamilton GF. Volume measuring of the severely injured hand. *Am J Occup Ther.* 1968;22(1):16–18.

172. King TI. The effect of water temperature on hand volume during volumetric measurement using the water displacement method. *J Hand Ther.* 1993;6(3):202–204.

173. Leard J, Breglio L, Fraga L, et al. Reliability and concurrent validity of the figure-of-eight method of measuring hand size with hand pathology. *J Orthop Sports Phys Ther.* 2004;24(6):335–340.

174. Pellecchia GL. Figure-of-eight method of measuring hand size: reliability and concurrent validity. *J Hand Ther.* 2003;16(4):300–304.

175. Maihafer GC, Llewellyn MA, Pillar WJ Jr, Scott KL, Marino DM, Bond RM. A comparison of the figure-of-eight method and water volumetry in the measurement of hand and wrist size. *J Hand Ther.* 2003;16(4):305–310.

176. Richard RL, Miller SF, Finley RK Jr, Jones LM. Comparison of the effect of passive exercise v static wrapping on finger range of motion in the burned hand. *J Burn Care Rehabil.* 1987;8(6):576–578.

177. Humphrey C, Richard RL, Staley MJ. Soft tissue management and exercise. In: Richard R, Staley MJ, eds. *Burn Care and Rehabilitation: Principles and Practice.* Philadelphia, Pa: FA Davis; 1994: 334.

178. Feller I, Jones CA. *Nursing the Burned Patient.* Ann Arbor, Mich: Institute for Burn Medicine; 1973: 73, 151.

179. Adkins P. Postoperative care. In: Kasdan ML, ed. *Occupational Hand and Upper Extremity Injuries and Diseases.* 2nd ed. Philadelphia, PA: Hanley & Belfus, Inc; 1998: 441.

180. Gordon M, Goodwin CW. Burn management: initial assessment, management, and stabilization. *Nurs Clin North Am.* 1997;32(2):237–249.

181. Beasly RW. Secondary repair of burned hands. *Clin Plast Surg.* 1981;8(1):141–162.

182. Chapman TT. Burn scar and contracture management. *J Trauma.* 2007;62(suppl 6):S8.

183. Brush KA. Abdominal compartment syndrome: the pressure is on. *Nursing.* 2007;37(7):36-41.

184. Gordon MD, Gottschlich MM, Hevlig EI, Marvin JA, Richard RL. Review of evidence-based practice for the prevention of pressure sores in burn patients. *J Burn Care Rehabil.* 2004;25(5):388–410.

185. Tymec AC, Pieper B, Vollman K. A comparison of two pressure-relieving devices on the prevention of heel pressure ulcers. *Adv Wound Care.* 1997;10(1):39–44.

186. Banwell PE. Topical negative pressure therapy in wound care. *J Wound Care.* 1999;8(2):79–84.

187. Atiyeh BS, Gunn SW, Hayek SN. State of the art in burn treatment. *World J Surg.* 2005;29(2):131–48.

188. Wolf S, Herndon DN, eds. *Burn Care.* Austin, Tes: Landes Bioscience; 1999: 9.

189. Blackbourne LH. *Surgical Recall.* 4th ed. Philadelphia, Pa: Lippincott Williams & Wilkins; 2005: 562.

190. Bull JP, Fisher AJ. A study of mortality in a burns unit: a revised estimate. *Ann Surg.* 1954;139(3):269–274.

191. Muller MJ, Herndon DN. The challenge of burns. *Lancet.* 1994;343:216–220

192. Burke JF, Bondoc CC, Quinby WC. Primary burn excision and immediate grafting: a method shortening illness. *J Trauma.* 1974;14(5):389–395.

193. Pietsch JB, Netscher DT, Nagaraj HS, Groff DB. Early excision of major burns in children: effect on morbidity and mortality. *J Pediatr Surg.* 1985;20(6):754–757.

194. Munster AM, Smith-Meek M, Sharkey P. The effect of early surgical intervention on mortality and cost-effectiveness in burn care, 1978–1991. *Burns.* 1994;20(1):61–64.

195. Jurkiewicz MJ, Krizek TJ, Mathes SJ, Ariyan S. Wound closure. In: Jurkiewicz MJ, ed. *Plastic Surgery: Principles and Practice.* Vol 1. Saint Louis, Mo: Mosby; 1990: 22.

196. Venturi ML, Attinger CE, Mesbahi AN, Hess CL, Graw KS. Mechanisms and clinical applications of the vacuum-assisted closure (VAC) device: a review. *Am J Clin Dermatol.* 2005;6(3):185–194.

197. Hartford CE. Surgical management. In: Fisher SV, Helm PA, eds. *Comprehensive Rehabilitation of Burns.* Baltimore, Md: Williams & Wilkins; 1984.

198. McCarthy JG. Facial burns. In: McCarthy JG, May JW, Littler JW, eds. *Plastic Surgery.* Vol 3. Philadelphia, Pa: Saunders; 1990: 2200.

199. Rheinwald JG, Green H. Serial cultivation of strains of human epidermal keratinocytes: the formation of keratinizing colonies from single cells. *Cell.* 1975;6(3):331–344.

200. Pittelkow MR, Scott RE. New techniques for the in vitro culture of human skin keratinocytes and perspectives on their use for grafting of patients with extensive burns. *Mayo Clin Proc.* 1986;61(10):771–777.

201. Heimbach D, Luterman A, Burke J, et al. Artificial dermis for major burns: a multi-center randomized clinical trial. *Ann Surg.* 1988;208(3):313–320.

202. Clarke JA. HIV transmission and skin grafts. *Lancet.* 1987;1:983.

203. Lawrence JC. Allografts as vectors of infection. *Lancet.* 1987;1:1318.

204. Haberal M, Oner Z, Bayraktar U, Bilgin N. The use of silver nitrate-incorporated amniotic membrane as a temporary dressing. *Burns Incl Therm Inj.* 1987;13(2):159–163.

205. Sawhney CP. Amniotic membrane as a biological dressing in the management of burns. *Burns.* 1989;15(5):339–342.

206. Hunt JL, Purdue GF, Zbar RIS. Burns: acute burns, burn surgery, and postburn reconstruction. *Selected Readings in Plast Surg.* 2000;9(12):7.

207. McHugh TP, Robson MC, Heggers JP, Phillips LG, Smith DJ Jr, McCollum MC. Therapeutic efficacy of Biobrane in partial- and full-thickness thermal injury. *Surgery.* 1986;100(4):661–664.

208. Grabb WC, Smith JW, Aston SJ, Beasley RW, Thorne C. *Grabb and Smith's Plastic Surgery.* 5th ed. Philadelphia, PA: Lippincott-Raven Publishers; 1997: 19.

209. Wood RJ, Peltier GL, Twomey JA. Management of the difficult split-thickness donor site. *Ann Plast Surg.* 1989;22(1):80–81.

210. Sood R, Achauer BM. *Achauer and Sood's Burn Surgery: Reconstruction and Rehabilitation.* Philadelphia, Pa: Saunders Elsevier; 2006.

211. Barillo D, Paulsen S. Management of burns to the hand. *Wounds.* 2003;15(1):4–9.

212. Giuliani CA, Perry GA. Factors to consider in the rehabilitation aspect of burn care. *Phys Ther.* 1985;65(5):619–623.

213. Firoz EF, Firoz BF, Williams J, Henning JS. Allergic contact dermatitis to mafenide acetate: a case series and review of the literature. *J Drugs Dematol.* Aug 2007;6(8):825–828.

214. Whitmore JJ, Burt MM, Fowler RS, Halar E, Bernie R. Bandaging the lower extremity to control swelling: figure-8 versus spiral technique. *Arch Phys Med Rehabil.* 1972;53(10):487–490.

215. Vitale M, Fields-Blache C, Luterman A. Severe itching in the patient with burns. *J Burn Care Rehabil*. 1991;12(4):330–333.

216. Field T, Peck M, et al. Postburn itching, pain, and psychological symptoms are reduced with massage therapy. *J Burn Care Rehabil*. 2000;21(3):189–193.

217. Van Zuijlen PP, Kreis RW, Vloemans AF, Groenevelt F, Mackie DP. The prognostic factors regarding long-term functional outcome of full-thickness hand burns. *Burns*. 1999;25(8):709–714.

218. Gibson T, Kenedi RM. Biomechanical properties of skin. *Surg Clin North Am*. 1967;47(2):279–294.

219. Lanir Y. The fibrous structure of the skin and its relation to mechanical behavior. In: Marks R, Payne PA, eds. *Bioengineering and the Skin: Based on the Proceedings of the European Society for Dermatological Research Symposium, Held at the Welsh National School of Medicine, Cardiff, 19–21 July 1979*. Boston, Mass: MTP Press; 1981: 93–96.

220. Oxlund H, Manschot J, Viidik A. The role of elastin in the mechanical properties of skin. *J Biomech*. 1988;21(3):213–218.

221. Gibson T, Kenedi RM. The structural components of the dermis and their mechanical characteristics. In: Bently JP, Dobson RL, Montagna W, eds. *The Dermis; Proceedings of a Symposium on the Biology of Skin held at Salishan Lodge, Gleneden Beach, Oregon, 1968*. New York, NY: Appleton-Century-Crofts; 1970.

222. Bartell TH, Monafo WW, Mustoe TA. A new instrument for serial measurements of elasticity in hypertrophic scar. *J Burn Care Rehabil*. 1988;9(6):657–660.

223. Clark JA, Cheng JCY, Leung KS, Leung PC. Mechanical characteristics of human postburn hypertrophic skin during pressure therapy. *J Biomech*. 1987;20:397–406.

224. Richard RL, Staley MJ. Biophysical aspects of normal skin and burn scar. In: Richard R, Staley MJ, eds. *Burn Care and Rehabilitation: Principles and Practice*. Philadelphia, Pa: FA Davis; 1994:49–69.

225. Koepke GH. The role of physical medicine in the treatment of burns. *Surg Clin North Am*. 1970;50(6):1385–1399.

226. Arem AJ, Madden JW. Effects of stress on healing wounds: I. Intermittent noncyclical tension. *J Surg Res*. 1976;20(2):93–102.

227. Viidik A. On the rheology and morphology of soft collagenous tissue. *J Anat*. 1969;105:184.

228. Escoffier C, de Rigal J, Rochefort A, Vasselet R, Lévêque JL, Agache PG. Age-related mechanical properties of human skin: an in vivo study. *J Invest Dermatol*. 1989;93(3):353–357.

229. Wilhelmi BJ, Blackwell SJ, Mancoll JS, Phillips LG. Creep vs. stretch: a review of the viscoelastic properties of skin. *Ann Plast Surg*. 1998;41(2):215–219.

230. Minns RJ, Soden PD, Jackson DS. The role of the fibrous components and ground substance in the mechanical properties of biological tissue: a preliminary investigation. *J Biomech*. 1973;6(2):153–165.

231. Richard R, Miller S, Staley M, Johnson RM. Multimodal versus progressive treatment techniques to correct burn scar contractures. *J Burn Care Rehabil*. 2000;21(6):506–512.

232. Andersen KN, ed. *Mosby's Medical, Nursing, and Allied Health Dictionary*. 4th ed. Saint Louis, Mo: Mosby; 1994: 1469.

233. Coppard BM, Lohman H, eds. *Introduction to Splinting*. Saint Louis, Mo: Mosby; 2001.

234. Richard R, Chapman T, Dougherty M, Franzen B, Serghiou M. *An Atlas and Compendium of Burn Splints*. San Antonio, Tex: Reg Richard, Inc; 2006.

235. Boscheinen-Morrin J, Conolly WB, eds. *The Hand: Fundamentals of Therapy*. Boston, MA: Butterworth-Heinemann; 2001.

236. Madden JW, Enna CD. The management of acute thermal injuries to the upper extremity. *J Hand Surg [Am]*. 1983;8:785–788.

237. Peacock EE Jr. *Wound repair*. 3rd ed. Philadelphia, Pa: WB Saunders; 1984.

238. Hartford CE, Kealey GP, Lavelle WE, Buckner H. An appliance to prevent and treat microstomia from burns. *J Trauma*. 1975;15(4):356–360.

239. Yeakel M. Occupational therapy. In: Artz CP, Moncrief JA, Pruitt Jr BA, eds. *Burns: a Team Approach*. Philadelphia, Pa: Saunders; 1979: 507.

240. Willis B. A follow-up. The use of orthoplast isoprene splints in the treatment of the acutely burned child. *Am J Occup Ther*. 1970;24;187–191.

241. Malick MH, Carr JA. Halo neck splint. In: Malick MH, Carr JA, eds. *Manual on Management of the Burn Patient: Including Splinting, Mold and Pressure Techniques*. Pittsburgh, Pa: Harmarville Rehabilitation Center; 1982: 55–56.

242. Perkins K, Davey RB, Wallis KA. Silicone gel: a new treatment for burn scars and contractures. *Burns Incl Them Inj*. 1983;9(3):201–204.

243. Braddon RL, Boe L, Flowers L, Johnson-Vann T. The physical treatment and rehabilitation of burn patients. In: Hummel RP, ed. *Clinical Burn Therapy: a Management and Prevention Guide*. Boston, Mass: Wright/PSG; 1982: 287.

244. Lavore JS, Marshall JH. Expedient splinting of the burned patient. *Phys Ther*. 1972;52(10):1036–1042.

245. Palm L, Reming RL, Moylan JA. A method for splinting the upper extremity of thermally injured patients. *Proc Am Burn Assoc*. 1972;4:91.

246. Daugherty M, Carr-Collins J. Splinting techniques for the burn patient. In: Richard RL, Staley MJ, eds. *Burn Care and Rehabilitation: Principles and Practice*. Philadelphia, Pa: FA Davis; 1994: 287–291.

247. Hogan L, Uditsky T. *Pediatric Splinting: Selection, Fabrication, and Clinical Application of Upper Extremity Splints*. San Antonio, TX: Therapy Skill Builders; 1998: 18.

248. Brand P. The forces of dynamic splinting: ten questions before applying a dynamic splint to the hand. In: Mackin E, Callahan A, Skirven T, Schneider L, Osterman A, eds. *Rehabilitation of the Hand and Upper Extremity*. 5th ed. Saint Louis, MO: Mosby; 2002.

249. Fess EE, Philips CA. *Hand Splinting: Principles and Methods*. 2nd ed. Saint Louis, Mo: Mosby; 1987.

250. Shah M, Lopez JK, Escalante AS, Green DP. Dynamic splinting of forearm rotational contracture after distal radius fracture. *J Hand Surg [Am]*. 2002;27(3):456–463.

251. Quick CD. Dorsal Wrist Extension Fulcrum Splint. Available at: http://www.burntherapist.com/images/SplintQuarter1-07/1stQuarter07Submission.pdf. Accessed January 14, 2009.

252. Colditz JC. Splinting peripheral nerve injuries. In: Hunter JM, Schneider LH, Mackin EJ, Callaghan AD, eds. *Rehabilitation of the Hand: Surgery and Therapy*. 3rd ed. Saint Louis, Mo: Mosby; 1990: 647–657.

253. Colditz JC. Splinting for radial nerve palsy. *J Hand Ther*. 1987;1:18–23.

254. Schultz-Johnson KS. Splinting: a problem-solving approach. In: Stanley BG, Tribuzi SM, eds. *Concepts in Hand Rehabilitation*. Philadelphia, Pa: FA Davis; 1992: 238–271.

255. Schultz-Johnson K. Static progressive splinting. *J Hand Ther*. 2002;15(2):163–178.

256. Flowers KR. A proposed decision hierarchy for splinting the stiff joint, with an emphasis on force application parameters. *J Hand Ther*. 2002;15(2):158–162.

257. Griffin A. Therapist's management of the stiff elbow. In: Mackin E, Callahan A, Skirven T, Schneider L, Osterman A, eds. *Rehabilitation of the Hand and Upper Extremity*. 5th ed. Saint Louis, Mo: Mosby; 2002.

258. Bennett GB, Helm P, Purdue GF, Hunt JL. Serial casting: a method for treating burn contractures. *J Burn Care Rehabil.* 1989;10(6):543–545.

259. Johnson J, Silverberg R. Serial casting of the lower extremity to correct contractures during the acute phase of burn care. *Phys Ther.* 1995;75(4):262–266.

260. Colditz JC. Plaster of Paris: the forgotten hand splinting material. *J Hand Ther.* 2002;15(2):144–157.

261. Ridgway CL, Daugherty MB, Warden GD. Serial casting as a technique to correct burn scar contractures. A case report. *J Burn Care Rehabil.* 1991;12(1):67–72.

262. Staley M, Serghiou M. Casting guidelines, tips, and techniques: proceedings from the 1997 American Burn Association PT/OT Casting Workshop. *J Burn Care Rehabil.* 1998;19(3):254–260.

263. Heimbach DM, Engrav LH. *Surgical Management of the Burn Wound.* New York, NY: Raven Press; 1984: 83–98.

264. Johnson CL, O'Shaughnessy EJ, Ostergren G. *Burn Management.* New York, NY: Raven Press; 1981: 79.

265. Nothdurft D, Smith PS, LeMaster J. Exercise and treatment modalities. In: Fisher SV, Helm PA, eds. *Comprehensive Rehabilitation of Burns.* Baltimore, Md: Williams & Wilkins; 1984: 6–147.

266. Covey MH. Application of CPM devices with burn patients. *J Burn Care Rehabil.* 1988;9(5):496–497.

267. Salter RB. The biologic concept of continuous passive motion of synovial joints. The first 18 years of basic research and its clinical application. *Clin Orthop Relat Res.* 1989;242:12–25.

268. Peters WJ. Heterotopic ossification: can early surgery be performed, with a positive bone scan? *J Burn Care Rehabil.* 1990;11(4):318–321.

269. Edlich RF, Horowitz JH, Rheuban KS, Nichter LS, Morgan RF. Heterotopic calcification and ossification in the burn patient. *J Burn Care Rehabil.* 1985;6(4):363–368.

270. Roberts ML, Pruitt BA. Nursing care and psychological considerations. In: Artz CP, Moncrief JA, Pruitt Jr BA, eds. *Burns: a Team Approach.* Philadelphia, Pa: Saunders; 1979: 370–389.

271. Harnar T, Engrav LH, Marvin J, Heimbach D, Cain V, Johnson C. Dr. Paul Unna's boot and early ambulation after skin grafting the leg: a survey of burn centers and a report of 20 cases. *Plast Reconstr Surg.* 1982;69(2):359–360.

272. Duncan CE. Use of a ramp surface for lower extremity exercise with burn-injured patients. *J Burn Care Rehabil.* 1989;10(4):346–349.

273. Kisner C, Colby LA. *Therapeutic Exercise: Foundations and Techniques.* 3rd ed. Philadelphia, Pa: FA Davis; 1996.

274. Richard RL, Staley MJ. Burn patient evaluation and treatment planning. In: Richard RL, Staley MJ, eds. *Burn Care and Rehabilitation: Principles and Practice.* Philadelphia, Pa: FA Davis; 1994.

275. Light KE, Nuzik S, Personius W, Barstrom A. Low-load prolonged stretch vs. high-load brief stretch in treating knee contractures. *Phys Ther.* 1984;64(3):330–333.

276. Helm P, Herndon DN, DeLateur B. Restoration of function. *J Burn Care Res.* 2007;28(4):611–614.

277. Trees D, Ketelsen C, Hobbs JA. Use of modified tilt table for preambulation strength training as an adjunct to burn rehabilitation: a case series. *J Burn Care Rehabil.* 2003;24(2):97–103.

278. Schmitt MA, French L, Kalil ET. How soon is safe? Ambulation of the patient with burns after lower-extremity skin grafting. *J Burn Care Rehabil.* 1991;12:33–37.

279. Burnsworth B, Krob MJ, Langer-Schnepp M. Immediate ambulation of patients with lower-extremity grafts. *J Burn Care Rehabil.* 1992;13:89–92.

280. Goodman CC, Boissonnault WG, Fuller KS. *Pathology: Implications for the Physical Therapist.* 2nd ed. Philadelphia, Pa: Saunders; 2003.

281. Davis C. *Complementary Therapies in Rehabilitation: Evidence for Efficacy in Therapy, Prevention, and Wellness.* Thorofare, NJ: SLACK; 2004.

282. *ACSM's Guidelines for Exercise Testing and Prescription.* 5th ed. Philadelphia, Pa: Lippincott, Williams & Wilkins; 1995.

283. Cronan T, Hammond J, Ward CG. The value of isokinetic exercise and testing in burn rehabilitation and determination of back-to-work status. *J Burn Care Rehabil.* 1990;11(3):224–227.

284. Austin KG, Hansbrough JF, Dore JF, Noordenbos J, Buono MJ. Thermoregulation in burn patients during exercise. *J Burn Care Rehabil.* 2003;24(1):9–14.

285. Wetzel JL, Giuffrida C, Petrazzi A, et al. Comparison of measures of physiologic stress during treadmill exercise in a patient with 20% lower extremity burn injuries and healthy matched and nonmatched individuals. *J Burn Care Rehabil.* 2000;21(4):359–366.

286. Pedretti LW. Activities of daily living. In: Pedretti LW, Zoltan B, eds. *Occupational Therapy: Practice Skills for Physical Dysfunction.* 3rd ed. Baltimore, Md: Mosby; 1990: 230–271.

287. Cheng S, Rogers JC. Changes in occupational role performance after a severe burn: a retrospective study. *Am J Occup Ther.* 1989;43(1):17–24.

288. Rivers EA, Fisher SV. Rehabilitation for burn patients. In: Krusen FH, Kottke FJ, Lehmann JF, eds. *Krusen's Handbook of Physical Medicine and Rehabilitation.* Philadelphia, Pa: Saunders; 1990: 1070–1101.

289. Wagner MM. *Care of the Burn-Injured Patient: a Multidisciplinary Involvement.* Littleton, Mass: PSG Publishing; 1981: 151–153.

290. Hales RE, Travis TW. Exercise as a treatment option for anxiety and depressive disorders. *Mil Med.* 1987;152(6):299–302.

291. Friedmann J, Shapiro J, Plon L. Psychosocial treatment and pain control. In: Achauer BM, ed. *Management of the Burned Patient.* Norwalk, Conn: Appleton & Lange; 1987: 244–262.

292. Tobiasen JM, Hiebert JM. Burns and adjustment to injury: do psychological coping strategies help? *J Trauma.* 1985;25(12):1151–1155.

293. Cromes FG Jr. Psychosocial aspects. In: Fisher SV, Helm PA, eds. *Comprehensive Rehabilitation of Burns.* Baltimore, Md: Williams & Wilkins; 1984: 330–352.

294. Watkins PN, Cook EL, May SR, Ehleben CM. Psychological stages in adaptation following burn injury: a method for facilitating psychological recovery of burn victims. *J Burn Care Rehabil.* 1988;9(4):376.

295. Summers TM. Psychosocial support of the burned patient. *Crit Care Nurs Clin North Am.* 1991;3(2):237–344.

296. Benson H. *Beyond the Relaxation Response: How to Harness the Healing Power of Your Personal Beliefs.* New York, NY: Times Books; 1984: 150.

297. Rivers EA. Rehabilitation management of the burn patient. In: Eisenberg MG, Grzesiak RC, eds. *Advances in Clinical Rehabilitation.* New York, NY: Springer; 1987: 177–214.

298. Krach LE, Fisher SV, Butzer SC, et al. Electrical injury: longterm outcome [abstract]. *Arch Phys Med Rehabil.* 1979;60:533.

299. Resick PA, Monson CM, Chard KM. *Cognitive Processing Therapy: Veteran/Military version*. Washington DC: US Department of Veterans Affairs; June 2007.

300. Blumenfield M, Schoeps M. Reintegrating the healed burned adult into society: psychological problems and solutions. *Clin Plas Surg*. 1992;19(3):599–605.

301. Adams RB, Tribble GC, Tafel AC, Edlich RF. Cardiovascular rehabilitation of patients with burns. *J Burn Care Rehabil*. 1990;11(3):246–255.

302. Thompson TL, Steele BF. The psychological aspects of pain. In: Simons RC, ed. *Understanding Human Behavior in Health and Illness*. 3rd ed. Baltimore, Md: Williams & Wilkins; 1985: 60–67.

303. American Medical Association. *Guides to the Evaluation of Permanent Impairment*. Chicago, Ill: AMA; 1984.

304. Sheridan R. Burn Rehabilitation. eMedicine from WebMD. Available at: http://emedicine.medscape.com/article/318436-overview. Accessed January 13, 2009.

305. Blakeney P, Partridge J, Rumsey N. Community integration. *J Burn Care Res*. 2007:28(4):598–601.

306. Haley J. *Uncommon Therapy: The Psychiatric Techniques of Milton H. Erickson, M.D.* New York, NY: WW Norton; 1973.

307. Bogaerts F, Boeckx W. Burns and sexuality. *J Burn Care Rehabil*. 1992;13(1):39–43.

308. Varghese G. Musculoskeletal considerations. In: Fisher SV, Helm PA, eds. *Comprehensive Rehabilitation of Burns*. Baltimore, MD: Williams & Wilkins; 1984: 242–248.

309. DeLisa JA. Rehabilitation of the patient with burns. In: *Rehabilitation Medicine: Principles and Practice*. Phildelphia, Pa: Lippincott; 1988: 821–839.

310. Artz CP, Moncrief JA, Pruitt BA. Burns: a team approach. Philadelphia, Pa: Saunders; 1979.

311. Young A. Rehabilitation of burn injuries. *Phys Med Rehabil Clin N Am*. 2002;13(1):85–108.

312. Banovac K, Gonzalez F, Renfree KJ. Treatment of heterotopic ossification after spinal cord injury. *J Spinal Cord Med*. 1997;20(1):60–65.

313. Shafer DM, Bay C, Caruso DM, Foster KN. The use of eidronate disodium in the prevention of heterotopic ossification in burn patients. *Burns*. 2008;34(3):355–360.

314. Yang SC, Chen AC, Chao EK, Yuan LJ, Lee MS, Ueng SW. Early surgical management for heterotopic ossification about the elbow presenting as limited range of motion associated with ulnar neuropathy. *Chang Gung Med J*. 2002;25(4):245–252.

315. Crawford CM, Varghese G, Mani MM, Neff JR. Heterotopic ossification: are range of motion exercises contraindicated? *J Burn Care Rehabil*. 1986;7(4):323–327.

316. Stover SL, Hataway CJ, Zeiger HE. Heterotopic ossification in spinal cord-injured patients. *Arch Phys Med Rehabil*. 1975;56(5):199–204.

317. Yowler CJ, Mozingo DW, Ryan JB, Pruitt BA Jr. Factors contributing to delayed extremity amputation in burn patients. *J Trauma*. 1998;45(3):522–526.

318. Viscardi PJ, Polk HC Jr. Outcome of amputations in patients with major burns. *Burns*. 1995;21:526–529.

319. García-Sánchez V, Gomez Morell P. Electric burns: high- and low-tension injuries. *Burns*. 1999;25(4):357–360.

320. Hussman J, Kucan JO, Russell RC, Bradley T, Zamboni WA. Electrical injuries—morbidity, outcome and treatment rationale. *Burns*. 1995;21(7):530–535.

321. Mann R, Gibran N, Engrav L, Heimbach D. Is immediate decompression of high voltage electrical injuries to the upper extremity always necessary? *J Trauma*. 1996;40(4):584–589.

322. Rai J, Jeschke MG, Barrow RE, Herndon DN. Electrical injuries: a 30-year review. *J Trauma*. 1999;46(5):933–936.

323. Tredget EE, Shankowsky HA, Tilley WA. Electrical injuries in Canadian burn care: identification of unsolved problems. *Ann N Y Acad Sci*. 1999;888:75–87.

324. Vadalouca A, Siafaka I, Argyra E, Vrachnou E, Moka E. Therapeutic management of chronic neuropathic pain: an examination of pharmacologic treatment. *Ann N Y Acad Sci*. 2006;1088:164–186.

325. Braddom RL. Rehabilitation of patients with burns. In: Braddom RL, Buschbacher RM, eds. *Physical Medicine and Rehabilitation*. 2nd ed. Philadelphia, Pa: Saunders; 2000: 1321–1342.

326. Helm PA. Neuromuscular considerations. In: Fisher SV, Helm PA, eds. *Comprehensive Rehabilitation of Burns*. Baltimore, Md: Williams & Wilkins; 1984: 235–241.

327. Hettrick HH, O'Brien K, Laznick H, et al. Effect of transcutaneous electrical nerve stimulation for the management of burn pruritus: a pilot study. *J Burn Care Rehabil*. 2004;25(3):236–240.

328. Prigerson HG, Maciejewski PK, Rosenheck RA. Combat trauma: trauma with highest risk of delayed onset and unresolved posttraumatic stress disorder symptoms, unemployment, and abuse among men. *J Nerv Ment Dis*. 2001;189(2):99–108.

329. Fauerbach JA, McKibben J, Bienvenu OJ, et al. Psychological distress after major burn injury. *Psychosom Med*. 2005;69(5):473–482.

330. Vasterling JJ, Proctor SP, Amoroso P, Kane R, Heeren T, White R. Neuropsychological outcomes of Army personnel following deployment to the Iraqi war. *JAMA*. 2006;296(5):519–529.

331. Faber AW, Klasen HJ, Sauër EW, Vuister F. Psychological and social problems in burn patients after discharge. A follow-up study. *Scand J Plast Reconstr Surg*. 1987;21(3):307–309.

332. Smith M, Doctor M, Boulter T. Unique considerations in caring for a pediatric burn patient: a developmental approach. *Crit Care Nurs Clin North Am*. 2004;16(1):99–108.

333. Howard SK, Rosekind MR, Katz JD, Berry AJ. Fatigue in anesthesia: implications and strategies for patient and provider safety. *Anesthesiology*. 2002;97(5):1281–1294.

334. Lydic R, Baghdoyan HA. Sleep, anesthesiology, and the neurobiology of arousal state control. *Anesthesiology*. 2005;103(6):1268–1295.

335. Zadra A, Pilon M, Donderi DC. Variety and intensity of emotions in nightmares and bad dreams. *J Nerv Ment Dis*. 2006;194(4):249–254.

336. Grace JB, Holmes J. The management of behavioural and psychiatric symptoms in delirium. *Expert Opin Pharmacother*. 2006;7(5):555–561.

337. Tuunainen A, Wahlbeck K, Gilbody S. Newer atypical antipsychotic medication in comparison to clozapine: a systematic review of randomized trials. *Schizophr Res*. 2002;56(1-2):1–10.

338. Hollander AC, Ekblad S, Mukhamadiev D, Muminova R. The validity of screening instruments for posttraumatic stress disorder, depression, and other anxiety symptoms in Tajikistan. *J Nerv Ment Dis*. 2007;195(11):955–958.

339. Kessler RC, Sonnega A, Bromet E, Hughes M, Nelson CB. Posttraumatic stress disorder in the National Comorbidity Survey. *Arch Gen Psychiatry*. 1995;52(12):1048–1060.

340. Browne G, Byrne C, Brown B, et al. Psychosocial adjustment of burn survivors. *Burns Incl Therm Inj*. 1985;12(1):28–35.

341. Pivar IL, Field NP. Unresolved grief in combat veterans with PTSD. *J Anxiety Disord*. 2004;18(6):745–755.

342. Cahners SS, Bernstein NR. Rehabilitating families with burned children. *Scand J Plast Reconstr Surg*. 1979;13(1):173–175.

343. Shelby J, Sullivan J, Groussman M, Gray R, Saffle J. Severe burn injury: effects on psychologic and immunologic function in noninjured close relatives. *J Burn Care Rehabil*. 1992;13(1):58–63.

344. Langeland W, Hartgers C. Child sexual and physical abuse and alcoholism: a review. *J Stud Alcohol*. 1998;59(3):336–348.

345. Burd A, Huang L. Hypertrophic response and keloid diathesis: two very different forms of scar. *Plast Reconstr Surg*. 2005;116(7):150e–157e.

346. Cummings GS, Crutchfield CA, Barnes MR. *Soft Tissue Changes in Contractures*. In: Orthopedic physical therapy series. Atlanta, Ga: Stokesville Publishing; 1983.

347. Greenhalgh DG, Staley MJ. Burn wound healing. In: Richard RL, Staley MJ, eds. *Burn Care and Rehabilitation: Principles and Practice*. Philadelphia, Pa: FA Davis; 1994: 70–102.

348. Deitch EA, Wheelahan TM, Rose MP, Clothier J, Cotter J. Hypertrophic burn scars: analysis of variables. *J Trauma*. 1983;23(10):895–898.

349. Rudolph R. The effect of skin graft preparation on wound contraction. *Surg Gynecol Obstet*. 1976;142(1):49–56.

350. Staley MJ, Richard RL. Scar management. In: Richard RL, Staley MJ, eds. *Burn Care and Rehabilitation: Principles and Practice*. Philadelphia, Pa: FA Davis; 1994: 381.

351. Linares HA. Hypertrophic healing: controversies and etiopathogenic review. In: Carvajal HF, Parks DH, eds. *Burns in Children: Pediatric Burn Management*. Chicago, Ill: Year Book Medical Publishers; 1988: 305–323.

352. Shakespeare PG, van Renterghem L. Some observations on the surface structure of collagen in hypertrophic scars. *Burns Incl Therm Inj*. 1985;11(3):175–180.

353. Berman B, Zell D, Perez O. *Keloid and Hypertrophic Scar*. eMedicine from WebMD. Available at: http://emedicine.medscape.com/article/1057599-overview. Accessed January 12, 2009.

354. Yamaguchi Y, Brenner M, Hearing VJ. The regulation of skin pigmentation. *J Biol Chem*. 2007;282(38):27557–27561.

355. Rauschuber E. Scar Management, Therapy Skills Builders Course. San Antonio, Tex: The Psychological Corporation; 1998.

356. Jewell L, Guerrero R, Quesada AR, Chan LS, Garner WL. Rate of healing in skin-grafted burn wounds. *Plast Reconstr Surg*. 2007;120(2):451–456.

357. Costa AM, Peyrol S, Pôrto LC, Comparin JP, Foyatier JL, Desmoulière A. Mechanical forces induce scar remodeling. Study in non-pressure-treated versus pressure-treated hypertrophic scars. *Am J Pathol*. 1999;155(5):1671–1679.

358. Davey RB. The place of "contact media" in a burn scar management programme. *Eur J Plast Surg*. 1998;21(1):24–27.

359. Ahn ST, Monafo WW, Mustoe TA. Topical silicone gel: a new treatment for hypertrophic scars. *Surgery*. 1989;106(4):781–787.

360. Mustoe TA. Evolution of silicone therapy and mechanism of action in scar management. *Aesthetic Plast Surg*. 2008;32(1):495–500.

361. Cuccurullo SJ. *Physical Medicine and Rehabilitation Board Review*. New York, NY: Demos; 2004.

362. Wust KJ. A modified dynamic mouth splint for burn patients. *J Burn Care Res*. 2006;27(1):86–92.

363. Robertson CF, Zuker R, Dabrowski B, Levison H. Obstructive sleep apnea: a complication of burns to the head and neck in children. *J Burn Care Rehabil*. 1985;(6):353–357.

364. Leung KS, Cheng JC, Ma GF, Clark JA, Leung PC. Complications of pressure therapy for post-burn hypertrophic scars. Biochemical analysis based on 5 patients. *Burns Incl Therm Inj*. 1984;10(6):434–438.

365. Bruster JM, Pullium G. Gradient pressure. *Am J Occup Ther*. 1983;37(7):485–488.

366. Kealey GP, Jensen KL, Laubenthal KN, Lewis RW. Prospective randomized comparison of two types of pressure therapy garments. *J Burn Care Rehabil*. 1990;11(4):334–336.

367. Allely R, Van-Buendia LB, Jeng JC, et al. Laser Doppler imaging of cutaneous blood flow through transparent face masks: a necessary preamble to computer-controlled rapid prototyping fabrication with submillimeter precision. *J Burn Care Res*. 2008;29(1):42–48.

368. Smith K, Owens K. Physical and occupational therapy burn unit protocol–benefits and uses. *J Burn Care Rehabil*. 1985;6(6):506–508.

369. Malick MH, Carr JA. *Manual on Management of the Burn Patient: Including Splinting, Mold and Pressure Techniques*. Pittsburgh, Pa: Harmarville Rehabilitation Center, Educational Resource Division; 1982.

370. Van den Kerchhove E, Boeckx W, Kochuyt A. Silicone patches as a supplement for pressure therapy to control hypertrophic scarring. *J Burn Care Rehabil*. 1991;12(4):361–369.

371. Quinn KJ. Silicone gel in scar treatment. *Burns Incl Therm Inj*. 1987;13(suppl):S33–S40.

372. American Society of Plastic Surgeons. Reconstructive surgery: procedures at a glance. Available at: http://www.plasticsurgery.org/patients_consumers/procedures/ReconstructiveSurgery.cfm. Accessed August 23, 2007.

373. Achauer BM. *Burn Reconstruction*. New York, NY: Thieme Medical Publishers; 1991.

374. Salisbury RE, Bevin AG. *Atlas of Reconstructive Burn Surgery*. Philadelphia, Pa: Saunders; 1981: 164.

375. Monafo WW, Creekmore H. Electrical injuries of the scalp. In: Wachtel TL, Frank DH, eds. *Burns of the Head and Neck*. Philadelphia, PA: Saunders; 1984; 29: 94–111.

376. Achauer BM. Reconstructing the burned face. *Clin Plast Surg*. 1992;19(3):623–636.

377. Ben-Simchon C, Tsur H, Keren G, Epstein Y, Shapiro Y. Heat intolerance in patients with extensive healed burns. *Plast Reconstr Surg*. 1981;67(4):499–504.

378. Roskind JL, Petrofsky J, Lind AR, Paletta FX. Quantitation of thermoregulatory impairment in patients with healed burns. *Ann Plast Surg*. 1978;1(2):172–176.

379. Shapiro Y, Epstein Y, Ben-Simchon C, Tsur H. Thermoregulatory responses of patients with extensive healed burns. *J Appl Physiol*. 1982;53(4):1019–1022.

380. US Army Human Resources Command. Army Physical Disability Evaluation System Web site. Available at: https://www.hrc.army.mil/site/active/tagd/pda/pdesystem.htm. Accessed January 14, 2009.

381. US Department of the Army. *Physical Evaluation for Retention, Retirement, or Separation*. Washington, DC: DA; 2006. Army Regulation 635-40, Para 1-1.

382. US Office of the Surgeon General, Medical Command, Patient Administration Division. Medical Evaluation Board Overview Brief. Available at: http://www.cs.amedd.army.mil/APDES/docs/CommandTeamInformation/MEB_OVERVIEW_BRIEF_(2).ppt. Accessed January 14, 2009.

383. Blakeney PE, Rosenberg L, Rosenberg M, Faber AW. Psychosocial care of persons with severe burns. *Burns*. 2008;34(4):433–440.

Chapter 14

HEARING IMPAIRMENT AMONG SOLDIERS: SPECIAL CONSIDERATIONS FOR AMPUTEES

DEBRA J. WILMINGTON, PhD*; M. SAMANTHA LEWIS, PhD†; PAULA J. MYERS, PhD‡; FREDERICK J. GALLUN, PhD§; AND STEPHEN A. FAUSTI, PhD¥

*Research Investigator, National Center for Rehabilitative Auditory Research, Portland VA Medical Center, 3710 SW US Veterans Hospital Road, Portland, Oregon 97207; Assistant Professor, Department of Otolaryngology, Oregon Health & Science University, 3181 SW Sam Jackson Park Road, Portland, Oregon 97239

†Research Investigator, National Center for Rehabilitative Auditory Research, Portland VA Medical Center, 3710 SW US Veterans Hospital Road, Portland, Oregon 97207; Assistant Professor, Department of Otolaryngology, Oregon Health & Science University, 3181 SW Sam Jackson Park Road, Portland, Oregon 97239

‡Chief, Audiology Section, Department of Audiology and Speech Pathology, James A. Haley Veterans Hospital, 13000 Bruce B. Downs Boulevard, Tampa, Florida 33612; formerly, Pediatric Audiologist, All Children's Hospital, Saint Petersburg, Florida

§Research Investigator, National Center for Rehabilitative Auditory Research, Portland VA Medical Center, 3710 SW US Veterans Hospital Road, Portland, Oregon 97207; Assistant Professor, Department of Otolaryngology, Oregon Health & Science University, 3181 SW Sam Jackson Park Road, Portland, Oregon 97239

¥Director, National Center for Rehabilitative Auditory Research, Portland VA Medical Center, 3710 SW US Veterans Hospital Road, Portland, Oregon 97207; Professor, Department of Otolaryngology, Oregon Health & Science University, 3181 SW Sam Jackson Park Road, Portland, Oregon 97239

INTRODUCTION

Injuries to the ear were the single most common injury type reported among Marines during Operation Iraqi Freedom (OIF) through 2004, accounting for 23% of all injuries.[1] One third of soldiers returning from Operation Enduring Freedom (OEF) and OIF were referred to audiologists for hearing evaluations because of exposure to acute acoustic blasts; 72% of those sustained hearing loss. Auditory disabilities represent one of the most prevalent service-connected disabilities, resulting in over one billion dollars in annual compensation. Acute blast trauma and resultant traumatic brain injury (TBI) make up 90% of the injuries seen at the Department of Veterans Affairs (VA) polytrauma rehabilitation centers, and an additional 11% to 28% of OEF and OIF troops may have mild TBI from blast exposure.[2] Polytrauma patients require care for hearing impairment, vestibular pathology, vision loss, nerve damage, multiple bone fractures, wounds, psychological problems, and amputations.[3] Soldiers with amputations and hearing impairment present significant challenges because their injuries affect multiple systems, often impairing communication and cognition. In addition, each patient has distinctive psychosocial requirements that greatly impact pain management, adjustment to disability, body image perception, movement through the military disability system, and reintegration into the community or back to active-duty status.[4] Furthermore, sensorineural hearing loss, unlike many other injuries, will continue to progress, creating greater impairment for the injured soldier. Early identification and treatment of hearing loss and vestibular impairment is essential to developing treatment strategies, ultimately leading to reduced cognitive deficits and improved rehabilitation outcomes and quality of life.[5]

TYPES OF HEARING LOSS

For service members with limb loss, the types of hearing damage sustained are not fundamentally different from those that could accompany any other type of injury. Hearing loss can result from a blast injury, from explosion or weapon firing (acoustic trauma), or from ototoxic medications used to treat injuries. The combined effect of trauma, noise exposure, and ototoxic agents (such as solvents or medications) can also result in hearing loss or vestibular impairment. Complex polytrauma patients commonly have hearing and balance deficits, which are often initially overlooked. TBI patients with hearing loss can also be misdiagnosed as unresponsive.[6] Clinical complaints from hearing-loss patients rarely occur until a communication problem becomes significant, indicating reduced audibility within the frequency range important for speech understanding (less than 8 kHz). Also, vestibular problems can be misdiagnosed in patients with lower limb amputation because impaired balance may be attributed to the limb loss. It is essential that auditory and vestibular deficits be identified early for possible intervention and so medical care and rehabilitation can be facilitated. Otologic consultation or, at the minimum, an audiometric hearing evaluation should be performed on the basis of exposure, regardless of symptoms. Damage to the outer or middle ear results in a conductive hearing loss, which can usually be corrected medically or surgically. Inner ear damage can result in permanent sensorineural hearing loss. Some otologic symptoms, such as tinnitus and hearing loss, may be permanent consequences of a blast injury, and their effects on quality of life may be substantial.[7]

Noise-Induced Hearing Loss

Sounds of a sufficient intensity and duration can cause temporary or permanent threshold shifts due to vascular, metabolic, and chemical changes of the hair cells of the cochlea and swelling of the auditory nerve endings. The stiffness of hair cell stereocilia can also decrease, which reduces the coupling of sound energy.[8] Recovery from temporary threshold shifts can occur if the noise exposure is not prolonged, although short exposures to sounds of sufficient intensity (such as explosions) can cause immediate, permanent hearing loss. Harmful noise exposure results in cell death by necrosis and apoptosis (programmed cell death), and eventually leads to the degeneration of the corresponding nerve fiber. Acoustic trauma typically produces a unilateral hearing loss without associated middle ear damage. The susceptibility to noise-induced hearing loss between individuals varies as much as 30 to 50 dB, possibly due to differences in ear anatomy and physiology, prior exposure to noise, and interactions with medications.[8]

Noise-induced hearing loss can occur as a result of steady-state or intermittent exposure to loud noise or from a single, impulsive exposure to a loud sound, such as an explosion (acoustic trauma). Steady-state exposure is usually symmetric, leading to bilateral sensorineural hearing loss, while some impulse noises, such as gunshots, can produce an asymmetric loss. Both steady-state and impulse noise exposure cause excessive oxidative stress and the production of free radicals (molecules that exist independently in an unstable state). To stabilize itself, a free radical takes available electrons from adjacent molecules, leaving them oxidized and therefore damaged. These changes lead to permanent cell damage in the inner ear. In addition, concurrent exposure to other agents, such as tobacco, solvents, or heavy metals, may have a synergistic effect on cell damage.[9] Soldiers in tactical situations who sustain acute noise-induced hearing loss may initially be unaware of it or delay reporting it because of the complexity of other injuries they have sustained, stress, fatigue, or the shock of the explosion.

Ototoxicity

Therapeutic drug regimens for infectious diseases and cancer can be ototoxic; nearly 200 prescription and over-the-counter drugs are recognized as having ototoxic potential and result in auditory or vestibular dysfunction. Ototoxicity causes irreversible cochlear damage and can occur in 60% to 70% of patients, often exacerbating preexisting hearing loss.[10] Clinical symptoms of ototoxicity are those commonly associated with hearing loss, such as tinnitus and difficulty understanding speech in noise. Hearing loss due to ototoxic medications is sensorineural, bilateral, and usually initially presents at high frequencies, subsequently progressing to the lower frequencies.[11–14] In addition, the effects of ototoxic drugs can continue well after cessation of therapeutic treatment. Previous noise exposure, almost universal in patients with blast injuries, increases the risk of ototoxicity.[15] Some ototoxic drugs commonly used to treat amputees for drug-resistant organisms (eg, gentamicin or vancomycin) can damage the vestibular system, causing instability and dizziness (dizziness, which includes vertigo, imbalance, and lightheadedness, can manifest with nausea, vomiting, a recurrent tendency to stumble or fall, floating feeling, mild unsteadiness, or faintness).[16]

Variations in the behavioral hearing threshold and number of frequencies affected suggest that individual susceptibility to ototoxicity is determined by multiple biochemical, physiologic, and genetic factors.[17] This individual susceptibility makes it difficult to determine which patients will experience ototoxic hearing changes and when the changes will occur. Therefore, high-frequency audiometry is essential to accurately identify and monitor ototoxic-induced hearing changes.

Audiologic Injury from Blast Exposure

Between 2003 and 2005, 68% of combat injuries in Afghanistan and Iraq were caused by explosions.[6] When exposed to the blast wave of an explosion, the auditory system is vulnerable to both peripheral and central damage from the pressure wave itself, and from the secondary and tertiary effects of blown objects impacting the body and the blown body impacting stationary objects (Figure 14-1). Blast trauma usually lasts longer and is more intense than acoustic trauma and typically affects both ears. The extent of damage from the primary blast injury is usually inversely proportional to the distance away from the blast. Due to the physics of blast waves, location within an environment may change the severity of injury, regardless of distance. Gases heated within a confined space may also result in a sustained period of positive pressure, and therefore prolonged injury. In general, closed-space blast injuries result in a higher incidence of primary blast injury, greater mortality, and greater injury severity.[18] Also, blast waves that are directed laterally to the head impact the auditory ear canal with a greater amount of energy, increasing the likelihood of ear injury. Permanent, pure sensorineural hearing loss is the most prevalent type of auditory impairment, occurring in 35% to 54% of blast injuries.[19]

One of the hallmark symptoms of unprotected blast exposure is injury to the tympanic membrane (TM) and, less frequently, to the ossicular chain. A ruptured TM indicates that a patient has undergone significant blast exposure and that further examination is warranted. The most common otologic complaints immediately following a blast are otalgia, tinnitus, aural fullness, dizziness, loudness sensitivity, distorted hearing, and hearing impairment. These complaints may last several minutes to several days. Hearing-related complaints may be due to a temporary threshold shift if present less than a month, or considered a permanent threshold shift if present over a month. Peripheral and central auditory system injury can combine to produce complex symptoms. The type of acoustic trauma, proximity, orientation of the ear to the blast, environment (open or closed space), and degree of ear shielding should be noted, when possible, in a patient's audiological case history.

Primary blast waves can cause concussions or mild TBI without a direct blow to the head by producing shock wave effects on the brain.[20] Concussions can cause audiologic symptoms, such as hearing loss, dizziness, and central deficits. Computed tomography scans and magnetic resonance imaging can detect pathology in the internal auditory canal, membranous

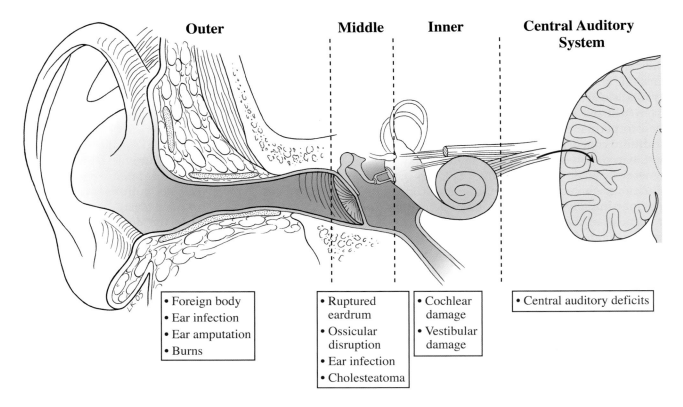

Outer

Middle **Inner**

Central Auditory System

- Foreign body
- Ear infection
- Ear amputation
- Burns

- Ruptured eardrum
- Ossicular disruption
- Ear infection
- Cholesteatoma

- Cochlear damage
- Vestibular damage

- Central auditory deficits

Figure 14-1. Blast injuries to the ear.
Drawing: Courtesy of Lynn H. Kitagawa, Veterans Affairs Medical Center, Portland, Oregon.

labyrinth, and bony labyrinth, and can characterize petrous apex lesions. Temporal bone fractures often cause loss of audiovestibular function. Auditory brain areas in the temporal lobe, corpus collosum, and thalamus are vulnerable to damage from exposure to the mechanisms of blast injury. Dizziness and sensitivity to sound can be symptoms of vestibular, peripheral, and central abnormality; posttraumatic stress disorder; concussion; and mild TBI. A thorough, multidisciplinary evaluation by specialists in neurology, otolaryngology, audiology, neuropsychology, physical therapy, and other related areas can facilitate appropriate diagnosis and treatment for patients with blast injuries and amputations. Long-term observation is important in all cases of blast-related auditory injuries because symptoms may be delayed. Postural instability and inner ear dysfunction may be evident up to 6 months or longer after blast trauma.[21]

Outer Ear Injury

The pinna can be damaged from flying debris and bomb fragments. Burns, contaminated debris, and purulent otorrhea in the ear canal are also frequently seen after exposure to blasts.[22,23] In addition, blasts can cause inner ear damage because of the impulse sound, location, and environment, leaving a patient with conductive, mixed, or sensorineural hearing loss. Alternatively, when the pinna is burned without associated noise-induced hearing loss or penetrating trauma, normal hearing sensitivity is often preserved. Burn patients, who are usually treated with antibiotics, are at risk for ototoxic sensorineural hearing loss and should be monitored accordingly.

Middle Ear Injury

Tympanic Membrane Perforation

When the primary shock wave reaches the end of the external auditory canal, it stretches and displaces the TM medially. Ruptured eardrums indicate that a patient has been exposed to peak pressure levels that far exceed those needed to produce damage to the inner ear, resulting in extensive hearing loss. The ear is much more sensitive to rupture pressure than other organs, with ruptures occurring in 50% of adults at 5 lb/in.² (approximately 185 dB peak pressure level) depending on the noise spectra and duration.[2,24,25] In contrast, pressure gradients of 56 to 76 lb/in^2 are needed to cause damage to other organs.[26] The improvised explosive devices causing injury in OIF and OEF produce pressures exceeding 60 lb/in^2, reaching peak pressure in about 2.5 to 50 milliseconds.

TM perforation is the most common injury to the middle ear, occurring during the positive phase of a blast. Typically, TM ruptures occur in the pars tensa, vary in appearance from linear tears to subtotal defects, and may have a protective effect because they reduce sound energy transmission to the inner ear.[23] TM rupture is also a clinical indicator that a patient has undergone a significant exposure, and it has been recommended as a diagnostic tool for determining whether or not a blast survivor has sustained life-threatening injuries. It may also be used as a potential marker for concussive injury.[22] However, the absence of TBI should not be assumed when TMs are intact.[27]

Clinical reports of TM rupture associated with ear infections range from 4% to 79% for explosion casualties.[1,28–30] Most TMs heal without surgical intervention, except in cases of resultant middle ear infection or when blast causes total TM perforation.

When the overpressure of a primary blast wave ruptures the eardrum, it sends small fragments of the squamous epithelium into the middle ear cavity. These cells may still be viable and grow into cholesteatomas that can infect or erode ossicles. Cholesteatomas usually present with conductive hearing loss and dizziness. Muscle weakness on the affected side can also occur. Careful surgical debridement is recommended for treatment, as is close follow up (10%–20% of cholesteatomas recur). Complications of cholesteatoma can include nerve damage and deafness.

Ossicular Disruption

The ossicles attach to the TM and transmit its vibrations to the cochlea, where the vibrations are converted into neural impulses via tiny hair cells. Overpressure can cause ossicle distortion and fracture. Ossicular damage is rare, usually occurring only with more severe blast trauma. Blasts that cause inner ear damage but spare the ossicular bones have been reported. A study of individuals exposed to blasts by explosive devices reported that ossicular damage occurred in 16% of patients, while 79% experienced TM perforations.[31] Injury to the middle ear structures usually results in relatively minor conductive hearing loss, compared to the extensive sensorineural hearing loss that can accompany exposure to impulsive

pressure waves. In addition, ossicular-chain disruption may absorb some of the incoming energy of the blast wave, sparing the sensory structures of the inner ear. In a small study of patients with ossicular-chain disruptions, subjects regained much of their hearing at the lower frequencies following surgical repair of the ossicles.[32]

Inner Ear Injury

Cochlear Injury

The cochlea at the Organ of Corti is less resilient than the ossicles. This delicate system is overwhelmed by the amplification of blast and sound waves, causing loss of structural integrity with damage of the inner and outer hair cells. The result is the development of conductive and sensorineural hearing loss[33] because the basilar membrane displacement tears and mechanically injures the sensory cells in the cochlea. Inner ear damage following explosions results from the combination of the blast wave and the subsequent impulse sound. Signs of otologic injury are usually present at the time of the blast and should be suspected in anyone presenting with hearing loss, tinnitus, otalgia, vertigo, bleeding from the external ear canal, TM rupture, or mucopurulent otorrhea. Immediately following a blast, casualties may experience temporary hearing loss and tinnitus; some may sustain permanent damage to the Organ of Corti.[7] Disruption of the oval or round window can cause permanent hearing loss.[22]

The risk of acoustic trauma exists at sound pressure levels exceeding 140 dB. In a blast injury, pressure levels may exceed 160 dB, subjecting the ear to both the pressure effect and the acoustic wave. The structures of the inner ear are exposed to mechanical forces exceeding the elastic compliance of the tissue. At lower sound pressure levels, the effects are thought to be conveyed via metabolic disturbances in the inner ear, which lead to subsequent sensory and neuronal damage.[34] Exposure to blasts in excess of 200 dB results in substantial TM and ossicular damage, but sensorineural hearing loss can be variable, with most losses having a recoverable temporary threshold shift. In general, sustained high-intensity noise causes more sensorineural damage than a single high-intensity blast.[32]

Pure sensorineural hearing loss is the most prevalent type of auditory impairment following blast injury.[19] Recent literature suggests that 35% to 100% of blast victims present with hearing loss.[7,33,35–37] Walter Reed Army Medical Center reported that 64% of blast injured patients seen in 2005 had ongoing hearing loss.[6] The audiometric configuration and degree of the hearing loss varied from normal hearing (typical of those who had shielding during the blast, such as headphones or earplugs), to high-frequency hearing loss at one or more frequencies (most likely presentation), to flat configurations from mild to severe hearing loss (primarily conductive or sensorineural), and in rare cases, profound deafness. Initial presentation can be mixed hearing loss (conductive element of TM perforation and mucosal lacerations of the middle ear and the sensorineural element due to mechanical injury). Although patients who have noise-induced hearing loss usually present with a 4 kHz "noise notch," or a decrease in hearing sensitivity around 4 kHz, those with blast injuries have a sloping high-frequency hearing loss that often affects frequencies below 8 kHz.

Vestibular Injury

Labyrinthine Damage

To maintain balance and postural stability, the vestibular system in the inner ear provides the brain with information about head movement via communication with the sensory organs (semicircular canals and otolith organs) and the eye, neck, arm, and leg muscles. Nerve connections from the semicircular canals and otoliths send information about head movement to the brain, resulting in eye movements that keep vision stable when the head moves. Similarly, nerve connections from the vestibular sensory organs to the brain send information to the neck, trunk, arms, and legs, resulting in posture changes that maintain balance. For the soldier with blast injury and amputation, it is possible that vestibular pathology, visual impairment, central pathology, certain medications, and proprioceptive changes all contribute to dizziness. The incidence of dizziness with mild head injuries ranges from 15% to 78%,[38,39] and is most often due to pathologies affecting the peripheral vestibular system, central nervous system (CNS), or cervical structures. In one of the few long-term studies on untreated patients with mild head trauma, vertigo persisted in 59% of patients after 5 years of recovery.[40] Compensation results from changes that occur within the CNS, rather than from changes in the peripheral vestibular system.[41] Following blast trauma, 27% of soldiers with amputation reported experiencing dizziness, and 18% reported experiencing vertigo.[16]

A primary care physician should rule out nonvestibular causes (orthostatic hypotension, postconcussive syndrome, TBI, ototoxic drugs, and visual impairment) of dizziness and an audiologist, otolaryngologist, and physical therapist can determine if dizziness is related to otovestibular pathology, such as peripheral disequilibrium, vertigo, or posttraumatic Ménière's disease.

TM injury can be complicated by a perilymph fistula, an often under-diagnosed condition in which a tear between the membranes of the inner and middle ear causes a perilymph leak that produces vertiginous symptoms.[39] Labyrinthine damage may also occur after blast injuries, resulting in complaints of vertigo.

Although blast injury often affects vestibular function, it is less common and the symptoms less defined than other auditory damage sustained during an explosion. Vestibular testing can typically determine the presence of a vestibular pathology, yet the cause of the vestibular disorder may remain unknown. In general, vestibular damage can occur to one or both ears, and may affect the sensory organs (semicircular canals or otoliths), the vestibular nerve, or its connections. The most common causes of vestibular disorders include benign paroxysmal positioning vertigo (BPPV), Ménière's disease, labyrinthitis, vestibular neuritis, and ototoxicity.

Head trauma as a result of blast injury is one of the most frequent causes of BPPV.[21] BPPV is characterized by brief (a few seconds to a minute), severe vertigo associated with changing head positions, such as looking up or rolling over in bed. Ménière's disease (or endolymphatic hydrops) results from an increase in the fluid of the inner ear and can be traumatically induced. It is characterized by attacks of vertigo, ringing or roaring in the ears, a feeling of pressure or fullness in the ear, and hearing loss. Attacks typically last several hours, but can vary in length and frequency.

Some acoustic trauma and dizziness studies also suggest that noise exposure may result in vestibular disturbance.[42] Asymmetric exposure to extremely intense (140 dB or above) sounds leads to a greater likelihood of producing vertigo. Finally, ototoxicity can cause temporary or permanent balance loss, hearing loss, or both. Individuals who lose unilateral peripheral vestibular information must depend on other components of the sensory system (visual and proprioception), further complicating the rehabilitation process for patients with visual field deficits and lower limb loss, particularly if they have uncompensated unilateral peripheral vestibular loss or bilateral vestibular loss.[41]

Central Vestibular Damage

Otologic effects of blast injuries can include centrally mediated symptoms. TBI as a result of the primary blast wave or subsequent blow to the head may lead to central vestibular pathology, peripheral vestibular pathology, or both. Central vestibular trauma may be due to postconcussive syndrome or cerebral or brainstem injuries.[43,44] Central vestibular pathology is less common than peripheral pathology in patients following head injury[45] and blast exposure.[37] In some cases, there may be evidence of both central and peripheral vestibular dysfunction.[45]

Central Auditory System Damage

While the presence of a ruptured TM is an obvious physical finding of blast exposure, the most detrimental effects of a blast may be less obvious and harder to treat. It is likely that patients with amputations resulting from blast exposure were either hit by flying objects (secondary damage) or were picked up by the blast wave and thrown into a stationary object, such as a vehicle or a wall (tertiary damage). In either case, there is a significant chance that the brain was also impacted. It is not known what proportion of those exposed to blasts sustained damage to the central auditory system; however, it has been well established that when an impact causes the brain to move to the extent that it impacts bone, contusions (hemorrhage and edema) occur, and the auditory processing areas of the temporal lobe are most commonly impacted.[46] Additionally, shearing, stretching, and angular forces of blast waves cause swelling and disconnection of axons in the central auditory system.[46] Damage to the CNS after an explosion has been increasingly attributed to the direct effects of the blast.[22] Inhalation of toxic chemicals (including materials such as paint and some industrial organic chemicals) may also affect the CNS and may present as vertigo or unsteadiness.[42]

There are a significant number of people who have normal hearing sensitivity following blast exposure, yet still complain of hearing difficulty. Central auditory dysfunction may contribute to these complaints, but diagnosis and treatment is challenging because the link between neural structures and function in central auditory processing (CAP) disorders has not been fully discerned. The lower brainstem nuclei, such as the inferior colliculus, are involved with comparing stimuli arriving from the ears ("binaural" processing). For this reason, only sensitivity to binaural relationships is affected by unilateral brainstem damage (bilateral lower brainstem damage is generally fatal). The thalamic nuclei in the upper brainstem can be damaged by shearing or stretching forces, resulting in deficits in determining the location or duration of sounds. Binaural "unmasking" refers to the ability to determine time and level differences at each ear to improve detection of speech and other important sounds in noisy environments. Essentially, listeners can "cancel out" noise coming from a location that differs from that of the signal to be detected.[47] Although exactly where such binaural unmasking occurs is still a matter of debate, it is possible that the binaural information extracted by the early brainstem is used for binaural unmasking operations that actually occur at the level of the auditory cortex.

At the cortical level, bilateral damage to the superior temporal gyrus (primary auditory cortex) can result in immediate and ongoing insensitivity to all sounds. The extent to which attentional and behavioral processes underlie these deficits is not yet well understood.[48] In addition to "cortical deafness," which often recovers over time, there are a number of additional processing deficits associated with damage to auditory cortical areas that may impact speech comprehension, appreciation and discrimination of music, and identification and discrimination of environmental sounds. These diverse "agnosias" may stem from difficulties analyzing spectrotemporal patterns in sounds.[49]

Providing clinical data that relates specific damage to discrete behavioral deficits will provide a better understanding for a clinician and corroborative evidence for the spectrotemporal processing pathways that are being uncovered in animal studies. The relevance of diagnosing clinical disorders using animal models of cortical processing will likely only be appreciated when clinical and animal data are merged. Current trends suggest that the same basic units of analysis that exist in the mammalian cortices of cats and primates correlate with human perception of speech, music, and environmental sounds. If such a relationship could be clearly established, it would be possible to develop a set of standardized diagnostic tests that specifically target the perception of patterns in frequency, time, level, and spatial position. A more detailed discussion of diagnostic testing has been provided below.

Tinnitus

Damage to hearing due to excessive noise exposure in acoustic trauma is frequently accompanied by tinnitus. Noise-induced tinnitus can be characterized by a high-pitched buzzing or ringing sound that lasts longer than 5 minutes and may produce annoyance, behavioral changes, and depression.[50,51] Damage to neural networks, association pathways, associated cortical regions, the limbic system, and the prefrontal cortex may be involved in the generation of tinnitus.[52] Tinnitus symptoms resulting from blast or impulse noise exposure often resolve over time. Persistent symptoms can occur in some tinnitus patients, many of whom report disability equal to or greater than that associated with hearing loss.[50] Although tinnitus is a symptom associated with many forms of hearing loss, it can also be a symptom of other health problems, such as stress, use of certain medications, allergies, tumors, metabolic factors, and vascular disease (especially that involving vessels in the jaw and neck).

DIAGNOSTIC TESTS

It is often difficult to assess for otovestibular injury in a polytrauma patient in a timely manner because of consciousness level, contraindications to testing (c-spine precaution, ventilator use, bed rest orders, pain), and multiple priority appointments at other clinics. Testing protocols are commonly modified based on the complexity of an injury. For example, many polytrauma patients have burns or severe injuries to their skulls, so some testing equipment, such as earphones or bone conduction headsets, is contraindicated. There is currently no standard method for diagnosing otologic, otovestibular, and CAP disorders in patients with blast injury and amputation. When possible, the following protocol is recommended until ongoing clinical research identifies factors to aid in the development of more sensitive tests to assess blast-injury amputees for peripheral, central, and otovestibular pathology.

Patient Questionnaires

Polytrauma patients should complete case history and standardized questionnaires that assess the impact of hearing loss, tinnitus, and dizziness. The audiologic case history questionnaire should elicit information about a patient's medical history, including cognitive functioning, visual history before and after the blast, audiologic history before and after the blast (including exposure to potentially damaging noise), and tinnitus history (if applicable). Patients should also be asked to provide detailed information about the blast exposure, describing the nature of the blast, proximity to the blast, use of hearing protection, and loss of consciousness at the time of injury. The Hearing Handicap Inventory for Adults consists of two subscales and assesses the emotional and social consequences of hearing loss.[53] The Tinnitus Handicap Inventory is used to assess self-perceived handicap related to tinnitus, and the Dizziness Handicap Inventory assesses handicap by quantifying the functional, emotional, and physical effects of dizziness and unsteadiness.[54,55] Screenings for posttraumatic stress disorder and mild TBI should be administered when appropriate. TBI screening was created for VA clinicians to screen all OEF and OIF veterans receiving medical care within the Veterans Health Administration. The screening allows clinicians to offer further evaluation and treatment to those who test positive.

Comprehensive Audiometric Evaluation

Otoscopy should be performed prior to audiometric evaluation. If otoscopy reveals occluding or impacted cerumen or otherwise abnormal pathology, patients should be referred to an otolaryngologist. Monaural air- and bone-conduction thresholds should be measured in each ear to determine the type and degree of peripheral hearing impairment. Because many patients with blast-related limb loss may be taking ototoxic medications, air-conduction hearing thresholds should be measured at frequencies up to 12,000 Hz, or to the frequency limits of the individual's hearing.[56] Monaural speech-recognition testing, including reception thresholds for speech and speech intelligibility for one-syllable words, should be conducted in quiet. To further rule out or confirm the presence of conductive or retrocochlear pathology, immittance audiometry, including tympanometry, ipsilateral and contralateral acoustic reflex thresholds, and contralateral acoustic reflex decay should be completed in each ear. If pure tone testing reveals conductive or mixed hearing loss or if tympanometry results are abnormal, the patient should be referred to an otolaryngologist for evaluation. Otoacoustic emissions should be used to confirm other test findings. Additionally, auditory brainstem response testing and auditory steady-state response testing should be considered when a patient is unable to undergo conventional behavioral audiometry.

Ototoxic Monitoring Protocol

For patients on ototoxic medications, comprehensive baseline testing should supply information about pretreatment hearing levels. Baseline measures will provide a reference for comparison to determine if hearing levels have changed. This testing should be done as soon as possible after patients have been identified as needing ototoxic medication. For patients treated with aminoglycoside antibiotics, baseline testing should occur prior to the start of medication or within 72 hours of the first dose administered. Patients receiving loop diuretics should be seen sooner than 72 hours after the first dose. For patients receiving cisplatin or carboplatin, baseline testing should be evaluated within 24 hours of the first dose.

Minimum baseline evaluation should consist of bilateral pure tone air-conduction thresholds from 250 to 8,000 Hz. This should include the half octaves of 3,000 and 6,000 Hz. Whenever possible, high-frequency thresholds above 8,000 Hz should be tested (9,000, 10,000, 11,200, 12,500, 14,000, 16,000, 18,000, and 20,000 Hz). Intrasession reliability should also be evaluated by retesting some frequencies to measure for consistent results. A reliable test should show responses that are within or equal to 5 dB HL. If hearing loss is present from 250 to 4,000 Hz, bone conduction should also be performed. Testing should be as thorough as possible; however, if a patient is too sick for a comprehensive evaluation, testing may need to be modified or may need to occur over multiple sessions. If a patient is unable to complete behavioral testing, electrophysiological testing may be performed.

Ototoxicity monitoring is based on a patient's drug therapy schedules. For patients receiving aminoglycosides, otoscopy and pure tone air conduction tests in the normal and high-frequency ranges should occur at least once a week. Cisplatin patients should be monitored within 24 hours preceding each dose. For ototoxic medication monitoring, speech audiometry, bone conduction, and immittance testing should be performed if there is a change in hearing. If a change in hearing occurs, a retest should take place within 24 hours to confirm threshold change. Reevaluation should occur at approximately 3 and 6 months after treatment to assess any residual effects of drug treatment. If a decrease in hearing threshold is noted, weekly tests should take place until changes cease.

Ototoxic monitoring protocols at military facilities and VA hospitals must institute best practice policies for situations in which baseline measures are not available, concomitant medications are being used, septic patients require immediate therapy, and when bedside testing must be made available for patients that cannot be transferred for testing. In addition, ototoxicity monitoring should include patient counseling and education.

Assessment of the Vestibular System

If a patient reports problems with dizziness or unsteadiness, a multisensory balance evaluation is indicatied. The comprehensive balance evaluation should include a vestibular, visual, somatosensory, and brain integration system assesment. Clinicians working with soldiers with blast trauma and amputation need to consider several causes of postural instability, including TBI, orthostatic hypotension, cervical vertigo, visual deficits, possible side effects of ototoxic drugs, and vestibular pathology. Vertigo is often related to a vestibular balance disorder; however, imbalance and lightheadedness may or may not be related to inner ear damage. Some other causes of imbalance or lightheadedness include neurological impairments, vascular flow or pressure changes, cardiac problems, certain medications, or systemic disorders, such as diabetes. Screening tests typically administered by physical therapists during the vestibular portion of the blast evaluation include a cervical range-of-motion and cervicalgia assessment, oculomotor evaluation, postural stability tests, gait assessments, and ver-

tebral artery tests to assess for potential vertebral insufficiency and vascular causes of dizziness. The passive dynamic visual acuity test and head thrust test performed bilaterally assess the vestibular ocular reflex. Contraindications to these screenings include cervical instability, fractures preventing cervical range-of-motion assessments, and use of medical equipment that precludes communication, such as a jugular line or ventilator.[16] Screening tests are not sensitive enough to detect all vestibular abnormalities and do not provide quantitative data to determine the presence or absence of vestibular lesions.

Patients showing signs of vestibular pathology should be further evaluated to determine if dizziness or balance problems are related to a vestibular disorder. Vestibular tests can help characterize the deficits a patient has and guide the development of appropriate rehabilitative techniques. Videonystagmography is a battery of tests that evaluates the horizontal semicircular canals (one of the inner ear balance organs), its nerve connections, and the eye movement systems. Because the vestibular system is connected to the eye muscles, vestibular function is measured by recording eye movement. If electrodes are used, the test battery is typically called electronystagmography. The videonystagmography test can identify an inner ear balance disorder that can occur in one or both ears and is related to the horizontal semicircular canal and its nerve. The Dix-Hallpike maneuver, often performed as part of the videonystagmography/electronystagmography test battery, can determine if the symptoms of vertigo are related to BPPV and can identify which semicircular canal is involved.

Vestibular-evoked myogenic potentials assess the saccule (one of the otolith organs) and its nerve connections to the neck muscles to evaluate vestibular function. The rotary chair test evaluates the horizontal semicircular canals and their connection to the eye muscles and is used to monitor vestibular loss in patients on ototoxic medications. Finally, computerized dynamic posturography evaluates a patient's ability to integrate vestibular, visual, and somatosensory cues to maintain balance. This test is helpful for patients with lower extremity issues (eg, amputation, paralysis, etc) to monitor their risk of falls and retrain them for better stability and balance.

More recent best practices have begun to incorporate the computerized dynamic visual acuity test and the subjective visual vertical test during off-axis rotation to assess utricle function in the blast-injured population. The computerized dynamic visual acuity test measures visual acuity during head movement to assess vestibular deficits.[57,58] Monitoring an amputee with vestibular symptoms is essential and can be accomplished by outcome questionnaires, physical screens, repeating tests that had initial positive findings, and assessing and modifying management strategies on an ongoing basis.

Assessment of Central Auditory Processing Disorders

Deficits in CAP refer to "difficulties in the perceptual processing of auditory information in the CNS," as demonstrated by poor performance in one or more of the following skills: (a) auditory performance in the presence of competing acoustic signals (eg, dichotic listening); (b) temporal aspects of audition (eg, temporal integration, temporal discrimination, temporal ordering, temporal masking); (c) auditory pattern recognition; (d) auditory discrimination; (e) auditory performance with degraded acoustic signals; and (f) sound localization and lateralization.[10] Unfortunately, central deficits can be mistaken for posttraumatic stress disorder, mental health issues, and cognitive deficits, and therefore may be overlooked. With the increased incidence of TBI, CAP function must be assessed to ensure that remediation strategies can be devised and implemented. Currently, no standard CAP assessment protocol exists. A CAP test battery should be chosen for a given patient based on specificity, reliability, and validity. Tests should be selected that measure different central processes, and both verbal and nonverbal stimuli should be used. Some potential test measures an audiologist may include in a CAP assessment battery are provided below.

Auditory Temporal Processing and Patterning Tests

Auditory temporal processing and patterning tests are designed to assess a patient's ability to analyze acoustic events over time. An example of such a test is the Gaps-in-Noise Test.[59]

Dichotic Speech Tests

Dichotic speech tests are designed to assess a patient's ability to either separate or integrate different auditory stimuli presented to the ears simultaneously. One such test, the Dichotic Digits Test, requires a patient to listen to numbers presented to both ears simultaneously and indicate what was heard in each ear.[60] This test has demonstrated sensitivity to CNS pathology while remaining relatively resistant to mild-to-moderate high-frequency cochlear hearing loss.[61]

Monaural Low-Redundancy Speech Tests

Monaural low-redundancy speech tests assess a patient's ability to recognize degraded speech stimuli. Many audiologists use a speech-in-noise test to assess this component of central auditory processing. An example of such an assessment is the Quick Speech-in-Noise Test.[62] This test can be used with patients that have either normal or impaired hearing.

Binaural Interaction Tests

Binaural interaction assessments, such as the masking-level difference test, evaluate binaural processes depending on intensity or time difference of acoustic stimuli. In the masking-level difference test, binaural thresholds for pure tones (typically 500 Hz) or speech are determined in the presence of binaural masking noise. The tone or speech signal is presented in-phase to the ears and the noise is presented either in-phase or out-of-phase between the ears. Normal binaural processing is associated with an improved detection threshold for the out-of-phase noise. A 500-Hz masking-level difference test is clinically available and can be used for this assessment.[63]

Electrophysiologic Tests

Electrophysiologic tests measure electrical potentials that reflect activity generated by the CNS in response to auditory stimulation. The middle-latency response and the late-latency response have been shown to assess central auditory dysfunction. Putative neural generators for the middle-latency response include the auditory thalamocortical pathways, the mesencephalic reticular formation, and the inferior colliculus. The middle-latency response consists of a series of positive and negative peaks that fall in the latency range of 10 to 80 milliseconds after onset of the stimulus. Putative neural generators for the late-latency response, on the other hand, include thalamic projections into the auditory cortex, the primary auditory cortex, the supratemporal plane, the tempoparietal association cortex, and the lateral frontal cortex. In general, an averaged late-latency response wave is composed of contributions from multiple structures and can reflect brain functions such as attention, cognition, discrimination, and integration. The recorded wave consists of a series of positive and negative peaks that occur from 70 to 500 milliseconds after onset of the stimulus. These electrophysiologic tests, in conjunction with the auditory brainstem response, can help pinpoint where in the auditory system deficits might exist.

CAP assessment is controversial and complex,

especially with the polytrauma population, because variables such as motivation, attention, cooperation, cognition, neuronal loss, noise toxicity, metabolic and circulatory changes, working memory, and other comorbid factors can confound test interpretations and cause misdiagnosis. Because CAP deficits can be mistaken for myriad other disorders, it is essential that this assessment be done as part of a comprehensive team approach. An audiologist should work closely with professionals in mental health, neuropsychiatry, speech-language pathology, physical and occupational therapy, and other related specialties.

Tinnitus Evaluation

Patients presenting with complaints of tinnitus should undergo evaluation to assess symptoms and to identify treatment options. The Tinnitus-Impact Screening Interview and the Tinnitus Handicap Inventory questionnaire should be completed to determine the severity of symptoms. Sound tolerance measures can determine the presence of hyperacusis, or reduced loudness tolerance.[64] In addition, psychoacoustic measures, such as loudness and pitch matching,[65] allow for full characterization of a patient's tinnitus if it is problematic and requires treatment. An assessment of tinnitus maskability, or the minimum masking level necessary to render the patient's tinnitus inaudible, has been shown to correlate with treatment efficacy.[66] Finally, if measures of otoacoustic emissions have not already been performed, they should be done at this time to provide objective evidence of cochlear dysfunction (even if normal pure tone thresholds), and to provide frequency-specific information, which may be associated with the frequency region of the tinnitus.[67]

Reevaluation

The long-term effect of blast exposure on peripheral and central auditory functioning is not yet known and needs to be investigated more fully. The current recommendation, therefore, is to reassess patients in 6 months (or sooner if indicated) and annually thereafter.

TREATMENT AND REHABILITATION

Treatment and rehabilitation of auditory and vestibular injury in the amputee often require a multidisciplinary approach, focusing on otolaryngology, neurology, audiology, occupational therapy, and physical therapy. The type of auditory deficit present in a patient will determine treatment options, including medical and surgical interventions, technological considerations, and auditory training and counseling. Audiologists must make special considerations for service members with severe injuries to their extremities as a result of blast exposure. Those with concurrent hearing impairment must adjust to life with prosthetic limbs as well as prosthetic hearing aids and assistive listening devices.[68] Additionally, many soldiers with amputation have concurrent TBI and require accommodating rehabilitative approaches. Providers may need to give examples to go with new ideas and concepts, reduce visual and auditory distractions, and give step-by-step directions to reduce confusion. It is also important to demonstrate and explain information in more than one modality. Brain injury can cause cognitive impairments, such as problems with orientation, attention, concentration, perception, comprehension, learning, thought organization, executive function, problem solving, and memory. Additionally, up to 28% of all blast-exposed soldiers have significant eye injuries. Visual field deficits must be taken into consideration when providing aural rehabilitation and amplification device instructions. Furthermore, behavioral issues, including aggression, agitation, mental trauma, and adjustment to disabilities may interfere with treatment plans at early stages of recovery.[3]

Audiologists must be knowledgeable about managing problems specific to a patient's amputation and work with the treatment team to reduce this impact. For example, upper limb amputees that require hearing aids need to learn how to independently place an aid using a prosthesis. These challenges become compounded if an individual also has a TBI, vision loss, or loss of more than one limb. It is imperative that an audiologist actively participates as part of the rehabilitation team.

Peripheral Hearing Loss

Hearing aids deliver an amplified signal to the ear and are recommended when their use can significantly improve a patient's ability to communicate. When effective medical treatment can be implemented to restore normal hearing, or when hearing-aid use would exacerbate a disease or interfere with treatment, amplification is not used. Hearing aids are classified by their style, size and placement, or technological features. The most important developments in hearing aids in the past decade have been the introduction of digital programmable hearing aids, ranging in size from completely in the ear canal to behind the ear, and the increasing popularity of directional microphones. Directional microphones provide the greatest amount of amplification for signals arriving from the front, where speech typically emanates, and places nulls (areas of reduced amplification) for signals from the sides and back, which are the usual locations for noise sources.

When selecting a hearing aid for today's polytrauma patient, there are multiple factors to consider. For instance, some returning soldiers with hearing impairment have body-image issues stemming from multiple scars, burns, and amputation requiring prosthetic limbs, and may prefer a completely in-the-canal hearing aid versus a larger style. Additionally, it is important to consider possible alternatives when it is difficult or impossible for the patient to manually insert the hearing aid. This is especially true if the patient has lost or significantly impaired one or both upper limbs. The use of remote control options to adjust the volume and program settings (for quiet and noisy environments, telecoil or frequency modulation [FM] use) is likely to be a good option for these patients. Automatic hearing aids that adjust to different acoustic environments without human intervention are also available as needed, especially for those with significant cognitive impairment.

Unfortunately, traditional hearing aids, even those equipped with directional-microphone technology, may provide only limited improvement in speech perception in everyday listening environments where there is noise and reverberation. One well-recognized technology to improve speech perception in listeners with hearing loss is FM systems. With an FM system, the speaker's voice is picked up by a wireless microphone and the signal is transmitted via FM radio waves to the receiver. The close proximity of the FM microphone minimizes the negative effects of reverberation, distance, and noise on speech perception.[69]

In addition to FM technology, a host of other assistive listening devices could be considered for this patient population. Some of these options include captioning for television viewing, teletext or volume-control telephones, and alerting devices that employ flash-visual or vibrotactile signals to warn of acoustical environmental events. Many of these devices are available at no cost to the veteran through the VA or the state in which the veteran resides.

Vestibular Problems

Treatment of vestibular problems should be specific to the patient and to the deficit, and physicians and physical therapists should collaborate on patient treatment. Depending on diagnostic test results, vestibular treatment options can include vestibular rehabilitation therapy; physical therapy; canalith repositioning therapy; change in activity levels, medication, and diet; treatment for underlying disease that may be contributing to the balance disorder; and surgery.

Vestibular rehabilitation therapy is the treatment of choice for many types of vestibular disorders. Vestibular rehabilitation therapy is exercise therapy that includes head and eye movement and balance and walking tasks that are designed to help the brain compensate for vestibular problems. Vestibular rehabilitation therapy, postural stability training, and gait training are usually provided by a physical therapist.

Canalith repositioning therapy is the preferred treatment for BPPV. The goal of canalith repositioning therapy is to move the displaced particles (otoconia) through the semicircular canal and back to the vestibule that houses the otolith organs. This is achieved by placing the patient in a series of head positions and observing eye movement. It may be performed by an audiologist, otolaryngologist, or physical therapist.

Central Auditory Processing Deficits

Treatment options for CAP deficits are currently under investigation by the research community. Current clinical guidelines recommend a two-step approach that includes auditory training and general management.[10] Auditory training is designed to capitalize on the plasticity of the auditory system by altering the neural encoding of sound and subsequent timing of brainstem responses. Studies have linked the neurophysiologic changes seen after training to perceptual changes.[70–72] Subjects can learn to interpret sounds as speech that could not be discriminated before training. It is recommended that training occur soon after injury to maximize the plasticity of the brain, and training should be patient specific and focused on the deficit areas noted on the CAP assessment. General management strategies include environmental tactics, like the use of an FM system, and teaching compensatory strategies. These treatment options may be provided by a speech-language pathologist, an audiologist, and an occupational and physical therapist. Specific remediation activities (deficit specific), such as phonological awareness and discrimination training (speech-to-print skills), auditory closure, and prosody training, can be provided by a speech-language pathologist. Speechreading and auditory training exercises can be provided by an audiologist, and occupational and physical therapists can use cross-modality activities to improve interhemispheric transfer of information.

Tinnitus

The majority of patients who present with tinnitus following blast exposure experience a resolution of symptoms over time and do not require any audiologic intervention.[19] Of the approximately 20% of tinnitus patients that have clinically significant symptoms, rehabilitation needs vary from simple education about the condition to counseling and treatment.[19] Because no treatment has been effective in directly reducing tinnitus symptoms, the goal of treatment is to lessen their impact.[9] Tinnitus treatments include medication, masking therapy, Tinnitus Retraining Therapy, Neuromonics Tinnitus Treatment and other sound therapy and directed counseling, psychological therapy (such as cognitive-behavioral therapy), and hearing aids.[50] The type of intervention for tinnitus patients can vary significantly, and clinical management methods do not adhere to any standards at this time.[67]

PREVENTION

Because of the many types of ear injuries incurred by soldiers, multiple strategies must be employed to prevent hearing loss in this population. Physical barriers to sound, pressure, and debris, such as headphones and earplugs, prevent injury to the external and middle ear. In addition, monitoring hearing thresholds while patients are receiving ototoxic medications provides early identification of hearing loss, allowing for possible changes in treatment. Finally, systemic compounds for otoprotection may prevent damage at the cellular level. The optimal treatment for soldiers may be a combination of all these approaches to ultimately minimize hearing impairment.

Hearing Conservation

Headphones and hearing protectors offer significant shielding and protection from otologic injury by protecting the ear from excessive noise, flying debris, and the pressure wave associated with a blast. Technological advances have enabled hearing protectants to be equipped with microphones so users can maintain hearing sensitivity. For those wearing hearing protection, the risk of hearing loss is minimized and the incidence of ruptured TM is significantly reduced. In several blast incidents, soldiers using hearing protection did not sustain ear injuries, whereas those without ear protection suffered ear damage and hearing loss.[73,74] Military personnel assigned to light armored vehicles as commanders, gunners, and drivers wear protective helmets, but personnel in the rear of these vehicles do not generally wear protection and are therefore most susceptible to ear blast injuries.[1] Greater than 20% of the blast-injured soldiers traveling in light armored vehicles in various military conflicts presented with ear injury, mostly ruptured TMs.[1] In contrast, eye injuries are extremely uncommon for these soldiers, presumably due to the ballistic eye protection soldiers wear when traveling in light armored vehicles.[1] It is essential to adopt hearing protection standards to shield service members at risk for blast or excessive noise exposure.

Otoprotectants

Otoprotective agents may be capable of preventing noise-induced and ototoxic hearing loss by reducing the damaging effects of noise or medications on the hair cells of the cochlea. In addition, some otoprotectants may be able to rescue damaged cells once injury has occurred, thereby minimizing hearing loss. There have been numerous studies of various compounds used to protect hearing, including antioxidants that scavenge free radicals, agents that increase blood flow, and drugs that block cell-death-pathway–signaling factors. Despite the potential of these compounds, the translation of animal studies of otoprotectants to clinical treatment has been limited. Clinical trials are needed to delineate the effects of these protective compounds. Effective preventative therapies may ultimately require a combination of compounds that employ multiple mechanisms to combat cell damage in the inner ear.

SUMMARY

The escalating use of explosive devices in warfare, combined with the excessive noise of ballistic weapons, has created an unprecedented number of hearing impairments among soldiers, many of whom also sustain amputations, further complicating rehabilitation efforts. A comprehensive interdisciplinary evaluation of peripheral, central, and vestibular components of the auditory system must be completed in polytrauma patients to ensure that all injury is accurately diagnosed and appropriate rehabilitation can be devised. Furthermore, the implementation of hearing conservation strategies—including physical ear protection, preventative therapy with otoprotectants, and implementation of early detection and monitoring programs—may significantly reduce the number of patients with disabling hearing impairments. Effective treatment and hearing loss protection programs can also reduce the potential for the medical, legal, and socioeconomic consequences of hearing loss, and ultimately allow patients to retain a better posttreatment quality of life.

REFERENCES

1. Gondusky JS, Reiter MP. Protecting military convoys in Iraq: an examination of battle injuries sustained by a mechanized battalion during Operation Iraqi Freedom II. *Mil Med*. 2005;170:546–549.

2. Zoroya G. Military prodded on brain injuries; memo cites gaps in spotting cases. *USA Today*. March 8, 2007:A1.

3. Cornis-Pop M. Blast injuries: a new kind of patient speech-language pathologists. *Am Speech Lang Hear Assoc Leader*. 2006;11:6–7,28.

4. Pasquina PF. Optimizing care for combat amputees: experiences at Walter Reed Army Medical Center. *J Rehabil Res Dev*. 2004;41:vii–xii.

5. Arlinger S. Negative consequences of uncorrected hearing loss—a review. *Int J Audiol*. 2003;42(Suppl 2):17–20.

6. Chandler D. Blast-related ear injury in current U.S. military operations. *Am Speech Lang Hear Assoc Leader*. 2006;11:8–9,29.

7. Mrena R, Pääkkönen R, Bäck L, Pirvola U, Ylikoski J. Otologic consequences of blast exposure: a Finnish case study of a shopping mall bomb explosion. *Acta Otolaryngol*. 2004;124:946–952.

8. Noise and hearing loss. *Consens Statement*. 1990;8:1–24.

9. Bilski B. Interaction between noise and ototoxic agents in the work environment [in Polish]. *Med Pr*. 2003;54:481–485.

10. American Speech-Language-Hearing Association. Guidelines for the audiologic management of individuals receiving cochleotoxic drug therapy. *Am Speech Lang Hear Assoc Leader*. 1994;36:11–19.

11. Fausti SA, Henry JA, Schaffer HI, Olson DJ, Frey RH, McDonald WJ. High-frequency audiometric monitoring for early detection of aminoglycoside ototoxicity. *J Infect Dis*. 165;1992:1026–1032.

12. Fausti SA, Henry JA, Schaffer HI, Olson DJ, Frey RH, Bagby GC, Jr. High-frequency monitoring for early detection of cisplatin ototoxicity. *Arch Otolaryngol Head Neck Surg*. 1993;119:661–665.

13. Fausti SA, Larson VD, Noffsinger D, Wilson RH, Phillips DS, Fowler CG. High-frequency audiometric strategies for early detection of ototoxicity. *Ear Hear*. 1994;15:232–239.

14. MacDonald MR, Harrison RV, Wake M, Bliss B, Macdonald RE. Ototoxicity of carboplatin: comparing animal and clinical models at the Hospital for Sick Children. *J Otolaryngol*. 1994;23:151–159.

15. Bokemeyer C, Berger CC, Hartmann JT, et al. Analysis of risk factors for cisplatin-induced ototoxicity in patients with testicular cancer. *Br J Canc*. 1998;77:1355–1362.

16. Scherer M, Burrows H, Pinto R, Somrack E. Characterizing self-reported dizziness and otovestibular impairment among blast-injured traumatic amputees: a pilot study. *Mil Med*. 2007;172(7):731–737.

17. Myers SF, Blakley BW, Schwan S, Rintelmann WF, Mathog RH. The "plateau effect" of cis-platinum-induced hearing loss. *Otolaryngol Head Neck Surg*. 1991;104:122–127.

18. Leibovici D, Gofrit ON, Stein M, et al. Blast injuries: bus versus open-air bombings—a comparative study of injuries in survivors of open-air versus confined-space explosions. *J Trauma*. 1996;41;1030–1035.

19. Lew HL, Guillory SB, Jerger J, Henry JA. Auditory dysfunction in traumatic brain injury and blast related injury. *J Rehabil Res Dev*. 2007;44(7):921–928.

20. American College of Emergency Physicians. *Emergency Medicine: a Comprehensive Study Guide.* Tintinalli JE, Kelen GD, Stapczynski JS, eds. 5th ed. New York, NY: McGraw-Hill; 2000:1275–1277.

21. Cohen JT, Ziv G, Bloom J, Zikk D, Rapoport Y, Himmelfarb MZ. Blast injury of the ear in a confined space explosion: auditory and vestibular evaluation. *Isr Med Assoc J.* 2003;4:559–562.

22. DePalma RG, Burris DG, Champion HR, Hodgson MJ. Blast injuries. *N Engl J Med.* 2005;352:1335–1342.

23. Helling ER. Otologic blast injuries due to the Kenya embassy bombing. *Mil Med.* 2004;169:872–876.

24. Kronenberg J, Ben-Shoshan J, Modan M, Leventon G. Blast injury and cholesteatoma. *Am J Otol.* 1988;9:127–130.

25. Zajtchuk JT, Philips YY. Effects of blast overpressure on the ear. *Ann Otol Rhinol Laryngol.* 1989;140:1–60.

26. Katz E, Ofek B, Adler J, Abramowitz HB, Krausz MM. Primary blast injury after a bomb explosion in a civilian bus. *Ann Surg.* 1989;209:484–488.

27. Xyadkis MS, Bebarta VS, Harrison CD, Conner JC, Grant GA, Robbins AS. Tympanic-membrane perforation as a marker of concussive brain injury in Iraq. *New Engl J Med.* 2007;357:830–831.

28. Roth Y, Kronenberg J, Lotem S, Leventon G. Blast injury of the ear [in Hebrew]. *Harefuah.* 1989;117:297–310.

29. Leibovici D, Gofrit ON, Shapira SC. Eardrum perforation in explosion survivors: is it a marker of pulmonary blast injury? *Ann Emerg Med.* 1999;34:168–172.

30. de Ceballos JP, Turégano-Fuentes F, Perez-Diaz D, Sanz-Sanchez M, Martin-Llorente C, Guerrero-Sanz JE. 11 March 2004: The terrorist bomb explosions in Madrid, Spain—an analysis of the logistics, injuries sustained and clinical management of causalities treated at the closest hospital. *Crit Care.* 2005;9:104–111.

31. Lucić M. Therapy of middle ear injuries caused by explosive devices [in Serbian]. *Vojnosanit Pregl.* 1995;52(3):221–224.

32. Chandler DW, Edmond CV. Effects of blast overpressure on the ear: case reports. *J Am Acad of Audiol.* 1997;8:81–88.

33. US Department of Health and Human Services, Agency for Healthcare Research and Quality. Pediatric terrorism and disaster preparedness: a resource for pediatricians. Available at: http://www.ahrq.gov/research/pedprep/. Published October 2006. Accessed August 15, 2008.

34. Ylikoski J. Acoustic trauma [in Finnish]. *Duodecim.* 1993;109:1370–1371.

35. Persaud R, Hajioff D, Wareing M, Chevretton E. Otological trauma resulting from the Soho Nail Bomb in London, April 1999. *Clin Otolaryngol Allied Sci.* 2003;28:203–206.

36. Perez R, Gatt N, Cohen D. Audiometric configurations following exposure to explosions. *Arch Otolaryngol Head Neck Surg.* 2000;126:1249–1252.

37. van Campen LE, Dennis JM, Hanlin RC, King SB, Velderman AM. One-year audiologic monitoring of individuals exposed to the 1995 Oklahoma City bombing. *J Am Acad Audiol.* 1999;10:231–247.

38. Fitzgerald DC. Head trauma: hearing loss and dizziness. *J Trauma.* 1996;40(3):488–496.

39. Bergemalm P, Borg E. Long-term objective and subjective audiologic consequences of closed head injury. *Acta Otolaryngol.* 2001;121:724–734.

40. Berman JM, Fredrickson JM. Vertigo after head injury—a five year follow-up. *J Otolaryngol.* 1978;7(3):237–245.

41. Herdman SJ. Advances in the treatment of vestibular disorders. *Phys Ther.* 1997;77:602–618.

42. Alberti PW. Noise induced hearing loss. *BMJ*. 1992;304:522.

43. Furman JM, Whitney SL. Central causes of dizziness. *Phys Ther*. 2000;80:179–187.

44. Hoffer ME, Gottshall KR, Moore R, Balough BJ, Wester D. Characterizing and treating dizziness after mild head trauma. *Otol Neurotol*. 2004;25:135–138.

45. Davies RA, Luxon LM. Dizziness following head injury: a neuro-otological study. *J Neurol*. 1995;242(4):222–230.

46. Taber KH, Warden DL, Hurley RA. Blast-related traumatic brain injury: what is known? *J Neuropsychiatry Clin Neurosci*. 2006;18:141–145.

47. Colburn HS, Durlach NI. Models of binaural interaction. In: Carterette EC, Friedman MP, eds. *Hearing*. Vol. 5. In: Carterette EC, Friedman MP, eds. *Handbook of Perception*. New York, NY: Academic Press; 1978: 467–518.

48. Petkov CI, Kang X, Alho K, Bertrand O, Yund EW, Woods DL. Attentional modulation of human auditory cortex. *Nat Neurosci*. 2004;7:658–663.

49. Griffiths TD, Rees A, Green GGR. Disorders of human complex sound processing. *Neurocase*. 1999;5:365–378.

50. Mrena R, Savolainen S, Kuokkanen JT, Ylikoski J. Characteristics of tinnitus induced by acute acoustic trauma: a long-term follow up. *Audiol Neurootol*. 2002;7:122–130.

51. Henry JA, Dennis KC, Schechter MA. General review of tinnitus: prevalence, mechanisms, effects, and management. *J Speech Lang Hear Res*. 2005;48:1204–1235.

52. Jastreboff PJ. Tinnitus retraining therapy. *Br J Audiol*. 1999;33:68–70.

53. Newman C, Jacobson G, Spitzer J. Development of the Tinnitus Handicap Inventory. *Arch Otolaryngol Head Neck Surg*. 1996;122:143–148.

54. Henry JA, Zaugg TL, Myers PJ, Schechter MA. The role of audiologic evaluation in progressive audiologic tinnitus management. *Trends Amplif*. 2008;12(3):170–187.

55. Jacobson G, Newman C. The development of the Dizziness Handicap Inventory. *Arch Otolaryngol Head Neck Surg*. 1990;116:424–427.

56. Fausti SA, Erickson DA, Frey RH, Rappaport BZ, Schechter MA. The effects of noise upon human hearing sensitivity from 8000 to 20000 Hz. *J Acoust Soc Am*. 1981;69:1343–1347.

57. Herdman SJ, Tusa RJ, Blatt P, Suzuki A, Venuto PJ, Roberts D. Computerized dynamic visual acuity test in the assessment of vestibular deficits. *Am J Otol*. 1998;19:790–796.

58. Herdman SJ, Schubert MC, Tusa RJ. Contribution of central pre-programming to visual acuity during head movements in patients with vestibular hypofunction. *Arch Otolaryngol Head Neck Surg*. 2001;127:1205–1210.

59. Musiek F, Shinn J, Jirsa R, Bamiou D, Baran J, Zaida E. GIN (Gaps-In-Noise) test performance in subjects with confirmed central auditory nervous system involvement. *Ear Hear*. 2005;26:608–618.

60. Musiek F. Assessment of central auditory dysfunction: the Dichotic Digits Test revisited. *Ear Hear*. 1983;4:79–83.

61. Musiek FE, Gollegly KM, Kibbe KS, Verkest-Lenz SB. Proposed screening test for central auditory disorders: follow-up on the Dichotic Digits Test. *Am J Otol*. 1991;12(2):109–113.

62. Killion M, Niquette P, Gundmundsen G, Revit L, Banjeree S. Development of a quick speech-in-noise test for measuring signal-to-noise ratio loss in normal-hearing and hearing-impaired listeners. *J Acoust Soc Am*. 2004;116:2395–2405.

63. Wilson RH, Moncrieff DW, Townsend EA, Pillion AL. Development of a 500-Hz masking-level difference protocol for clinical use. *J Am Acad Audiol*. 2003;14(1):1–8.

64. Jastreboff MN, Jastreboff PJ. Decreased sound tolerance and tinnitus retraining therapy (TRT). *Aust N Z J Audiol*. 2002; 24:74–81.

65. Henry JA, Zaugg TL, Schecter MA. Clinical guide for audiologic tinnitus management II: Treatment. *Am J Audiol*. 2005;14(1):49–70.

66. Jastreboff PJ, Hazell JW, Graham RL. Neurophysiological model of tinnitus: dependency of the minimal masking level on treatment outcome. *Hear Res*. 1994;80:216–232.

67. Henry JA, Jastreboff MM, Jastreboff PJ, Schechter MA, Fausti SA. Assessment of patients for treatment with tinnitus retraining therapy. *J Am Acad Audiol*. 2002;13:523–544.

68. Fihn SD. Does VA health care measure up? *N Engl J Med*. 2000;343:1963–1965.

69. Crandell C, Smaldino J, Flexer C. *Sound-Field FM Amplification: Theory and Practical Applications*. Independence, Kans: Thomson Learning; 1995.

70. Kraus N, McGee T, Carrell T, Sharma A. Neurophysiologic bases of speech discrimination. *Ear Hear*. 1995;16:19–37.

71. Tremblay K, Kraus N, Carrell TD, McGee T. Central auditory system plasticity: generalization to novel stimuli following listening training. *J Acoust Soc Am*. 1997;102:3762–3773.

72. Tremblay K, Kraus N, McGee T. The time course of auditory perceptual learning: neurophysiological changes during speech-sound training. *Neuroreport*. 1998;9:3557–3560.

73. Schulz TY. Troops return with alarming rates of hearing loss. *Hear Health*. 2004;20(3):18–21.

74. Fallon E. Army audiologists on duty in Iraq. In: Fabry D, ed. *Front Line News & Information for Government Audiologists*; 2005.

Chapter 15

TRAUMATIC BRAIN INJURY

LOUIS M. FRENCH, PsyD*; MARIA MOURATIDIS, PsyD†; BRAD DICIANNO, MD§; AND BRADLEY IMPINK, BSE¥

INTRODUCTION

DEFINITION OF TRAUMATIC BRAIN INJURY

BASIC PATHOPHYSIOLOGY OF TRAUMATIC BRAIN INJURY

BLAST EFFECTS

NEUROBEHAVIORAL SEQUELAE OF TRAUMATIC BRAIN INJURY AND POST-CONCUSSIVE DISORDER

TRAUMATIC BRAIN INJURY IN THE AMPUTEE

TREATMENT OF TRAUMATIC BRAIN INJURY

ACUTE MEDICAL CARE

REHABILITATION

SUMMARY

*Director, TBI Program, Departments of Orthopaedics and Rehabilitation, Walter Reed Army Medical Center, Military Advanced Training Center, Building 2A, 6900 Georgia Avenue, NW, Washington, DC 20307; Assistant Professor of Neurology, Uniformed Services University of the Health Sciences, 4301 Jones Bridge Road, Bethesda, Maryland 20814

†Command Consultant and Subject Matter Expert for Traumatic Brain Injury and Psychological Health, National Naval Medical Center, 8901 Wisconsin Avenue, Bethesda, Maryland 20889

§Assistant Professor, Human Engineering and Research Labs, VA Pittsburgh Healthcare System, 7180 Highland Drive, 151R1-H, Building 4, 2nd Floor East, Pittsburgh, Pennsylvania 15206

‡Predoctoral Fellow, Human Engineering Research Laboratories, VA Pittsburgh Healthcare System, 7180 Highland Drive, 151R1-H, Building 4, 2nd Floor East, Pittsburgh, Pennsylvania 15206; formerly, Graduate Student Researcher, Department of Bioengineering, University of Pittsburgh, Pittsburgh, Pennsylvania

INTRODUCTION

Traumatic brain injury (TBI) is a global public health issue that is the leading cause of death and disability in young adults in the United States. The Centers for Disease Control and Prevention (CDC) estimates that 1.4 million individuals in the United States sustain TBI annually; 50,000 of those injuries are fatal.[1] Around 80,000 to 90,000 individuals per year sustain permanent disability as a result of TBI. The CDC estimates the monetary cost of TBI to the public to be almost $50 billion annually when treatment costs, lost wages, disability, and death are considered.[2,3]

TBI can significantly impair functioning and may negatively impact an individual's relationships, health, and happiness. Military service, even during peacetime, increases the risk of brain injury. In wartime, combat operations add to that risk. The incidence of TBI in young female service members is similar to that of young adult male civilians, the group with the highest rate of TBI in the civilian population.[4] TBI impacts the military as a whole by compromising the health and well-being of service members and their families and hindering operational readiness.

The survival rate for those injured in Operation Iraqi Freedom (OIF) and Operation Enduring Freedom (OEF) is much higher than in past wars. The current ratio of wounded to killed in Iraq is over nine to one,[5] compared to a ratio of fewer than three to one in Vietnam and Korea and about two to one in World War II.[6] This rate of survival is related to numerous factors, including advanced in-theater medical care, rapid evacuation, and advanced protective equipment. Concurrent with these survival rates, the military has observed an increased number of those who may have experienced TBI. The most common causes of injury in OEF and OIF are roadside bombs, improvised explosive devices, and explosively formed projectiles. The resultant blast wave from these weapons may cause TBI either through the direct blast effect or the secondary or tertiary effects (impact of an object against a person or a person against an object, respectively). Additionally, many service members deployed in support of OIF and OEF have been exposed to a multitude of blasts. Although a specific injury may be attributed to one of these events, the effect on the brain by cumulative blast exposures has not yet been clearly elucidated. Therefore, it is important that all healthcare providers who work with injured military service members be aware of the potential for existing TBI.

TBI is typically identified soon after injury. However, delayed recognition, especially when the injury is relatively mild, is not uncommon. These "silent injuries," whether occurring in a military or civilian setting, typically resolve without long-term consequences. Under some circumstances though, they have implications for functioning and may significantly impact the recovery and rehabilitation of other, more visible injuries.

As of March 31, 2008, Defense and Veterans Brain Injury Center sites reported 6,602 US service members have sustained TBI related to the global war on terror since January 1, 2003. The majority of those (1,523) were seen at Walter Reed Army Medical Center. Thirty-two percent of those arriving via air from Iraq and Afghanistan were diagnosed with TBI, often in association with another injury. Of all US service members medically evacuated from Iraq or Afghanistan, 25% reportedly sustained injuries to the head or neck.[7] Additionally, military screening of service members returning from deployment (not medically evacuated) have determined 10% to 20% sustained a concussion or mild TBI (MTBI) at some time during their tour.[8]

DEFINITION OF TRAUMATIC BRAIN INJURY

TBI is described as either closed or penetrating injury. A penetrating brain injury occurs when a foreign object or bone penetrates the dura surrounding the brain. In a military setting, this is most commonly a bullet or metal fragment, but it can involve bone from the skull or other foreign bodies, such as stones. Although the dura is not penetrated in a closed TBI, large external forces may act on the head, leading to significant brain damage. Although there is some variability in the definition of TBI, especially with respect to defining milder injuries, most accepted definitions (those advanced by the CDC, American Congress on Rehabilitation Medicine, American Psychological Association, and the World Health Organization) share common elements. The Department of Defense's current definition was drafted in 2007 by a consensus panel of experts (Exhibit 15-1, Table 15-1).

BASIC PATHOPHYSIOLOGY OF TRAUMATIC BRAIN INJURY

The severity of closed TBI is typically characterized by the duration of loss of consciousness; duration of posttraumatic amnesia; and initial, postresuscitation Glasgow Coma Scale score. In addition to these criteria,

---

EXHIBIT 15-1

DEPARTMENT OF DEFENSE CONSENSUS ON TRAUMATIC BRAIN INJURY DEFINITION

The Department of Defense Consensus on Traumatic Brain Injury (TBI) defines TBI as a traumatically induced structural injury or physiological disruption of brain function as a result of an external force that is indicated by new onset or worsening of at least one of the following clinical signs immediately following the event:

- any period of loss of or decreased level of consciousness;
- any loss of memory of events immediately before or after the injury;
- any alteration in mental state at the time of the injury (eg, confusion, disorientation, slowed thinking);
- neurological deficits (eg, weakness, balance disturbance, praxis, paresis/plegia, change in vision, other sensory alterations, aphasia) that may be transient; or
- intracranial abnormalities (eg, contusions, diffuse axonal injury, hemorrhages, aneurysms).

External forces include the following:

- an object striking the head;
- the head striking an object;
- the brain undergoing an acceleration or deceleration movement without direct external trauma to the head;
- a foreign body penetrating the brain;
- forces generated from an event such as a blast or explosion; or
- other forces yet to be defined.

Sequelae of TBI may resolve quickly, within minutes to hours after the neurological event, or they may persist. Some sequelae of TBI may be permanent. Most signs and symptoms will manifest immediately following the event; however, other signs and symptoms may be delayed from days to months (eg, subdural hematoma, seizures, hydrocephalus, and spasticity). Signs and symptoms may occur alone or in varying combinations and may result in functional impairment. The following signs and symptoms are not better explained by preexisting conditions or other medical, neurological, or psychological causes, except in cases of an exacerbation of a preexisting condition:

- cognitive (eg, attention, concentration, memory, speed of processing, new learning, planning, reasoning, judgment, executive control, self-awareness, language, or abstract thinking);
- physical (eg, headache, nausea, vomiting, dizziness, blurred vision, sleep disturbance, weakness, paresis/plegia, sensory loss, spasticity, aphasia, dysphagia, apraxia, balance disorders, coordination disorders, or seizure disorders); and
- emotional/behavioral (eg, depression, anxiety, agitation, irritability, impulsivity, or aggression).

Cognitive, physical, or emotional/behavioral manifestations that cannot be better explained by another process may be casually related to the blast event, even when there is no identifiable evidence of structural brain injury on imaging studies or altered brain function immediately following the event. Further study is needed to determine if an episode of altered brain function at the time of the trauma is required for a diagnosis of TBI resulting from an explosion or blast.

Injury severity is determined at the time of the injury. Although this severity level has some prognostic value, it does not necessarily reflect the patient's ability to function. Serial assessments of the patient's cognitive, emotional/behavioral, and social functioning are required. The patient is classified as mild, moderate, or severe (see Table 15-1).

Data source: US Department of Defense Consensus Traumatic Brain Injury Definition. Developed at: DoD Force Health Protection and Readiness TBI Consensus Meeting; 2007.

---

neuroimaging results also play a role in injury severity. For example, an individual who loses consciousness or sustains posttraumatic amnesia consistent with MTBI will be classified as having a moderate injury if abnormality is evident on brain images because those individuals have similar outcomes.[9,10] Current definitions and designations of TBI only describe the severity of the brain injury itself, and do not neces-

TABLE 15-1

BRAIN INJURY SEVERITY LEVELS

Level	Structural Imaging	Loss of Consciousness	Alteration of Consciousness	Posttraumatic Amnesia
Mild	Normal	0–30 min	a moment–24 hrs	0–1 day
Moderate	Normal or abnormal	> 30 min–24 hrs	24 hrs; severity based on other criteria	1–7 days
Severe	Normal or abnormal	> 24 hrs	24 hrs; severity based on other criteria	> 7 days

Data source: US Department of Defense Consensus Traumatic Brain Injury Definition. Developed at: DoD Force Health Protection and Readiness TBI Consensus Meeting; 2007.

sarily correlate with resultant symptomatic sequelae, clinical outcomes, or functionality. There is generally a greater chance for persistent problems in those with severe injuries, but it is not uncommon for individuals diagnosed with severe TBI to have a better functional recovery than those diagnosed with MTBI, who may have resultant catastrophic changes in personal, social, and occupational functioning. Fortunately, such poor outcomes are relatively rare and are often mediated by a variety of factors.[11] Further research is required to determine if the typical outcomes seen in a civilian population, especially in the case of recovery from MTBI, are similar to those seen in the combat-injured population. Contextual issues, such as the high rate of comorbid medical, physical, or psychological problems, may also significantly impact TBI recovery in this patient population.

The two most common injury mechanisms associated with TBI are contact and acceleration/deceleration. A third mechanism, blast, has become the subject of increasing debate given the large number of blast casualties returning from OEF and OIF. Blast injuries may have some different characteristics than those resulting from contact or acceleration/deceleration injuries. TBI, regardless of its severity, can result in damage to the structure and function of the brain. Contact injuries can result in focal brain damage, such as lacerations, contusions, skull fractures, penetration wounds, and intracranial hemorrhage. Acceleration/deceleration injuries can result in diffuse brain damage, such as diffuse axonal injury and cerebral edema.[12–16] Immediately following TBI, cerebral blood

flow regulation and glucose metabolism are impaired. Cerebral blood flow may decrease significantly, and cerebral ischemia is common.[17–25] Cerebral metabolism is often diminished following TBI, which is related to mitochondrial dysfunction and reduced production of adenosine triphosphate. Reduced cerebral blood flow causes an ischemic-like state wherein anaerobic glycolysis leads to lactic acid accumulation. Anaerobic glycolysis cannot provide sufficient energy for cellular function and, because of adenosine triphosphate depletion, the energy-dependent membrane ion pumps fail. This results in a secondary pathophysiological response, which includes membrane depolarization, excessive neurotransmitter release, and ion flux.[12,26] The primary excitatory neurotransmitter released is glutamate, which over-stimulates ionotropic glutamate receptors, resulting in Ca^{2+}, Na^+, and K^+ fluxes. This leads to a catabolic state, increasing the intracellular concentrations of toxic products, such as free fatty acids and free radicals. Ultimately, the activation of various enzymes (proteases, peroxidases, phospholipases, caspases, translocases, and endonucleases) leads to membrane degradation, blood–brain barrier breakdown, necrosis, and apoptosis. Breakdown of the cerebral-vascular barrier results in increased cell membrane permeability, ultimately resulting in cerebral edema, which may further exacerbate the ischemic state.[27,28] This process is more pronounced as the severity of the trauma increases.[29]

While not considered TBI in itself, secondary brain insults, like systemic hypotension and hypoxia, reportedly worsen outcomes in patients with TBI.[30]

BLAST EFFECTS

In 20th-century military conflicts such as Vietnam, the focus of attention in combat-related brain injuries

has been on the penetrating craniocerebral injury.[31] In the current global war on terror, concussive forces and resultant MTBI have proven challenging. A recent report states that 88% of injuries seen at an echelon II medical unit during OIF were due to explosions.[32] This figure is generally consistent with official reports on mechanism of injury in US troops in Iraq, in which 80% of casualties were due to blast.[33] Sophisticated body armor and protection against penetrating head wounds allow US troops to survive explosive attacks they would not have survived in previous wars. Because of the frequency of TBI and its impact on service members, the military has increased its efforts to screen for MTBI.

Levi and colleagues reported on a series of head-injured patients during the 1982–1985 Lebanese war and found the majority of TBI reported was penetrating.[34,35] One subset (n = 17) of the patients who suffered blast injury were identified. Blast was defined as "a) primary—due to the air blast, b) secondary—due to the impact of blast energized debris (either on the victim or vice versa), and c) tertiary—due to the effects of fire, gases or collapse of a building."[35(p555)] The authors commented on the high frequency of pathology identified by computed tomography, including diffuse brain injury. They concluded that there was a "unique character of head injuries sustained during explosion."[34] In one study of injuries in the Balkan conflicts, 30% of the blast injured had long-term (greater than 1 year) symptoms reflecting central nervous system disorders, as compared to just 4% of the non-blast–injured patients.[36] Building on experience with soldiers, Cernak et al conducted animal studies in the laboratory to examine blast wave effects on the central nervous system. The studies showed structural, biochemical, and cognitive impairments in rat brains after either whole-body or local (chest) overpressure while the head was protected. Both groups of animals showed neuronal injury in the hippocampus. The whole-body–exposed group showed significant decline in performance on a previously learned task that persisted at least 5 days. In the local (chest overpressure) group, there was also a significant drop in performance, but with normalization by 1 day after injury. There was a significant linear relationship between blast injury severity and decline in task performance in each group.[37]

Interest in combat-blast–related injury in the central nervous system dates back to at least World War I and is again discussed in the scientific literature of the World War II era.[38,39] The effects of physical and psychological injuries on soldiers' symptom presentation and functioning was often debated. A more modern understanding fully appreciates the relationship between cognitive functioning and emotional stress; it has been shown that combat exposure puts individuals at higher risk for health-related problems, partly because of potential TBI.[40]

Whether blast-induced brain injury demonstrates a different course of illness and recovery than more traditional causes of TBI is the subject of ongoing investigation, as is whether cognitive and emotional profiles affect outcomes. It has been suggested that differences may result from the effect of the blast wave itself, the added emotional factors associated with military service and combat, and the potential that blasts may cause greater overall extracranial injury. In a study of victims of terror-related activities, Peleg and colleagues showed that gunshot wounds and injuries from explosions differ in the body regions of injury, distribution of severity, hospital length of stay, and length of stay in the intensive care unit.[41] In the blast victims, it was reported that multiple body regions were more often affected. The blast victims also had more critical and fatal injuries compared to the gunshot victims. Traumatic vasospasm has also been reported in a substantial number of patients with severe blast neurotrauma (80.8%–86.7% of those injured). Additionally, it was noted that clinical outcomes were worse for those with this condition.[6] TBI was noted in 56% of patients seen in the Veterans Affairs polytrauma system. Those with blast-related TBI demonstrated unique patterns of injury. Soft tissue, eye, oral and maxillofacial, otologic, and penetrating brain injuries; symptoms of posttraumatic stress disorder (PTSD); and auditory impairments were more common in blast-injured patients than in those with other war-related injuries. Despite these differences in injury profiles, functional outcome was not predicted by the mechanism of the injury.[42]

NEUROBEHAVIORAL SEQUELAE OF TRAUMATIC BRAIN INJURY AND POSTCONCUSSIVE DISORDER

Neurobehavioral changes are a common consequence of TBI. The characteristics, extent, and duration of these changes are dependent on a multitude of factors, including the type and location of injury, genetic predisposition, environment, and psychosocial support system. Psychosocial functioning has also been shown to be affected by TBI. The extent of these functional limitations is related to the demographics of the population injured, existing comorbid injuries, and severity of the head injury itself. As would be expected, more severe head injuries are associated with poorer outcomes, including greater reliance on family and social subsidy systems, greater unemployment, and lower income. The severity of the TBI is also more closely related to objective indices of psychosocial outcome (eg, employment) than to self-perceived psychosocial limitations.[43]

Cognitive changes are among the most frequently reported difficulties following TBI and can be the most debilitating. In at least one study, physical deficits were not related to the ability to return to employment, but the presence of cognitive, behavioral, and personality changes was significantly related to work failure.[44] The extent of cognitive difficulties is based largely on the nature and extent of damage to the brain, especially the severity of the diffuse axonal injury suffered.[45] Potential cognitive difficulties are wide ranging and encompass disruptions in various aspects of attention, learning and memory, language, and executive functioning (the ability to plan, organize, and self-monitor). These key aspects of executive functioning, which are necessary for the execution of goal-directed activities in daily life, are increasingly disrupted with anterior brain lesions because of the anatomic localization of these critical neural substrates in the anterior forebrain.[46]

In general, MTBI is unlikely to cause persistent, significant cognitive difficulties. In a study of MTBI, Belanger and colleagues conducted a metaanalysis of the relevant literature based on 39 studies involving 1,463 cases of MTBI and 1,191 control cases to determine the impact of MTBI across nine cognitive domains (global cognitive ability, attention, executive functions, fluency, memory acquisition, delayed memory, language, visuospatial skill, and motor functions).[47] The overall effect of MTBI on neuropsychological functioning was moderate, and was found to correlate with patient characteristics, time since injury, and the cognitive domain affected. Acute (less than 3 months after injury) effects of MTBI were greatest for delayed memory and fluency. In unselected or prospective groups of patients, the overall analysis revealed no residual neuropsychological impairment by 3 months after injury. In contrast, clinic-based groups of patients and those groups including participants in litigation were associated with greater cognitive sequelae of MTBI. In another study by the same investigators, a metaanalysis of sports concussion literature from 1970 to 2004 found 21 studies meeting inclusion criteria, leading to a total of 790 cases of MTBI and 2,016

control cases.[48] TBI only modestly effected cognitive functioning, with delayed memory, memory acquisition, and global cognitive functioning showing the greatest effects acutely. No residual effects were found from the group tested over 1 week after injury. Iverson illustrated that moderate and severe TBI have a significant, negative effect on cognition, but, after the acute recovery period, MTBI has essentially no measurable effect.[29] Larger effects were observed in conditions such as depression, bipolar disorder, and attention deficit hyperactivity disorder than from MTBI.

A World Health Organization analysis of MTBI outcomes concluded that although acute symptoms are common, MTBI symptoms resolve in the vast majority of individuals by 3 months after injury, often sooner.[11] However, the authors acknowledge that a subset of those with MTBI continue to manifest persistent symptoms. This has also been clinically observed in both military and civilian settings. In a review article on outcomes from MTBI, Iverson et al report that postconcussion symptoms are common in healthy subjects, including those without history of TBI. These findings have important implications for symptom attribution and recovery.[49] In some cases, without education about recovery and expected course of illness, patients who have suffered MTBI (ie, concussion) may attribute symptoms related to the combat environment or the challenges of everyday life to the effects of a remote brain injury.

The issues surrounding persistent symptoms after MTBI, especially as related to military deployment, has led to debate. The first controversy relates to the scope of the problem itself. Although it has been reported that 10% to 20% of those with MTBI will develop chronic persistent symptoms, it is likely that this figure is closer to 5%.[49] An equally controversial topic is the theoretical cause of persistent symptoms after MTBI. Various authors have attributed MTBI symptoms to different causes, some believing they are related to the type and location of injury, others purporting a multicausal etiology, influenced by premorbid personality characteristics, social-psychological factors, and exaggeration of symptom manifestation (either conscious or unconscious).

TRAUMATIC BRAIN INJURY IN THE AMPUTEE

For those who have sustained limb amputation as a result of combat operations, there is concern about other conditions that may be a consequence of combat exposure, such as TBI, acute stress, and PTSD. Hoge et al surveyed four US combat infantry units either before their deployment to Iraq or 3 to 4 months after their return from combat duty in Iraq or Afghanistan.

Those who had been deployed to Iraq reported a high number of combat experiences, with more than 90% reporting being shot at and a high percentage reporting handling dead bodies, knowing someone who was injured or killed, or killing an enemy combatant.[50] Soldiers who served in Afghanistan reported lower but still substantial rates of similar combat experiences.

The percentage of individuals whose responses met the screening criteria for major depression, PTSD, or alcohol misuse was significantly higher among soldiers after deployment than before deployment. Among service members in OIF, the prevalence of PTSD increased with the number of firefights during deployment, reaching 19.3% for those involved in more than five firefights. Additionally within this group, it was found that the rates of PTSD were associated with having been wounded or injured (odds ratio for those deployed to Iraq was 3.27; odds ratio for those deployed to Afghanistan was 2.49). This latter finding is consistent with Koren's study of PTSD rates in injured Israeli war veterans.[51] In that study, findings indicated that bodily injury is a risk factor for PTSD, with odds of developing PTSD following traumatic injury approximately eight times higher than following injury-free emotional trauma.

Although myriad factors influence the overall functional outcome of a service member with a major limb amputation, it is clear that both emotional and cognitive factors play a significant role in recovery. The presence of disorders such as depression or anxiety is associated with greater overall use of healthcare resources.[52] There is limited literature on the predictive value of mental disturbances and cognitive impairments on functional outcome in an amputee population. In general, and representative of the war-injured population, younger men have more difficulties adjusting to amputations, presumably because of concerns over body image, social stigma, or other related factors.[53] These concerns may contribute to the high rates of self-reported sexual problems in those with lower extremity amputations.[54]

In a study of the physical, mental, and social predictors of functional outcome in geriatric, unilateral lower limb amputees, Schoppen et al reported that memory ability was the most important of the mental predictors for functioning after leg amputation,[55] suggesting that good memory may be important for relearning daily tasks. Depression level 2 weeks after amputation was also found to be predictive of outcome at 1 year. In another study of geriatric amputees, records of 2,375 lower extremity amputees treated in Veterans Affairs hospitals were examined to determine which patient factors may influence the prescription of a prosthesis.[56] Those with high cognitive Functional Independence Measure (FIM) scores were 1.67 times more likely to be prescribed a prosthesis than those in the lowest FIM category (the FIM, a widely accepted functional measure in the research community, is an 18-item, 7-level ordinal scale intended to be sensitive to change in an individual over the course of a comprehensive inpatient medical rehabilitation program). Taylor et al investigated the relationship between a variety of preoperative clinical characteristics after major lower limb amputation and postoperative functional outcome.[57] Among other factors, the presence of dementia was significantly associated with failure to maintain independent living status. Because TBI may disrupt cognitive functioning, some aspects of amputee rehabilitation may be complicated, such as learning new tasks, remembering appointments, and regaining independence.

TREATMENT OF TRAUMATIC BRAIN INJURY

Because the majority of TBI that occurs in the civilian and military settings is mild, symptoms can generally be expected to improve over time and, in most cases, completely resolve.[29] MTBI is characterized by immediate physiological changes in the brain, but in the first week after injury, the brain undergoes a dynamic restorative process. This is often seen in athletes, who are typically able to return to preinjury functioning (cognitive and self-report) within 2 weeks after a concussion. Trauma patients usually take longer to return to preinjury functioning because of factors such as preexisting psychiatric or substance abuse problems, poor general health, concurrent orthopaedic injuries, pain, or various psychosocial problems.[29] The clinical team should communicate the expectation of a full recovery with the patient while simultaneously assessing the patient's symptom complex and providing treatment as indicated. The extent of intervention or rehabilitation required will be determined by a patient's comorbid injuries rather than the degree of brain injury.[42]

Symptom treatment for MTBI includes four areas of focus: pharmacological management, educational interventions, rest and return to duty decisions, and targeted therapies. Evidence for the efficiency of various pharmacologic interventions is prolific.[58,59] Pharmacological interventions are often indicated for sleep regulation,[60] headache,[61,62] pain,[63] and depression.[64] Treating these associated conditions improves quality of life and rehabilitation outcomes.

Educational and psychological therapies have also proven effective in treating MTBI. Mittenberg compared two groups of patients with MTBI. Group I (n = 29) participated in a cognitive-behavioral model of symptom maintenance and treatment, learned techniques for reducing symptoms, received printed educational manuals, and met with a therapist prior to hospital discharge to review the nature and incidence of expected symptoms and instructions for gradual resumption of premorbid activities.[65] The control group (n = 29) received routine hospital treatment and discharge instructions. After 6 months, Group I reported significantly shorter average symptom duration (33 compared to 51 days) and significantly fewer symptoms at follow-up. The conclusion was that brief, early psychological interventions are effective in reducing the incidence of postconcussive symptoms. Ponsford et al have shown similar results.[66] Individuals seen 1 week after injury and given informational material reported fewer symptoms overall and were significantly less stressed at 3 months after the injury than a group that did not receive the same education. A number of educational materials are available from public and private sources, including the Defense and Veterans Brain Injury Center.[67]

ACUTE MEDICAL CARE

Emergency preadmission care is aimed at preventing hypoxia and hypotension, which can lead to secondary neurological injury.[68] When admitting a patient for neurosurgical services, care is geared toward stabilizing the patient, treating infection, and detecting operable lesions that may prevent further neurological deterioration. The role of decompressive craniectomy remains controversial because it does not result in improved outcomes in all cases. Once the patient is stabilized, treatment is focused on creating an environment in which the brain has the best chance of neural recovery; this involves managing temperature, intracranial pressure, and perfusion and oxygenation; glycemic control; and early nutrition.[68,69] Drug-based neuroprotection is one aspect of the acute management of TBI. Medications, such as N-methyl-D-aspartate antagonists, are being studied in clinical trials and have shown potential long-term benefit.[69]

The risk of posttraumatic seizures is high in some subpopulations, especially those with war injuries.[70] Steroid therapy has not been shown to have any beneficial effect on seizures.[69] It is also clear from the literature that long-term use of anticonvulsants, such as phenytoin, does not prevent late seizures.[69] Managing early seizures with anticonvulsant therapy remains controversial. One study showed that late-seizure risk factors include brain contusion with subdural hematoma, skull fracture, loss of consciousness or amnesia (lasting > 1 day), and being older than 65 years.[70] However, in another study by four National Institute on Disability and Rehabilitation Research model system sites, bilateral parietal contusion, penetration of the dura, and multiple intracranial operations resulted in the highest risks for late seizures.[71]

Heterotopic ossification (HO), defined as pathologic ectopic bone formation in the soft tissue surrounding the joints, often afflicts patients after TBI, and this can have a significant impact on the rehabilitation and recovery of the amputee. The incidence of HO in TBI varies from approximately 10% to 70%, with a clinically significant incidence reported in the range of 10% to 20%.[72–75] HO typically causes pain and limits range of motion. Larger joints, like the hips, knees, and elbows, are most commonly affected. The pathogenesis of HO is unknown, but several risk factors have been identified, including prolonged coma after TBI, spasticity, immobilization, and increased serum alkaline phosphotase levels. HO is best diagnosed using sonography, three-phase bone scanning, or plain radiography. Range-of-motion therapy is often used to prevent HO. Although there is little evidence to support this theory, some believe active range-of-motion therapy may promote HO, therefore passive range-of-motion therapy is often recommended. Surgical excision, when indicated, is typically delayed until bone fully matures (typically 12–18 months). This waiting period is thought to reduce the risk of reoccurrence, but recent data suggests that early excision may be better and that recurrence is unlikely.[72] Literature concerning HO treatment is generally limited to surgical case studies without control groups.

Preventing and treating deep venous thrombosis (DVT) in patients with TBI can be complicated by concerns for intracranial bleeding. However, many recent studies show that chemical prophylaxis can help prevent DVT in certain populations that are at increased risk of bleeding. The importance of screening for DVT in these populations by ultrasound, computed tomography, and now by D-dimer testing (despite its high false-positive rates) remains critical because the risks of DVT and subsequent fatal pulmonary embolism are high, especially for those with blast injuries.[76] Although there is no consensus on national clinical practice guidelines,[77] Walter Reed Army Medical Center has developed its own guidelines specific to trauma patients.[76]

Diffuse spasticity is a relatively common complication in individuals with severe TBI. Management can often be challenging, but begins with a well-structured and consistent program of stretching and range-of-motion exercises administered by trained therapists. Family members can often be taught how to help facilitate range-of-motion exercises. Oral medications, such as tizanidine[78] or baclofen (which is more effective at managing lower limb tone),[79] may also be helpful. Unfortunately, oral management may be limited by side effects, such as sedation. For focal spasticity, interventional injections with botulinum toxin can be efficacious.[80] Intrathecal baclofen pumps have also proven to be effective in a number of trials for more diffuse spasticity and may also be useful in managing dysautonomia (the inability to regulate the autonomic nervous system).[69] Dysautonomia can manifest with tachycardia, tachypnea, fever, or hypertension. This process is less well understood, but a collection of case studies suggests that beta blockers, morphine, chlorpromazine, or midazolam may be effective treatments. Caution is needed any time such sedation medications are used in patients with TBI.[69]

REHABILITATION

When discussing TBI rehabilitation, it is important to note that "we have really only recently begun to evaluate the efficacy of approaches being used and the development of alternatives to optimize functional outcomes for TBI."[70] As noted earlier in this chapter, given the heterogeneity of the patient population with TBI and the complexity of the brain, it is difficult to categorize patients with TBI into clear diagnostic groups. Moreover, because recovery is dependent on a multitude of factors (eg, mechanism, location and circumstances surrounding the injury, an individual's premorbid constitution, environmental and psychosocial issues), examining outcomes in this patient population is challenging. These challenges are compounded when trying to evaluate optimal rehabilitation strategies to care for the military service member who sustains TBI in association with other combat-related injuries.

TBI rehabilitation begins with a careful evaluation of an individual's injuries. This evaluation should include a thorough cognitive, neurologic, motor, and extremity examination, as well as a full assessment of any sensory difficulties in vision, hearing, balance, and sense of smell.[81,82] It is also important for all rehabilitation disciplines to perform a thorough functional assessment of the patient, determining areas of function in hygiene, eating, mobility, dressing, toileting, and communication. This thorough, multidisciplinary evaluation facilitates the development and implementation of a comprehensive treatment approach. Assessment and treatment approaches that focus on the entire person, including physical, psychological, cognitive, social, occupational, academic, and spiritual aspects will have the greatest potential for maximizing a patient's functioning and quality of life. A multidisciplinary treatment team is necessary to treat complex patients recovering from polytraumatic injuries, such as those returning from OEF and OIF. Rehabilitation teams may include:

- physiatrists,
- rehabilitation nurses,
- prosthetists,
- neuropsychologists,
- rehabilitation psychologists,
- clinical psychologists,
- health psychologists,
- deployment health psychologists,
- marriage and family therapists,
- psychiatrists,
- neurologists,
- speech pathologists,
- occupational therapists,
- physical therapists,
- rehabilitation engineers,
- rehabilitation counselors,
- vocational rehabilitation therapists,
- clinical social workers,
- nurse case managers,
- substance abuse counselors, and
- chaplains.

In some cases, this team, combined with a patient's community and case managers, will be needed to provide care across the lifespan of the injured individual. In addition to the challenges presented immediately after TBI, symptom complexes may change over time. Symptoms of depression and reduced motor or cognitive function may result from a variety of life factors, such as the development of cardiovascular disease, arthritis, and dementia. Therefore it is important to provide individuals with TBI life-long coordinated health services and access to healthcare to promote the highest quality of life.[83] This is especially relevant for polytrauma patients who have multiple comorbid injuries, such as TBI, traumatic amputation, visual impairment, and psychological illness.[84] Polytrauma patients require an integrated treatment approach whereby patients receive care for all injuries simultaneously, as opposed to sequentially.

The role physical therapists play in assessing and treating TBI-related deficits is wide-ranging.[85] Physical therapy has proven effective in treating pain,[63] balance impairment, and postural instability, which are common symptoms in polytrauma patients with TBI.[86] Physical therapy is also helpful in assessing and treating motor impairments, especially those associated with severe TBI.[87] Paresis, ataxia, postural instability, tandem gait disturbances, and other motor neuron abnormalities are common and can be addressed through physical therapy interventions.

In addition to helping build independence in activities of daily living, occupational therapy has demonstrated efficacy in improving self-awareness after TBI.[88] Its role as part of a long-term strategy in more severe TBI patients is also well established.[89] Occupational therapists are critical to managing upper limb and hand spasticity positioning and functioning in those with motor deficits. They are also valuable partners to vocational rehabilitation experts, performing work assessments and helping integrate assistive technology to facilitate independence in the workplace.[90]

Evidence suggests that early rehabilitative interventions after TBI improve outcomes.[91,92] Polytrauma patients often have treatment targets in various domains. For example, if an injury was severe enough to require amputation, other areas of the patient's health may also have been affected. Blast-exposed patients may sustain TBI and psychological injuries in addition to the blast injury. Considering all of these factors, a patient's impairments, strengths, and functioning must be assessed to enhance the rehabilitation outcome from a major limb amputation.

Because so many patients undergoing rehabilitation for amputation suffer from brain injury, it is important to explore the particular needs and approaches for treating this dual condition. The presence and severity of TBI can have significant implications on the rehabilitation process. Patients with TBI may have restricted awareness of their injuries or limitations, may process information differently, and are likely to have difficulty participating in treatment at the same pace as amputees without TBI. An undiagnosed TBI or a treatment plan that is not modified based on a patient's cognitive impairment is likely to result in poor treatment response.

A complete neuropsychological evaluation not only reveals if a patient sustained cognitive deficits secondary to blast-related brain injury or other mechanisms, but also identifies the patient's strengths. For the purposes of this discussion, the term "neuropsychological evaluation" means the administration, scoring, and interpretation of empirically validated and normed neuropsychological tests by a neuropsychologist.

Cognitive and psychological function reciprocate and share several mechanisms. Identifying the origin of a symptom will inform the treatment approach. For example, if a patient has poor motivation, it is important to determine if that symptom is primarily due to

frontal lobe dysfunction or to depression. In addition, MTBI and PTSD share a similar cognitive dysfunction profile. Trudeau et al have suggested that blast patients may suffer from a complex chronic concussive disorder with overlapping cognitive deficits, depression, and PTSD. Neuropsychological testing can help tease apart these symptoms.[93]

A comprehensive neuropsychological evaluation comprises empirically validated cognitive testing and a complete mental health evaluation. Recommended cognitive testing includes a survey of all major domains of cognitive functioning (Table 15-2). Some caution is warranted when using inventories or questionnaires that have been developed for use in a civilian TBI population. There may be differences in the demographics (eg, education, employment status, etc) or the circumstances of the injury (eg, combat and related emotional factors) in military patients as compared to their civilian counterparts.

The recommended mental health assessment portion of a neuropsychological evaluation includes a review of the patient's personal history, including academic, occupational, military, social, family, medical (especially history of prior TBI or concussion), substance use and family substance abuse, mental health, deployment, and combat history. Patients with amputations may suffer from a number of mental health disorders, not likely limited to PTSD. Among the disorders of concern are depression and possible narcotic dependence secondary to overuse of pain medications. Clinical interviews focus on how amputees and their families are adjusting to daily living, as well as on the patient's strengths and resilience factors. Gathering a thorough history and performing a complete mental health examination is necessary in order to approximate a patient's baseline and to appropriately interpret results from the neuropsychological evaluation.

The results of the neuropsychological evaluation inform the treatment plan, and there are several ways in which the results from a neuropsychological evaluation can be clinically applied. They can be used to modify rehabilitation strategies based on a patient's cognitive abilities, or used to directly treat cognitive dysfunction and psychological injuries. They can also facilitate adjustment to amputation.

In order for many patients to effectively participate in the physical aspects of their rehabilitation, their cognitive deficits must be recognized and addressed. Patients with cognitive deficits often have difficulty participating in "treatment as usual." Many patients are considered "treatment failures" when the expected treatment outcome is not obtained. However, cognitive deficits often interfere with patients' abilities to

TABLE 15-2

DOMAINS OF COGNITIVE FUNCTIONING AND REPRESENTATIVE NEUROPSYCHOLOGICAL TESTS

Cognitive Function	Test
Verbal memory: immediate and delayed	California Verbal Learning Test II
Visual memory: immediate and delayed	Rey-Osterrieth Complex Figure, copy and delayed visual reproduction subtests from the Wechsler Memory Scale III
Executive functioning	Stroop Test, Wisconsin Card Sorting Test, Trail Making Test (part B)
Attention	Conners' Continuous Performance Test, Paced Auditory Serial Addition Test, digit span subtest from the Wechsler Adult Intelligence Scale III
Psychomotor speed	Trail Making Test (part A), finger tapping test, grooved pegboard test
General intellectual functioning	Wechsler Abbreviated Scale of Intelligence
Psychological functioning	Clinical interview, collateral interview, Personality Assessment Inventory, Detailed Assessment of Posttraumatic Stress
Effort/motivation	Test of Memory Malingering, Word Memory Test

understand and follow directions, follow sequences or schedules, practice on their own, remember what they have learned, manage their behavior, maintain sufficient motivation, or work cooperatively with others. Substance abuse, dementia, and stroke literature discuss the value of modifying patients' treatment plans in accordance with their cognitive deficits. Several studies address either comprehensive rehabilitation of patients with cognitive deficits or interventions for specific cognitive deficits.[70] Such approaches also show strong support from the brain injury advocacy community.[94] Treating psychological injuries that occurred with a traumatic event is important for overall clinical improvement. Similarly, as a patient begins to make gains in physical rehabilitation, improvements in mental health symptoms are often observed.

The experience and management of pain also appears to be related to mental health and, more specifically, to PTSD. Patients with depression experience higher subjective pain levels,[95] and pain-related variables have been shown to be significant predictors of PTSD symptom cluster scores in both male and female veterans.[96] These findings suggest that managing pain for the amputee may improve mental health prognosis. Similarly, treating mental health symptoms may improve an amputee's ability to engage in physical rehabilitation because of decreased pain perception. Facilitating patient and family adjustment to TBI and amputation, the rehabilitation process, and return to daily life are integral to patients being able to maintain treatment gains, achieve the highest level of independent functioning, and maximize quality of life.

SUMMARY

In times of peace and during times of active military operations, TBI is a significant and important health issue for US military service members. Even with the best efforts at prevention, a relatively large number of service members can be expected to sustain TBI each year. To optimize treatment and rehabilitation, the complicated interplay between physiologic insult to the brain, the disruption of the mind, and the injury to the body must be better understood. An assessment and appreciation of how these factors act together to ameliorate or hinder an individual's functioning is necessary to maximize outcomes and promote recovery across a patient's lifespan.

REFERENCES

1. Langlois JA, Rutland-Brown W, Thomas KE. Traumatic brain injury in the United States: emergency department visits, hospitalizations, and deaths. Atlanta, Ga: Department of Health and Human Services, Centers for Disease Control and Prevention; 2004.

2. Lewin ICF. *The Cost of Disorders of the Brain*. Washington, DC: The National Foundation for the Brain; 1992.

3. Thurman DJ. Traumatic Brain Injury in the United States: a Report to Congress. Atlanta, Ga: Centers for Disease Control and Prevention; 2001.

4. Ommaya AK, Ommaya AK, Dannenberg AL, Salazar AM. Causation, incidence, and costs of traumatic brain injury in the U.S. military medical system. *J Trauma*. 1996:40(2):211–217.

5. US Department of Defense. Casualty Update Web page. Available at: http://www.defenselink.mil/news/casualty.pdf. Accessed May 16, 2007.

6. Armonda RA, Bell RS, Vo AH, et al. Wartime traumatic cerebral vasospasm: recent review of combat casualties. *Neurosurgery*. 2006;59(6):1215–1225.

7. Xydakis MS, Fravell MD, Nasser KE, Casler JD. Analysis of battlefield head and neck injuries in Iraq and Afghanistan. *Otolaryngol Head Neck Surg*. 2005;133(4):497–504.

8. US Department of the Army. Traumatic Brain Injury (TBI) Task Force report. Available at: http://www.armymedicine.army.mil/prr/tbitfr.html. Published January 2008. Accessed May 7, 2008.

9. Williams DH, Levin HS, Eisenberg HM. Mild head injury classification. *Neurosurgery*. 1990;27(3):422–428.

10. Hsiang J, Yeung T, Yu AL, Poon WS. High-risk mild head injury. *J Neurosurg*. 1997;87(2):234–238.

11. Carroll LJ, Cassidy JD, Peloso PM, et al. Prognosis for mild traumatic brain injury: results of the WHO Collaborating Centre Task Force on Mild Traumatic Brain Injury. *J Rehabil Med*. 2004;43:84–105.

12. Werner C, Engelhard K. Pathophysiology of traumatic brain injury. *Br J Anaesth*. 2007;99:4–9.

13. Baethmann A, Eriskat J, Stoffel M, Chapuis D, Wirth A, Plesnila N. Special aspects of severe head injury: recent developments. *Curr Opin Anaesthesiol*. 1998;11:193–200.

14. Marshall LF. Head injury: recent past, present, and future. *Neurosurgery*. 2000;47:546–561.

15. McIntosh TK, Smith DH, Meaney DF, Kotapka MJ, Gennarelli TA, Graham DI. Neuropathological sequelae of traumatic brain injury: relationship to neurochemical and biochemical mechanisms. *Lab Invest*. 1996;74:315–342.

16. Nortje J, Menon DK. Traumatic brain injury: physiology, mechanisms, and outcome. *Curr Opin Neurol*. 2004;17:711–718.

17. Dietrich WD, Alonso O, Busto R, et al. Posttraumatic cerebral ischemia after fluid percussion brain injury: an autoradiographic and histopathological study in rats. *Neurosurgery*. 1998;43:585–593.

18. Dietrich WD, Alonso O, Busto R, et al. Widespread hemodynamic depression and focal platelet accumulation after fluid percussion brain injury: a double-label autoradiographic study in rats. *J Cereb Blood Flow Metab*. 1996;16:481–489.

19. Bouma GJ, Muizelaar JP, Choi SC, Newlon PG, Young HF. Cerebral circulation and metabolism after severe traumatic brain injury: the elusive role of ischemia. *J Neurosurg*. 1991;75:685–693.

20. von Oettingen G, Bergholt B, Gyldensted C, Astrup J. Blood flow and ischemia within traumatic cerebral contusions. *Neurosurgery*. 2002;50:781.

21. Marion DW, Darby J, Yonas H. Acute regional cerebral blood flow changes caused by severe head injuries. *J Neurosurg.* 1991;74:407–414.

22. Bouma GJ, Muizelaar JP, Stringer WA, Choi SC, Fatouros P, Young HF. Ultra-early evaluation of regional cerebral blood flow in severely head-injured patients using xenon-enhanced computerized tomography. *J Neurosurg.* 1992;77:360–368.

23. Coles JP, Fryer TD, Smielewski P, et al. Defining ischemic burden after traumatic brain injury using ^{15}O PET imaging of cerebral physiology. *J Cereb Blood Flow Metab.* 2004;24:191–201.

24. Inoue Y, Shiozaki T, Tasaki O, et al. Changes in cerebral blood flow from the acute to the chronic phase of severe head injury. *J Neurotrauma.* 2005;22:1411–1418.

25. Overgaard J, Tweed WA. Cerebral circulation after head injury. Part 4: Functional anatomy and boundary-zone flow deprivation in the first week of traumatic coma. *J Neurosurg.* 1983;59:439–446.

26. Madikians A, Giza CC. A clinician's guide to the pathophysiology of traumatic brain injury. *Indian J Neurotrauma.* 2006;3:9–17.

27. Marmarou A, Fatouros PP, Barzó P, et al. Contribution of edema and cerebral blood volume to traumatic brain swelling in head-injured patients. *J Neurosurg.* 2000;93:183–193.

28. Marmarou A, Signoretti S, Fatouros P, Portella G, Aygok GA, Bullock MR. Predominance of cellular edema in traumatic brain swelling in patients with severe head injuries. *J Neurosurg.* 2006;104:720–730.

29. Iverson GL. Outcome from mild traumatic brain injury. *Curr Opin Psychiatry.* 2005;18(3):301–317.

30. Barton CW, Hemphill JC, Morabito D, Manley G. A novel method of evaluating the impact of secondary brain insults on functional outcomes in traumatic brain-injured patients. *Acad Emerg Med.* 2005;12(1):1–6.

31. Salazar AM, Schwab K, Grafman JH. Penetrating injuries in the Vietnam war. Traumatic unconsciousness, epilepsy, and psychosocial outcome. *Neurosurg Clin N Am.* 1995;6(4):715–726.

32. Murray CK, Reynolds JC, Schroeder JM, Harrison MB, Evans OM, Hospenthal DR. Spectrum of care provided at an echelon II medical unit during Operation Iraqi Freedom. *Mil Med.* 2005;170:516–520.

33. Brookings Institution. *Iraq Index: Tracking Reconstruction and Security in Post-Saddam Iraq.* Available at: http://www.brookings.edu/saban/iraq-index.aspx. Accessed September 26, 2008.

34. Levi L, Borovich B, Guilburd JN, et al. Wartime neurosurgical experience in Lebanon, 1982–85. I: Penetrating craniocerebral injuries. *Isr J Med Sci.* 1990;26(10):548–554.

35. Levi L, Borovich B, Guilburd JN, et al. Wartime neurosurgical experience in Lebanon, 1982-85. II: Closed craniocerebral injuries. *Isr J Med Sci.* 1990;26(10):555–558.

36. Cernak I, Savic J, Ignjatovic D, Jevtic M. Blast injury from explosive munitions. *J Trauma.* 1999;47(1):96–104.

37. Cernak I, O'Connor C, Vink R. Activation of cyclo-oxygenase-2 contributes to motor and cognitive dysfunction following diffuse traumatic brain injury in rats. *Clin Exp Pharmacol Physiol.* 2001;28(11):922–925.

38. Mott FW. The effects of high explosives upon the central nervous system. *Lancet.* 1916;4824:331–338.

39. Cohen H, Biskind GR. Pathologic aspects of atmospheric blast injuries in man. *Arch Pathol.* 1946;42:12–34.

40. Bryant RA. Disentangling mild traumatic brain injury and stress reactions. *N Engl J Med.* 2008;358(5):525–527.

41. Peleg K, Aharonson-Daniel L, Michael M, Shapira SC. Patterns of injury in hospitalized terrorist victims. *Am J Emerg Med.* 2003;21(4):258–262.

42. Sayer NA, Chiros CE, Sigford B, et al. Characteristics and rehabilitation outcomes among patients with blast and other injuries sustained during the Global War on Terror. *Arch Phys Med Rehabil*. 2008;89(1):163–170.

43. Dikmen SS, Ross BL, Machamer JE, Temkin NR. One year psychosocial outcome in head injury. *J Int Neuropsychol Soc*. 1995;1(1):67–77.

44. Brooks N, McKinlay W, Symington C, Beattie A, Campsie L. Return to work within the first seven years of severe head injury. *Brain Inj*. 1987;1(1):5–19.

45. Katz DI, Alexander MP. Traumatic brain injury. Predicting course of recovery and outcome for patients admitted to rehabilitation. *Arch Neurol*. 1994;51(7):661–670.

46. Lux WE. A neuropsychiatric perspective on traumatic brain injury. *J Rehabil Res Dev*. 2007;44(7):951–962.

47. Belanger HG, Curtiss G, Demery JA, Lebowitz BK, Vanderploeg RD. Factors moderating neuropsychological outcomes following mild traumatic brain injury: a meta-analysis. *J Int Neuropsychol Soc*. 2005;11(3):215–227.

48. Belanger HG, Vanderploeg RD. The neuropsychological impact of sports-related concussion: a meta-analysis. *J Int Neuropsychol Soc*. 2005;11:345–357.

49. Iverson GL, Zasler N, Lange RT. Post-concussive disorder. In: Zasler ND, Katz DI, Zafonte RD, eds. *Brain Injury Medicine: Principles and Practice*. New York, NY: Demos Medical Publishing; 2006: 373–405.

50. Hoge CW, Castro CA, Messer SC, McGurk D, Cotting DI, Koffman RL. Combat duty in Iraq and Afghanistan, mental health problems, and barriers to care. *N Engl J Med*. 2004;351:13–22.

51. Koren D, Norman D, Cohen A, Berman J, Klein EM. Increased PTSD risk with combat-related injury: a matched comparison study of injured and uninjured soldiers experiencing the same combat events. *Am J Psychiatry*. 2005;162:276–282.

52. Simon G, Ormel J, VonKorff M, Barlow W. Health care costs associated with depressive and anxiety disorders in primary care. *Am J Psychiatry*. 1995;152(3):352–357.

53. Rybarczyk B, Nyenhuis DL, Nicholas JJ, Cash SM, Kaiser J. Body image, perceived social stigma, and the prediction of psychosocial adjustment to leg amputation. *Rehabil Psychol*. 1995;40(2):95–110.

54. Bodenheimer C, Kerrigan AJ, Garber SL, Monga TN. Sexuality in persons with lower extremity amputations. *Disabil Rehabil*. 2000;22(9):409–415.

55. Schoppen T, Boonstra A, Groothoff JW, de Vries J, Göeken LN, Eisma WH. Physical, mental, and social predictors of functional outcome in unilateral lower-limb amputees. *Arch Phys Med Rehabil*. 2003;84(6):803–811.

56. Kurichi JE, Kwong PL, Reker DM, Bates BE, Marshall CR, Stineman MG. Clinical factors associated with prescription of a prosthetic limb in elderly veterans. *J Am Geriatr Soc*. 2007;55(6):900–906.

57. Taylor SM, Kalbaugh CA, Blackhurst DW, et al. Preoperative clinical factors predict postoperative functional outcomes after major lower limb amputation: an analysis of 553 consecutive patients. *J Vasc Surg*. 2005;42(2):227–235.

58. Warden DL, Gordon B, McAllister TW, et al. Guidelines for the pharmacologic treatment of neurobehavioral sequelae of traumatic brain injury. *J Neurotrauma*. 2006;23(10):1468–1501.

59. Lee HB, Lyketsos CG, Rao V. Pharmacological management of the psychiatric aspects of traumatic brain injury. *Inter Rev Psychiatry*. 2003;15(4):359–370.

60. Thaxton L, Myers MA. Sleep disturbances and their management in patients with brain injury. *J Head Trauma Rehabil*. 2002;17(4):335–348.

61. Walker WC, Seel RT, Curtiss G, Warden DL. Headache after moderate and severe traumatic brain injury: a longitudinal analysis. *Arch Phys Med Rehabil*. 2005;86(9):1793–1800.

62. Lew HL, Lin PH, Fuh JL, Wang SJ, Clark DJ, Walker WC. Characteristics and treatment of headache after traumatic brain injury: a focused review. *Am J Phys Med Rehabil*. 2006;85(7):619–627.

63. Young JA. Pain and traumatic brain injury. *Phys Med Rehabil Clin N Am*. 2007;18(1):145–163.

64. Alderfer BS, Arciniegas DB, Silver JM. Treatment of depression following traumatic brain injury. *J Head Trauma Rehabil*. 2005;20(6):544–562.

65. Mittenberg W, Tremont G, Zielinski RE, Fichera S, Rayls KR. Cognitive-behavioral prevention of postconcussion syndrome. *Arch Clin Neuropsychol*. 1996;11(2):139–145.

66. Ponsford J, Willmott C, Rothwell A, et al. Impact of early intervention on outcome following mild head injury in adults. *J Neurol Neurosurg Psychiatry*. 2002;73:330–332.

67. Defense and Veterans Brain Injury Center. Traumatic brain injury education Web site. Available at: http://www.dvbic.org/cms.php?p=Education. Accessed October 8, 2008.

68. Maas AI, Stocchetti N, Bullock R. Moderate and severe traumatic brain injury in adults. *Lancet Neurol*. 2008;7(8):728–741.

69. Gordon WA, Zafonte R, Cicerone K, et al. Traumatic brain injury rehabilitation: state of the science. *Am J Phys Med Rehabil*. 2006;85(4):343–382.

70. Annegers JF, Hauser WA, Coan SP, Rocca WA. A population-based study of seizures after traumatic brain injuries. *N Engl J Med*. 1998;338(1):20–24.

71. Englander J, Bushnik T, Duong TT, et al. Analyzing risk factors for late posttraumatic seizures: a prospective, multi-center investigation. *Arch Phys Med Rehabil*. 2003;84(3):365–373.

72. Melamed E, Robinson D, Halperin N, Wallach N, Keren O, Groswasser Z. Brain injury-related heterotopic bone formation: treatment strategy and results. *Am J Phys Med Rehabil*. 2002;81(9):670–674.

73. Garland DE. Clinical observations on fractures and heterotopic ossification in the spinal cord and traumatic brain injured populations. *Clin Orthop*. 1996;233:86–101.

74. Garland DE. A clinical perspective on common forms of acquired heterotopic ossification. *Clin Orthop Relat Res*. 1991;263:13–29.

75. Sazbon L, Najenson T, Tartakovsky M, Becker E, Grosswasser Z. Widespread periarticular new-bone formation in long-term comatose patients. *J Bone Joint Surg Br*. 1981;63-B:120–125.

76. Colombo CJ, Mount CA, Popa CA. Critical care medicine at Walter Reed Army Medical Center in support of the global war on terrorism. *Crit Care Med*. 2008;36(7 Suppl):S388–394.

77. Carlile MC, Yablon SA, Mysiw WJ, Frol AB, Lo D, Diaz-Arrastia R. Deep venous thrombosis management following traumatic brain injury: a practice survey of the traumatic brain injury model systems. *J Head Trauma Rehabil*. 2006;21(6):483–490.

78. Meythaler JM, Guin-Renfroe S, Johnson A, Brunner RM. Prospective assessment of tizanidine for spasticity due to acquired brain injury. *Arch Phys Med Rehabil*. 2001;82(9):1155–1163.

79. Meythaler JM, Clayton W, Davis LK, Guin-Renfroe S, Brunner RC. Orally delivered baclofen to control spastic hypertonia in acquired brain injury. *J Head Trauma Rehabil*. 2004;19(2):101–108.

80. Pavesi G, Brianti R, Medici D, Mammi P, Mazzucchi A, Mancia D. Botulinum toxin type A in the treatment of upper limb spasticity among patients with traumatic brain injury. *J Neurol Neurosurg Psychiatry*. 1998;64(3):419–420.

81. Goodrich GL, Kirby J, Cockerham G, Ingalla SP, Lew HL. Visual function in patients of a polytrauma rehabilitation center: a descriptive study. *J Rehabil Res Dev*. 2007;44(7):929–936.

82. Lew HL, Jerger JF, Guillory SB, Henry JA. Auditory dysfunction in traumatic brain injury. *J Rehabil Res Dev.* 2007;44(7):921–928.

83. Lew HL, Poole JH, Guillory SB, Salerno RM, Leskin G, Sigford B. Persistent problems after traumatic brain injury: the need for long-term follow-up and coordinated care. *J Rehabil Res Dev.* 2006;43(2):vii–x.

84. Keel M, Trentz O. Pathophysiology of polytrauma. *Injury.* 2005;36(6):691–709.

85. Hellweg S, Johannes S. Physiotherapy after traumatic brain injury: a systematic review of the literature. *Brain Inj.* 2008;22(5):365–373.

86. Pickett TC, Radfar-Baublitz LS, McDonald SD, Walker WC, Cifu DX. Objectively assessing balance deficits after TBI: role of computerized posturography. *J Rehabil Res Dev.* 2007;44(7):983–990.

87. Walker WC, Pickett TC. Motor impairment after severe traumatic brain injury: a longitudinal multicenter study. *J Rehabil Res Dev.* 2007;44(7):975–982.

88. Goverover Y, Johnston MV, Toglia J, Deluca J. Treatment to improve self-awareness in persons with acquired brain injury. *Brain Inj.* 2007;21(9):913–923.

89. Parish L, Oddy M. Efficacy of rehabilitation for functional skills more than 10 years after extremely severe brain injury. *Neuropsychol Rehabil.* 2007;17(2):230–243.

90. Murphy L, Chamberlain E, Weir J, Berry A, Nathaniel-James D, Agnew R. Effectiveness of vocational rehabilitation following acquired brain injury: preliminary evaluation of a UK specialist rehabilitation programme. *Brain Inj.* 2006;20(11):1119–1129.

91. Mazaux JM, De Sèze M, Joseph PA, Barat M. Early rehabilitation after severe brain injury: a French perspective. *J Rehabil Med.* 2001;33(3):99–109.

92. Wagner AK, Fabio T, Zafonte RD, Goldberg G, Marion DW, Peitzman AB. Physical medicine and rehabilitation consultation: relationships with acute functional outcome, length of stay, and discharge planning after traumatic brain injury. *Am J Phys Med Rehabil.* 2003;82(7):526–536.

93. Trudeau DL, Anderson J, Hansen LM, et al. Findings of mild traumatic brain injury in combat veterans with PTSD and a history of blast concussion. *J Neuropsychiatry Clin Neurosci.* 1998;10(3):308–313.

94. Brain Injury Association of America Web site. Available at: http://www.biausa.org/. Accessed October 8, 2008.

95. Carter LE, McNeil DW, Vowles KE, et al. Effects of emotion on pain reports, tolerance and physiology. *Pain Res Manag.* 2002;7(1):21–30.

96. Asmundson GJ, Wright KD, Stein MB. Pain and PTSD symptoms in female veterans. *Eur J Pain.* 2004;8(4):345–350.

Chapter 16

SPINAL CORD INJURY REHABILITATION

STEPHEN P. BURNS, MD[*]; BARRY GOLDSTEIN, MD, PhD[†]; JELENA SVIRCEV, MD[‡]; STEVEN STIENS, MD[§]; KENDRA BETZ, MSPT, ATP[¥]; JAMES W. LITTLE, MD, PhD[¶]; and MARGARET C. HAMMOND, MD[**]

[*]Staff Physician, VA Puget Sound Health Care System, SCI (128), 1660 South Columbian Way, Seattle, Washington 98108; Associate Professor, Department of Rehabilitation Medicine, 1959 NE Pacific, Seattle, Washington 98195

[†]Associate Chief Consultant, Spinal Cord Injury/Disorders Services, Department of Veterans Affairs; VA Puget Sound Health Care System, SCI (128N), 1660 South Columbian Way, Seattle, Washington 98108; Professor, Department of Rehabilitation Medicine, 1959 NE Pacific, Seattle, Washington 98195

[‡]Staff Physician, VA Puget Sound Health Care System, SCI (128), 1660 South Columbian Way, Seattle, Washington 98108; Acting Instructor, Department of Rehabilitation Medicine, University of Washington, 1959 NE Pacific, Seattle, Washington 98195

[§]Staff Physician, VA Puget Sound Health Care System, SCI (128), 1660 South Columbian Way, Seattle, Washington 98108; Associate Professor, Department of Rehabilitation Medicine, 1959 NE Pacific, Seattle, Washington 98195

[¥]SCI Clinical Specialist, Veterans Health Administration, Prosthetic & Sensory Aids (113), 810 Vermont Avenue, NW, Washington, DC 20006

[¶]Assistant Chief, VA Puget Sound Health Care System, SCI (128), 1660 South Columbian Way, Seattle, Washington 98108; Professor, Department of Rehabilitation Medicine, 1959 NE Pacific, Seattle, Washington 98195

[**]Chief Consultant, Spinal Cord Injury/Disorders Services, Department of Veterans Affairs; Chief, Spinal Cord Injury Service, VA Puget Sound Health Care System, SCI (128N), 1660 South Columbian Way, Seattle, Washington 98108; Professor, Department of Rehabilitation Medicine, 1959 NE Pacific, Seattle, Washington 98195

415

INTRODUCTION

Spinal cord injury (SCI) among the US civilian population occurs at the rate of 11,000 new injuries per year. The most recent data from US National SCI Statistical Center indicate that young men are the most common demographic to sustain SCI (78% of the total injured are males). Although the most frequent age at injury is 19, the mean age at injury is 38. Impacts at high velocity are the most common cause of SCI. Motor vehicle collisions are responsible for 50%, falls for 24%, acts of violence for 11%, and sports for 9% of SCIs.[1,2] Low-velocity gunshot injuries are responsible for most acts of violence that result in SCI; other penetrating injuries account for 0.9%, and blasts account for 0.1%.[3] The most common SCI site is the cervical cord (54% of cases), followed by the thoracic cord (36%), and the lumbar cord (10%). The most common neurological category is incomplete tetraplegia (34.1% of all injuries; the term "tetraplegia" replaced "quadriplegia" to indicate a cervical neurological level, and "paraplegia" refers to a thoracic, lumbar, or sacral neurological level).[1] About 253,000 Americans (roughly 0.1% of the US population) are traumatic SCI survivors.

The demographic profile of war-injured SCI survivors is less well documented. In Vietnam, 0.9% of those admitted to US Army hospitals had sustained SCI, and 3.8% of those patients died during initial hospitalization.[4] In various Israeli wars, the percentage of those injured by gunshots to the spinal cord varied between 0.2% during the War of Independence in 1948–1949 and 1.1% in the Sinai Campaign of 1956.[5] As of December 31, 2008, 432 active duty US service members serving during Operations Enduring Freedom and Iraqi Freedom sustained SCI and received treatment in Department of Veterans Affairs SCI units. Of these individuals, 141 were injured in theater.

From the time the first recorded description of SCI was written on Egyptian papyrus until World War II, SCI was viewed as "an ailment not to be treated." Death following SCI commonly ensued from uncontrollable urinary tract infections (UTIs) and pressure ulcers. During the Balkan Wars of 1912–1913, 95% of soldiers with SCI died within a few weeks. During World War I, 80% of overseas American troops with SCI died before they could return to the United States.[6]

During World War II, the attitude of fatalism toward the spinal cord injured began to change. Advances in anesthesia, surgical techniques, blood transfusions, and antibiotics all contributed to increased survival. Teams of physicians, nurses, and therapists in Great Britain established SCI units and developed procedures for meticulous care and rehabilitation of the injured.[7] These protocols not only allowed the injured to survive, but in many cases made it possible for them to return to their communities.

At the conclusion of World War II, the US government, following the British model, established the first comprehensive SCI unit at Hines Veterans Administration Hospital in suburban Chicago. Over 75% of the paraplegics from World War II were alive 20 years later, and of the 2,500 American paraplegics from that war, over half returned to the job force. The first federally designated SCI care system center (part of the national Model SCI System) for civilians in the United States opened in 1970, and additional regional centers were developed through the 1970s. Fourteen centers are currently funded through the National Institute on Disability and Rehabilitation Research to provide comprehensive care for individuals with new, traumatic SCI; contribute data to the National SCI Statistical Center; and conduct SCI research.

With improved care, particularly of urologic and skin complications, late mortality (ie, after initial rehabilitation) from SCI also declined. Late mortality was 1.7 times higher for those injured in the 1940s than for those injured in the 1960s.[8] For those injured at age 20 and with minimal paralysis, life expectancy is only reduced by about 6 years. With more than minimal paralysis, life expectancy is progressively reduced across higher injury levels, with life expectancy of about 43 years for a person who becomes ventilator dependent at age 20 and survives for the first year following injury.[9] As mortality has declined, the focus of SCI care has gradually shifted. Initially, the target was defining and adopting procedures and practices to control the often fatal sequelae. Now the focus also includes retraining individuals for independence, return to community, a lifetime of healthy behaviors, and full quality of life.

PATHOPHYSIOLOGY OF SPINAL CORD INJURY

The two primary types of traumatic SCI mechanisms are penetrating and nonpenetrating injuries. Penetrating injuries typically result from a bullet, fragment, or knife blade directly lacerating the spinal cord. Penetrating injury accounts for only 17% of traumatic SCI in the civilian population, and nearly all of these are due to gunshots. Nonpenetrating injuries commonly result from bone or herniated disk material compressing the spinal cord or cauda equina, or from traction from spinal dislocation. In the civilian population, automobile and motorcycle crashes, falls, and sports injuries are the primary causes of nonpenetrating SCI. Blast injuries cause SCI through secondary effects (eg, fragments that penetrate the spinal canal) or tertiary effects (eg, nonpenetrating injuries from acute angulation or loading of the spine due to blast wind, structural collapse, or deceleration after being thrown by a blast).[10] Penetrating and nonpenetrating SCI may involve vertebral fracture with displacement of bony fragments into the spinal canal, or ischemia due to disruption in the blood supply to the cord. Nonpenetrating injuries often result in ligament disruption, with instability and resulting vertebral malalignment. Individuals with narrow spinal canals, either congenital or acquired due to degenerative changes, are at greater risk for cord injury, even from relatively minor trauma.

Penetrating and nonpenetrating injuries may compromise gray matter, white matter, and nerve roots. Gray matter contains motor neurons that provide output to muscles and interneurons that receive descending motor and segmental reflex input. Gray matter is thought to be more vulnerable to mechanical trauma than white matter because it is relatively more vascular. Gray matter damage typically extends one or two segments rostral and caudal to the cord injury, but may be more extensive if the cord blood supply has been disrupted. All segments involved compose the "zone of injury." Damage to gray matter causes segmental changes with denervation, muscle atrophy, and impaired reflexes. White matter is comprised of ascending and descending fibers at the periphery of the cord. Pathologic studies of cord trauma show greater gray than white matter involvement.[11-13] Damage to white matter is more disabling because it results in loss of motor control and sensory input at and below the injury site, and hypertonia and hyperreflexia accompany weakness and sensory loss with such white matter involvement. Nerve root injury often results in an asymmetric level of injury.

Spinal cord damage can also arise indirectly from vascular disruption. Thus, cross clamping of the thoracic aorta or disruption of the artery of Adamkiewicz or a vertebral artery can result in cord ischemia or infarction.[14-16] Another type of ischemic cord injury is decompression sickness, in which hyperbaric exposure (as in underwater diving) followed by sudden decompression results in gas bubble formation and bubble emboli that occlude blood vessels.[17,18]

In the majority of cases, the spinal cord is not completely transected anatomically, and secondary processes contribute to the degree of neurological deficit. These processes include ischemia, edema, hematomyelia, demyelination, persisting mechanical pressure, lactic acidosis, intracellular influx of calcium, increase of lipid peroxidation, and free radical formation.[19-22] Various early treatments, such as hyperbaric oxygen, cord cooling, naloxone, thyrotropin-releasing hormone, and osmotic diuretics, have been proposed to minimize this secondary neurologic injury.[22] Methylprednisolone has been investigated in three multicenter trials as a neuroprotective agent following acute SCI,[23-25] and it may modestly improve neurological outcomes when given within 8 hours of nonpenetrating SCI. However, trial findings have been questioned,[26] and there are concerns about increased infection rates with use of methylprednisolone. GM-1 gaglioside showed promising results as a neuroprotective agent in an early trial, but a multicenter trial with 760 subjects failed to show any benefit in the primary neurologic outcome.[27] Another intervention to promote recovery is late (ie, 1–12 months after SCI) anterior decompression. This procedure reportedly allowed functional recovery in subjects with incomplete SCI, and residual cord or root compression for those whose recovery had plateaued for 4 weeks or more.[28]

Animal models of incomplete SCI demonstrate that much of the spontaneous neurologic recovery is mediated by spared white matter axons that substitute for those pathways that have degenerated, rather than by resolution of conduction block, remyelination or resolution of ischemia, or edema. The mechanisms that allow for this substitution of function by spared pathways likely include rapid-acting denervation supersensitivity and slower-acting synaptogenesis. When spared, descending white matter pathways and spinal reflex pathways undergo trauma-induced reactive synaptogenesis, which may result in both motor recovery and spinal hyperreflexia. The slow pace of this motor recovery and the gradual onset of spasticity may be explained by the slowness of synaptogenesis. Because neural activity seems to be a necessary condition for such recovery, one way to enhance this process may be to increase the activity in the spared neural pathways.[29] In animal models of stroke, administration of central nervous system stimulants (eg, amphetamine), combined with exercise, has enhanced recovery. These observations suggest that remobilization of the patient and active exercise are essential factors in optimizing recovery of function after SCI.

Medications and growth factors are unexplored methods of regulating activity in the cord's spared neural pathways. The optimal treatment for minimizing developing spasticity during this period of recovery is also unresolved. With stroke patients, some advocate reflex facilitation during strengthening exercises to enhance motor recovery; however, this may result in greater spasticity. Alternatively, aggressive early treatment with medication and physical modalities may suppress the development of spasticity, but it may not optimize recovery of motor function. Resolving these issues will allow more effective rehabilitation of acute, incomplete SCI in the future.

In contrast to white matter or long-tract recovery, zone-of-injury recovery involves recovery of lower motor neurons (gray matter recovery) and roots at the site of injury.[30,31] Mechanisms to explain zone-of-injury recovery include resolution of conduction block, reactive synaptogenesis by descending pathways in the spinal cord, motor axon sprouting by lower motor neurons,[32] and muscle fiber hypertrophy. These recovery mechanisms mitigate upper and lower motor neuron weakness, both of which can be identified electrophysiologically.[33] The optimal rehabilitation interventions for these two types of weakness are not yet known.

NEUROLOGICAL ASSESSMENT AND CLASSIFICATION

The methods described in the *International Standards for Neurological Classification of Spinal Cord Injury* are the most widely used ways of classifying SCI.[34,35] Commonly referred to as "the American Spinal Injury Association (ASIA) classification," this assessment requires manual muscle testing of 10 key muscles bilaterally (Table 16-1), sensory testing for light touch and sharp/dull discrimination in all dermatomes, and a rectal exam for sensation and presence of voluntary anal contraction. These tests are used to classify injury levels and ASIA Impairment Scale (AIS) grade (Figure 16-1). The sensory level is the most caudal level with normal light touch and sharp/dull discrimination (provided that all rostral levels are normal), and is defined separately for the right and left sides. Motor level is defined as the most caudal level that is grade 3 or greater with all rostral levels normal (grade 5), and it is also defined separately for the right and left sides. If the sensory level falls in a segment where there are no corresponding limb muscles to test (levels C2–C4, T2–L1, or S2–S4/5), the motor level is assumed to be the same as the sensory level. A single neurological level can be derived from the four levels (right and left motor, right and left sensory) by taking the most rostral of the four; however, motor level is more closely associated with functional capacity.

The AIS grade is a measure of the completeness of SCI. A complete injury is one in which no sensory or motor signals traverse the entire zone of cord injury. Because sparing of sensation or motor is most likely to occur in the sacral segments, the classification has been standardized to examine neurologic function in this region for the purpose of classifying injury completeness. An AIS score of *A* indicates a complete SCI and is defined as the absence of sensory and motor function in segments S4–5. AIS *B* is an incomplete SCI, with preservation of sensory function but not motor function below the injury level (patients may have some motor function in the segments adjacent to the neurological level, but it does not extend more than three segments below the neurological level). AIS *C* indicates an incomplete SCI, with motor function preserved below the neurological level and the majority of muscles below the neurological level having less than grade 3 strength. AIS *D* indicates an incomplete SCI, with motor function preserved below the neurological level and at least half the muscles below the neurological level with muscle grade 3 or greater. AIS *E* indicates the patient had an SCI but made a complete neurologic recovery for all sensory and motor functions used in this classification. The exam required for this classification system does not involve deep tendon reflexes or muscle spasticity, and the muscles selected for the examination are not necessarily those

TABLE 16-1

NEUROLOGIC EVALUATION: MYOTOMAL LEVELS

Level	Area of Sensation
C-1,-2,-3	Trapezius, SCM, upper cervical paraspinals, prevertebral neck muscles
C-4	Diaphragm
C-5	*Biceps brachii*, brachialis
C-6	*Extensor carpi radialis longus*
C-7	*Triceps brachii*
C-8	*Flexor digitorum profundus* (3rd digit)
T-1	*Abductor digiti minimi*, 1st dorsal interosseus
T-6,-7,-8,-9,-10	Beevor's sign*
L-2	*Iliopsoas*, hip adductors
L-3	*Quadriceps femoris*
L-4	*Tibialis anterior*
L-5	*Extensor hallucis longus*, hip abduction
S-1	*Gastrocnemius, soleus*
S-2,-3,-4	Anal sphincter

*Beevor's sign represents upward movement of the umbilicus when the patient attempts a sit-up from supine lying.
SCM: sternocleidomastoid
The italicized muscles are the standard muscles used by the American Spinal Cord Injury Association for classifying injury level.[1] These muscles are innervated by more than one root level, but reduction to a representative level is useful for injury classification.
(1) American Spinal Injury Association. *International Standards for Neurological Classification of Spinal Cord Injury.* Chicago, Ill: ASIA; 2000.

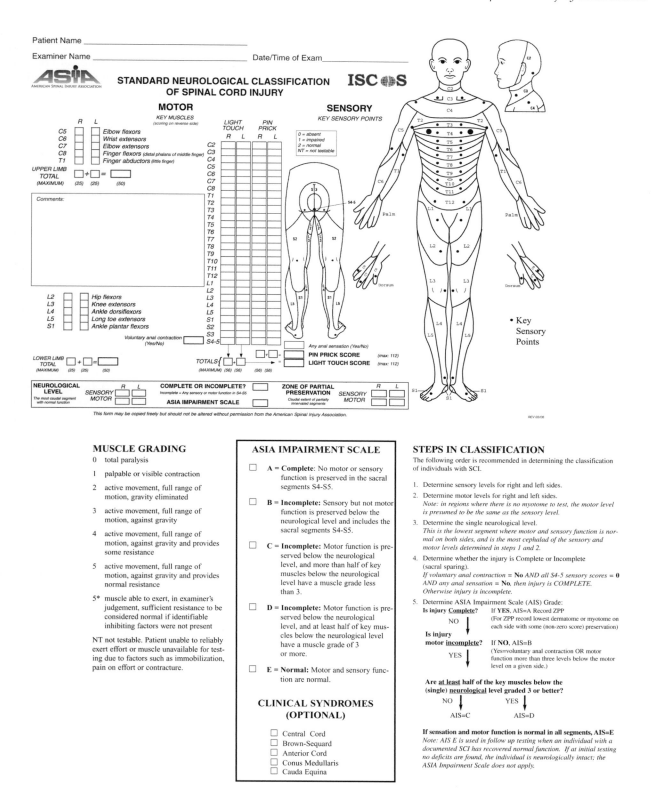

Figure 16-1. Standard neurological classification of spinal cord injury worksheet produced by the American Spinal Injury Association.

Reproduced with permission from: American Spinal Injury Association. *International Standards for Neurological Classification of SCI.* Chicago, Ill: ASIA; 2002.

of the most functional importance.

It has been reported that early neurological classification reliably predicts the classification of civilian SCI at follow up. Earlier studies focused on the examination 3 to 7 days after injury, but it appears the initial emergency department examination has high predictive value when distracting facts, like intoxication or brain injury, have been removed.[36] For example, of patients with initial AIS *A* injuries and no distracting factors, 6.7% converted to AIS *B* and none converted to AIS *C* or *D* at 1 year following initial examination. In the presence of factors affecting the exam reliability, 17.4% of those with initial AIS *A* scores converted to AIS *B*, and 13% converted to AIS *C*. Sparing of sharp/dull discrimination in sacral dermatomes is favorable for motor recovery to a degree that allows ambulation, possibly due to a similar location of corticospinal and spinothalamic tracts within the spinal cord.[37] The prognosis for improvement in AIS grade is much better for those initially classified AIS *B*, with 54% converting to AIS *C* or *D*. Patients initially classified AIS *C* or *D* often show large improvements in neurologic function; a trace of toe movement in the first few days after injury is highly favorable for functional recovery. Motor function typically descends at least one level between the acute exam and 1-year follow-up. Nearly all muscles near the injury level that initially show grade 1 on manual muscle test will regain at least grade 3 strength by follow-up.[31]

Various SCI clinical syndromes have been described (Table 16-2).[38] Several relate to the presumed extent of the cord injury in the transverse plane, such as Brown-Séquard, central cord, and anterior cord syndromes. Brown-Séquard syndrome is attributed to a cord hemisection and is often the result of a penetrating injury, such as a knife or gunshot wound. The prognosis for return of functional ambulation and voluntary bladder control following Brown-Séquard syndrome is good.[39,40] Central cord syndrome is a cervical-level, motor-incomplete injury with greater weakness in upper versus lower limbs. Central cord syndrome often occurs from a cervical hyperextension injury in the presence of an underlying narrow cervical canal, either from congenital or acquired stenosis. Bony fractures or instability are often absent. Anterior cord syndrome typically results from a cervical burst fracture or disk herniation, impinging on the anterior spinal artery, anterior cord, or both. It is not known whether direct mechanical pressure or disruption of arterial blood flow is the major cause. The likelihood of a return of lower limb function in anterior cord syndrome is reduced.

Cauda equina syndrome results from injury below the termination of the spinal cord (levels L-1–L-2), damaging the anterior and posterior roots, but sparing the cord itself. Midline lumbar disk herniations and major trauma (eg, gunshot wounds or seatbelt injuries) are common causes of cauda equina injury. Prognosis for functional recovery is good because the roots are less vulnerable to mechanical trauma than the spinal

TABLE 16-2

SPINAL CORD INJURY CLINICAL SYNDROMES

	Clinical Features	Prognosis
Central Cord	Common; greater weakness of upper limbs than lower limbs	Often recover bladder and bowel function/control and ambulation
Brown-Séquard	Common; unilateral impaired pain and temperature sensation contralateral to the more paretic side; unilateral impaired vibration and position sense ipsilateral to the paretic side	Usually recover bladder and bowel function/control and ambulation
Anterior cord	Uncommon as pure syndrome; loss of motor, pain, and temperature, with preserved vibratory and proprioception	Functional recovery uncommon
Posterior cord	Rare; absent position and vibratory sensation; intact pain and temperature sensation	Usually recover bladder and bowel function/control and ambulation
Cauda equina	About 10% of all cord injuries; often motor incomplete and with asymmetric deficits	Commonly recover bladder and bowel function/control and ambulation
Conus medullaris	Mixed upper motor neuron and lower motor neuron findings through lumbar and sacral myotomes	May recover ambulation; less likely to recover bladder and bowel control

cord. In addition, motor axons have some capacity for regeneration to proximal muscles and to the bladder.[41] Conus medullaris syndrome involves damage to the spinal cord at the lumbar or sacral segments, resulting in bowel, bladder, and sexual dysfunction, with some upper motor neuron findings present due to sparing of the terminal portion of the conus, and lower motor neuron findings due to root injury or direct compression of lower motor neuron cell bodies. In cases where the entire conus has been injured at its termination at level L-1 or level L-2, the clinical findings are identical to cauda equina syndrome.

"Spinal shock" represents depressed spinal reflexes and weakness caudal to an SCI. This is likely caused by loss of normal tonic descending facilitation because a block of conduction in suprasegmental pathways results in hyperpolarization of cord neurons.[42] Spinal

reflexes gradually return over days to months, typically becoming hyperactive leading to spasticity, flexor and extensor spasms, and hypertonia.[43,44] Some reflex activity may return as early as 24 hours after complete SCI, such as the bulbocavernosus reflex or the tibial H-reflex, even though tendon reflexes usually return weeks or months later in patients with complete injuries. In those with incomplete SCI, tendon reflexes and spasticity may appear within days of the injury.[45] Spinal shock is not observed if the myelopathy develops gradually, as is often seen with a cord tumor, cervical stenosis, or syringomyelia. Presumably, hyperactive reflexes, such as a Babinski sign and ankle clonus, develop before overt weakness because mechanisms of neuroplasticity (such as sprouting by reflex afferents and spared descending pathways) mediate hyperreflexia and spared voluntary movement.

INITIAL REHABILITATION

Functional Outcome

Rehabilitation goals vary according to the level of injury and the extent of damage to the spinal cord. When the injury is motor-complete (AIS *A* or *B*), the functional outcome depends to a large degree on the level of injury. The lower the injury is on the cord, the more voluntary movement is preserved and the greater the expectations for independence. Expected functional outcomes for the average person with SCI may be found in recent clinical practice guidelines.[46]

Mobility

Mobility is essential to resuming life outside the hospital. In teaching mobility, self-care, and other functional tasks, the following general principles apply: (*a*) start with the simple and move toward the more complex; (*b*) break tasks down into components, beginning with discrete units that can be learned separately and then combined into completed units; and (*c*) teach patients to substitute for weakened or absent muscles with head motions, momentum, and preserved muscles. The expected optimal outcome for a given patient, based on the level and the completeness of the injury, dictates how and which muscles should be trained (Table 16-3).[46]

Mobility encompasses a spectrum of movement, including bed mobility (ie, turning from side to side, moving from supine to sitting), sitting balance, wheelchair transfers (ie, from wheelchair to bed, wheelchair to car, and wheelchair to floor), standing balance, and ambulation (wheelchair or walking). Each task is mastered in physical therapy.

Wheelchair Use

One of the first objectives of therapy for the spinal cord injured is to get the patient sitting upright, a task usually attended to by physical therapists and nurses. During this procedure, the patient is monitored closely for orthostatic hypotension (OH), a common condition brought on by prolonged bed rest and the deficient vasoconstriction that accompanies disruption of the sympathetic nervous system. Tilt tables and reclining wheelchairs can aid in achieving upright posture. Progressively increasing the verticality of a tilt table challenges the cardiovascular system, which eventually improves systolic blood pressure and cerebral blood flow in the upright sitting and standing positions. For expected wheelchair users, the same can be achieved at the bedside in a reclining wheelchair with elevating leg rests; therapy staff can immediately recline the chair if a patient develops symptomatic hypotension.

As the patient regains mobility, spinal alignment and neurologic status may be affected. If this is suspected, frequent radiographs and neurologic examinations are required to be certain that gravity, postural changes, and muscular forces do not compromise alignment.

The wheelchair is a patient's key to mobility, and helping the patient select the correct chair is a complex task. The chair should be custom fit according to the user's pelvis width, trunk height, and leg, thigh, and forearm length. A clinician must review the wheelchair setup and make appropriate adjustments to ensure proper posture and seating. The chair should be efficient, appropriately stable, maneuverable, and matched to the strength and coordination of the user; a manual wheelchair that is configured to allow one

TABLE 16-3

EXPECTED FUNCTIONAL OUTCOME FOR COMPLETE SPINAL CORD INJURY

Cord Level	Preserved Muscle	Eating	Dressing	Transfers	Mobility Indoor	Outdoor	Writing
C-1, -2	Trapezius, sternocleidomastoid	D	D	D lift or pivot	I Power WC Sip and puff	I	I Computer Sip and puff
C-3, -4	Diaphragm, neck flexor/extensor	D	D	D lift or pivot	I Chin control	I	I Mouth stick
C-5	Deltoid, biceps	I cuff	D	D lift or pivot	I Power WC	I	I cuff
C-6	Serratus anterior, extensor carpi radialis	I	I?	I? loops sliding board	I (+/– power WC)	I?	I
C-7	Triceps	I	I reachers adapted clothes	I	I Manual WC	I	I
C-8 to T-1	Hand intrinsics	I	I	I	I Manual WC	I	I
T-2 to T-6	Intercostals, paraspinals	I	I	I	I Manual WC	I	I
T-7 to T-12	Abdominals	I	I	I	I Manual WC	I	I
L2	Iliopsoas	I	I	I	I (+ manual WC)	I	I
L-3	Quadriceps	I	I	I	I (+/– manual WC)	I	I
L-4, -5	Tibialis anterior, extensor hallucis longus	I	I	I	I Crutches	I AFOs	I
L-5 to S-1	Hamstrings, gluteus medius	I	I	I	I AFOs	I AFOs	I
S-1, -2	Gluteus maximus, gastrocnemius-soleus	I	I	I	I	I	I
S-3, -4	Anal/urethral sphincters	I	I	I	I	I	I

AFO: ankle-foot orthosis
cuff: universal cuff
D: dependent

I: independent
I?: possibly independent
lift: hydraulic lift transfer

pivot: quad pivot transfer
WC: wheelchair

patient to negotiate a curb with a "wheelie" may put another at risk for a dangerous fall. Extra features to consider include antitip devices, lap trays, arm rests, and foot and leg supports. Aesthetics and cost must be considered as well. Proper training is essential for long-term protection of the upper extremities.[47]

An individual with tetraplegia as high as the C-5 level may be able to propel a manual wheelchair. Propulsion for individuals with C-5 level cervical injuries is possible by using the biceps brachii, brachialis, and anterior deltoid muscles in a closed kinetic chain to convert the regular elbow–shoulder flexion to elbow

extension when the hand is fixed on a wheelchair handrim by friction. The benefits to operating a manual wheelchair include greater upper limb and cardiovascular exercise, having a backup means of mobility in the event that a power wheelchair malfunctions, and the ability to travel in a passenger car without a wheelchair lift or ramp. Despite this, most C-5 level manual wheelchair users will require a power chair for outdoor mobility involving distances, rough terrain, or grades. For many of these individuals, power wheelchairs are the only feasible means of mobility. Fit and function should be considered when selecting power chairs as

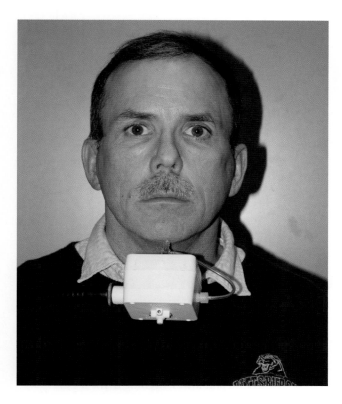

Figure 16-2. A chin joystick controller can be mounted on a boom attached to the chair frame (as shown) or on a plastic yoke placed over the sternum. In addition to driving the power wheelchair, it can be used to operate a tilt-in-space mechanism or environmental control unit.

well, as should the method of control (eg, manual joystick, chin, sip-and-puff straw, mouth stick, or tongue; Figure 16-2). For these patients, reclining mechanisms are essential to minimize the risk of skin breakdown. Two such mechanisms are the zero-shear mechanism and the tilt-in-space recline. The latter is less likely to elicit extensor spasms (Figure 16-3).

Walking

Some patients will progress from sitting to walking. Ambulation goals differ depending on the level of the SCI and whether the cord injury is complete or incomplete. For motor-complete SCI in the absence of lower limb movement, the goals are exercise and short-distance mobility on level surfaces. Those with complete injuries at the T-6 level or below with no other major medical complications are the usual candidates for this training. Contraindications include limited lumbar spine extension or limited hip, knee, and ankle joint motion. Initially, patients are taught to stand between parallel bars and maintain balance without arm

support, using temporary knee-ankle-foot orthoses. They then learn to walk with a swing-through gait, using the parallel bars for support. With this gait, upper body center of gravity must be behind the axis of rotation of the hip joint to maintain hip extension (Figure 16-4). The energy expended for this type of walking can be as much as 800% of that of able-bodied walking and manual wheelchair propulsion.[48] Swing-through walking also requires considerable motor coordination and can place excessive loads across the upper limb joints. Previously, this form of ambulation was considered a goal for all young patients with new paraplegia, but that has changed in recent years because most patients did not continue to ambulate after discharge from the hospital. Only those who demonstrate progress and sustained motivation with temporary bracing should be fitted with custom knee-ankle-foot orthoses and proceed to learning a swing-through gait, which requires use of forearm crutches.

For individuals with some preserved lower limb movement, the goals vary from assisted standing-pivot transfers to long-distance ambulation, depending on the extent of motor and proprioceptive function and the degree of spasticity. For those with considerable sparing and rapid recovery, therapy is primarily the reconditioning of muscles that have atrophied from disuse. Those with little sparing and slow recovery require months of spontaneous healing, strengthening, and functional training. For the latter, recovery is less complete and spasticity often interferes with movement, although extensor spasms can aid standing.

Activity-Based Therapy

In past years, there has been a relatively static view of neuroplasticity and neurologic recovery following SCI. Most interventions were pharmacologic and surgical, with the intention of minimizing the primary injury and secondary effects, such as edema. As general knowledge of plasticity and remodeling in the central nervous system has grown, there is renewed interest in developing therapies to stimulate these processes and enhance functional recovery. Physical rehabilitation strategies have recently been employed for these purposes.

Activity-based therapy is now advocated by many rehabilitation centers throughout the world. The general approach is to use neuromuscular activity below the level of an incomplete SCI to stimulate neuroplasticity and promote recovery of function. Locomotor training is the most well-developed activity-based therapy.[49,50,51] Bodyweight support

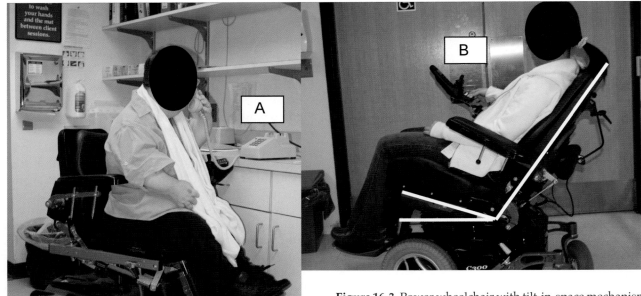

Figure 16-3. Power wheelchair with tilt-in-space mechanism for relieving pressure on the skin near the ischial tuberosities. The chair is driven using a joystick controller. (**a**) The seat elevation feature can be used to allow a user to reach high objects. (**b**) Seat tilt and recline help prevent pressure ulcers, reduce discomfort, and lower swelling in the legs.

and a treadmill, overground ambulation with upper limb aids, electrical stimulation during walking to activate the neuromuscular system, and functional electrical stimulation bikes are used for locomotor training.

Spinal Cord Injury Complicated by Concomitant Traumatic Amputation

Review of data from Operations Iraqi Freedom and Enduring Freedom reveals that the incidence of SCI and amputation is low, albeit with a high functional impact. In addition to managing the multitude of medical issues associated with both SCI and amputation, specific attention must be directed toward identifying and managing heterotopic ossification (HO), which is a known complication after SCI[52] and combat amputations.[53]

The functional impact of SCI complicated by amputation depends on the level of SCI, AIS grade, and the anatomic location of the amputation. When amputation level can be elected, consideration should be given to preserving length in individuals without SCI. An individual with SCI who will be a full-time

wheelchair user will be affected differently by an amputation than an individual with SCI presentation consistent with partial or full-time ambulation. For the wheelchair user, a lower limb amputation must be considered relative to the prescribed seating system because a unilateral amputation is likely to cause postural compromise. Specific modifications may be needed to provide postural support and skin protection. The functional impact of lower extremity amputation can be minimized for wheelchair users who acquire compensatory techniques to optimize balance and stability while performing self-care tasks and mobility skills. For individuals with SCI who can stand and walk, the impact of lower limb amputation is a greater challenge because the individual may desire to use a prosthetic leg despite impaired neuromuscular function in the residual limb and trunk. Given the known significant physical requirements for prosthetic limb use and the additional demands resulting from SCI-related impairments, part-time or intermittent wheelchair use should be considered. Upper limb amputation in individuals with SCI creates significant self-care and mobility challenges and indicates a high risk for upper limb pain and injury due to repetitive strain of the intact arm. Clinical interventions and patient education must be targeted toward optimizing functional skills while preserving remaining upper limb function, as

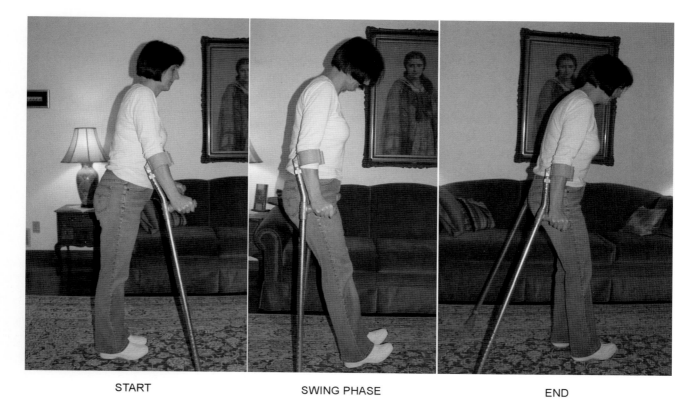

START   SWING PHASE   END

Figure 16-4. Swing-through gait.

supported by published clinical practice guidelines.[47] This may be partially addressed by providing a power wheelchair with power seat functions. Regardless of level of SCI, AIS, or amputation location, maintaining normal range of motion across all joints, maximizing strength of innervated muscles, developing efficient mobility skills, and learning joint preservation techniques are critical to optimize functional outcomes and long-term quality of life.

Driver's Training and Community Mobility

Automobiles usually provide the greatest convenience and flexibility for accessing the community and participating in vocational and avocational activities. Some patients with motor-complete (AIS *A* or *B*) injuries as high as level C-5 can learn to drive with hand controls, although even at the C-6 level, a specialized van with sensitized steering and braking is often required. Those with SCI at level C-7 or lower can often use a passenger car with hand controls, provided they have the ability to transfer themselves and stow their wheelchairs independently. Vision, including visual scanning (the absence of which can sometimes be compensated for with panoramic

and side mirrors), reaction time, absence of seizures, adequate spasm control, cognitive awareness, hand function, transfer skills, and a financial source for the necessary equipment and insurance are additional factors determining whether or not a patient is a candidate for driver's training. Adaptations may include hand controls for brakes and gas, steering wheel attachments, power seats, and vans with wheelchair lifts or ramps.

Self-Care

Along with increasing mobility, minimizing the need for assistance in self-care is a major step toward independence for those with SCI. Self-care includes feeding, bathing, dressing, grooming, and toileting. Those with motor-complete injuries at the C-7 level or below can usually achieve independence in all of these activities. Occupational therapists and rehabilitation nurses work with patients to master new techniques for accomplishing these tasks. Alternate strategies, such as using a tenodesis grip (which uses wrist extension to passively flex fingers) for holding eating utensils or writing implements, must be learned and mastered. A wrist-driven, flexor-hinge splint improves the strength of a tenodesis grip. Other special equipment such as reachers, universal cuffs, built-up handles on utensils, and tub benches also aid independence. Tendon transfers[54] or implantable functional electrical stimulators[55] may achieve a more functional pinch, but costs and training time are considerable. Full independence and self-management of the neurogenic bladder and bowel is a goal for patients with a motor level of C-7 or caudal.

Partial independence may be achieved with level C-6 or level C-5 motor-complete injury. For those tasks that require assistance, the patient is shown how to teach others to complete the task and a caregiver is instructed in how to help with the activity. For example, the assistance needed for self-feeding may include fitting a universal cuff and utensil on a patient, positioning food, opening containers, and cutting meat. With similar assistance, some grooming and hygiene tasks, such as combing hair, brushing teeth, shaving, and washing face and upper body, may be mastered. With motor-complete injury at a C-4 level or rostral, a person will typically be dependent for all self-care activities.

Living Skills

Living skills (eg, meal preparation, shopping, check writing, housekeeping, etc) are necessary tasks of everyday life and must be relearned and adapted to a patient's needs. These skills are often reacquired with the help of occupational therapists. Again, reachers and other specialized equipment are used as aids and spared muscles substitute for paretic muscles, a motor learning task that requires practice. These tasks can usually be managed by patients with injuries sparing level C-7 or more. Those with higher injuries need assistance, including environmental control systems and computers. These can be accessed via mouth stick, sip-and-puff, tongue touch pads, eye movements, or voice. Environmental control systems allow the use of telephones, appliances, sound equipment, intercoms, televisions, lights, and door openers—all items that can be accessed by remote control. The complexity of the system will vary according to the extent of the impairment and the patient's financial resources. The use of a computer, accessed through the keyboard using hand or mouth sticks, head controls, or voice activation, allows a degree of control and a range of communication, vocation, and recreation options.

Vocational and Avocational Pursuits

Tools to help patients explore available vocational and avocational opportunities include psychological testing, vocational counseling, assessing physical

---

EXHIBIT 16-1

EXAMPLES OF ACTIVITIES AVAILABLE TO INDIVIDUALS WITH SPINAL CORD INJURIES

- archery
- boating
- football
- camping
- hunting
- flying
- golf
- scuba diving
- swimming
- sailing
- basketball
- table tennis
- weight lifting
- tennis
- horseback riding
- wheelchair racing
- wheelchair dancing
- sit skiing

---

capacities, vocational remediation and training, identifying sources of financial assistance to support training and education, peer counseling, and job-seeking guidance. Rehabilitation staff can also communicate with potential employers. Hiring an individual with a disability can raise issues about physical accommodations for a disabled person and the psychology of responding to someone who is permanently disabled. Providing technical assistance for workspace modifications and information about disability can also aid patients in their employment pursuits.

Healthcare providers should organize and encourage outings for SCI patients, such as attending sporting and cultural events, eating at restaurants, and shopping. Many individuals with SCI will want to return to a form of physical exercise or sport, although they may initially be apprehensive. They should be made aware that numerous activities have been successfully pursued by people with SCI (Exhibit 16-1).

Patient and Family Education

Families are critical to helping patients adjust to disability. Initially, the concerns of the patient and family often center on prognosis for neurological and functional recovery. Response to these concerns should respectfully acknowledge the uncertainty and difficulty a patient may have in accepting new limitations.

Hope, even if based on an improbable outcome, helps patients cope with the initial grief that accompanies disability. Acceptance of the new reality generally comes with time. Patients and their families can be convinced of the need to learn alternate methods of mobility and self-care.

The focus during rehabilitation is to educate the patient, family, and caregivers on the nature of SCI, maximizing health, and accessing community resources. Educational topics include the following:

- level and completeness of the SCI, which determine the anatomic and physiological correlates;
- prognosis for motor recovery and spasticity;
- current research on spinal cord regeneration and new technology;
- care of neurogenic bladder and bowel;
- prevention of skin breakdown;
- management of autonomic dysreflexia (AD), if applicable;
- psychological adjustment to disability;
- attendant care management;
- sexuality, impaired sexual function, and fertility;
- vocational and educational options;
- avocational outlets, such as wheelchair sports;
- finances; and
- housing.

Various educational tools can be used, such as patient manuals for instruction and reference, weekly class discussions, peer interaction, and one-on-one instruction provided by each member of the rehabilitation team. Intake and discharge meetings with the rehabilitation team further complement instruction. The intake meeting defines specific goals for the hospitalization and addresses specific questions related to prognosis and course of treatment. The discharge meeting discusses plans for follow up, equipment needs, and accessing community resources. Family members and other caregivers of partially dependent patients need to be instructed in their roles. Onsite independent-living apartments allow patients and their caregivers to rehearse tasks, such as shopping, meal preparation, transfers, toileting, and bathing, with staff backup. Day and weekend passes can also be granted once a patient is medically stable and sufficiently trained in self care and mobility. Patients can practice their recently acquired mobility and self-care skills by participating in community outings organized by a recreation therapist. These outings typically include activities such as taking public transportation, visiting shopping malls, going to movies, grocery shopping, banking, and eating in restaurants.

Housing, Finances, and Community Reintegration

Social workers can help patients understand social security disability, Veterans Affairs and Medicare/Medicaid benefits, separation from the military, accessible housing, housing modifications, advocacy groups for the disabled, and legal resources and protections. Occupational therapists can help patients understand accessibility features, such as ramp inclines and door widths.

PREVENTING AND MANAGING SPINAL CORD INJURY COMPLICATIONS

Mortality and morbidity due to SCI are higher in patients with tetraplegia than paraplegia and complete injuries compared to incomplete injuries, both acutely and chronically. Medical complications associated with SCI commonly occur during the first few months following the injury, and patients are frequently rehospitalized to treat acute medical conditions, particularly during the first year postinjury. Many need early diagnosis and treatment to minimize long-term sequelae.

Some conditions occur more frequently in the first several years following injury, such as hydronephrosis, spasticity, and contractures. Suicides are also more common during this time. Other complications become more prevalent with increasing time (eg, musculoskeletal problems), and some complications are most closely associated with the patient's age (eg, cardiovascular complications) or neurological classification (eg, pneumonia, AD). The most common causes of death after the first year following injury are respiratory disorders (22% of deaths), cardiovascular disorders (21%), cancer (11.9%), and sepsis (9.8%).[9] More than 75% of respiratory-related deaths following SCI are due to pneumonia. Urologic causes, which were previously the leading causes of death following SCI, now account for only 2.3% of deaths.

Pulmonary Complications

The inspiratory phase of breathing requires active muscle contraction and depends primarily on the diaphragm innervated at the C-3, C-4, and C-5 levels. Resting expiration is passive and depends on the viscoelastic properties of the lung and chest wall; forced expiration is active, as in a cough for clearing secretions from the lungs—an action requiring rapid contraction by the abdominal muscles innervated at the T-6 to L-1 levels and the thoracically innervated intercostals. If they are not paralyzed, the clavicular portion of the pectoralis major and the latissimus dorsi can contribute to active expiration.[56] Impairment of the inspiratory phase of breathing and forced expiration cause most SCI pulmonary complications.[57]

Acute Respiratory Failure

The earliest pulmonary complication to manifest in SCI patients is acute respiratory failure. This condition develops most commonly in those with cervical cord injury at the C-5 level or rostral. It may appear immediately after the injury or develop over hours to days as respiratory muscles fatigue. Close monitoring is needed to detect muscle fatigue and avoid emergent intubation. Oxygen saturation may not be a sensitive marker for respiratory failure, especially in patients who are receiving supplemental oxygen, so the vital capacity and partial pressure of carbon dioxide need to be closely monitored. Attention must be directed to aggressive pulmonary toilet and early detection and treatment of atelectasis and pneumonia, which occur in 50% of all patients with motor-complete SCI during the first month following injury.[58,59] The majority of patients who have initial ventilatory failure will eventually wean from the ventilator over a period of days to months. Forced vital capacities in patients with mid-cervical level tetraplegia typically improve over a period of months, presumably due to a combination of inspiratory muscle strengthening and changes in the stiffness of the ribcage. Tracheostomy is usually performed early if rapid weaning is not anticipated (prolonged endotracheal intubation has been associated with airway complications, such as subglottic stenosis). A tracheostomy tube can also allow for direct tracheal suctioning, oral intake of food, and leak speech, in which the tracheostomy cuff is deflated and larger ventilator volumes are delivered, enabling air to leak around the tracheostomy tube and upward through the larynx.[60]

Communication can be a major problem for intubated individuals. Initially, tongue clicking or exaggerated eye blinks can be used for "yes" and "no" signaling, but head nodding may not be possible because of spine instability or neck muscle paralysis with injuries at the C-1 or brainstem levels. Communication can also be pursued through lip reading, communication board, or computer. Eventually, as pulmonary status stabilizes, patients can use leak speech. Ventilator-dependent patients must always carry a suction device for clearing secretions and a self-inflating bag valve mask in the event of ventilator failure.

Atelectasis, Pneumonia, Aspiration, Impaired Cough

Pneumonia is the leading cause of death for both acute and chronic SCI.[61] Almost all SCI patients, with the exception of those with lesions at a low thoracic level or below, have impaired cough because of the loss of abdominal muscle strength. Those with tetraplegia and higher-level paraplegia have impaired inspiratory effort as well. Impaired cough and impaired inspiration predispose a patient to atelectasis. Mucous hypersecretion and hyperviscosity, along with impaired cough, contribute to mucous plugging. All of these factors predispose a patient to pneumonia; those most vulnerable are patients with high cervical cord injuries. The site of pneumonia during the acute phase is most often the left lower lobe, where the sharper angle of the left mainstem bronchus makes suctioning more difficult.[59]

The following strategies promote clearing secretions and reduce the risk of pneumonia: (*a*) turn the patient at least every 2 hours to promote gravity-assisted postural drainage; (*b*) offer incentive spirometry; (*c*) assist cough by manually compressing the abdomen in synchronization with the patient's cough (ie, quad cough; this is contraindicated in the presence of an inferior vena caval filter); (*d*) consider use of a mechanical insufflator-exsufflator, which delivers $+ 40$ cm H_2O pressure, then rapidly switches to $- 40$cm H_2O pressure, producing an airflow that approximates a normal cough and mobilizes bronchial secretions. Fever, increased purulent sputum, altered auscultation of the lungs, and change in chest radiographs suggest pneumonia. Treatment for pneumonia involves more frequent and more aggressive pulmonary hygiene and antibiotics.

An additional pulmonary problem is aspiration. Those with SCI at level T-10 or above are less able to cough effectively and clear their airways if they aspirate. Major risk factors for dysphagia in patients with recent SCI include tracheostomy and recent anterior cervical surgery.[62,63] Precautions to minimize aspiration risk include restricting oral intake, gastric decompression by nasogastric tube for those with gastroparesis or ileus, upright or side-lying for eating, and avoiding assisted coughing by manual abdominal compression immediately after meals. Patients with suspected aspiration should have a swallowing evaluation that compares the effects of various consistencies, amounts, and techniques and develops optimal feeding strategies. Hyperextension of the neck in a cervical brace can make it easier for a patient to aspirate. Family members and caregivers should be trained to perform the Heimlich maneuver on someone who is lying down or sitting.

Certain interventions should be taken to reduce the long-term risk of respiratory complications in individuals with SCI, including smoking cessation and pneumococcal and annual influenza vaccination. When a patient has achieved a stable neurological exam and is free of acute respiratory disease, pulmonary function tests should be performed to establish a baseline. For patients with reduced vital capacity, an arterial blood gas test should also be performed as part of the baseline assessment.

Cardiovascular Complications

A variety of cardiac complications can compromise acute and chronic health for the spinal cord injured. Cervical and upper thoracic cord lesions disrupt sympathetic outflow to the heart and blood vessels, and the heart is influenced by unopposed parasympathetic activity. Abnormalities in sympathetic outflow manifest as arrhythmias (including bradycardia and asystole), postural hypotension, and AD. Loss of tonic arteriolar vasoconstriction results in vascular pooling and a lower baseline blood pressure; the expected blood pressure for a person with tetraplegia is around 90/60 mmHg. In addition, decreased muscle activity in the lower extremities leads to venous stasis and the compromise of venous return. Reduced physical function as a result of motor paralysis and lipid dysfunction contribute to long-term cardiovascular risk.

Bradycardia and Cardiac Arrest

Bradycardia that leads to cardiac arrest is a serious early complication of SCI; its incidence in those with tetraplegia is greatest in the first 5 weeks after injury.[64,65] Tetraplegic injuries impair cardiac sympathetic outflow arising at the T-1 to T-4 levels, which normally accelerates the heart. The remaining cardiac innervation is parasympathetic; vagal input slows heart rate. If deceleration is severe, cardiac arrest may result. Tracheal suctioning or hypoxemia can trigger such a bradyarrhythmia, presumably via a vagovagal reflex. Oxygen and atropine can be administered prior to suctioning to inhibit the cholinergic receptors of the vagal efferents to the heart. Patients may occasionally require transvenous cardiac pacing.

Succinylcholine is a depolarizing paralytic medication rarely given as an adjunct to general anesthesia, but in patients with recent SCI, it can result in profound hyperkalemia with cardiac arrest because the neuromuscular junction is hypersensitive to cholinergic agents.[66] Succinylcholine is contraindicated in SCI patients.

Deep Venous Thrombosis, Pulmonary Embolus

Another common and potentially fatal complication of acute SCI is deep venous thrombosis (DVT) with consequent pulmonary emboli. More than 50% of individuals with acute SCI develop DVT if they do not receive prophylaxis. DVT usually develops within the first 3 months following injury, peaking at 10 to 14 days; it occurs less commonly thereafter. Known predisposing factors are venous stasis, a hypercoagulable state following trauma, and venous intimal damage. All of these factors are commonly present in SCI patients. Preventive measures include performing a baseline venous Doppler examination to exclude early DVT, prescribing subcutaneous heparin (typically using low-molecular–weight heparin) and applying venous sequential compression pumps to the lower extremities.[67,68,69] In patients whose thromboprophylaxis has been delayed for more than 72 hours after injury, tests should be performed to exclude the presence of DVT prior to applying venous sequential compression pumps. D-dimer has limited utility as a screening test in this population because of a high false-positive rate. Regular thigh and calf circumference measurements aid early detection of DVT. If a sudden increase or asymmetry in lower extremity circumference develops, or if a patient experiences unexplained low-grade fever or sudden onset dyspnea or chest pain, DVT or pulmonary embolism must be suspected and prompt action taken.[70] The differential diagnosis for lower limb findings can include lower extremity fracture or hemorrhage, HO, dependent edema, or cellulitis. DVT can be diagnosed with ultrasound and, if inconclusive, contrast venogram. DVT is treated with low-molecular–weight heparin, transitioning to oral warfarin for at least 3 months. Bed rest, without lower extremity range-of-motion exercises, is recommended for 48 to 72 hours, until medical therapy is implemented.[67] If anticoagulation therapy is contraindicated or if pulmonary emboli occur despite anticoagulation, an inferior vena cava filter should be considered. The routine placement of inferior vena cava filters in all patients with SCI is discouraged because their placement precludes the practice of quad coughing and their presence may lead to long-term complications. For patients with short-term contraindications to anticoagulation, a temporary filter can be placed and then removed once anticoagulation has been started.

Autonomic Dysreflexia

AD is a delayed sequela of high thoracic or cervical cord injury.[71] This unique manifestation of SCI at or above the T-6 level presents after the resolution of spinal (neurogenic) shock, typically no sooner than 8 weeks after injury. AD occurs in response to a noxious stimulus below the level of injury, most often due to overdistension of a hollow viscus, such as a bladder or bowel. Loss of supraspinal control results in unmodulated norepinephrine release and exaggerated vasoconstriction of arterioles receiving sympathetic innervation from below the level of the cord injury. Resultant blood pressure elevation may be moderate (140–160/90–100 mm Hg) or severe (> 180/110 mm Hg). In order to compensate for the elevated blood pressure, parasympathetic stimulation to the heart is increased via the vagus nerve and often causes bradycardia.[72] Symptoms of AD include pounding headache, flushing, and diaphoresis. Severity varies among patients; in some, there are no manifestations besides these symptoms, while in others, hypertension can lead to retinal or intracerebral hemorrhage, seizures, and death.[73,74] These symptoms result from high and potentially life-threatening systolic hypertension. To treat the condition, the head of the patient's bed should be promptly elevated to promote dependent blood pooling and to lower the risk of intracerebral bleed, then the noxious triggering agent should be identified and eliminated (adequate bladder drainage can be ensured by catheterizing the bladder, flushing or replacing a possibly clogged indwelling catheter, or untwisting a condom catheter, and bowel impaction can be removed by digital evacuation; lidocaine jelly may be used as a rectal anesthetic to avoid further aggravating the condition). Other triggers of AD may include peptic ulcer, cholecystitis, appendicitis, bowel obstruction, rectal fissure, ureteral stone, UTI, ingrown toenail, fracture, or labor and delivery. If hypertension persists, nitroglycerine paste or oral hydralazine (10 mg) can be administered. Other antihypertensive medications are also used, including phenoxybenzamine, prazosin, mecamylamine, and clonidine.[75] Patients are encouraged to carry an AD treatment card to facilitate prompt and appropriate treatment by health professionals less familiar with complications of SCI.

Orthostatic Hypotension

An early and occasionally chronic problem that is less threatening but nonetheless disabling is symptomatic OH. With OH, patients complain of dizziness, lightheadedness, and fainting when in an upright position. OH is most severe in patients with higher lesions (typically cervical and high thoracic SCI), complete injuries, and after prolonged periods of bed rest. Several factors contribute to OH, including impaired sympathetically-mediated vasoconstriction and consequent blood pooling in the lower limbs and splanchnic bed, decreased sympathetic drive to the heart, and relative volume depletion. Tetraplegic patients who typically run blood pressures of 90/60 mm Hg are at highest risk for developing OH. These patients often become orthostatic when first sitting in the morning. To minimize these episodes, patients can be fitted with an abdominal binder, lower limb compression stockings, and elastic wraps. Liberal salt and fluid intake and elevating leg rests may also help avert orthostasis. Patients may also require midodrine or ephedrine sulfate administered 30 minutes before sitting. In patients with acute SCI, OH improves with repeated sitting trials; individuals with tetraplegia are known to have high renin and aldosterone levels, which presumably compensate for orthostasis. Late worsening of OH could suggest development of posttraumatic syringomyelia or a silent myocardial infarction.

Cardiovascular disease

Cardiovascular disease has emerged as a leading cause of mortality in individuals with chronic SCI.[76] Risk factors include hyperlipidemia, obesity, diabetes, sedentary lifestyle, and reduced physical function. As individuals with SCI live longer, cardiovascular disease has become a major source of morbidity and mortality, and is likely related to increased incidence of obesity, diabetes, and lowered high-density lipoprotein levels after SCI.[77,78] Another cardiac complication for the cervical-cord injured is silent myocardial infarction. Cardiac ischemia and infarction in this population may be painless because the cardiac afferents course along cardiac-sympathetic nerves and enter the spinal cord at the T-1 to T-4 levels. In such cases, the clinical manifestations of myocardial infarct may be subtle and nonspecific, such as hypotension, dyspnea on exertion, orthopnea, or increased pedal edema.

Gastrointestinal Complications

SCI disrupts central nervous system coordination and direct nerve supply to the gastrointestinal tract. Consequences are addressed by region below.

Oral Cavity

The prevalence of periodontal disease and caries increases rapidly with age after SCI. A few of the major causes include failure of patients to control plaque, diet, deficits in saliva production, smoking, and problems with tooth occlusion.[79] Plaque removal is affected by upper extremity function, habit, and caregiver commitment for those who require assistance. Saliva production is often reduced by anticholinergic medications, such as those used to treat depression or detrusor overactivity. In addition, smoking deactivates salivary leukocytes, further promoting plaque formation and caries. Removing plaque once or twice per day with a fluoride toothpaste and integrating dental care into personal or attendant responsibilities reduces risk for tooth loss.

Esophagus

Dysphagia and esophagitis are the most common problems with the esophagus after SCI. The esophagus can be damaged by traumatic injury or surgery; perforation can cause mediastinitis, and local manipulation to place spine stabilization hardware can damage nerve supply, reducing sensation and peristalsis. Further iatrogenic contributions to swallowing problems include forced supine position, tong traction, and halo-vest immobilization. Dysphagia after acute cervical SCI occurs in up to 20% of cases, and half of the patients are asymptomatic. Predictors include age, tracheostomy, and anterior approach for cervical spinal surgery.[80] Early specific diagnosis can be accomplished with bedside examination by a speech pathologist. Fiberoptic endoscopic examination and videofloroscopic study of swallowing provide further objective evidence of swallowing capabilities. Elevating the trunk to 30° or more for drinking and eating reduces aspiration risk. Interdisciplinary treatment of severe dysphagia can reduce up to 90% of symptoms and can prevent pnemonia.[63] Reflux esophagitis is common after SCI because of abdominal distention, recumbent position, and altered peristaltic patterns. Low-amplitude esophageal contraction, a motility disorder commonly found in neurologically intact patients with gastroesophageal reflux disease, is highly prevalent among people with SCI.[81,82] Patients should be queried for symptoms of heartburn or sour eructation. Mild symptoms should be managed with antacids, and persistent symptoms should be treated with acid-suppressing medication.

Stomach

For the first few weeks following SCI, there is a risk for incomplete gastric emptying and vomiting, particularly in patients with lesions above the T-1 level. Slow gastric emptying can persist into chronic SCI.[83] Acute treatment with intravenous metoclopramide (5–10 mg per dose) or bethanechol (25 mg 30 min before meals) is effective.[84] Without prophylaxis, stress gastritis or peptic ulcers occur in 5% to 20% of acute SCI patients[85,86]; risk increases with age and in lesions above the T-5 level. Parasympathetic stimulation of acid secretion is unopposed because of reduced sympathetic tone, increasing the acidity of gastric juice. Additional sources of gastric

lining irritation are corticosteroids (which decrease mucosal resistance), gastric distention, hypotension, and sepsis. Mechanical ventilation and anticoagulation with heparin are also independent risk factors for gastrointestinal bleeding. All these risks can be reduced with preventive use of H_2 blockers, proton pump inhibitors, and stool fecal occult blood surveillance for gastrointestinal bleeding. Continuous suction via a nasogastric tube prevents gastric overdistension, and periodically monitoring gastric secretions for occult blood reduces risk and can detect gastric bleeding early. If prophylaxis is inadequate, upper gastrointestinal endoscopy or angiography (if the cervical spine is unstable) will locate gastrointestinal bleeding and facilitate treatment.

Duodenum

Superior mesenteric artery syndrome is attributed to intermittent functional obstruction of the third segment of the duodenum between the superior mesenteric artery and the aorta. The syndrome is more common in patients with tetraplegia.[87] The diagnosis can be confirmed with a barium upper gastrointestinal series. Findings include dilatation of the proximal duodenum and a "cut off" of the transverse duodenum, blocking barium flow. Sitting the patient up reduces the superior mesenteric forces on the duodenum and facilitates gravity flow in the gut.

Pancreas

Sympathetic–parasympathetic imbalance may result in hyperstimulation of the sphincter of Oddi, leading to stasis of secretions and pancreatic damage.[88] Pancreatitis may appear as early as 3 days after injury, but its presence may be masked because of a patient's loss of sensory, motor, and reflex functions.[89] A pancreatitis diagnosis is supported by increases in amylase and lipase over three times the upper limit of normal.

Gallbladder

Imbalances in parasympathetic and sympathetic nervous system innervation and modulation of gallbladder activity after SCI may reduce contractility and lead to cholestasis. The gallbladder receives sympathetic innervation from the T-7 through T-10 levels. The development of cholelithiasis during acute SCI has been related to acute trauma, decreased gut motility, reduction in food intake, intravenous hyperalimentation, parenteral nutrition, rapid weight loss, and mobilization of peripheral fat stores.[90,91] Gallstones are most prevalent in individuals with SCI and can affect 20% to 30% of chronic populations.[92] In spite of sensory deficits, patients with SCI usually present with symptoms that allow for acute diagnosis and cholecystectomy.[93] The rate of complication following cholecystectomy is not significantly greater in individuals with SCI than in the neurologically intact population[94]; therefore, gallstones detected by ultrasound or other imaging should be documented and considered when patients present with nausea and right upper quadrant pain.

Ileum

Abdominal distention is common during the first few days to weeks after SCI. This is often attributed to nonmechanical intestinal obstruction or paralytic adynamic ileus. Loss of gastrointestinal motility is noted in 63% of SCI patients for several days, and occasionally for weeks, after acute SCI.[89] Several risk factors for loss of gastrointestinal mobility are common in people with SCI, including major trauma, surgery, anesthesia, and severe medical illness.[95] Evaluation requires a careful check for the presence of bowel sounds and focal tenderness (if sensation is present). An abdominal radiograph can gauge severity by revealing nonspecific gas patterns or dilated loops of intestine and air fluid levels, as seen in obstruction or severe ileus. Upright sitting and lateral decubitus position films screen for air, which indicates perforation, under the diaphragm or the abdominal wall. Management includes reviewing amylase levels, electrolytes, and complete blood counts. Hyponatremia and hypochloremia should be treated with intravenous electrolyte therapy. The intestines can be decompressed by placing a nasogastric tube and running it to suction. Symptoms typically improve in days. If not, intravenous metoclopramide is helpful in resolving prolonged gastroparesis or ileus.[96]

Colon

Neurogenic bowel is a term that relates colon dysfunction (constipation, incontinence, and discoordination of defecation) to a lack of nervous system control. There are two basic patterns of dysfunction. Upper motor neuron bowel results from a spinal cord lesion above the conus medullaris and typically manifests as fecal distention of the colon, overactive segmental peristalsis, hypoactive propulsive peristalsis, and a hyperactive holding reflex with spastic external anal sphincter constriction (requiring mechanical or chemical stimulus to trigger reflex defecation). Lower motor neuron bowel results from a lesion that affects the parasympathetic and somatic pudendal cell bodies or axons at the conus, cauda equina, or inferior splanchnic nerve and the pudendal nerve. Lower motor neuron bowel results in low descending colon wall tone and

flaccid pelvic floor and anal sphincter. No spinal cord mediated reflex peristalsis occurs. Slow stool propulsion is coordinated by the myenteric plexus alone, and incontinence is common with movement. The denervated colon produces a drier, rounder stool because the prolonged transit time results in increased absorption of moisture from the stool.[97]

Obstipation, Fecal Impaction, Pseudoobstruction, Megacolon

Decreased colonic motility, increased colonic compliance, and anal sphincter spasticity in those with chronic SCI may result in obstipation and fecal impaction.[98] Key elements of a bowel management program include the following: (*a*) adequate fluid intake (1,500–2,000 mL/day); (*b*) high fiber diet (40–60 gm/day); (*c*) bulk cathartics, such as psyllium hydrophilic mucilloid; (*d*) regular mealtimes; and (*e*) timed bowel programs, with evacuations scheduled for every day or every other day, using rectal suppositories (glycerin or bisacodyl) and digital stimulation. Evacuation intervals of more than 3 days increase the risk of impaction and incontinence. The goal of a good program is continence, with focus on techniques that minimize mechanical damage and irritation to the colon and promote long-term health.[99]

Patients reporting poor results with a bowel care program may manifest nausea, vomiting, abdominal distension, early satiety, and shortness of breath from compromised diaphragm descent. Reviewing the elements of the bowel program and ensuring that patients are not on medications that slow gut motility (eg, anticholinergics, narcotics, tricyclics, clonidine, etc) are the first steps to remediation. In addition, patients may require periodic hyperosmotic laxatives (milk of magnesia, lactulose, sorbitol). If these are unsuccessful, saline or phosphosoda enema or whole gut irrigation can be tried. Because enemas tend to stretch the bowel, causing a loss of muscle tone and perhaps AD, they should be used judiciously. In severe cases, nasogastric decompression, with or without a rectal tube, may be required. Rarely, colonoscopy or surgical decompression must be considered if cecal diameter is greater than 12 cm. For those with recurrent bowel obstruction or markedly prolonged bowel programs, refractory to conservative measures, colostomy may be a desirable solution.[100]

Acute abdomen

Acute abdomen is often diagnosed late, with a resulting high morbidity and mortality in patients with SCI. Patients with injury at level T-10 or rostral and resultant impaired sensation do not perceive abdominal pain or report poorly localized pain at a later stage of acute abdomen.[101,102] The physician caring for the SCI patient must maintain a high index of suspicion for acute abdomen and be alert to its minimal manifestations in SCI patients, which may be limited to tachycardia, increased spasticity, and AD.

Endocrinologic Complications

SCI can directly and indirectly contribute to endocrine and metabolic disorders. One neurologic mechanism for determining endocrine function is via sympathetics that innervate the pancreas, adrenal medulla, and juxtaglomerular apparatus of the kidney and originate from the spinal cord at the T-5 through T-12 levels.[103] Sympathetic activity inhibits insulin secretion, while parasympathetic activity stimulates insulin secretion. Reduced sympathetic activity, as occurs with SCI, elevates plasma renin, which can lead to production of angiotensin II, a potent vasoconstrictor. Aldosterone promotes sodium retention and potassium release.

Acute complications

Within days after SCI, antidiuretic hormone secretion is reduced, resulting in diuresis that can continue for a few days. Adrenocorticotrophic hormone is normally secreted in a diurnal pattern that disappears soon after SCI, causing a drop in blood pressure. Clinicians should be prepared for hypothalamic and pituitary abnormalities following SCI, as well. Stress can contribute to impaired release of growth hormone, which can lead to weakness. At the time of injury, the stress response triggers release of corticotrophin, and resultant release of hormone from the hypothalamus. Adrenocorticotrophic hormone is released and stimulates cortisol production. The syndrome of inappropriate antidiuretic hormone can contribute to free-water retention and electrolyte dilution.

Hypercalcemia, though uncommon, occurs most often in the first months after injury in adolescent males with complete tetraplegia and spinal shock. In addition to gender and youth, risk factors include complete neurologic injury, high cervical injury, and prolonged immobilization. Symptoms and signs are subtle and include malaise, anorexia, nausea, vomiting, constipation, polydipsia, and polyuria. Left untreated, hypercalcemia can progress to lethargy and coma. Treatment includes intravenous saline with furosemide and remobilization. Additional measures may be needed to inhibit osteoclast-mediated bone resorption, such as administering bisphosphonates (eg,

etidronate or pamidronate), calcitonin, mithramycin, glucocorticoids, and gallium nitrate.[104]

Osteoporosis

Fracture risk increases with injury duration in individuals with chronic SCI. In general, there is no demineralization in bones above the SCI level. The major contributors to mineral loss after SCI include the amount of paralyzed muscle, lower limb weight-bearing status, presence of spasticity, age, sex, and the time elapsed since injury. Long bones lose more calcium than the axial skeleton, and trabecular bone is more affected than cortical bone. The efficacy of preventive treatments used in the general population has not been conclusively demonstrated in nonambulatory individuals with SCI.

Insulin-Dependent Diabetes Mellitus

SCI can produce profound metabolic consequences that result in disorders of carbohydrate and lipid metabolism.[77] Abnormal glucose tolerance and hyperinsulinemia are common following SCI. SCI complicates the management of diabetes mellitus in two ways. First, individuals with SCI are prone to increased insulin resistance because of decreased muscle mass and obesity that can result from limited mobility. Second, those with tetraplegia fail to exhibit adrenergic hypoglycemic symptoms (diaphoresis and tachycardia). For the latter, clinicians must develop an increased awareness of the neuroglycopenic symptoms (drowsiness or impaired mental status).

Dermatologic Complications

Pressure Ulcers

Pressure ulcers remain a major cause of morbidity and mortality after SCI. Pressure ulcers in individuals with acute SCI commonly delay remobilization, full participation in rehabilitation, and discharge to the community. A clinical practice guideline on the prevention and treatment of pressure ulcers in people with SCI was published in 2000 to improve the quality and consistency of care.[105]

Pressure ulcers are common in the acute care phase, during rehabilitation, and when living in the community.[106–109] Despite efforts to prevent pressure ulcers, there is little evidence that the overall incidence or prevalence of pressure ulcers in people with SCI is decreasing. In addition to medical complications, prolonged bed rest, and loss of function, the cost of treating pressure ulcers is high, estimated to be $3 to \$5 billion per year in the United States.[110,111] Braun and colleagues reported that the cost to heal a severe, full-thickness pressure ulcer is \$70,000.[112]

A common misconception is that pressure ulcers must first involve the skin; however, most severe pressure ulcers develop in deep body wall tissues over bony prominences and on areas of the body that have little body fat. This includes areas over the ischial tuberosity, sacrum, greater trochanter, heel, scapula, vertebra, malleolus, and occiput. The pathophysiology of pressure ulcers has been related to sustained high loads without pressure relief. Deep, severe pressure ulcers typically start at the bone-muscle interface. Frictional and shear injuries can result in more superficial ulcers.

External forces that result in pressure ulcers include unrelieved direct perpendicular pressure, skin shearing, and friction. Risk factors that predispose an individual to developing pressure ulcers are prolonged sitting, severe spasticity, contractures, edema, anemia, poor nutrition, bruises and skin damage from falls or scrapes, worn or inadequate cushions, urinary or fecal incontinence, excessive sweating, and smoking.[113,114] Some conditions that put acute SCI patients at risk of developing pressure ulcers are anesthetic skin, immobility from paralysis, hypotension, spine immobilization, poor nutrition and subsequent weight loss, febrile illness, urinary and fecal incontinence, flexor spasm, and altered mental status, such as coma, depression, or chronic alcohol use. From 20% to 40% of patients develop pressure ulcers during the first month after SCI.[105,115] Education, awareness, and behavioral change can minimize the risk of developing pressure ulcers. Optimizing equipment, posture, and seating are also critical to prevention, as is avoiding trauma and injury during activities of daily living.

Risk should be assessed comprehensively and systematically, and is high with acute SCI and a significant degree of paralysis. Risk can be decreased by avoiding prolonged immobilization, periodically relieving pressure, using pressure-reducing support surfaces, preventing moisture accumulation, and applying pillows and cushions to pad-contacting surfaces. Use of bed-positioning devices and periodic turns while in bed are also important preventive measures. Pressure-reducing bed support surfaces can be used for at-risk individuals during acute hospitalization, rehabilitation, and in the instance of acute illness.

Specialized wheelchair cushions and mattresses should be used for all people with SCI who are at high risk for skin breakdown. Interface pressures should be evaluated when using foam, gel, and air cushions in a wheelchair. Foam, static air, alternating air, gel, and water mattresses are common pressure-reducing tools. In people with one or more pressure ulcers, pressure-reducing bed support surfaces are an important consideration for healing and preventing ulcers on other surfaces.

Regardless of predisposing factors, pressure ulcers are caused by prolonged pressure or shear sufficient to cause underlying skin and muscle necrosis from ischemia. Yet the exact timing of pressure reliefs (ie, relieving pressure on a periodic basis while sitting in a wheelchair or lying in bed) is still the subject of debate. It is reasonable to turn patients in bed every 2 hours during their acute stay and during rehabilitation. When sitting, body weight is distributed over a smaller surface, so it is recommended that pressure be relieved for at least 15 seconds every 15 minutes.

Pressure can be relieved while sitting in a wheelchair by cushions that distribute weight optimally. Well-fitted wheelchairs with solid (rather than sling) seats; high-quality foam, gel, or air cushions; and pressure releases are standard preventative equipment.[116] The region over the ischial tuberosities is generally at greatest risk when an individual is seated, although postural abnormalities and incorrect seating can put excessive pressure on the sacrum or greater trochanters.

Patients and caregivers must be taught to check the skin daily. If redness or skin breakdown is noted, patients must alter their positions and routines to keep the affected areas free of pressure until redness disappears or the skin heals. For pressure ulcers in regions that receive high pressure while seated, this usually requires strict bed rest. Patients should be made aware that burns can occur by dropping cigarette ash on anesthetic skin, using hot water bottles, placing hot plates or mugs on the thighs, sitting too close to fires or radiators, and bathing in water that is too hot (greater than 98°F or 36.5°C). To avoid skin breakdown, condom catheters or leg straps should not be applied too tightly, feet and nails should be cared for, and shoes should fit well or loosely and be checked for sharp objects before donning. To avoid scrotal breakdown, men must routinely reposition the scrotum forward after transferring to a wheelchair or sitting surface.

Following onset of a pressure ulcer, it is important to assess and describe the ulcer so appropriate treatment can be promptly initiated. Several parameters should be described, including anatomical location, general appearance, size (length, width, and depth of the wound area), stage, exudate, odor, necrosis, undermining, sinus tracts, healing, wound margins, surrounding tissue, and signs of infection. Staging ulcers is an important part of pressure ulcer assessment (Table 16-4).[117]

Superficial pressure ulcers may heal with conservative treatment; deeper wounds may require surgical intervention. Pressure ulcer treatment involves debrid-

TABLE 16-4

NATIONAL PRESSURE ULCER ADVISORY PANEL PRESSURE ULCER STAGES

Suspected Deep Tissue Injury	Purple or maroon localized area of discolored intact skin or blood-filled blister due to damage of underlying soft tissue from pressure or shear. The area may be preceded by tissue that is painful, firm, mushy, boggy, warmer, or cooler as compared to adjacent tissue.
Deep Tissue Injury	Purple or maroon localized area of discolored intact skin or blood-filled blister due to damage of underlying soft tissue from pressure or shear.
Stage I	Intact skin with nonblanchable redness of a localized area usually over a bony prominence. Darkly pigmented skin may not have visible blanching; its color may differ from the surrounding area.
Stage II	Partial thickness loss of dermis presenting as a shallow open ulcer with a red pink wound bed, without slough. May also present as an intact or open/ruptured serum-filled blister.
Stage III	Full thickness tissue loss. Subcutaneous fat may be visible but bone, tendon, or muscle are not exposed. Slough may be present but does not obscure the depth of tissue loss. May include undermining and tunneling.
Stage IV	Full thickness tissue loss with exposed bone, tendon, or muscle. Slough or eschar may be present on some parts of the wound bed. Often include undermining and tunneling.
Unstageable	Full thickness tissue loss in which actual depth of the ulcer is completely obscured by slough (yellow, tan, gray, green or brown) or eschar (tan, brown, or black) in the wound bed.

Adapted from: National Pressure Ulcer Advisory Panel. Updated Staging System Web site. Available at: http://www.npuap.org/pr2.htm. Accessed September 15, 2008.

ing necrotic tissue, cleaning the wound bed at each dressing change, and applying appropriate dressings. Dressings that maintain a continuously moist ulcer bed and keep the surrounding intact skin dry are generally preferred. Other important considerations include controlling exudate and filling wounds that have tracks and undermining. Many comorbid conditions may interfere with wound healing. Cardiac, pulmonary, and metabolic (eg, diabetes mellitus) diseases should be stabilized. Nutritional status requires optimization, and tobacco cessation should be strongly encouraged. Wound infection and osteomyelitis will interfere with healing and should be treated. Other issues related to SCI that may interfere with pressure ulcer healing include incontinence, spasticity, HO, and UTI.

Surgical intervention is made when an ulcer is too large to heal with conservative measures, a deep soft tissue or bone infection must be surgically debrided, there are nonhealing tracts, or a bony deformity must be corrected. Myocutaneous or fasciocutaneous flaps are the standard surgical treatment, preceded by inspection of bony prominences and debridement of osteomyelitis (Figure 16-5). A pedicle flap with the suture line away from the area of direct pressure releases skin and underlying muscle while preserving blood supply, repositioning it over the ulcer. The most common examples of pedicle flaps are gluteus maximus rotation flaps to cover sacral or ischial ulcers, hamstring V-Y advancement flaps to cover ischial ulcers, and tensor fascia lata, vastus lateralis, or rectus abdominus flaps to cover trochanteric ulcers. Skin grafts can be used over granulated tissue, but they are not very durable over weight-bearing areas. The possibility for future surgeries should be considered when tissue sites are chosen.

Postoperative care requires rigorous attention to keep

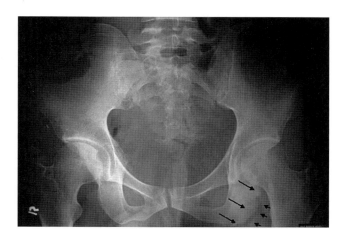

Figure 16-5. With deeper ischial pressure ulcers, the ischial tuberosity commonly develops osteomyelitis. This pelvic radiograph shows an area of marked sclerosis, with a wide zone of transition and cortical irregularity involving the left ischial tuberosity (thin arrow). Areas of lucencies are seen in the adjacent soft tissue (arrowheads).

pressure off the surgical site and allow healing. Following surgery, patients should remain on an air-fluidized bed for a period of 3 to 6 weeks. During this time, tension on flap incisions should be avoided. For patients with spasms, this may mean increased spasmolytic medication and positioning to minimize hip flexor spasms. After 3 to 6 weeks, if the flap is healing well, the patient progresses to a regular hospital bed and lower extremity range-of-motion exercises are allowed, with direct observation of the flap suture lines. Later, the patient is gradually remobilized in a fitted wheelchair. Using progressively longer flap-sitting times over several weeks has been successful following surgery. It is important to reinforce the need to perform regular pressure releases and twice-daily skin checks.

Pressure ulcers may result in complications such as cellulitis and osteomyelitis, which frequently originate through the direct spread of infection. The common presenting symptoms of cellulitis are swelling, redness, local warmth, and fever. The symptoms of osteomyelitis include fever, shaking chills, and purulent drainage. Laboratory findings in both include leukocytosis, elevated erythrocyte sedimentation rate, and positive blood cultures. A radiograph may show periosteal reaction or lytic lesions. Bone scans are of limited use because they are usually positive below a pressure ulcer, whether the underlying bone is infected or not. Magnetic resonance imaging (MRI) findings are somewhat more specific, but false positive tests are still possible. Definitive diagnosis of osteomyelitis is possible through bone biopsy and histologic confirmation, with more reliable results obtained through a needle biopsy or at the time of operative treatment of an ulcer. Cellulitis is treated with oral or parenteral antibiotics (usually taken for 10 to 14 days). Osteomyelitis is usually treated with 6 weeks or more of antibiotic administration and requires bone debridement. Other complications of pressure ulcers that require treatment include wound infection, AD, and malnutrition.

Musculoskeletal Disorders

Musculoskeletal disorders are common among individuals with SCI. Many types of musculoskeletal problems have been reported, including soft tissue and osseous injuries at the time of SCI; traumatic injuries after SCI; unique musculoskeletal disorders precipitated by SCI; and chronic upper limb disorders related to repetitive use, poor biomechanics, and aging. The impact of musculoskeletal problems on the overall function and well-being of a person with SCI cannot be overstated. Even relatively minor musculoskeletal pathologies can result in significant secondary disabilities and new limitations.

Fractures

Fractures at the time of SCI are common and directly related to extrinsic factors (eg, force of injury) and intrinsic factors (eg, bone density). Fractures of vertebrae, limb girdles, and long bones are most common. A high index of suspicion and use of imaging studies are necessary to identify fractures below the neurologic level of injury.

Fractures also commonly occur after SCI (Figure 16-6). The incidence of long bone fractures in the lower limb has been estimated to be 4% to 7%.[118] Fractures are related to osteoporosis that occurs within months after injury below the level of injury. The injury that results in fracture may be minor as bone mineral density decreases and less force is required to produce failure in the bone. The Model SCI System has reported fracture rates based on time following SCI, with cumulative

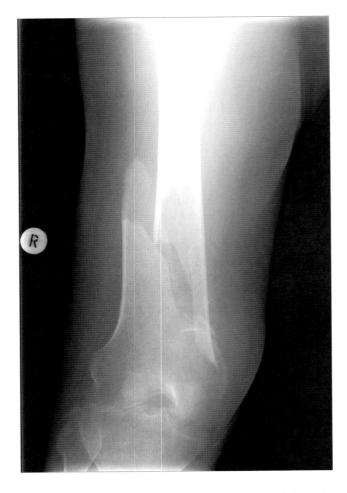

Figure 16-6. Supracondylar fracture in osteoporotic bone in a male with long-standing paraplegia. The fracture occurred secondary to a fall from a gurney.

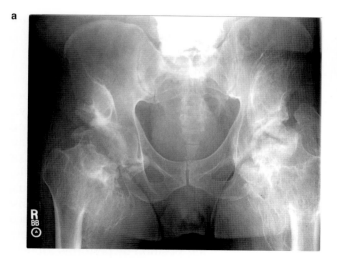

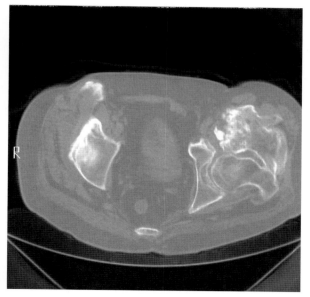

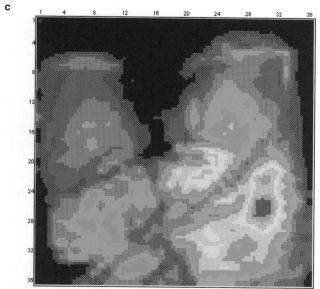

Figure 16-7. (**a**) Radiograph showing severe heterotopic ossification involving bilateral hips. (**b**) Computed tomography scan shows large mass of bone anterior to the left acetabulum. (**c**) Heterotopic ossification can indirectly cause pressure ulcers through restriction of joint range of motion, which results in pelvic obliquity when seated. In this patient with severely limited left hip flexion, a seating interface pressure transducer map placed between the patient and wheelchair cushion demonstrates increased pressure (yellow and red colors) posterior to the right greater trochanter.

incidences of 14% at 5 years, 28% at 10 years, and 39% 15 years after injury.[119]

Managing fractures includes immobilizing the limb and preventing complications. AD may occur in individuals with SCI at level T-6 and above. Other potential complications include DVT, increased spasticity, and the development of pressure ulcers. Well-padded, bivalved casts allow frequent inspection of skin. Delayed union, malunion, and nonunion are common problems after fracture in SCI. Functional consequences, such as difficulty transferring, must be anticipated and addressed.

Heterotopic Ossification

HO is the development of ectopic bone within periarticular soft tissues and is a well-described complication of SCI and traumatic brain injury. Although HO may develop around any joint or within muscle below the level of SCI, it develops most commonly about the hips (Figure 16-7). Onset is typically within the first 5 weeks after SCI, although it may not become clinically apparent for an additional few weeks. The prevalence is thought to be approximately 20% to 30%, although only about half the cases are clinically significant. Between 3% and 8% develop complete ankylosis of the involved joint.[120,121]

Diagnosing hip and shoulder HO may be challenging because the periarticular structures are not as easy to examine as more superficial joints (eg, knee and elbow). HO may present with erythema, swelling, warmth, decreased range of motion, increased spasticity, pain, and fever. Bone scintigraphy and MRI are more sensitive diagnostic tests than plain film radiographs, which may not be helpful if the HO matrix is not yet calcified. Complications include decreased range of motion affecting transfers and seating, skin breakdown, increased spasticity, and DVT.

The mainstay of treatment for HO has been pharmacologic. Bisphosphonates, such as etidronate disodium, and nonsteroidal antiinflammatories (eg, indomethacin) have been used to treat HO. Low-dose radiation, manipulation, and surgical excision are also reportedly useful for treating HO that does not respond to medications.[122,123]

Contractures

Progressive shortening (contracture) of muscles, tendons, ligaments, and joint capsules results in stiffness, movement limitation, and deformity. Contractures limit self-care, transfers, bed positioning, standing, sitting, and walking. Finger flexion deformities compromise hand function and skin care. Ankle plantar flexion contractures may lead to pressure ulcers and limit footwear. Knee and hip flexion contractures increase the energy cost of standing and walking. Hip adductor contractures limit perineal care. Preventing contractures involves daily range-of-motion exercise, which may be complicated by spasticity. Early contracture may be reversed with stretching with or without heat treatments, such as ultrasound diathermy. Severe contractures may require surgical release.

Chronic Upper Limb Disorders

Upper limb pain and dysfunction are common following SCI. Using the upper limbs for weight-bearing purposes over decades creates biomechanical challenges for limbs that are designed primarily for prehension and mobility. Rotator cuff disease, tendonitis, epicondylitis, arthritis, and carpal tunnel syndrome are all common upper limb problems. Recommendations in *Preservation of Upper Limb Function Following Spinal Cord Injury* address biomechanical stressors, techniques, equipment, musculoskeletal health, and the environment.[47] Most address well-established ergonomic associations between strenuous tasks and musculoskeletal disorders. Minimizing the force and frequency of tasks, such as wheelchair pushing, is achieved by optimizing equipment (eg, wheelchair weight and setup) and technique. Optimizing technique includes education and training in performing tasks (eg, transfer, wheelchair propulsion) and avoiding extreme limb postures. Equipment, technological, and environmental interventions are effective. For example, an elevated wheelchair seat, standing position, or lowered environment prevents repetitive overhead reaching.

Neurological Disorders

A variety of secondary neurologic complications can develop following SCI, including spasticity,

neuropathic pain, posttraumatic syringomyelia, and peripheral nerve entrapment.

Spasticity

Spasticity develops in individuals with upper motor neuron damage and spared reflex pathways, with hyperactive phasic stretch reflexes mediated by 1A afferents from the muscle spindle. The 1A afferents respond to rapid stretch, as in a tendon tap, or rapid passive movement of a joint. Clinically, spasticity manifests as hyperactive tendon reflexes, clonus, velocity-dependent hypertonus, and extensor spasms. The latter are commonly elicited by the passive stretch of hip flexors, for example, as the patient moves from sitting to supine-lying position or performs a push-up pressure release. Extensor spasms may interfere during transfers, although some patients use them to aid standing. Flexor spasms can interfere with prone or supine positioning in bed, bed mobility, transfers, and walking; they can also interfere with sleep and contribute to pressure ulcers.

Spasticity and other hypertonus require treatment only if they interfere with function, cause discomfort or poor sleep, hinder caregivers' tasks, or contribute to medical complications, as with pressure ulcer formation.[124] Treatment benefits must always be weighed against the possible beneficial effects of spasticity, such as positioning extremities or aiding standing transfers and walking.

Once spasticity is determined to be more detrimental than beneficial and nociceptive sources such as UTI, renal stone, or fecal impaction have been ruled out, various treatments may be undertaken. The least invasive is daily passive stretching of hypertonic muscles, which reduces tone and spasms for several hours and maintains joint range of motion. Oral medications, such as baclofen, tizanidine, or diazepam most commonly, gabapentin or dantroline rarely, must often be administered. If these prove insufficient, invasive techniques should be considered. Focal spasticity can often be treated with percutaneous injection of botulinum toxin, phenol, or alcohol. Generalized and severe spasticity usually responds to continuous intrathecal baclofen delivered via a subcutaneous pump. Surgical options, such as tenotomy or rhizotomy, are rarely required for severe spasticity that fails to respond to other treatments.

Pain

About one third of individuals with chronic SCI experience severe pain, and up to 80% experience at least some pain on a regular basis. Pain is far more common in the spinal cord injured than in the general population,[125] and it frequently contributes to lower psychological functioning, interferes with daily activities, and hinders social integration.

Pain usually originates centrally within the spinal cord. It presents with any combination of burning, tingling, or lancinating unaffected by neck movements or posture, and is thought to represent spontaneous discharge of neurons in the ascending pain pathways. Individuals with cauda equina injury experience a series of stabbing pains that radiate down one or both lower limbs every few seconds to minutes. These shock-like pains may be continuously present or appear intermittently. Another type of pain presents as a segmental hyperesthesia over one or two dermatomes at the level of injury. This hypersensitivity to light touch may only be a minor inconvenience and often does not require treatment. Central pain has been treated with a variety of agents, including nonnarcotic analgesics (acetaminophen, acetylsalicylic acid, ibuprofen); anticonvulsants (gabapentin, phenytoin, clonazepam); tricyclic antidepressants (amitriptyline, doxepin); and opioids. Chronic opioid use (eg, methadone and sustained-release morphine) should be administered only in a highly structured setting in which the patient's compliance and psychological status can be carefully monitored.

It is essential to distinguish central dysesthetic SCI pains from pain arising due to mechanical causes, such as persisting cord or nerve root impingement, an enlarging posttraumatic syrinx, or a number of common musculoskeletal conditions. These latter types of pain are generally aggravated by spinal movements or postural changes and may be clinically distinguishable from central pain. Treatment involves addressing the underlying cause of mechanical pain, if possible.

Posttraumatic Syringomyelia

Symptomatic posttraumatic syringomyelia is an uncommon but potentially severely disabling complication of SCI.[126,127] The prevalence of clinically significant posttraumatic syringomyelia has been estimated at 4.5% for tetraplegia and 1.7% for paraplegia. Posttraumatic syringomyelia results from a syrinx at the level of the cord injury (Figure 16-8). It can cause progressive spinal cord damage by extending rostrally or caudally from the injury site, and can extend the length of the spinal cord up to the brainstem. Syringomyelia may develop within months after SCI, but more typically develops over many years.

The earliest symptoms of syringomyelia may be subtle. They include pain, often aggravated by postural change; altered spasticity; sweating; worsening OH;

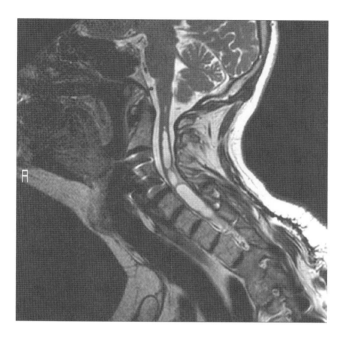

Figure 16-8. Nine months following a motor vehicle accident with upper thoracic fractures and level T-3 complete paraplegia, this patient presented with an ascending sensory level and increasing left hand weakness. Magnetic resonance imaging demonstrated a posttraumatic syrinx extending from the C-1 level through the conus.

ascending loss of pain and temperature sensation; and ascending loss of segmental reflexes. Ascending weakness is a late manifestation, the appearance of which often indicates that the condition is advanced and may not be reversible. MRI is definitive for diagnosing posttraumatic syringomyelia, but up to 60% of all SCI patients have at least a small intramedullary cystic structure at their level of injury. Careful serial clinical examinations and MRI are useful for determining whether a syrinx is causing neurologic deterioration. Treatment may include minimizing Valsalva maneuvers and spine movements, surgical decompression with syringosubarachnoid, syringopleural or syringoperitoneal shunting of syrinx fluid, or duraplasty. For those with complete cord injury, cordectomy is an alternative.

Peripheral Nerve Entrapment

Upper limb peripheral nerve entrapment is highly prevalent in individuals with SCI because of the physical demands placed on the upper limbs during functional tasks.[128] Predisposing factors include increased use of the upper extremities for transfers and wheelchair propulsion, resulting in an increased incidence of carpal tunnel syndrome; absent pain sensation, particularly in posttraumatic syringomyelia, resulting in ulnar nerve entrapment; and proximal compression of motor neurons and motor axons in the presence of cervical spondylosis. Radial nerve entrapment, as in Saturday Night Palsy and thoracic outlet syndrome, also occurs with increased frequency. Preventive measures include use of wheelchair gloves, optimized wheelchair setup and propulsion technique, and avoidance of direct pressure to the ulnar groove. New sensory loss, weakness, or loss of function should prompt electrodiagnostic studies to rule out nerve entrapment. Wrist splints, elbow pads, and surgical decompression are common treatments.

Genitourinary Complications

Morbidity and mortality due to urosepsis and renal failure in individuals with SCI have decreased significantly since the 1940s because of improved management principles and techniques. Understanding how the level of the cord lesion relates to bladder function aids in anticipating possible urinary dysfunctions.[129,130] Upper motor neuron/spastic bladder dysfunction is generally associated with fractures at the T-12 vertebral level and above (ie, cervical and thoracic fractures). For patients with these conditions, voluntary control from the brain is disrupted, but reflex activity recovers after spinal shock dissipates. SCI patients with upper motor neuron lesions rostral to and sparing the conus (S-2 through S-4 neurological levels, located at the L-1 vertebral body) usually develop reflex bladder emptying after the resolution of spinal shock. Many of these patients also develop detrusor-sphincter dyssynergia, in which the reflex detrusor contraction occurs simultaneously with external urethral sphincter contraction.[131–133] The result is high bladder pressures that may lead to detrusor muscle hypertrophy, vesicoureteral reflux, hydroureter, hydronephrosis, and renal failure. This process is often clinically silent and needs to be regularly monitored. Lower motor neuron/flaccid/areflexic bladder dysfunction generally occurs when the bony injury is at level L-1 and below and affects the conus medullaris or cauda equina. Individuals do not regain reflex contraction; the bladder remains flaccid and overfills. Mixed dysfunctions may occur with injuries at the T-12 or L-1 vertebral levels, with a variable degree of upper and lower motor neuron dysfunction and less predictable effects on voiding.

Goals for bladder management in individuals with SCI include urinary continence, complete bladder emptying, maintaining safe vesicular pressures during storage and voiding, and minimizing the need for physical assistance. Factors predisposing individuals with SCI to chronic renal failure include high-pressure voiding

with reflux nephropathy, nephrolithiasis from urea-splitting bacteria, chronic pyelonephritis, and amyloidosis from chronic pressure ulcers and osteomyelitis.

Bladder Management Techniques

During the initial period of spinal shock, before reflex emptying develops, bladder drainage is managed with an indwelling Foley catheter until fluid intake can be regulated to less than 2 L per day. If they have adequate hand function to perform self-catheterization, patients may be transitioned to intermittent catheterization every 4 to 6 hours to keep maximal bladder distension to less than 500 mL. Fluid intake must be limited to prevent the need for more frequent catheterizations. After several months, reflex detrusor contractions develop in patients with upper motor neuron/spastic bladder; this can be anticipated in those with preserved bulbocavernosus and anal reflexes. When spontaneous reflex bladder emptying develops, anticholinergics may be needed to prevent incontinence between catheterizations. In individuals whose hand function is inadequate to perform self-catheterization, long-term use of an indwelling Foley catheter or suprapubic catheter may be considered. In males with SCI, the use of a condom catheter in conjunction with sphincterotomy or urethral stents may be a reasonable bladder management option. Post-void residuals should be less than 100 mL to prevent bacterial colonization in the bladder from achieving a concentration that will cause symptoms. The less common lower motor neuron bladder (in which the S-2, S-3, S-4 reflex arc is interrupted) can be managed with intermittent catheterization. Although voiding into a condom catheter can sometimes be achieved with prolonged direct compression over the bladder (Crede's maneuver), this can lead to vesicoureteral reflux and hydronephrosis and is therefore discouraged.[134]

Pharmacological treatment can be used to improve urinary continence. Anticholinergic drugs bind to muscarinic receptors in the bladder. Medications, including oxybutinin and tolterodine, are used to decrease detrusor contractility and increase bladder compliance. Side effects are dry mouth, decreased sweating, and constipation. Alpha antagonists (eg, prazosin, terazosin, doxazosin) can occasionally allow patients with incomplete injuries to initiate voiding. Side effects may include hypotension and dizziness. Injections with botulinum toxin have been used to control detrusor hyperactivity.[135]

Surgery is sometimes used to manage neurogenic bladder.[136] Surgeries for hyperreflexic bladder include bladder augmentation with or without urinary diversion (ie, continent ileal conduit diversion and catheterization via an abdominal stoma) or cystoplasty and detrusor myectomy. In instances of areflexic bladder, outlet resistance may be enhanced by artificial sphincters or bladder neck procedures. Additionally, periurethral injections and fascial slings have been used to achieve continence. Newer strategies are arising to manage hyperreflexic bladder.[136] Electrode stimulation involves surgical posterior rhizotomy of the sacral nerve roots and electrode placement at the anterior nerve roots. Stimulation of the anterior roots causes contraction of the detrusor and voiding.

Renal function should be regularly monitored and compromise detected and treated early. A yearly urologic examination is recommended for individuals with chronic SCI, although there is no consensus on the examination components.[136] The exam often includes an evaluation of the upper (via ultrasound, renal scan, computed tomography [CT] scan, or intravenous pyelogram) and lower (via urodynamics, cystogram, or cystoscopy) tracts.

Urinary Tract Infection

Bacteriuria (> 100,000 organisms per mL) is a nearly inevitable consequence of neurogenic bladder.[137] Bacteriuria is not treated if it is asymptomatic. Symptoms of UTI prompting antibiotic treatment may include fever, shaking chills, leukocytosis, hematuria, pyuria, and unexplained increase in spasticity. Preventing UTI may involve ensuring adequate bladder drainage with a low postvoid residual, perineal hygiene, cleaning the drainage tube and bag, clean catheterization (washing hands and catheter with soap and water for those on intermittent catheterization), and eliminating urinary tract stones.[138] The role of prophylactic antibiotics in preventing recurrent UTIs has not been clarified because of concerns about promoting multidrug-resistant organisms.[137] High fevers and shaking chills suggest urosepsis, which requires broad antibiotic coverage (including antipseudomonal coverage), placement of an indwelling catheter to assure bladder drainage, and a renal ultrasound to rule out upper tract obstruction. If the patient fails to respond to antibiotics within 48 to 72 hours or sustains septic shock, an abdominal CT scan should be performed to rule out perinephric abscess.

Bladder and Renal Calculi

Bladder stones may cause bladder spasms or urinary sediment and are often removed by transurethral cystolithectomy. Renal stones are most commonly infection-associated struvite stones caused by vesicoureteral reflux and urea-splitting organisms, such as *Proteus mirabilis*. Another risk factor for stone for-

mation in recently injured patients is hypercalciuria in response to paralysis. If stones are large enough to obstruct the ureter, SCI patients must be closely monitored until treated because upper tract obstruction may be relatively silent in patients with impaired sensation until urosepsis develops. Upper tract stones may be removed by extracorporeal shock wave lithotripsy or percutaneous procedures.

Bladder Carcinoma

SCI patients with long-term indwelling catheters have an increased risk of bladder carcinoma.[139] There is no consensus on appropriate screening, although some advocate for yearly cystoscopy and biopsy of the bladder for those who have had indwelling catheters for more than 10 years.

Sexual Function and Fertility

Individuals with SCI need to be reassured of their ability to express their sexuality, and they may need to be provided with information about techniques and devices they can use to assist them with that expression. Individuals should be encouraged to consider how increased physical dependency will play a role in their feelings of control or powerlessness and desirability. Sexual activities and barriers to sexual expression should be identified and addressed.

Individuals with SCI should be provided with information on sexual function and made aware that sexual desires are psychological and hormonal, not affected by nerve damage. Pleasurable sexual experience may be realized by focusing on skin, lips, and other areas where sensation is intact. Information about manual stimulation, oral–genital sex, positioning, and effects of spasticity can be discussed.

Despite absent sensation below the level of injury, many males, particularly those with neurologic lesions above the S-2 to S-4 levels or incomplete lower lesions, are sometimes able to achieve and maintain erections (the overall rate is 50% for all categories of injury). Oral medications (ie, phosphodiesterase type 5 inhibitors), external appliances, intracavernosal injections (eg, prostaglandin E, papaverine), and implanted penile prostheses are additional options to maintain sexual function. Although many men with SCI are able to achieve erections, most are unable to ejaculate. Vibration-induced ejaculation or electroejaculation can yield sperm for artificial insemination in some individuals. AD is a small risk with these procedures in men with injuries at or above level T-6. Fertility in men diminishes to less than 5% with clinically complete injuries. Semen quality declines rapidly after SCI, possibly because of recurrent UTIs and increased testicle temperature. Nonetheless, artificial insemination with semen obtained by electroejaculation or more invasive techniques has resulted in pregnancies and healthy live births.

For females, loss of sensation and lack of vaginal lubrication are the primary sexual changes after SCI. Many women with SCI are able to achieve orgasm, although the perception of orgasm may be altered from preinjury experience.[140] Use of a vibrator and lubricants can be helpful when engaging in sexual activity. Emptying the bladder by catheterization and decreasing fluid intake prior to intercourse can help reduce the chance of bladder incontinence.

Female fertility returns to preinjury level once the body has recovered from the initial trauma and menses return. Oral contraceptives and intrauterine devices carry extra risks for women with SCI, making foam and condoms better birth control choices. The physiology of labor is unaltered by SCI; however, impaired sensation may lead to undetected labor pains and presentation in later stages of labor, or, rarely, unsupervised birth. Prolonged or mechanically assisted labor (due to compromised ability to push), and AD in those with SCI above level T-7 are additional risks of pregnancy and childbirth in this population.

Because of the extraordinary physical and emotional demands on patients following SCI, sexual and marital counseling should be offered during rehabilitation. It is essential that the rehabilitation team respect individuals' values and approach this topic with sensitivity.

Psychological Issues

Assessment and support are the two major psychological services offered to individuals with SCI. Assessment is the evaluation of the individual's potential to learn, think, and interact with the environment and others. Standardized tests that measure psychosocial function and intelligence are used for assessment. These tests provide a clear picture of an individual's potential for rehabilitation and suggest appropriate guidelines for educational and vocational pursuits.

The other major psychological service to SCI patients, support, should extend to patients and family members. It should be grounded in knowledge of the patient's history, disposition, values, limitations, and potential. In addition to psychologists, members of the rehabilitation team, particularly social workers, vocational counselors, and recreation therapists, also contribute to a patient's psychosocial adjustment to SCI.

Denial or inability to accept SCI is common and can interfere with rehabilitation, although expectations for recovery may be a source of motivation. Patients are counseled to focus on current rehabilitation issues without destroying hopes of recovery. Confronting a patient's denial can destroy the physician–patient relationship. Eventually, many patients accept their conditions and approach their physicians for information on prognosis.

Associated Traumatic Brain Injury

A significant percentage of SCI patients incur traumatic brain injuries at the time of SCI or have a prior history of traumatic brain injury.[141–143] Resulting agitation, impulsiveness, impaired judgment, and impaired new learning may all impact rehabilitation.

Premorbid Personality

Premorbid factors affect rehabilitation outcomes and should be considered during acute rehabilitation. Risk-taking behavior and drug and alcohol abuse are associated with some cases of SCI and affect adjustment to disability after SCI. More preinjury education is associated with greater likelihood of employment after SCI; among those with less than 12 years of education, only 38% returned to work after SCI, compared to 93% of those with 16 or more years of education.[43]

Reactive Depression and Suicide

A depressed mood is common following SCI. When depression is extreme or prolonged, it can interfere with rehabilitation and precipitate suicide. Suicide rates are higher in individuals with SCI than in a matched general population.[144] Risk factors for suicide include chronic pain and alcohol or drug abuse.

Marital Adjustment and Discord

Divorce is common after SCI. Factors that may contribute to divorce are altered family roles, dependence on a caregiver–spouse (with subsequent burnout), and impaired sexual function.

Health Maintenance

Periodic comprehensive evaluations of medical and functional status are recommended for individuals with SCI after initial rehabilitation. Although the optimal frequency for each type of assessment has not been determined, it is standard practice to perform comprehensive evaluations annually. In addition to a general history and physical examination, the assessment should evaluate the neurologic system, skin, urogenital system and

neurogenic bladder management, functional status, and equipment needs. The patients' psychosocial and vocational adjustments should also be assessed.

ORGANIZATION OF A SPINAL CORD INJURY UNIT

Acute trauma facilities, including those used by the US military, usually lack comprehensive SCI units. Rather, they have orthopedists, neurosurgeons, physiatrists, physical and occupational therapists, psychologists, social workers, and skilled nurses who can decompress the spinal cord, establish spine stability, prevent acute medical complications, and begin the initial process of rehabilitation. As soon as patients are medically stable, they are transferred to specialized SCI rehabilitation facilities. The US military has a long-standing agreement with the US Department of Veterans Affairs to transfer patients to one of 23 Veterans Affairs SCI centers. A comprehensive SCI facility employs physiatrists, urologists, orthopaedic surgeons, neurosurgeons, internists, plastic surgeons, rehabilitation nurses, physical and occupational therapists, psychologists, social workers, vocational counselors, orthotists, recreation therapists, respiratory

therapists, and dietitians. Specialized facilities in an SCI unit include urodynamics with videofluoroscopy, advanced neuroimaging, a physical and occupational therapy gym, and a wheelchair-accessible pool. All patient care space must be wheelchair and gurney accessible. An independent living apartment, where SCI patients can live with spouse or attendant support, is particularly useful when the patient's ability to return to the community is uncertain.

Compared to a medical, surgical, or general rehabilitation ward, a specialized SCI unit can anticipate and minimize complications and enhance functional outcomes, which results in shorter hospitalizations, fewer rehospitalizations, and less economic cost. Expertise, unique team relationships, and specialized equipment and facilities contribute to the efficiency of an SCI unit. Specialized SCI centers allow clinical and applied basic research to further improve SCI care.

SUMMARY

Prior to World War II, SCI was usually fatal. Now, most SCI patients survive, return home completely or partially independent, have only modestly reduced life expectancy, and achieve satisfactory quality of life. For most SCI patients, these favorable outcomes can be expected if the emergency, acute, and rehabilitative interventions during the first 6 months following injury are appropriate. SCI leads to multiorgan dysfunction, partially mediated by autonomic dysfunction, and loss of somatic sensation, making diagnosis challenging. Strength, sensation, blood pressure control, bladder and bowel emptying, and sexual function are often

impaired in individuals with SCI. Life-threatening or disabling conditions that affect organ systems, such as pressure ulcers, DVT with pulmonary embolism, AD, OH, HO, posttraumatic syringomyelia, depression, and suicide, must be prevented or diagnosed and treated early. In addition, SCI patients must undergo extensive training in order to resume maximum function. Specialized training and adaptive equipment is required for mobility and independent self care. Guidance and instruction is required for psychological, social, financial, vocational, and avocational adjustment to disability.

REFERENCES

1. Stover SL, Fine PR, eds. *Spinal Cord Injury: the Facts & Figures*. Birmingham, Ala: University of Alabama; 1986.

2. Jackson AB, Dijkers M, DeVivo MJ, Poczatek RB. A demographic profile of new traumatic spinal cord injuries: change and stability over 30 years. *Arch Phys Med Rehabil*. 2004;85(11):1740–1748.

3. National Spinal Cord Injury Statistical Center. The 2006 Annual Statistical Report for the Model Spinal Cord Injury Care Systems Web site. Available at: http://images.main.uab.edu/spinalcord/pdffiles/NSCIC%20Annual%2006.pdf. Accessed August 23, 2007.

4. Hardaway RM III. Viet Nam wound analysis. *J Trauma*. 1978;18(9):635–643.

5. Ohry A, Rozin R. Acute spinal cord injuries in the Lebanon war, 1982. *Isr J Med Sci*. 1984;20:345–349.

6. Yashon D. *Spinal Injury*. New York, NY: Appleton-Century-Crofts; 1978.

7. Griffin JW, Tooms RE, Mendius RA, Clifft JK, Vander Zwaag R, el-Zeky F. Efficacy of high voltage pulsed current for healing of pressure ulcers in patients with spinal cord injury. *Phys Ther*. 1991;71(6):433–444.

8. Whiteneck GG, Charlifue SW, Frankel HL, et al. Mortality, morbidity, and psychosocial outcomes of persons spinal cord injured more than 20 years ago. *Paraplegia*. 1992;30(9):617–630.

9. DeVivo MJ, Krause JS, Lammertse DP. Recent trends in mortality and causes of death among persons with spinal cord injury. *Arch Phys Med Rehabil*. 1999;80(11):1411–1419.

10. DePalma RG, Burris DG, Champion HR, Hodgson MJ. Blast injuries. *N Engl J Med*. 2005;352(13):1335–1342.

11. Jellinger K. Neuropathology of spinal cord injuries. In: Vinken PJ, Bruyn GW, eds. *Handbook of Clinical Neurology*. New York, NY: Wiley Interscience Division; 1976: 43–121.

12. Kakulas BA. The clinical neuropathology of spinal cord injury. A guide to the future. *Paraplegia*. 1987;25(3):212–216.

13. Schneider H. Acute and chronic pathomorphological reactions to cord injury. In: Schramm J, Jones S, eds. *Spinal Cord Monitoring*. Berlin, Germany: Springer-Verlag; 1985: 103–120.

14. Eltorai IM, Juler G. Ischemic myelopathy. *Angiology*. 1979;30:81–94.

15. Foo D, Rossier AB. Anterior spinal artery syndrome and its natural history. *Paraplegia*. 1983;21:1–10.

16. Sliwa JA, Maclean IC. Ischemic myelopathy: a review of spinal vasculature and related clinical syndromes. *Arch Phys Med Rehabil*. 1992;73:365–372.

17. Francis TJR, Pearson RR, Robertson AG, Hodgson M, Dutka AJ, Flynn ET. Central nervous system decompression sickness: latency of 1,070 human cases. *Undersea Biomed Res*. 1989;15:403–417.

18. Melamed Y, Shupak A, Bitterman H. Medical problems associated with underwater diving. *N Engl J Med*. 1992;326:30–35.

19. Braughler JM, Hall JD. Central nervous system trauma and stroke. *Free Radic Biol Med*. 1989;6:289–301.

20. Papadopoulos SM. Spinal cord injury. *Curr Opin Neurol Neurosurg*. 1992;5:554–557.

21. Waxman SG. Demyelination in spinal cord injury and multiple sclerosis: what can we do to enhance functional recovery. *J Neurotrauma*. 1991;9:S105–117.

22. Young W. Pharmacologic therapy of acute spinal cord injury. In: Errico TJ, Bauer RD, Waugh T, eds. *Spinal Trauma*. Philadelphia, Pa: JB Lippincott; 1991: 415–433.

23. Bracken MB, Shepard MJ, Collins WF, et al. A randomized, controlled trial of methylprednisolone or naloxone in the treatment of acute spinal cord injury. *N Engl J Med*. 1990;322:1405–1411.

24. Bracken MB, Collins WF, Freeman DF, et al. Efficacy of methylprednisolone in acute spinal cord injury. *JAMA*. 1984;251:45–52.

25. Bracken MB, Shepard MJ, Holford TR, et al. Administration of methylprednisolone for 24 or 48 hours or tirilizad mesylate for 48 hours in the treatment of acute spinal cord injury. Results of the third national acute spinal cord injury randomized controlled trial. National Acute Spinal Cord Injury Study. *JAMA*. 1997;277(20):1597–1604.

26. Coleman WP, Benzel D, Cahill DW, et al. A critical appraisal of the reporting of the National Acute Spinal Cord Injury Studies (II and III) of methylprednisolone in acute spinal cord injury. *J Spinal Disord*. 2000;13(3):185–199.

27. Geisler FH, Coleman WP, Greico G, Poonian D. The Sygen multicenter acute spinal cord injury study. *Spine*. 2001;26(24 Suppl): S87–98.

28. Anderson PA, Bohlman HH. Anterior decompression and arthrodesis of the cervical spine: long-term motor improvement. Part II: improvement in complete traumatic quadriplegia. *J Bone Joint Surg Am.* 1992;74(5):683–691.

29. Little JW, Harris RM, Lerner SJ. Immobilization impairs recovery after spinal cord injury. *Arch Phys Med Rehabil.* 1991;72:408–412.

30. Wu L, Marino RJ, Herbison GJ, Ditunno JF Jr. Recovery of zero-grade muscles in the zone of partial preservation in motor complete quadriplegia. *Arch Phys Med Rehabil.* 1992;73:40–43.

31. Ditunno JF Jr, Stover SL, Freed MM, Ahn JH. Motor recovery of the upper extremities in traumatic quadriplegia: a multicenter study. *Arch Phys Med Rehabil.* 1992;73(5):431–436.

32. Marino RJ, Herbison GJ, Ditunno JF Jr. Peripheral sprouting as a mechanism for recovery in the zone of injury in acute quadriplegia: a single-fiber EMG study. *Muscle Nerve.* 1994;17(12):1466–1468.

33. Little JW, Powers RK, Michelson P, Moore D, Robinson LR, Goldstein B. Electrodiagnosis of upper limb weakness in acute quadriplegia. *Am J Phys Med Rehabil.* 1994;73(1):15–22.

34. American Spinal Injury Association. *International Standards for Neurological Classification of Spinal Cord Injury.* Chicago, Ill: ASIA; 2000.

35. American Spinal Injury Association. Scoring, scaling, and classification. In: *Reference Manual for the International Standards for Neurological Classification of Spinal Cord Injury.* Chicago, Ill: ASIA; 2003: 46–60.

36. Burns AS, Lee BS, Ditunno JF Jr, Tessler T. Patient selection for clinical trials: the reliability of the early spinal cord injury examination. *J Neurotrauma.* 2003;20(5):477–482.

37. Crozier KS, Graziani V, Ditunno JF Jr, Herbison GJ. Spinal cord injury: prognosis for ambulation based on sensory examination in patients who are initially motor complete. *Arch Phys Med Rehabil.* 1991;72:119–121.

38. McKinley W, Santos K, Meade M, Brooke K. Incidence and outcomes of spinal cord injury clinical syndromes. *J Spinal Cord Med.* 2007;30(3):215–224.

39. Little JW, Halar E. Temporal course of motor recovery after Brown-Sequard spinal cord injuries. *Paraplegia.* 1985;23:39–46.

40. Roth EJ, Park T, Pang T, Yarkony GM, Lee MY. Traumatic cervical Brown-Sequard and Brown-Sequard-plus syndromes: the spectrum of presentations and outcomes. *Paraplegia.* 1991;29(9):582–589.

41. Little JW, DeLisa JA. Cauda equina injury: late motor recovery. *Arch Phys Med Rehabil.* 1986;67:45–47.

42. Barnes CD, Joynt RJ, Schottelius BA. Motorneuron resting potentials in spinal shock. *Am J Physiol.* 1961;203:1113–1116.

43. Burke D. Spasticity as an adaptation to pyramidal tract injury. *Adv Neurol.* 1988;47:401–423.

44. Krause JS. Employment after spinal cord injury. *Arch Phys Med Rehabil.* 1992;73:163–169.

45. Ashworth B. Preliminary trial of carisoprodol in multiple sclerosis. *Practitioner.* 1964;192:540–542.

46. Consortium for Spinal Cord Medicine, Paralyzed Veterans of America. *Outcomes Following Traumatic Spinal Cord Injury: Clinical Practice Guidelines for Health-Care Professionals.* Washington, DC: Paralyzed Veterans of America; 1999.

47. Consortium for Spinal Cord Medicine, Paralyzed Veterans of America. *Preservation of Upper Limb Function Following Spinal Cord Injury: A Clinical Practice Guideline for Health-Care Professionals.* Washington, DC: Paralyzed Veterans of America; 2005.

48. Waring WP, Maynard FM. Shoulder pain in acute traumatic quadriplegia. *Paraplegia.* 1991;29:37–42.

49. Barbeau H, Wainberg M, Finch L. Description and application of a system for locomotor rehabilitation. *Med Biol Eng Comput.* 1987;25:341–344.

50. Martin J, Plummer P, Bowden MG, Fulk G, Behrman AL. Body weight support systems: considerations for clinicians. *Phys Ther Reviews.* 2006;11:143–152.

51. Behrman AL, Bowden MG, Nair PM. Neuroplasticity after spinal cord injury and training: an emerging paradigm shift in rehabilitation and walking recovery. *Phys Ther.* 2006;86:1406–1425.

52. Banovac K, Sherman AL, Estores IM, Banovac F. Prevention and treatment of heterotopic ossification after spinal cord injury. *J Spinal Cord Med.* 2004;27(4):376–382.

53. Potter BK, Burns TC, Lacap AP, Granville RR, Gajewski DA. Heterotopic ossification following traumatic and combat-related amputations. Prevalence, risk factors, and preliminary results of excision. *J Bone Joint Surg Am.* 2007;89(3):476–486.

54. Johnstone BR, Jordan CJ, Buntine JA. A review of surgical rehabilitation of the upper limb in quadriplegia. *Paraplegia.* 1988;26:317–339.

55. Peckham PH, Keith MW, Freehafer AA. Restoration of functional control by electrical stimulation in the upper extremity of the quadriplegic patient. *J Bone Joint Surg Am.* 1988;70:144–148.

56. De Troyer A, Estenne M, Heilporn A. Mechanism of active expiration in tetraplegic subjects. *N Engl J Med.* 1986;314:740–744.

57. Carter RE. Respiratory aspects of spinal cord injury management. *Paraplegia.* 1987;25:262–266.

58. Schmitt J, Midha M, McKenzie N. Medical complications of spinal cord disease. *Neurol Clin.* 1991;9:779–795.

59. Fishburn MJ, Marino RJ, Ditunno JF Jr. Atelectasis and pneumonia in acute spinal cord injury. *Arch Phys Med Rehabil.* 1990;71(3):197–200.

60. Consortium for Spinal Cord Medicine, Paralyzed Veterans of America. *Respiratory Management Following Spinal Cord Injury: A Clinical Practice Guideline for Health-Care Professionals.* Washington, DC: Paralyzed Veterans of America; 2005.

61. DeVivo MJ, Stover SL. Long term survival and causes of death. In: Stover SL, DeLisa JA, Whiteneck GG, eds. *Spinal Cord Injury: Clinical Outcomes for the Model Systems.* Gaithersburg, Md: Aspen Publications; 1995: 289–316.

62. Kirshblum S, Johnston MV, Brown J, O'Connor KC, Jarosz P. Predictors of dysphagia after spinal cord injury. *Arch Phys Med Rehabil.* 1999;80(9):1101–1105.

63. Wolf C, Meiners TH. Dysphagia in patients with acute cervical spinal cord injury. *Spinal Cord.* 2003;41(6):347–353.

64. Krassioukov A, Claydon VE. The clinical problems in cardiovascular control following spinal cord injury: an overview. *Prog Brain Res.* 2006;152:223–229.

65. Lehmann KG, Lane JG, Piepmeier JM, Batsford WP. Cardiovascular abnormalities accompanying acute spinal cord injury in humans: incidence, time course and severity. *J Am Coll Cardiol.* 1987;10:46–52.

66. Frankel HL, Hancock DO, Hyslop G, et al. The value of postural reduction in the initial management of closed injuries of the spine with paraplegia and tetraplegia. *Paraplegia.* 1969;7:179–192.

67. Consortium for Spinal Cord Medicine, Paralyzed Veterans of America. *Prevention of Thromboembolism in Spinal Cord Injury.* Washington, DC: Consortium for Spinal Cord Medicine; 1997.

68. Green D, Lee MY, Lim AC, et al. Prevention of thromboembolism after spinal cord injury using low-molecular–weight heparin. *Ann Intern Med.* 1990;113:571–574.

69. Kulkarni JR, Burt AA, Tromans AT, Constable PD. Prophylactic low dose heparin anticoagulant therapy in patients with spinal cord injuries: a retrospective study. *Paraplegia*. 1992;30:169–172.

70. Weingarden SI, Weingarden DS, Belen J. Fever and thromboembolic disease in acute spinal cord injury. *Paraplegia*. 1988;26:35–42.

71. Colachis SC III. Autonomic hyperreflexia with spinal cord injury. *J Am Paraplegia Soc*. 1992;15:171–186.

72. Consortium for Spinal Cord Medicine, Paralyzed Veterans of America. *Acute Management of Autonomic Dysreflexia: Adults with Spinal Cord Injury Presenting to Health-Care Facilities*. Washington, DC: Consortium for Spinal Cord Medicine; 1997.

73. Eltorai I, Kim R, Vulpe M, Kasravi H, Ho W. Fatal cerebral hemorrhage due to autonomic dysreflexia in a tetraplegic patient: case report and review. *Paraplegia*. 1992;30:355–360.

74. Kursh ED, Freehafer A, Persky L. Complications of autonomic dysreflexia. *J Urol*. 1977;118:70–72.

75. Braddom RL, Rocco JF. Autonomic dysreflexia. A survey of current treatment. *Am J Phys Med Rehabil*. 1991;70:234–241.

76. Myers J, Lee M, Kiratli J. Cardiovascular disease in spinal cord injury: an overview of prevalence, risk, evaluation, and management. *Am J Phys Med Rehabil*. 2007;86:142–152.

77. Bauman WA, Spungen AM, Raza M, et al. Coronary artery disease: metabolic risk factors and latent disease in individuals with paraplegia. *Mt Sinai J Med*. 1992;59:163–168.

78. Yekutiel M, Brooks ME, Ohry A, Yarom J, Carel R. The prevalence of hypertension, ischemic heart disease and diabetes in traumatic spinal cord injured patients and amputees. *Paraplegia*. 1989;27:58–62.

79. Schluger S. *Periodontal Diseases: Basic Phenomena, Clinical Management, and Occlusal and Restorative Interrelationships*. Philadelphia, Pa: Lea & Febiger; 1990: 759.

80. Brady S, Miserendino R, Statkus D, Springer T, Hakel M, Stambolis V. Predictors to dysphagia and recovery after cervical spinal cord injury during acute rehabilitation. *J Appl Res*. 2004;4:1–11.

81. Katzka DA. Motility abnormalities in gastroesophageal reflux disease. *Gastroenterol Clin North Am*. 1999;28:905–915.

82. Stinneford JG, Keshavarzian, A, Nemchausky BA, Doria, MI, Durkin M. Esophagitis and esophageal motor abnormalities in patients with chronic spinal cord injuries. *Paraplegia*. 1993;31:384–392.

83. Fealey RD, Szurszewski JH, Merritt JL, DiMagno EP. Effect of traumatic spinal cord transection on human upper gastrointestinal motility and gastric emptying. *Gastroenterology*. 1984;89:69–75.

84. Stiens SA, Fajardo NR, Korsten MA. The gastrointestinal system after spinal cord injury. In: Lin VW, ed. *Spinal Cord Medicine: Principles and Practice*. New York, NY: Demos; 2003.

85. Albert TJ, Levine MJ, Balderston RA, Cotler JM. Gastrointestinal complications in spinal cord injury. *Spine*. 1991;16(Suppl10):522–525.

86. Kewalramani LS. Neurogenic gastroduodenal ulceration and bleeding associated with spinal cord injuries. *J Trauma*. 1979;19:259–265.

87. Roth EJ, Fenton LL, Gaebler-Spira DJ, Frost FS, Yarkony GM. Superior mesenteric artery syndrome in acute traumatic quadriplegia: case reports and literature review. *Arch Phys Med Rehabil*. 1991;72:417–420.

88. Carey ME, Nance FC, Kirgis HD, Young HF, Megison LC Jr, Kline DG. Pancreatitis following spinal cord injury. *J Neurosurg*. 1977;47:917–922.

89. Berlly MH, Wilmot CB. Acute abdominal emergencies during the first four weeks after spinal cord injury. *Arch Phys Med Rehabil*. 1984;65:687–690.

90. Apstein MD, Dalecki-Chipperfield K. Spinal cord injury is a risk factor for gallstone disease. *Gastroenterology.* 1987;92:966–968.

91. Nino-Murcia M, Burton D, Chang P, Stone J, Perkash I. Gallbladder contractility in patients with spinal cord injuries: a sonographic investigation. *AJR Am J Roentgenol.* 1990;154:521–524.

92. Moonka R, Stiens SA, Resnick WJ, et al. The prevalence and natural history of gallstones in spinal cord injured patients. *J Am Coll Surg.* 1999;189:274–281.

93. Tola VB, Chamberlain S, Kostyk SK, Soybel DI. Symptomatic gallstones in patients with spinal cord injury. *J Gastrointest Surg.* 2000;4:642–647.

94. Moonka R, Stiens SA, Eubank WB, Stelzner M. The presentation of gallstones and results of biliary surgery in a spinal cord injured population. *Am J Surg.* 1999;178:246–250.

95. Frost F. Gastrointestinal dysfunction in spinal cord injury. In: Yarkony G, ed. *Spinal Cord Injury: Medical Management and Rehabilitation.* Gaithersburg, Md: Aspen Publishers; 1994: 27–38.

96. Miller F, Fenzl TC. Prolonged ileus with acute spinal cord injury responding to metaclopramide. *Paraplegia.* 1981;19:43–45.

97. Stiens SA, Bergman SB, Goetz LL. Neurogenic bowel dysfunction after spinal cord injury: clinical evaluation and rehabilitation management. *Arch Phys Med Rehabil.* 1997;78:S86–102.

98. Glick ME, Meshkinpour H, Haldeman S, Hoehler F, Downey N, Bradley WE. Colonic dysfunction in patients with thoracic spinal cord injury. *Gastroenterology.* 1984;86:287–294.

99. Consortium for Spinal Cord Medicine, Paralyzed Veterans of America. *Neurogenic Bowel Management in Adults with Spinal Cord Injury.* Washington, DC: Consortium for Spinal Cord Medicine; 1998.

100. Stone JM, Wolfe VA, Nino-Murcia M, Perkash I. Colostomy as treatment for complications of spinal cord injury. *Arch Phys Med Rehabil.* 1990;71:514–518.

101. Bond W. Acute abdomen in spinal cord injured patients. In: Lee BY, Ostrander LE, Cochran GVB, Shaw WW, eds. *The Spinal Cord Injured Patient: Comprehensive Management.* Philadelphia, Pa: WB Saunders; 1991: 18–23.

102. Juler GL, Eltorai IM. The acute abdomen in spinal cord injury patients. *Paraplegia.* 1985;23:118–123.

103. Schmitt JK, Schroeder DL. Endocrine and metabolic consequences of spinal cord injuries. In: Lin VW, Cardenas DD, Cutter NC, et al, eds. *Spinal Cord Medicine: Principles and Practice.* New York, NY: Demos; 2002.

104. Nance PW, Schryvers O, Leslie W, Ludwig S, Krahn J, Uebelhart D. Intravenous pamidronate attenuates bone density loss after acute spinal cord injury. *Arch Phys Med Rehabil.* 1999;80:243–251.

105. Consortium for Spinal Cord Medicine, *Paralyzed Veterans of America. Pressure Ulcer Prevention and Treatment Following Spinal Cord Injury: a Clinical Practice Guideline for Health Care Professionals.* Washington, DC: Paralyzed Veterans of America; 2000.

106. Richards JS. Pressure ulcers in spinal cord injury: psychosocial correlates. *SCI Digest.* 1981;3:11–18.

107. Mawson AR, Biundo JJ Jr, Neville P, Linares HA, Winchester Y, Lopez A. Risk factors for early occurring pressure ulcers following spinal cord injury. *Am J Phys Med Rehabil.* 1988;67(3):123–127.

108. Young JS, Burns PE. Pressure sores and the spinal cord injured. *SCI Digest.* 1981;3:9–25.

109. Yarkony GM, Heinemann AW. Pressure ulcers. In: Stover SL, DeLisa JA, Whiteneck GG, eds. *Spinal Cord Injury: Clinical outcomes from the Model Systems.* Gaithersburg, Md: Aspen Publishing; 1995.

110. Edberg EL, Cerny K, Stauffer ES. Prevention and treatment of pressure sores. *Phys Ther*. 1973;53:246–252.

111. Knight AL. Medical management of pressure sores. *J Fam Pract*. 1988;27:95–100.

112. Braun JA, Silvetti A, Xakellis G. What really works for pressure sores? *Patient Care*. 1992;26:63–76.

113. Lamid S, El Ghatit AZ. Smoking, spasticity and pressure sores in spinal cord injured patients. *Am J Phys Med*. 1983;62:300–306.

114. Thiyagarajan C, Silver JR. Aetiology of pressure sores in patients with spinal cord injury. *Brit Med J (Clin Res Ed)*. 1984;289:1487–1490.

115. Woolsey RM. Rehabilitation outcome following spinal cord injury. *Arch Neurol*. 1985;42:116–121.

116. Garber SL. Wheelchair cushions for spinal cord-injured individuals. *Am J Occup Ther*. 1985;39:722–725.

117. National Pressure Ulcer Advisory Panel. Updated Staging System Web site. Available at: http://www.npuap.org/pr2.htm. Accessed September 12, 2008.

118. Ragnarsson KT, Sell GH. Lower extremity fractures after spinal cord injury: a retrospective study. *Arch Phys Med Rehabil*. 1981;62:418–423.

119. Garland DE, Steward CA, Adkins RH, et al. Osteoporosis after spinal cord injury. *J Orthop Res*. 1992;10:371–378.

120. Garland DE. A clinical perspective on common forms of acquired heterotopic ossification. *Clin Orthop Relat Res*. 1991;263:13–29.

121. Stover SL. Heterotopic ossification after spinal cord injury. In: Bloch RF, Basbaum M, eds. *Management of Spinal Cord Injuries*. Baltimore, Md: Williams & Wilkins; 1986: 284–302.

122. Banovac K, Gonzalez F. Evaluation and management of heterotopic ossification in patients with spinal cord injury. *Spinal Cord*. 1997;35:158–162.

123. Biering-Sørensen F, Tøndevold E. Indomethacin and disodium etidronate for the prevention of recurrence of heterotopic ossification after surgical resection. Two case reports. *Paraplegia*. 1993;31:513–515.

124. Little JW, Micklesen P, Umlauf R, Britell C. Lower extremity manifestations of spasticity in chronic spinal cord injury. *Am J Phys Med Rehabil*. 1989;68:32–36.

125. Jensen MP, Hoffman AJ, Cardenas DD. Chronic pain in individuals with spinal cord injury: a survey and longitudinal study. *Spinal Cord*. 2005;43:704–712.

126. Williams B. Post-traumatic syringomyelia, an update. *Paraplegia*. 1990;28:296–313.

127. Rossier AB, Foo D, Shillito J, Dyro FM. Posttraumatic cervical syringomyelia. Incidence, clinical presentation, electrophysiological studies, syrinx protein and results of conservative and operative treatment. *Brain*. 1985;108:439–461.

128. Gellman H, Sie I, Waters RL. Late complications of the weight-bearing upper extremity in the paraplegic patient. *Clin Orthop Relat Res*. 1988;233:132–135.

129. Fam B, Yalla SV. Vesicourethral dysfunction in spinal cord injury and its management. *Semin Neurol*. 1988;8:150–155.

130. Kaplan SA, Chancellor MB, Blaivas JG. Bladder and sphincter behavior in patients with spinal cord lesions. *J Urol*. 1991;146:113–117.

131. Perkash I. Pressor response during cystomanometry in spinal injury patients complicated with detrusor-sphincter dyssynergia. *J Urol*. 1979;121:778–782.

132. Wyndaele JJ. Urethral sphincter dyssynergia in spinal injury patients. *Paraplegia*. 1987;25:10–15.

133. Yalla SV, Blunt KJ, Fam BA, Constantinople NL, Gittes RF. Detrusor-urethral sphincter dyssynergia. *J Urol*. 1977;118: 1026–1029.

134. Tempkin A, Sullivan G, Paldi J, Perkash I. Radioisotope renography in spinal cord injury. *J Urol*. 1985;133:228–230.

135. Schurch B, Stöhrer M, Kramer G, Schmid DM, Gaul G, Hauri D. Botulinum-A toxin for treating detrusor hyperreflexia in spinal cord injured patients: a new alternative to anticholinergic drugs? Preliminary results. *J Urol*. 2000;164:692–697.

136. Consortium for Spinal Cord Medicine, Paralyzed Veterans of America. *Bladder Management for Adults with Spinal Cord Injury: a Clinical Practice Guideline for Health-Care Professionals*. Washington, DC: Paralyzed Veterans of America; 2006.

137. Lloyd LK. New trends in urologic management of spinal cord injured patients. *Cent Nerv Syst Trauma*. 1986;3:3–12.

138. Sanderson PJ, Rawal P. Contamination of the environment of spinal cord injured patients by organisms causing urinary-tract infection. *J Hosp Infect*. 1987;10:173–178.

139. Bickel A, Culkin DJ, Wheeler JS Jr. Bladder cancer in spinal cord injury patients. *J Urol*. 1991;146:1240–1242.

140. Jackson AB, Wadley V. A multicenter study of women's self-reported reproductive health after spinal cord injury. *Arch Phys Med Rehabil*. 1999;80:1420–1428.

141. Davidoff GN, Roth EJ, Richards JS. Cognitive deficits in spinal cord injury: epidemiology and outcome. *Arch Phys Med Rehabil*. 1992;73:275–284.

142. Richards JS, Brown L, Hagglund K, Bua G, Reeder K. Spinal cord injury and concomitant traumatic brain injury. Results of a longitudinal investigation. *Am J Phys Med Rehabil*. 1988;67:211–216.

143. Roth E, Davidoff G, Thomas P, et al. A controlled study of neuropsychological deficits in acute spinal cord injury patients. *Paraplegia*. 1989;27:480–489.

144. DeVivo MJ, Black KJ, Richards JS, Stover SL. Suicide following spinal cord injury. *Paraplegia*. 1991;29:620–627.

Chapter 17

PHYSICAL THERAPY FOR THE POLYTRAUMA CASUALTY WITH LIMB LOSS

ROBERT S. GAILEY, PhD, PT[*]; BARBARA A. SPRINGER, PhD, PT, OCS, SCS[†]; AND MATTHEW SCHERER, PT, MPT, NCS[‡]

[*]Director, Functional Outcomes Research and Evaluation Laboratory, Miami Veterans Affairs Healthcare System, 1201 NW 16th Street, Miami, Florida 33125 and Associate Professor, Department of Physical Therapy, University of Miami Miller School of Medicine, 5915 Ponce de Leon Boulevard, Plumer Building, Coral Gables, Florida 33146
[†]Colonel, Medical Specialist Corps, US Army; Director, Propency Office for Rehabilitation & Reintegration, Office of The Surgeon General, Falls Church, Virginia 22041; formerly, Chief, Integrated Physical Therapy Service, National Naval Medical Center, 8901 Rockville Pike, Bethesda, Maryland and Walter Reed Army Medical Center, 6900 Georgia Avenue, NW, Washington, DC
[‡]Captain, Medical Specialist Corps, US Army; Doctoral Student, Department of Rehabilitation Science, University of Maryland at Baltimore, 111 South Greene Street, Baltimore, Maryland 21212; formerly, Amputee Physical Therapy Section Chief, Physical Therapy Service, Department of Orthopaedics and Rehabilitation, Walter Reed Army Medical Center, 6900 Georgia Avenue, NW, Washington, DC

INTRODUCTION

Service members (SMs) that are wounded during active duty often present with multiple injuries. Some of the most devastating wounds can result in the loss of one or more limbs in addition to concomitant injuries. Care of the injured SM is a complex process that requires a team effort that begins at the time of injury continuing throughout all stages of care including postsurgical rehabilitation and frequently persists after discharge. Physical therapists and physical therapy assistants have a central role in ensuring that these SMs with limb loss achieve the maximum possible level of functional ability permitting them to resume their recreational and occupational goals.

SMs who sustain traumatic amputations are generally young and otherwise healthy. They were very active up to the moment of injury, and then suddenly their lives were dramatically changed. As devastating as their wounds may be, they do not want to stop living active and productive lives that include work, sports, and recreational activities. Because of the SMs' pursuit of highly physical activities they are often referred to as "tactical athletes." Therefore, the main focus of rehabilitation in this patient population is application of the orthopaedic sports medicine model to return wounded SMs to optimal levels of physical function. This chapter will present the US military's four-phase program of functional progressive rehabilitation for SMs with lower limb loss.

Rehabilitation should begin as soon after the amputation(s) as possible. Following a comprehensive physical evaluation the physical therapists and physical therapy assistants progress those amputees through the four-phase rehabilitation program:

(1) initial management,
(2) preprosthetic,
(3) prosthetic/ambulation, and
(4) progressive activities/return to active duty.

Individual progression through these phases is a fluid process and will depend on tissue healing, surgical procedures, complications, and individual functional readiness. Patients who undergo further surgery, for example, will return to the earlier phases of rehabilitation. (For an in-depth outline of the Military Amputee Rehabilitation Protocol see attachment at the end of this chapter.) Functional outcome measures are administered at regular intervals to determine and document rehabilitation progress toward short- and long-term goals.

The physical therapist's role in prosthetic training is 3-fold. First, the amputee must be physically prepared for prosthetic gait training and educated about residual limb care before being fitted with the prosthesis. Second, the amputee must learn how to use and care for the prosthesis. Prosthetic gait training can be the most frustrating, yet rewarding phase of rehabilitation for all involved. The amputee must be reeducated in the biomechanics of gait while learning how to use a prosthesis. Once success is achieved, the amputee may look forward to resuming a productive life. Third, the therapist should introduce the amputee to higher levels of activities beyond learning to walk. The amputee may not be ready to participate in sport and recreational activities immediately; however, this is an anticipated goal within the military program. The current rehabilitation program includes higher level training as a standard and most, if not all amputees, are expected to participate as their injuries permit. For those amputees that may receive early discharge, contact information for support and disabled recreational organizations should be provided so they can participate when ready.

Physical Therapy Evaluation

The initial physical therapy evaluation is typically performed at bedside to assess mobility, strength, range of motion, and pain. Amputees with polytrauma will present with secondary injuries other than limb loss that will be evaluated and considered as the rehabilitation plan is prepared.

Physical and occupational therapists can work together with acute patients to eliminate redundancy in the evaluation and cotreatment of mobility and activities of daily living (ADLs). Many ADLs can be evaluated and practiced during occupational therapy and physical therapy evaluations. For example, physical therapists can assess mobility, range of motion, and balance as occupational therapists evaluate and teach dressing activities. Adaptive clothing with tear-away access is helpful to have during an occupational therapist's assessment and to protect patients' modesty as they venture from their room. Every opportunity should be taken to encourage early supervised transfer training with a wheelchair provided when appropriate to allow mobility off the ward and enhance independence. Transfers and wheelchair training activities are examples of early mobility training. The initial evaluation can also be an opportunity to educate the patient and family members about the goals and course of rehabilitation and to develop initial rapport. SMs wounded in the global war on terror will consider their future plans but should be assured that every feasible opportunity will be made available to them if their goal is to remain on active duty. The wounded SM's goals, which largely determine the long-term rehabilitation plan of care, are important to update as he or she progresses through rehabilitation.

Bedside Management

Generally, the goals of postoperative treatment for the new amputee are to reduce edema, promote healing, prevent loss of motion, increase cardiovascular endurance, and improve strength. Functional skills must also be introduced as early as possible to promote independence in bed mobility, transfers, and ambulation. Further independence and prevention of complications may be addressed with education in the self-care of the residual limb and intact limbs. Moreover, each rehabilitation team member should be aware of the need to assist the patient with the psychological adjustment to limb loss.

PHASE I. INITIAL MANAGEMENT PHASE

The protective healing phase is the first phase of amputee rehabilitation that corresponds with the acute inpatient stay and on average ranges from 1 to 2 weeks depending on the severity and complexity of injury. Patient management strategies for the interdisciplinary team during the first phase include surgical management often with repeated irrigation and debridement of concomitant residual limb(s), wounds, or management of other comorbid conditions. Rehabilitation providers concurrently work together to promote early functional skills, provide patient and family member education, and initiate early conditioning activities as tolerated by the patient.

Functional Activities

Bed Mobility

The importance of good bed mobility extends beyond simple positional adjustments for comfort or to get in and out of bed. The patient must acquire bed mobility skills to maintain correct bed positioning to prevent contractures or excessive friction of the sheets against the suture line(s), scar tissue, or frail skin secondary to burns and other surface wounds. If the patient is unable to perform the skills necessary to maintain proper positioning, then assistance must be provided. Promoting independence as soon as possible is always encouraged because adequate bed mobility is a basic skill required for bed to wheelchair transfers. Independent transfer to a wheelchair is the first step in providing a sense of freedom from the hospital bed and allows the patient to begin moving freely throughout the rehabilitation ward and interact with fellow amputees.

Transfers

Transfer ability is essential during early assessment especially when the rehabilitation team is determining discharge planning from the acute care setting. Independence or limited assistance with transfers makes it possible for the amputee to gain independence quickly and develop a sense of belonging with peers during rehabilitation.

Once bed mobility is mastered, the patient must learn to transfer from the bed to a chair or a wheelchair and then progress to more advanced transfer skills such as toilet, tub, and car transfers. In cases where an immediate postoperative or temporary prosthesis is utilized, weight bearing through the prosthesis can assist the patient in the transfer and provide additional safety. For transtibial amputees who are not ambulatory candidates, a light-weight transfer prosthesis may facilitate more independent transfers. This prosthesis is typically fit when the residual limb is healed and the patient is ready for training. Bilateral amputees that are not fitted with an initial prosthesis transfer in a "head on" manner where the patient slides forward from the wheelchair onto the desired surface by lifting the body and pushing forward with both hands.

Wheelchair Management

The primary means of mobility during early rehabilitation for the majority of amputees will be the wheelchair. Therefore, wheelchair skills should be taught as a part of the early rehabilitation program. Bilateral amputees with complex injuries may require greater use of the wheelchair, while unilateral amputees will be more likely to choose other assistive devices when not ambulating with their prosthesis. Because of the loss of body weight anteriorly when sitting, the bilateral amputee will be prone to tipping backward during propulsion with a standard wheelchair. Amputee adapters set the axle approximately 5 centimeters back, thus moving the center of mass posteriorly to prevent tipping, especially when ascending ramps or curbs. However, this strategy may limit mobility of active wheelchair users by making propulsion less efficient. An alternative method to prevent tipping would be the addition of anti-tippers (simple devices attached to the back of the wheelchair that prevent it from accidentally tipping over backward) in place of or in addition to the amputee wheel adapters. Transtibial amputees will also require an elevating leg rest or residual limb board designed to maintain the knee in extension, thus preventing prolonged knee flexion and reducing the dependent position of the limb to control edema. Finally, it is recommended that the wheelchair be fitted with removable armrests to enable ease of transfer to or from either side of the chair.

Flexibility

Range of Motion

Prevention of decreased range of motion (ROM) and contractures is a major concern. The best way to prevent loss of ROM is to remain active and ensure full available ROM of affected joints. Unfortunately, not all amputees have this option, and therefore proper limb positioning as previously described must be maintained, especially during the 6 months after amputation. A functional assessment of gross upper limb and sound lower limb motions should be made. A measurement of the residual limb's ROM should be recorded for future reference.

Contracture Prevention/Positioning

Contractures are a complication that can greatly hinder the amputee's ability to ambulate efficiently with a prosthesis; thus extra care should be made to avoid this situation. The most common contractured position for the transfemoral amputee is hip flexion, external rotation, and abduction, and knee flexion is the most frequently seen contracture in the transtibial amputee. During ROM assessment the therapist should determine whether the patient has a fixed contracture or just muscle tightness from immobility that can be corrected with stretching in the near term.

To reduce the risk of contractures, the transfemoral amputee, when in a supine position, should place a pillow laterally along the residual limb to maintain neutral rotation with no abduction. If the prone position is tolerable during the day or evening, then a pillow is placed under the residual limb to maintain hip extension. Transtibial amputees should avoid knee flexion for prolonged periods when sitting or reclining. A stump board will help maintain knee extension when using a wheelchair.

Strengthening

Strength of the major muscle groups should be assessed by manual muscle testing of all limbs including the residual limb and the trunk core stabilizers.

Adequate muscle strength will help the patient's functional skill level when performing activities such as transfers, wheelchair management, and ambulation with and without the prosthesis.

Therapeutic Exercise (Bedside and/or Mat)

Lower limb strengthening is imperative to prepare the legs for prosthetic gait training and mitigate the effects of potentially prolonged periods of nonweight bearing secondary to healing of the residual limb(s). Therapeutic exercise progresses from early isometric and active exercise to progressive resistive strengthening and closed kinetic chain (CKC) exercises. During Phase I, specific surgical techniques and healing requirements may dictate the selection of strengthening methods. For example, isometric strengthening may be selected for longer durations where a myodesis was performed and adherence to the bone is required. If there are fewer surgical restrictions, patients may be progressed from isometric strengthening to open kinetic chain and CKC exercises as strength increases permit. Table 17-1 contains a list of early postoperative rehabilitation guidelines. All times annotated are from date of final closure (skin closure with sutures).

Core Stabilization

As soon as bed or mat exercises can be tolerated, the patient with amputation(s) learns the basics of core (lumbopelvic) stabilization, which focuses on intervertebral control, lumbopelvic orientation, and whole body equilibrium, via strengthening of the transversus abdominis and multifidus muscles.[1]

Strengthening this core musculature may minimize or prevent the negative effects following lower limb amputation (eg, low back pain, gait dysfunction, and functional impairments).[2–9] Theoretically, core strengthening can enhance transfer activities, balance, and ambulation because it has been used in athletic and therapeutic settings to enhance neuromuscular pathways, strength, proprioception, and balance and aids in coordination of synergistic and stabilizer muscles.[10–12] Additionally, it has been shown to improve athletic performance and prevent low back pain.[13–15] The transversus abdominis, which is the deepest abdominal muscle, is believed to be a key stabilizer of the lumbopelvic region. It is a thin muscle running horizontally around the abdomen, attaching to the transverse processes of the lumbar vertebrae via the thoracolumbar fascia.[16] The muscle orientation is hoop-like and, when contracted, creates a rigid cylinder resulting in enhanced stiffness of the lumbar spine that creates lateral tension

TABLE 17-1

EARLY POSTOPERATIVE REHABILITATION GUIDELINES

Level(s)	Postoperative Dressing	Weight-bearing Guidelines	Surgical Considerations	Therapeutic Exercise Guidelines
Partial Foot	Fit with shrinker as soon as possible upon removal of sutures or when cleared by orthopaedic surgeon.	Heel pad weight bearing allowed when cleared by orthopaedic surgeon.	N/A	CKC rehabilitation to tolerance.
Symes	Patients casted for 2 to 3 weeks to permit stabilization of heel pad.	NWB for additional 3 weeks after the cast is removed for a total of 5 weeks NWB.	Heel pad and Achilles tendon sutured to tibia.	CKC exercises are appropriate once casted (however, no distal end bearing in cast). Expect delayed prosthetic fitting.
Transtibial	Dressing, figure 8 wrapping. Shrinker sock when sutures are removed.	NWB at distal limb near suture line until sutures removed and cleared by orthopaedic surgeon.	If myodesis is tenuous, the patient may be casted in knee flexion.	Mat CKC exercise may begin immediately if stabilization point on bolster is proximal to the myodesis. Hamstring stretching is restricted for 2 weeks in patients with tenuous myodesis. No other exercise restrictions.
Knee Disarticulation	Postoperative dressing per protocol.	NWB at distal limb near suture line until sutures removed and cleared by orthopaedic surgeon.	Patellar tendon is sutured into the ACL during surgery.	Straight leg raise is restricted to no weights for 2 weeks after surgery. No restrictions thereafter. No restrictions to abduction or adduction movement.
Transfemoral	Hip spica configuration for wrapping with progression to shrinker socks when cleared by the orthopaedic surgeon.	NWB at distal limb near suture line until sutures removed and cleared by the orthopaedic surgeon.	Myodesis of adductor magnus tendon is secured to the lateral femur during surgery.	No active adduction strengthening exercises for 4 weeks. No active abduction strengthening past neutral for 2 weeks (abduction to neutral from adducted posture with supervision). No hip flexion for 2 weeks s/p myodesis to protect distal insertion. Bridging in supine is permitted when performed with bolster under the distal residual limb.
Hip Disarticulation	Hip spica configuration for wrapping. Shrinkers may be ordered to capture hip and provide compression.	Patient may weight bear as tolerated at suture site (ie, sitting) unless restricted for other comorbidity (eg, pelvic or acetabular fractures).	No muscle attachments stressed with end bearing/ sitting on the hip disarticulation.	No exercise restrictions once wound healing complete for end bearing.

ACL: anterior cruciate ligament
CKC: closed kinetic chain

NWB: nonweight bearing
s/p: status post

through the transverse processes.[16,17] Bilateral contraction of the transversus abdominis can contribute to lumbopelvic control by tensioning the fascial structures of the lumbar region via intra-abdominal pressure.[18–20] This helps limit translational and rotational movements in the lumbar spine for which transfemoral and hip disarticulation amputees are extremely vulnerable. The other key deep core stabilizer is the multifidus, which is the largest and most medial of the lumbar muscles.[21] This muscle co-contracts with the transversus abdominis via the thoracolumbar fascia and its functions are to reduce anterior shear force, stabilize the trunk, and act as a primary trunk extensor.[22]

The goals of core stabilization are to control, prevent, or eliminate low back pain; increase patient education and kinesthetic awareness; increase strength, flexibility, coordination, balance, and endurance; and develop strong trunk musculature to enhance upper and lower limb functional activities.

Co-contraction of these deep muscles for core stabilization is a difficult task to learn. Education and training are essential to achieving core stability. Illustrations of the specific muscles and explanations of the exercises are provided to the amputees before practice. Once visualization is established patients are taught how to maintain a neutral spine (the position of most comfort) and how to correctly "draw in" or correctly contract the muscles of the lower abdominal region. Usually this is first attempted in the "hooklying" position, but may need to be taught in the quadruped position using gravity for stretch reflex assistance. It is also important to explain that these muscles are predominantly type 1 muscle fibers providing the longer endurance-type contractions that are important for proper posture. Following instruction and practice, rehabilitative ul-

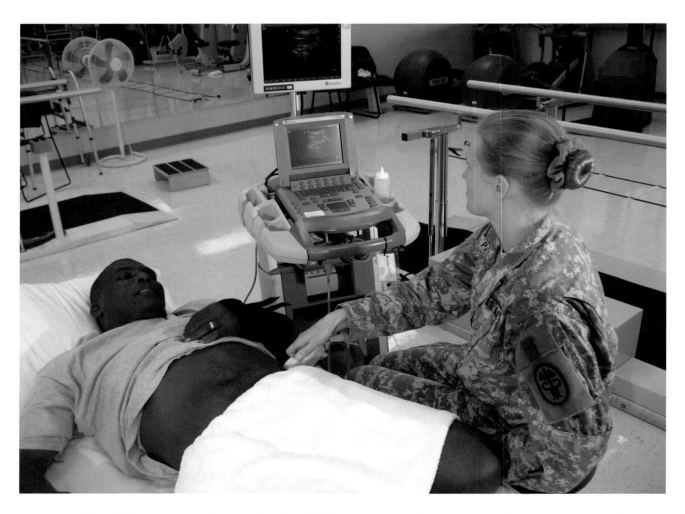

Figure 17-1. Elizabeth Painter uses ultrasound to identify the transverse abdominis muscle of Gregory Gadson and provide visual feedback for muscle reeducation.

trasound imaging may be utilized to provide further biofeedback and record direct outcome measures of the resting and contracted size of the transversus abdominis as illustrated in Figure 17-1.

Once the basics of neutral spine and proper muscle contraction are learned, amputees will perform a basic core stabilization exercise program. Throughout the training program patients must be reminded to maintain neutral spine, "draw in," or contract the lower abdomen, and gradually increase time spent performing the exercise. Examples of early/level-1 exercises include the following:

- Hooklying: raising hands over head, alternating hands to knees(s), bridging with one leg, crunches, and leg circles;

- Prone: one arm, one leg, alternate arm, and leg lifts;
- Quadruped (if able): one arm, one leg, or alternate arm and leg lifts; and
- Sitting: arms overhead, one leg out, alternate hands to knee.

Advancement occurs by progressing from stable to unstable surfaces (ball, disc), large simple to smaller more complex movements, one plane of movement to multiple/combined planes, short lever arm to longer lever arm, no weights to weights, and slow to fast speed. It is important to maintain the neutral spine during the exercise. Figure 17-2 shows examples of advancing a bilateral transfemoral amputee through a prone back extension progression on a variety of surfaces.

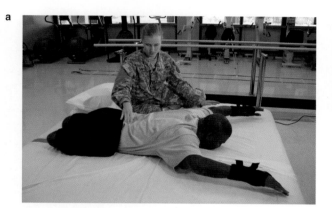
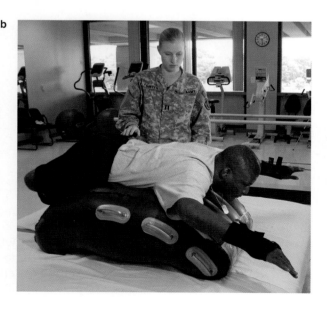
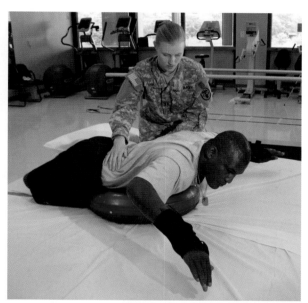
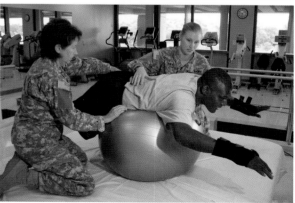

Figure 17-2. (a–d) Elizabeth Painter and Barbara Springer assist Gregory Gadson, a bilateral transfemoral amputee, with exercises to advance through a prone back extension progression on a variety of surfaces.

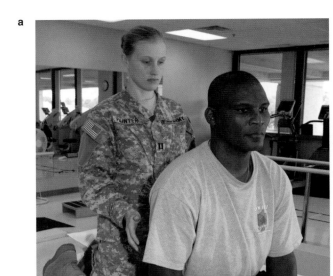

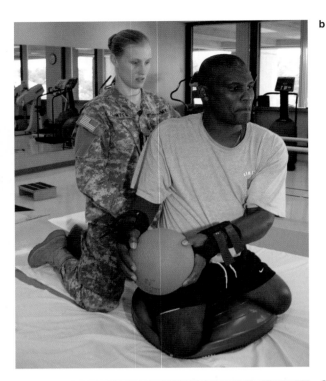

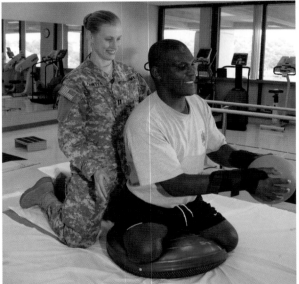

Figure 17-3. (a–c) Elizabeth Painter assists Gregory Gadson, a bilateral transfemoral amputee, with sitting balance training.

Cardiovascular Endurance

Aerobic training typically begins immediately after surgery while increasing sitting tolerance and early ambulation. However, specific attention to improving aerobic fitness should be incorporated into the rehabilitation program and remain as a part of the amputee's general fitness long after discharge. Bedside calisthenics are an excellent form of exercise when transfers to the rehabilitation gym are limited. Educating family members to assist with simple movement exercises is always suggested to help engage them into the amputee's early recovery and introduce the need to reduce the number of sedentary hours each day. The three most beneficial exercises are the (1) upper body ergometer (UBE), (2) lower body ergometer, and (3) the treadmill.

Initially, the UBE can be introduced and safely performed with most people.[23–25] The UBE, which has been shown to quickly elevate the heart rate and is also good early conditioning for hand crank cycling, has become popular in the young, active, athletic, and competitive traumatic amputee population.[26,27] Once balance and strength return, lower body ergometry may be per-

formed at first with only the sound limb progressing to use of the prosthetic limb when appropriate. Over time and when the level of fitness improves other equipment may be used such as treadmills, stair climbing machines, and rowing machines. Amputees can enjoy the same activities as the nonamputee population. As a result, swimming and walking are still the ideal exercises for general fitness regardless of age or athletic ability.[28]

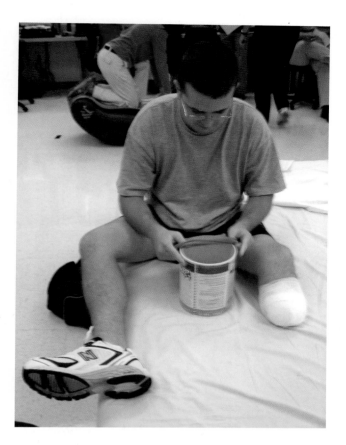

Figure 17-4. Andrew Forney, a transfemoral amputee, prepares the shrinker sock over the donning tube.

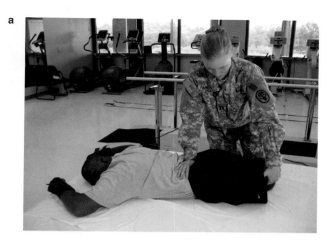

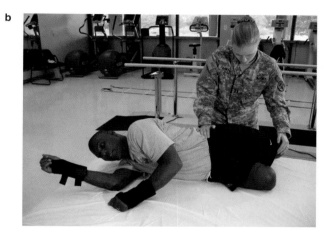

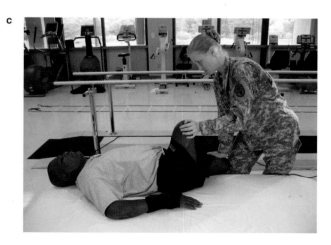

Figure 17-6. Elizabeth Painter assists Gregory Gadson, a bilateral transfemoral amputee, as he stretches the hip while maintaining a neutral spine for increasing or maintaining range of motion for the (**a**) hip flexors prone, (**b**) hip flexors side lying, and (**c**) hip extensors.

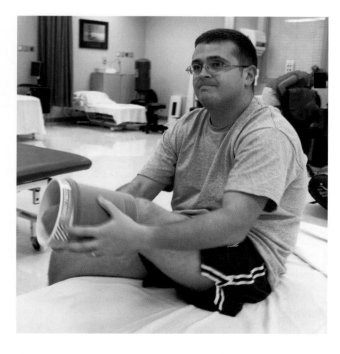

Figure 17-5. Andrew Forney dons a shrinker sock with a donning tube.

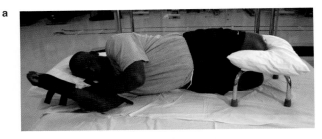
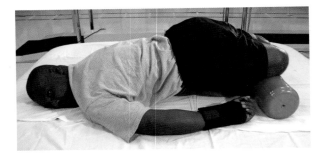
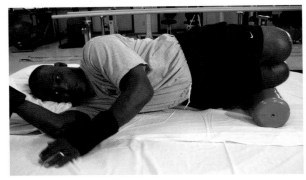
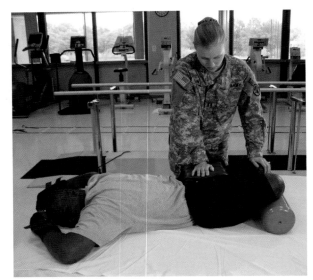

Figure 17-7. Elizabeth Painter assists Gregory Gadson, a bilateral transfemoral amputee, as he performs dynamic stump exercises that are designed to strengthen (**a**) hip adductors, (**b**) hip abductors, (**c**) hip flexors against gravity, and (**d**) hip flexors against manual resistance.

Balance

After the loss of a limb, the decrease in body weight will alter the body's center of mass (COM). Sitting balance is practiced first and then progressed to single limb balance. To maintain the single limb balance necessary during stance without a prosthesis, ambulating with an assistive device, or single limb hopping, the amputee must shift the COM over the base of support (BOS), which in this case is the foot of the sound limb. As amputees become more secure in their single limb support, there is greater difficulty in reorienting the amputee to maintaining the COM over both the sound and prosthetic limbs.[29] Ultimately, amputees must learn to maintain the COM and their entire body weight over the prosthesis. Once comfortable with weight bearing equally on both limbs, the amputee can begin to develop confidence with independent standing and eventually with ambulation.

Sitting Balance

Sitting balance is instrumental for providing the stability required for standing and ambulation. Often the time spent in bed and sitting in a chair can contribute to the deconditioning of the trunk and pelvic muscula-

ture. The early rehabilitation period is an excellent time to introduce core stability strengthening exercises and to educate the amputee on the importance of maintaining the strength of the trunk and pelvic musculature often referred to as the core stabilizers. Many of these exercises can be performed in the supine, prone, and sitting positions and when properly prescribed can prove to be extremely challenging and beneficial for even the strongest of amputees. A well-constructed exercise program can provide a foundation of strength and stability that will ease the transition from sitting to standing and walking and create a positive rehabilitation experience. An example of sitting balance training for a bilateral transfemoral amputee is shown in Figure 17-3.

Single Leg Balance

In preparation for ambulation without a prosthesis all amputees must learn to compensate for the loss of weight of the amputated limb by balancing the COM over the sound limb. Although this habit must be broken when learning prosthetic ambulation, single limb balance must be learned initially to provide confidence

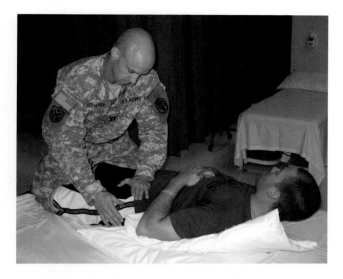

Figure 17-8. Matthew Scherer performs a semisupine resisted pelvic rotation drill on Joshua Bleill.

during stand pivot transfers, ambulation with assistive devices, and eventually hopping, depending on the amputee's skill level.[30]

Ambulation with Assistive Devices

All single limb amputees will need an assistive device when they choose not to wear a prosthesis or on occasions when they are unable to wear a prosthesis due to edema, skin irritation, or a poor prosthetic fit. Bilateral transfemoral amputees usually require some form of an assistive device while ambulating with their prostheses.

Ambulate in Parallel Bars

Safety is the primary factor when selecting the appropriate assistive device; however, mobility is a secondary consideration that cannot be overlooked. As a result, initial ambulation training without prosthesis should begin early within the parallel bars. This provides the security of sturdy support while learning the prescribed gait pattern and simultaneously allows the therapist to evaluate the amputee's ambulation potential.

Ambulate with Assistive Devices

The criteria for selection in the early phases and throughout rehabilitation should include the following:

- the ability for unsupported standing balance,
- the degree of upper limb strength,

- coordination and skill with the assistive device, and
- cognition.[31]

A walker is chosen when an amputee has fair to poor balance, strength, and coordination. If balance and strength are good to normal, Lofstrand (Canadian) or regular crutches may be used for ambulation with or without a prosthesis. A cane may be selected to ensure safety when balance is questionable while ambulating with a prosthesis.

A traditional evaluation of the amputee's potential for ambulation includes the following:

- strength of the sound lower limb and both upper limbs,
- single limb balance,
- coordination, and
- mental status.

The selection of an assistive device should meet with the amputee's level of skill, considering that with time the assistive device may change. For example, initially an individual may require a walker during early healing, especially if balance is altered from traumatic brain injury (TBI), but with proper training Lofstrand crutches may prove more beneficial within a short period of rehabilitation and as a long-term assistive device.

Teaching the amputee to negotiate uneven terrain, ramps, curbs, and stairs with assistive devices early in the rehabilitation process is essential. As mobility increases, the freedom and opportunity to independently travel throughout the rehabilitation center and into the community also increases. Often the amputee

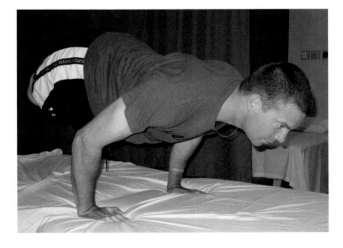

Figure 17-9. Joshua Bleill, a bilateral transfemoral amputee, performs unsupported push-ups.

a

b

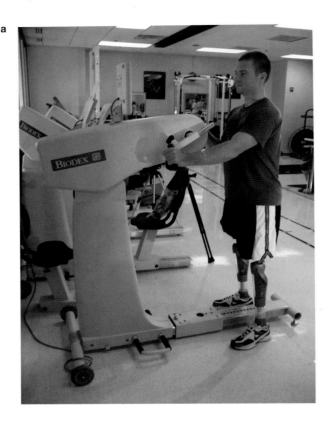
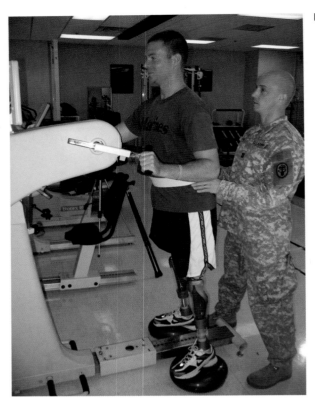

Figure 17-10. Joshua Bleill, a bilateral transfemoral amputee, performs upper limb ergometry on a (**a**) compliant surface and a (**b**) noncompliant surface assisted by Matthew Scherer.

embraces this ability to demonstrate the beginning levels of independence and the ability to spend time with family members and friends away from the hospital environment during weekly community outings.

Patient and Family Education

Compression Dressing

Management of edema and postoperative swelling is critical to an amputee's rehabilitation progression. There are numerous methods for controlling edema and avoiding skin compromise of the residual limb. Early rigid dressings, semirigid dressings, compression wrapping, or the use of shrinker garments for the residual limb can have several positive effects. They can (*a*) decrease edema, (*b*) increase circulation, (*c*) assist in shaping, (*d*) provide skin protection, (*e*) reduce redundant tissue problems, (*f*) reduce phantom limb pain/sensation, and (*g*) desensitize the residual limb. Rigid dressings with transtibial amputees casted in extension will prevent knee flexion contractures and aid in greater confidence with early bed mobility.[32] In the case of transfemoral residual limbs, there may be some value in counteracting contracture forces

with specific compression wrapping techniques.

Controversy does exist around the use of traditional compression wrapping versus the use of stump shrinker socks. Currently, many institutions prefer commercial shrinkers for their ease of donning. Advocates of compression wrapping state that they provide more control over pressure gradients and tissue shaping.[33] The use of a shrinker sock within 10 days after amputation has been found to be an equally and potentially more effective means to reduce time from amputation to prosthetic casting from those amputees using wrapping methods.[34] Likewise, even shorter time to prosthetic casting has been observed with transtibial amputees receiving semirigid and rigid dressings.[33,34] Compression therapy can begin with wraps or rigid dressings and progress to shrinkers after the suture line has healed.

Because this is a controversial area, each rehabilitation team should determine the best course for their respective clients and utilize a consistent method among team members. All compression techniques must be performed correctly and in a consistent manner to prevent (*a*) circulation constriction, (*b*) poor residual limb shaping, and (*c*) edema. Likewise, compliance is considered to be an intricate part of the compression

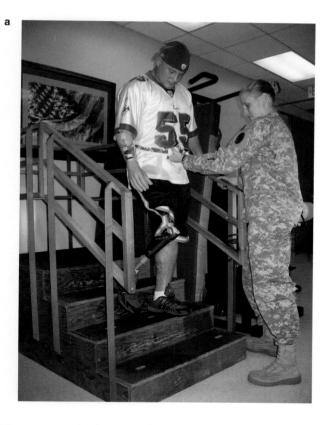

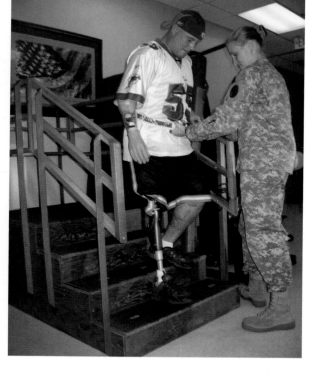

Figure 17-11. (a–c) Elizabeth Painter assists Luke Shirley, a unilateral transfemoral amputee, with descending stairs step-over-step.

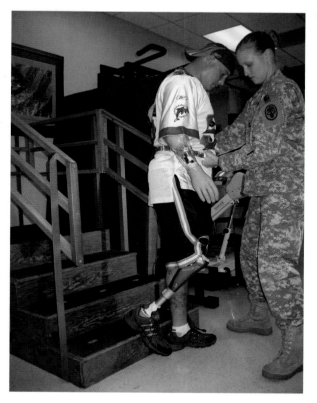

program. All methods of wrapping or shrinker sock use should be routinely checked or reapplied several times per day. A transfemoral amputee preparing the shrinker sock over the donning tube is shown in Figure 17-4. Figure 17-5 illustrates the donning of a shrinker sock with a donning tube.

Goals for Progression to Phase II

Patient and provider goals for the first phase of rehabilitation include but are not limited to the following:

- achieve independent bed mobility (turning over and sitting up),
- acquire the ability to correctly contract transversus abdominis and perform level-1 exercises for at least 3 minutes,
- maintain independent sitting balance for at least 1 minute,
- prevent contractures and other complications, and
- perform at least 10 minutes of cardiovascular exercise.

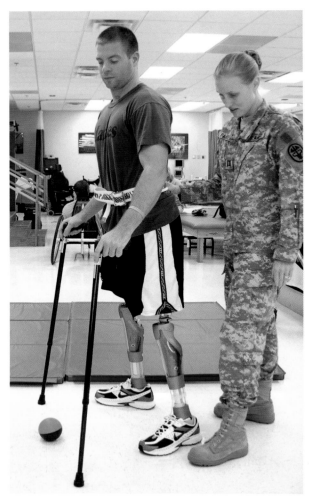
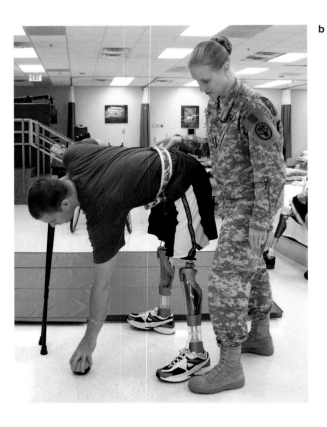
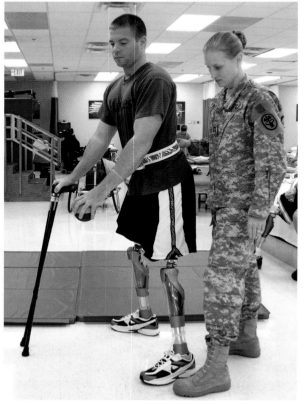

Figure 17-12. (**a–c**) Elizabeth Painter assists as Joshua Bleill, a bilateral transfemoral amputee, picks an object off the floor using cane support.

PHASE II. PREPROSTHETIC PHASE

The preprosthetic phase is the second phase of amputee rehabilitation and typically begins when the patient is discharged to an outpatient status and is characterized by independence with mobility and ADLs. The patient has usually undergone final closure of the residual limb(s) and prosthetic casting pending the removal of sutures.

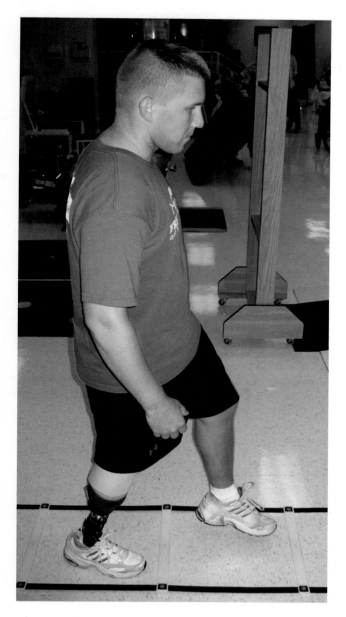

Figure 17-13. Christopher Millward, a transtibial amputee, performs ladder walking drills.

Functional Activities

Encouraging community reintegration activities as soon as possible after amputation surgery helps speed recovery in several ways. First, it will offset the negative effects of immobility by promoting movement through the joints, muscle activity, and increased circulation. Second, the amputee may begin to reestablish his or her independence, which may be perceived as threatened because of the loss of limb. Third, the psychological advantage derived from activity and independence will impact the amputee's motivation throughout rehabilitation.

Flexibility

Amputees who have already lost ROM may benefit from many of the traditional therapy procedures such as passive ROM, active ROM, contract-relax stretching, soft tissue mobilization, myofascial techniques, joint mobilization, and other methods that promote increased ROM. Daily ROM and stretching exercises should be performed at the beginning of each rehabilitation session so that the routine is developed and carried over after discharge. Few differences exist between stretching activities for lower limb amputees and those stretches prescribed to nonamputees. The shorter residual limb—especially with transfemoral amputees—allows the amputee to hold the limb and move into the stretch position. Handling of the residual limb also can help to desensitize the limb while maintaining joint motion.[35]

Hip flexor tightness must be addressed aggressively with bilateral transfemoral amputees to minimize restriction of hip extension. A sustained stretching program coupled with the core strengthening exercises described previously will help maintain a neutral pelvis. Figure 17-6 shows examples of stretching a bilateral transfemoral amputee's hip while maintaining a neutral spine.

Strengthening

Dynamic Stump Exercises

Dynamic stump exercises only require a towel roll and step stool.[29,36] These exercises offer additional benefits aside from strengthening, such as desensitization, improving bed mobility, and maintaining joint ROM. While lying on an exercise mat the patient is asked to depress the residual limb into the towel roll by raising his or her pelvis off the surface for 10 seconds. The

four postural positions that strengthen the hip musculature include (1) prone for the hip extensors, (2) side
lying for hip abductors, (3) side lying opposite side
for adductors, and (4) supine for hip flexor muscles.
As strength improves, resistance can be increased by
placing cuff weights over the patient's hip or have
him or her wear a weighted vest.[35] Figure 17-7 shows
examples of dynamic stump exercises for a bilateral
transfemoral amputee.

Patients with transtibial limb loss can initially
perform short arc quad exercises with or without the
addition of resistance such as a cuff weight. Other
exercises for the hip and knee musculature include
performing a straight leg raise in prone, supine, and
side-lying positions. Again, as strength improves
a cuff weight can be used to increase resistance.
Implementation of CKC strengthening for the prosthetic side limb musculature can be difficult before
receiving a prosthesis. Electrical stimulation can be
used to enhance quadriceps muscle reeducation and
recruitment.

As the amputee progresses, strengthening must be
performed in multiple planes of motion. For example,

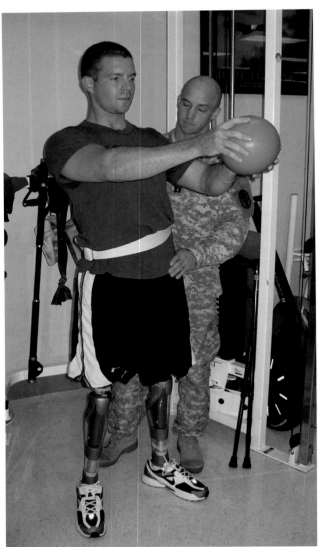

Figure 17-15. Joshua Bleill, a bilateral transfemoral amputee,
performs weighted ball swings to promote standing dynamic
balance assisted by Matthew Scherer.

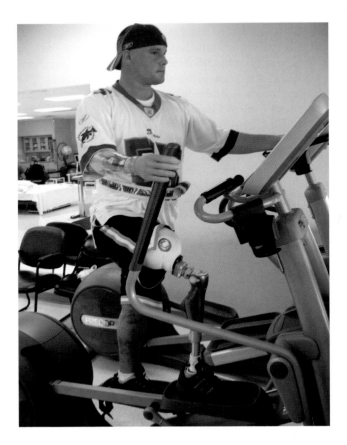

Figure 17-14. Luke Shirley, an upper and lower limb amputee, uses the elliptical trainer.

the patient can perform hip strengthening exercises for
abduction, extension, flexion, and adduction incorporating components of both isometric and isotonic
contractions in the standing position. Resistance can
be applied to the exercise leg with manual resistance,
resistive bands, or cable/pulley weight machines.
Progressive resistance exercises may be augmented
by having the patient perform isometric contractions
at end range to facilitate fatiguing of the contracting
muscle group. The stance limb will also benefit from
this mode of strengthening because stability must be
achieved through the stance limb as the contralateral
exercising limb performs the resisted movements. This

and counter resistance during the return phase of movement. To initiate the drill, the patient is cued to actively and forcefully rotate the anterior superior iliac spine into the therapist's anterior hand placements, allowing the patient to train disassociation of pelvic rotation with respect to shoulder girdle rotation (shoulders are still supported and stabilized by the mat and pillows allowing the pelvis to rotate freely). When the patient has overcome applied resistance through the complete range, counter cueing will be applied posterior to the ipsilateral iliac crest to initiate movement along the same rotational axis back to the starting position. Multiple repetitions of this drill performed with prosthetic limb(s) on or off can provide the patient with effective motor cues immediately before resistive gait training in the parallel bars and can be very effective in teaching patients who have difficulty with pelvic rotation during gait. A semisupine resisted pelvic rotation drill is illustrated in Figure 17-8.

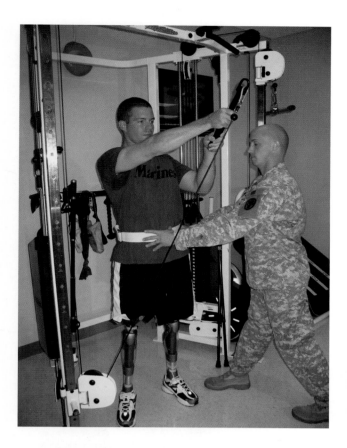

Figure 17-16. Joshua Bleill, a bilateral transfemoral amputee, performs resisted diagonal patterns to promote standing dynamic balance assisted by Matthew Scherer.

mode of training is particularly useful in promoting functional stability in the patient with transfemoral limb loss.

Semisupine Resisted Pelvic Rotation Drills

Early preparation for resistive pelvic rotation during gait can be performed using resisted pelvic rotation drills. For proper execution of this drill, the patient should assume a semisupine position with his or her back partially supported with pillows or a bolster and the torso rotated to about 45 degrees between supine and side lying. The patient's pelvis should remain free and not blocked with pillows to allow movement within the full range of rotation at the hips. In the correct starting position, the patient will be facing the therapist who is kneeling next to him or her. The therapist will assume hand placement at the anterior superior iliac spine on the side of the pelvis to be trained (the side not in direct contact with the treatment table, see Figure 17-8). The therapist's other hand will prepare for positioning posterior to the iliac crest to provide cueing

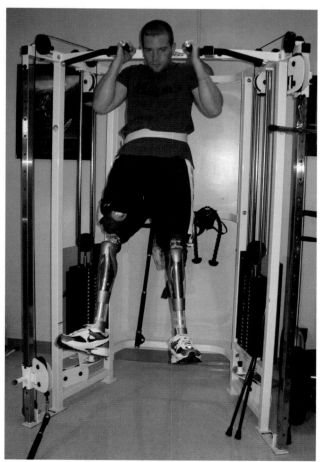

Figure 17-17. Joshua Bleill, a bilateral transfemoral amputee, performs pull-ups to promote upper body strength.

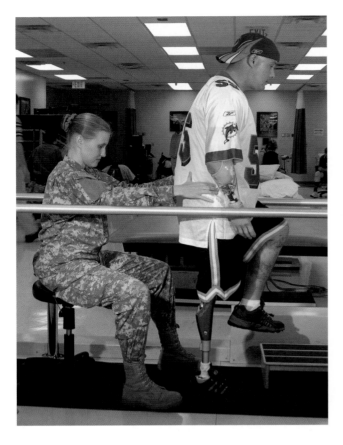

Figure 17-18. Elizabeth Painter assists Luke Shirley, a transfemoral amputee, with performing a stool stepping exercise to promote single limb standing balance.

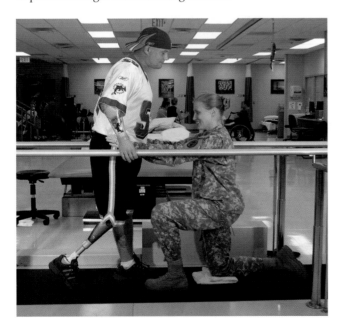

Figure 17-19. Elizabeth Painter assists Luke Shirley, a transfemoral amputee, with resisted gait training to promote pelvic rotation.

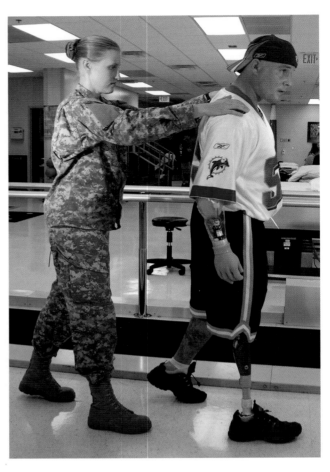

Figure 17-20. Elizabeth Painter assists Luke Shirley, a transfemoral amputee, with passive trunk rotation to improve balance during ambulation.

Progressive Resistive Exercise for Uninvolved Limbs

Access to isotonic strengthening equipment can be a tremendous advantage because of the numerous benefits derived from these forms of strengthening. There are few modifications in patient positioning on the weight machines and with most free weight programs. Moreover, this form of strengthening is very familiar to amputees who lifted weights before their injuries. When prescribing a program it is important to include the amputees in the exercise selection and choose familiar exercises. When they are ready, let them perform their general strengthening program with other amputees as they typically would with their unit. The sense of independence and ownership in their rehabilitation program can have lasting effects well beyond general strength increases. Figure 17-9 illustrates a bilateral transfemoral amputee performing unsupported push-ups.

Core Stabilization

Amputees are not always able to rely on proprioceptive feedback, ankle strategies, knee strategies, or sometimes hip strategies to help them stand, balance, and ambulate. They must rely on visual, somatosensory, vestibular, and lumbopelvic stability cues to effectively function. It continues to be important in this phase to progress core stabilization exercises to maintain trunk strength, decrease the possible risk of back pain, and assist in the reduction of gait deviations associated with the trunk.

Progression of core stabilization exercises occurs when level-1 exercises are mastered; endurance has improved; and the patient can perform at least one

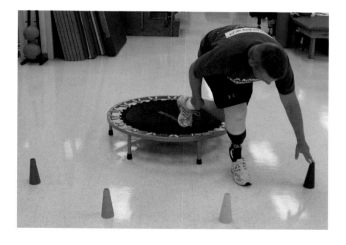

Figure 17-22. Christopher Millward, a transtibial amputee, works on rotational stability and eccentric lower limb control while on a dynamic surface.

level-1 exercise for 3 minutes with good form/neutral spine, minimal cueing, and loaded postures are tolerated. Examples of more challenging core stabilization exercises include the following:

- sitting on dynamic disc and moving arms/legs,
- therapist performing rhythmic stabilization,
- prone superman,
- supine "dead bug,"
- advanced exercise ball bridging,
- prone with heavier weights, and
- medicine ball drills.

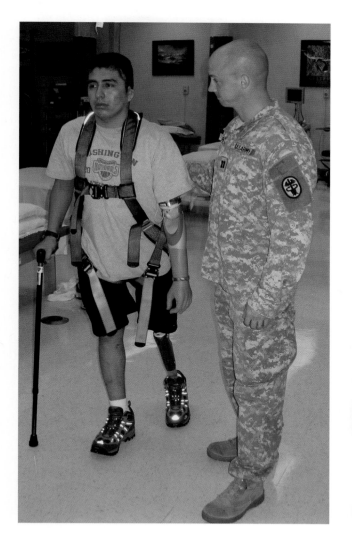

Figure 17-21. A ceiling suspension device is used during ambulation with Marco Robledo, a transfemoral amputee who is first learning to walk with a cane assisted by Matthew Scherer.

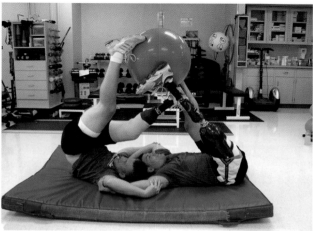

Figure 17-23. Two amputees, Christopher Millward and Chad Watson, work as partners to develop dynamic core stability and lower limb control.

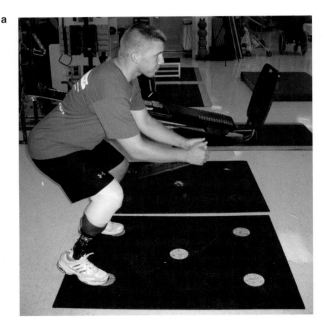
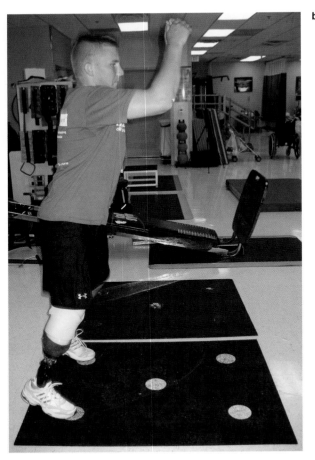

Figure 17-24. (a–e) Christopher Millward, a transtibial amputee, performs plyometric spot drills performed to increase lower limb strength, speed, and agility.

Cardiovascular Endurance

Because of the severity of injuries many SMs sustain and the deconditioning that occurs as a result of the prolonged postoperative periods, cardiovascular conditioning is compromised in many of the lower limb amputees. Cardiovascular endurance training can have a direct effect on the functional walking capabilities with regard to distance and assistive device required to ambulate.[37–39] The ability to improve overall ambulation capabilities with aerobic training applies to all levels of amputation.[39] Throughout the rehabilitation program cardiovascular fitness should be incorporated into every treatment plan. Progressing the amputee from the UBE to the lower limb ergometer can begin as early as their sitting balance and wounds permit. Once the ability to stand with the prosthesis(es) is achieved, balance training can be incorporated by standing on a compliant surface while working the arms with the UBE (Figure 17-10). Often single limb cycling with the nonamputated limb is introduced early in the rehabilitation program. Swimming, hand

cycling, and rowing can also be encouraged once the wounds are healed and the amputee is ready for more dynamic training away from the rehabilitation gym.

Goals for Progression to Phase III

Patient and provider goals for the second phase of rehabilitation include but are not limited to the following:

- independence with prescribed therapeutic exercises in strengthening, core stability, balance, and cardiovascular conditioning;
- functional range of motion of the lower limb joints to allow optimal gait training with the use of prosthetic device(s); and
- independence with ambulation with appropriate assistive device (without prosthesis).

PHASE III. PROSTHETIC/AMBULATION PHASE

The prosthetic/ambulation phase is the third phase of rehabilitation and begins when the amputee receives his or her prosthesis(es) and is medically cleared by the

physician to begin weight bearing on the amputated limb. Healing of the residual limb permits the amputee to begin weight bearing as tolerated. Initially the amputee focuses

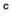

c

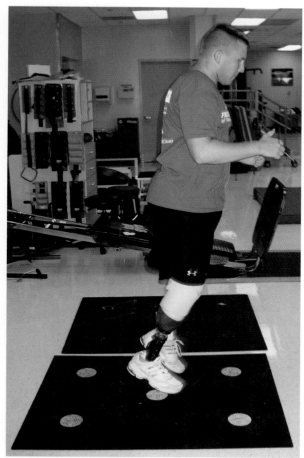

d

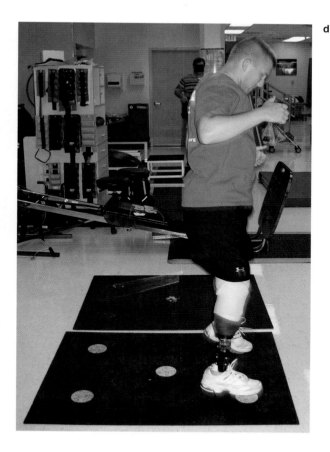

e

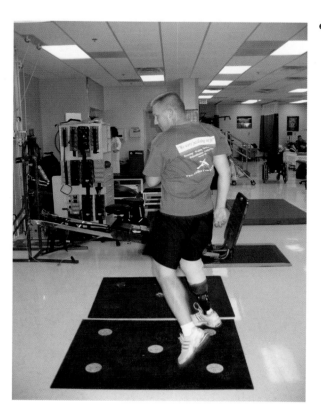

on reestablishing standing balance that would include the ability to transfer weight equally between both limbs and maintain single limb stability over the prosthetic limb(s). Prosthetic gait training includes movement re-education for a symmetrical gait and ambulation with the appropriate assistive device. As proficiency with the prosthesis improves, functional activities such as stairs, curbs, ramps, and uneven terrain may be introduced.

Functional Activities

Falls/Recovery

Falling or lowering oneself to the floor is an important skill to learn not only for safety reasons, but also as a means to perform floor level activities. During falling the amputee must first discard any assistive device to avoid injury. Amputees should land on their hands with the elbows slightly flexed to dampen the force and decrease the possibility of injury. As the elbows flex, the amputee should roll to one side, further decreasing the impact of the fall.

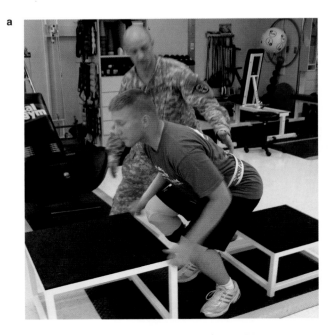

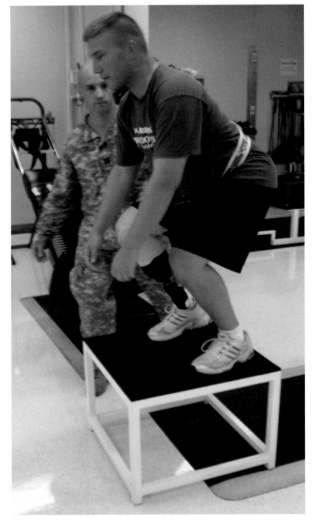

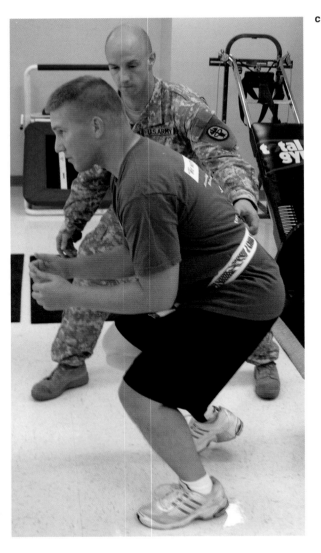

Figure 17-25. (a–c) Matthew Scherer assists Christopher Millward, a transtibial amputee, with plyometric depth jumps to increase lower limb power and prosthetic control.

Lowering the body to the floor in a controlled manner is initiated by squatting with the sound limb followed by gently leaning forward onto the slightly flexed upper limbs. From this position the amputee has the choice of remaining in quadruped or assuming a sitting posture.

Floor to Standing. Many techniques exist for teaching amputees how to rise from the floor to a standing position. The fundamental principle is to use the assistive device for balance and the sound limb for power as the body begins to rise. Depending on the type of amputation and the level of skill, the amputee and therapist must work closely together to determine the most efficient and safe manner to successfully master this task.

Stairs

Ascending and descending stairs is most safely and comfortably performed one step at a time (step-by-step). A few exceptional transfemoral amputees can descend stairs step-over-step. Most transtibial amputees have the option of either method, although hip disarticulation and hemipelvectomy amputees are limited to the step-by-step method.

Step-by-Step. This method is essentially the same for all levels of amputees. When ascending stairs, the body weight is shifted to the trailing prosthetic limb as the leading sound limb firmly places the foot on the stair. The trunk is slightly flexed over the sound limb as the knee extends raising the prosthetic limb to the same step. The same process is repeated for each step. One of the primary goals for ascending stairs step-over-step is to increase the ascent speed. To decrease the effort and increase safety, the easiest method to increase ascent speed is to skip a step. The amputee simply skips a stair with the leading sound limb and raises the body placing the prosthetic limb on the same step.

When descending stairs, the body weight is shifted to the sound limb as the prosthetic limb is lowered to the step below by eccentrically flexing the knee of the sound limb. Once the prosthetic limb is securely in place, the body weight is transferred to the prosthetic limb and the sound limb is lowered to the same step.

Transfemoral Amputees: Step-over-Step. Timing and coordination become critical factors in executing stair climbing step-over-step. As the transfemoral amputee approaches the stairs, the prosthetic limb is the first to ascend the stairs by rapid acceleration of hip flexion to clear the step. With the prosthetic foot firmly on the step, the residual limb must exert a great enough force to fully extend the hip so that the sound foot may advance to the step above. As the amputee advances to the next step, the sound side hip extends and the prosthetic side hip must once again flex at an accelerated speed to achieve sufficient knee flexion to place the prosthetic foot on the next step above.

Descending stairs is achieved by placing only the heel of the prosthetic foot on the stair below, then shifting the body weight over the prosthetic limb, thus, passively flexing the knee. The sound limb must quickly reach the step below in time to catch the body's weight. The yield rate control of the prosthetic knee will dictate the speed of descent, but the key to most knee systems is maintaining body weight over the prosthesis. The process is repeated until a rhythm is achieved.[29] Most transfemoral amputees who have mastered this skill descend stairs at a fast pace, so the therapist should consider if the speed of descent is safe for each individual (Figure 17-11).

Transtibial Amputees: Step-over-Step Stairs. When ascending stairs transtibial amputees that do not have the ability to dorsiflex their foot/ankle assembly must generate a stronger concentric contraction of the knee and hip extensors to successfully transfer their body weight over the prosthetic limb.

Descending stairs is very similar to normal descent with one exception: only the prosthetic foot heel is placed on the stair. This compensates for the lack of dorsiflexion within the foot/ankle assembly.[29]

Picking up Objects

Single limb balance and bending to pick objects off the floor is taught during the early stages of rehabilitation for crutch walking, hopping, and other skills. Single limb squatting is considerably more difficult but can help improve balance and strength. When first attempting this skill, half squats with a chair underneath the amputee are recommended. Progression from picking larger objects off the floor to smaller objects requires deeper or lower squats (Figure 17-12).

Core Stabilization, Closed Kinetic Chain Exercises, and Balance/Proprioception

Core stabilization exercises in Phase III may be progressed to include standing and more challenging balance activities. The same principles apply: maintain neutral spine, correctly draw in the lower abdominal wall, and work on endurance. Core strengthening occurs while also performing CKC strengthening and balance exercises. Examples in this phase follow:

- standing on foam or DynaDiscs (Exertools, Rohnert Park, Calif);
- cone walking;
- single leg balance on either limb/steamboats;
- medicine ball exercises in standing, sitting, prone, or supine exercise ball progression;
- Plyoback (Exertools, Rohnert Park, Calif) training with increasing weight;
- wall squats;
- quadrant and plane stepping activities;
- ball rolling with sound limb;
- ladder walking drills (Figure 17-13); and
- elliptical trainer or stair stepper (Figure 17-14).

Bilateral lower limb amputees will benefit from standing and dynamic balance activities. Therapeutic interventions designed to improve core stability in standing include diagonal movements with resistance cables or medicine balls (Figure 17-15, Figure 17-16, and Figure 17-17). Functional challenges may include similar activities performed outside on grassy surfaces.

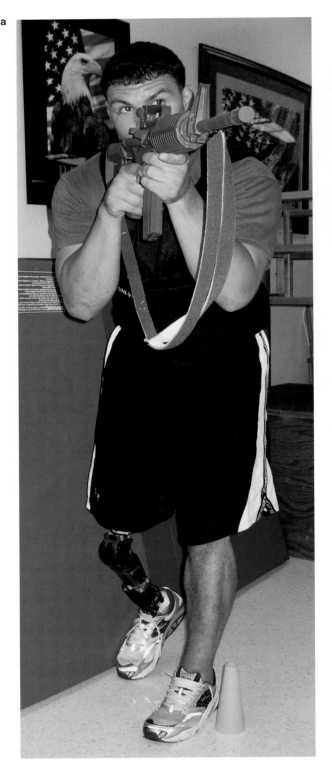

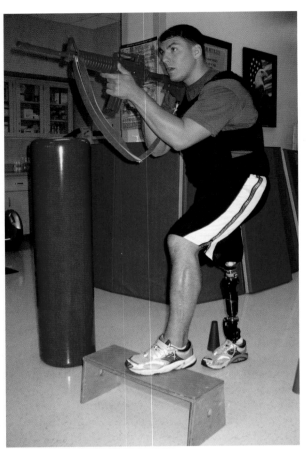

Figure 17-26. (a–e) Chad Watson, a transfemoral amputee, performs a series of weapon drills to prepare to return to active duty.

Weight-Shifting Progression

Orientation of the COM over the BOS to maintain balance requires that the amputee become familiar with these terms and aware of their relationship. Learning to shift the COM over one foot and then the other will assist with lateral displacement of the COM. As the displacement from side to side increases, amputees should take their sound side hand off the parallel bars and eventually both hands off the parallel bars. Increased weight bearing will be a direct result of improved COM displacement and will establish a firm foundation for actual weight shifting during ambulation.[29]

Standing Progression with Prosthetic Limb

Single limb balance over the prosthetic limb while advancing the sound limb should be practiced in a controlled manner so that when called to do so in a dynamic situation, such as walking,

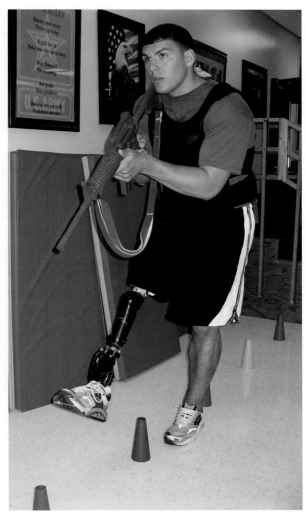

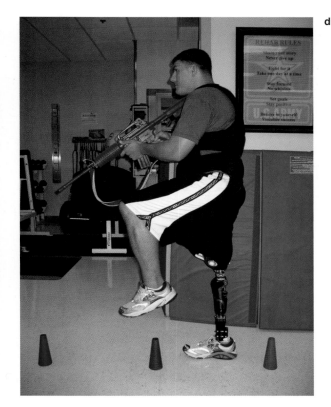

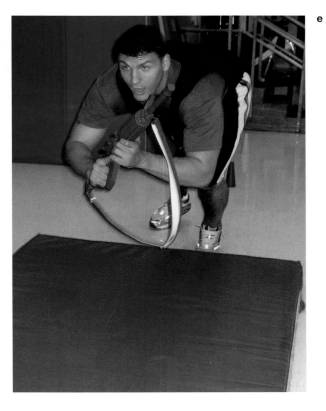

this skill can be used with relatively little difficulty. The stool stepping exercise is an excellent method in which this skill may be learned.[32] The amputee should stand in the parallel bars with the sound limb in front of a 10- to 20-centimeter high stool (or block). The height depends on the ability level. The amputee should step slowly onto the stool with the sound limb while using bilateral upper limb support on the parallel bars (Figure 17-18). To further increase these weight-bearing skills, the amputee should remove the sound side hand from the parallel bars and then eventually the other hand. Initially, the speed of the sound leg will increase when upper limb support is removed. However, with practice the speed will become slower and more controlled, thus promoting increased weight bearing on the prosthesis.[29]

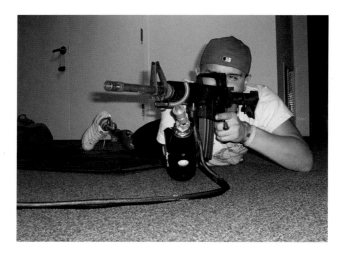

Figure 17-27. A transfemoral/transradial amputee performs prone position weapons training in the firearms training simulation center to prepare to return to duty.

Ambulation

Once the amputee has the base strength and balance, resistive gait training techniques are implemented to reeducate the amputee to the normal gait movements necessary to maximize prosthetic performance and promote economy of gait.[29,40] Advanced gait training exercises are also offered to assist the amputee to negotiate environmental conditions that require multidirectional movements and superior dynamic balance.

Pelvic Rotation

To restore the correct pelvic motion, resistive gait training for lower limb amputees has been demonstrated to improve balance and normalize gait.[29,40] Restoration of pelvic rotation requires that the therapist use rhythmic initiation through the anterior superior iliac spines, giving the amputee the feeling of rotating the pelvis forward as passive flexion of the prosthetic knee occurs. The amputee will gradually begin to actively rotate his or her pelvis during this time. The therapist can gradually progress from active assistive motions to resistive while continually facilitating proper motion of the pelvis and prosthesis (Figure 17-19). Once the therapist is satisfied with pelvic motions, the amputee progresses to the swing phase of gait stepping forward and backward with the prosthetic limb.

When both the therapist and the amputee are comfortable with the gait demonstrated in the parallel bars, the same procedure as described above is practiced out of the parallel bars with the amputee initially using the therapist's shoulders as support and progressing to both hands free when appropriate. The therapist may or may not continue to provide proprioceptive input to the pelvis.

Trunk Rotation and Arm Swing

During human locomotion, the trunk and upper limb rotate opposite to the pelvic girdle and lower limb. Trunk rotation is necessary for balance, momentum, and symmetry of gait. Arm swing, which provides balance, momentum, and symmetry of gait, is directly influenced by the speed of ambulation.[29,41] As the walking speed of gait is accelerated, arm swing increases, thus permitting a more efficient gait.

Many amputees have a decreased trunk rotation and arm swing, especially on the prosthetic side. This may be the result of fear or lack of confidence when walking with the prosthesis. Returning trunk rotation and arm swing is easily accomplished by utilizing rhythmic initiation or passively cueing the trunk as the amputee walks. The therapist stands behind the amputee with one hand on either shoulder. As the amputee walks the therapist gently rotates the trunk. When the left leg steps forward the right shoulder is rotated forward and vice versa. Once the amputee feels comfortable with the motion, he or she can actively take over the motion[29] (Figure 17-20).

Stride Length, Width, and Cadence

As the amputee begins to ambulate independently, verbal cueing may be necessary as a reminder to keep the sound foot away from mid-line to maintain the

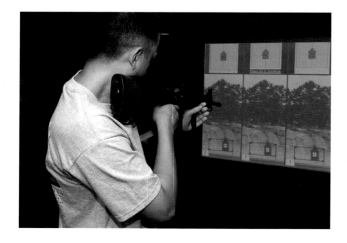

Figure 17-28. Computerized simulation allows amputees to begin preparation for weapons-related activities.

a

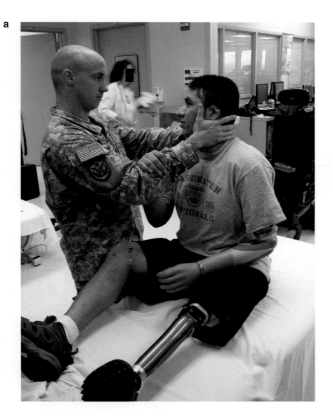

b

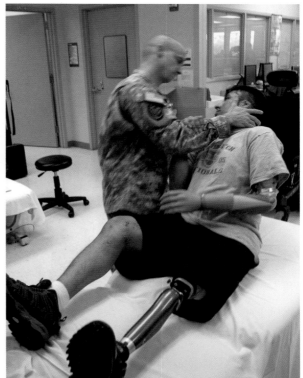

c

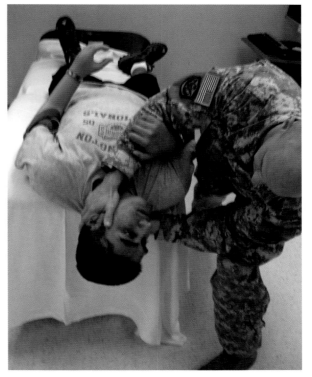

Figure 17-29. (a–c) Matthew Scherer performs a Dix-Hallpike maneuver on Marco Robledo, an amputee with benign paroxysmal positional vertigo.

proper BOS. Maintenance of equal stride length may not be immediately forthcoming because many amputees tend to take a longer step with the prosthetic limb than the sound limb. When adequate weight bearing through the prosthetic limb has been achieved, the amputee should begin to take longer steps with the sound limb and slightly shorter steps with the prosthetic limb. This principle also applies when increasing the cadence. When an amputee increases his or her speed of ambulation, the prosthetic limb often compensates by taking a longer step, thus increasing the asymmetry. By simply having the amputee take a longer step with the sound limb and a moderate step with the prosthetic limb, increased speed of gait is accomplished without increased asymmetry. As balance and confidence and symmetry in stride length improve, the amputee's cadence will increase.[29]

Assistive Devices and Gait Training

Amputees who will be independent ambulators and those who will require an assistive device can benefit from the above systematic rehabilitation program. Most patients can be progressed to the point of ambulating out of the parallel bars. At that time, the amputee must practice ambulating with the chosen

a

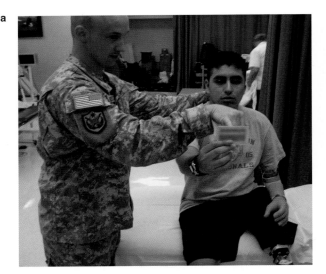

Figure 17-30. (**a–b**) Marco Robledo is a traumatic brain injury patient with a unilateral transradial amputation and a unilateral transfemoral amputation.

b

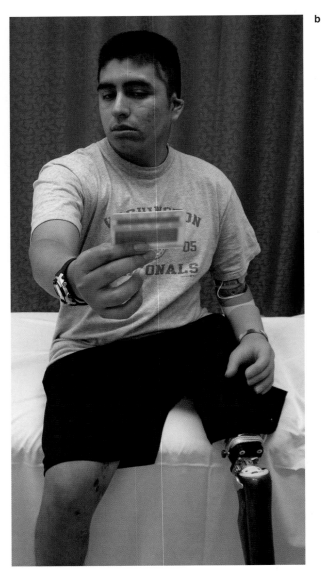

assistive device and maintaining pelvic rotation, adequate BOS, equal stance time, and equal stride length, all of which can have a direct influence on the energy cost of walking. Trunk rotation would be absent with amputees utilizing a walker as an assistive device; however, those ambulating with crutches or a cane should be able to incorporate trunk rotation into their gait. Amputees will also find ceiling suspension tracks useful for early ambulation when developing confidence with the prosthesis and assistive device (Figure 17-21).

Resistive Rollover Drills

Inability to roll over the prosthetic foot during late stance phases can lead to asymmetrical gait patterns. Therapists can facilitate more efficient rollover on the prosthetic foot by cueing the patient to push into a cane held in both hands at waist level by both the therapist and the patient. During this drill, the therapist and patient face one another with the therapist's back to the direction of movement. The therapist applies mild to moderate resistance to the cane beginning at mid-stance on the prosthetic side. The patient must overcome this resistance while maintaining upright posture throughout the late stance. The therapist can vary resistance to the patient during the rollover phase, thereby enhancing proprioceptive feedback in the residual limb, core recruitment, and balance.

Excessive Lateral Trunk Movement

Patients with knee disarticulation and transfemoral amputations commonly present with excessive lateral trunk lean over the prosthetic side limb(s) during ambulation. Decreased force production by the hip abductors secondary to decreased length of femur may be compensated for by increased lateral trunk lean over the prosthetic stance limb. Strengthening the hip musculature with emphasis on the hip abductors may increase single leg stance stability. CKC exercises and resistive gait training may help reduce lateral trunk lean over the prosthetic side limb.

Multidirectional Movements—Sidestepping

Sidestepping, or walking sideways, can be introduced to amputees at various times throughout their rehabilitation. Amputees can begin with simple weight shifting in the parallel bars and later perform higher level activities such as unassisted sidestepping around tables or a small obstacle course that requires many small turns. During early rehabilitation this skill provides amputees with a functional exercise for strengthening the hip abductors, and later in the rehabilitation process, an opportunity to progress into multidirectional movements.

Multidirectional Movements—Backward Walking

Walking backward is not difficult for transtibial amputees but it does pose a problem for amputees requiring a prosthetic knee because they cannot actively flex the knee for adequate ground clearance. The most comfortable method of backward walking is by vaulting upward (plantarflexing) on the sound foot to obtain sufficient height so that the prosthetic limb that is moving posteriorly can clear the ground.

Goals for Progression to Phase IV

Patient and provider goals for the third phase of rehabilitation include but are not limited to the following:

- able to tolerate progressive weight-bearing and weight-shifting activities;
- independent with Phase III rehabilitation drills and exercises;
- minimal gait deviations that are not worsened with higher level activity;
- independent with falls recovery;
- progressing ambulation to modified independence or independence with appropriate assistive device over level surfaces, inclines, and stairs;
- able to transition from standard foot to a high energy foot for those with transtibial amputation; and
- able to start pre-running drills in free swing mode (microprocessor knee) with progression to running drills in mechanical knee for those with a transfemoral amputation.

PHASE IV. PROGRESSIVE ACTIVITIES /RETURN TO ACTIVE DUTY PHASE

The progressive activities/return to active duty phase is the fourth phase in which amputees specifically train for and return to recreational and sporting activities, and for those who wish to remain on active duty. The active duty military population will typically set goals of achieving the highest level of physical function possible regardless of the extent of their injuries. Their unique qualities include young age, good health before injury, and high motivation. As a result, many SMs have raised the bar of expectations traditionally held by rehabilitation professionals for young people with limb loss.

Walter Reed Amputee Patient Care team policy stipulates that patients undergo a total body Dexa Scan (hip, spine, residual limb) to assess overall fracture risk (osteopenia/osteoporosis) due to rapid bone loss in proximal amputated limb (proximal portion of an amputated limb) or other extremities that have been partial or nonweight bearing for prolonged periods of time (eg, from external fixaters). The bone density must be within normal limits before receiving an advanced running prosthesis.

Recreational/Sports Activities

Agility, sports-specific drills, and strength training continue to be an important part of rehabilitation. The sports medicine model is used to prepare amputees for an active lifestyle. Agility drills and strengthening exercises that are geared toward specific sports or recreation are practiced individually or in group sessions. In addition, training for hand crank cycling, SCUBA, and kayaking are provided to those who wish to participate.

Core Stabilization

By Phase IV, core stabilization should be incorporated into all agility, sports-specific drills, strength training, plyometrics, balance, and proprioception activities (Figure 17-22). Plyometrics begin when the residual limb(s) can withstand the forces during this training for power enhancement. Rotational drills with medicine balls are frequently performed with a partner or as group exercises (Figure 17-23). Other advanced core stabilizing exercises in this phase include balancing while standing on a DynaDisc (Exertools, Rohnert Park, Calif), using an exercise ball during single leg wall sits, single leg balance with perturbations, plyometric jumps, and other higher level exercises (Figure 17-24 and Figure 17-25). Amputees are verbally reminded to maintain a strong core by sustaining a regular exercise program to help prevent secondary health conditions such as low back pain and to enhance physical performance.

Military Task Training/Military Operations

Although not every amputee wishes to return to active duty, those that do will have the option of participating in military specific tasks before returning to their units. Performing military specific tasks and drills with a prosthesis(es) can be difficult initially; however, learning the "tricks" of prosthetic use can often make the difference for success. Amputees must meet the established criteria for a warrior and successfully perform common tasks to remain on active duty. The training requirements and preparation will be even greater for those amputees who seek to return to an operations type unit. Examples of military task training that can be incorporated into rehabilitation include but are not limited to the following:

- road marching;
- rescues and buddy carries;
- reaction drills;
- site picture drills and room clearing drills; and
- physical fitness test training such as push-ups, sit-ups, and running.

Road Marching

Tasking an amputee to march with a weighted rucksack over a prescribed distance challenges dynamic postural stability, ambulation tolerance, cardiovascular reserves, residual limb integrity, and prosthetic capabilities. Distance and cadence should be progressed as tolerated by the amputee.

Rescues and Buddy Carries

Amputees can be challenged to carry or extract fellow SMs using various carrying or extraction techniques to simulate such tasks in an operational environment. Drills with weights and heavy sacks should be practiced initially to develop movement skills with the prosthesis(es), progressing to live maneuvers with a partner when appropriate.

Immediate Action Drills and Reacting to Contact

Reaction drills require quick transitions from standing to kneeling, kneeling to supine, back up to standing, and advancing with a simulated weapon.

Site Picture Drills and Room Clearing Drills

Site picture drills and room clearing drills simulate movement in tactical environments to include urban terrain with a simulated weapon either aimed or "at

the ready" in preparation for deployment. These basic drills can be progressed by challenging an amputee's ability to negotiate uneven terrain, compliant surfaces, and obstacles while maintaining an operational posture and efficient and effective continuous forward movement (Figure 17-26).

Firearms Training Simulator Centers

Firearms training simulator centers, which are located within military training facilities, allow amputees the opportunity to reestablish firearms qualifications with various weapons using video simulation (Figure 17-27 and Figure 17-28). Physical therapists work closely with occupational therapists and the firearms training simulator trainer to promote ADLs by training amputees who stay on active duty and/or have the vocational/leisure interest in recreational activities such as hunting or skeet shooting. Specialized terminal devices, adaptive techniques, and hand or eye dominance retraining can all be incorporated for enhanced experiences. Improving basic firearm skills with these modifications allows amputees to succeed and improve their confidence.

Special Considerations for Amputees with Comorbidities and Multiple Limb Loss

Comorbidity Considerations

Overcoming the challenges of limb loss can be complicated by the effects of comorbidities including soft tissue injuries and abdominal injuries, fractures, peripheral nerve injuries, vestibular pathology, and TBI. Varying degrees of severity of these conditions can significantly affect early weight bearing, mobility, tolerance for rehabilitation, and potentially even the ability to concentrate and follow commands. All interdisciplinary team members have a role in evaluating, treating, and advising their colleagues on comorbid conditions, the resultant level of the patient's functionality, and how this clinical picture should be best managed.

Abdominal/Visceral Trauma

Patients with external stomas will require the assistance of a wound care nurse for initial patient and family member education. They will not be allowed prone for stretching or conditioning exercises. Therefore, great care must be taken to ensure that transfemoral amputees use alternate hip flexor stretching techniques (side lying or supine with leg off edge of bed) in preparation for gait training.

Fractures

Patients with fractures in one or more limbs, the pelvis, or vertebrae will likely have weight-bearing restrictions that will affect their mobility and ability to participate in certain types of therapeutic exercise. It is not uncommon for polytrauma patients to bear weight on their prosthetic side before their fractured contralateral lower limb. Although devices such as external fixators may stabilize comminuted fractures and allow for earlier weight bearing, they are often painful and require diligent pin care to guard against infection. Those patients with fractured upper limbs will be limited in the use of their upper limbs for transfers, ADLs, and upper limb muscular endurance and resistance training. Fractures in the pelvis or the vertebrae will limit the patient's ability to sit, participate in gait training, and perform CKC strengthening and conditioning.

Peripheral Nerve Injuries

Patients with limb loss may have to contend with the effects of peripheral nerve injuries in residual upper or lower limbs. For example, deep and superficial fibular nerve injuries from blast shrapnel on the "sound side" limb can cause difficulty or the inability to effectively dorsiflex the foot during gait, necessitating the use of an ankle foot orthosis. Similarly, upper limb injuries to the radial, median, or ulnar nerves can affect a patient's ability to perform ADLs, transfer independently, or even operate a power wheelchair.

Vestibular Insult

Although the incidence of vestibular pathology across the broad spectrum of polytrauma patients is unknown, blast injury survivors with limb loss often present with vestibular deficits such as benign paroxysmal positional vertigo and vestibular hypofunction.[42] Vestibular dysfunction can diminish rehabilitation tolerance, affect static and dynamic balance, and increase risk of falls during ambulation. Early management of these conditions may include use of the Canalith Repositioning Maneuver for benign paroxysmal positional vertigo or adaptation, substitution, and habituation exercises for unilateral or bilateral vestibular hypofunction. Early and aggressive static and dynamic balance training and gait training can help patients compensate for vestibular deficits as they work through vestibular rehabilitation. Figure 17-29 demonstrates the Dix-Hallpike maneuver being performed on an amputee with benign paroxysmal positional vertigo.

Traumatic Brain Injury

Amputees with TBI must be assessed for the severity of their brain injury before the initiation of the standard rehabilitation protocol. Patients' ability to attend to tasks and participate in therapy usually dictates whether they are appropriate candidates for polytrauma rehabilitation immediately or whether they should be first managed by the Veterans Affairs Healthcare System for more intensive neurological rehabilitation and neuropsychological needs. Amputees with mild TBI may present with balance deficits, vestibular pathology, difficulty with learning (or relearning) motor tasks, and changes in affect. These deficits can complicate the typical course of rehabilitation and interventions should be incorporated into the overall plan of care to address them. Although numerous other conditions complicate a patient's ability to participate in full spectrum amputee and polytrauma rehabilitation, the aforementioned are among the most common. It is imperative to document all pathologies, impairments, and functional limitations so that they can be prioritized and addressed in the interdisciplinary plan of care. Figure 17-30 shows a patient with a TBI, a unilateral transradial amputation, and a unilateral transfemoral amputation undergoing physical therapy.

Special Considerations for the Patient with Multiple Limb Loss

Since the initiation of hostilities in Iraq and Afghanistan the incidence of bilateral lower limb loss is 18%.[43] For patients with bilateral lower limb loss prosthetic and rehabilitation management continues to improve because of increased attention to this population of amputees. The attachment at the end of this chapter displays the bilateral transfemoral amputee protocol.

The altered anatomy of a bilateral lower limb amputee offers additional considerations when planning a standing and gait training program. For example, the physical therapist may observe increased lordosis during standing, loss of balance strategies, and altered postural stability. These considerations can contribute to reduced standing or dynamic balance and the increased possibility of falls. Thus, the importance of initiating core and postural stability exercises early in the rehabilitation program is even more pronounced for the bilateral lower limb amputee. Furthermore, it is essential to perform thorough vestibular assessments and TBI screening to document and address any neurologic impairments that may contribute to balance reduction.

The use of low profile prosthesis or "stubbies" can assist bilateral transfemoral amputees with learning to use their hip and trunk musculature. Stubbies by design lower the COM closer to the BOS, therefore requiring less muscular effort to maintain standing balance. Although body image can be an issue for some patients, the early bipedal locomotion and increased mobility in most instances outweigh the body image issues. Other benefits identified with use of stubbies include facilitating early weight-bearing activities in the parallel bars, achieving improved weight shifting during ambulation, assisting in the development of core stability and postural stability, and decreasing the risk of falls with early ambulation training in the clinic.

SUMMARY

Rehabilitative care of SMs with limb loss has evolved from the elementary goal of healing wounds and returning home to a comprehensive rehabilitative philosophy: restoration of function to the highest possible degree. The multifaceted rehabilitation programs go beyond daily activities and mobility training to include the opportunity to train for return to duty, vocational preparation, sports, or other leisure activities. The US military's four-phase program of functional progressive rehabilitation for wounded SMs with lower limb loss presented in this chapter is designed to promote a rehabilitation philosophy of treating the amputee as a "tactical athlete" applying the highest level training similar to that of sports medicine rehabilitation. The four-phase rehabilitation program includes (1) initial management, (2) preprosthetic, (3) prosthetic/ambulation, and (4) progressive activities/return to active duty. Within each phase of rehabilitation evidence-based rehabilitation techniques and innovative exercise applications are applied with the goal of maximizing the rehabilitation potential of every amputee. The information in this chapter presents the most current rehabilitation techniques and philosophy in an ever evolving process of providing the best care possible.

Acknowledgments

The authors would like to thank the following individuals for their valuable assistance in writing the clinical protocols and their contributions to this chapter: Janet Papazis, Justin LaFerrier, Greg Loomis, Bo Bergeron, Jacqueline Coley Moore, Don Gajewski, Brandon Goff, and Stuart Campbell.

The authors would also like to thank the following for their participation as patient models for the figures included in this chapter and more importantly for their service to the United States: Joshua Bleill, Andrew Forney, Gregory Gadson, Christopher Millward, Marco Robledo, Luke Shirley, and Chad Watson.

REFERENCES

1. Hodges PW, Julls GA. Motor relearning strategies for the rehabilitation of intervertebral control of the spine. In: Liebenson C, ed. *Rehabilitation of the Spine: A Practitioner's Manual.* 2nd ed. Baltimore, Md: Lippincott Williams & Wilkins; 2003.

2. Ehde DM, Smith DG, Czerniecki JM, Campbell KM, Malchow DM, Robinson LR. Back pain as a secondary disability in persons with lower limb amputations. *Arch Phys Med Rehabil.* 2001;82:731–734.

3. Friberg O. Biomechanical significance of the correct length of lower limb prostheses: a clinical and radiological study. *Prosthet Orthot Int.* 1984;8:124–129.

4. Friel K, Domholdt E, Smith DG. Physical and functional measures related to low back pain in individuals with lower-limb amputation: an exploratory pilot study. *J Rehabil Res Dev.* 2005;42:155–166.

5. Hagberg K, Branemark R. Consequences of non-vascular trans-femoral amputation: a survey of quality of life, prosthetic use and problems. *Prosthet Orthot Int.* 2001;25:186–194.

6. Sjodahl C, Jarnlo GB, Persson BM. Gait improvement in unilateral transfemoral amputees by a combined psychological and physiotherapeutic treatment. *J Rehabil Med.* 2001;33:114–118.

7. Smith DG, Ehde DM, Legro MW, Reiber GE, del Aguila M, Boone DA. Phantom limb, residual limb, and back pain after lower extremity amputations. *Clin Orthop Relat Res.* 1999;361:29–38.

8. Kulkarni J, Gaine WJ, Buckley JG, Rankine JJ, Adams J. Chronic low back pain in traumatic lower limb amputees. *Clin Rehabil.* 2005;19:81–86.

9. Marshall HM, Jensen MP, Ehde DM, Campbell KM. Pain site and impairment in individuals with amputation pain. *Arch Phys Med Rehabil.* 2002;83:1116–1119.

10. Bartonietz K, Strange D. The use of Swiss balls in athletic training: an effective combination of load and fun. *Track Coach.* 1999;1:49.

11. Smith K, Smith E. Integrating Pilates-based core strengthening into older adult fitness programs: implications for practice. *Top Geriatr Rehabil.* 2005;21:57–67.

12. Rutherford OM, Jones DA. The role of learning and coordination in strength training. *Eur J Appl Physiol Occup Physiol.* 1986;55:100–105.

13. Donachy JE, Brannon KD, Hughes LS, Seahorn J, Crutcher TT, Christian EL. Strength and endurance training of an individual with left upper and lower limb amputations. *Disabil Rehabil.* 2004;26:495–499.

14. Thompson C, Blackwell J, Kepesidis I, Myers-Cobb K. Effect of core stabilization training on fitness, swing speed, and weight transfer in older male golfers. *Med Sci Sport Exer.* 2004;36:S204.

15. Gundewall B, Liljeqvist M, Hansson T. Primary prevention of back symptoms and absence from work. A prospective randomized study among hospital employees. *Spine.* 1993;18:587–594.

16. Hodges PW. Abdominal mechanism and support of the lumbar spine and pelvis. In: Richardson CA, Hodges PW, Hides JA, eds. *Therapeutic Exercise for Lumbopelvic Stabilization. A Motor Control Approach for the Treatment and Prevention of Low Back Pain.* New York, NY: Churchill Livingstone; 2004.

17. Richardson CA, Hides JA. Stiffness of the lumbopelvic region for load transfer. In: Richardson CA, Hodges PW, Hides JA, eds. *Therapeutic Exercise for Lumbopelvic Stabilization. A Motor Control Approach for the Treatment and Prevention of Low Back Pain.* New York, NY: Churchill Livingstone; 2004.

18. Hodges PW, Eriksson AE, Shirley D, Gandevia SC. Intra-abdominal pressure increases stiffness of the lumbar spine. *J Biomech.* 2005;38:1873–1880.

19. Hodges PW, Cresswell AG, Daggfeldt K, Thorstensson A. In vivo measurement of the effect of intra-abdominal pressure on the human spine. *J Biomech.* 2001;34:347–353.

20. Hodges PW, Kaigle Holm A, Holm S, et al. Intervertebral stiffness of the spine is increased by evoked contraction of tranversus abdominis and the diaphragm: in vivo porcine studies. *Spine.* 2003;28:2594–2601.

21. Macintosh JE, Valencia F, Bogduk N, Munro RR. The morphology of the human lumbar multifidus. *Clin Biomech.* 1986;1:196–204.

22. Hides JA. Paraspinal mechanism and support of the lumbar spine. In: Richardson CA, Hodges PW, Hides JA, eds. *Therapeutic Exercise for Lumbopelvic Stabilization. A Motor Control Approach for the Treatment and Prevention of Low Back Pain.* New York, NY: Churchill Livingstone; 2004.

23. Currie D, Gilbert D, Dierschke B. Aerobic capacity with two leg work versus one leg plus both arms work in men with peripheral vascular disease. *Arch Phys Med Rehabil.* 1992;73:1081–1084.

24. Davidoff GN, Lampman RM, Westbury L, Deron J, Finestone HM, Islam S. Exercise testing and training of persons with dysvascular amputation: safety and efficacy of arm ergometry. *Arch Phys Med Rehabil.* 1992;73:334–338.

25. Finestone HM, Lampman RM, Davidoff GN, Westbury L, Islam S, Schultz JS. Arm ergometry exercise testing in patients with dysvascular amputations. *Arch Phys Med Rehabil.* 1991;72:15–19.

26. Kang J, Chaloupka EC, Mastrangelo MA, Angelucci J. Physiological responses to upper body exercise on an arm and a modified leg ergometer. *Med Sci Sports Exerc.* 1999;31:1453–1459.

27. Lai AM, Stanish WD, Stanish HI. The young athlete with physical challenges. *Clin Sports Med.* 2000;19:793–819.

28. Gailey RS. Recreational pursuits of elders with amputation. *Top Geriatr Rehabil.* 1992;8:39–58.

29. Gailey RS, Gailey AM. *Prosthetic Gait Training for Lower Limb Amputees.* Miami, Fla: Advanced Rehabilitation Therapy Inc; 1989.

30. Gailey RS, McKenzie A. *Balance, Agility, Coordination and Endurance for Lower Extremity Amputees.* Miami, Fla: Advanced Rehabilitation Therapy Inc; 1994.

31. American Academy of Orthopaedic Surgeons. In: Smith DG, Bowker JH, Michael JW, eds. *Atlas of Amputations and Limb Deficiencies: Surgical, Prosthetic, and Rehabilitation Principles.* 3rd ed. Rosemont, Ill: Mosby Company; 2004.

32. Burgess EM. Immediate postsurgical prosthetic fitting: a system of amputee management. *Phys Ther.* 1971;51:139–143.

33. May BJ. Stump bandaging of the lower-extremity amputee. *Phys Ther.* 1964;44:808–814.

34. Condie E, Jones D, Treweek S, Scott H. A one-year national survey of patients having a lower limb amputation. *Physiotherapy.* 1996;82:14–20.

35. Gailey RS, McKenzie A. *Stretching and Strengthening for Lower Extremity Amputees.* Miami, Fla: Advanced Rehabilitation Therapy Inc; 1994.

36. Eisert O, Tester OW. Dynamic exercises for lower extremity amputees. *Arch Phys Med Rehabil.* 1954;33:695–704.

37. Cruts H, De Vries J, Zilvold G, Huisman K, Van Alste J, Boom HB. Lower extremity amputees with peripheral vascular disease: graded exercise testing and results of prosthetic training. *Arch Phys Med Rehabil.* 1987;68:14–19.

38. Perry J, Shanfield S. Efficiency of dynamic elastic response prosthetic feet. *J Rehabil Res Dev.* 1993;30:137–143.

39. Ward K, Meyers M. Exercise performance of lower-extremity amputees. *Sports Med.* 1995;20:207–214.

40. Yigiter K, Sener G, Erbahceci F, Bayar K, Ulger OG, Akdogan S. A comparison of traditional prosthetic training versus proprioceptive neuromuscular facilitation resistive gait training with trans-femoral amputees. *Prosthet Orthot Int.* 2002;26:213–217.

41. Murray MP, Drought AB, Kory RC. Walking patterns of normal men. *J Bone Joint Surg Am.* 1964;46:335–360.

42. Scherer M, Burrows H, Pinto R, Somrack E. Characterizing self-reported dizziness and otovestibular impairment among blast-injured amputees: a pilot study. *Mil Med.* 2007;172:731–737.

43. Amputee Patient Care Database. Washington, DC: Walter Reed Army Medical Center. Updated December 17, 2007.

ATTACHMENT: MILITARY AMPUTEE REHABILITATION PROTOCOL

Note: Each surgeon has preferred methods or guidance that may deviate from the below stated recommendations based on the specifics of the case or other parameters. This protocol should not be used in lieu of clear and regular communication between attending surgeon and the patient's physical therapist.

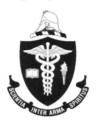

PHYSICAL THERAPY SECTION
WALTER REED ARMY MEDICAL CENTER
6900 Georgia Ave NW, Wash. D.C.
(202) 782-6371

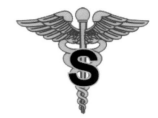

AMPUTEE REHABILITATION

Revised May 2007

Phase I: Protective Healing (Post-op Days 1–7)

Note: Exercise prescription is dependent upon the tissue healing process and _individual_ functional readiness in _all_ stages. If any concerns or complications arise regarding the progress of any patient, physical therapy will contact the orthopedist or physiatrist.

Immediate post-operative therapy focuses on bed mobility, transfers, wheelchair management and/or ambulation with appropriate assistive device (AD), therapeutic exercise for deconditioning, contracture avoidance, pain management assistance, and self-care.

Goals:
1. Restore functional mobility/basic ambulation
    Bed mobility
    Transfers (bedside chair/wheelchair)
    Ambulation with appropriate AD
    Wheelchair management
2. Teach appropriate residual limb management and self-care
3. Maintain/restore baseline conditioning and balance
4. Assist with pain management
5. Institute range of motion (ROM) and stretching exercises to avoid contractures
6. Address any potential barriers to rehabilitation at earliest opportunity

Cardiovascular
- Upper body ergometer
- Seated calisthenics

Functional Activities
- Bed mobility
- Rolling
- Transfers
- Wheelchair management/mobility

Range of Motion *(see addendum for stretching and ROM restrictions during Phase I)*
- Contracture avoidance/stretching program (static, contract relax)
- Passive ROM
- Active Assistive ROM (AAROM) to tolerance
- Active ROM (AROM) as needed for activity

Strengthening *(see Phase I addendum for restrictions by level during Phase I)*
- Isometrics—Quadriceps, Gluteals, Hamstrings
- Ankle pumps
- 3- or 4-way hip/sliding board (Abduction, Adduction, Flexion) Prone hip extension
- Lumbar stabilization (initiate instruction on Transversus Abdominis contraction)

Balance
- Seated mat
- Shifting on mat
- Sit to stand
- Stand in parallel bars
- Single leg balance

Gait
- Ambulate in parallel bars
- Ambulate with appropriate AD on level surfaces
- Ambulate with appropriate AD on unlevel surfaces

Phase I Addendum: Post Surgical Restrictions

During the acute phase of rehabilitation patients will need to be carefully monitored to ensure appropriate healing of the myodesis/surgical repair. The following are guidelines established by the PT AMP section in accordance the primary lower extremity amputee surgeon.

Note that each surgeon has preferred methods or guidance that may deviate from the below stated recommendations based on the specifics of the case or other parameters. This protocol should not be used to the exclusion of clear communication between attending surgeon and the patient's physical therapist.

1. Partial foot amputations:
   - Heel Weight Bearing permissible.
   - Fit with shrinker ASAP to control swelling
   - No therapeutic exercise restrictions

2. Symes amputations:
   - Patients are casted x 2-3 weeks to stabilize the heel pad which is secured into the tibia. Non weight bearing for additional 3 weeks after the cast is removed (5 weeks NWB total).
   - Closed Kinetic Chain Exercises appropriate once casted (no distal end bearing in cast)
   - Expect delayed prosthetic fitting.

3. Transtibial amputations:
   - If myodesis is tenuous, the patient may be casted in knee flexion.
   - Hamstring stretching restricted x 2 weeks with tenuous myodesis. Otherwise, no therex restrictions.
   - CKC immediately if stabilization point on bolster is proximal to the myodesis.

4. Knee Disarticulation:
   - Patellar tendon is sewn into the ACL during surgery
   - Straight Leg Raise without weight x 2 weeks s/p surgery. No restrictions thereafter.
   - No restrictions to abduction or adduction therex.

5. Transfemoral amputations:
   - Myodesis of adductor magnus tendon secured to lateral femur during surgery.
     i. No active adduction strengthening exercises x 4 weeks,
     ii. No active abduction strengthening past neutral x 2 weeks (abduction to neutral from adducted posture is permissible)
     iii. No forward flexion x 2 weeks s/p myodesis to protect distal HS attachment
     iv. Bridging in supine is authorized (distal HS attachments are stabilized with proximal placement of bolster)

6. Hip Disarticulation:
   - No muscle attachments stressed with endbearing/sitting on the hip disarticulation
   - No therex restrictions once wound healing complete for end bearing.

Phase II: Preprosthetic Training (Weeks 2–10)

Patient is likely recovering from final closure and emphasis is on preparation for the prosthesis. Phase II concentrates on continued limb management to include wrapping, don and doff shrinker, contracture avoidance, desensitization/pain management, cardiovascular endurance, balance and coordination, and ambulation with AD or wheelchair activities as appropriate.

Goals: 1.   Independent with Phase I and Phase II exercises in the following areas of rehabilitation:
                  Strengthening
                  Core stability/lumbar stabilization
                  Balance
                  Cardiovascular conditioning
      2.   Independent with residual limb care and volume management
      3.   Sufficient ROM to allow optimal gait training with use of prosthetic device(s)
      4.   Independent with mobility and ambulation with appropriate AD(s)
      5.   Continue to assist with pain management

Cardiovascular
- Upper body ergometer
- Well leg bike
- Aquatic physical therapy when wounds well healed

Functional Activities
- Bed mobility
- Transfers
- Fall training
- Community re-integration
- Household activities

Range of Motion
- ROM progression as tolerated without other contraindications
- Continue contracture avoidance/stretching program
- Prone positioning, prone on elbows to prone press ups
- Scar massage

Strengthening/Lumbar Stabilization
- Isometrics
- Progressive resistive exercise of uninvolved extremities
- 4-way hip with weight progression
- Short arc quadriceps exercise with weight progression (if have painfree knee)
- Bridging
- Sky divers
- Crunches (with Transversus Abdominis contraction)
- Total gym squats
- Controlled dips
- Standing 4-way hip

Balance
- Sitting with PNF patterns (ball, resisted)
- Balance board or disk sitting
- Medicine ball catch
- Bolster under base of LE support
- Weight shift arms and legs
- Add perturbation or unstable base (Swiss Ball)
- Trunk stabilization
- Quadruped/Biped to push up (can use large round bolster)
- Wand trunk rotations with/without weights
- Diagonal movements

Gait
- Ambulation with assistive device
- Unlevel surfaces, uneven terrain, ramps

Phase III: Prosthetic Training (Weeks 11– 20)

During this phase the patient learns to use the prosthesis. Initially the amputee focuses on weight shifting and weight bearing, normalizing mechanics of available joints and motion (trunk, pelvic, hip), and ambulation with various assistive devices and prosthesis.

Goals: 1. Progressive weight bearing and weight shifting activities
2. Independent with Phase III rehab drills and exercises
3. Normalize gait
4. Progress gait to modified independence or independence with appropriate AD

Cardiovascular
- Upper body ergometer
- Calisthenics
- Bike
- Swim
- Circuit training
- Treadmill walk
- Stairmaster/Elliptical Trainer

Functional Activity
- Prosthesis management
- Picking up objects
- Stepping up curbs/ramps/hills/stairs
- Floor to chairs, floor to stand, stand to floor transfers
- Falling/ falls recovery strategies

Range of Motion
- Contracture avoidance
- HEP stretching program

Strengthening
- Upper/Lower extremity progressive resistive exercise and general strength conditioning
- Closed chain: wall squats, step ups, quadrant and plane stepping activities, steamboats, ball rolling with sound limb, trunk stabilization
- Isokinetics

Balance
- Sitting Swiss ball with activities
- Standing with prosthesis: weight shift forward, backward, lateral with progression to diagonal
- Weight shifting on soft surface
- Rocker board
- Ball rolling with sound limb
- Balance recovery
- Single leg stepping
- Single leg balance

Gait
- Component training: pelvic rotation, knee flexion
- Single leg to well leg step
- Stride width, length, cadence
- Trunk rotation
- Ambulate in parallel bars
- Ambulate with walker/crutches/canes level surfaces
- Treadmill walk

Progression
- Sideways walk
- Tandem walk
- Backward walk
- Multiple prostheses (C-leg, mechanical)

Phase IV (Months 3 – 6)

Return to progressive activities is where patients return to recreational activities and prosthetic use. For most of our population active duty military have a high level of activity prior to amputation. For others return to prior activity level may be household and family daily activities.

Goals: 1. Return to high level/high impact conditioning activities (agility drills, lower extremity plyometrics and ladder drills)
2. Initiate the return to run protocol (Transfemoral/Transtibial)
3. Return to organized and individualized sport activity utilizing developed conditioning, balance and running training base.
4. Return to vocation or MOS specific skill and task training

Cardiovascular
- Activity specific
- Walking
- Upper body ergometer
- Bike/Stairmaster/Elliptical Trainer

ROM
- Home exercise program for maintenance
- Stretching

Strengthening
- Progressive resistive exercise for overall strengthening program
- Closed chain with prosthesis
- Trunk and core strengthening

Balance
- Bilateral standing on rocker board
- Single leg standing with progressive perturbation, unlevel surfaces with ball/bodyblade
- Single leg hops
- Agility drills
- Climbing

Gait
- Progressive run/walk

Functional and Sport Specific Drills
Plyometrics
Military Skills

OUTCOME MEASURES/ FUNCTIONAL INDEX MEASURES

Gait Lab Analysis with Prosthesis
AMPPRO/AMPnoPRO
Timed Up and Go
6 Minute Walk Test (distances marked on veranda)
Transversus Abdominis Measurements
Sensory Organization Test (NeuroCom Balancemaster)
Oswestry Disability Index (ODI) for low back pain related disability
WRAMC Blast Injury Questionnaire (for blast related sequallae)

No sports until goals are met

BARBARA A. SPRINGER, PhD, PT, OCS, SCS
COL, SP
Chief, Physical Therapy Service
Integrated Department of Orthopaedics and Rehabilitation
National Naval Medical Center
Walter Reed Army Medical Center

DONALD GAJEWSKI, MD
LTC, MC
Orthopaedic Surgery Service
Integrated Department of Orthopaedics and Rehabilitation
National Naval Medical Center
Walter Reed Army Medical Center

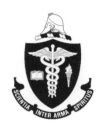

PHYSICAL THERAPY SECTION
WALTER REED ARMY MEDICAL CENTER
6900 Georgia Ave NW, Wash. D.C.
(202) 782-6371

AMPUTEE REHABILITATION ADDENDUM
BILATERAL TRANSFEMORAL PROTOCOL

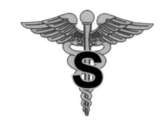

Revised May 2007

Days 1–5 on Short Prostheses

Goals:
1. Independently don/doff liners and short prostheses & liners
2. Independently roll prone/supine and transition to long sitting
3. Independently transfer in and out of wheelchair wearing prostheses
4. Independently transfer down to and up from 15 inch bench and/or bolster
5. Transfer to and from floor with stand by assist (SBA)
6. Stand in parallel bars on prosthesis x 30 minutes with no skin break down
7. Stand in parallel bars and perform tennis ball circles x 60 seconds each leg
8. Independently ambulate in parallel bars x 50 feet
9. Step up and off 3 inch step in parallel bars forward and laterally x 30 repetitions
10. Ambulate in clinic with 2 canes x 160 feet with contact guard assist (CGA)
11. Ambulate backward and laterally with 2 canes x 30 feet with CGA

Activities:
1. Don/doff liners and prostheses
2. Bed mobility/Transfers with wheelchair, bolster, to/from floor
3. Standing in parallel bars (add tennis ball circles, trunk rotation with medicine ball)
4. Ambulation in/out of parallel bars forward/backward
5. Stepping up/down from 3 inch step
6. Ensure aggressive HF stretching to allow full extension at bilateral hips
7. Patient education on importance of neutral pelvis, flat back and the role of postural alignment in functional bilateral gait

Days 5 – 15 on Short Prostheses

Gait/Stairs Goals:
1. Take prostheses home to increase wear time and tolerance to 4 hours per day
2. Ambulate with one cane x 30 feet
3. Ambulate forward with 2 canes x 600 feet with supervision s. restbreak
4. Ambulate backward and laterally with 2 canes x 50 feet with CGA and theraband around legs
5. Ambulate with one cane x 400 feet and CGA
6. Step up and off 6 inch step in parallel bars forward and laterally
7. Ascend and descent 4 steps using hands and railings with CGA

Balance/Strength Goals:
1. Perform standing chopping movements with weighted ball in parallel bars
2. Standing throw and catch weighted ball in parallel bars with supervision
3. Standing throws with weighted ball against rebounder
4. Stand on 2 dynadisks in parallel bars 1-2 minutes x 4 repetitions
5. Standing 4 way open kinetic chain hip exercises with theraband in parallel bars (can hold bars with one hand)
6. Standing upper body ergometer in prostheses x 10 minutes
7. Standing cone reaching/cone lifting in semicircle
8. Standing chest and arm exercises with universal cable pulley weights
9. Perform supine bicycle core strengthening exercise 3 x 60 seconds in prostheses
10. Perform Pelvic Girdle PNF patterns to facilitate pelvic rotation in semi-supine

Activities:
1. Increase wear time of prostheses
2. Ambulation progression (see goals)
3. Stepping progression (see goals)
4. Standing balance (see goals)

Days 16-30: Raise pylon ½ length/Add microprocessor knee if 8-10 inches clearance

Goals (reset from days 5-15 at increased height):
1. Tolerate wear of prostheses 4-6 hours per day
2. Independently ambulate with one cane x 1000 feet without rest break
3. Independently ambulate with one cane x 100 feet holding weighted ball
4. Perform weighted ball throws against rebounder standing on one dynadisk (progress to one under each foot)
5. Independently ambulate without assistive device x 50 feet

Activities:
1. Increase wear of prostheses to 4–6 hours per day (use for daily functional activities, eg, going to dining hall)
2. Ambulation progression (see goals)
3. Standing balance (see goals)

Days 31-40: Progress to bilateral microprocessor knee prostheses with one microprocessor knee locked in extension

Goals (reset from days 5-30 at increased height):
1. Stair-climbing using one microprocessor knee prosthesis to ride down step with CGA
2. Use microprocessor knee correctly (hit toe load) 95% of time during ambulation

Activities: Ambulation/balance/functional activity progression (see goals)

Note: Only after meeting all above goals will patient be progressed to bilateral fully programmed and functioning prostheses with microprocessor knee.

Days 41+: Progress to bilateral microprocessor knees prostheses with one microprocessor knee in second mode for free swing as tolerated
1. Aggressively pursue heel strikes, single leg step ups, terminal knee extension drills to develop quick contractile hamstring and gluteus maximus musculature.
2. Pursue return to running drills with one mechanical knee and one pylon when able to perform single leg step up to a 14" step x 10 repetitions or 20 unilateral LE repetitions on the total gym on level 10 with each lower extremity.

BARBARA A. SPRINGER, PhD, PT, OCS, SCS
COL, SP
Chief, Physical Therapy Service
Integrated Department of Orthopaedics and Rehabilitation
National Naval Medical Center
Walter Reed Army Medical Center

Chapter 18

OCCUPATIONAL THERAPY FOR THE POLY-TRAUMA CASUALTY WITH LIMB LOSS

LISA M. SMURR, MS, OTR/L, CHT[*]; KATHLEEN YANCOSEK, MS, OTR/L, CHT[†]; KRISTIN GULICK, OTR/L, BS, CHT[‡]; OREN GANZ, MOT, OTR/L[§]; SCOTT KULLA, MS, OTR[¥]; MELISSA JONES, PhD, OTR/L[¶]; CHRISTOPHER EBNER, MS, OTR/L[**]; AND ALBERT ESQUENAZI, MD[††]

[*]Major, Medical Specialist Corps, US Army; Assistant Chief of Occupational Therapy, Brooke Army Medical Center and Officer in Charge of Occupational Therapy, Center for the Intrepid, Brooke Army Medical Center, 3851 Roger Brooke Drive, Fort Sam Houston, Texas 78234; formerly, Chief of Occupational Therapy, Orthopaedic Podiatry, Schofield Barracks Health Clinic, Tripler Army Medical Center, 1 Jarrett White Road, Tripler Army Medical Center, Hawaii

[†]Major, Medical Specialist Corps, US Army; Graduate Student, Department of Rehabilitation Science, University of Kentucky, 923 Forest Lake Drive, Lexington, Kentucky 40515; formerly, Chief of Amputee Section of Occupational Therapy Service, Walter Reed Army Medical Center, 6900 Georgia Avenue, NW, Washington, DC

[‡]Occupational Therapist; formerly, Director of Therapy Services, Advanced Arm Dynamics, 123 West Torrance Boulevard, Suite 203, Redondo Beach, California

[§]Occupational Therapist, Department of Orthopaedics and Rehabilitation/Occupational Therapy Services, Amputee Section, Walter Reed Army Medical Center, 6900 Georgia Avenue, NW, Washington, DC 20307

[¥]Captain, Medical Specialist Corps, US Army; Chief, Department of Occupational Therapy, HHC 121 Combat Support Hospital, Box 238, APO AP 96205; formerly, Chief, Amputee Services, Department of Occupational Therapy, Center for the Intrepid, Brooke Army Medical Center, 3851 Roger Brooke Drive, Fort Sam Houston, Texas

[¶]Lieutenant Colonel (Retired), Medical Specialist Corps, US Army; formerly, Research Coordinator, Department of Orthopaedics and Rehabilitation, Walter Reed Army Medical Center, 6900 Georgia Avenue, NW, Washington, DC

[**]Occupational Therapist, Department of Orthopaedics and Rehabilitation, Brooke Army Medical Center, Center for the Intrepid, 3851 Roger Brooke Drive, Fort Sam Houston, Texas 78234; formerly, Occupational Therapist, Department of Orthopaedics and Rehabilitation, Brooke Army Medical Center, Fort Sam Houston, Texas

[††]Chair, Physical Medicine and Rehabilitation, Chief Medical Officer, MossRehab/Einstein at Elkins Park, 60 East Township Line Road, Elkins Park, Pennsylvania 19027

INTRODUCTION

As stated by Dillingham "the care of amputees is a major problem facing any Army during wartime."[1] Historically, trauma experienced in battle results in substantial numbers of upper and lower extremity amputees that far exceed those seen in civilian medicine. For this reason, amputee care in the military must remain at the forefront of rehabilitation and technology while simultaneously maintaining readiness to assume the full care of treating service members (SMs) with limb loss.[1]

Since the beginning of Operation Enduring Freedom/Operation Iraqi Freedom, over 904 patients with major limb amputations have been managed in the military healthcare system.[2] The causes of injuries include mortars, gun munitions, improvised explosive devices, vehicle-borne improvised explosive devices, and rocket-propelled grenade launchers. Given the nature of these explosive and thermal injuries, the heavily contaminated wounds are left open to allow for multiple debridements and washouts in the operating room. Frequently, multiple extremities are involved and although injury patterns may be similar, no two patients are alike. As a result of the high force velocity and high temperatures at the time of injury concomitant injuries often occur. These range from traumatic brain injury (TBI) to visual loss, hearing loss, massive soft tissue loss, fractures, burns, and nerve and vascular damage. The severity and complexity of these polytrauma injuries in addition to amputation(s) complicate rehabilitation. Occupational therapy (OT) is critical in the treatment of patients with upper limb amputation. The focus of OT is on the patient's ability to engage in purposeful and meaningful activities. Human occupations may be work, leisure, or self-care related. Most occupations are performed with the hands and thus the role of the occupational therapist is to assist the amputee to perform these occupations with and without a prosthesis through the use of compensatory strategies or adaptive and durable medical equipment.

To address the rehabilitation needs of those individuals who have sustained complex polytrauma injuries in addition to upper limb amputation(s), a standardized, comprehensive, and multidimensional four-phase protocol of care was developed with a focus of achieving maximum reintegration into the community and resuming previous or assuming new occupational roles. The development of this protocol was most influenced by the *Model of Human Occupation* by Gary Kielhofner.[3] This theoretical framework facilitates understanding of the impairments, activity limitations, and participant restrictions resulting from limb loss, especially when accompanied by the comorbidities experienced by many patients.[3]

The *Model of Human Occupation* addresses the acquisition of preliminary and advanced performance skills, the underlying volition or motivation of patients required to engage in occupation, and the habituation required for use of the prosthesis while engaging in multiple roles and daily routines in their social and physical environments.[3] The goal of OT intervention for patients with limb loss is returning them to their potential for maximum performance of daily occupations that lead to a meaningful and satisfying life. OT provides the patient the necessary skills and tools to reintegrate back into the military unit or to civilian life physically, psychologically, and socially. Inherent in this overall goal is for SMs to successfully integrate the use of a prosthesis into their basic motor skill set if they so choose. The authors have termed the successful integration of the prosthesis as prosthetic acceptance or prosthetic integration.

The environments for amputee rehabilitation at the military amputee centers of excellence, such as Brooke Army Medical Center, Walter Reed Army Medical Center, and Naval Medical Center San Diego, are ideal settings because occupational therapists and prosthetists specializing in upper extremity amputee rehabilitation and prosthetics, respectively, are on site working jointly in the care and management of upper extremity amputees. Additionally, SMs stay on the campus of each facility while they undergo comprehensive rehabilitation and reintegration into the community with their prosthesis.

FOUR-PHASE UPPER LIMB AMPUTEE PROTOCOL OF CARE

As previously stated, the goal of OT intervention is for patients with limb loss to return to their highest potential for performance of daily occupations that lead them to a meaningful and satisfying life. To meet this objective a four-phase upper limb rehabilitation protocol is used. Phase one addresses initial management and protective healing; phase two marks the introduction of preprosthetic training; phase three addresses intermediate prosthetic training; and phase four focuses on advanced prosthetic training. Throughout each phase, discharge planning and community reintegration are incorporated and addressed to meet the patients' needs. Overlap occurs between each phase that is bidirectional to allow flexibility of patient progression based on severity of injuries, wound healing, and patient tolerance. The patient may regress in the protocol because of secondary problems of wound infection and delayed closure, heterotropic ossification, residual limb hypersensitivity, or other conditions resulting from concomitant injuries. Throughout each phase care is individualized to meet the needs of each patient, and as the patient becomes medically stable occupation-based goals are established. Also phases are repeated as necessary with each prosthesis that the patient acquires. With training of subsequent prosthetic use, the user's ability to master the foundational skills and perform functional tasks is rapid.

PHASE ONE: INITIAL MANAGEMENT AND PROTECTIVE HEALING

The primary overarching rehabilitation goals of this phase are to promote wound closure and educate the patient and family (Exhibit 18-1). This phase begins immediately after the injury and continues until all wounds have successfully closed and are free of infection. The time in this phase varies depending on the extent of the injury, but generally lasts from 1 to 3 weeks after admission. Patients and family members are introduced to rehabilitative and prosthetic services in the early stage of this phase. It is imperative that these interventions begin early to reduce uncertainties and fears, provide support throughout the grieving and recovery processes, and engage the patient and family with the rehabilitative team. The components of this phase include comprehensive evaluation, wound healing, edema control, desensitization and scar management, pain control, exercise, flexibility, gross motor activity, and psychological support. Basic activities of daily living (ADLs) include those activities that are involved in personal body care.[4]

Evaluation

A comprehensive evaluation of the patient is administered in a holistic and multidisciplinary approach to obtain baseline information about functional status, background, abilities, and future goals. This complete evaluation provides the rehabilitation team with a

---

EXHIBIT 18-1

PHASE ONE: BASIC REHABILITATION GOALS

Goals: 1 to 3 Weeks after Admission

1. All open wounds will be clean, dry, and free from infection.
2. Patient will perform self-feeding, oral hygiene, and toilet hygiene with the use of adaptive equipment and set up as necessary.
3. Patient will wear a form of compressive limb wrap 24 hours a day that extends above the most distal joint.
4. Patient will elevate the limb(s) as appropriate.
5. Patient will visually inspect residual limb.
6. Patient will tolerate tactile input on residual limb.
7. Patient will demonstrate independence in desensitization home exercise program.
8. Patient will tolerate scar massage.
9. Patient will assist in massage.
10. Patient will have functional active range of motion in bilateral extremities.
11. Patient will perform therapeutic exercise daily to prevent de-conditioning.
12. Patient will perform postural exercises with a focus on body symmetry.
13. Patient will receive support from the therapist through discussion of future function, which may include video of other prosthetic users.
14. Patient and the patient's family will receive information about the prosthetic rehabilitation process.
15. Patient and the patient's family will receive information about available types of prostheses and their differences.
16. Patient and the patient's family will receive information about the stages of grieving the loss of a limb and change in body image.

comprehensive assessment of the patient's physical and emotional baseline status.

The patient's medical history is obtained with special attention to all injuries that impact care and long-term goals. Current medications and the patient's response to these medications are documented. The evaluation includes an indepth information-gathering interview with the patient and family members to identify premorbid lifestyle and occupational roles, hand dominance, educational level, vocation, and recreational interests. Given the military's mobile nature, the patient's current living situation is reviewed to determine the level of family support available and any physical or environmental limitations within the current home environment that may be problematic once the patient returns home.

It is critical to screen each patient's psychosocial status. Information is gathered on the patient's current emotional state and his or her premorbid emotional resiliency. This helps the therapist to prepare for the next therapy session because it provides an understanding of where the patient came from and what he or she is going through emotionally. If possible, current knowledge, thoughts, and fears regarding amputation are also assessed. An understanding of the patient's previous exposure to amputees informs the therapist of the patient's possible perception of their injury. At the end of the evaluation, depending on the mental and emotional status and interest of the patient, a discussion is initiated regarding prosthetic rehabilitation and prosthetic options.

The objective components of the evaluation include the following:

- basic ADLs,
- upper quadrant range of motion (ROM) on the intact side,
- bilateral manual muscle testing,
- limb volume measurement,
- wound description,
- scar evaluation,
- pain (phantom and residual limb pain), and
- sensation of the residual and intact limb.

It is important for the therapist and prosthetist to assess residual limb sensation because areas of hyposensitivity or hypersensitivity are necessary considerations in the fabrication and fitting of the prosthetic socket. The evaluation includes a thorough assessment of pain of the residual limb, phantom pain, and its differentiation from phantom sensation.

A functional evaluation is completed to assess baseline basic ADL performance in bathing/showering, bowel and bladder management, toilet hygiene,

upper and lower body dressing, personal hygiene and grooming, eating, sleep/rest, and functional transfers to include bed, chair, wheelchair, toilet, and shower transfers. Each area is assessed to determine the amount of physical and/or cognitive assistance that is required to complete the task. A rating of modified independent is given if the patient can complete the task with increased time or the use of adaptive equipment; a rating of supervision is given if the patient requires supervision to safely complete the task; a rating of minimal assistance is given if the patient requires contact guard-25% assistance to complete the task; moderate assistance if the patient requires 25% to 50% assistance; maximum assistance if the patient requires 50% to 75% assistance; and total assistance if the patient requires 75% to 100% assistance. All aspects of this ADL evaluation may be completed in one or several days depending on the patient's tolerance.

Prehension evaluations are performed as appropriate for each patient. Although no standardized evaluation for prehension deficits is identified in this population, it is necessary to determine baseline function of the remaining limb because the intact limb will be responsible for conducting all fine motor and dexterity tasks for vocational, leisure, and occupational purposes. Useful evaluations include the Jebson Taylor test of hand function; Minnesota Rate of Manipulation Test, Boxes and Blocks; and Nine Hole Peg tests.

Activities of Daily Living

The evaluation findings and assessment provide a foundation on which to build the treatment program. One of OT's major goals is to help the individual gain independence in self-care. This is a critical component that should be addressed very early when working with an amputee because a sense of dependence can lead to feelings of helplessness. This sense of helplessness is a common response after the loss of a limb; however, the degree of helplessness tends to be greater in the bilateral upper limb amputee. Therefore, it is essential for the rehabilitation team to assist the patient in gaining a sense of independence and control over his or her environment as soon as possible, preferably while still in the acute phase. Three ADLs that the occupational therapist should address in the first treatments include (1) toilet hygiene, (2) self-feeding, and (3) oral hygiene. These are some of the most rudimentary basic ADLs that can help the patient feel some sense of independence. Such adaptive equipment as toilet hygiene devices, use of foot-operated bidet, universal cuffs, and pump bottles can improve self-sufficiency in these tasks for the unilateral amputee.

Depending on the severity of injuries and medical

stability of the patient, performance in additional basic ADLs may not be appropriate. Areas such as dressing, showering, and facial hygiene are addressed in phase two. However, if patients are medically stable and wounds are healed, phase two ADL training may be initiated earlier. Patients whose wounds and medical status do not allow progression to these ADLs are encouraged to wear loose-fitting pullover shirts, athletic shorts or pants, and slip-on shoes with traction on the sole to prevent falls. Adaptive equipment, such as a reacher and a dressing stick, is issued to patients as appropriate. Patients who are unable to use adaptive equipment require creativity on the part of the occupational therapist to achieve maximal independence in one-handed dressing strategies. See "Activities of Daily Living, Adaptive Equipment, and Change of Dominance" under phase two for some of these additional strategies.

Wound Healing

Wounds are left open for operative washouts and to avoid closed-space infections and tissue loss. Various procedures to promote healing are utilized depending on the type and size of the wound. If allograft soft tissue is used for skin coverage, drains are placed as appropriate. Wounds greater than 5 cm in depth are kept free from infection through intraoperative placement of antibiotic beads that are replaced surgically as necessary. Another strategy involves the use of vacuum-assisted closure systems, or negative pressure wound therapy. This technique is designed to promote the formation of granular tissue in the wound bed through intraoperative placement of sterile foam dressing with an evacuation tube placed over the dressing via an adhesive barrier creating an airtight seal around the wound. Negative pressure is applied by way of the evacuation tube, which is attached to an external canister to collect the wound exudate. The negative pressure therapy system is maintained until the wound enters the granulation stage and the wound edges draw closer together.

During initial residual limb wound healing, occupational therapists perform wound care and dressing changes according to physician guidelines. Also, a figure-of-eight wrap is used for distal to proximal compression and shaping over the healing distal aspect of the residual limb. Once the wound stops draining, the patient progresses to a sewn Compressogrip sleeve (AliMed, Dedham, Mass) or the use of Tubegrip (Valco Cincinnati Inc, Cincinnati, Ohio), which is tapered at the distal end of the residual limb. As the wound closes and the mature scar tissue forms, the patient and the family are instructed in the application and wear of a silicone liner that provides continuous force compression with the added benefit of minimizing hypertrophic scar tissue formation.

One of the goals for the patient, or his or her family member as appropriate, is to be able to independently don and doff compression garments. The compression garments are changed frequently throughout the day to maintain consistent concentric pressure from the distal to proximal margins of the residual limb. Edema control measures are implemented to assist in decreasing limb volume to prepare for fitting a preparatory prosthesis.

Desensitization

Desensitization is initiated promptly through the use of the aforementioned compression techniques. When the wound progresses to the granulation stage and drainage ceases, antibacterial ointment is applied to the wound bed for use with gentle massage and wound debridement, if necessary. As the wound closes, desensitization is initiated through tapping and the use of texture bins for immersion of the hypersensitive limb. Desensitization is critical and is performed daily as the patient's skin and scar tolerates. Reduction in residual limb hypersensitivity improves tolerance to wearing the prosthetic socket. Desensitization training is tailored for each patient depending on level of hypersensitivity and wound status. Patients and family members are also instructed in limb massage and desensitization to continue therapy outside of the clinic because this is critical for success.

Upper Limb Flexibility, Body Symmetry, and Exercise

The weeks immediately postamputation are the most critical in terms of implementing a comprehensive exercise program. The specific exercise program goals are established with physician guidance and coordinated between occupational, physical, and recreational therapies. The exercise program focuses on four main components: (1) flexibility, (2) body symmetry with exercise, (3) incorporation of the residual limb into activity to assist with desensitization and increase residual limb tolerance to pressure, and (4) muscle strengthening, the latter being addressed in phase two.

Daily maintenance of upper limb flexibility following amputation is critical to prepare the residual limb for prosthetic use. Initially, mat exercises should be utilized to promote independent upper limb mobility. Low load prolonged stretch to the shoulder flexors, abductors, and rotators as well as the scapular protractors and retractors is a priority because limitation of shoulder motion may result in rejection of the prosthesis.[5] The patient is then instructed to consistently increase the duration and daily frequency of the stretch. Each stretch should be performed for a minimum of five repetitions and held for 30 seconds in each joint direction. If self-stretches are not successful, then manual assisted stretching must be implemented with possible augmentation through facilitatory techniques. Good success has been achieved using proprioceptive neuromuscular facilitation techniques of contract-relax and slow-reversal for those patients demonstrating significant muscle guarding.[6] Pain medication, hydrotherapy, ultrasound, and other physical modalities may also be incorporated into the stretch program.

Incorrect postures may lead to cumulative trauma or overuse injuries of the upper limbs, neck, or back; therefore, emphasis is placed on proper body mechanics and awareness of body symmetry during activity. Visual feedback is the technique of choice for body symmetry awareness training and instruction often begins with observation of static postures in front of a mirror. Training quickly progresses to performance of dynamic therapeutic activities in front of a mirror. Additionally, the therapist provides verbal and tactile cues as necessary to maintain proper body symmetry. The patient is educated and encouraged to check his or her posture regularly when in front of a mirror during routine daily activities such as oral hygiene.

Patients with transradial level amputations or longer should be able to bear some weight directly through their residual limb. Early weight-bearing activities can reduce complaints of residual and phantom limb pain and prepare the residual limb for prosthetic usage.

Amputees must develop improved aerobic fitness levels because of the increased demands associated with prosthetic use. Exercise after limb loss is further enhanced through patient participation in physical therapy to address core strengthening and cardiovascular endurance (see Chapter 17, Physical Therapy for the Polytrauma Casualty With Limb Loss).

Pain Management Strategies throughout Rehabilitation

Amputee associated pain is broken into two distinct categories: (1) phantom limb pain and (2) residual limb pain. Phantom limb pain is described as pain in an absent limb or portion of a limb.[7] Residual limb pain is described as pain in the part of the limb remaining after the amputation.[8] These types of pain are acknowledged as two separate entities and have both common and unique treatment approaches for management.

Nonpharmacological pain management in the immediate postoperative period includes appropriate therapeutic interventions based on the type and origin of the pain. Treatment modalities include transcuta-

neous electrical nerve stimulation, ice, heat, contrast baths, massage, functional tasks to encourage normal motor pattern of the painful extremity, desensitization, and continuous psychological support in addition to psychiatric and pain management services. In some cases, an individual with a severely hypersensitive residual limb may benefit from desensitization 20 minutes five times per day until the sensitivity improves.[9] The use of a mirror box, in which the uninvolved side is visually reflected as the missing side, has been shown to decrease phantom pain in some cases.[10,11] Interventions for pain control are continuous through the multiple phases of the rehabilitation program.

Phantom sensation is any nonpainful sensory phenomenon in an absent limb.[7] Phantom sensation is frequently experienced after limb amputation and can be a concern to patients; therefore, it is important to reassure them that this is normal. The patient's experience of phantom limb sensation may change over time; research suggests that use of a prosthesis may improve phantom limb pain.[12,13]

Psychological Support

Psychological support is essential for successful rehabilitation and begins during the first interaction with the patient. Psychological support offered by OT during this phase encompasses patient and family education that facilitates coping and management of limb loss.

Psychological issues frequently seen in an amputee population include (*a*) fear of the unknown, (*b*) loss of self-esteem, (*c*) loss of self-confidence, (*d*) change in body image, (*e*) fear of rejection, and (*f*) loss of occupational roles. In the initial stage, patients are supported appropriately as their needs change. Intervention is provided by the entire interdisciplinary team. The goal is to successfully transition the patient to "real life" after hospitalization. Methods of psychological support include the following:

- education on the rehabilitative process to allay fears of the unknown,
- reinforcement of the patient's personal style,
- reassurance of normalcy of the patient's response to amputation,
- involvement in preventative medical psychiatry,
- engagement in empathetic interaction with both the patient and family,
- development of confidence and self-esteem,
- promotion of success in tasks and activities,
- encouragement to develop his or her identity, and
- engagement in weekly therapeutic outings.

PHASE TWO: PREPROSTHETIC TRAINING

Approximately 2 to 3 weeks after injury, depending on the patient's medical circumstances and concomitant injuries, he or she progresses into phase two of the protocol (Exhibit 18-2). The goal of this phase is to prepare the patient and the limb to receive a well-fit prosthetic socket and functional prosthesis. This phase begins at wound closure and ends with acquisition of a preparatory prosthesis, or an early postoperative prosthesis. Time spent in this phase varies depending on limb volume, sensitivity, ROM, physical condition of the residual limb, and the patient's psychological status. Therefore, portions of phase one continue as necessary to address these deficits.

Psychological Support through the Grieving Process to Acceptance

Patients entering the second phase may require additional psychological support from therapy as they progress emotionally from combat survival mode, through the awareness that they have survived a combat-related injury, to the realization that they will have to live with an altered body. Psychological support is continued and modified as necessary to appropriately respond to the patients' rapidly changing needs as they advance through the grieving process. As the patient demonstrates signs of acceptance of the injury, he or she is informed about the many

---

EXHIBIT 18-2

PHASE TWO: PREPROSTHETIC TRAINING: UNILATERAL AND BILATERAL AMPUTEE REHABILITATION GOALS

Rehabilitation Goals Specific to Unilateral Amputee

Goals: 1 to 4 Weeks after Admission

1. Patient will be independent in dressing using one-handed techniques.
2. Patient will be independent in light hygiene and showering with use of adaptive equipment as necessary.
3. Patient will be independent in donning compressive garment.
4. Patient will demonstrate in-hand manipulation without dropping items.
5. Patient will demonstrate functional prehensile patterns with an eating utensil.
6. Patient will demonstrate functional prehensile patterns with a writing utensil in the residual hand.
7. Patient will demonstrate proper position of body and paper for writing.
8. Patient will sign his or her name.
9. Patient will write a sentence.

Rehabilitation Goals Specific to Bilateral Amputee

Goals: 1 to 4 Weeks after Admission

1. Patient will receive adaptive equipment and technique training to maximize independence in self-feeding, oral hygiene, toileting, and dressing.

Common Unilateral and Bilateral Amputee Rehabilitation Goals

1. Patient will tolerate a compressive garment on the residual limbs 24 hours a day.
2. Once full range of motion is achieved, patient will tolerate a resistive upper body strengthening program.
3. Patient will be able to isolate two opposing myosites (ie, flexors and extensors).
4. Patient will be able to equally co-contract two opposing myosites.
5. Patient will tolerate myosite training daily.
6. Continue phase one goals as necessary (ie, scar management and desensitization).

possibilities of function with a prosthesis. Patients who choose to wear a prosthesis are educated on the reality of prosthetic function because individuals have varying perceptions of a prosthesis ranging from that of a picture of Captain Hook to the opposite extreme of a superhuman bionic arm. Adding peer support or a peer visitor significantly helps the patient. A peer support with a similar level of amputation can help educate about realistic expectations, provide a real life perspective of living with such an injury, and may potentially become a support with whom the patient can relate to throughout recovery. These peer visitors are trained individuals accessed through organizations such as the Amputee Coalition of America in Knoxville, Tennessee.

Patients may also participate in the Promoting Amputee Life Skills program, an 8-week course designed to teach persons with limb loss the skills to help them deal with problems they may encounter. The goals of the course are to reduce pain, depression, and anxiety, and to improve each person's ability to problem solve, communicate with family and friends, and improve overall quality of life.

Peak performance training, developed at the Center of Enhanced Performance at the US Military Academy, provides a method to effectively train individuals to develop mental and emotional attributes to efficiently operate in a fluid and ambiguous environment. The specific topics introduced include (*a*) confidence building, (*b*) goal setting, (*c*) attention control, (*d*) stress and energy management, and (*e*) visualization and imagery. Education and training to develop each skill is provided with the goal of the individual being able to ultimately achieve self-awareness, mental agility, and adaptability to overcome and thrive in demanding environments throughout recovery and future challenges.[14] This training may assist amputees to overcome the psychological hurdles throughout their emotional recovery and rehabilitation.[14]

It has been the experience of this rehabilitation team that the patient rapidly progresses through grieving during phase two. The supportive psychological services available, the therapeutic milieu, participation with other individuals with limb loss, and the performance of ADLs in an environment promoting recovery provide the basis to achieve psychological adjustment. Patients who successfully negotiate the grieving process frequently begin to verbalize or display their injury in a humorous light. For example, patients purchase and wear various clothing paraphernalia with sayings such as "dude where's my leg," or "IEDs suck." Although many of the statements are a crude representation of humor, they provide a valuable clinical sign that the individual has "broken through" the grieving process, entered the acceptance phase of recovery, and can project humor in regards to amputation.

Activities of Daily Living, Adaptive Equipment, and Change of Dominance

During phase two the patient becomes more independent with basic ADLs as the wounds heal. Independence in toileting, self-feeding, and oral hygiene is achieved during phase one, and the patient progresses to showering, dressing, personal hygiene, grooming, sexual activity, functional mobility, and laundry activities during phase two. The patient is introduced to various adaptive aids and compensatory techniques for one-handed ADL performance. Adaptive equipment offered includes (*a*) modified long-handled sponges, (*b*) one-handed nail clippers, (*c*) nail brush, (*d*) wash mitt, and (*e*) any other additional equipment necessary to achieve independence. In addition, custom adaptive equipment is fabricated as necessary for the patient to return to one-handed ADL independence. Data obtained through patient report revealed that the most helpful adaptive aids include the following:

- one-handed nail clipper and nail brush,
- modified long-handled sponges,
- elastic shoe laces,
- wash mitts,
- pump bottles,
- rocker knives or Knorks (Phantom Enterprises Inc, North Newton, Kans), and
- one-handed cutting boards.

Most patients prefer to minimize the number of adaptive aids because of the constrictions that equipment may pose for flexibility in task performance in different environments.

The bilateral upper limb amputee requires special attention to complete basic ADLs. Techniques and modifications listed in Table 18-1 (also shown in Figure 18-1) are basic ideas to assist the individual in achieving independence in ADLs. This table is not an exhaustive list. Once patients receive ADL training, they may continue to modify techniques and the environment to meet their individual needs. Many bilateral upper limb amputees become adept at using the environment, body movements, their mouths, and their lower extremities to assist themselves. However, significant use of the mouth is discouraged to prevent damage to the teeth and jaw. It is reasonable to expect that patients with bilateral transradial amputations will be independent with all ADLs and active in their chosen occupations. A patient with bilateral shoulder

TABLE 18-1

BILATERAL UPPER EXTREMITY ACTIVITY OF DAILY LIVING TASK SAMPLE TECHNIQUE OPTIONS AND CONSIDERATIONS

ADL Task	Sample Technique Options	Considerations
Toileting	• Use of a bidet. • Squatting down and using one's heel that is covered with toilet paper or hygienic wipes. • Placing toilet paper that is folded back on itself repeatedly on the toilet seat with the tail of the toilet paper dropped into the water to secure it.	• The prosthetic device must have wrist flexion and rotation if the prosthetic user is to perform toilet hygiene without other aids. This ability is patient dependent. • It is helpful for patients to try to develop a regular bowel program so that they can plan to be in a location where the environment is ideal for them to care for themselves. Otherwise it can be helpful to carry a supply of hygienic wipes when they are out in public.
Feeding	• Use of Dycem (Dycem Limited, Warwick Central Industrial Park, RI) or some nonskid material secures the plate or bowl and prevents sliding. • Use of a rocker knife or Knork (Phantom Enterprises Inc, North Newton, Kans) for cutting. When in a restaurant the person can ask for meat to be pre-cut before being brought to the table. • Use of a straw for liquids. • Use of a plate with a rim or a broad bowl to allow for ease in loading the utensil. • Some patients are comfortable bringing their mouth to the tabletop.	• A prosthesis that supports maximal elbow flexion, wrist rotation, and wrist flexion will allow patients to feed themselves with unmodified utensils. • Finger foods are often the most difficult due to the significant amount of ROM required to get to the mouth without the added length of the utensil.
Dressing	**Upper body dressing** • Pullover clothing should be placed at a higher height to allow patients to easily bend over and use their residual limbs in concert with their mouth to get the shirt over their limbs and head. At this point using body motion will assist in getting the shirt down over the torso. If patients have difficulty getting the shirt over their torso, have them lie down and maneuver on a bed. • Open-front shirts can be donned while hanging from a hook or hanger, again using the lower extremities to hold the tails of the shirt or the mouth to hold the collar to adjust the fit. • Jackets are donned easier if the cuffs are loose. • Buttons can be fastened using hook terminal devices or a button hook, or they can be modified by applying Velcro (Velcro USA Inc, Manchester, NH) closures. Buttons higher up at the neck are the most challenging. • Zippers can be more easily fastened with stable catches and a good pull tab or added string or monofilament line pull. • Pretied ties are the easiest to don.	• The patient with bilateral upper limb loss may find that loose-fitting clothing with limited fasteners will be easier to manage.

(**Table 18-1** *continues*)

Table 18-1 *continued*

ADL Task	Sample Technique Options	Considerations
	Lower body dressing	
	• Garments with elastic waists will ease lower body dressing. Using a non-skid material like Dycem (Dycem Limited, Warwick Central Industrial Park, RI) mounted on the wall slightly below waist height can be used to assist in raising or lowering lower body garments.	
	• Socks with loose cuffs that have been rolled down facilitate donning. Sock aids are useful to some patients.	
	• Donning shoes is made easier by using slip-on shoes, Velcro (Velcro USA Inc, Manchester, NH) closures, elastic laces, or a variety of lace holders.	
	• Preplacing a belt in the loops before donning pants makes donning a belt easier.	
	• The hooks mounted on a donning stand or in a wall can be helpful for various aspects of dressing.	
Bathing	• Bathing may be performed by using elastic shower mitts over the end of the residual limb or by using a suction-mounted brush or scrubbing material.	• It is critical to ensure a safe environment during bathing because a fall, when one does not have upper limbs to protect oneself, can be devastating. Using a nonskid mat in the tub provides secure footing in a slippery environment. Some patients may prefer to use a tub bench. A floor-to-ceiling pole can assist with getting in or out of a tub if a patient has one transradial length limb.
	• Soap and shampoo can be applied from a wall-mounted soap dispenser or from pump dispenser type of bottles.	
	• Drying oneself can be done easily with a terry cloth type of robe that hangs allowing ease of donning.	
	• Drying can also be done with a wall or countertop-mounted hairdryer.	
Hygiene	• Shaving is more easily performed with an electric shaver. A modified gooseneck with a clamp that is mounted to the wall can hold the shaver and be moved to access areas of the face (Figure 18-1). Women can sit and use a prosthetic device to shave their lower extremities. Women can consider laser hair removal, waxing, or electrolysis as an option for hair removal.	• Performing hygiene activities independently can be done with use of prosthetic devices, adaptive equipment, modifications to the environment, and use of many products made for the general public.
	• Brushing teeth can be performed with prosthetic devices or a mounted extension with a clamp. Using an electric toothbrush can facilitate better oral hygiene.	
	• Trimming toenails can be done with a larger nail clipper mounted on a suction board. This can be operated with a prosthesis or the other foot depending on dexterity.	
	• Use of a gooseneck arm with a clamp that is wall mounted can be useful to hold shavers, toothbrushes, and hair dryers. Commercially available hair dryer holders are helpful as well.	

ADL: activity of daily living
ROM: range of motion

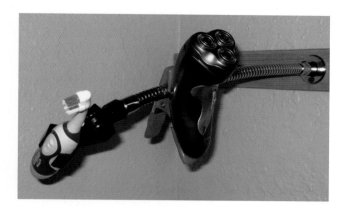

Figure 18-1. An example of a modified gooseneck clamp mounted to a wall. It provides a versatile method for a patient with bilateral limb loss to perform a variety of activities of daily living tasks independently.

disarticulation amputation will most likely require some assistance for certain ADLs despite the use of prosthetic devices and environmental modifications.

As a bilateral upper limb amputee becomes more independent in some basic ADLs, the learned skills necessary to achieve independence in these tasks will transfer when learning more complex daily living tasks. Initial training will require the therapist to be creative and the patient to be willing to try various approaches to a task to identify the best option. Once an ideal approach is identified repetition is necessary to habituate the new skill set into the motor repertoire to become more efficient in task performance. Additionally, learning more complex tasks will often occur with less frustration and more ease. Ultimately, each patient chooses the method(s) and equipment that work most effectively for him or her.

As mastery in basic ADLs is achieved the patient begins to explore instrumental ADLs, which are those activities that are complex and involve interaction with the physical and cognitive environment.[4] Instrumental ADLs addressed during phase two include the use of communication devices, light meal preparation and cleanup, financial management, mobility in the community, and safety and emergency response procedures. Depending on the patient's circumstances additional adaptive equipment recommendations are made in preparation for discharge.

In addition to progression toward instrumental ADLs, change of hand dominance training is introduced as necessary. Some patients perform this task with hesitation because they hope to use the prosthesis to perform writing tasks. However, based on the limitation of fine motor prehension and dexterity capabilities of any available prosthesis, it is impor-

tant to transfer hand dominance for writing skills to reestablish independence in written communication. Fine motor activities include using tweezers, pumping spray bottles, twisting caps on and off, twisting nuts on and off of bolts, performing lacing activities on a vertical surface, and rolling putty balls. These activities encourage radial digit coordination, separation of radial and ulnar sides of the hand, and wrist extension. These are necessary motor components of handwriting. The patient learns rote penmanship exercises through progressive motor writing activities culminating in sentences with at least one character each from the alphabet: "The quick brown fox jumped over the lazy dogs." Bilateral upper limb amputees are encouraged to use a terminal device (TD) of their choice in order to gain the necessary skills for writing with a prosthesis.

At some point during the second phase of the protocol, most patients may be discharged from inpatient status, depending on medical status, comorbidities, and ability to perform self-care in a controlled living environment, such as a hotel on the military campus. This event marks a transition in the patient's recovery as he or she leaves the structure and safety of the hospital environment and is encouraged and successfully challenged to regain full independence. Evaluations similar to home evaluation are performed as necessary in this new living environment to ensure competence and confidence in ADL performance and reinforce the family members' caregiving responsibilities.

Postural Exercises and Strengthening

During phase two upper quadrant flexibility, postural exercises for body symmetry, residual limb weight bearing, and physical therapy are continued. Once the patient is medically stable and pain is controlled, early mobilization, general progressive strengthening and muscular endurance exercises are initiated with emphasis on the shoulder girdle and proximal residual limb to prevent joint contractures. Strengthening of the remaining upper limb musculature is aggressively pursued to prepare the patient for the weight and upper body strength demands of the donned prosthesis. Specificity of training is the preferred method to emphasize the remaining limb strength and function.

Strengthening exercises include isometric and isotonic contraction with modification to allow for use of the residual limb. Individuals who receive a body-powered prosthesis must strengthen the muscles that control shoulder flexion and scapular protraction, retraction, and depression because these gross body movements are used to control the prosthesis.

Rote practice of these movements early in rehabilitation will encourage muscle memory of those motions allowing for easier training once the patient receives the prosthesis.

The muscles that stabilize the gleno-humeral and scapulo-thoracic joints include the trapezius, serratus anterior, rotator cuff, and deltoid groups. These muscles play an important role in functional activity; therefore, a balance in muscle strength between these groups is critical to optimize prosthetic use. Scapular protraction, shoulder shrugging, and seated push-ups will help ensure proper scapular positioning for smooth gleno-humeral rhythm.[15] A spectrum of internal and external rotation up to 90 degrees in the scapular plane will maintain proper humeral head depression during shoulder elevation motions. Additionally, elbow stability should be maintained through bicep and tricep strengthening. Various therapeutic equipment and tools utilized for strengthening include Thera-Band and Baltimore Therapuetic Equipment (BTE Technologies, Hanover, Md). As the patient's endurance and residual limb tolerance to pressure improves, resisted exercises and weight-lifting activities involving the upper extremities should be considered. Trunk stability and core strengthening are also emphasized.

Myosite Testing and Training

Due to the rapid medical evacuation of an SM from the battlefield to the medical center, early and aggressive prosthetic rehabilitation is possible. For this reason, SMs are fitted with electric prosthetic systems that create less shear force and end-bearing forces on the healing residual limb. In instances where early prosthetic fitting is not possible, the residual limb may require further preparation for either a body-powered or electric prosthesis. Many SMs are fit with an activity-specific prosthesis that allows them to participate in meaningful leisure and recreational activities.

Research has demonstrated that individuals in the general amputee population fit with a prosthesis within 30 days of amputation exhibited a 93% rehabilitation success rate with a 100% return to work rate within 4 months of injury. Those fit beyond 30 days exhibited a 42% rehabilitation success rate with a 15% return to work rate within 6 to 24 months. This 30-day period is termed the "golden window."[16] The extensive polytrauma incurred during combat complicates the rehabilitation team's ability to achieve initial prosthetic fitting on combat-injured patients within this golden window. The impact of this problem has been managed through the use of training technology. Within 2 to 3 weeks postinjury, patients treated begin socket electrode site identification and training necessary

for operation of a myoelectric prosthesis. The goals of this early intervention training are to identify, instruct, and train the patient to independently, correctly, and efficiently use specific residual limb musculature to activate and perform basic myoelectric prosthesis functions resulting in the ability to immediately operate the myoelectric prosthesis at first fitting.

Electrode site identification occurs in OT with use of socket electrodes (Figure 18-2) hooked up to a biofeedback unit, such as the MyoBoy (Otto Bock, Minneapolis, Minn), or the MyoLabII (Motion Control, Inc, Salt Lake City, Utah). Site selection involves multiple factors and requires the specialized skill of trained therapists and prosthetists to determine the proper and best available sites. The sites located in the training are used to identify the correct placement of the electrodes within the future prosthetic socket. The rehabilitation team works closely together during this stage to identify the best possible electrode placement and the most effective control scheme for each patient's particular abilities and needs.

Many factors affect the optimal muscle site selection. Ideally a flexor muscle—used to operate TD closing and pronation—and an extensor muscle—used to operate TD opening and supination—are identified. However, many patients do not have two available sites or have undergone reconstruction resulting in nonanatomic tissue presentation of the residual limb. These cases require team creativity and individual encouragement. Other issues to consider include (*a*) scar and graft site locations because the signal is not as easily transmitted through dense tissue, (*b*) identification of an appropriate superficial muscle site for a stronger signal, and (*c*) continuous contact between the skin and electrode at the selected myosite throughout the maximum ROM of the residual limb. The latter requires special attention during this process. For

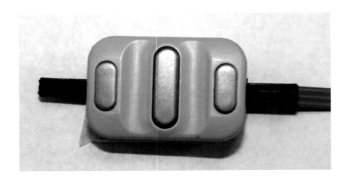

Figure 18-2. Socket electrode used for myoelectric training. This same type of electrode is placed within the myoelectric prosthetic socket.
Photograph courtesy of Otto Bock.

example, if an electrode is placed over a proximal residual limb muscle that is activated during an activity such as reaching, the individual will perform inadvertent operation of the prosthesis and experience frustration. A quality muscle signal is characterized by an adequate electromyogram output that is isolated from the antagonist muscle. Once the best sites are identified, motor training begins.

Motor training takes place using computer-based MyoSoft software attached to the MyoBoy hardware (Otto Bock, Minneapolis, Minn) and the socket electrodes. On an electromyogram-like screen, the patient can visualize color-coded signals, representative of each of the selected electrode site muscles, as they are activated for the corresponding TD operation (Figure 18-3). Initially, the focus of training is on independent activation of each muscle. When the patient is able to demonstrate separation of these muscle signals, the concept of proportional control is introduced. Proportional control is a term used to describe the proportional relationship of the elicited strength of the selected muscle contraction to the speed and grip force of the TD. Many myoelectric components use this type of control. It is more physiologic and predictable for the patient than previously used digital control systems. Depending on the manufacturer of the system, the

gain (sensitive) of the electrodes may be manually adjusted. This allows the therapist to amplify or dampen the strength of the received signal from the muscle contraction to modulate prosthetic output. Changes in the gain may need to be made frequently as the individual develops mastery of control and increased muscle strength.

The initial myosite training takes place with the upper limb in a relaxed position at or near midline. As the patient develops control in this plane, introduction of limb placement in various positions is initiated to

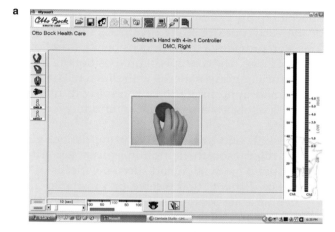

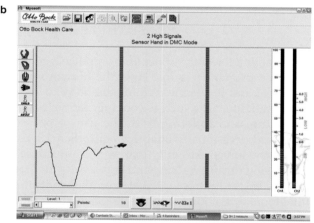

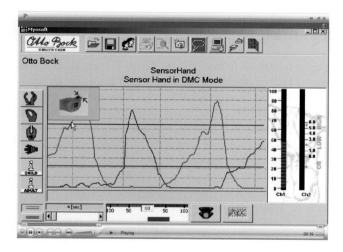

Figure 18-3. MyoBoy software (Otto Bock, Minneapolis, Minn) computer screenshot demonstrating a patient performing signal separation. For example, signal 1 (blue line) represents the flexor muscle or the muscles identified to most commonly perform terminal device closing and pronation; signal 2 (red line) represents the extensor muscles or the muscles identified to most commonly perform terminal opening and supination. The goal is for the patient to be able to activate each muscle signal (1 and 2) separately without co-contracting the other muscle (1 or 2).
Courtesy of Otto Bock.

Figure 18-4. Various games are available on the MyoBoy software (Otto Bock, Minneapolis, Minn) package. **(a)** The object of the virtual hand game is for the patient to exercise the proper force of contraction to grasp and release the ball. **(b)** In this example, the car represents one of the two muscle signals used to control the terminal device. The object of this game is for the patient to master accuracy with contraction force and to increase contraction endurance to navigate the car over the wall without crashing. This game can be further graded with the addition of a second simultaneous car representing the opposing muscle used for terminal device operation.

simulate reaching to heights, across midline, and to the floor. Use of an isolated muscle in such a way, especially following major trauma, is foreign and fatiguing; therefore, the individual's endurance should be considered during initial training. The MyoSoft offers programs with a virtual hand that respond to muscle signal as a myoelectric TD would and a car game that uses accuracy and a score for the competitive at heart (Figure 18-4). The excitement of success and the involvement of competition in the training process are contagious, but must be monitored to prevent fatigue and subsequent overuse.

The electrodes used for the myosite training can be attached to the patient's actual TD before fabrication of the early postoperative prosthesis (Figure 18-5). This step provides a three-dimensional perception of the prosthesis. The concepts of pre-positioning for the most efficient grasp patterns with different shapes of objects and appropriate force control with different densities of objects are effectively introduced during this stage.

The skills and knowledge that the patient gains during the preprosthetic training phase are critical to continued motivation and success with his or her prosthesis. Patients that receive preprosthetic training demonstrate some initial success at first fitting. This phase promotes motivation, gain of function in the residual limb, and a preliminary sense that the

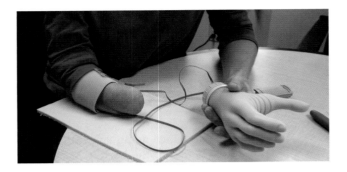

Figure 18-5. The socket electrodes attached to the actual terminal device are placed on the corresponding myosites. The patient is instructed to activate each muscle to perform the specified terminal device function. This approach provides three-dimensional, real-time feedback to the patient.

patient will once again have control over his/her life. The earlier the individual learns these valuable principles, the easier it is to transition to actual prosthetic use and refrain from poor ergonomic postures during prosthetic use that may lead to cumulative trauma disorders. For those individuals with limited muscle site access or injury-related denervation, other options are available. The use of one site to control mechanisms can be explored or the use of nonmyoelectric tension control systems can be very useful.

PHASE THREE: INTERMEDIATE PROSTHETIC TRAINING

Rehabilitation of the upper limb amputee is complex for three primary reasons. First, the human mind is powerful and it quickly retrains the body to accomplish daily life tasks such as cooking, eating, bathing, grooming, and toileting with the use of only one hand and occasionally adaptive equipment. Second, unlike the lower extremity that serves a purpose for propulsion during walking and balance during standing, the upper limb is extremely complex in its many functional operations at multiple joints and requires many integrated motions to accomplish preferred occupational tasks. Third, by comparison to the human limb, current prosthetic systems are heavy, bulky, and uncomfortable, and they require unfamiliar motor pattern performance to produce a simulated function that is rudimentary. Overall, it is a challenge to return an upper limb amputee, who quickly adapts to one-handed living, to a contrived two-handed world with one intact limb and one artificial limb.

A valid question often posed by the upper limb amputee, especially younger ones, is "Why do I have to wear a prosthesis?" As previously mentioned, it is true that most unilateral amputees can function independently with the use of one hand. The prosthesis will never truly replace the loss of a human limb. Instead, a prosthesis is a primitive facsimile of the original arm, which can be clumsy and uncomfortable and feel foreign to the wearer. However, with early, skilled prosthetic training the improvement in independent functional performance cannot be understated.

Phase three marks a major turning point in the rehabilitative care of the upper limb amputee. Phases one and two lay the foundation for success in phase three. Phase one and two wound healing, strengthening/endurance training, desensitization, residual limb shaping, and myosite testing and training provide the foundation for actual practice and prosthesis use. The focus during phase three is for the patient to master and habituate the mechanical actions required for prosthetic limb control, integrate prosthesis use in activity performance, and ultimately achieve independence in all purposeful and meaningful daily life activities. The goals of phase three training include (*a*) knowledge on the operation and performance of the prosthesis, (*b*) initiation of controls training, and (*c*) initiation of ADL training (Exhibit 18-3).

EXHIBIT 18-3

PHASE THREE: INTERMEDIATE PROSTHETIC TRAINING: UNILATERAL AND BILATERAL AMPUTEE GOALS FOR MYOELECTRIC AND BODY-POWERED PROSTHESIS

Unilateral Goals: 2 to 8 Weeks after Receiving Prosthesis
Bilateral Goals: 4 to 10 Weeks after Receiving Prosthesis

Common Unilateral and Bilateral Transradial and Transhumeral Amputee Rehabilitation Goals

1. Patient will be independent donning and doffing select prosthesis (M, B).
2. Patient will know, understand, and demonstrate compliance with the prosthetic wear schedule as directed by therapist (M, B).
3. Patient will independently perform limb hygiene daily (M, B).
4. Patient will be able to perform basic care of the prosthesis (M, B).
5. Patient will progress to tolerate prosthetic wear 6 to 8 hours per day (M, B).
6. Patient will be able to change the cable system (B).
7. Patient will be able to adjust the harnessing system (B).
8. Patient will be able to identify components and understand terminology of select prosthesis (M, B).
9. Patient will be able to change the TD independently (M, B).
10. Patient will be able to open and close the TD through the full range (M, B).
11. Patient will be able to open and close the TD to 1/3, 1/2, and 3/4 ranges (M, B).
12. Patient will be able to operate the wrist flexion component if applicable (M, B).
13. Patient will be able to operate the wrist rotation unit (M, B).
14. Patient will be independent in the battery change and charge process (M).
15. Patient pre-positions TD without verbal cueing (M, B).
16. Patient will become modified independent, using prosthesis, in basic ADLs within a reasonable time period with minimal extraneous movement and energy expenditure (M, B).

Specific Elbow Disarticulation and Transhumeral Rehabilitation Goals *(in addition to goals 1 - 16)*

1. Patient will demonstrate locking/unlocking of the elbow unit (M, B).
2. Patient will be able to position the elbow at 1/3, 1/2, and 3/4 range with and without weight (M, B).
3. Patient will demonstrate free swing if available (M, B).
4. Patient will demonstrate simultaneous control of the elbow unit and the TD concurrently (M).
5. Patient will position turn table component for internal/external rotation (B).
6. Patient pre-positions elbow unit without verbal cueing (M, B).

Specific Shoulder Disarticulation or Scapulo-thoracic Rehabilitation Goals *(in addition to goals 1 - 16, and Elbow Disarticulation and Transhumeral Goals)*

1. Patient will demonstrate unlocking/locking of the shoulder unit (M, B).
2. Patient will demonstrate free swing of the shoulder unit (M, B).
3. Patient pre-positions shoulder unit without verbal cueing (M, B).

Common Advanced Control Training Goals for Unilateral and Bilateral, Transradial, and Transhumeral Amputee *(Initiate once all above goals have been achieved)*

1. Patient will demonstrate simultaneous control of the TD concurrent with elbow unit operations (and shoulder unit if applicable) (M, B).
2. Patient will demonstrate proficiency in grasping and releasing objects in various planes away from midline (M, B).
3. Patient will demonstrate proficiency in proportional control when grasping objects without crushing (M, B).

(Exhibit 18-3 continues)

Exhibit 18-3 *continued*

Additional Bilateral Advanced Control Training Goals *(in addition to common goals 1 - 3)*

1. Patient will be able to operate one prosthesis without inadvertently operating the other prosthesis.
2. Patient will be able to operate prostheses simultaneously or in isolation.

ADLs: activities of daily living
B: body-powered
M: myoelectric
TD: terminal device

Operational Prosthetic Knowledge and Performance

Initially, most patients receive a myoelectric prosthesis. However, in some instances fabrication of a body-powered prosthesis may be prescribed. A body-powered prosthesis, also known as a conventional or cable-driven prosthesis, is powered by the patient's own body motions. Depending on the amputation level more cables are attached for control from the prosthetic harness system to the TD and if necessary the elbow joint. Gross muscle movements of the residual limb, shoulder, scapula, and chest are captured by the prosthetic harness system, and the force produced through these motions generates tension on the cable(s) affording prosthetic use.

There are two main types of prehensile TD systems available for body-powered systems: (1) voluntary open and (2) voluntary close. In the voluntary open system, the TD remains in the closed position until the user exerts specific gross body motions to open the TD. The force to sustain prehensile grasp is produced by elastic bands or springs on or in the TD. With the voluntary close system, the TD remains open until the user produces gross body movements to close the TD around an object. Springs within the TD provide the force to sustain grip in this system.

As previously mentioned, ROM and upper body strengthening of the intact proximal muscle groups improve the overall condition of the upper body and aid the prosthetic user in achieving full functional use of his or her prosthesis without the need for additional prosthetic and environmental modifications. The gross body movements used to control the body-powered prosthesis include (*a*) shoulder flexion, abduction, and extension; (*b*) scapular protraction, retraction, and depression; and (*c*) chest expansion.[17-19]

Scapular Protraction, Retraction, and Shoulder Flexion

Opening and closing of the body-powered TD is controlled primarily through shoulder and scapular movements depending on the type of TD system.

Protraction (or retraction in a voluntary open system) of one or both shoulder blades and forward flexion of the residual limb causes the contralateral side to stabilize the harness at the axilla and shoulder, thereby producing tension across the control cable, which is attached between the harness and TD. In a voluntary open system, scapular protraction will cause the TD to open and scapular relaxation/retraction will cause the TD to close. In a voluntary close system, scapular protraction will cause the TD to close and relaxation/retraction of the scapula will cause the TD to open. Forward flexion is also used to flex and extend the forearm of an above elbow prosthesis when the elbow is in unlocked position.[17-19]

Scapular Depression and Shoulder Extension and Abduction

Unlocking and locking of the elbow for an above elbow prosthesis is controlled through scapular depression and shoulder extension and abduction. The combination of the movements lengthens the attachment between the harness and elbow unit and in turn activates the locking mechanism of the elbow. When the elbow is unlocked the forearm can be controlled through shoulder movements.[17-19]

Chest Expansion

Although this motion provides less excursion force than shoulder and scapular movements, chest expansion can be helpful to provide improved prosthetic control to patients with high-level amputations, nerve involvement, or other comorbid injuries. Modifications in harness design may be needed to capture this motion.[17-19]

Regardless of the type of prosthesis, it is critical that the individual obtain and demonstrate knowledge of component terminology, a general understanding of how the components make up the prosthesis, and instructions on how to perform basic maintenance on the prosthesis. This education affords the patient a basic vocabulary to effectively articulate with the rehabilitation team any mechanical difficulties or operational malfunctions of the prosthesis. Ability to articulate malfunctions using correct terminology greatly assists the prosthetist in diagnosing and fixing any repair issues. The prosthetist provides equipment education and reinforces it during therapy. Each patient should possess common terminology including—but not limited to—the following:

- socket and harnessing design,
- component terminology care,
- types of TD(s),
- type of control system(s) used, and
- basic mechanics of the prosthesis.

The patient must communicate with the prosthetist when maintenance is required. When basic repairs are necessary, the goal is for the patient to have enough knowledge to perform such maintenance. The patient is expected to be able to perform the following:

- socket maintenance to include daily cleaning and inspection of the socket;
- battery charging and component maintenance to include routine cleaning and application of lubricant; and
- harness adjustment, rubber band replacement, and cable system changes, as needed.

Patients are provided with this education for use in settings where a prosthetist may not be available. The occupational therapist is responsible for ensuring that patients receive ample functional training to make them efficient and proficient in functional maintenance performance and prosthetic care in various environmental and physical circumstances relative to their everyday operational environment. Also, the occupational therapist is responsible for considering any other existing injuries that may hinder efficient performance of maintenance tasks and identifying ways for the patient to perform these tasks independently. For example, a patient that wants to return to the theater of operation would practice—while participating in OT—prosthetic maintenance under simulated conditions to mimic such an environment.

Residual Limb Tolerance/Care

With traumatic amputation, the limb continues to heal beneath the surface of the skin well beyond wound closure and that makes the limb more susceptible to pathology. Frequent inspection of the residual limb(s) should become a daily ritual for all prosthetic users. If the skin integrity of the residual limb is compromised

the patient's ability to wear the prosthesis is hindered. Buried fragments, development of heterotropic ossification, peripheral nerve injuries, or the development of a neuroma are several type of injuries that may make the residual limb more susceptible to skin disruption. The rehabilitation team should inform the patient about the signs and symptoms of potential significant changes related to these areas.

Along with inspection of the residual limb, establishing a wearing schedule for the prosthesis is also important. Initially the prosthesis should be worn for no more than 15 to 30 minutes, 2 to 3 times daily. Upon doffing of the prosthesis, the residual limb should be thoroughly inspected for any skin redness, irritation, and breakdown. If no signs of ill fit are evident, the user can increase the wearing time by 30-minute increments, 2 to 3 times daily. Improper socket fit must be immediately addressed by the prosthetist. Inspection of the residual limb should continue to be a daily routine even after the patient has progressed to all-day wear and use of the prosthesis. Along with limb inspection, proper hygiene of the residual limb is also essential. This includes daily washing of the residual limb with mild soap followed by thorough drying before donning the prosthesis.

Donning/Doffing Prosthesis

The eventual goal is for the prosthetic user to be able to tolerate approximately 8 hours of prosthesis wear and use within 1 to 2 weeks from the start of training. Therefore, early independence in donning and doffing is important to achieve. The patient must be able to independently don and doff the full prosthetic system that includes (*a*) residual limb sock, (*b*) prosthetic donning liner, (*c*) prosthetic socket, and (*d*) harnessing(s) as appropriate.

There is a range of different methods for donning/doffing each type of prosthesis. When training the patient on donning and doffing the myoelectric prosthesis, the Reduced Friction Donning System (Advanced Arm Dynamics, Inc, Redondo Beach, Calif) is used (Figure 18-6). With the use of a special donning sock and socket design, the limb is placed into the socket and the sock is pulled out of the socket. The result is secure soft tissue placement within the socket trim lines ensuring optimum electrode contact. Individuals with a transhumeral amputation use the same donning system for application of the myoelectric prosthesis. However, on the socket a prosthetic valve is added to create a suction or semisuction fit of the socket on the limb. Once the sock is removed from the socket the excess air is removed at the touch of a button allowing for a vacuum seal. In the transradial socket, valves are

a

b

c

d

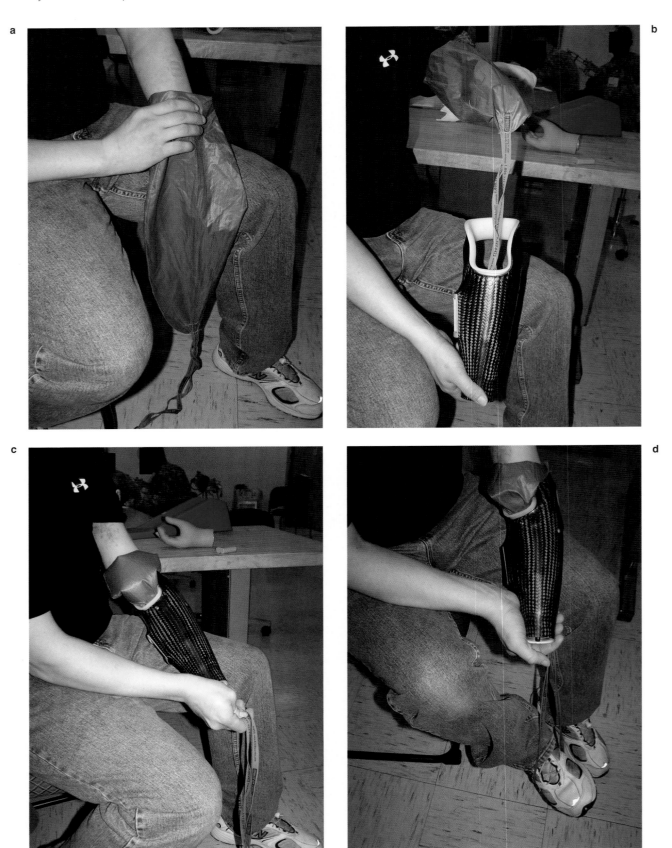

e

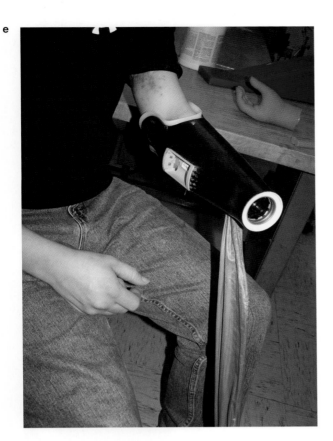

Figure 18-6. The patient is trained to don the myoelectric prosthesis with the use of a limited friction donning sock with a lanyard secured to the end. (**a**) The sleeve is inverted over the residual limb. (**b**) The lanyard is dropped through a pull tube that is located in the distal end of the socket. (**c**) The sock-covered limb is placed in the prosthesis. The patient places tension on the lanyard to begin to pull the sock through the socket, thus pulling the limb into the socket. (**d**) Additional tension to pull the sock is achieved by placing the loop of the lanyard around the foot and subsequently pulling the sock out of the socket while the residual limb provides counterforce to the prosthetic socket. (**e**) The sock is pulled through the tube via the lanyard gently bringing the soft tissue into the socket.

rarely used because the sockets are typically suspending via bony anatomy.

When training to don the body-powered prosthesis the patient is instructed in the pullover method, where the harness is donned over the head, or the jacket method, where the harness is donned over one extremity and then the other (Figure 18-7 and Figure 18-8). The methods for donning and doffing the prosthetic system for bilateral amputees vary significantly based on level of amputation. However, the end goal is for the patient to perform this task independently. Additional creativity on the part of the therapist and patient is

required to achieve this goal. Sample technique options for donning and doffing the prosthesis are listed in Table 18-2 and Figure 18-9. All patients are informed about the most appropriate method for them and they may even develop their own technique.

Initiation of Controls Training

Learning to use any type of prosthesis is similar to learning the operation of other multicomponent mechanical devices. For example, when beginning to drive, the first step is learning to control the individual components required for operating a vehicle. This includes turning it on and off; adjusting the mirrors and seats; and operating the gear shift, gas, and brake. These components are eventually combined into the actual performance of driving a vehicle. Similarly, when an amputee begins his or her prosthetic training, the first step is to learn how to control the individual components to operate the prosthesis. Subsequent steps in the newly learned motor patterns are combined to accomplish tasks creating a hierarchy of progression through the controls training. The goal is to achieve smooth movement of the prosthesis with minimal amount of delays and awkward motions in daily activity task performance.[20]

The tasks used to achieve mastery of each control skill depend on the therapist's creativity. Media appropriate for training include objects of various shape, texture, density, and weight, such as 1-inch wood square blocks, round blocks, cotton balls, Styrofoam cups, or a cup filled with water. This type of media provides various different ways to grade the task at hand to achieve mastery of control. Initial training is frequently rote. However, with mastery of each skill, motions are combined resulting in performance of an activity. A multisensory approach is also useful. Verbal, tactile, and visual cues can be helpful to attain success. The progression through the hierarchy of body-powered and myoelectric prosthetic controls training described by each level of upper limb amputation is depicted in Figure 18-10 and Figure 18-11, respectively.

Patients performing controls training with the use of a preliminary myoelectric prosthesis may find that the gains of the imbedded electrodes require adjustment to perform the task at hand. The prosthetist can more specifically set the electrode sensitivity with customizing software that is specific to each manufacture.

Activities of Daily Living Prosthetic Training

The final stage of phase three is to apply the skills learned during the controls training portion to begin functional use of the prosthesis. The user may become

511

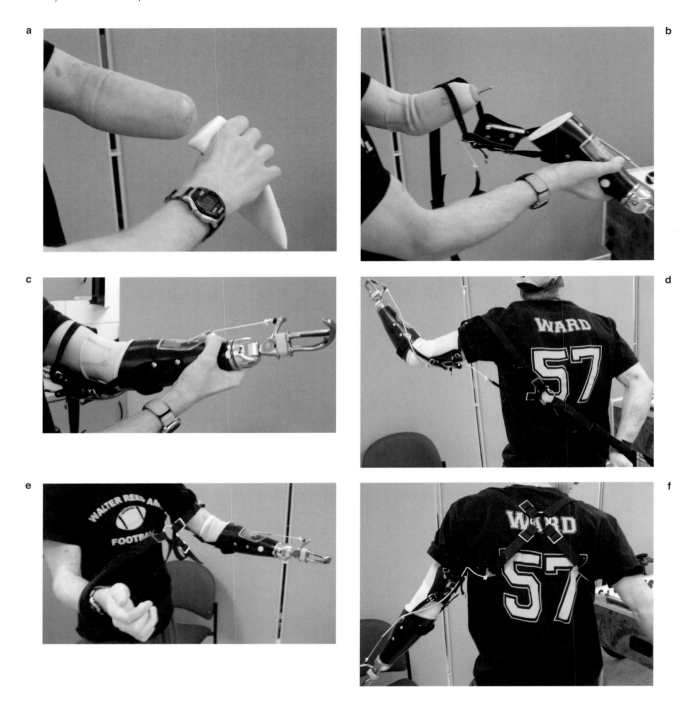

Figure 18-7. Sample donning methods for a transradial amputee with a body-powered pin lock suspension prosthetic system. (**a**) The roll on silicon liner is inverted and rolled onto the residual limb. (**b**) The residual limb is placed through the harness (note the locking pin at the distal end of the liner). (**c**) The limb is guided into the socket with slight pressure to secure the pin into the pin lock within the socket. This creates a secure relationship between the patient and the prosthesis to allow for more aggressive activities or for reduced harnessing. This type of suspension has been found to be necessary for the activity level in this population. (**d**) Instructing in the jacket method of donning, the harness is pulled across the back and the residual limb is placed through the remaining figure-of-eight harness. (**e**) Instructing in the over the head method, the residual limb is placed through the figure-of-eight harness anteriorly before guiding the harness overhead. (**f**) The completed figure-of-eight body-powered prosthetic system is donned. It is important that the patient adjust the placement of the figure-of-eight ring when donning this system to ensure the harness is centered both medially and laterally and distally and proximally between the scapulae.

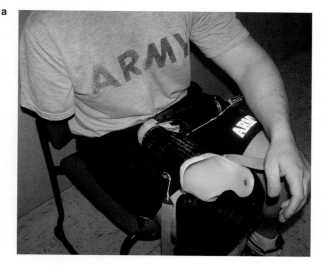

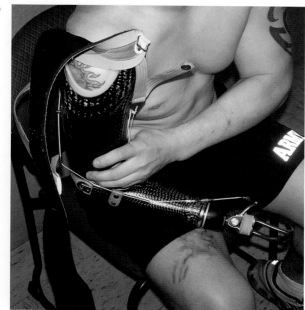

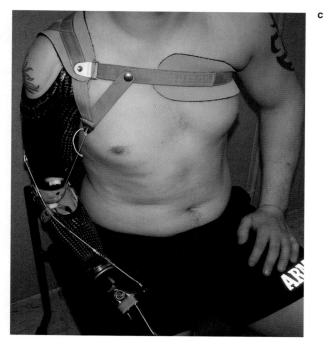

Figure 18-8. Sample donning method for a transhumeral amputee. (**a**) Preparation for donning a suction socket prosthesis using the jacket method, the elbow is locked into 90 degrees flexion and the prosthesis is laid out with the harness system toward the outside of the body. (**b**) The residual limb is placed into the socket using downward force with the prosthesis stabilized using the remaining limb. (**c**) The harness is donned across the back and under the residual arm. The harness is secured to the anterior portion of prosthesis with snaps, buckles, or Velcro (Velcro USA Inc, Manchester, NH).

more frustrated because of the awkward and artificial nature of a prosthesis. In addition, those with unilateral amputation quickly learn to adapt to one-handed task performance that can become habitual. The rehabilitation team must continue to provide support and encouragement during basic daily living skills to help the individual use a prosthesis.

Rating guides developed by Atkins titled "Unilateral Upper Extremity Amputation: Activities of Daily Living Assessment" (Figure 18-12) provide a comprehensive list of activities the patient should be able to perform with the use of the prosthesis.[20] A rating guide is also available for bilateral upper limb amputations. The patient is observed performing the identified tasks and is graded on task performance using a zero to three scale; zero identifies tasks that are impossible for the individual to complete; one identifies tasks that are accomplished with much strain or many awkward motions; two identifies tasks that are somewhat labored, or few awkward motions; and three identifies tasks that are performed smoothly, with minimal amount of delays or awkward motions. With the permission of Diane Atkins through direct communication, these rating guides were modified to include tasks relevant to military duties. It is unreasonable to expect a unilateral amputee to use a prosthesis to the same extent because he or she spontaneously uses the preexisting sound limb.

The level of difficulty in training and the amount of training time needed may vary from one prosthetic user to another. Factors that may influence this include the level of amputation (ie, transhumeral vs transradial), unilateral versus bilateral amputation, and the type of prosthetic device fitted to the user (ie, body-powered vs myoelectric prosthesis). Additional

TABLE 18-2

BILATERAL UPPER EXTREMITY PROSTHETIC SAMPLE DONNING AND DOFFING STRATEGIES AND CONSIDERATIONS

Strategies	Body Powered	Myoelectric	Considerations
Donning prostheses: This will be dependent on the type of prostheses and the harnessing system used. Donning methods vary based on the suspension system and whether the prosthetic devices are harnessed independently or connected through harnessing.	• If each prosthesis has an independent harness system, the longer of the residual limbs is donned first. This prosthesis is then used to assist with donning the second prosthesis. • If the prostheses are connected by harnessing, the shorter residual limb prosthesis will be donned first. The two most common methods of donning attached prostheses is to don the prostheses as you would a coat or to place both limbs simultaneously in the prostheses and don them overhead like a T-shirt.	• Self-suspending sockets are often donned using a reduced friction donning sock. The patient will use the lower extremities or the other prosthesis to pull the sock through the pull tube that pulls the soft tissue into the socket providing an intimate fit with skin traction. • Suction sockets are donned using an evaporative moisture technique, such as Cal Stat (Steris Corporation, Mentor, Ohio), or other products. Air is expelled through the valve as the limb is pushed into the socket creating a suction fit.	• A donning stand may be helpful for high-level amputee patients (Figure 18-9). Additionally, patients with high-level amputations will require more creativity from the prosthetic team for independence in donning.
Doffing prostheses: Doffing is often easier than donning.	• If the prosthesis is donned using the jacket or T-shirt method, the prosthesis is doffed using the method in reverse.	• To doff a self-suspending type of prosthesis, patients will typically use their lower extremities or the environment to assist in removing the prosthesis. In the case of a suction suspension, patients will often use an object in their environment to assist them to press the button on the valve that will release the suction. The donning stand can also be used as needed.	

factors include the individual's (*a*) motivation, (*b*) cognitive and emotional status, and (*c*) physical condition and comorbid conditions. The ultimate goal is for the patient to achieve maximum independence in the performance of ADLs and instrumental ADLs through the integration and use of the prosthesis.

Although using a prosthesis to perform ADLs is supported, patients are also encouraged to master independence in one-handed ADLs because there will be times when the prosthesis is unavailable. The patient must master one-handed ADL performance

independently, efficiently, and ergonomically correctly to avoid the possibility of developing cumulative trauma disorders. The patient is taught the signs and symptoms of various cumulative trauma disorders and encouraged to seek initial medical attention early if they develop. Little information has been published on the prevalence of over-use injuries in the upper limb amputee population; however, a small study published by Jones and Davidson found over-use injuries were more common in the unilateral amputee population than the nonamputee population.[21]

Muscle Strengthening and Endurance

The patient should be independent with a postoperative self-stretching program of the same frequency and duration as previously discussed. The patient can incorporate the prosthesis into the stretching program. The therapist emphasizes strict adherence to this program because many patients neglect joint stretching once they begin to reach their goal of ADL independence. However, the patient remains at risk for shoulder and elbow contractures because scar and surgical incisions continue to mature.

Muscle endurance training and strengthening require a more demanding, yet specific mode. The patient continues to participate in a regular cardiovascular program with physical therapy and is encouraged to incorporate the use of the prosthesis during such physical activity. Supervised progressive strengthening is initiated through weight training. Programs begin conservatively for 15 to 20 minutes at low resistance with minimal distal end weight bearing of the residual limb. There is no published set protocol for progressing resistance training for the upper limb amputee. Skin and residual limb tolerance are the confounding factors when progressive upper limb conditioning is initiated. During weight training the patient must have a properly fitting socket with adequate suspension and a TD that will allow completion of the weight-lifting task. A snug prosthesis will increase total surface area contact and thus reduce the incidence of skin trauma from shearing or abnormal forces. Weight lifting may not be well tolerated in the transradial amputee or the amputee with a self-suspending socket because abnormal leverage or the traction of tissues, respectively, coupled with the need for full elbow extension as part of an exercise may increase socket pressure in

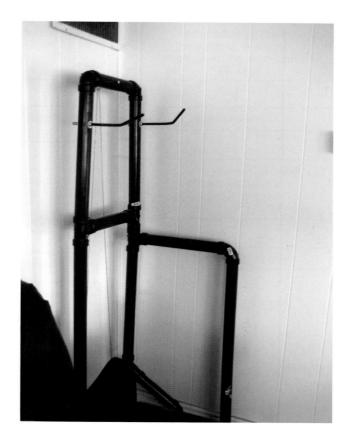

Figure 18-9. An example of a donning stand that may allow a patient with bilateral upper extremity limb loss independence in the donning and doffing of a body-powered prosthesis.

the antecubital region or the condyles. A safety point as weight lifting increases is to secure the weight to the TD.

PHASE FOUR: ADVANCED PROSTHETIC TRAINING

Phase four begins approximately 8 to 16 weeks after the initiation of rehabilitation (Exhibit 18-4). This time frame is not fixed, however, and it depends on the patient's medical and rehabilitation progress. Individuals who reach this stage can accomplish all basic skills from phase three. They can don and doff the prosthesis independently, tolerate a full day's wearing schedule, and are proficient in basic operations of the prosthesis. The goals of this phase are for the patient to complete basic and advanced daily tasks incorporating the prosthesis efficiently and demonstrating a natural motor pattern. The outcome of this phase is for the patient to save body energy, decrease biomechanical stress to the intact limb, and learn the best approach

to tasks without extraneous body movements and the reliance on adaptive equipment.

Five characteristics of advanced prosthetic rehabilitation are available to guide therapists during this phase. The first characteristic is that advanced rehabilitation is highly individualized. Overall, successful rehabilitation of upper limb amputees involves knowing the whole person and what meaningful occupations they previously selected; however, phases one, two, and three follow more of a predictable therapy guide to treatment activities. When the patient progresses to phase four, therapy becomes more individualized, incorporating his or her particular vocational and avocational goals. The second characteristic is that this phase most as-

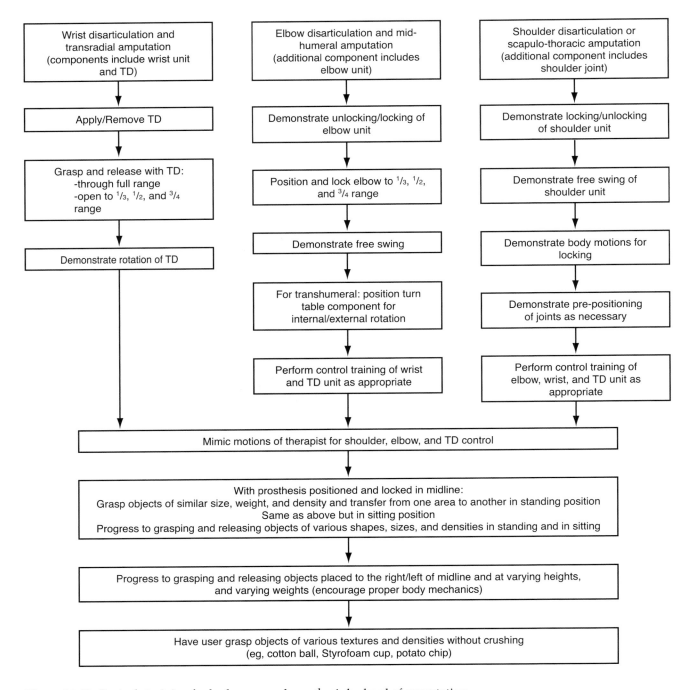

Figure 18-10. Controls training for body-powered prosthesis by level of amputation.
TD: terminal device

suredly requires the use and operation of a tool, or interaction with an object, such as a carpenter's tool, a musical instrument, a cooking utensil, or a machine. The third characteristic is that advanced training involves completing a multistepped complex task with many required bimanual movements. In the language of the occupational therapist, it could best be said that advanced prosthetic training is "occupation-based." Treatment activities in this phase are less static and generally challenge the therapist to remove the patient from the clinic setting. In this way, the advanced rehabilitation is not a series of similar, repetitive movements such as moving one object after another to the same location, as would be the case for phase three training.

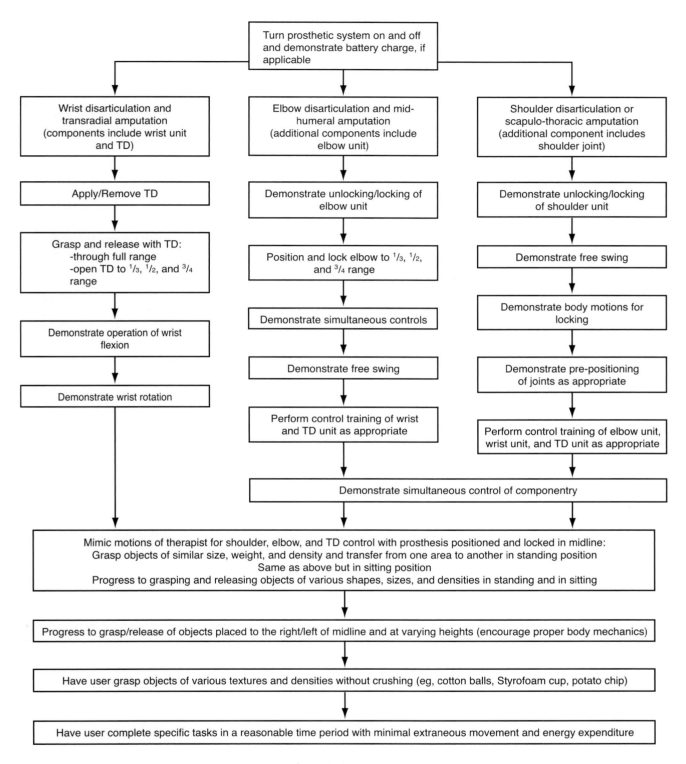

Figure 18-11. Controls training for myoelectric prosthesis by level of amputation.
TD: terminal device

The fourth characteristic is that this type of training should involve the prosthesis of choice for the patient. Users are encouraged to try different TDs during activity performance to determine which device best meets their needs. Whether the individual self-selects the myoelectric or body-powered prosthesis as his or her preferred

Name:		Age:	Occupation:		Date of Test:
Therapist:		Sex:	Type of terminal device:		

RATING GUIDE KEY:

0 Impossible	1 Accomplished with much strain, or many awkward motions	2 Somewhat labored, or few awkward motions	3 Smooth, minimal amount of delays and awkward motions

ACTIVITIES OF DAILY LIVING	0	1	2	3	ACTIVITIES OF DAILY LIVING	0	1	2	3
PERSONAL NEEDS:					**GENERAL PROCEDURES:**				
Don/doff pull-over shirt					Turn key in lock				
Dress button-down shirt: cuffs and front					Operate door knob				
Manage zippers and snaps					Place chain on chain lock				
Don/doff pants					Plug cord into Wan outlet				
Don/doff belt					Set time on watch				
Lace and tie shoes					**HOUSEKEEPING PROCEDURES:**				
Don/doff pantyhose					Perform laundry				
Tie a tie					Fold clothes				
Don/doff bra					Set up ironing board				
Don/doff glove					Iron clothes				
Cut and file finger nails					Hand wash dishes				
Polish finger nails					Dry dishes with a towel				
Screw/unscrew cap of toothpaste tube					Load and unload dishwasher				
Squeeze toothpaste					Use broom and dustpan				
Open top of pill bottle					Operate vacuum cleaner				
Set hair					Use wet and dry mop				
Take bill from wallet					Make bed				
Open pack of cigarettes					Change garbage bag				
Light a match					Open/close jar				
Don/doff prosthesis					Open lid of can				
Perform residual limb care					Cut vegetables				
EATING PROCEDURES:					Peel vegetables				
Carry a tray					Manipulate hot pots				
Cut meat					Thread a needle				
Butter bread					Sew a button				
Open milk carton					**USE OF TOOLS:**				
DESK PROCEDURES:					Saw				
Use phone and take notes					Hammer				
Use pay phone					Screw drivers				
Sharpen pencil					Tape measure				
Use scissors					Wrenches				
Use ruler					Power tools: drill, sander				
Remove and replace ink pen cap					Plane				
Fold and seal letter					Shovel				
Use paper clip					Rake				
Use stapler					Wheelbarrow				
Wrap package					**CAR PROCEDURES:**				
Use computer: typing, access Internet					Open and close doors, trunk and hood				
Demonstrate handwriting					Perform steps required to operate vehicle				
COMMENTS:					*COMMENTS:*				

Figure 18-12 (left page). The "Unilateral Upper Extremity Amputation: Activities of Daily Living Assessment" is a rating guide that provides a comprehensive list of activities of daily living that a unilateral amputee should be able to accomplish.
Adapted with permission from Atkins DJ, Meier RH. *Comprehensive Management of the Upper-Limb Amputee.* New York, NY: Springer-Verlag; 1989.

prosthesis, the advanced training should be geared toward fine-tuning the operation and control of that prosthesis as needed to engage in the appropriate tasks at this level of rehabilitation. The fifth characteristic is that there is a meaningful product or outcome upon task completion. For example, the patient would have built the frame, weeded the garden, assembled the weapon, dug the hole, or repaired the engine. It is helpful to encourage patients to complete a "prosthesis thesis" as a capstone assignment from this phase of training. Several individuals have completed carpentry projects, leather belt or wallet projects, and complex stained glass or wood-burning crafts (Figure 18-13).

Phase four includes a variety of advanced tasks that patients perform once they demonstrate proficiency with the prosthesis in phase three. Additionally, these advanced activities are specific to the patient's interests, hobbies, family, and work goals. Patients are trained on tasks such as military warrior tasks, yard work, home repair and maintenance, shopping, meal preparation, child care, pet care, and recreational and sports activities. Tasks within these general categories challenge the individual to complete the task successfully with the prosthesis. The patient who passes the rigors of this level of training is often identified by the rehabilitation staff as "integrator" because of his or her success at integrating the prosthesis into the motor skill repertoire, thereby attaining the goal of this phase of rehabilitation. Overall, the patient's movements should be coordinated, smooth, and precise with accurate and consistent control of the operations of the prosthesis using ergonomically sound postures proximally. Patients who elect to not utilize a prosthesis should be able to perform these tasks as independently as possible or have an identified plan to complete such tasks with the assistance of others as necessary.

Military Warrior Tasks

The military warrior tasks category includes tasks specific to basic warfighter skills such as assembling and disassembling, firing, repairing, and cleaning a military service weapon; donning and doffing a gas mask; using a military radio; and assembling a ruck-

---

EXHIBIT 18-4

PHASE FOUR: ADVANCED PROSTHETIC TRAINING: UNILATERAL AND BILATERAL, ALL LEVELS

Goals: 4 to 10 Weeks after Prosthetic Delivery

1. Patient will be able to perform self-selected advanced prosthetic activities with smooth movements, minimal amount of operational delays, or awkward motions and postures.
2. Patient will be able to identify community resources for prosthetic needs.
3. Patient will be able to identify resources for vocational planning.

---

sack with all appropriate military gear. Many SMs are interested in completing these tasks because they solidify their compromised identity. Furthermore, those who wish to remain on active duty can demonstrate that they can meet the minimum standards of required skills for military service.

Yard Work, Home Repair, and Maintenance

The responsibilities of yard work and home maintenance are complex and varied and the patient must work with a variety of tools to complete the identified task. Yard work activities are performed outside of the clinic utilizing gardening tools such as spades, shovels, hedge clippers, and wheelbarrows. These tasks require movements in many planes with various tools that require difficult postures and much upper body and trunk muscle strength. As the patient identifies his or her previous home responsibilities or predicts those of a future living environment, the therapist may set up simulated tasks in a functional apartment. The individual may perform tasks such as taking garbage out, fixing a leaky sink, replacing a light bulb, changing bed sheets, running the vacuum, unloading groceries into the pantry, and replacing the bathroom shower curtain liner. Whatever the task, the patient gains self-confidence to return to independence in a home environment through practice of "real-life" chores.

Shopping

Shopping is its own distinct category of training because of the many functional obstacles to overcome in the commercial market square. The

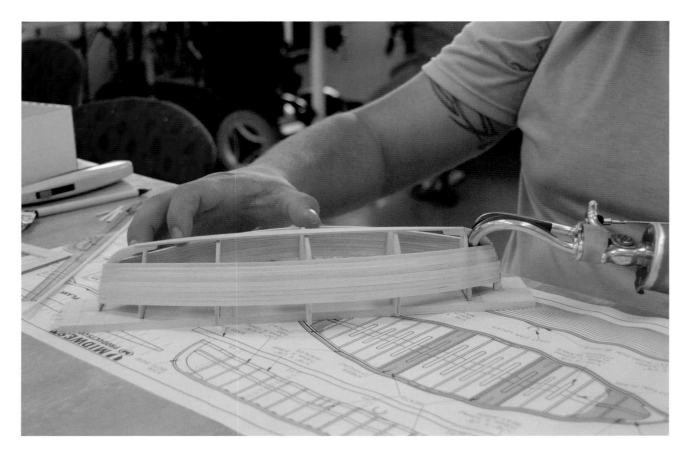

Figure 18-13. This patient is using the body-powered prosthesis to assemble a sailboat made of wood. This project requires fine-tuned prosthetic skill and control; these skills are addressed during advanced prosthetic training.

individual must shop for groceries and be able to reach many types of packages from shelves of variable heights. Now that most supermarkets have self-service check-out lanes, the patient must train to complete the entire gamut of tasks related to purchasing, scanning, bagging, and paying for groceries. The final money transaction should be practiced using the automated credit card machine and the automated cash machine.

Shopping for clothes and shoes must be addressed for the specifics inherent in such tasks. For example, upper limb amputees who choose to use elastic shoe laces must be aware of the difficulty they will have when shoe shopping. This makes the case for learning to tie one's shoes one-handed or using a prosthesis, even if the individual often relies on elastic shoe laces. For clothes shopping, it can be awkward and tiresome for an upper limb amputee to shop for shirts that accommodate the prosthesis and possible harnessing systems if a body-powered system is the individual's preferred prosthesis.

Meal Preparation

Meal preparation makes up a special category of this phase of rehabilitation. Throughout the patient's rehabilitation, he or she participates in a weekly cooking group. This group is the individual's first exposure to one-handed adaptive equipment such as one-handed cutting boards, can openers (Dycem Limited, Warwick Central Industrial Park, RI), and electric mixers. When the patient reaches this phase of training, he or she must complete the entire meal preparation process from cooking to serving to cleaning. There are many challenges and rewards in cooking. Completion of this high-level training gives the individual a sense of accomplishment and a strong sense of independence.

Child Care and Pet Care

Child care and pet care are addressed at this phase of rehabilitation. The tasks in this category are numerous, changing, and varied. The patient must identify his or her responsibilities related to child and pet care, and the therapist must perform careful task analysis to offer detailed training. The use of therapy dogs allows for training in pet care to be realistic. It is best to address child care training as it relates to the specifics of the patient's own children. Therapists have often used a doll to practice diapering, holding, bathing, swaddling, and to improve the confidence of the individual who can be apprehensive about hurting or dropping his or her own child while using the prosthesis.

Introduction to Driver's Training

It is not uncommon for an SM returning from combat to experience some amount of difficulty acclimating to driving again. Some SMs have informally reported physical incompatibilities to driving while others identify issues with hyper-vigilance that left them uncomfortable and unsure about returning to it. SMs have informally reported that the following situations made them the most nervous while driving: (*a*) potholes, (*b*) traveling under or over bridges or overpasses, (*c*) unexpected sudden flashes or sounds out of the periphery of vision, and (*d*) vehicles quickly approaching from the rear.

The rehabilitation team may use a cursory treatment as necessary to prepare the patient for driver's training utilizing driving simulators within the military training facility. The driver's training simulator provides an opportunity for cursory exploration of possible modifications to assist the SM in physically operating his or her vehicle and a method to assist in desensitizing the SM to driving again. Various scenarios are introduced in a progressive desensitization method with the goal of returning confidence and comfort with driving. Reaction time and appropriateness of the reaction can be documented and recorded allowing for subjective and objective data to determine progress. This process also is a method to demonstrate and mitigate safety concerns that the SM or treatment team may have about returning to the road.

During rehabilitation, once the SM has acclimated and is ready to progress to community driving, he or she is enrolled in driver's training evaluation at local Veterans Affairs (VA) facilities. VA-certified driver's training is a multidisciplinary program and links the patient with available VA benefits related to driving. These specialists identify appropriate vehicle modification equipment used as needed to assist the patient in performing driving tasks and provide training on this equipment. They also assist in acquiring the necessary vehicle modifications. OT in the military training facility is not responsible for performing this evaluation.

Vocational Planning and Training

The vocational training category is specific to the individual's particular occupational pursuit. Those patients who choose to remain on active duty may be faced with learning new skills to complete their current military occupational specialty (MOS), consider changing their MOS, and learning new skills. Others may choose to leave the service and pursue a new or familiar civilian occupation. This decision can be further complicated by the addition of a prosthesis(es).

The occupational therapist must help patients sort through the various tasks associated with their particular occupational pursuits or MOS demands. To facilitate this all patients should receive an initial screen to determine appropriateness for a functional capacity evaluation (FCE). This evaluation may be completed to determine an individual's ability to perform work-related activities through assessment of strength, flexibility, endurance, cardiovascular function, and maintenance of certain positions. This is an intense evaluation performed by the occupational therapist and includes, but is not limited to, assessment of the following:

- repetitive heavy lifting,
- carrying,
- pushing/pulling,
- repetitive squatting,
- stair climbing,
- ladder climbing,
- kneeling,
- bending, and
- overhead work.

Completion of an FCE may take anywhere between 3 to 5 hours over 1 to 2 days, depending on the individual and his or her specific diagnosis(es).

Flexibility of the FCE allows variation in the prosthesis utilized during testing. For example, therapists may choose to test an upper limb amputee in his or her ability to utilize both a body-powered and a myoelectric prosthesis in various functional tasks including lifting, carrying, and positional tolerance tasks. Individual prosthetic manufacturer recommendations for maximum weight guidelines should be carefully considered to ensure patient safety while performing lifting and carrying tasks.

Occupational therapists also may choose to design individualized custom FCE protocols to objectively measure a patient's ability to perform basic military warrior tasks. In addition, custom FCE protocols may be established to objectively measure a patient's ability to perform the specific tasks in his or her MOS/area of concentration (AOC). Further identification of a patient's vocational and educational interests may be necessary if an individual does not wish to or is unable to remain in the military secondary to physical and/or cognitive deficits.

Findings from FCE testing may be used to support a patient's medical evaluation board or physical evaluation board. Specifically, data obtained during the FCE testing may be used to determine an individual's fitness to return to duty. Furthermore, individualized retraining may be necessary to enable an individual to remain in his or her current MOS or AOC or preparation for transition to a new MOS or AOC.

If the SM decides to leave the military and pursue a civilian occupation, he or she is linked with a vocational rehabilitation counselor and resources through the Department of Veterans Affairs (VA). To facilitate this relationship, it is recommended that the VA vocational rehabilitation counselor be colocated with the OT service in the military training facility. Once linked to the VA vocational rehabilitation counselor, patients undergo appropriate evaluation if necessary and may see a VA occupational therapist for an FCE. Additionally, VA rehabilitation counselors provide software and training packages to all eligible beneficiaries.

Whether or not the patient decides to remain on active duty, therapists should research vocational resources and plan for future vocational pursuits with patients. For example, those who elect to pursue a welding career in their hometown may benefit from individualized research and planning with the therapist to ensure that they have a formidable plan to meet this vocational pursuit. An example is identifying a local welding union and locating what companies may have job openings.

Adaptive Equipment and Environmental Modifications

To maximize independence and function in ADLs, wounded SMs may require various adaptive equipment and environmental adaptations. Assessment is made early for adaptive equipment or environmental modification needs and continues until patients prepare for discharge and transition into their future occupational and home environment. OT serves a significant role in this assessment. While still an inpatient the therapist can assess the SM's current use of electronics and help him or her acquire the resources to begin this process. Once determination is made on needs and previous premorbid use of electronics, items may be ordered. SMs may be trained and begin using

these devices to assist in return to duty or eventual discharge to the VA system.

Programs, such as the Computer/Electronic Accommodations Program (CAP) offered through Tricare, offer SMs various types of adaptive equipment to enhance independence in vocational activities. CAP equipment can be obtained to increase independence for individuals with vision loss, low vision, or are deaf or hard of hearing, and those with cognitive, communication, and dexterity disabilities, which frequently occur as a result of combat. As the patient progresses through the final phase of rehabilitation, he or she explores vocational options. If adaptive equipment facilitates independence in work-related tasks, a CAP assessment is initiated as soon as possible. Patients who elect to transition to civilian occupations should initiate a CAP assessment as early as possible in their final phase of rehabilitation to facilitate a rapid and seamless transition to the VA vocational rehabilitation counselors.

Environmental modifications necessary within the home are acquired through the VA. A therapist certified in adaptive technology from the regional VA Medical Center completes the necessary assessments of various environmental modifications needed within the home.

Exercise Prescription Considerations

For those who enjoy activities of low to moderate intensity, fishing, gardening, walking, golf, biking, and swimming are exercise options. Swimming, in particular, is ideal recreational activity secondary to its relatively low overload on skin, muscles, and joints as well as its accessibility and no requirement to use an activity-specific prosthesis. Cardiovascular demands vary because the sport can be geared to target heart ranges as low as 50% of maximum heart rate. Intensity begins with 5- to 15-minute exercise sessions that follow established target heart ranges for the individual. Progression to a continuous exercise session lasting 30 to 40 minutes will guarantee sport-specific aerobic conditioning while in the water.

The amputee seeking moderate to high activity levels of exercise has even greater recreation choices including sports such as running, aerobic dance, weight lifting, and skiing as well as racquet and team sports to address these needs. Those who choose to exercise with their prosthesis must have a proper fit because of the significant shear forces experienced during these activities. A prosthetist may be consulted regarding sport-specific prosthetic options and special prosthetic modifications before engaging in a sport.

Recreational and Sports Activities

Recreational and sports activities during this phase of training are appealing to young active SMs. Various recreational choices exist for low to moderate and moderate to high levels of exercise intensity. Many customized prostheses and TDs are available on the commercial market to facilitate the return to previously enjoyable activities.

The roles of the amputee clinical team are interdependent when attempting to train the patient for recreational and sport activities. The occupational and/or recreational therapist interviews the patient to determine his or her leisure history or recreational interests and conveys this information to the rehabilitation team to ensure future treatment is targeted at achieving the physical demands of the chosen activity within a timely manner. The physical and occupational therapists should train the patient in the prerequisite conditioning components of the sport. In addition, the team prosthetist is consulted to determine appropriate prosthetic adaptations necessary for proficiency in the identified task. These devices are purchased and/or modifications are completed and the occupational therapist trains the amputee accordingly with the new equipment. Once all minimal physical and adaptive needs are met, the recreational therapist begins the sport- or activity-specific training with other clinicians acting as consultants. Often a patient's love of and desire to resume a certain leisure interest or sport serves as a reward for participation during previous phases of the protocol to advance to this category of training.

COMMUNITY REENTRY AND REINTEGRATION

The community reentry and reintegration processes are a significant component of life that any individual recovering from trauma must face. No matter how well an individual is prepared for interactions in the community, the demands of the community cannot be re-created within the confines of the clinic. Furthermore, a challenging first experience without support can result in a major setback for the patient, whereas a positive and supportive first experience typically leads to more. Although these experiences may be overwhelming and frightening for the patient, they are invaluable in recovery.

Occupational and physical therapists coordinate programs for injured SMs with input from all interdisciplinary team members. The program, which is an important part of recovery, is an early reminder of the crux of the entire program—to return the patient to the highest attainable level of participation in life. The goal is to get the patient back into the community—at some level—very early in recovery. This alleviates the fear and stress of reentry that is common following a devastating and physically altering injury such as limb loss.

To participate in the therapeutic outing the patient must be medically cleared. He or she must be off contact precautions, be able to tolerate sitting in a wheelchair for at least 2 hours, and be allowed to stop intravenous medications for 2 hours. The patient may still require wound vacuums, but they are portable. The patient does not have to be able to complete transfers independently because therapists and nurses can assist with them. Wheelchair accessible transportation is utilized for the therapeutic outings. The patient also must be psychologically ready to encounter the world outside the hospital and be willing to participate in the therapeutic outing. The entire team believes that the sooner the patient overcomes the fear of reentry into the community, the easier each subsequent trip becomes.

Early in their rehabilitation patients tend to manage better on a small trip, such as to a local shopping mall or restaurant. These are often the most meaningful trips for the therapists because they accompany the patient across a new threshold toward independence outside of the hospital.

For most patients, it has been some time since they have been back in the United States, so the readjustment to life outside the combat zone must be addressed. Patients often comment that they are "lost without their weapon" and feel unsafe without having the protection of "being armed." As discussed previously in the "Introduction to Driver's Training" section, patients become frightened or anxious on bridges or underpasses while traveling on the busy highways in a bus or van. Patients also may feel a sense of powerlessness and panic in crowded places, such as restaurants and malls. The hyper-vigilance while riding in a vehicle and the lack of tolerance for public places are often other sources of anxiety because patients did not expect to feel this way once they returned home. Patients need to be reassured by accompanying staff that this is a normal part of community reentry and their feelings and concerns should be openly discussed and addressed. The therapist discourages the patient from isolation, avoidance of public places, and traveling while reassuring the patient that his or her emotions and reactions will get easier with each subsequent outing.

The community reentry and reintegration program has gained much support from outside not-for-profit organizations. These organizations have made phenomenal opportunities available to patients allowing them to engage in all types of sports such as golfing, fishing, bowling, wheelchair basketball, snow and water skiing, canoeing, and horseback riding. Also, a program created through the American Red Cross in the national capitol region establishes tours around such sites as the White House, FBI building, US Treasury Department, US Capital building, Pentagon, and the Spy Museum. The therapist is encouraged to seek out local community opportunities for participation.

Therapists plan and coordinate the outings well in advance. Due to patient volume and patients' individual needs and demands when participating coupled with the community reentry program's growth, there are often two or more trips each week. This demands astute attention by team members that care for these patients and therefore community reintegration is a topic at the weekly team meetings. The interdisciplinary team is interested in knowing how the patient tolerates the community outing because this provides valuable information about the psychosocial status of the recovering patient.

The Adaptive Sports Program: An Extension of Community Reentry

Occupational therapists understand disability and have the skill set to address all areas of performance with special consideration to the patient factors and context of sport. The use of therapeutic sports as part of community reentry addresses all patient factors including (a) sensory, (b) neuromuscular skeletal, (c) cardiovascular, and (d) mental. Sports can generally be adapted to meet the patients where they are along a continuum of skill level.[22] The physical task demands of balance, strength, dexterity, and endurance inherent in sports continually prove challenging to the military patient population. Therapists understand that satisfaction in life is directly related to one's ability to participate fully in life, with as few restrictions as possible. In this way, therapists use sports to place the spotlight on the ability while de-emphasizing the disability.[22]

Therapeutic recreation has long been used to promote the achievement of optimal health through sports and leisure.[23] Adaptive sports consist of any sporting activity that has been modified to enable participation by someone with a disability. The Adaptive Sports Program (ASP) raises the performance bar from basic ADLs to extreme sports of all kinds. The engagement in sports as a therapeutic medium increases motivation, eases feelings of idleness, and alleviates loneliness and depression.[23] Sports naturally promote high-level skills, so occupational and physical therapy staff work in tandem to prepare patients for participation in sports.

Occupational and physical therapists utilize government and private organizations that offer adaptive sports opportunities. The Disabled American Veterans (Cold Spring, Ky) and Paralyzed Veterans of America (Washington, DC) offer opportunities to the military patients. The National Veterans Wheelchair Games are one of many sporting opportunities sponsored by the Paralyzed Veterans of America. Private nonprofit organizations such as the Disabled Sports USA (Rockville, Md) and Project Healing Waters (Washington, DC) are two of many organizations that also contribute to the mission of integrating sports into the recovery plan of the war-wounded SMs. Many of these organizations were established by veterans of prior and current conflicts to aid in the recovery of injured SMs returning from Operation Enduring Freedom/Operation Iraqi Freedom.

Overall, participation in the ASP facilitates the intrinsic motivation of the competitive and athletic military patient population. Patients learn adaptive skiing and snowmobiling in various Colorado cities; they learn adaptive kayaking in Maryland and Virginia; and they learn adaptive fly fishing in Montana. Some take on more physical challenges through participation in the Baton Death March, the Army Ten Miler, or National Veterans Wheelchair Games where they compete for medals in wheelchair sports such as quad rugby, basketball, skeet shooting, and softball.[24]

Through the ASP, the energy of the military culture physical competition and camaraderie is harnessed. The ASP simulates a familiar culture of competitiveness, in which the young, active, and adrenaline-seeking military patients thrive. The built-in activity demands of sports allow therapists to transcend the traditional activities of cones, blocks, and pegs that are familiar and necessary to most OT clinics. Moreover, the ASP represents "the doing" that defines so much of the therapeutic process innate to OT resulting in an evolution of recovery of function that can lead the SM to an active lifestyle following a disabling injury. This active lifestyle might likely include an adapted sporting activity.

DISCHARGE PLANNING

Before the global war on terror, the options for SMs with limb loss were more limited. Now SMs can requalify for active duty or pursue civilian careers. Whether or not the SM has the desire or the ability to return to active duty, the goal of the rehabilitation team is to help each patient achieve maximal function and the highest quality of life possible.

The discharge plan begins on the day the rehabilitation team is introduced to the injured patient. As is true with civilian patients undergoing rehabilitation, the information gathered during the initial evaluation serves as the foundation for discharge planning. The intent of a discharge plan is to provide a smooth transition from one level of care to another.

Discharge planning is best performed by a multidisciplinary team, along with the patient and the family. The medical members of this team may consist of a physiatrist who acts as coordinator for medical and surgical subspecialists, nurses, occupational and physical therapists, prosthetists, social workers, psychologists, dieticians, pharmacists, and psychiatrists. This group may also include a physical evaluation board liaison officer and a VA counselor to assist with the military medical disability system. It is suggested that this team meet weekly through team conferences and outpatient amputee clinics to ensure communication for quality and efficient care of every patient.

Many injured SMs have severe concomitant injuries in addition to an upper limb amputation that affect the choices that they must make about the lifestyle they will strive to live. Understanding the individual's lifestyle before admission will give insight into possible future goals. Knowledge about the patient's preexisting family/support system, physical condition, emotional/cognitive status, educational level, vocation, and avocations cannot be understated. The patient's culture and primary language—if other than English—also will impact discharge planning.

Follow-up Care

Many combat-injured military personnel will need provision for ongoing medical care that includes—at minimum—regular follow-ups with a physiatrist who will act as a coordinator for any specialty care required. Ongoing medical care includes regular follow-up visits with a prosthetist, psychologist, and/or psychiatrist, and intervention as needed with occupational and physical therapy, vocational rehabilitation, social work, and subspecialty medicine.

Resources

Providing the patient with resources to support ongoing rehabilitation is critical. For persons who have undergone rehabilitation in a protected hospital environment with significant support systems in place, transitioning to care outside the hospital is a very turbulent time. Transitions to different levels of care outside of this support system bring new stresses that frequently go understated in discharge planning. The individual does not often recognize these stresses until after the transition has occurred. To reduce the occurrence of feelings of isolation, the rehabilitation team introduces patients to numerous resources in preparation for discharge including the (a) Amputee Coalition of America (Knoxville, Tenn), (b) peer support, (c) local support groups, and (d) specialty interest groups for amputees. A number of nonprofit organizations for disabled veterans as well as for civilians with a disability provide recreational opportunities and other types of support. Paralyzed Veterans of America and Disabled American Veterans are two groups that support wounded veterans. Publications such as *InMotion* magazine (Amputee Coalition of America, Knoxville, Tenn) and *Challenge* magazine (Disabled Sports USA, Rockville, Md) can be great resources for both military and nonmilitary persons.

REHABILITATION FACTORS

Concomitant Injuries

As stated throughout this text, individuals who have sustained combat injuries frequently have concomitant injuries that must be considered when planning the rehabilitation process. Such injuries may influence available treatment options, treatment progress, and progression through rehabilitation phases. It is critical that the team communicate at least weekly on patient progress to ensure that all care the patient receives meets his or her needs. Additionally, communication among facilities actively engaged in the provision of treatment to those individuals who require highly specialized treatment in conditions, such as TBI, visual loss, or burns, is critical. Highly specialized centers may be located throughout the United States and communication may be facilitated through video teleconferencing or telephone conferences.

Once medically stable, those individuals with TBI are rehabilitated through one of five VA hospitals across the United States. Coordination of care is through the accepting physician and team and also through visual and administrative patient handoff between the gaining and losing facilities. The same process is repeated once the patient completes his or her TBI rehabilitation and returns to the gaining amputee center of excellence. The patient initiates the phase of amputee rehabilitation as appropriate. Depending on the severity of his or her TBI, rehabilitation must be adjusted according to the patient's needs.

Other factors that must be addressed or considered throughout rehabilitation include burns or skin grafts, infections, multiple organ injuries or failures, visual deficits, hearing and/or vestibular deficits, multiple extremity amputations, fractures, shrapnel injuries, peripheral nerve injuries, neuroma(s) development, heterotropic ossification, and risk of joint contracture. Psychosocial injuries and posttraumatic stress disorder also play a factor in rehabilitation. The impact of comorbid injuries sustained in combat adds to the complexity and intensity of rehabilitation but must be addressed appropriately to achieve a successful patient outcome.

Bilateral Upper Limb Amputee Training Considerations

Although any upper limb amputation challenges a person's physical and emotional self, a patient who loses both upper limbs will require more inner strength, patience, and willingness to persevere. A solid support system will augment the inner strength required during some of the challenges of rehabilitation. Additionally, the needs of a patient with bilateral upper limb loss requires an experienced team that can blend all of the current technology and creativity required to maximize the patient's independence and performance in his or her desired occupational performance areas. As soon as the team deems appropriate, a visit from a trained, matched peer visitor can be crucial to enhancing the patient's hope and vision for his or her future.

All areas of care previously described in this chapter apply to the bilateral limb loss amputee. However, some applications are unique to the bilateral limb loss amputee that would not be used by the unilateral limb loss amputee. In general, the traumatic bilateral upper limb loss amputee will usually choose to use at least one prosthesis to gain independence in ADLs. Also, he or she will require more adaptive equipment and

environmental modification, and will have a stronger tendency to use the environment to achieve the most efficient task performance possible.

Another significant factor that influences a bilateral upper limb amputee's decision to use a prosthesis is the length of the residual limbs. Length significantly impacts a patient's ability to function independently and influences his or her choice of prostheses and adaptive devices. A patient with longer residual limbs can utilize the available sensory feedback area on the residual limb to oppose each limb during functional grasping. Length is also a critical factor in determining limb dominance. Typically the longer residual limb will become the chosen dominant side because of the increased functionality of either the prosthesis or the increased sensory area and sound joints available to engage in activities. Therefore, in general, the longer the length of the residual limb(s), the more independent the person will be and fewer environmental modifications will be necessary. Patients with congenital bilateral limb loss develop unique motor patterns at a young age, such as the use of foot skills. Therefore, prosthetic use varies more as compared to those with traumatic limb loss.

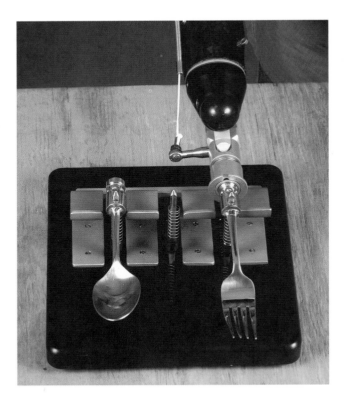

Figure 18-14. This is an example of a hands-free tool changing station.
Photograph courtesy of Texas Assistive Devices.

Of note regarding specific types of prosthetic componentry, for the bilateral upper limb prosthetic user wrist flexion is a benefit that allows the user to gain closer access to midline and to the facial area. This is critical for ADLs in which patients will use their prostheses. Certain prosthetic componentry and modified TD attachments can assist in providing increased degrees of freedom or task-specific function. Manufacturers have begun to fabricate componentry including the Five Function Wrist unit from Texas Assistive Devices (www.n-abler.org) that increases the patient's options for wrist positioning. Texas Assistive Devices (Brazoria, Tex) and TRS Inc (TRS Inc, Boulder, Colo) manufacture TD attachments that are task or activity specific, such as wrench sets, knives, hygiene items, and sports equipment. Texas Assistive Devices manufactures a hands-free tool changing station that allows a bilateral upper limb amputee to independently change the TD tool (Figure 18-14).

Many household items designed to address weakened grasp or pinch for the general population are useful to a bilateral upper limb loss amputee. A few examples include lever door handles, number pad key locks, motion sensor lighting, touch pad light switches, particular drawer pulls and handles, liquid bottle dispensers, refrigerators with in-door water dispensers, robotic vacuum cleaners, and computer controlled environments. Thanks to the evolution of computers and computer search engines, many options for bilateral limb loss amputees can be found through the Internet. As patients develop the ability to problem solve tasks that are specifically related to their needs, they begin to formulate their own solutions or ideas for problematic or difficult tasks.

RECENT ADVANCEMENTS IN PROSTHETIC DEVELOPMENT: IMPACT ON TREATMENT

In the 1980s Malone et al demonstrated that upper limb amputees fit with a prosthesis within 30 days had higher rehabilitation success.[25] This was supported by Fletchall's work evaluating "the value of specialized rehabilitation of trauma and amputation" in 2005.[26] Research and development in prosthetics are rapidly evolving, providing more prosthetic options with improved functional abilities for upper limb loss amputees.

Advances in prosthetic technology for partial hand and finger amputation levels, which have moved beyond traditional cosmetic and passive prosthesis, provide more functional joint components and incorporate remaining functionality of the residual hand and/or finger. Access to various finger prosthetic devices requires greater lead time than most other prostheses. Prosthetic options range from devices that are connected to a wrist-hand orthosis, utilization of the X-finger (Didrick Medical Inc, Naples, Fla), customized orthosis, and cosmesis that take advantage of residual active digit motion for increased function. Furthermore, future developments are underway as a result of research funded through the global war on terror to allow greater prosthetic fine motor control. These advances and others will influence future rehabilitation approaches and possibly a new rehabilitation standard of care will evolve.

Targeted reinnervation is a surgical option to provide an increased number of myosites by utilizing remaining distal peripheral nerves that are surgically placed over motor end points on healthy proximal denervated musculature of the residual limb. Ultimately, this procedure provides additional available muscle sites to control componentry necessary for prosthetic control for a high-level amputee. Another benefit of this procedure is the potential of sensory feedback from the skin over the reinnervated areas. SMs interested in this procedure are considered for eligibility once they have demonstrated proficiency with both a body-powered and a myoelectric prosthesis and have intact cognitive abilities to properly control and operate the prosthesis. It takes a minimum of 6 months to recover. During this time the SM is educated in scar management and followed as needed by OT. After recovery, the residual limb is evaluated to determine reinnervation of the newly created myosites. It is expected that by month six, reinnervation is complete and the SM should be able to be refit with the prosthesis and begin training with the new myosites and prosthesis. Once reinnervation occurs, prosthetic retraining is initiated in the same manner as described in this protocol but faster as the patient tolerates (see chapter 27, Future of Artificial Limbs, for more details).

Although engineering and electronic developments for the mass market continue to influence prosthetic technology development, federal and military sources have significantly increased their support for development of upper limb prosthetic technology. The Defense Advanced Research Projects Agency (Arlington, Va) Revolutionizing Prosthetics initiative is an example of this type of support. There are two programs under this initiative: (1) Revolutionizing Prosthetics 2007 and (2) Revolutionizing Prosthetics 2009. The intent of Revolutionizing Prosthetics 2007 is to develop a robotic prosthesis that looks and performs like a human arm. The prosthesis will perform functional range of motion at the shoulder, elbow, wrist, and digits; have a cosmetic cover that is durable and appears like skin; and weigh less than 8 pounds, the weight of the human arm.[27] Revolutionizing Prosthetics 2009 program will provide the upper limb prosthetic user with proprioceptive, sensory, temperature, and vibratory sensations.[28] Furthermore, the prosthetics that result from both Defense Advanced Research Projects Agency programs will be controlled through a neural interface, meaning they will be controlled through the user's brain as opposed to myosites.[27]

Research Updates

At the established centers of excellence across the country, the recent influx of polytrauma patients managed and treated has provided research opportunities that will result in the advancement of medical care and rehabilitation of these patients. Multiple studies have been proposed and are in various stages of research. A review of completed and current studies as well as discussion for future research will be presented in the following paragraphs.

Firearm Training Simulator

In 2004 the Telemedicine and Advanced Technology Research Center funded a study to assess the use of a virtual reality training simulator called the Firearm Training System (FATS). FATS is a projection-based type of virtual reality (VR) that uses a computer-generated image that creates a virtual environment to allow the patient to be part of a scenario in three dimensions, a virtual world. FATS has distinct weapons that look and feel authentic to SMs; however, instead of live ammunition, carbon dioxide discharges from the muzzle, which mimics the recoil of an actual weapon. Through FATS, patients work on weapons marksmanship. In the scenarios generated through FATS VR, patients complete training to replicate a live-firing range or select participation in a situation that places them in the middle of a simulated battle. The use of VR in physical rehabilitation can bring the complexity of the real world to rehabilitation while eliminating the associated risks.[29] The funded study enrolled 35 patients, two female and 33 male, with upper limb amputation or severe peripheral nerve, bone, or soft tissue injury.[30] The purpose of the study was to assess the number of patients that—with guided training—would achieve a basic proficiency status of "qualified" to fire a military service weapon. The patients had a choice of weapon selection. Six patients shot the M-9, 20 patients shot the M-4, and nine patients shot the M-16.

Eighteen failed to qualify with their chosen weapon on the initial marksmanship test; and in surprising contrast, 17 did qualify on the initial weapons fire.[30] By the conclusion of the study, all but one qualified with a military service weapon, yielding an overwhelmingly successful outcome of the FATS study. The patients were able to remaster a basic military skill that would not have been possible to train for safety reasons using real weapons at a live-fire range. The average time spent training was 9 hours; 23 SMs completed the recommended 10 hours of training.[30] Seventeen of the study participants were upper limb orthopaedic patients. They averaged 69% of targets hit on their initial marksmanship score and 88% of targets hit on their exit score, an average increase of 19%.[30] Eighteen participants were upper limb amputees. Eight of the study participants were transradial amputees, three of whom lost their dominant hand and therefore learned to shoot cross-dominance. The transradial amputees averaged 71% of targets hit on their initial marksmanship score and 84% of targets hit on their exit score, an average increase of 13%.[30]

Ten of the study participants were classified as transhumeral amputees and two were shoulder disarticulation amputees. Six of the participants lost their dominant arm. They averaged 68% of targets hit on their initial marksmanship score and 82% of targets on their exit score, an average increase of 14% (Table 18-3). Therapists believed that the patient's premorbid skill and training level, strong intrinsic motivation to return to soldier skills, and keen interest in VR aided in the pilot study's success. Many reported that the skills learned through FATS training were beneficial to their overall rehabilitation. Based on feedback from therapists and patients who were involved in the pilot study, the use of VR for weapons training offered identity-restoring therapeutic benefits, as well as the inherent task demands of eye-hand coordination and motor control. FATS is a standard treatment in OT for combat-wounded veterans.

Voice Recognition Software

Assistive technology offers a modern day portal to independence for people with disabilities.[31] Voice recognition technology is a type of assistive technology that allows a patient with compromised use of one or both upper limbs the opportunity to control voice-sensitive electronic devices that respond to human speech. Computer assistive technology systems called environmental control units enable the patient to control such items as lights, doors, and home appliances. Some less complicated systems based on computer software allow human speech to operate a personal computer. The technology of voice recognition software offers a viable alternative

TABLE 18-3

FIREARMS TRAINING SIMULATOR DATA: PERCENTAGE CHANGE FROM INITIAL TO FINAL WEAPONS TESTING BASED ON TYPE OF INJURY SUSTAINED BY PARTICIPATING SERVICE MEMBER

Injury Type	Average Targets Hit on Initial Test	Average Targets Hit on Final Test	Percentage Change
Upper extremity orthopaedic	69%	88%	19%
Transradial amputation	71%	84%	13%
Transhumeral amputation	68%	82%	14%

Source: Yancosek K, Daugherty SE, Cancio L. Treatment for the service member: a description of innovative interventions. *J Hand Ther.* 2008;21:189–195.

for standard computer keyboard operation that may be disrupted by the loss of function with one or both hands. In 1990 Lazzaro suggested that technology may serve as an electronic bill of rights to the physically challenged.[31]

The Telemedicine and Advanced Technology Research Center funded a qualitative pilot study that evaluated the functional outcome of training patients on voice recognition software for basic computer operation. The objective of this study was to determine the usefulness of integrating voice recognition software training into a comprehensive rehabilitation program for individuals with upper limb amputation(s) or orthopaedic injuries impairing upper limb function. Patients referred for OT services meeting inclusion criteria were considered for the study.[30] Fifteen patients, 13 male and 2 female, participated in this study. The software utilized was Dragon Naturally Speaking (DNS) version 7.0. Resources for assistive technology were provided through CAP.[32] Training occurred in three phases and included (1) instruction on software use, (2) command memorization, and (3) the opportunity to take a laptop out of the clinic for personal use and practice time.[30] Software training was conducted by a certified software instructor over the course of five class rotations with four separate class dates composed of 2 hours of training per class.[30] Participants in each of the five class rotations received a minimum of 8 hours of instruction. Investigators tracked the number of hours each person spent training on the software. This intervention was provided in addition to the standard rehabilitation care plan, and the patient consented to the time commitment inherent in study participation. All of the subjects included participated throughout the study.[30]

A post-training survey was mailed to participants after completion of their individual Medical Evaluation Board. The survey obtained qualitative data related to the ultimate usefulness of the software

and the training. Questions sought to determine the subject's final occupational outcome (ie, did he or she remain in the military, enroll in a college, or obtain employment) and whether he or she utilized the DNS software. Of the 15 follow-up surveys sent to participants, 9 were completed and returned. The six participants that did not reply were unable to be contacted by telephone or e-mail. The average training time of the nine participants who returned the survey was 7.25 hours. Of the nine surveys returned, six of the study participants had enrolled in college and four stated they used DNS version 7.0 to write all of their papers and long e-mails and to surf the Internet. The two remaining participants went to college but did not use DNS. One explained that despite having been trained on the software it was easier to "hunt-and-peck" and the other "nonuser" stated the orthopaedic condition that had rendered him unable to type during rehabilitation had resolved. Therefore, he was able to type. Three participants who completed the follow-up surveys did not go to college and all reported continued use of DNS for e-mails and word processing for employment and personal tasks. A quote from a survey by one of these three participants reads, "Voice makes it easier to navigate my PC and also increases my speed with writing letters and e-mail." Another participant commented, "Dragon was outstanding for me. It enabled me to continue to enjoy the computer. I don't feel like it's a challenge anymore." Another participant wrote, "Voice, on a daily basis, makes tasks that used to be difficult seem easy. It helped make things with PCs easier, faster, and less complicated once I became familiar with the software."[30]

The resounding positive comments of the participants and training results indicated that this training was effective. For patients with permanent disability to one or both upper limbs, the learning investment of training and utilizing voice recognition software is worth the benefit of being able to replace typing with voice activation text entry.[33] Additionally, the ability to interact with a computer is important to younger persons because they regularly engage in interactive communication to connect with others through the Internet or e-mail. These reasons provide credence to using voice recognition software in the standard rehabilitation care plan.[33]

Targeted Muscle Reinnervation

In collaboration with Brooke Army Medical Center and Walter Reed Army Medical Center, the Rehabilitation Institute of Chicago conducted a study titled "Targeted Reinnervation in Upper Limb Amputees to Improve Myoelectric Prosthesis Function." The goal of the study was to improve myoelectric prosthetic control for high-level upper limb amputees through targeted reinnervation surgery. A successful surgery may result in the availability of additional myoelectric control sites in the residual limb, the ability to control motion at multiple joints simultaneously creating a more natural motor pattern with prosthetic use, and a sensory feedback mechanism.

Recruited subjects who met inclusion and exclusion criteria were tested before the surgery with their current prosthesis. Both objective and subjective evaluations were performed on the subjects. The objective tests completed consisted of a modified version of the Box and Blocks Test, Clothes Pin Relocation Test, and Cubicle Reach Test. Subjective evaluations included a series of timed commonly performed ADL tasks that were designed to incorporate multiple joint movements of the upper limb in both standing and seated positions. Subjects underwent surgical intervention targeted at reinnervation of residual limb musculature using nerves remaining in the upper extremity. This technique is called targeted reinnervation.

Following surgery, patients were given approximately 5 to 8 months to heal before fitting of the dedicated targeted reinnervation prosthesis. The socket was modified to accommodate any changes that may have occurred in the residual limb shape and to incorporate additional myosites as a result of the targeted reinnervation surgery. Once the subject healed and fitting was completed the patient re-engaged in prosthetic training with OT to further enhance control of the myoelectric prosthesis with the additional myosites. Upon completion of prosthetic training and the patient's demonstration of adequate prosthetic control, the aforementioned tests were repeated. Follow-up evaluation was completed at 4 months and 8 months to measure and compare performance with the surgically created myosites.

The Type of Prosthesis and Its Effect on Functional Activities

The overall success of prosthetic users is still a highly debated issue. What makes a user prefer a body-powered over a myoelectric over no prosthesis use? This question remains unanswered. To provide further insight, a research project is underway to examine differing functional capabilities with a body-powered versus a myoelectric device. The purpose of the current study titled "The Effect of Upper Limb Prostheses Type on Functional Activity" is to determine the effectiveness of upper limb body-powered prostheses versus myoelectric prostheses when performing functional activities to more accurately assess an SM's potential to return to his or her MOS or AOC. The goal is to provide prosthetic engineers and therapists with pertinent data regarding the effectiveness of body-powered and myoelectric prostheses currently being provided to Operation Enduring Freedom/Operation Iraqi Freedom SMs. This study will promote a better understanding of body mechanics and pre-positioning techniques used by SMs when performing MOS/AOC relevant tasks while wearing an upper limb prosthesis.

Military upper limb amputation rehabilitation programs will benefit from the results of this study because SMs and therapists will be better prepared to select prostheses that best support SMs in their return to a specific MOS. Also, prosthetists will gain insight regarding prosthetic mechanical failures. This knowledge will aid in the development of prostheses that are effective and reliable in a field environment, allowing SMs to meet the physical demands of their MOS/AOC.

Community Reintegration Survey

Community reintegration is a critical component in rehabilitation. These activities provide motivation while simultaneously providing an opportunity to challenge and integrate the SM into everyday life, sports, and the workplace. To address difficulty in defining the parameters of community reintegration and measuring its success for a patient, a survey tool is being developed. It will aid in goal setting and prioritizing events/activities in which the SM may select to participate. Survey questions will address physical abilities and psychosocial status, both of which are important.

Multiple Exposure/Progressive Desensitization

Many SMs returning from combat have combat stress reaction and posttraumatic stress that influence rehabilitation. Graded treatment approaches have been developed and implemented to address the influence of these disorders on return to certain activities. The use of virtual simulators during firearms training and driver's training simulators provides excellent media to grade shooting and driving, respectively. SMs are provided the opportunity to gradually reacclimate and desensitize themselves from the associated trauma while engaging in these activities. It has been the rehabilitation team experi-

ence that SMs participating in these forms of therapy have improved their confidence. The FATS study has presented a solid basis for virtual simulators to help with reintegrating weaponry skills for patients with a prosthesis. However, future research to determine whether the virtual simulators make a difference in the SM's ability to recover and reintegrate into the military or at a minimum cope better with his or her future environment is warranted.

SUMMARY

Providing an environment to attempt previous activities or new challenges can lead to some of the most rewarding experiences. A wide variety of activities can be made available to support SMs before discharge from the hospital. Members of the armed forces are young, athletic, and competitive, so harnessing this desire has been incredibly successful. Some popular programs are snow skiing, water skiing, rafting and kayaking, hunting and shooting, and rock climbing. Providing resources and contacts to enable the patient to pursue or continue new activities in his or her home community can be a critical component to full

reintegration.

Life is forever changing and challenging. Providing dynamic, supportive, and skilled upper limb loss rehabilitation through a comprehensive approach beginning with the medical model and progressing to an occupation-based model in a controlled living environment provides the amputee with a solid foundation. Ultimately, the upper limb amputee rehabilitation efforts are designed to provide patients with fundamental upper limb prosthetic skills to live balanced and productive lives both in and out of the military system.

Acknowledgments

The authors would like to acknowledge Harvey Naranjo, COTA, and Ibrihim Kabbah, COTA, for their effort and dedication to the development of the Walter Reed Army Medical Center Amputee Program. In addition, they also would like to acknowledge Colonel (Retired) William J. Howard, III, OTR/L for his enthusiastic leadership, unwavering support, and his extraordinary vision for the Walter Reed Army Medical Center Amputee Program.

REFERENCES

1. Dillingham TR. Rehabilitation of the upper limb amputee. In: Dillingham TR, Belandres PV, eds. *Rehabilitation of the Injured Combatant.* Vol 1. In: Zajtchuk R, Bellamy RF, eds. *Textbooks of Military Medicine.* Washington, DC: Department of the Army, Office of The Surgeon General, Borden Institute; 1998:33–77.

2. Walter Reed Army Medical Center. Amputee Monthly Statistics. Washington, DC: Walter Reed Army Medical Center Amputee Program; Updated July 1, 2009.

3. Kielhofner G. *Model of Human Occupation: Theory and Application.* 4th ed. Conshohocken, Pa: Lippincott Williams & Wilkins; 2007.

4. Pendleton HM, Schultz-Krohn W. The occupational therapy practice framework and the practice of occupational therapy for people with physical disabilities. In: Pendleton HM, Schultz-Krohn W, eds. *Pedretti's Occupational Therapy: Practice Skills for Physical Dysfunction.* 6th ed. St. Louis, Mo: Mosby Elsevier; 2006:6–7.

5. Esquenazi A, Wikoff E, Lucas M. Amputation rehabilitation. In: Grabois M, Garrison SJ, eds. *Physical Medicine and Rehabilitation: The Complete Approach.* Ames, Iowa: Blackwell Science; 2000.

6. Esquenazi A, DiGiacomo R. Exercise prescription for the amputee. In: Shankar K, ed. *Exercise Prescription.* Philadelphia, Pa: Hanley & Belfus; 1999.

7. Huston C, Dillingham TR, Esquenazi A. Rehabilitation of the lower limb amputee. In: Dillingham TR, Belandres PV, eds. *Rehabilitation of the Injured Combatant*. Vol 1. In: Zajtchuk R, Bellamy RF, eds. *Textbooks of Military Medicine*. Washington, DC: Department of the Army, Office of The Surgeon General, Borden Institute; 1998:79–159.

8. Jefferies GE. Pain management: post-amputation pain. *InMotion*. Knoxville, Tenn: Amputee Coalition of America; 2007.

9. Walsh MT, Muntzer E. Therapists management of complex regional pain syndrome (reflex sympathetic dystrophy). In: Hunter MC, ed. *Rehabilitation of the Hand and Upper Limb*. 5th ed. St. Louis, Mo: Mosby; 2002.

10. Ramachandran VS, Hirstein W. The perception of phantom limbs: the D.O. Hebb lecture. *Brain*. 1998;121:1603–1630.

11. Ramachandran VS, Rogers-Ramachandran D. Synaesthesia in phantom limbs induced with mirrors. *Proc Biol Sci*. 1996;263:377–386.

12. Weiss T, Miltner WH, Adler T, Bruckner L, Taub E. Decrease in phantom limb pain associated with prosthesis-induced increased use of an amputation stump in humans. *Neurosci Lett*. 1999;272:131–134.

13. Lotze M, Grodd W, Birbaumer N, Erb M, Huse E, Flor H. Does use of a myoelectric prosthesis prevent cortical reorganization and phantom limb pain? *Nat Neurosci*. 1999;2:501–502.

14. Lifelong Peak Performance Program student workbook. Peak Performance Training, 2007.

15. Esquenazi A. Upper limb amputee rehabilitation and prosthetic restoration. In: Braddom RL, ed. *Physical Medicine and Rehabilitation*. 3rd ed. Philadelphia, Pa: Saunders Elsevier; 2007.

16. Bowker JH. The art of prosthesis prescription. In: Smith DG, Michael JW, Bowker JH, eds. *Atlas of Amputations and Limb Deficiencies: Surgical, Prosthetic, and Rehabilitation Principles*. 3rd ed. Rosemont, Ill: American Academy of Orthopaedic Surgeons; 2004: 742.

17. Atkins DJ. Prosthetic training. In: Smith DG, Michael JW, Bowker JH, eds. *Atlas of Amputations and Limb Deficiencies: Surgical, Prosthetic, and Rehabilitation Principles*. 3rd ed. Rosemont, Ill: American Academy of Orthopaedic Surgeons; 2004.

18. Heinze A. *The Use of Upper-Extremity Prostheses*. Thief River Falls, Minn: Dynamic Rehab Videos and Rentals; 1988.

19. Leavy JD. *It Can Be Done: An Upper Extremity Amputee Training Handbook*. Quincy, Calif: Feather Publishing Company; 1977.

20. Atkins DJ. *Comprehensive Management of the Upper-Limb Amputee*. New York, NY: Springer-Verlag; 1989.

21. Jones LE, Davidson JH. Save that arm: a study of problems in the remaining arm of unilateral upper limb amputees. *Prosthet Orthot Int*. 1999;23:55–58.

22. Occupational therapy practice framework: domain and process. *Am J Occup Ther*. 2002;56:609–639.

23. Wardlaw FB, McGuire FA, Overby Z. Therapeutic recreation: optimal health treatment for orthopaedic disability. *Orthop Nurs*. 2000;19:56–60.

24. Paralyzed Veterans of America Web site. *Sports & Recreation*. Available at: www.pva.org. Accessed July 1, 2008.

25. Malone JM, Fleming LL, Roberson J, et al. Immediate, early, and late postsurgical management of upper-limb amputation. *J Rehabil Res Dev*. 1984;21:33–41.

26. Fletchall S. Returning upper-extremity amputees to work. *The O&P Edge*. 2005;28– 33.

27. Beard J. DARPA's bio-revolution: an array of programs aimed to improve the safety, health, and well-being of the military and civilians alike. Arlington, Va: Defense Advanced Research Projects Agency; 158–160. Available at: http://www.darpa.mil/Docs/Biology-biomedical_services_200807171322092.pdf - 2008-08-20. Accessed July 12, 2009.

28. Defense Advanced Research Projects Agency. DARPA fact sheet. Arlington, Va: DARPA; 2008. Available at: www. darpa.mil/Docs/prosthetics_f_s3_200807180945042.pdf - 2008-08-20. Accessed July 12, 2009.

29. Rose FD, Attree EA, Johnson DA. Virtual reality: an assistive technology in neurological rehabilitation. *Curr Opin Neurol.* 1996;9:461–467.

30. Yancosek K, Daugherty SE, Cancio L. Treatment for the service member: a description of innovative interventions. *J Hand Ther.* 2008;21:189–195.

31. Lazzaro JJ. Opening doors for the disabled. *BYTE.* 1990:258–268.

32. Military Health System. Computer/Electronic Accommodations Program, February 13, 2007.

33. Goette T, Marchewka JT. Voice recognition technology for persons who have motoric disabilities. *J Rehabil Med.* 1994;60:38–41.

Chapter 19

GAIT ANALYSIS AND TRAINING OF PEOPLE WITH LIMB LOSS

JASON M. WILKEN, PhD, PT[*]; AND RAUL MARIN, MD[†]

[*]Director, Military Performance Laboratory, Department of Orthopaedics and Rehabilitation, Center for the Intrepid, Brooke Army Medical Center, 3851 Roger Brooke Drive, Fort Sam Houston, Texas 78234
[†]Colonel (Retired), Medical Corps, US Army; Physician, Center for the Intrepid, Brooke Army Medical Center, 3851 Roger Brooke Drive, Fort Sam Houston, Texas 78234; formerly, Medical Director, GaitLab, Physical Medicine and Rehabilitation Teaching Staff, and Chair, Internal Review Board, Department of Orthopaedics and Rehabilitation, Walter Reed Army Medical Center, 6900 Georgia Avenue, NW, Washington, DC

INTRODUCTION

The systematic study of human ambulation began in the mid-1800s with the appearance of photography and observation-based studies.[1] Subsequently, kinetic (forces)[2] and kinematic (joint movement)[3] studies began near the onset of World War II. The large number of amputees resulting from this conflict became a catalyst for the use of technology for the assessment of amputee gait. Inman and his colleagues introduced the use of movies in the coronal, sagittal, and transverse planes, as well as the use of force plates and electromyography (EMG) into the evaluation of able-bodied and amputee gait.[4]

The intent of amputee gait assessment is the identification of gait parameters that deviate or differ from able-bodied gait (ie, from "normal"). This identification, in turn, provides an opportunity to develop corrective strategies designed to enhance the efficiency, comfort, and cosmesis of amputee gait. Attainment of "normality" is not an end in itself, but rather a guide toward the optimization of function.

This chapter reviews the terminology of gait assessment and discusses both observational and computerized gait assessment. The authors' current understanding of able-bodied gait and documentation of gait performance observed in current military amputees is presented. Also included is a discussion of several special considerations about amputee gait and how gait laboratory assessment translates into effective therapeutic interventions.

TERMINOLOGY OF GAIT ASSESSMENT

A clear understanding of the terminology used in the description and evaluation of gait is essential prior to the assessment of patient performance. A clear or well-defined "common language" among the various disciplines forms the foundation on which a systematic and reliable assessment is built. Such assessment, in turn, leads to the effective planning and execution of interventions. Furthermore, common language facilitates a systematic tracking of progress because it allows for consistent pre- and postintervention comparison and monitoring.

The gait cycle consists of one stride that is divided into two periods known as stance and swing periods. During stance, the primary responsibility of the limb is to support the superincumbent body weight, while during swing, the task of limb advancement is accomplished. Figure 19-1 provides a visual representation of the gait cycle.[5] Note that double support forms 20% to 30% of the gait cycle and that the terminology for describing the phases of gait has changed in recent years. To account for the frequent absence of heel strike in pathologic gait and to allow for a more consistent framework for discussing gait deviations, the classic terminology of heel strike, foot flat, midstance, heel-off, toe-off; and early, mid, and terminal swing is used less frequently. Rather, initial contact, loading response, midstance, terminal stance, and pre-swing are commonly used to describe the stance phase. Initial, middle, and late swing are used to characterize the swing phase.

One of the easiest temporal and spatial parameters to measure quantitatively is walking speed (meters/ second). This parameter is critical because velocity strongly influences the loading, motion, and alignment of the different joints throughout the gait cycle. Furthermore, each individual selects his or her natural rate of walking so that the speed selected minimizes energy expenditure.[4] When the gait efficiency of an individual is plotted against various walking speeds ranging from very slow to very fast, a parabolic curve is displayed demonstrating that speeds slower or faster than the self-selected walking velocity (SSWV) will increase energy expenditure.[6]

There are several other temporal and spatial measurements that are used in the assessment of gait. Step length is the distance between a person's heels during the double support phase of gait. Stride length is the distance traveled by the heel from initial contact of one foot to the subsequent initial contact of the same foot. One stride length contains two step lengths. The number of steps that occur within a given period of time (typically per minute) is known as cadence. Cadence can be multiplied by the individual's stride length to determine walking velocity.[5]

Bipedal human locomotion is the result of evolutionary changes that allowed—among other things—the freeing of the upper limbs. This evolutionary change from quadruped to biped locomotion involved changes in the action of forces across levers responsible for locomotion. Torque from application of force distant to the axis of rotation that results in motion about the axis of rotation (if not opposed) is referred to in this chapter as a joint moment or simply moment. The convention of internal joint moments will be used throughout this chapter. Internal joint moments are commonly used because they are associated with the internal (typically muscular) forces that are necessary to produce or resist rotational motion at a given joint. These forces are in direct response to external moments, which are generated by the forces

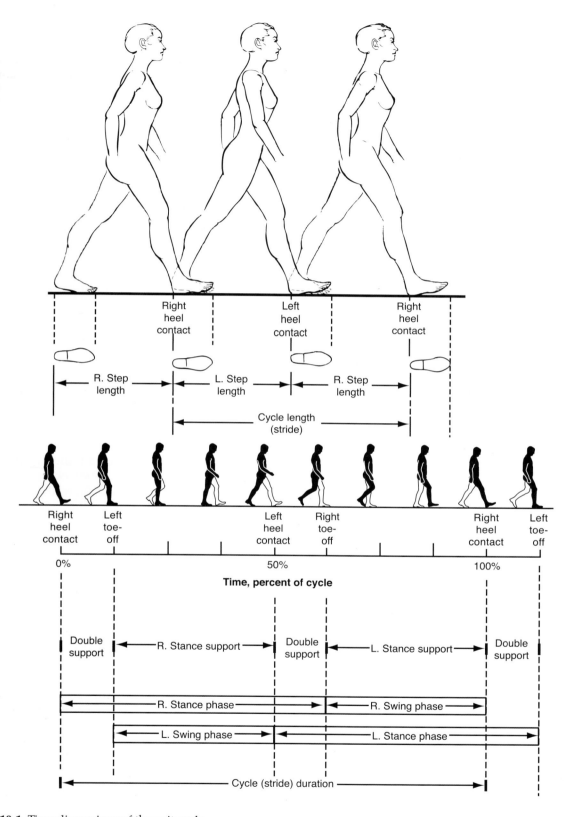

Figure 19-1. Time dimensions of the gait cycle.
Reproduced with permission from: Rose J, Gamble JG, Eds. *Human Walking*. Baltimore, Md: Lippincott Williams & Wilkins; 2005:26.

that push against the body (eg, ground reaction force). In standard reporting of gait laboratory data the term moment refers to net or resultant joint internal moment or torque produced by muscular, ligamentous, or bony force.

To the clinician performing an observational gait assessment, the temporal and spatial components of gait are—at most—approximations of observed deviations from what an expected symmetric gait should be. Computerized gait assessment, however, provides for precise quantifiable measurements of these variables.

OBSERVATIONAL GAIT ASSESSMENT

In the military setting a wide range of tools is available to assess amputee gait performance. These tools range from the brief informal visual assessment commonly used in the clinic to the application of advanced motion capture technologies. Selection of the most appropriate assessment approach is based primarily on the desired outcome of that particular evaluation session, which is determined using the patient's and therapist's rehabilitation goals, as well as the standardized assessment protocols at each facility. Observational assessment is—by its very nature—prone to inaccuracies. When a patient is walking, the speed at which motion occurs is commonly faster than what can be processed by the observing clinician. Intuitively, one would think that this limitation can be addressed by the presence of multiple observers under the belief that what one observer may miss may be caught by another observer. However, Krebs et al noted that single observer observational gait analysis is more consistent than multiple observer gait analysis and that this consistency could be increased for both methods by video recording, particularly if the replayed video was in slow motion.[7]

If computerized gait analysis is used as the gold standard by which observational gait analysis is to be compared, then it is apparent that—although convenient—observational gait analysis lacks adequate sensitivity. Saleh and Murdoch demonstrated that visual observers recorded only 22% of the gait laboratory-determined gait deviations with the measurement system detecting 3.4 times more deviations than visual observation alone.[8]

Although the above discussion makes a strong case for the application of computerized gait analysis, the complexity, cost, and limited availability of this methodology significantly hampers its clinical utility. Thus, the average clinician is left with his or her observations to assess the degree of pathology and the intervention required to address that pathology. A report by Gage in 2004 recommends that a systematic and well-organized observational gait analysis recording form be used for all such evaluations.[5] The Rancho Los Amigos full body observational gait analysis form is perhaps the most well-known tool to accomplish this evaluation.[9]

COMPUTERIZED GAIT ASSESSMENT

Gait laboratory assessment in the military setting typically consists of video-based observational analysis in combination with quantitative assessment of temporal-spatial, kinematic, and kinetic parameters. This assessment differs significantly from the typical evaluation performed in the clinic in that it provides quantitative information that can be used to identify gait deviations, provide insight into joint loading and torques, and objectively track progress through pre- and postintervention comparisons. Computerized gait analysis is the standard of care for military amputees and is part of a regular assessment plan. Clinical experience suggests that the best results are obtained in cases where the gait pattern is complex or deviations are subtle, the altered gait pattern is believed to be the source of decreased function or pain, and the patient is highly motivated and follows the resulting treatment plan.

Data Collection

To allow data sharing, facilitate troubleshooting, and support collaborative research projects, the Military Advanced Training Center and the Center for the Intrepid military amputee patient care sites use similar assessment tools for quantifying gait performance.

To provide an accurate assessment of amputee gait kinematics (motion), both sites use passive marker-based optoelectronic motion tracking systems. Passive tracking systems rely on the placement of small (9 mm) reflective markers on the patient's body to accurately track joint and segment positions in three-dimensional space. To independently monitor the three-dimensional motion of each segment, a minimum of three tracking markers is placed on each segment. These tracking markers are supplemented with additional markers that are used to identify bony landmarks and define the orientation of each segment (eg, thigh). The total number of markers used during a session can range from 6 to 70, depending on the type of assessment being performed.

Between 12 and 26 motion capture cameras emit infrared light that is reflected off the surface of the tracking markers and then recorded on the camera's image sensor. Image processing is performed within the camera to identify the centroid—or center—of the marker as a two-dimensional coordinate (vertical and medial-lateral position). The information from each camera is then sent to a central data collection computer. By combining two-dimensional images from the cameras, the system can triangulate the three-dimensional position of the marker with an accuracy of 0.7 millimeters. These marker position data are then used to quantify the magnitude and direction of motion that occur at individual joints and are presented in graphical format for interpretation by the clinical staff.

Force plates are used in all amputee center gait laboratories to assess gait kinetics (or forces). Typically eight force plates are embedded in the main walkway allowing the ability to measure location, direction, and magnitude of force applied at the foot floor interface. Although ground reaction force data are useful as an independent assessment tool, the force data are typically combined with marker data to calculate joint moments as well as power generation and absorption. Insight into the compensatory responses exhibited by amputees is provided using an approach called inverse dynamics. When using this method, joint position, segment motion, mass properties, orientation, and external forces acting on the segment are used to estimate lower extremity joint reaction forces, moments, and powers. Although not providing direct information regarding activation of individual muscles, the approach provides insight into the net effect of muscle activation at each joint of interest.

Because of the large effect of walking velocity on gait performance, gait kinetics in particular, patients are asked to walk along the laboratory walkway at both controlled and SSWV during standard clinical assessment. Collecting gait data at controlled speeds allows the opportunity to determine whether deviations from normal self-selected gait are a result of the amputation or simply the result of changes in walking velocity as compared to uninjured individuals.

Energy Expenditure

Metabolic cost assessment, another assessment technique that can provide insight into gait performance, is commonly used to assess the effectiveness of prosthetic components (as well as training interventions). Metabolic cost assessment is typically performed as patients ambulate on a treadmill while walking velocity is incrementally increased. Patients are typically tested at three to six controlled walking velocities approximately centered about the individual's SSWV. Such assessment allows the ability to determine the patient's gait efficiency and his or her ability to accommodate ambulation at multiple speeds.

Electromyography

EMG can be used to provide insight into the timing, magnitude, and patterns of muscular activation used by amputees. Use of surface electrodes allows the ability to quantify muscle activation while minimizing the risk of discomfort and infection that can be associated with indwelling electrodes. Although challenges such as appropriate normalization of EMG data and reduced access to residual limb musculature must be overcome, the assessment of muscle activation provides insight that other approaches cannot. Unlike the inverse dynamic approach that is unable to account for co-contraction and force production by passive structures (bony or ligamentous restraint), EMG allows the ability to directly record the timing and magnitude of muscle activation.

ABLE-BODIED ("NORMAL") GAIT

In 1985 Perry described four essential requirements for normal gait that—when absent in part or in whole—produce deviations from the norm.[10] These requirements are (1) symmetric or proportionate step length, (2) stance stability, (3) swing clearance, and (4) adequate foot position before initial contact. Gage added energy conservation as a fifth essential requirement in 1991.[11]

Energy conservation during ambulation is multifactorial in nature. The body is designed to be able to take advantage of the ground reaction force for joint stability and efficiency. Efficiency is also increased by the predominant use of eccentric muscle contractions during movement. Furthermore, when the less efficient concentric contractions occur, the muscle begins from a stretched or elongated position to allow the recovery of kinetic energy stored in elastic connective tissues. Energy conservation also occurs through muscles crossing two joints that serve the function of linking and transferring forces across body segments.

The phases of the gait cycle depicted in Figure 19-1 are helpful in understanding the sequence of events that is characteristic of a normal gait cycle. Human walking can be described as a process of alternating acceleration and deceleration of the center of mass, with the bulk of energy utilization occurring at the beginning and at the end of the stance periods. As such, during loading response the quadriceps and tibialis anterior muscles contract eccentrically to allow controlled knee flexion and ankle plantarflexion resulting in a net absorption of force and subsequent deceleration of the body. During midstance the momentum generated by the above described muscle actions takes the body's center of gravity over the weight-bearing leg as the contralateral leg swings like a pendulum with minimal energy utilization. During terminal stance and pre-swing, there is ipsilateral force generation and acceleration via the concentric contraction of the gastroc-soleus complex and similar response of the gluteus maximus in the contralateral side.

Evolutionary changes in human anatomy and biomechanics have ensured that human ambulation occurs with the greatest efficiency at self-selected walking speeds. In 1953 Saunders et al proposed the six determinants of gait as a way of explaining how the body's displacement of the center of mass within a 5-cm sinusoidal pattern of horizontal and vertical displacement conserves energy expenditures during walking.[12] Saunders et al's six determinants of gait follow:

1. Pelvic tilt: in the frontal plane, during stance the weight-bearing gluteus medius allows a drop of the contralateral swing side iliac crest, thus decreasing the rise in the center of mass during single limb support.
2. Pelvic rotation: in the horizontal plane during double limb support, pelvic rotaion allows increased step length while minimizing the drop of the center of mass.
3. Knee flexion at loading response and during stance: reduces the rise of the center of mass as the body transitions over the stance limb.
4. Ankle dorsiflexion at initial contact: effectively elongates the limb allowing a smooth transition onto the stance limb preventing a

drop of the center of mass.
5. Ankle plantarflexion at terminal stance/pre-swing: effectively elongates the limb allowing a smooth transition off of the stance limb by preventing a drop of the center of mass.
6. Side-to-side pelvic displacement from stance to stance: shifts the center of mass from one weight-bearing leg to the other.

For decades, these six determinants of gait were believed to effectively characterize the major factors that serve to minimize energy expenditure in human ambulation under the premise that they minimized the excursion or displacement of the center of gravity. Although evidence supports the association between vertical displacement of the center of mass and energy consumption, other studies have questioned the premise that the six determinants of gait (in combination or independently) are the sole factors responsible for controlling the center of mass displacement and thus energy expenditure.[13]

As early as 1983, in a study measuring mechanical cost at three different walking speeds (slow, self-selected, fast), Winter found that energy cost decreases as knee extension increases during stance with a significant positive correlation between energy cost and the degree of knee flexion.[14] In a series of articles, Kerrigan and her co-investigators found that heel rise from foot flat to pre-swing significantly raises the center of mass when it is at its lowest point during the gait cycle with the end result of reducing its overall displacement. They also found that pelvic rotation contributes no more than 12% of the total reduction of the vertical displacement of the center of mass.[15,16] Likewise, other investigators have documented that although knee flexion reduces the center of mass vertical excursion, it significantly increases the energy costs, and that heel rise from foot-flat to pre-swing is responsible for two-thirds of the reduction in the center of mass vertical excursion.[17-19]

It appears then that the six determinants do not have the same influence in reducing the center of mass excursion and that perhaps other as-of-yet to be identified determinants must be contributing to the energy cost savings resulting from the minimization of the center of mass displacement.

GAIT DEVIATIONS IN THE LOWER LIMB AMPUTEE

As in the civilian setting, lower limb military amputees typically demonstrate characteristic gait deviations as a result of the partial loss of lower limb function. Gait deviations observed in the amputee patient are commonly attributed to the following:

- loss of active torque generation;
- loss of somatosensory feedback and limb position awareness;
- additional degrees of freedom added by the mobile interface between the residual limb

540

- and socket;
- pain;
- limitations of current prosthetic devices (foot, socket, and knee if applicable); and
- functional impairments in the contralateral limb.

Fortunately, with adequate training, prosthetic care, and patient motivation, these factors can be minimized or compensated for, yielding a very functional gait pattern that is nearly indistinguishable from that of uninjured individuals.

Many factors influence the maximal gait performance patients attain before discharge from treatment. In military amputees, the frequent presence of significant injury to multiple areas of the body plays an important role in determining the maximal gait performance attained after completion of therapy. Patients often experience significant bony and soft tissue injury to the nonamputated limb at the time of injury, which can result in a nonamputated side that is less functional than the amputated side. In some instances the amputated side is referred to as the "good" or more functional side. Because other injuries vary widely in their impact on the patient's overall gait performance, the current discussion will focus on what is currently deemed the maximal gait performance exhibited by the highest functioning patients and then on commonly observed deviations from that gait pattern.

When assessing gait performance it is important to consider the potential long-term impact of individual gait deviations. Although the patients and clinicians may wish to minimize all gait deviations until they are not readily noticeable, efforts should first be focused on facilitating the most functional and efficient gait while identifying and addressing the source of gait deviations that are most likely to produce long-term morbidity such as osteoarthritis, low back pain, and other commonly observed problems.

STANDARDIZED GAIT ASSESSMENT

To provide a consistent and thorough assessment of amputee gait, a standardized approach is used for the interpretation of gait performance. A comprehensive assessment typically begins with the assessment of temporal-spatial parameters such as walking velocity, step length, step width, stride length, and other gait parameters that allow the rapid detection of gross asymmetries and other deviations from normal. Information such as walking velocity is particularly valuable when interpreting kinematic and kinetic data that are influenced by walking velocity. Kinematic data are then assessed using what is commonly known as a "bottom-up" approach, beginning with the examination of ankle and foot motion and progressing up the kinematic chain. These measures are compared with that of uninjured individuals and high functioning patients that are thought to demonstrate maximal or "optimal" gait performance. After completing the assessment of kinematic data, torque production at the ankle, knee, and hip is assessed in a similar manner, beginning at the ankle and ending at the hips. This is followed by assessment of joint power data before providing a comprehensive assessment of the patient's overall gait pattern and final report generation.

TRANSTIBIAL AMPUTEE GAIT

Due to their relatively young age and high fitness level, service members who have experienced transtibial amputation with adequate residual limb length and minimal contralateral involvement are typically able to achieve a gait pattern that is indistinguishable from uninjured individuals. The highest functioning individuals demonstrate gait patterns that are fluid, functional, and approximate the gait of uninjured individuals in terms of gait kinematics and kinetics: their gait patterns are used as the benchmark against which other amputees are compared. For this reason, deviations from normal gait that are demonstrated by patients with maximal or "optimal" gait performance will be presented before discussing additional deviations that are addressed with training or prosthetic management. Despite the extensive study of amputee gait, the "optimal" gait pattern has yet to be defined.

Initial Contact through Midstance

For most transtibial amputees, the stance phase begins with the lower limb positioned in a manner nearly identical to that of uninjured individuals. The ankle is in a neutral position, the knee is nearly fully extended, and the hip is flexed to between 25 degrees and 35 degrees. Differences from normal gait are, however, observed as soon as the patient begins to bear weight on and control motion of the involved limb and prosthesis.

Ankle Kinematics and Kinetics

State-of-the-art prosthetic feet currently provided to military amputees function—mechanically speaking—in a manner that is significantly different from the physiologic ankle. Shock absorption and "ankle" motion after initial contact are achieved by compression of the heel component rather than through true plantarflexion rotation about a physiologic ankle joint. Observed motion is, therefore, primarily an artifact of proximal displacement of the heel relative to the forefoot resulting in rotation of the shoe relative to the shank. However, meaningful information can be gained from the interpretation of "ankle" kinematic and kinetic data as will be established during presentation of specific gait deviations associated with prosthetic alignment, foot category, and training.

During loading response most high functioning patients are able to reproduce sagittal plane ankle kinematics that are indistinguishable from uninjured individuals. Although they produce normal kinematics, most patients demonstrate dorsiflexion torque that is increased in both duration and magnitude.[20,21] This is due—in part—to the frequently observed increase in double limb support time, which is believed to impart additional stability, and compression of the prosthetic heel, which results in patients spending a significant amount of time on the heel. Once patients reach a stable foot flat position and transition off the heel component, ankle kinematics and kinetics are nearly identical to that of uninjured individuals until pre-swing. As loading shifts from the heel to the forefoot due to forward rotation of the tibia associated with progression of the trunk over the stance limb, gradual dorsiflexion motion and an increasing plantarflexor moment are observed. Resulting sagittal plane ankle kinematics and kinetics (moment and power) during midstance are commonly normal with respect to both pattern and peak magnitude.

Knee Kinematics and Kinetics

Consistent with the broader amputee population, high functioning patients typically display decreased knee flexion from loading response until pre-swing.[20,22,23] Although knee flexion during the stance phase is present, it is both decreased and delayed relative to nonamputee gait.[22] Although nonamputee gait is commonly seen as ideal, a convincing case has not been made to indicate that decreased knee flexion during stance phase is detrimental and not an effective compensatory strategy. There are several potential explanations why patients choose to decrease knee flexion. First, this altered gait pattern may compensate for the functional loss of leg length because of the distal translation of the residual limb within the socket and compression of the prosthetic foot and shock absorber (if present).[24-29] Second, decreased knee flexion during midstance

may assist in the gradual storage of energy in the prosthetic forefoot that can be released for propulsion. With an extended knee the body moves as an inverted pendulum. Forward movement of the body over the fixed foot and rotation of the extended leg result in gradual dorsiflexion of the prosthetic foot and storage of energy that can be returned during pre-swing. In this manner, amputees are also able to effectively utilize the rollover characteristics of the prosthetic foot.[30,31] Third, co-contraction may be used as a strategy to stabilize the mobile bone–socket interface and decrease the degrees of freedom of the residual limb.[24,26-29] Increased activation of the quadriceps muscle, despite an extended knee position, has been previously identified as a strategy to stabilize the knee.[21,22] Although this strategy likely serves to control the knee, it may also be in response to knee flexor torque produced by activation of the biarticular gastrocnemius muscle and an overall stiffening of the limb. Activation has been identified as a strategy to stabilize the bone–socket interface by increasing the stiffness of the soft tissue in the residual limb.[32] Although sagittal plane kinematics of the knee is altered, as previously reported net joint torques are minimally affected.[22]

Hip Kinematics and Kinetics

Sagittal plane kinematics and kinetics of the hip have been identified as the primary source of compensation in civilian transtibial amputees, but are relatively unaffected in high functioning military amputees.[20,21] Hip flexion is occasionally increased at initial contact and toe-off but this does not significantly alter joint torques or powers. The increased hamstring activation associated with reported co-contraction at the knee and other reported changes in muscle activation are either not present or have little effect on the sagittal plane kinematics and net sagittal plane hip moments for military amputees. In the highest functioning transtibial amputees the most frequent deviation in hip kinematics is an occasional increase in hip flexion at initial contact.[21]

Trunk and Pelvic Kinematics

A unique characteristic of very high functioning military transtibial amputees is the ability to produce frontal plane trunk and pelvic kinematics that are similar to that of uninjured individuals. Deviations in frontal plane kinematics are documented in other populations but are typically most evident early in the rehabilitation process for military amputees.[33] This deviation is apparently reduced through the combination of extensive training using manual and verbal feedback in combination with proper prosthetic management. Although normal kinematics can be replicated in high functioning transtibial amputees, as a general rule patients demonstrate increased frontal plane motion at the trunk and pelvis during gait.

Pre-Swing

Gait kinematics and kinetics during pre-swing and swing in the military population are similar to those of civilian amputees with a few key exceptions. For all amputees using dynamic energy storing and return feet, the peak dorsiflexion angle that is achieved is determined by a combination of foot stiffness, alignment, and the ankle joint torque produced by the patient due to loading of the trail limb. As observed in previous studies, with appropriate prosthetic management patients are able to attain normal plantarflexor torque and motion at terminal stance. Patients demonstrate a remarkable ability to control the rate of energy returned from the foot and as a result are able to achieve nearly normal power output at the ankle. This observation is in sharp contrast to literature indicating "marked reduction in energy generating capabilities compared to the normal gastrocnemius-soleus."[20,21,34-36] Although the exact mechanism by which normal ankle powers are achieved is unknown, current explanations focus on training to sustain loading of the trail leg until just before the foot is lifted from the floor. The ability to produce normal ankle power is particularly impressive given that current prosthetic feet only return to the neutral alignment position (typically in slight dorsiflexion) when unloaded.

Swing

With the exception of ankle kinematics, few differences exist between the swing phase kinematics of high functioning transtibial amputees and uninjured individuals. Toe clearance (1–2 cm) is the most important aspect of the swing phase in transtibial amputees. The loss of active control of ankle motion prevents patients from using dorsiflexion during midswing to aid in clearing the toe. This is particularly relevant when considering the effective increase in leg length that occurs due to distal translation of the socket relative to the residual limb during swing.[37] Although microprocessor controlled prosthetic foot and ankle systems are available to aid with toe clearance, they have not been widely accepted by the patients. Instead patients use nearly imperceptible compensatory changes at more proximal joints that allow adequate clearance.

Additional Kinematic and Kinetic Deviations in the Transtibial Amputee

Deviations in ankle kinematics and kinetics are most commonly observed early in the rehabilitation process as patients are beginning to walk or are accommodating to new prosthetic components. In the authors' experience, ankle kinematics and kinetics are primarily influenced by the stiffness (grade) of the prosthetic foot and training to control loading of the prosthetic foot.

Initial Contact Through Midstance

One of the most commonly observed deviations in transtibial military amputees includes ankle plantarflexion motion and ankle dorsiflexion torques that are increased in duration and magnitude relative to other transtibial amputees.[20,21] These deviations are primarily attributed to a prosthetic foot that is too soft or too excessive and poorly controlled loading early in stance phase. In the case of a soft foot, the heel undergoes significant compression resulting in increased time in loading response. Rather than gradually moving from the heel during loading response to foot flat, this transition is delayed as the patient compresses the prosthetic heel. The aforementioned deviations in ankle kinematics and kinetics are typically accompanied by deviations at more proximal joints. Knee flexion is decreased or nearly absent resulting in a gait pattern similar to that of high functioning transfemoral amputees. As the heel compresses, patients lean toward the stance limb resulting in frontal plane rotation of the trunk and pelvis toward the stance limb.

In contrast, some individuals demonstrate an opposite response in which ankle plantarflexion motion and ankle dorsiflexion torques are decreased in duration and magnitude.[21] This is typically observed in patients with a prosthetic foot that is too stiff and/or in cases where patients are experiencing anterior-distal pain or have a poor tolerance for loading early in stance phase. In both instances, patients tend to move quickly to a foot flat position following initial contact. In the case of a foot that is too stiff, it appears as though patients avoid the unstable position of balancing on a firm heel and instead quickly move to a more stable foot flat position. For patients with a painful residual limb, a compensatory response of a foot flat landing and decreased time on the heel is reasonable given the current understanding of limb–socket dynamics. At initial contact a significant anterior and inferiorly directed force is applied at the bone–socket interface resulting in distal translation of the limb within the socket and loading along the anterior aspect of the socket. By landing in a foot flat position, patients are able to decrease the shear force during loading response and direct force along the axis of the residual limb into the soft tissue bulk instead of focusing it on the anterior-distal end. Due to the inability to actively control ankle orientation to bring the forefoot to the floor, patients use increased knee and hip flexion motion to lower the foot to the floor in a controlled manner.[21] Knee extensor torque is not, however, typically increased in military amputees because of efforts to minimize anterior shear forces in the painful patient.

Pre-Swing

Improper stiffness (grade), alignment of the prosthetic foot, or poor muscular control also results in gait deviations during pre-swing. As previously mentioned, the alignment and stiffness of the foot can significantly influence the peak dorsiflexion angle and response of the foot during pre-swing. A forefoot that is too soft or is aligned in excessive dorsiflexion can allow excessive peak dorsiflexion motion and is com-

monly accompanied by patient reports of insufficient foot length or energy return. Rather than exhibiting increased peak dorsiflexion, patients commonly accommodate by decreasing loading of the trail limb, which has the negative consequence of decreased plantarflexor power. Although compensations such as increased knee and hip extension are additional strategies that may be used to accommodate a prosthetic foot that is too soft, such responses are not consistently observed.

A forefoot that is too stiff or is aligned in excessive plantarflexion does not allow sufficient dorsiflexion motion and is accompanied by increased knee extension during mid and late stance.[21] This is due to increased resistance to forward rotation of the tibia over the foot. Rather than increasing the loading on the forefoot to attempt to deflect the foot, patients typically compensate by extending the knee. As a result, dorsiflexion motion is decreased, which leads to decreased peak plantarflexor power as the foot is unloaded at terminal stance.[21]

TRANSFEMORAL AMPUTEE GAIT

The combined loss of ankle and knee function and a dynamic bone–socket interface results in more pronounced gait deviations in patients that have undergone transfemoral amputation or knee disarticulation procedures. Although military transfemoral amputees have access to the latest prosthetic technologies and training, they typically have gait deviations that are readily apparent to an untrained observer. Appropriate prosthetic and physical therapy management is essential to allow restoration of a functional, efficient gait pattern. Contracture prevention, strength training, and appropriate socket fit are critical to provide patients the range of motion, strength, and control of the prosthesis necessary to produce a good gait pattern.

Initial Contact Through Midstance

Ankle Kinematic and Kinetic Data

Sagittal plane ankle kinematics and kinetics of the high functioning transfemoral amputee closely mimic those of the transtibial amputee. They typically demonstrate near normal sagittal plane ankle kinematics but exhibit the frequently observed pronounced dorsiflexion moment at loading response.[38-40]

Knee Flexion Kinematic and Kinetic Data

Sagittal plane knee kinematics differs significantly from that of uninjured individuals. Like most civilian

amputees, military transfemoral amputees have little if any knee flexion and exhibit knee flexor torques throughout the stance phase.[38-41] This is primarily attributed to a training philosophy that encourages patients to utilize hip extensor activation to stabilize the prosthetic knee by pushing it into full extension during stance. There are three perceived benefits of this training. First, by not relying on the 10 degrees to 15 degrees of stance flexion allowed by most prosthetic knees, there is a greater margin for error when performing challenging tasks such as ambulating on uneven terrain. If patients land on an object that serves to push their knee into flexion, they are already actively creating stability rather than relying on the response of the prosthesis. If the knee begins to buckle, the muscles are already tensioned leading to a faster response time and decreased likelihood of falling. Second, it encourages activation of hip extensor musculature for propulsion decreasing demand on the contralateral limb and easing the transition to high-level activities, such as running, during which hip extensor torque is a primary means of propulsion. Third, the repeated activation of residual limb musculature that is encouraged with this approach is thought to reduce muscle atrophy (maintain muscle volume) and provide a more rigid limb–socket interface.

Although stance flexion was thought to play an important role in minimizing center of mass excursion and therefore metabolic cost, its value has recently been questioned. More recently the focus on stance flexion has revolved around its role as a shock absorbing mechanism. Although likely useful for some patients, in the authors' experience, stance flexion is not necessary because of adequate shock absorption provided by the inclusion of rotation and shock absorbers, deflection of the prosthetic heel, and the bone–socket displacement that occurs in current prosthetic socket designs.[30] This ability to adequately absorb impact forces is clearly evident in ground reaction force curves that typically lack the pronounced vertical impact peaks observed in normal gait.[9]

Hip Kinematic and Kinetic Data

As a result of the closed kinematic chain present during stance, altered kinematics of the knee results in deviations in hip kinematics. Unlike normal gait in which the hip flexion angle changes little during the first 5% to 10% of the gait cycle, transfemoral amputees commonly demonstrate a more constant hip extension velocity (straight line on kinematic curve) from initial contact until peak hip extension. In uninjured individuals the minimal changes in hip flexion angles during early stance are the result of stance flexion moving the entire limb into a more flexed position resulting in a delayed transition toward extension at the hip. In transfemoral amputees, the absence of stance flexion results in a consistent hip extension velocity as the pelvis progresses over the fully extended leg.

Trunk and Pelvic Kinematics

Typically only high functioning amputees with well-fitting sockets are able to minimize deviations in frontal, sagittal, and transverse plane pelvic and trunk kinematics that are commonly seen in civilians.[33,42-44] It is unclear whether deviations in pelvic motion are the result of limitations in prosthetic technology, training, or both. Although the use of ischial containment socket designs allows freedom of hip and pelvic motion not otherwise attainable with an ischial weight-bearing quadrilateral socket, most patients demonstrate a compensated gluteus medius gait pattern. Rather than the contralateral side of the pelvis decreasing in height during loading response, the contralateral shoulder and pelvis elevate resulting in trunk and pelvis rotation toward the stance limb.[42,44] This altered trunk and pelvic motion, which is commonly the most visually apparent gait deviation, is readily recognized by the untrained observer. Two primary causes of this increase in motion are believed to be (1) hip abductor weakness and the (2) mobility of the femur within the socket.[30,45] By bringing the

center of mass over the hip joint center the hip abductor moment is decreased, thus reducing the torque requirements of the gluteus medius. Similarly, frontal plane trunk and pelvic rotation toward the stance limb allows the patients to axially load through the socket rather than relying on compression of the lateral soft tissues or co-contraction of thigh muscles to stabilize the femur in the socket.

Although some patients are able to achieve normal pelvic orientation (15 degrees anterior pelvic tilt) and excursions (approximately 5 degrees) throughout the gait cycle, a majority of patients demonstrate increased anterior pelvic tilt and sagittal plane motion.[33] Commonly, patients move into a position of increased anterior pelvic tilt during late stance as they approximate hip end range of motion and then rapidly posteriorly tilt the pelvis to help initiate swing. Because of the perceived increased risk of low back pain associated with increased sagittal plane motion of the pelvis and lumbar spine, efforts are under way to more effectively train patients to decrease this motion.

Terminal Stance Heel Strike

Although transfemoral amputees approximate the nearly normal sagittal plane ankle motion and torque exhibited by transtibial amputees, subtle differences result in ankle joint power peaks that are consistently less than that exhibited by high functioning transtibial amputees.[38,40] It is, however, unclear whether this difference is due to the loss of active control of the knee that alters loading of the foot, or the use of low profile feet that tend to be less dynamic.

During terminal stance, the knee joint angle rapidly moves from the extended position during midstance to approximate normal peak flexion angles during swing.[38,40] The rapid transition from extension into flexion is controlled by extensor torque produced by resistance within the prosthetic knee resulting in a burst of negative power that peaks around toe off.

Because it is the only source of active power generation in the involved limb, deviations are commonly seen in hip kinematics and kinetics. It is common for patients to demonstrate increased hip extension motion and increased hip flexor torque in late stance as compared to uninjured individuals. The most commonly observed deviation in sagittal plane pelvic motion is rapid motion into anterior pelvic tilt during terminal stance. Rather than isolating the motion to the hip joint they extend through the lumbar spine. Although functional, this motion pattern is discouraged because it is believed to contribute to the high prevalence of low back pain in amputees.

SPECIAL CONSIDERATIONS

Energy Expenditure

The energy expenditure of an amputee is influenced by extrinsic factors such as prosthetic malalignment, leg length discrepancies, and the limb–socket interface mismatches previously discussed.

Intrinsic factors are those inherent to the amputee such as age and the presence of vascular disease. In addition, amputee specific gait deviations that result from the loss of sensory perception in the amputated limb (particularly proprioception), loss of the shock absorbing and propulsion properties of the foot and ankle (for transfemoral and transtibial amputees), and loss of the loading response at the knee (transfemoral amputee) lead to unavoidable deviations from the energy-efficient gait pattern of nonamputees. These losses can result in deviations that result in an increase in energy expenditure. As stated previously, although changes in the six determinants of gait have been used to explain these changes, some of these may actually have no influence and other factors yet to be identified may be more influential. Table 19-1 shows the percent increase in energy cost for the different levels of lower limb amputation.[46] Note that these average values will increase when pathological deviations exist. The end result shows that to minimize these average energy cost increases, the amputee slows down the ambulation speed. Thus, just as in able-bodied individuals, the U-shaped curve seen when gait efficiency is plotted against various walking speeds is also seen in the amputee, although at a higher baseline. That is, the amputee consumes more energy when walking at slower or faster speeds than the SSWV with the energy expenditure of that SSWV being higher than in able-bodied individuals.[47] As a general rule, appropriate prosthetic management of the amputee aims to keep the energy costs of ambulation at or below the values listed in Table 19-1 by minimizing previously discussed gait deviations.

In a review of the influence of prosthetic alignment and prosthetic components on energy expenditure, Schmalz et al found that malalignments affect transfemoral more than transtibial amputee gait.[48] Furthermore, it was also found that there were no differences in energy expenditure when different prosthetic feet were worn by transtibial amputees and that microprocessor controlled knees reduced energy costs when compared to conventional hydraulic knees. Buckley et al also found that microprocessor knees tend to lower energy costs when compared to conventional pneumatic knees.[49] Taylor et al found that although energy cost differences exist between these two prosthetic types at slower or SSWVs, there were energy cost savings when walking at higher speeds.[50] Barth et al found no differences in metabolic costs among different feet in transtibial amputees although significant differences in temporal-spatial, kinetic, and kinematic parameters were found among the various feet tested.[51] Furthermore, vascular amputees had higher metabolic costs than traumatic amputees. However, these studies had small sample sizes and lacked randomization or stringent controls. Large sample comprehensive randomized studies with stringent controls are needed to fully and conclusively assess the purported advantages of currently available advanced prosthetic components.

Effect of Prosthetic Mass

As shown in Table 19-1, the average energy costs of prosthetic ambulation increase as the level of limb loss increases. This reality, with the evidence showing that adding weight to the lower extremities of nonamputees increases metabolic costs of walking, has triggered the development of lightweight prosthetic components over the past decade.[52]

The concerted effort to decrease prosthetic weight so as to decrease the metabolic costs of amputee gait, however, appears to have little scientific basis. Investigators have consistently demonstrated that no relationship exists between metabolic costs and prosthetic limb mass,[53-56] while others have also shown that no relationships exist between prosthetic mass and temporal-spatial gait parameters such as stride length, stride frequency, or self-selected walking speed.[55,57,58]

Selles et al found that although variations in prosthetic mass do not seem to affect joint angles (ie, kinematics), changing limb mass does influence the forces being applied across the joints (ie, kinetics).[59] Gitter et

TABLE 19-1

AVERAGE ENERGY COSTS OF PROSTHETIC AMBULATION

	Percentage Increase
Unilateral transtibial	9%–28%
Unilateral transfemoral	40%–655%
Bilateral transtibial	41%–100%
Bilateral transfemoral	280%
Transtibial plus transfemoral	75%
Unilateral hip disarticulation	82%
Hemipelvectomy	125%

al explained these changes in the kinetics of gait, however, in 1997 when they demonstrated that although an increase in the mechanical energy occurs across the prosthetic side hip joint during the pre-swing and swing phases of gait to accelerate the heavier prosthesis into swing, there is also a net absorption of energy during the terminal swing phase.[57] Thus, the force needed to accelerate the heavier prosthesis during swing is counteracted by an equal degree of energy recovery as the limb decelerates during terminal swing with a net effect of zero loss of energy.

To best serve the patient, the clinician should consider the location of the mass of the prosthesis rather than concentrate on the actual total weight of any given prosthesis. Lehmann et al demonstrated that the economy of gait decreases when the center of mass of the prosthesis is located distally.[55] Furthermore, investigators have also determined that intermediate center of mass locations were the most energy-efficient locations for the prosthetic center of mass.[52,56]

Effect of Prosthetic Components

In an extensive review of the literature, van der Linde et al classified all the studies evaluating the effect of prosthetic components on amputee gait using established quality assessment criteria.[60] The literature was divided into three categories:

1. A-level studies: studies meeting the most stringent criteria, thus defining these as studies of the highest quality.
2. B-level studies: studies partially meeting the selection criteria, thus defining these as studies of moderate quality.
3. C-level studies: studies not meeting most of the criteria, thus defining them as studies of low-level quality.

A total of 40 of the 356 articles identified met the criteria warranting full assessment. These studies were then divided into prosthetic foot, prosthetic knee, prosthetic socket, and prosthetic mass focus studies. Within the prosthetic foot studies, one met the A-level criteria, 15 met the B-level criteria, and 5 met the C-level criteria. As a whole, foot type did not influence the SSWV among individuals with traumatic transtibial and transfemoral amputation. There were few foot-specific effects on gait performance and the few foot-specific effects that were observed occurred when energy-storing feet were compared with the Solid Ankle Cushion Heel foot. In general, although variability existed resulting from study group selection bias, the energy-storing feet appeared to provide

for a higher SSWV. However, the evidence for a slight decrease in oxygen consumption is not convincing. Likewise, the evidence for a higher degree of patient satisfaction with the energy-storing feet is not fully convincing.

In this review, the authors also reported that as a whole, prosthetic knees offering advanced swing control (pneumatic, microprocessor-controlled, hydraulic) provide improved symmetry and gait velocity when compared to constant friction mechanical knees, particularly in active amputees. For the geriatric and more sedentary amputee, however, a locked knee with circumduction or hip hiking during swing may be more efficient because it provides improved knee stability required for this type of patient who is at risk of falls.[60]

Although van der Linde et al's literature review used stringent criteria to select methodologically sound articles in their final analysis, only five manuscripts were included addressing the prosthetic knee, two of which were from the early 1980s, two from the mid 1990s, and one from 2000. Furthermore, their conclusions compared the pneumatic, hydraulic, and microprocessor knees versus the constant friction knee. Studies comparing microprocessor-controlled knees versus mechanical pneumatic or hydraulic knees and studies comparing various types of microprocessor-controlled knees were thus not included in their review.[60]

In an assessment of the C-Leg (Otto Bock Healthcare, Minneapolis, Minn) versus two hydraulic-based mechanical knees utilizing 10 amputees, Kastner et al reported that when using the C-Leg, amputees had the most normal kinematic parameters at various speeds and their walk was more efficient as demonstrated by having the fastest time in a 1,000-meter walk test.[61] A more recent eight-subject study compared two microprocessor-controlled knees (C-Leg; RHEO KNEE, Ossur, Aliso Viejo, Calif) and a commonly used hydraulic mechanical knee (Mauch SNS, Ossur, Aliso Viejo, Calif).[38] The outcome measures included (a) metabolic cost, (b) kinetic and kinematic data, and (c) EMG and accelerometer data. The investigators found that metabolic costs decreased the most with the RHEO KNEE followed by the C-Leg. Furthermore, the microprocessor-controlled knees demonstrated biomechanical advantages in several kinetic and kinematic parameters.[38] EMG analysis revealed that there was decreased muscular activity of the gluteus medius on the affected side with the RHEO KNEE compared to the Mauch SNS and C-Leg. Finally, accelerometer data demonstrated smoother transitions from swing to stance and vice versa with the microprocessor knees.[38] Although these studies seem to demonstrate differences among the knees studied, these results need further corroboration. This is highlighted by the current self-selection of conventional hydraulic knees by military amputees.

In regards to the prosthetic socket, only one C-level study was found that suggested increased symmetry of gait with vacuum versus suction sockets. The methodology of this study, however, was poor with no control for other prosthetic components. The literature analysis dealing with prosthetic mass supported the points already discussed in the section above.[60]

In summary, when it comes to prosthetic prescription guidelines, the clinician must rely on a consensus team decision and patient input due to the current paucity of scientific evidence for the prescription of prosthetic devices to injured service members.

Effect of Gait Training

A review of the Ovid database over the past 10 years revealed only two articles on this topic, both by the same investigators.[62,63] Both papers originate from the same research with the first paper describing the effect of a gait reeducation program on self-selected walking speed and pain-free or adaptive equipment free ambulation. The second paper described the effects of the gait reeducation program on sagittal plane kinetic and kinematic variables.

The sample size for both papers was 9 transfemoral trauma or tumor-related amputees with a mean age of 33 years. All had worn their respective prosthesis for 18 months. Measurements were made at baseline (before the start of training), at the conclusion of the training program, and at 6 months follow-up. The training program averaged 10 months and incorporated traditional motor skills based gait training with a psychologically based self-awareness and confidence building outreach component. Training sessions occurred weekly for 1 to 2 hours.

The investigators reported that the gait re-education program led to improvements in SSWV, gait symmetry, and an associated increase in the amount of muscle work on the amputated side. Three subjects were able to walk without walking aids, seven subjects learned to jog, and all had either a decrease or a disappearance of pre-training low back pain. These findings persisted until the 6-month follow-up. Although the findings described in these two studies are promising, more studies are needed in this area.

GAIT LABORATORY DEPENDENT THERAPEUTIC INTERVENTIONS

Although rarely implemented in the past, the use of advanced technologies holds great promise for rehabilitation of the military amputee.[64,65] The combined resources of real-time feedback and virtual reality are being implemented with the goal of improving gait performance. Current efforts are based on promising work that suggests that improved symmetry of loading and decreased metabolic cost can be attained in a relatively short period of time using visual feedback.[64,65] It is anticipated that the use of the virtual reality and a real-time feedback could be effective in accelerating the rehabilitation process, especially with gait training. This method also could prove valuable in prosthetic device modifications, gait strategies used by amputees, and selection of an environment to achieve optimal efficient prosthetic gait.

SUMMARY

This chapter has attempted to provide the reader with an overview of the terminology of gait, as well as observational and computerized gait assessment. The able-bodied "normal" gait has been discussed as a construct from which to understand gait deviations in the amputee. An indepth discussion of transtibial and transfemoral amputee gait has been provided with specific discussions concerning kinematic and kinetic parameters of joints throughout the gait cycle. Further discussion of specific considerations in amputee gait such as energy expenditure and prosthetic mass effect has also been provided. The chapter concludes with a discussion of how gait laboratory evaluation assists in the management of lower extremity amputees.

REFERENCES

1. Weber W, Weber E. *Mechanik du Meschlichen*. Gottingen, Germany: Gehwerkzeugen; 1836.

2. Schwartz RP, Heath AL, Misiek W, Wright JN. Kinetics of human gait: the making and interpretation of electrobasographic records of gait. *J Bone Joint Surg Am*. 1934;16:343–350.

3. Bernstein NA. Biodynamics of locomotion. In: Whiting HTA, ed. *Human Motor Actions: Bernstein Reassessed*. Amsterdam, The Netherlands: North-Holland; 1984.

4. Inman VT, Ralston HJ. Human walking. In: Lieberman JC, ed. *Human Walking*. Baltimore, Md: Williams and Wilkins; 1981.

5. Gage JR. A quantitative description of normal gait. In: Gage JR, ed. *The Treatment of Gait Problems in Cerebral Palsy*. 2nd ed. London, England: Mac Keith Press; 2004.

6. Rose J, Ralston HJ. Energetics of walking. In: Rose J, Gambel JG, eds. *Human Walking*. Baltimore, Md: Williams and Wilkins; 1994.

7. Krebs DE, Edelstein JE, Fishman S. Reliability of observational kinematic gait analysis. *Phys Ther.* 1985;65:1027–1033.

8. Saleh M, Murdoch G. In defence of gait analysis. Observation and measurement in gait assessment. *J Bone Joint Surg Br.* 1985;67:237–241.

9. Perry J. Gait analysis systems. In: Perry J, ed. *Gait Analysis: Normal and Pathological Gait*. Thorofare, NJ: Slack; 1992.

10. Perry J. Normal and pathologic gait. In: Bunch WH, ed. *Atlas of Orthotics*. St. Louis, Mo: Mosby; 1985.

11. Gage JR. *Gait Analysis in Cerebral Palsy*. London, England: Mac Keith Press; 1991.

12. Saunders JB, Inman VT, Eberhart HD. The major determinants in normal and pathological gait. *J Bone Joint Surg Am.* 1953;35:543–558.

13. Kerrigan DC, Viramontes BE, Corcoran PJ, LaRaia PJ. Measured versus predicted vertical displacement of the sacrum during gait as a tool to measure biomechanical gait performance. *Arch Phys Med Rehabil.* 1995;74:3–8.

14. Winter DA. Knee flexion during stance as a determinant of inefficient walking. *Phys Ther.* 1983;63:331–333.

15. Kerrigan DC, Della Croce U, Marciello M, Riley PO. A refined view of the determinants of gait: significance of heel rise. *Arch Phys Med Rehabil.* 2000;81:1077–1080.

16. Kerrigan DC, Riley PO, Lelas JL, Della Croce U. Quantification of pelvic rotation as a determinant of gait. *Arch Phys Med Rehabil.* 2001;82:217–220.

17. Della Croce U, Riley PO, Lelas JL, Kerrigan DC. A refined view of the determinants of gait. *Gait Posture.* 2001;14:79–84.

18. Gard SA, Childress DS. The influence of stance-phase knee flexion on the vertical displacement of the trunk during normal walking. *Arch Phys Med Rehabil.* 1999;80:26–32.

19. Ortega JD, Farley CT. Minimizing center of mass vertical movement increases metabolic cost in walking. *J Appl Physiol.* 2005;99:2099–2107.

20. Seroussi RE, Gitter A, Czerniecki JM, Weaver K. Mechanical work adaptations of above-knee amputee ambulation. *Arch Phys Med Rehabil.* 1996;77:1209–1214.

21. Winter DA, Sienko SE. Biomechanics of below-knee amputee gait. *J Biomech.* 1988;21:361–367.

22. Powers CM, Rao S, Perry J. Knee kinetics in transtibial amputee gait. *Gait Posture.* 1998;8:1–7.

23. Sanderson DJ, Martin PE. Lower extremity kinematic and kinetic adaptations in unilateral below-knee amputees during walking. *Gait Posture.* 1997;6:126–136.

24. Commean PK, Smith KE, Vannier MW. Lower extremity residual limb slippage within the prosthesis. *Arch Phys Med Rehabil.* 1997;78:476–485.

25. Erikson U, Lemperg R. Roentgenological study of movements of the amputation stump within the prosthesis socket in below-knee amputees fitted with a PTB prosthesis. *Acta Orthop Scand*. 1969;40:520–529.

26. Grevsten S, Erikson U. A roentgenological study of the stump-socket contact and skeletal displacement in the PTB-Suction Prosthesis. *Up J Med Sci*. 1975;80:49–57.

27. Grevsten S, Eriksson U. Stump-socket contact and skeletal displacement in a suction patellar-tendon bearing prosthesis. *J Bone Joint Surg Am*. 1974;56:1692–1696.

28. Lilja M, Johansson T, Oberg T. Movement of the tibial end in a PTB prosthesis socket: a sagittal X-ray study of the PTB prosthesis. *Prosthet Orthot Int*. 1993;17:21–26.

29. Narita H, Yokogushi K, Shii S, Kakizawa M, Nosaka T. Suspension effect and dynamic evaluation of the total surface bearing (TSB) transtibial prosthesis: a comparison with the patellar tendon bearing (PTB) transtibial prosthesis. *Prosthet Orthot Int*. 1997;21:175–178.

30. Convery P, Murray KD. Ultrasound study of the motion of the residual femur within a transfemoral socket during gait. *Prosthet Orthot Int*. 2000;24:226–232.

31. Hansen AH, Sam M, Childress DS. The effective foot length ratio: a potential tool for characterization and evaluation of prosthetic feet. *J Prosthet Orthot*. 2004;16:41–45.

32. Kegel B, Burgess EM, Starr TW, Daly WK. Effects of isometric muscle training on residual limb volume, strength, and gait of below-knee amputees. *Phys Ther*. 1981;61:1419–1426.

33. Michaud SB, Gard SA, Childress DS. A preliminary investigation of pelvic obliquity patterns during gait in persons with transtibial and transfemoral amputation. *J Rehabil Res Dev*. 2000;37:1–10.

34. Czerniecki JM, Gitter AJ, Beck JC. Energy transfer mechanisms as a compensatory strategy in below knee amputee runners. *J Biomech*. 1996;29:717–722.

35. Gitter A, Czerniecki JM, DeGroot DM. Biomechanical analysis of the influence of prosthetic feet on below-knee amputee walking. *Am J Phys Med Rehabil*. 1991;70:142–148.

36. Postema K, Hermens HJ, de Vries J, Koopman HF, Eisma WH. Energy storage and release of prosthetic feet. Part 1: Biomechanical analysis related to user benefits. *Prosthet Orthot Int*. 1997;21:17–27.

37. Board WJ, Street GM, Caspers C. A comparison of transtibial amputee suction and vacuum socket conditions. *Prosthet Orthot Int*. 2001;25:202–209.

38. Johansson JL, Sherrill DM, Riley PO, Bonato P, Herr H. A clinical comparison of variable-damping and mechanically passive prosthetic knee devices. *Am J Phys Med Rehabil*. 2005;84:563–575.

39. Segal AD, Orendurff MS, Klute GK, et al. Kinematic and kinetic comparisons of transfemoral amputee gait using C-Leg and Mauch SNS prosthetic knees. *J Rehabil Res Dev*. 2006;43:857–870.

40. van der Linden ML, Solomonidis SE, Spence WD, Li N, Paul JP. A methodology for studying the effects of various types of prosthetic feet on the biomechanics of transfemoral amputee gait. *J Biomech*. 1999;32:877–889.

41. Boonstra AM, Schrama JM, Eisma WH, Hof AL, Fidler V. Gait analysis of transfemoral amputee patients using prostheses with two different knee joints. *Arch Phys Med Rehabil*. 1996;77:515–520.

42. Cappozzo A, Figura F, Gazzani F, Leo T, Marchetti M. Angular displacements in the upper body of AK amputees during level walking. *Prosthet Orthot Int*. 1982;6:131–138.

43. Macfarlane PA, Nielsen DH, Shurr DG, Kenneth M. Gait comparisons for below-knee amputees using a flex-foot (TM) versus a conventional prosthetic foot. *J Prosthet Orthot*. 1991;3:150–161.

44. Tazawa E. Analysis of torso movement of trans-femoral amputees during level walking. *Prosthet Orthot Int.* 1997;21:129–140.

45. Ryser DK, Erickson RP, Cahalan T. Isometric and isokinetic hip abductor strength in persons with above-knee amputations. *Arch Phys Med Rehabil.* 1988;69:840–845.

46. Shah SK. Cardiac rehabilitation. In: DeLisa J, Gans BM, Wash NE, eds. *Physical Medicine & Rehabilitation: Principles and Practice.* Philadelphia, Pa: Lippincott Williams & Wilkins; 2004.

47. Pagliarulo MA, Waters R, Hislop HJ. Energy cost of walking of below-knee amputees having no vascular disease. *Phys Ther.* 1979;59:538–543.

48. Schmalz T, Blumentritt S, Jarasch R. Energy expenditure and biomechanical characteristics of lower limb amputee gait: the influence of prosthetic alignment and different prosthetic components. *Gait Posture.* 2002;16:255–263.

49. Buckley J, Spence W, Solomonidis S. Energy cost of walking: comparison of "intelligent prosthesis" with conventional mechanism. *Arch Phys Med Rehabil.* 1997;78:330–333.

50. Taylor MB, Clark E, Offord EA, Baxter C. A comparison of energy expenditure by a high level trans-femoral amputee using the Intelligent Prosthesis and conventionally damped prosthetic limbs. *Prosthet Orthot Int.* 1996;20:116–121.

51. Barth DI, Schmacher L, Thomas SS. Gait analysis and energy cost of below-knee amputees wearing six different prosthetic feet. *J Prosthet Orthot.* 1992;4:63–75.

52. Skinner HB, Mote CD. Optimization of amputee prosthetic weight and weight distribution. *Rehabil Res Dev Programs Rep.* 1989;26(suppl):32–33.

53. Czerniecki JM, Gitter A, Weaver K. Effect of alterations in prosthetic shank mass on the metabolic costs of ambulation in above-knee amputees. *Am J Phys Med Rehabil.* 1994;73:348–352.

54. Gailey RS, Nash MS, Atchley TA, et al. The effects of prosthesis mass on metabolic cost of ambulation in non-vascular trans-tibial amputees. *Prosthet Orthot Int.* 1997;21:9–16.

55. Lehmann JF, Price R, Okumura R, Questad K, de Lateur BJ, Négretot A. Mass and mass distribution of below-knee prostheses: effect on gait efficacy and self-selected walking speed. *Arch Phys Med Rehabil.* 1998;79:162–168.

56. Lin-Chan SJ, Nielsen DH, Yack HJ, Hsu MJ, Shurr DG. The effects of added prosthetic mass on physiologic responses and stride frequency during multiple speeds of walking in persons with transtibial amputation. *Arch Phys Med Rehabil.* 2003;84:1865–1871.

57. Gitter AJ, Czerniecki J, Meinders M. Effect of prosthetic mass on swing phase work during above-knee amputee ambulation. *Am J Phys Med Rehabil.* 1997;76:114–121.

58. Hale SA. Analysis of the swing phase dynamics and muscular effort of the above-knee amputee for varying prosthetic shank loads. *Prosthet Orthot Int.* 1990;14:125–135.

59. Selles RW, Bussmann JB, Klip LM, Speet B, Van Soest AJ, Stam HJ. Adaptations to mass perturbations in trans-tibial amputees: kinetic or kinematic invariance? *Arch Phys Med Rehabil.* 2004;85:2046–2052.

60. van der Linde H, Hofstad CJ, Geurts AC, Postema K, Geertzen JH, van Limbeek J. A systematic literature review of the effect of different prosthetic components on human functioning with a lower-limb prosthesis. *J Rehabil Res Dev.* 2004;41:555–570.

61. Kastner J, Nimmervoll R, Kristen H, Wagner P. What are the benefits of the C-Leg? A comparative gait analysis of the C-Leg, the 3R45 and the 3R80 prosthetic knee joints. *Med Orth Tech.* 1999;119:131–137.

62. Sjödahl C, Jarnlo GB, Persson BM. Gait improvement in unilateral transfemoral amputees by a combined psychological and physiotherapeutic treatment. *J Rehabil Med.* 2001;33:114–118.

63. Sjödahl C, Jarnlo GB, Söderberg B, Persson BM. Kinematic and kinetic gait analysis in the sagittal plane of trans-femoral amputees before and after special gait re-education. *Prosthet Orthot Int.* 2002;26:101–112.

64. Davis BL, Ortolano (Cater) M, Richards K, Redhed J, Kuznicki J, Sahgal V. Realtime visual feedback diminishes energy consumption of amputee subjects during treadmill locomotion. *J Prosthet Orthot.* 2004;16:49–54.

65. Dingwell JB, Davis BL, Frazier DM. Use of an instrumented treadmill for real-time gait symmetry evaluation and feedback in normal and trans-tibial amputee subjects. *Prosthet Orthot Int.* 1996;20:101–110.

Chapter 20

LOWER LIMB PROSTHETICS

SUSAN KAPP, MEd, CPO, LPO[*]; AND JOSEPH A. MILLER, MS, CP, CPT[†]

[*]*Associate Professor and Director, Prosthetic and Orthotic Program, University of Texas Southwestern Medical Center at Dallas, 5323 Harry Hines Boulevard, Suite V5.400, Dallas, Texas 75390*

[†]*Captain, Medical Service Corps, US Army; Chief Prosthetic and Orthotic Service, Integrated Department of Orthopaedics and Rehabilitation, Walter Reed Army Medical Center, 6900 Georgia Avenue, NW, Building 2, RM3H, Washington, DC 20307, and the National Naval Medical Center, 8901 Rockville Pike, Bethesda, Maryland 20889; formerly, Deputy Chief, Prosthetic and Sensory Aids Service, Department of Veterans Affairs, Central Office, 50 Irving Street, NW, Washington, DC 20422*

INTRODUCTION

Lower extremity amputation is the most common level of amputation in both civilian and military populations. These two groups, although outwardly similar, have vastly differing etiologies that lead to amputation and have dramatically different rehabilitation and prosthetic concerns that exist throughout their lifetimes. A service member with lower extremity amputation will rely on a variety of prosthetic devices and components to maximize rehabilitation and integration to independence. The proper prescription, fitting, and training of lower extremity prosthetic devices are critical to successful usage and reintegration.

Military medical treatment facility (MTF) personnel, who specialize in amputee care, have designed programs based on a multidisciplinary team approach. The team is comprised of both medical professionals (surgeons, physiatrists, prosthetists, physical therapists, occupational therapists, nurses, physician assistants, psychiatrists, and physiologists) and nonmedical specialists (case managers, benefits counselors, and volunteers) who provide comprehensive services throughout the service members' rehabilitation.

The goals of providing lower extremity prosthetics devices are to allow the service member to achieve basic ambulation, to progress to a variety of advanced activities (eg, running, skiing), and, if warranted, to perform warrior tasks required to meet return-to-duty standards. These goals are best accomplished by using the comprehensive team approach to rehabilitation and prescribing multiple prosthetic limbs that include the use of technically advanced prosthetic devices. Use of advanced prosthetic limb components in this population is associated with successful rehabilitation outcomes. Experience has revealed that this group consistently outperforms the most advanced systems.

The purpose of this chapter is to identify the role of the prosthetist as a member of the comprehensive rehabilitation team, provide an overview of prosthetic components used at MTFs, and present the treatment protocol.

ROLE OF THE PROSTHETIST

Ideally, the rehabilitation team works in unison and complements each other's roles. Prescription formulation usually occurs during an interdisciplinary specialized clinic and is centered on the service member's needs and desires for prosthetic rehabilitation. Each member of the clinical team plays an important role. However, during prosthetic limb prescription formulation, the prosthetist takes center stage. The increasing complexity involved in prosthetics technology and the development of unique materials, computer programs, and fabrication techniques/applicability require the specialized knowledge of the prosthetist. The American Board for Certification in Orthotics, Prosthetics & Pedorthics (ABC) and the Board for Orthotic/Prosthetic Certification (BOC) provide benchmark certification levels for competency in the field. There are several pathways to certification, and it is important for each MTF to ensure that its prosthetists are appropriately certified. ABC, formed in 1946, requires that prosthetic education be obtained from institutions accredited by the Commission on Accreditation of Allied Health Education Programs and that prosthetists successfully complete a 1-year residency requirement per discipline (prosthetics and orthotics), as well as take subsequent board examinations. BOC requires 2 years of education, training, and/or work experience and 2 years of experience in providing direct patient care services.

Nearly all of the clinical specialties that comprise this interdisciplinary team are uniformed service members bridging both officer and enlisted ranks. The military occupational specialty classification for orthotist (originally code 42C) was eliminated in the mid-1990s. However, because of the global war on terror and the ensuing combat operations in Iraq and Afghanistan, the need for military prosthetists and orthotists is on the rise. To fill this gap, civilian orthotists and prosthetists have been employed at MTFs either through service contracts with companies or through hiring individual prosthetists as government service employees. It is important that prosthetists have a clear position within the military organizational system. This position has typically been classifed under the Department of Orthopaedics and Rehabilitation. In addition, it has not been uncommon for the Department of Defense to request that prosthetists help provide strategic and operational knowledge of prosthetic programs to allied governments, which has called into question the need for uniformed military prosthetists.

For example, during Operation Iraqi Freedom (specifically from January 2006 to June 2006), a five-man team of rehabilitation providers from the US Armed Forces Amputee Patient Care Program worked with Iraqi prosthetic and rehabilitation specialists to educate them on best practices in caring for patients with limb loss and complex trauma. The team instructed, assisted, and supervised Iraqi clinicians in the delivery of prosthetic and rehabilitation services to 124 patients (totaling more than 350 patient clinical visits). The clinic that they developed was transferred to the Iraqi Veterans Agency (in Baghdad, Iraq) and is now considered the premier prosthetics and rehabilitation clinic in Iraq.

The prosthetic mission was to educate Iraqi providers on state-of-the-art prosthetic care, with emphasis on enhancing provider clinical decision-making skills, improving tradecraft and bench skills, and enhancing the use of available technology. The primary goal was to shift Iraqi practice patterns from those of a semiskilled worker model to a more professional paradigm. Typically, Iraqi prosthetists are locally trained by the International Committee of the Red Cross or by nongovernmental organizations with support from the Iraqi Ministry of Health. Practitioners are often characterized as technicians working in "limb factories," as opposed to the Western model of an allied health professional performing clinical services. The assistance team trained local Iraqi prosthetists how to adopt an internationally recognized role as allied health providers in a community of rehabilitation

science experts. Clinically, this required a change in paradigm from fabricating, fitting, and delivering fair-to-adequate lower extremity prosthetic limbs to one of consistently producing reliable and comfortable prosthetic arms and legs in a reasonable and timely manner while optimizing the use of available technology [eg, computer-aided design (CAD)/computer-aided manufacturing (CAM) systems]. Additionally, their Iraqi counterparts were instructed in how to refine their clinical evaluation skills, clinical documentation techniques, and prosthetic fabrication abilities. On completion of formal training, the Iraqi prosthetic providers returned to full-time direct patient care.

The art and science of prosthetic care and rehabilitation of persons with limb loss and polytrauma by necessity accelerates during times of war. Clinicians have a strong moral imperative to share with our allies the lessons learned in caring for seriously wounded service members. Thus, the outcome of this mission was to demonstrate the importance of appropriate technology, emphasize a multidisciplinary approach to care, and describe the standard of care in a subsegment of the Iraqi population of war wounded.

OVERVIEW OF COMPONENTS

Prosthetic Feet

Function

Prosthetic feet are classified according to function and features. An understanding of prosthetic foot function and design will assist clinicians in selecting feet best suited to a patient's activities. The prosthetic foot is the interface between the patient and the ground, and ideally would emulate the anatomical foot perfectly. Achieving this, however, is difficult. Prosthetic feet range from simple to complex as they attempt to mimic anatomical function. Anatomical articulation at the ankle and midfoot greatly affects gait efficiency and smoothness. It can increase knee stability, and a multiaxial foot can increase the base of support by accommodating uneven terrain. Prosthetic joint simulation can be accomplished by true articulation of the prosthetic foot, as well as compression of the foot itself. Related to joint movement is shock absorption, another critical feature that the prosthetic foot must emulate. The foot must dampen the impact at loading response during gait. This is necessary to diminish forces transmitted to the residual limb. An example of this is the compressible heel of the foot. At loading response, the heel of the prosthetic foot compresses, emulating the eccentric contraction of the dorsiflexors. This is referred to as simulated or relative plantar flexion. Another less

functional, yet important, feature of prosthetic feet is appearance. This is more important to some individuals than others. If the patient intends to wear sandals, it is obvious that the cosmetic appearance of the foot must be good. With the exception of specialty feet designed for running or other activity, all feet have a cosmetic foot shell as a minimum. This shell protects the internal components from unnecessary wear and tear. The overall design of the prosthetic foot, its ability to articulate, and its material composition can have a significant effect on the foot's ability to emulate anatomical function. Generally, the greater the ability and activity of the patient, the more features the patient may be able to take advantage of during use.

Dynamic Response

The dynamic response foot has a deformable spring-type keel that provides a lively, responsive feel while the patient is walking. As the keel deforms under loading, it absorbs shock and then quickly returns to its original position once the load is removed. This type of design is often referred to as an energy storage and return (ESAR) design.[1] Suggested benefits of ESAR feet include the following: increased self-selected walking velocity, increased stride length, decreased sound side weight acceptance force, and increased prosthetic side propulsive force.[2,3] The spring-like keels are fabricated from carbon fiber, Delrin (E. I. du Pont de Nemours and Company, Wilmington, Del), or other materials. They deform as body weight is applied (Figure 20-1). Designs vary in configuration. Most have a forefoot keel and a hind foot keel that function as springs and deform primarily in the sagittal plane. The hind foot keel that projects posteriorly (a heel spring) deforms at loading response and simulates plantar flexion. From late midstance to toe off, the forefoot keel deforms under the increased load. As the patient begins to push off, the spring resists this motion while it yields slightly. As the load is being removed from the foot, the toe spring pushes back against the patient until it returns to its original shape. This yields a livelier feel for the patient. Some carbon keels are split longitudinally, which allows the toe spring to scissor slightly, thus simulating inversion and eversion. Dynamic response feet are designed to yield upon load application. Keel thickness and strength are based on the patient's weight and activity level. If either one increases, it is possible that the keel may fracture. A decrease in activity or weight may make the keel seem too rigid. Therefore, it is crucial that body weight and activity level be accurately assessed when selecting a dynamic response foot, given that keels are designed with a relatively narrow tolerance. With many carbon dynamic response feet, the keel continues to the distal socket that acts as both the foot and shank of the prosthesis. This increased carbon strut length provides more stored energy than those that terminate at the ankle. Patient height and residual limb length often will determine which style

of foot can be used. Dynamic response feet provide excellent stability. The composition may vary, but, in general, these feet are typically lightweight, durable, and covered with a cosmetic foot shell.

Dynamic Response With Vertical, Shock-Absorbing Pylons

Vertical, shock-absorbing pylons help to dampen the axial loading of the prosthesis and thereby decrease the shock transmitted to the residual limb.[4] Several designs are available; some are integrated into the foot using a side carbon strut (Figure 20-2) that supports

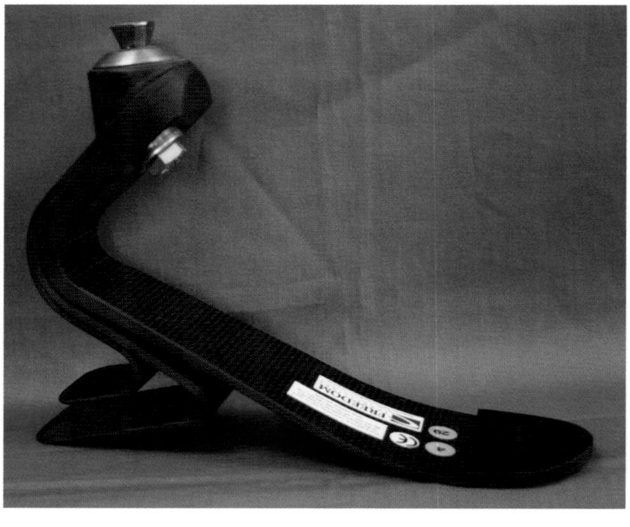

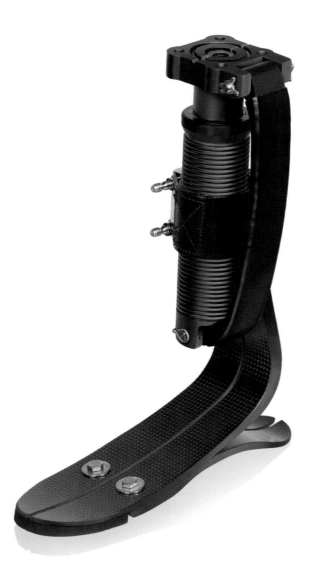

Figure 20-1. Renegade Prosthetic Foot (Freedom Innovations, Irvine, Calif).
Photograph: Used with permission from Freedom Innovations.

Figure 20-2. Re-Flex VSP prosthetic foot (Ossur Americas, Aliso Viejo, Calif).
Photograph: Courtesy of Ossur Americas, www.ossur.com.

the patient's weight and bows outwardly on weight bearing as the piston slides freely into and out of the cylinder. Other designs provide the user with the ability to adjust the resistance to vertical load by changing the psi in the unit (Figure 20-3), whereas other designs are separate components added to the standard pylon. These feet are available in standard and low profile heights to accommodate most limb lengths. Their ability to provide shock absorption can increase the patient's comfort significantly when stepping off a curb, going down stairs, or performing other high-impact activities. These feet are designed with a split keel and also offer simulated inversion and eversion.

Articulated. Commonly used articulated feet are multiaxis in the sagittal, coronal, and transverse planes. Articulating dynamic response feet possess the advantages of the multiaxis foot in terms of terrain accommodation and the liveliness of the dynamic response foot. These feet are intended to provide accommodation with the ground without sacrificing their ability to provide dynamic response. They articulate through either a joint or a deformable wedge. If the prosthetic foot has an actual joint axis about which it articulates (Figure 20-4), it is referred to as a true articulation. Almost any prosthetic foot with an axis of rotation

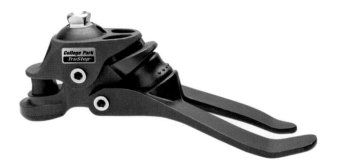

Figure 20-4. TruStep prosthetic foot (College Park Industries, Fraser, Mich).
Photograph: Courtesy of College Park Industries.

will require regular maintenance to lubricate the joint, which prevents wear and tear. Compressible bumpers are available with varying firmness (or durometer), allowing the prosthetist to adjust the plantar flexion resistance to accommodate the patient. Some designs also allow for dorsiflexion bumper exchange so that resistance to dorsiflexion may be adjusted until the foot hits the anterior stop.

Another method of providing articulation without moving parts, such as an axis, is to use an elastic bond of some sort between two dynamic response keels to provide ground conformance (Figure 20-5). A strap on the posterior aspect of the foot prevents excessive

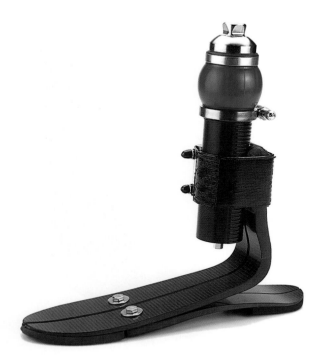

Figure 20-3. Ceterus prosthetic foot (Ossur Americas, Aliso Viejo, Calif).
Photograph: Used with permission from Ossur Americas, www.ossur.com.

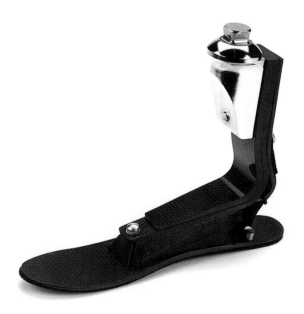

Figure 20-5. Talux prosthetic foot (Ossur Americas, Aliso Viejo, Calif).
Photograph: Courtesy of Ossur Americas, www.ossur.com.

elongation of the posterior section of the elastic bonding material as the patient rolls over onto the toe of the foot. Other dynamic response feet use a thick elastomeric material between carbon fiber keel plates. In this case, the bottommost keel readily accommodates to uneven terrain, while the more proximal keel may provide the typical energy-storing function. These types of feet are referred to as simulated articulation, because there is no true articulation (Figure 20-6).

Increased knee stability on the prosthetic side can be achieved by an articulated ankle. The knee flexion moment is reduced as the foot plantar flexes at loading response. The articulation can also increase knee stability as the patient walks down an incline. Plantar flexion resistance in the foot can be adjusted to accommodate the patient with compressible bumpers or wedges and through prosthetic alignment.

Additional Features

Heel Height Adjustability. Prosthetic feet are usually manufactured with a contour on the plantar surface. This is intended to match the patient's preferred heel height. Heel height is defined as the net difference between the thickness of the shoe sole at the ball of the foot (eg, ¼ inch) and the thickness of the heel at the posterior aspect of the shoe (eg, 1 inch). In this instance, the net difference is ¾ of an inch; a prosthetic foot with a ¾-inch heel rise would be appropriate. When placed in the shoe, the proper orientation of the prosthetic foot aligns the proximal surface of the foot horizontally, parallel to the floor. Feet are available that permit patients to adjust the foot's dorsiflexion/plantar flexion position, providing them with the freedom to wear shoes of varying heel heights.

Inversion/Eversion. Many carbon keels are split longitudinally (Figure 20-7), which allows the forefoot keel to scissor slightly, simulating inversion and eversion as the foot traverses uneven terrain. This increased ground conformance provides greater stability. Another way to accomplish inversion and eversion is with an articulated foot, which provides coronal plane motion about the joint and is dampened by stiff rubber bumpers.

Microprocessor Ankle/Foot. One foot incorporates microprocessor-controlled and motor-powered dorsiflexion and plantar flexion during the swing phase. It is designed to make navigation of inclines, stair ascent and descent, and sitting onto or rising from a chair easier. A combination of sensors acts together to replace the mechanoreceptor function and provide artificial proprioception via gait pattern recognition algorithms (Figure 20-8). It is especially useful when there is a range of motion limitation of the contralateral knee and/or ankle.

Knee Units

Axis

Single Axis. In addition to their other features, prosthetic knees can be categorized as single axis or polycentric. The single axis knee is a simple, low-maintenance hinge design generally lightweight and

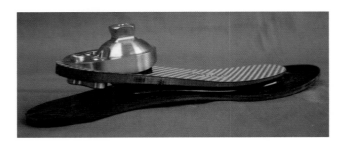

Figure 20-6. Axtion prosthetic foot (Otto Bock HealthCare, Minneapolis, Minn).
Photograph: Courtesy of Otto Bock HealthCare.

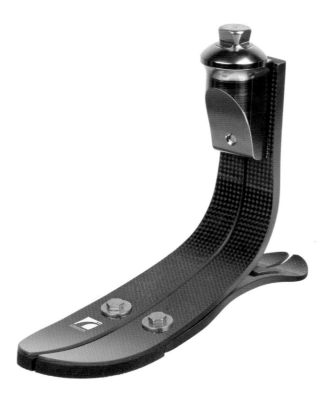

Figure 20-7. Vari-Flex prosthetic foot (Ossur Americas, Aliso Viejo, Calif).
Photograph: Courtesy of Ossur Americas, www.ossur.com.

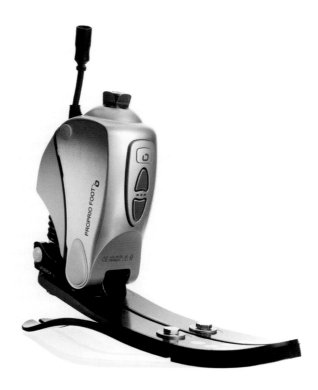

Figure 20-8. PROPRIO FOOT (Ossur Americas, Aliso Viejo, Calif).
Photograph: Courtesy of Ossur Americas, www.ossur.com.

low profile. Prosthetic knee stability with a single axis knee relies heavily on alignment of the knee in relation to the socket and foot, and on the volitional control of the patient. The single axis design is coupled with constant friction, fluid, and microprocessor or powered stride control features. It is used for any level of patient ability.

Polycentric. The polycentric design is more complex and yields multiple centers of rotation, much like the anatomical knee. Prosthetic polycentric knees simulate the rocking and gliding motions of the anatomical knee either by curved-bearing surfaces or by linkages. Location of the axis changes as the prosthetic knee moves through its available range of motion. This is referred to as an instantaneous center of rotation (ICR) and results in an inherently stable knee. The way that the ground reaction forces move about the ICR makes this design more stable early in stance when the patient needs it most. In addition, the polycentric design shortens the shank during the swing phase, thus helping the foot clear the ground. Because of reorientation of the linkages during flexion of the polycentric knee, the shin segment translates posteriorly, and the segment rotates differently than it would if it acted about a single axis. This action results in a relative dorsiflexion of the foot

as the knee flexes, which in turn creates increased toe clearance. The polycentric design also provides a more cosmetic appearance while sitting for those patients with long transfemoral amputations or knee disarticulations. The knee is designed so the shin folds back behind the socket at 90 degrees of flexion. This design minimizes the length discrepancy between the knees while sitting. The polycentric design is also ideal for patients with short residual limbs because the linkages place the axis of rotation proximal (closer to the workforce of the hip), requiring less hip extensor action, and the linkages also place the axis of rotation posterior to the weight line.[5]

Cadence Control

Constant Friction. Prosthetic knee joints should provide stability during stance and smooth, controlled knee extension during the swing phase. The most basic knee joint operates via a feature termed constant friction. A constant friction, single axis knee has a feature that provides continuous pressure / friction around the knee axis to control the velocity at which the shank and foot can swing to prevent excessive heel rise during flexion and terminal impact at full extension. The resistance to swing is adjustable, but not self-adjusting as velocity changes. For patients who do not alter the speed of their cadence, a constant friction knee is indicated because of its simplicity, durability, and ease of use. However, most individuals walk at varying speeds and will require a more gait-responsive knee.

Pneumatic/Hydraulic/Magnetorheologic. A fluid (or hydraulically)-controlled knee provides frictional resistance about the knee axis that will increase proportionally with speed. There are two basic types of fluid-controlled knees: (1) hydraulic or (2) pneumatic. Fluids include liquids, vapors, and gases. The major difference with fluids in prosthetic knees is that air is more easily compressible, and hydraulic fluids are not. Oil or air is forced through a small orifice or tube. Adjustment screws allow the size of the orifice to be changed to control the rate in which fluid flows through these ports. This permits fine-tuning of swing-phase resistance to individual needs. If air is used, the air under compression within the pneumatic cylinder also acts as an extension assist. The ability of air to compress gives pneumatic knees a springier feel to the patient. One knee functions with a magnetorheologic fluid (Figure 20-9). This fluid contains metallic particles that respond to an electrical charge affecting the viscosity of the fluid. Instead of flowing through valve-controlled ports, the fluid acts on the knee axis to provide braking friction by becoming more or less viscous. Here, too, sensors

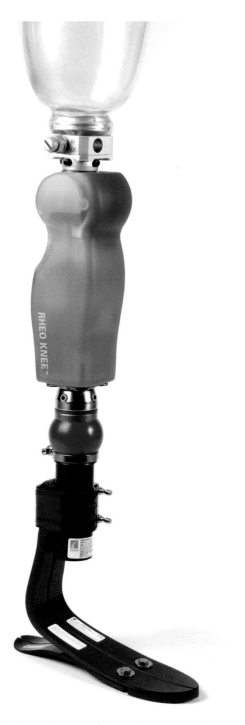

Figure 20-9. RHEO KNEE (Ossur Americas, Aliso Viejo, Calif).
Photograph: Courtesy of Ossur Americas, www.ossur.com.

send knee angle, velocity, and force data to the knee's microprocessor, which in turn adjusts a magnetic field around the fluid.

Microprocessor Knee

Microprocessor knees (Figure 20-10) are a class of knees that sense the conditions acting on the knee joint and can quickly make internal adjustments to safely meet those conditions. Joint angles and forces on the pylon are measured via sensors and are then sent to the microprocessor for rapid adjustment. Valves open or close electronically to increase or decrease fluid flow through the knee's internal ports, or the viscosity of the magnetorheologic fluid changes to vary resistance to knee flexion or extension. The advantage that microprocessor knees have over mechanical knees is that rapid input from the microprocessor makes them significantly more responsive to the patient's activity, whether walking, running, descending stairs, or stumbling.[6] These knees allow for manipulation of the computer program to vary the stability and safety of the knee as the patient progresses through rehabilitation. Stumble recovery is a significant feature of these knees.

Motorized Knee

Building on microprocessor technology, the motorized knee (Figure 20-11) provides flexion and extension to an externally powered motor-driven knee. The knee replaces lost muscle function. It is therefore possible for the user to climb stairs step by step, ascend inclines, and walk longer distances on level ground. Sensors are positioned on the sound side, which accurately measure motion, load, and position. This information is transmitted to the knee via Bluetooth technology, where the microprocessor analyzes the data and determines the response of the knee to the activity and the amount of power or force needed from the knee to generate the appropriate knee flexion or extension.

Additional Knee Features

Stance Flexion. Controlled prosthetic knee flexion under weight bearing is referred to as stance flexion. As the patient transfers weight onto the prosthesis in the early stance phase, the knee gradually yields to approximately 15 degrees, thereby cushioning the impact of weight bearing to the wearer. Stance flexion is adjustable and may be completely eliminated if the patient finds it disconcerting and fears that the knee may buckle, or it can be adjusted to allow up to 15 degrees of flexion. Although it requires some getting used to, this can be a very smooth knee mechanism for the patient to ambulate on because the stance flexion absorbs some of the shock transmitted to the socket during loading response.

Geometric Lock. The geometric lock feature, also

activities requiring maximum stability, this mechanism is ideal. Prolonged standing (ie, at a workbench) is one such example, as is traversing exceptionally rugged terrain. The patient simply flips a lever to engage the locking feature. A patient with bilateral amputations may occasionally need the stability of a locked knee. Ambulation with a locked knee compromises normal gait mechanics and should be carefully considered before being used for the purpose of daily ambulation. Locked knees are intended for activities beyond normal ambulation. Whereas mechanical knees are locked at full extension, one microprocessor knee can be adjusted through programming to lock the knee at any degree of knee flexion.

Other Components

Torsion

The rotation/torsion that occurs about the limb during gait can result in shear pressures if too much torsion is translated onto the limb.[7] Gel liners, feet with integrated ankles, and torsion adaptors can absorb

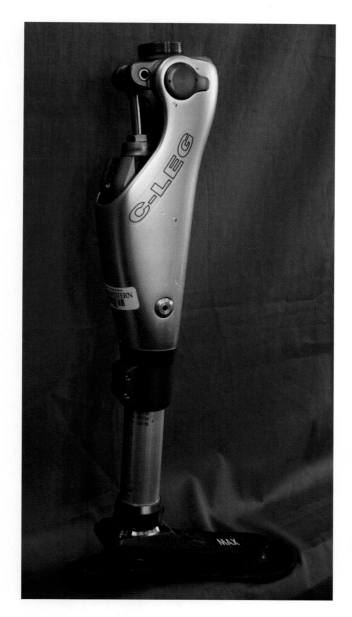

Figure 20-10. C-Leg (Otto Bock HealthCare, Minneapolis, Minn).
Photograph: Used with permission from Otto Bock Health-Care.

referred to as a mechanical stance phase lock, locks the knee on full extension (initial contact) and does not release it until the weight line passes over the forefoot and hyperextension of the knee unit occurs. This clever geometric design is engineered into a polycentric knee and provides excellent stability. The geometric lock can be convenient because it provides reliable stance control.

User-Activated Lock. A manual lock is available on some constant friction and fluid knees. For those

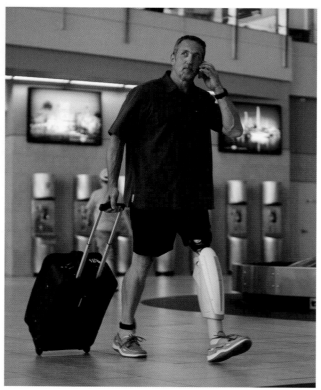

Figure 20-11. POWER KNEE (Ossur Americas, Aliso Viejo, Calif).
Photograph: Courtesy of Ossur Americas, www.ossur.com.

some of this torsion to decrease the rotational shear preventing skin abrasions and reducing stress on the knee joint. The torsion adaptor should be placed as proximal on the transtibial or transfemoral prosthesis as possible to minimize the perceived weight of the prosthesis by the patient. This feature is particularly helpful with activities that include a lot of pivotal movements (eg, golfing) in which patients experience a greater level of comfort. Axial motion occurs in the adaptor instead of between the socket and the skin. Some torsion adaptors have independent internal and external rotation adjustments.

Combined Torsion and Vertical Shock

Independent torsion and shock-absorbing units are available and can be paired with any foot. Interchangeable elastomer rods or adjustable springs provide dampening of vertical and rotational forces, thus reducing the strain on joints and soft tissues. Both torsion absorption and vertical shock dampening are inherent to some prosthetic feet (Figure 20-12).

Positional Rotators

A positional rotator (Figure 20-13) permits the patient to rotate the flexed knee and shank of the prosthesis out of the way for ease of movement. It enables

patients to sit cross-legged and swing the prosthesis away from the pedals while driving. This is an added convenience for patients with transfemoral or higher level amputations. Designed for non–weight-bearing activities only, the rotation is activated by pressing a button, and snaps back into place. Changing shoes and socks while wearing the prosthesis also becomes a much easier task.

Quick Release Couplings

Knees and feet can be easily interchanged by the patient under a well-fitting socket. A quick release coupler is available when varying activities necessitate such a change. Examples include the following: exchanging a microprocessor knee for a water-resistant knee and foot or temporarily removing components below the socket to maneuver about tight spaces.

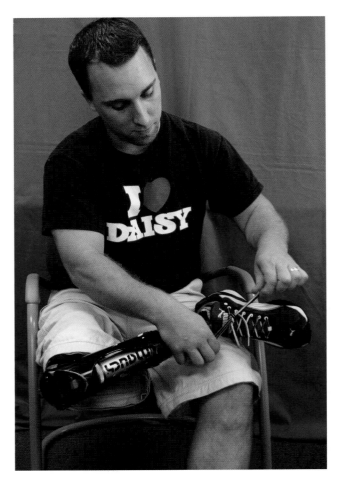

Figure 20-13. Positional Locking Rotator (Otto Bock Healthcare, Minneapolis, Minn).
Photograph: Used with permission from Otto Bock Healthcare.

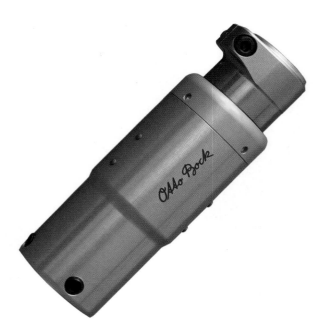

Figure 20-12. Delta Twist Shock Absorber (Otto Bock HealthCare, Minneapolis, Minn).
Photograph: Courtesy of Otto Bock HealthCare.

Socket Interfaces

Gel Liners

Cushioning and shear-reducing properties of gel liners make them ideal for all patients at any level of amputation. In addition, their compressive properties make them ideal as a shrinker during the early phase of rehabilitation. Gel liners can be used as a means of suspension, given their friction properties against the skin that prevents distal migration of the liner (Figure 20-14). They can be used for comfort in conjunction with any type of suspension. Patients exhibiting scar tissue will particularly benefit from the gel. Not only is shear greatly reduced, but also some liners slowly diffuse a medical-grade mineral oil or other emollient onto the skin. This aids in scar management by keeping the scar tissue soft and supple. Protection from socket pressures and shear has historically been treated with custom-made soft liners of high-density foams or with a combination of leather and silicone. Additionally, lack of protective sensation is another condition commonly managed with gel liners. Gel liners are available in 3-mm, 6-mm, and 9-mm thicknesses, with the latter being the most protective. They are available with or without fabric covering. Choosing a liner with a matrix embedded within the gel minimizes vertical displacement. The liners are available off the shelf in many sizes, durometers, and thicknesses. They are made of silicone, urethane, mineral oil, or a thermoplastic elastomer. Custom liners can be designed for atypical limb contours with varying durometers. Some liners are manufactured with a unique distal fabric weave to minimize elongation, and most are thinner posteriorly or rippled, thus facilitating comfortable knee flexion. Although the liners are relatively durable, they are not puncture-resistant or tear-resistant. Proper caution must be exercised to minimize damage. Longevity of the liners is very much dependent on the activity level of the patient and the care given to the liner. Heavy duty use, improper donning, lack of routine cleansing, or careless storage can shorten the life of a liner. Worn liners may abrade the skin and should be replaced. Given direct contact with the skin and the sealed environment, it is imperative that the liners be cleansed daily. They are designed to be hypoallergenic, and the occurrence of dermatitis or other skin irritations is rare. If a skin reaction does occur, it can be dealt with by switching to a gel liner made of another material and/or consulting with a physician. If the problem persists, a physician should be notified. Applying the liner correctly requires some degree of dexterity and cognitive function. Donning is achieved by turning the liner inside out, placing the end firmly against the limb, and rolling the liner up the limb. The inherent frictional (suspension) properties of the liners preclude them from being pulled on like a sock. Prosthetic socks can be worn over the liner to accommodate limb volume fluctuation.

Prosthetic Socks

Prosthetic socks are the interface materials between the residual limb and the socket. Even with the use of a gel liner, socks are still required to adjust the fit of the prosthesis. Generally, socks are

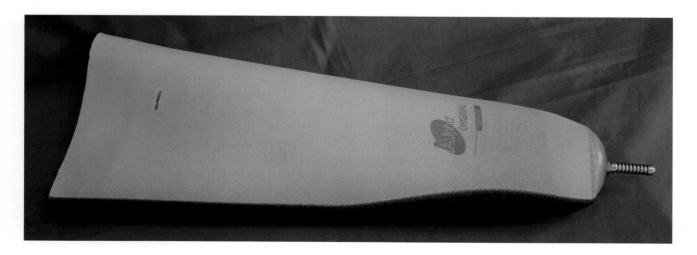

Figure 20-14. Original Alpha Liner (or gel liner; Ohio Willow Wood, Mt. Sterling, Ohio).
Photograph: Used with permission from Ohio Willow Wood.

provided in one-ply, three-ply, and five-ply thicknesses, and are combined to the desired thickness. They cushion the limb and wick away moisture when worn against the skin. In suction or vacuum suspension prostheses, they are necessary to wick air out of the system. Socks are knitted with wool, cotton, or any number of synthetic fibers. Some synthetic blends offer stretch, increased wicking ability of moisture away from the skin, and ease of care. When using a hard socket, oftentimes placing a prosthetic nylon sheath directly over the skin, followed by thicker prosthetic socks, reduces shear and increases comfort. As the patient's limb volume changes throughout the day, the addition or reduction of a few plies will maintain a comfortable fit. Temperature, activity, weight change, and diet all have an effect on socket fit.

Prosthetic socks for fit adjustment are placed over the liner and do not affect the function of the pin. A hole is required in the distal end of the sock to allow the pin to pass through to the locking mechanism. Sock ply can be adjusted without affecting pin suspension. Patients should always be reminded to pull up the sock completely onto the liner and not allow any sock material to remain over the area of the pin. If the fabric is pulled into the locking mechanism along with the pin, it may jam and prevent the disengagement of the pin. This action prevents removal of the prosthesis. If this happens, it may be necessary to dismantle the locking mechanism to free the pin.

Hard Sockets

Transtibial hard socket designs have the advantage of simplicity, less bulk, durability, and easy cleanability. The classic description indicates that only a sock interface is present. The popularity of gel liners makes the hard socket with socks only a less prescribed option. However, patients who choose not to wear a gel liner and who desire the low maintenance and simple socket style can use the hard socket with a sock interface. Because the socket is not as forgiving as one with a gel liner, a well-fitting socket is crucial, and the patient must be diligent in sock management to remain comfortable. Scar tissue and sharp bony prominences are contraindications for this socket style.

Transfemoral Flexible Inner Liner With Rigid Frame

The rigid frame provides socket stability, and the inner flexible socket provides comfort proximally in the transfemoral socket and also space for muscle expansion in both the transtibial and transfemoral sockets via specifically placed frame cutouts. If designed with large frame cutouts, the flexible inner socket might even provide added proprioceptive feedback through the socket wall when in contact with, for example, a chair edge while sitting. Postfabrication adjustments of socket contours are also more easily accomplished when there is a flexible inner liner. In the instance of heterotopic ossification, flexible inner liners can be removed, heat-expanded to provide relief, and placed back into the rigid frame.

SYME PROSTHESIS

Socket Design and Suspension

Although the Syme amputation is considered end bearing, the socket design and trimlines remain similar to that of the transtibial socket. The high socket trimline provides the same loading characteristics as that of the transtibial socket. This trimline also reduces the likelihood of edge pressure along the tibial crest during late stance. The prosthesis should spread the load over the entire limb. The Syme prosthesis generally resists axial rotation because of the elliptical contour at the level of the malleoli. Shock absorption is limited because of length constraints because no vertical shock units can be incorporated into the prosthesis. The calcaneal heel pad, however, provides padding and protects the distal limb.

Commonly used suspension designs are window designs placed medially, cut to the smallest size necessary to allow the malleoli to pass through, and are of tubular construction with no opening to weaken the design. The latter offers the greatest socket strength against compressive forces during gait and is therefore most desirable. The medial window design is most appropriate when the distal limb width is much greater than the width just proximal to the bulbous end. This commonly occurs when the flares of the malleoli are left intact and prominent. The tubular-styled prosthesis is donned by applying a thin pad placed just proximal to the widest part of the distal limb. Once the limb is seated firmly into the prosthesis, it is wedged into the socket. Secure suspension is achieved via pad thickness and sock ply. Occasionally, this pad may also be incorporated into a full polyethylene closed-cell foam liner. If the malleoli have been completely tapered and no flare at the distal limb exists, then the prosthesis cannot be self-suspended. In this case, a gel liner, outer sleeve, and one-way expulsion valve can be used to provide suction suspension.

Foot Options

The Syme amputation retains the talus and calcaneus, resulting in limited clearance between the limb and floor. Most prosthetic feet are too tall to fit under a Syme prosthesis without creating a limb length discrepancy. Low profile feet specifically designed for use with the Syme amputation are available. Many are of a carbon plate design. Bolted directly to the distal socket, they can also be affixed with epoxies or other adhesives.

Syme Biomechanics and Socket Strength

At loading response, the patient will feel pressure on the posterior proximal and anterior distal residual limb. At late-stance phase, the pressures occur in exactly the opposite locations: the anterior proximal and posterior distal residual limb. Pressures are greatest on the residual limb during this late-stance phase as the patient pushes off to propel forward. To decrease forces on the residual limb at this time, the foot can be slightly dorsiflexed or moved more posterior. This is also the rationale for keeping the socket trimline to the level of the patellar ligament, thereby preventing edge pressure along the tibial crest. Similarly, increasing toe-out to functionally reduce the toe lever will lower anterior proximal pressure on the limb. Increased toe-out can provide additional lateral stability.

The greatest forces on the socket occur in the sagittal plane. The anterior distal aspect of the socket is subject to high compressive loads during late stance and should be strengthened to prevent socket failure. This is most important when using a socket with a medial window. Extra layers of carbon fiber or fiberglass should be incorporated into the laminated socket in this area. Decreasing the anterior lever (toe lever) during alignment reduces the compressive loads on the anterior distal socket.

TRANSTIBIAL PROSTHESIS

Socket Design

Patellar Tendon Bearing

The patellar tendon-bearing (PTB)[8] socket consists of a laminated or thermoplastic socket that provides an intimate, total contact fit over the entire surface of the residual limb. The anterior wall of the socket extends proximally to encapsulate the distal third of the patella. Just below the patella, located at the middle of the patellar ligament, is an inward contour or bar that (via other biomechanical forces) converts the patellar tendon (ligament) of the residual limb into a weight-bearing surface. PTB is a misnomer, however, because the patellar tendon is not the only weight-bearing surface used by the PTB socket. The medial and lateral walls extend proximally to about the level of the adductor tubercle of the femur. Together, they serve to control mediolateral/rotary forces applied to the residual limb. The medial wall is modified with an undercut in the area of the medial flare of the tibia, a pressure-tolerant surface and primary weight-bearing area. The lateral wall provides relief for the head of the fibula and the cut end of the fibula. This wall applies pressure along the fibular shaft to enhance medial-lateral stability. In addition, the lateral wall acts as a counter pressure to the medial wall. The posterior wall is slightly higher than the patellar bar and is designed to apply an anteriorly directed force to maintain the patellar tendon on the bar. The posterior wall is flared proximally to allow comfortable knee flexion and is contoured to prevent pressure on the hamstring tendons. The total contact fit provides relief over nonpressure-tolerant areas and supports the body's weight over the pressure-tolerant areas of the limb. Total contact is necessary to prevent limb edema, but does not imply equal pressures throughout the socket. PTB socket design is appropriate for nearly all transtibial amputations, but is seen less often with introduction of the total surface-bearing socket. The PTB prosthesis is designed to maintain the residual limb in slight initial flexion (from 5 degrees to 10 degrees) to convert the patellar bar to a more horizontal supporting force. However, because the patellar bar is not completely horizontal, the residual limb still has a tendency to slide down posteriorly. This tendency must be counteracted by the posterior wall that is contoured to maintain the patellar tendon's position on the patellar bar.

Total Surface Bearing

The total surface-bearing (TSB) socket design is commonly used when a gel liner is prescribed. The gel dissipates pressures throughout the socket and relieves bony prominences. Different from the PTB socket, pressure is intended for global distribution over the entire limb, as opposed to pressure-tolerant areas only. Bone and other sensitive regions are cushioned by the gel liner. Socket contours are smooth and without any obvious reliefs or undercuts lowering peak pressures.[9] Similar to the PTB socket, this design also provides a total contact fit for comfort. The TSB socket significantly differs from PTB concepts in modification technique. In the PTB socket, plaster is removed over the patellar tendon, lateral pretibial group, the medial flare, and the popliteal region. Areas of plaster addition are the tibial tubercle, along the tibial crest, and the proximal and distal fibulae. TSB modification does not require buildups. The gel material dissipates pressures throughout the socket and relieves bony prominences. Patients with fragile soft tissues, burns, skin grafts, scarring, or bony residual limbs can benefit significantly from the extra protection offered by the gel liner and TSB design.[10,11]

Suspension

Suspension Sleeves

Suspension sleeves (Figure 20-15) are available in neoprene, gel, or a breathable elasticized fabric. A neoprene suspension sleeve provides simple, low profile, relatively effective suspension. Its ease of application makes it an ideal option as an auxiliary form of suspension for periods of increased activity. The sleeve is fitted to the proximal third of the prosthesis and onto the midthigh several inches past the prosthetic socks. A small puncture or tear in the neoprene or gel sleeve can significantly impact its effectiveness because it provides suspension through a snug fit, resulting in friction and negative pressure. Activities such as kneeling or other heavy duty use may easily cut through a sleeve, thus hindering the ability to provide partial suction. On occasion, a patient may be allergic to the material. Because sleeves fit snugly onto the thigh, the patient must have the strength and dexterity for proper application. If this is not the case, a more suitable suspension option should be sought. Heat buildup and perspiration are also concerns. Patients with upper extremity involvement may find the sleeve difficult to pull up onto the thigh. Sleeves do not provide sagittal or coronal stability.

Supracondylar/Supracondylar Suprapatellar Design

The supracondylar socket design affords the patient two primary benefits: (1) its high trimlines offer inherent suspension, and (2) it provides some control to a mildly unstable knee joint. The medial wall encompasses the femoral condyle and contours closely to the femur to purchase just past the level of the adductor tubercle, therefore creating a reduced proximal mediolateral dimension. This tight proximal configuration suspends the prosthesis over the femoral condyles. It is indicated primarily for individuals with short residual limbs to provide increased medial-lateral stability. It is

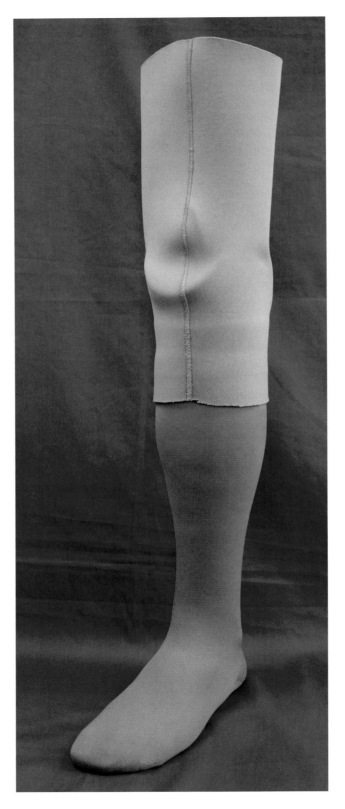

Figure 20-15. Neoprene suspension sleeve (Southern Prosthetic Supply, Alpharetta, Ga).
Photograph: Used with permission from Southern Prosthetic Supply.

contraindicated when knee instability requires more support. When a high anterior trimline—just past the proximal aspect of the patella—is added, then the socket becomes a supracondylar suprapatellar design. This area is referred to as the quadriceps bar. Encompassing the patella provides additional suspension, a kinesthetic reminder to limit knee extension, and prevents the medial and lateral brims from spreading.

Mechanical Lock Mechanisms

Mechanical locks are a positive locking system for suspension of the prosthesis. They are coupled with gel liners. The gel liner is rolled directly onto the skin and provides suspension through the mechanical lock. A variety of locks are available, some providing an audible clicking sound (ratchet style) that lets the patient know that the pin is engaged. Another lock style incorporates a clutch mechanism that allows the patient to manually draw the limb even deeper into

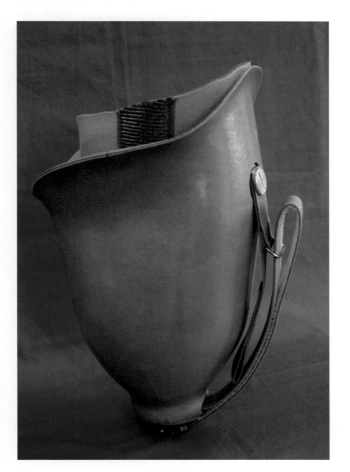

Figure 20-16. Lanyard-style suspension (KISS Technologies LLC, Baltimore, Md).
Photograph: Used with permission from KISS Technologies LLC.

the socket by turning a knob to eliminate any vertical displacement. A lanyard system is available when pin engagement is difficult because of mobile distal tissue or when a low profile lock is required to avoid making the prosthesis too long and creating a length discrepancy (Figure 20-16). Lock mechanisms can be very secure and less cumbersome forms of suspension, avoiding straps, belts, etc. To remove the prosthesis, a release pin is depressed that disengages the lock.

Suction

Suction suspension can be created by using a gel liner without the locking pin and by adding an airtight outer sealing sleeve. A one-way expulsion valve located at the distal socket removes air from the socket, thus creating a negative vacuum environment. With such a system, the patient can enjoy the benefits of suction suspension, minimal vertical displacement, and increased proprioception. Maintenance of an airtight seal is important for the system to function properly.

Sealing Liners

Similar to suction suspension with a knee sleeve, sealing liners have the added benefit of eliminating the knee sleeve by providing a hypobaric seal (Figure 20-17) between the liner and the socket. The seal is pressed against the socket wall, and suction is maintained below the level of the sealing ring. A thin sheath is worn below the seal to wick air out through a one-way, push-button release expulsion valve. Knee flexion is unrestricted because no additional sleeve is required. These liners are available prefabricated or can be customized to place the seal at any desired level.

Vacuum Assisted

Suction can be enhanced with a vacuum. The hypobaric environment is achieved and maintained via a telescoping mechanical vacuum pump (Figure 20-18) or an electric pump. With each step, air is actively drawn out of the socket, maintaining a consistent and

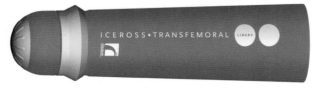

Figure 20-17. Iceross Transfemoral Seal-In Liner with DermoSil (Ossur Americas, Aliso Viejo, Calif).
Photograph: Courtesy of Ossur Americas, www.ossur.com.

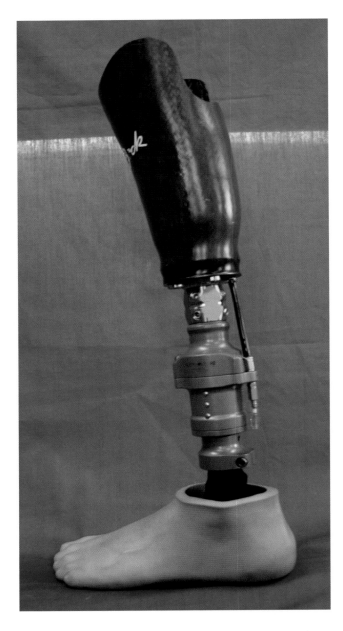

Figure 20-18. Harmony mechanical vacuum pump (Otto Bock HealthCare, Minneapolis, Minn).
Photograph: Used with permission from Otto Bock HealthCare.

comfortable level of vacuum. Additionally, the mechanical pump acts as a vertical shock absorber. The system consists of a gel liner covered by a sheath with a sealing sleeve placed over the prosthesis and rolled onto the thigh to create a sealed chamber. A tube exits the socket distally and routes into the vacuum pump. As with other suction systems, patients typically report increased proprioception.

Transtibial Biomechanics and Alignment (Endoskeletal Systems)

Biomechanics

The biomechanics of socket fit, alignment, foot function, and suspension are interrelated and highly dependent on each other. Socket biomechanics has already been partially covered in the section on socket design. To complete the discussion, dynamic forces and their relationship to the socket should also be explained. By placing the foot just medial (12 mm) to the socket midline, the medial flare and the shaft of the fibula are loaded during single limb support. These are both excellent, weight-tolerant areas, and foot placement is fine-tuned during dynamic alignment to maximize these regions of the limb. Contours to the pretibial region and the medial aspect of the tibia protect the distal end and crest of the tibia during loading response. At this time, the quadriceps are active, and distal tibial pressures can occur. Foot selection can alter gait and pressures within the socket. Articulated feet, feet with firm hind foot keels, or feet with shorter internal keels all have a different effect on a patient's comfort and gait efficiency. Inadequate suspension will result in a prosthesis that appears too long and will alter swing phase gait. The patient may vault on the sound side to clear the prosthesis. Shear within the socket may cause skin breakdown.

Prosthetic alignment refers to the fixed spatial relationship between the prosthetic socket and foot. With appropriate attachments, it is possible to reposition the foot in all planes. The foot can be moved in a linear fashion anteriorly or posteriorly and medially or laterally in relation to the socket. Prosthetic foot inversion or eversion and foot dorsiflexion or plantar flexion (socket flexion and extension) are also possible. All of these adjustments directly affect pressures within the socket as the patient ambulates.

Overall length of the prosthesis is determined by the length of the pylon used. Length of a transtibial prosthesis is correct when the medial tibial plateau of the residual limb is maintained at the same height as the medial tibial plateau on the sound side (as the patient stands with weight borne equally on both feet). The most convenient indication of correct height is through a comparison of the iliac crests (or the anterior superior iliac spines). If they are not the same level, then the height of the prosthesis should be corrected. This is a general rule, of course, and may not apply if the patient has scoliosis, pelvic obliquity, or congenital leg length discrepancy. Such cases must be taken individually, and often the best indicator of correct height is through gait analysis and patient comfort.

Proper foot rotation is important both cosmetically and functionally. Toe-out refers to the angle between the line of progression and the medial border of the prosthetic foot. A transtibial prosthesis is initially aligned with the medial border of the foot parallel to the line of progression. This position may need to be altered during static and dynamic alignment so that foot rotation on the prosthesis visibly matches that of the sound limb. In addition to appearance, foot rotation affects prosthetic function. How this occurs may be understood if the keel of the foot is viewed as a lever arm. During the stance phase, the tendency of the body to fall over the foot is resisted by the counter force of this lever arm. Therefore, rotation of the foot directly affects the length and direction of force exerted by the lever arm. The net effect of externally rotating the foot is to increase stability by widening the base of support. There is a cosmetic trade-off, of course, because the toe-out attitude of the prosthesis will not match that of the contralateral limb. Although it is rarely necessary to alter toe-out in this way, an awareness of the biomechanical effects of foot rotation is important.

Socket flexion was briefly discussed in the section on PTB design. To reiterate, pressures on the residual limb can be greatly influenced by the inclination of the supporting surfaces in contact with the limb. For example, if a prosthesis was fabricated with the patient's residual limb in 90 degrees of flexion, the shaft of the tibia would be horizontal in relation to the supporting surface of the socket, and the vertical force exerted by the socket would be equal to the weight of the body. The socket is placed in 5 degrees to 10 degrees of initial flexion to increase its supporting surface.

Alignment

Prosthetic alignment will change as the patient's range of motion, muscle strength, and balance improves, and as the patient gains confidence and becomes more physically comfortable in the prosthesis. Intervention by physical therapy is crucial during this early period to aid the patient in developing appropriate gait habits. Prosthetic alignment during early fitting, just after amputation, can be significantly different on the same patient one year later when the limb is well healed and the patient returns to high-level activity. As confidence and ability increase and limb contours change, the socket and/or foot will be replaced, resulting in a need for prosthetic alignment change. Initial static and dynamic alignment goals consider the patient's level of ability, limb length, stage of healing, range of motion, and muscle strength. Use

of instrumented gait evaluation has also been beneficial in optimizing prosthetic alignment. The goals in each plane during the first fitting/alignment visit are as follows:

Coronal

- Iliac crests are at the same level. Patient's gait is smooth and symmetrical with no excessive trunk lean to either side.
- Foot is inset loading the proximal-medial and distal-lateral aspects of the residual limb and encouraging an energy-efficient, narrow-based gait.
- Socket adduction or abduction matches the residual limb, resulting in a vertical pylon or a foot that is flat on the floor at midstance. On average, sockets are in 5 degrees of adduction, but some patients may actually require an abducted socket.
- There is less than 6 mm of socket displacement during the swing phase.

Sagittal

- No forced knee flexion or extension when standing. Shoe has even contact with floor and is bearing weight evenly.
- Presence of a smooth, energy-efficient gait pattern—including controlled knee flexion after initial contact-loading response—smooth rollover with no recurvatum tendency, or early dropoff at late stance.
- As previously described, an attitude of initial flexion increases the weight-bearing capacity of all load-tolerant areas. In addition to improving the weight-bearing characteristics, appropriate socket flexion also allows a smooth gait pattern by placing the quadriceps muscles on stretch. Because the knee is maintained in slight flexion, the quadriceps have a mechanical advantage to control the prosthesis. The constant attitude of knee flexion also lessens the possibility of hyperextension of the knee during midstance and terminal stance.

Transverse

- The degree of toe-out on the prosthesis should approximate that of the sound limb. The degree of toe-out should not decrease the patient's stance phase stability.

KNEE DISARTICULATION

Although the anatomical knee joint has been lost, the patient with a knee disarticulation amputation will be somewhat more functional than those with a higher level transfemoral amputation. The intact femur provides a long lever arm with good muscle control and strength because muscle insertions are not compromised. The asymmetrical shape of the distal end prevents socket rotation about the limb and provides a broad, partial weight-bearing surface. Another benefit of the knee disarticulation is that outward flaring of the femoral condyles can often be used to suspend the prosthesis. Control of the prosthetic knee is analogous to transfemoral principles. However, the full-length lever-arm, retention of thigh muscles, and center of rotation close to the knee center all enable the patient with a knee disarticulation amputation to have better control of the knee joint. The stable femur minimizes lateral socket shift and allows for abbreviated socket trimlines, resulting in increased comfort and range of motion. It is unlikely that hip flexion or hip abduction contractures will exist because the musculature remains balanced across the hip. When the prosthesis is removed, it is still possible for the patient to kneel because the residual limb can commonly withstand end bearing.

Socket Design

Socket design for knee disarticulation is often dictated by the degree to which distal weight bearing can be tolerated by the patient, as well as size of the femoral condyles in relationship to the thigh. Although knee disarticulation amputation is able to tolerate partial or full end bearing, the socket should provide total contact over the entire thigh to dissipate pressures over the greatest amount of surface area as possible. Ischial containment socket concepts remain the same, but trimlines and dimensions can be less aggressive than those of the transfemoral prosthetic design, even to the point of totally eliminating ischial containment. The proximal brim of the socket will be near round, terminating just distal to the ischium and pubic ramus to prevent impingement (similar to the old plug-fit transfemoral socket). Weight bearing will be distributed over the entire surface area of the residual limb contained in the socket, as well as over the distal end. Sockets are either thermoplastic or laminated and can include a gel liner or a flexible inner liner with a rigid outer frame. In weight bearing, a thin, firm, resilient pad provides the patient with a distal end pad to increase comfort under the bony condyles. During the early stance phase, the patient

stabilizes the prosthetic knee in much the same way as a person with a transfemoral amputation: by actively contracting the hip extensors. Therefore, the rotary forces occurring in the sagittal plane during this gait phase will be greatest over the anterior proximal aspect of the thigh and over the distal posterior end of the residual limb. Consequently, the proximal anterior brim of the socket should provide even, comfortable, counter pressure, and the distal posterior socket should provide total contact and comfortable loading. During midstance, the socket will rotate about the distal end of the knee disarticulation, thus generating counter pressure against the proximal tissues of the thigh. Although the long residual limb provides a greater surface area to disperse these forces, the direction of socket rotation concentrates pressures around the distal femur laterally and the proximal thigh medially. In light of these forces, socket design for this level should facilitate comfortable distal loading, the proximal brim should stabilize laterally, and the medial-proximal brim should flare generously to minimize tissue rolls and avoid painful pressure.

Suspension

The spared femoral condyles offer similar suspension options as the malleoli do in the Syme prosthesis. Supracondylar suspension is obtained with either a pad placed over the flares of the condyles to wedge the limb into the socket or a medial cutout in the distal socket that allows the widest points of the condyles to pass. The cutout is closed to hold the socket in place. A removable medial plate is locked in place over the opening with Velcro (Velcro USA, Inc, Manchester, NH) straps after the prosthesis is donned to securely hold the residual limb in place. A disadvantage of this design is that the opening weakens the structural strength of the socket, and care in fabrication to reinforce this area is necessary. This suspension method works well when the femoral condyles are prominent, but suspension can be compromised by excessive redundant soft tissue or postoperative edema. In such cases, some form of auxiliary suspension is needed. The medial window design is simple and easy to don. The pad or partial sleeve suspension design results in a strong, continuous socket and eliminates circumferential straps about the distal aspect of the socket. It consists of a split cylindrical pad that the patient slips over the lower femur proximal to the condyles, converting the residual limb to a cylindrical shape. Prosthetic socks are used to hold the pad in place. The patient then pushes into the socket until it is firmly seated. Compression of the pad and friction suspend the prosthesis. Because this method does not require a complete liner, no additional bulk is added around the bulbous distal end. Both designs require a socket interface, such as a gel liner, socks, or both. Suspension during swing is maintained by ensuring a tight fit via added sock plies or by increasing the thickness of the suspension pad. If the distal residual limb contours are captured well enough, this can provide suspension and rotational control because the rounded brim cannot be relied on to prevent rotation.

Knee Selection Considerations

The full length of the femur poses a challenge in that virtually any prosthetic knee joint will result in a lower knee center on the prosthetic side. Historically, outside knee joints were incorporated to minimize knee center discrepancy, but their many disadvantages—most importantly lack of swing phase control—make them rarely used today. The knees of choice at this level are those of the polycentric design, and some knees are designed specifically for the knee disarticulation amputation. They decrease the overall prosthetic length of the thigh section, while decreasing the length of the shin section. In addition, some knees incorporate a linkage that, when flexed to 90 degrees, translates posteriorly under the socket, thereby reducing the thigh section length. As the linkage folds up underneath the prosthetic socket during sitting, the foot will often rise off the floor. The thigh segment will still appear somewhat longer when compared with the sound side. These are common issues, and the patient should be made aware of them during the fitting process. The polycentric design also reduces the length of the shank section during swing, thus facilitating toe clearance.[12]

TRANSFEMORAL PROSTHESIS

Socket Design

Ischial Containment

In 1955, Radcliffe[13] described the biomechanics affecting lateral stabilization of the femur and pelvis in the transfemoral prosthesis. These principles are summarized as follows:

- During single limb support on the prosthetic side, the weight of the amputee's body, acting through the center of gravity, causes the pelvis to dip toward the sound side.
- Because of this tendency for the pelvis to rotate toward the sound side, the pelvis can be described as a lever with a fulcrum, or supporting point, located lateral of the ischium.
- The tendency for the pelvis to dip or rotate toward the sound side is resisted by contraction of the hip abductor (gluteus medius), which exerts a counteracting moment to the pelvic lever.
- For the gluteus medius to have maximum effectiveness, it should be maintained at its normal resting length.
- This can be achieved if the femur is kept in a normal position of adduction.
- For the person with a transfemoral amputation, the lateral wall of the socket must be shaped to maintain the femur in adduction because contraction of the gluteus medius causes the femur to stabilize against the lateral wall. Pressures thus generated must be distributed evenly, and excess pressure over the distal lateral end of the femoral shaft must be avoided.
- As a result of these forces acting against the lateral shaft of the femur, counter pressure is generated by the medial wall against the proximal medial tissues of the limb.

These principles have not changed, although the ongoing challenge of managing them has produced a gradual evolution toward ischial containment socket designs and changing theories of prosthetic alignment.

One of the primary goals of the ischial containment socket is to provide medial-lateral stability by controlling the lateral shift of the femur during stance. This is accomplished by the narrow medial-lateral design and closely fitting socket that encases the medial aspect of the ischial tuberosity and ramus.[14] Per its name, the ischial containment socket has the ischium within the socket itself. The socket is just wide enough at the level of the ischial tuberosity to allow the ischium to drop down inside the socket. The portion of the socket that extends proximally along the medial aspect of the ischial tuberosity and the ischial ramus is called the medial containment wall. This wall is angled to match the ischial ramus angle and does not follow the line of progression. Because the medial containment wall extends above the ischium, it will not allow the socket to migrate laterally. A tight dimension spanning the area just below the trochanter and at the medial aspect of the ischium maintains the bony structures snugly against the medial containment wall. In the transverse plane, the ischial containment socket tends to follow the anatomical shape of the proximal thigh.

It has been proposed that the ischial containment socket can provide a bony lock via a three-point force system and increase femoral stabilization in the socket during weight bearing. It is also believed that this three-point force system provides additional means for holding the femur in adduction. In 1989, a study by Gottschalk et al[15] demonstrated that socket design is not necessarily a primary determinant of femoral adduction. This work showed that there was no significant difference in femoral adduction in the socket when comparing quadrilateral or ischial containment designs. The postsurgical length of the adductor musculature had a much greater bearing on proper femoral adduction.

When the socket trimlines in the perineum are aggressively high to capture the ischium and posterior aspect of the ramus, using a flexible inner liner with a rigid frame is recommended. The frame needs only to support or control the bony structures, thus leaving the flexible plastic to contain the anterior ramus and soft tissues. The added feature of the frame cutouts provides comfort, room for expanding musculature, and some proprioceptive feedback.

Ischial Containment Variants

Once the concept of ischial containment was established, there have been varied iterations of this design. Some sockets accentuate and clearly define the functioning muscle bellies, allowing space for muscle contraction. Others lower the posterior aspect of the socket for sitting comfort. This minimizes gluteal support, but renders a better cosmetic result. Each of these designs follows the basic ischial containment principles with additional specific goals. Furthermore, each prosthetist will custom design any socket a bit differently, given the many contours and trimlines possible with the transfemoral socket.

Quadrilateral

If the ischial containment design is not successful, then the more historical quadrilateral socket may be considered. Quadrilateral refers to the four-sided shape of the socket when viewed transversely. As Radcliffe[13] states: "The four walls of the socket are designed to apply pressures and counter pressures to facilitate comfortable load bearing through soft tissue and underlying structures." The ischial tuberosity and gluteal musculature are used as primary weight-bearing structures and are supported by a posterior shelf. The ischium is maintained on the shelf or seat by the counter force of an inward contour (Scarpa's bulge) in the anteromedial socket located over the femoral triangle. Although the femoral triangle contains the femoral artery, vein, and nerve, years of clinical trials have demonstrated that correctly distributed pressure over these structures is well tolerated. A convex contour in the proximal anterolateral socket accommodates the bulk and the contraction of the quadriceps muscle group. The quadrilateral socket may be suspended in a number of ways, including use of suction, a Silesian belt, or a hip joint with a pelvic belt.

Suspension

Suction by Skin Contact

A suction socket offers intrinsic suspension and is held in place by a combination of negative air pressure, surface tension between the socket and the patient's skin, and muscular contraction against the socket walls. For the socket walls to be in direct contact with the patient's skin, no socks are worn. A valve, usually located at the distal-medial aspect of the socket, allows air to escape from the socket during weight bearing while preventing air entrance during the swing phase. The patient generally dons a suction socket by removing the valve, applying a donning sleeve over the residual limb, and feeding the loose end of the material through the valve hole. The material breaks the surface tension between the socket and the patient's skin, allowing the patient to pull the limb comfortably into the socket. By using the donning sleeve to help pull skin and soft tissue into the socket, the patient can usually minimize problems caused by tissue overhanging the socket brim. Patients with a long, muscular limb may choose to push directly into the socket with a small amount of skin lubricant. Either way, it is critical that no distal air pockets remain. If there is lack of total contact distally in a suction socket, the high negative pressures created in the air space can result in circulatory congestion and edema. There are many advantages to selecting suction suspension. The most apparent advantage is elimination of belts and liners. Thus, the patient enjoys an unencumbered, lightweight, and relatively simple-to-apply suspension. The socket is a total contact fit that minimizes the possibility of edema. Suction is a solid form of suspension because once the skin is drawn down into the socket, the residual limb is effectively trapped in the socket, thereby minimizing vertical displacement. Because the socket is firmly attached to the patient's residual limb, and rotational control is provided by the brim design, patients usually report that they have much better control of the prosthesis when using this form of suspension, especially during the swing phase.

One noted contraindication to a suction socket is that limb volume must remain stable to maintain a negative pressure environment. It is common for a patient's residual limb to change volume over time, especially within the first year postsurgery. Even the residual limb of a longtime wearer can decrease in volume over the course of the day. Slight fluctuations are normal and generally not problematic, but those seen just after surgery make this suspension option inappropriate. If the patient presents with scarring, which extends across the proximal tissues of the residual limb, it is possible that those scars will break the air seal around the proximal socket and allow air to enter. As a result, suction is not maintained. Donning the suction socket requires strength and balance. If the patient does not possess sufficient ability and endurance, or has upper extremity involvement, another suspension mechanism must be used.

Sealing Liners

Suction is the suspension of choice because it eliminates belts and buckles. To address some of the aforementioned contraindications, a sealing liner as presented in the transtibial section is a good choice. A gel liner with a hypobaric seal is rolled onto the limb and then pushed into the socket. The seal is pressed against the socket wall, and suction is maintained below the level of the sealing ring. A thin sheath is worn below the level of the ring to wick air out through a one-way, push-button release expulsion valve.

Locking Gel Liners

When the two previous suspensions cannot be used, gel locking liners may be considered. The locks can incorporate pins, lanyards, or buckles. The goals of the gel locking liner for the transfemoral design are similar to that of the transtibial socket, with a primary goal to suspend the prosthesis and distribute pressure over the entire surface of the residual limb. As in the transtibial prosthesis, the silicone or gel type liner can provide a significant amount of protection for the residual limb. Locking liners can be applied to virtually any length of transfemoral residual limb. If a locking liner is planned for a long transfemoral or knee disarticulation amputation level, then a lanyard-type suspension may be required. This does not require the use of a long locking mechanism and keeps the prosthetic knee center at or just slightly below the anatomical knee.

The most common advantage for the gel locking liner is an added measure of protection for the residual limb. The use of a liner can provide reduced shear on the residual limb and thus increased protec-

tion for fragile tissues. The liner can accommodate varying circumferences of the residual limb, thus ensuring total contact in the socket. As a result, the patient is much less likely to experience the failure of suspension because of suction loss. As an added benefit, donning the locking liner can be much easier than the skin suction socket because the patient is not required to lean over and pull into the socket. Typically, this locking liner suspension only requires that the patient engage the pin or pull up on a lanyard while stepping into the socket. Another significant advantage for the transfemoral patient, who tends to experience volumetric changes of the residual limb, is that the patient can apply prosthetic socks over the locking liner. The socks must have a hole at the distal end, which allows the pin to pass through and engage into the locking mechanism of the distal socket. As the patient's residual limb volume decreases, the sock ply can be increased accordingly and vice versa.

Silesian Belt

The Silesian belt is a simple, low-profile, belt-type suspension mechanism. Indication for its use is primarily the need for rotational control of the prosthesis. The Silesian belt can be used as an auxiliary to suction suspension and, the in the case of an individual with weak adductors, can even assist the adductor muscles during swing phase. The belt sits firmly over the sound side ilium and may not be as effective with the obese patient. Scarring about the pelvis can also prevent its use because the belt creates friction in this area. If the patient presents with severe mediolateral instability, the hip joint and belt are better choices. The Silesian belt can be easily used with prosthetic socks to suspend the prosthesis while also accommodating residual limb volume fluctuation. The Silesian bandage is an excellent auxiliary suspension for a suction socket fitting for shorter levels. Support of the belt helps to prevent the socket from slipping off when the patient is seated. It also provides additional security during any activity.

Elastic Belt

An elastic suspension belt is fabricated of Neoprene (or polychloroprene; DuPont Performance Elastomers LLC, Wilmington, Del) or similar elastic material. Typically, this kind of belt is fastened anteriorly by Velcro (Velcro USA, Inc, Manchester, NH). Because the belt is made of elastic material, it is not ideal as a primary suspensor. The belt can allow rotation and elongation of the prosthesis. Because of its simplicity, however, it is not uncommon for an elastic belt to be used as an intermediate form of suspension or as an auxiliary suspension (along with suction). If the patient is involved in high-level activities, there might be a concern, on occasion, of losing suction. For those high-level activities, the patient may choose to temporarily apply a belt to the prosthesis in the event that suction suspension is lost. With its simple Velcro closure, it is very easy to don.

Hip Joint and Pelvic Band

Whereas the Silesian belt is generally considered an auxiliary suspension, the pelvic belt is a primary suspension. This system includes a hip joint attached to the proximal lateral socket, a metal or plastic pelvic band contoured to the patient's pelvis just below the iliac crest, and a leather belt that encircles the patient's pelvis. The hip joint and pelvic band are typically considered a suspension means of last resort. Accurate placement is critical to proper function. If any other suspension can be successfully used, it should be explored first. A short transfemoral residual limb may be too short or may not generate enough abductor force during single limb support on the prosthetic side to provide a level pelvis. The added leverage offered by the hip joint and extension up to the pelvic band can usually provide adequate medial-lateral stability to the hip. This suspension system is very simple to use. If the patient can use an ordinary belt, then usually this form of suspension can be adequately donned, thus allowing the amputee to wear socks so that volumetric changes can be easily accommodated. The hip joint and pelvic band are obviously bulky and heavy. This can restrict hip range of motion and make sitting less comfortable.

Transfemoral Biomechanics and Alignment (Endoskeletal Systems)

The smooth and safe function of a transfemoral prosthesis is dependent on the relation between socket, suspension, knee, and foot. The socket is positioned in all planes for optimum function. Generally, 5 degrees of socket flexion will place the hip extensors at a mechanical advantage, ready to resist a knee flexion moment at heel contact. If a hip flexion contracture is present, additional socket flexion will be necessary. A flexion contracture of up to 25 degrees may be accommodated by prosthetic alignment. Anything beyond 25 degrees will cause excessive lumbar lordosis, leading to possible low back pain. Knee stability is determined by volitional control, the mechanics of the knee itself, and, most importantly, alignment. The knee is positioned

at or just behind a line connecting the trochanter and ankle (also known as the TA line). Moving the knee fore or aft, even a few millimeters, can have significant impact on the overall safety of the prosthesis. In the coronal plane, the adduction angle of the sound side is matched, unless there is a limitation at the hip preventing full adduction. The posterior brim of the socket is divided into thirds, and the foot is placed under the medial third mark. This provides good lateral loading of the femoral shaft during stance. A shorter limb or weak hip abductors might require that the foot be placed a bit more laterally under the midsocket to reduce the forces along the lateral aspect of the socket. In the transverse plane, the medial containment wall is rotated to follow the angle of the ramus. The prosthetic knee is set into 5 degrees of external rotation to the line of progression, and the foot is positioned to match the patient's sound side foot rotation. Alignment of prosthetic components can be refined by gait lab analysis using center of mass instead of the TA line.

Alignment

As described in the section on transtibial prostheses, the prosthetic alignment will change as the patient progresses through the first year postsurgery, especially during early therapy treatment. Improvements in strength, balance, comfort, and confidence will periodically make reassessment of alignment necessary. Much attention is given to knee stability. Not only does moving the knee in relation to the ground reaction line affect stability, but also internal knee adjustments to resistance can reduce the likelihood of unexpected knee collapse and yield a smooth and efficient gait pattern.

Initial static and dynamic alignment goals take into consideration the patient's level of ability, limb length, stage of healing, range of motion, and muscle strength. The goals in each plane during the first fitting/alignment visit are as follows:

Coronal

- Iliac crests are at the same level.
- Patient's gait is smooth and symmetrical with no excessive trunk lean to either side.
- Foot is inset-loading the lateral femur during stance, encouraging a narrow-based and energy-efficient gait.
- The foot/shoe has even contact with the floor and is bearing weight evenly.
- The socket is well suspended and does not drop away from the residual limb.

- There is no vaulting on the sound side.
- There is no abducted or circumducted gait.

Sagittal

- The prosthetic knee is stable at initial contact/loading response.
- During terminal stance, the foot rolls without dropping off or causing pelvic rise.
- The plantar flexion bumper of the articulated foot is firm and does not allow foot slap.
- Heel rise is not excessive.
- There is no terminal impact.

- Steps are equal.
- Lumbar lordosis is not excessive.

Transverse

- The degree of toe-out on the prosthesis should approximate that of the sound limb. The degree of toe-out should not decrease the patient's stance phase stability.
- There is no medial or lateral whip at terminal stance.
- There is no rotation of foot at initial contact/loading response.

HIP DISARTICULATION AND TRANSPELVIC AMPUTATION

These levels of amputation are almost always treated with the lighter weight endoskeletal prosthesis, given their lightweight properties, ease of fabrication, and postfabrication adjustability. Knee components, feet, and alignment are selected to enhance stability and ease of use. Energy required to ambulate with these prostheses is 200% times greater than normal.[16]

Hip Disarticulation Socket Design

Originally developed as the Canadian hip disarticulation prosthesis, this prosthesis incorporates both the sound and affected side iliac crest contours into the socket design. The socket is intended to bear weight on the ischium; however, this weight is shared along the anterior torso and the posterior gluteal muscle area by sloped anterior and posterior walls lifting the torso off the ischium to some degree. Primary suspension is provided over the affected side ilium. The contralateral ilium provides only minimal support during swing phase. Trimlines extend proximally above the ilium, and socket contours accentuate the narrower waist groove. During swing phase, the weight of the prosthesis is borne here. One socket feature that facilitates donning and doffing the prosthesis is a flexible lamination located about the posterior midline. Flexibility at this location allows the patient to spread the rigid, supporting socket open and wrap it around the pelvis. Because of the asymmetric contours of the pelvis and the intimate socket fit, rotational stability of the socket is good.

A two-piece socket design was developed at the University of California, Los Angeles.[17] By splitting the socket into two parts and fastening them together with a crisscrossing strap design posteriorly, this design can provide support and suspension during stance, as well as swing phase. During midstance, as the weight is borne into the socket, the strap system draws the inferior aspect of the sound side portion of the socket medially. This holds the patient firmly into the prosthetic socket while easing up on the iliac crest. During swing phase, the prosthesis attempts to move inferiorly on the patient's pelvis. The contralateral portion of the socket provides increased pressure over the iliac crest, increasing swing phase stability of the socket on the patient. This floating sound side design is more comfortable for the patient and is easier to fabricate for the prosthetist.

Transpelvic Socket Design

Transpelvic amputation is completed at the junction of the sacrum and ilium. The primary consideration with the transpelvic socket design is that the patient's weight is borne against the socket wall through soft tissues alone. The transpelvic socket extends to the body midline and encompasses the lower rib cage bilaterally, with the abdomen and the pelvis on the sound side. The socket may extend superiorly as high as the tenth rib. Inferiorly, the socket must clear the sound side limb and genitalia. On the sound side, the trimlines are brought inferior just proximal to the trochanter. In general, by encompassing more of the rib cage, the stability of the socket on the lower trunk is improved. There is generally less rotation of the pelvis and the socket because no ischial tuberosity exists that forms a fulcrum, as in the case of hip disarticulation. Raising the trimlines also increases the available surface area over which weight can be borne. The concave contour of the socket matches the convex contour of the residual limb. The socket wall generates forces oriented obliquely upward on soft tissue and the sound side pelvis.

Hip and Knee Joint Considerations

There are numerous endoskeletal components available to be used in the hip disarticulation prosthesis. Hip joints are single axis requiring an extension stop and extension assist. Single axis or polycentric knee units can be incorporated into the prosthetic design. A polycentric knee with a mechanical stance phase lock with extension aid in reaching full knee extension is a good choice for this prosthesis. The polycentric feature shortens the shank during swing phase, making it easier to clear the ground. In the polycentric design, the knee joint center resides more proximally than a single axis design. This provides the patient with an added biomechanical advantage in both initiating and resisting flexion because of the proximity of the instantaneous center of rotation to the anatomical hip joint center. Also ideal is a microprocessor knee. Both designs offer excellent stance phase stability. Careful consideration of overall prosthetic weight versus function and stability is necessary for optimal outcome.

Hip Disarticulation/Transpelvic Biomechanics and Alignment

The hip joint is placed far anterior on the socket relative to the normal hip joint location. The knee axis also falls considerably posterior to the anatomical knee. A combination of these two joint positions creates a significant knee extension moment. The knee hyperextends until an extension stop is contacted. This particular alignment provides an extremely secure knee, making it difficult for the knee to buckle inadvertently. If the center of gravity remains within boundaries formed by vertical reference lines placed at both the hip and knee centers, the hip and knee joints will remain stable. If the patient's center of gravity falls behind the posterior line located at the knee joint, this creates a knee flexion moment and causes the knee to buckle. If the center

of gravity falls anterior to the hip joint, this creates a hip flexion moment and causes the socket to flex at the hip joint.

Alignment

A line projected through the hip joint axis and the knee joint axis should intersect with the ground approximately 1½ inches posterior to the heel. The theoretical weight line begins at the point in the socket 1 inch anterior to the ischial tuberosity. It extends vertically to the ground passing ½ inch anterior to the knee center and intersects with the ground at approximately 7/16 of an inch anterior to the center of the prosthetic foot. In proper coronal plane alignment, one proposed method places the hip joint 10 mm lateral to the lateral ¼ mark. In the transverse plane, the hip joint should be externally rotated 5 degrees to 10 degrees for a more anatomical swing phase action of the thigh and shank. The length of the prosthesis should be approximately ½ inch shorter than the sound side to provide adequate clearance of the toe during gait.

Gait

The gait pattern for these individuals to properly ambulate requires that the patient use atypical motions to generate appropriate forces to advance the prosthetic limb. These forces include vaulting on the sound side, hip hiking on the prosthetic side during swing, and posterior tilting of the pelvis at late stance on the prosthetic side to initiate hip and knee flexion. As patients become more proficient, these motions are minimized, but nevertheless are present during gait. The gait of these individuals requires a great deal of energy expenditure to facilitate balance and advance the prosthetic limb. The energy costs can be twice that of normal human gait. Comfort is another issue for these individuals. Whether sitting, standing, or ambulating, it is important that socket contours and trimlines provide the greatest comfort to the patient.

COMORBIDITIES AFFECTING THE REHABILITATION PRESCRIPTION

Multiple Limb Loss

Bilateral lower extremity amputations require special consideration related to prosthetic design and alignment. Socket design remains the same; however, accommodative gel liners are recommended because the patient is not able to shift weight to a sound side foot. This is particularly important for the more bony transtibial amputation. Torsion adaptors reduce ana-

tomical knee and hip joint torque and shear at the skin/socket interface. Any additional components placed as close to the sockets as possible reduce the perceived weight of the prostheses. Constructing the prosthesis as light in weight as possible helps the patient keep energy costs down. An alignment that moves the feet slightly more lateral or increasing toe-out gives a wider base of support. This decreases the coronal plane forces placed on the limb during weight bearing. A wider base also results in additional stability. Foot selection can influence prosthetic knee stability and ground conformance. For bilateral transfemoral patients, articulated feet—or those with a softer heel or hind foot keel—move the weight line anterior to the knee joint more quickly, stabilizing the knee in early stance. Regardless of the level of amputations, identical foot components should be used for consistent gait mechanics. The use of stubby prostheses, sockets without knees, keeps the patient's center of gravity low to ground and helps the patient gain balance, strength, and confidence early on. Incremental height increases and the addition of knees, added one at a time if necessary, bring the patient to, or near to, preinjury height. If only one knee at a time is added, leaving the other side with a straight pylon, then the longer limb or the limb with better muscle control is fitted with a knee first. Progress requires commitment by the patient and an intense physical therapy regimen. To facilitate good posture and a well-placed base of support, feet may be articulated and perhaps mounted backward. Foot blocks with rocker design are also common. Knees for the bilateral transfemoral patient should offer good stability. Polycentric design, fluid control, and microprocessor control all offer stability and can be aligned for maximal safety. The polycentric knee shortens through swing phase, a useful feature, when the opposite limb is a transtibial amputation. Marking liners, socks, valves, etc, as right and left is helpful when donning.

When upper limb amputations are also present, the most pressing issue is one of independent donning. Donning devices can be designed for individual needs, and easy suspension options (eg, gel liners with locking pins or sealing liners) can be used.

Bone

Heterotopic ossification is a concern for amputations resulting from blast injuries.[18] Socket modifications, a soft gel interface, and/or socket replacement help to manage and accommodate the changing limb contours. External fixators on the amputated side or the contralateral limb do not preclude prosthetic fitting. The prosthetic management goal is to get the patient ambulatory quickly. Sockets can be modified to distribute weight away from the fixator, and/or cutouts can be made around the device. Prosthetic knees offering maximum stability will provide safer ambulation.

Soft Tissue

Shrapnel fragments, foreign bodies, and other detritus may migrate until they are just under the skin surface. Often they are expelled. This process requires close monitoring and ongoing socket modification. Neuromas are treated prosthetically in much the same way because they are painful and limit prosthetic use.

Skin

Grafted skin or excessive scar tissue can be a challenge, and a comfortable fitting socket can be difficult to achieve. Liners made of softer rather than firmer gel protect fragile skin. Alignment intended to reduce forces on the limb is also helpful. Pain as a result of fragments in the soft tissue and under the skin may be managed with soft gel liners as well. Occasionally, shrapnel can work its way through the skin.

Joint Function and Condition

Limited range of motion, contractures, and/or loss of muscle function require alignments and component selections that accommodate these situations. Fall prevention and socket comfort are the foremost considerations. If alignment alone does not produce the desired results, then components providing either additional range of motion (eg, articulated feet) or knee components with added stance control can be selected.

Blindness

Donning is a consideration when the patient is blind. Tactile markers on the prosthesis and its components help the patient to orient the gel liner, socks, or belt for proper donning. Ratcheted locking pins emit audible clicks as they engage into a shuttle lock confirming positive suspension.

THE PROSTHETIC REHABILITATIVE PROCESS

The prosthetic phases (preprosthetic, initial prosthetic, basic prosthetic, and advanced prosthetic) mirror the timelines set by the Physical Therapy Service for treatment protocols for amputees.

Phase I: Preprosthetic (Weeks 1–4)

Care typically includes prosthetic plan formulation, patient education, wound management, and volume control through the use of shrinker socks, silicone or equal liners, or elastic wraps.

Phase II: Initial Prosthetic (Weeks 2–10)

Care typically includes the provision of a prosthetic limb with multiple replacement sockets as warranted. The use of early postoperative prosthesis (EPOP) is common at military MTFs. EPOPs comprise custom-designed sockets fabricated from ThermoLyn PETG (Otto Bock HealthCare, Minneapolis, Minn) material attached to advanced prosthetic components. The components may consist of a C-Leg (Otto Bock HealthCare, Minneapolis, Minn) microprocessor knee unit for knee disarticulation level and higher, and a dynamic response or stored energy foot. EPOP sockets are replaced at an extraordinary rate. Standard practice is to maintain an appropriately fitting socket at all times. As service members progress through the rehabilitation process, their limbs undergo changes in size and shape. These changes are atypical when compared with the geriatric dysvascular amputee, in which shape and size reductions are typically uniform. For the service member who has sustained a blast injury, limb size and shape reduction are not uniform, in particular for those with heterotopic ossification.

CAD/CAM is an excellent tool to use in an acute care setting for a variety of reasons. It does not replace the skill and experience of the prosthetist; rather, it enhances prosthetic services by decreasing delivery times and increasing efficiency. It provides a way to objectively document limb morphology and volume and to track limb change. Residual limb shape capture is accomplished by noncontact scanners, digitized passive casts, measurements, or photos dependent on the particular CAD system used. The software to manipulate the shapes is intuitive and relatively easy to use. Output is to a milling machine for fabrication of a positive model. Standard fabrication procedures of the prosthetic socket are followed at that point.

Use of microprocessor knee units as first-fit systems are not uniform at all military MTFs. Safety is paramount, and the facilities rely on a team approach for prescription rationale of such devices. In general, all of the military MTFs are prescribing microprocessor units for those with bilateral lower extremity amputation and/or those with lower and upper extremity amputations.

Phase III: Basic Prosthetic (Weeks 11–20)

Care includes continued socket replacements, also the introduction of dynamic response or stored energy prosthetic feet as indicated. Progression to more dynamic feet should coincide with the patient's progress in physical therapy. Sockets may be fabricated from definitive materials (eg, carbon graphite and acrylic resin) as indicated.

Phase IV: Advanced Prosthetic (Months 3–6)

Care includes the design and delivery of specialty prostheses to include, but are not limited to, sport use prostheses. These prosthetic limbs should be fabricated from definitive materials.

ACTIVE DUTY MILITARY, LOWER LIMB PROSTHETIC PROTOCOLS

Recommendations for Daily Use Prosthesis

1. Sockets
   a. ThermoLyn or its equal until ready for definitive socket.
   b. Definitive socket materials (eg, carbon graphite and acrylic or epoxy resin) prior to high-level sporting/recreational activities.
   c. Definitive socket for transfemoral amputees: flexible socket with rigid frame.
   d. Hip disarticulation: start with socket; add custom liner/suspension system, depending on individual limbs; consider using three-dimensional modeling to help guide design as indicated, especially with secondary problems (eg, heterotopic ossification).

2. Suspension
   a. Suction suspension for all amputees unless meets criteria for pin lock or lanyard.
   b. Pin lock or lanyard for amputees with anticipated large-volume changes or when suction is contraindicated.
   c. Auxiliary suspension added as needed for higher level activities.

3. Feet
   In general, limit three different feet for each amputee during the first year. Integrate gait lab to augment clinical decisions.
   a. Transtibial
      i. Use soft, multiaxial, easy, rollover, and shock-absorbing properties to promote early weight bearing and weight

shifting (eg, Talux [Ossur Americas, Aliso Viejo, Calif] or TruStep [College Park Industries, Fraser, Mich]).

    ii. Progress to a higher energy returning foot, such as Ceterus (Ossur Americas, Aliso Viejo, Calif), Renegade (Freedom Innovations, Irvine, Calif), Re-Flex VSP (Ossur Americas, Aliso Viejo, Calif), Modular III (Ossur Americas, Aliso Viejo, Calif), or low-profile equivalents. Can have a second, high-energy returning foot if properties of new foot are different from existing foot.

    iii. Consider microprocessor foot or other advanced power prosthesis, depending on individual goals and activity levels after they have mastered above feet for a minimum of 3 months or as otherwise decided by the rehabilitation team.

  b. Transfemoral
    Same as transtibial level.

4. Specialty Prosthetic Limbs
Lower extremity amputees may also receive a water/swimming leg and running leg.

  a. The water leg may be used for bathing, as well as for other water activities. Modifications to be used for swimming may be added if the amputee expresses such interest.

  b. Running-specific legs will be prescribed when clinically appropriate for amputees who express the desire and motivation to return to more frequent and longer distance running than that accommodated through the use of the dynamic response foot. The primary goal will be to help the service member return to Army physical fitness standards. Providers must be aware that conditions such as osteoporosis, nerve injury, fractures, etc, might be contraindicated to aggressive running with a running specialty leg. Use of a dual-energy X-ray absorptiometry scan (or DEXA scan) is warranted to determine osteopenia. Furthermore, appropriate training with an experienced therapist is essential to successful and safe running on a running specialty leg. All running legs will be fabricated with a definite socket. Guidance is to start with a distance foot (eg, FlexRun [Ossur Americas, Aliso Viejo, Calif] or Cheetah [Ossur Americas, Aliso Viejo, Calif]) and progress to a sprint foot if the patient demonstrates proficiency.

5. Knees
One microprocessor; need to have gait assessment first with the C-Leg, then gait analysis after 4 weeks of training with the RHEO KNEE (Ossur Americas, Aliso Viejo, Calif) and/or the POWER KNEE (Ossur Americas, Aliso Viejo, Calif).

SUMMARY

This chapter focused on the prosthetist as a member of a comprehensive, clinical rehabilitation team at military MTFs. Also reviewed were the unique role of prosthetists during combat deployments, as well as the lower limb prosthetic technology provided to combat-injured service members who sustained an amputation. The prosthetist is an integral part of the multidisciplinary rehabilitation team, often working in unison with other team members, yet also taking center stage during formulation of the prosthetic limb prescription. During the global war on terror, prosthetists played a unique role in worldwide deployments. They provided strategic and operational knowledge to allied governments in the areas of prosthetic clinical education, clinical evaluation, and prosthetic fabrication techniques. The increasing complexity involved in prosthetics technology and the development of unique materials, computer programs, and fabrication techniques applicability require the specialized knowledge of the prosthetist. This chapter provided an overview of lower limb prosthetic technologies, ranging from classification of prosthetic feet, knee units, socket design, socket interfaces, and components to how these technologies related to the amputation levels of the lower limb. The prosthetic rehabilitation process used at military MTFs and the comorbidities affecting the rehabilitation prescription were also examined.

REFERENCES

1. Michael J. Energy storing feet: a clinical comparison. *Clin Prosthet Orthot.* 1987;11:154–168.

2. Gailey R. Functional value of prosthetic foot/ankle systems to the amputee. *J Prosthet Orthot.* 2005;17(4S):39–41.

3. Hafner BJ, Sanders JE, Czerniecki J, Fergason J. Energy storage and return prostheses: does patient perception correlate with biomechanical analysis? *Clin Biomech*. 2002;17:325–344.

4. Gard SA, Konz RJ. The effect of a shock-absorbing pylon on the gait of persons with unilateral transtibial amputation. *J Rehabil Res Dev*. 2003;40:109–124.

5. Greene M. Four bar knee linkage analysis. *Orthot Prosthet*. 1983;37:15–24.

6. Hafner BJ, Willingham LL, Buell NC, Allyn KJ, Smith DG. Evaluation of function, performance, and preference as transfemoral amputees transition from mechanical to microprocessor control of the prosthetic knee. *Arch Phys Med Rehabil*. 2007;88:207–217.

7. Flick KC, Orendurff MS, Berge JS, Segal AD, Klute GK. Comparison of human turning gait with the mechanical performance of lower limb prosthetic transverse rotation adapters. *Prosthet Orthot Int*. 2005;29:73-81.

8. Radcliffe C, Foort J. *The Patellar-Tendon-Bearing Below-Knee Prosthesis*. Berkeley, Calif: Biomechanics Laboratory, Department of Engineering, University of California; 1961.

9. Beil TL, Street GM. Comparison of interface pressures with pin and suction suspension systems. *J Rehabil Res Dev*. 2004;41:821–828.

10. Kahle J. Conventional and hydrostatic transfemoral interface comparison. *J Prosthet Orthot*. 1999;11:85–91.

11. Narita H, Yokogushi K, Shii S, Kakizawa M, Nosaka T. Suspension effect and dynamic evaluation of the total surface bearing (TSB) trans-tibial prosthesis: a comparison with the patellar tendon bearing (PTB) trans-tibial prosthesis. *Prosthet Orthot Int*. 1997;21:175–178.

12. Gard SA, Childress DS, Uellendahl JE. The influence of four-bar linkage knees on prosthetic swing-phase floor clearance. *J Prosthet Orthot*. 1996;8:34–40.

13. Radcliffe CW. Functional considerations in the fitting of above-knee prostheses. *Artif Limbs*. 1955;2;35–60.

14. Hoyt C, Littig D, Lundt J, Staats T. *The Ischial Containment Above-Knee Prosthesis: Course Manual*. 3rd ed. Version 1.3. Los Angeles, Calif: UCLA Prosthetics Education and Research Program; 1987.

15. Gottschalk F, Kourosh S, Stills M, McClellan B, Roberts J. Does socket configuration influence the position of the femur in above-knee amputation? *J Prosthet Orthot*. 1990;2:94–102.

16. Huang CT. Energy cost of ambulation with Canadian hip disarticulation prosthesis. *J Med Assoc State Ala*. 1983;52:47–48.

17. Littig DH, Lundt JE. The UCLA anatomical hip disarticulation prosthesis. *Clin Prosthet Orthot*. 1988;12:114–118.

18. Potter BK, Burns TC, Lacap AP, Granville RR, Gajewski DA. Heterotopic ossification following traumatic and combat-related amputations: prevalence, risk factors, and preliminary results of excision. *J Bone Joint Surg Am*. 2007;89:476–486.

Chapter 21

LOWER LIMB PROSTHETICS FOR SPORTS AND RECREATION

JOHN R. FERGASON, CPO[*]; AND PETER D. HARSCH, CP[†]

[*]Chief Prosthetist, Department of Orthopaedics and Rehabilitation, Brooke Army Medical Center, 3851 Roger Brooke Drive, Fort Sam Houston, Texas 78234
[†]Chief Prosthetist, C5 Combat Care Center Prosthetics, Naval Medical Center San Diego, 34800 Bob Wilson Drive, Building 3, San Diego, California 92134

INTRODUCTION

The value of sports and recreation continues to be a primary motivational factor for many service members with newly acquired lower limb amputations. Whether they were competitive prior to their amputations or not, they will become competitive to overcome their current physical limitations. The background and demographics of an active duty service member differ from the demographics of the majority of new civilian amputations that occur each year. Unlike the general population, every service member is preconditioned to train and work to pass mandatory physical fitness tests. Contrary to an elective amputation secondary to disease, trauma amputees have no time to prepare or process what it will be like to function with limb loss. They must be encouraged to challenge themselves to achieve new skills in activities that are unfamiliar to them that may be more appropriate to their new body, as well as continue to participate in their favorite sports. An informative survey conducted with disabled competitors in the 1996 Paralympic Games showed no mean differences in the results obtained in Goal Orientation, Competitiveness, and Desire-to-Win Scales when comparing men and women, onset of disability, adolescents and adults, and severity classifications.[1] This may suggest that the healthcare team does not have reliable predictors for who will excel; therefore, all competitors should be given the same opportunities. Participation in sports and recreation is universally beneficial not only for the demographic of an active duty service member, but also for the general population. Several publications[2–4] have made recommendations regarding the efficacy of regular physical activity to reduce disease concerns. Inactivity also increases the risk of many physical pathologies[5,6] and is the second most costly risk factor in cardiovascular disease.[7]

Physical activity has many specific benefits for the disabled population, including a decrease in self-reported stress, pain, and depression, as well as a general increase in the quality of life.[8] Participation in physical activity has shown a positive relationship with improved body image for many amputees.[9] For many active duty service members, the desire to continue in the Armed Forces is correlated to their physical ability to return to their previous military occupational specialty. Amputation of a lower limb does indeed constitute a major disability that can lead to functional and professional incapacities.[10] A commonly referenced survey (Kegel, 1985)[11] revealed that lower limb amputees had a strong interest in participating in sports and recreation. A majority of respondents indicated that their quality of life could be enhanced if the prosthesis did not limit their ability to move quickly and run.[11] A more recent survey showed that the 20- to 39-year-old age group had a similar distribution of interests between high-, moderate-, and low-energy-level activities; the survey reported a high ability to perform these activities while using a prosthesis.[12] This information suggests that the prosthesis is no longer the primary limiting factor when participating in desired activities. Given the opportunities for participation in sports that are currently offered to injured service members, the demand for new, innovative prosthetic designs is challenging the clinical and technical expertise of the prosthetist.

No artificial limb can replace what is lost in the trauma of conflict. However, aggressive rehabilitation and appropriate prosthetic provision will enhance the ability of injured individuals to pursue athletic activities once again. Understanding the biomechanics of the sport and the physical characteristics of the remnant limb are the first steps in determining what a prosthesis can provide. The following sections present principles involved in the design of prostheses suitable for sports and recreational activities.

WHEN TO PROVIDE A SPORTS-SPECIFIC PROSTHESIS

Because of the unique, comprehensive nature of military rehabilitation programs, high expectations are instituted early. Goal setting can be started by using the physical training fitness test as standard if the patient wants to remain on active duty. Encouragement from other patients with similar injuries can also be a significant motivating factor in the pursuit of recreational activity.

In addition, the general public has a heightened sense of awareness of the challenges involved in disabled sporting activities. Competition such as that seen in the Paralympic Games has gained wider exposure and has

demonstrated that high-activity goals are attainable. Although world-class athletes seen in the Paralympic Games are true inspirations, most individuals will not pursue this level of activity. Exposure to a variety of sporting activities is a more effective method to peak the interest of the injured and even to open up new possibilities for recreation or competition.

The prosthesis optimized for recreation is finely tuned both to the specific function required and to the capabilities of the user. Realistic goals should be set in context to the overall physical capabilities of the individual. It is more encouraging to reach a small goal

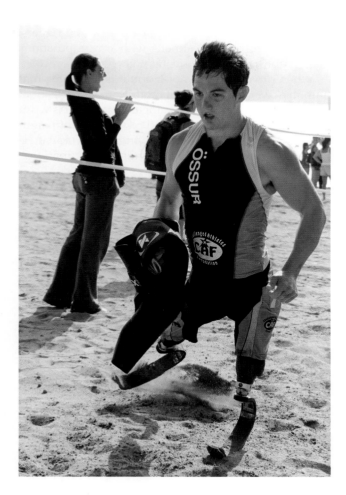

Figure 21-1. Exiting the water using short, nonarticulated prostheses provides stability and function during the triathlon transition.
Photograph: Courtesy of Terry Martin.

quickly and then set more ambitious goals as incremental steps are attained. During performance of the physical evaluation and patient history, two of the most important considerations include (1) the mechanism of amputation and (2) the physical factors associated with the injury (eg, if the patient has experienced prolonged bed rest, rehabilitation must begin with a focus on the deconditioned status). The polytrauma nature of military injury often complicates the intensity of the rehabilitation because the patient has not experienced any significant activity since the injury. For example, in patients with compromised skin and associated diminished sensation, excessive skin loading in early weight bearing can lead to ulcers and an interruption in the ability to progress in ambulation skill.

While weight-bearing capability is being established, a comprehensive program of physical rehabilitation should be in progress. In one study on physi-

cal fitness, amputee test subjects were significantly deconditioned when demographically matched to able-bodied subjects. After an endurance training program was completed, there was no significant difference from the able-bodied subjects, showing that individuals with limb loss are able to recover from a poorly conditioned state.[13] The patient must be educated to understand that the primary key to successful participation in sports is a combination of preparatory physical training and appropriate prosthetic design. The prosthesis is merely a tool that plays an increasingly important role in maximized performance once strength, stamina, and skill progress.

Depending on individual choice, patients can opt to participate in sports without a prosthesis. Swimming is one example of an activity in which use of a prosthesis is not always desired. The prosthesis can be used to reach the water and then removed on entry (Figure 21-1). In competition, the International Paralympic Committee

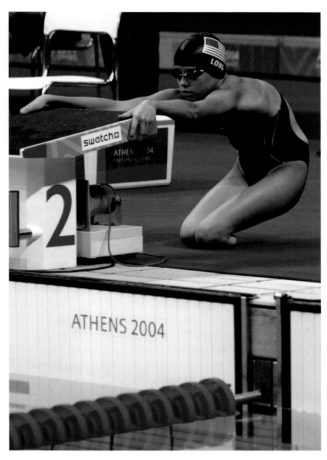

Figure 21-2. Bilateral transtibial amputee preparing for competition in the 2004 Paralympic Games.
Photograph: Courtesy of the US Paralympics, Colorado Springs, Colorado.

governs the use of assistive devices in the water. All prosthetics are removed prior to competition (Figure 21-2). The International Amputee Soccer Association requires that participants use bilateral forearm crutches with at least one amputated limb without a prosthesis. In these instances, it would be counterproductive for high-level competition to train with a prosthesis when it cannot be used in the competition. In contrast, the Paralympic alpine disciplines allow athletes with single

leg amputations to choose use of a single ski, outriggers, or prostheses; however, athletes with arm amputations usually compete without using poles.

When prostheses are not worn, it is advisable that amputees wear some form of protection on the residual limb. It can be as simple as using the liner that is worn with the prosthesis. If increased protection from high-impact falls is needed, a custom limb protector can be fabricated.

GENERAL-USE UTILITY PROSTHESIS

Although the residual limb is undergoing expected shape and volume changes, it is important to consider using the prosthesis for as many activities as possible. In most instances, prostheses that allow the amputee to participate in a wide range of activity, including selected sports, can be designed. Current options—such as elastomeric gel liners that provide socket comfort and skin protection—required during everyday ambulation can suffice for many recreational activities. Careful choice of the prosthetic foot allows the amputee to walk faster and achieve a more equal step length on both sides, thus facilitating recreation and routine walking.[14] The foot that has been aligned for comfort and efficiency during walking can still function adequately for intermittent, moderate bouts of higher activity. Although it has been shown that amputees find it difficult to accurately report their ac-

tivity level versus measured activity level, the clinician does not have to rush into sports-specific limbs during the early stages of rehabilitation.[15] Once the amputee commits to participation and training for a particular sport, a specific prosthesis or component may be necessary. When a single use prosthesis is provided, the optimized design facilitates full and potentially competitive participation in the desired activity.

Another approach is to utilize the current daily use socket with additional foot and/or knee combinations. The socket can be coupled with interchangeable distal components that have been selected to facilitate different tasks. A quick-release coupler can be provided to permit interchanging knee and foot/ankle components. This alternative, when appropriate, can be more time- and cost-effective than multiple individual prostheses.

SKIN TOLERANCE TO HIGH ACTIVITY

Identification of the functional demands the activity will place on the residual limb will help determine the design of the prosthetic socket. A prosthesis cannot fully replace complexities of the human leg, such as providing dynamic shock absorption, adaptation to uneven terrain, torque conversion, knee stabilization, limb lengthening and shortening to diminish the arc of the center of gravity, transfer of weight-bearing forces, and reliable weight-bearing support.[16] The significant difference in the activity is the nature and amount of impact and shear that will be placed on the residual limb. Long-term monitoring of ambulatory activity has indicated that our assumptions about the definition of high-activity level may not be correct.[17] Some sports (eg, running) require quick movement and many steps for a limited amount of time, whereas other sports (eg, golf) require many more steps over a period of several hours. The sports of running and golf could be considered high-activity levels, although with different durations. Understanding the functional demands is even more important. The runner's prosthesis must absorb the impact of loading response, support body weight

through midstance to allow a long stride length on the sound side, and provide a measure of propulsive thrust at the end of stance. The golfer using a prosthesis endures long time periods of standing; maintains overall stability when twisting during swings; and ambulates safely over uneven terrain, slopes, and inclines.

Once the demands of the activity are understood, a careful evaluation will identify the weight-tolerant regions, as well as the skin sensitivity of the limb. A simple 10-g monofilament used to test foot sensation can be used to identify regions of the limb that lack protective sensation. This information should be relayed to the patient so that the individual has a full understanding of the importance of periodic visual skin evaluation during at-risk activity.

The greater the shear forces generated with a prosthesis, the lower the pressure required to cause tissue breakdown.[18] The cyclic shear stress that inevitably occurs within a prosthetic socket can cause a blister to form within the epidermis or can create an abrasion on the skin surface. When there is adherent scar tissue present, which is common following traumatic amputations, shear stress adjacent to the area results in skin tension that can cause blanching or even cell rupture.[19] Investigation of an instrumented patella tendon-bearing prosthetic socket demonstrated that maximal pressure and resultant shear stresses shifted locations between the loading phase of stance and the latter phases of the gait cycle.[20] This is a result of the dynamic movement of the residual limb within the socket. The planar force coupling that results in these measurement differences will be increased as directional activity changes with variations in movement of the prosthesis during sports.

As the individual's activity level increases, the pressure and shear forces can easily rise to levels that cause soft-tissue damage. An increase in activity can also be associated with a rise in the incidence of skin problems.[21] Common skin problems associated with prosthetic use include ulcers, irritations, inclusion cysts, calluses, contact dermatitis, hyperhidrosis, and infections.[22,23] When these complications occur, medical management and prosthetic adjustments are often necessary. Controlled prosthetic use while treating ulcerations, for example, can still allow the patient to be ambulatory and the ulcer to heal satisfactorily.[22]

GENERAL ALIGNMENT CONSIDERATIONS FOR SPORTS

Several studies demonstrate that alignment is not as critical as volume change in affecting skin stress on the residual limb.[24–26] In the context of this evidence, it still remains a critical aspect of optimal sports performance. Alignment of the socket and shank of a lower limb prosthesis critically affects the comfort and dynamic performance of the person it supports by altering the manner in which the weight-bearing load is transferred between the supporting foot and the residual limb. Furthermore, alignment of the lower extremity prosthesis for sports activities may

be significantly different than what is optimal for other activities of daily living. Water and snow skiing are good examples of sports requiring increased ankle dorsiflexion. However, when the prosthesis is optimally aligned for these sports, it will not function well for general ambulation (Figure 21-3). In these instances, either a special-use prosthesis or interchangeable components will be necessary. If the user intends to interchange components, education must be instituted carefully to protect the limb from misalignment.

GENERAL COMPONENT CHOICES FOR FORCE REDUCTION IN SPORTS

When the multidirectional forces that give rise to pressure and shear stresses are expected to increase because of athletic activity, a socket liner made from an elastomeric gel is often recommended. Patients with conditions such as skin grafts or adherent scars will have a reduced tolerance for shear.[27] For transfemoral limbs, special consideration should be given to the ischial tuberosity area and the proximal tissue along the socket brim. Patient comfort can be increased by the use of a flexible plastic inner socket supported by a rigid external frame. This combination maintains the structural weight supporting the integrity of the socket while increasing the range of hip motion from the flexibility of the proximal socket.

The heels of prosthetic feet can dissipate significant amounts of energy during loading.[28] Feet were shown to be capable of dissipating up to 63% of the input energy. Once a running shoe was added, the dissipation capacity increased to 73%. Even with the encouraging capability of the foot to absorb energy, once it has reached its limit, the forces are transferred to the socket and then ultimately the limb. Shock-absorbing pylons can be added between the socket and foot if additional impact reduction is desired. They may be an independent component or part of a foot/ankle/

shin integrated system. Some shock-absorbing pylon systems are pneumatic and easily adjusted by the user; other systems must be adjusted by the prosthetist to provide the optimal amount of vertical travel. The addition of a shock-absorbing pylon may show few

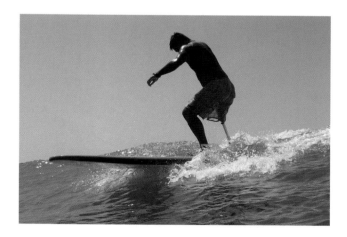

Figure 21-3. Upright control while surfing is enhanced when using straight pylons on the transfemoral prosthesis. Photograph: Courtesy of Joseph Gabunilas.

quantitative kinetic or kinematic advantages in how someone walks, but pylons do show a force reduction during loading response and a report of increased comfort, particularly at higher speeds.[29,30] It is important to consider that, when negotiating stair and step descent, the transfemoral amputee may gain added effect from an energy-absorbing pylon because of the increased lower extremity stiffness secondary to a lack of shock-absorbing knee flexion of a mechanical knee.

A prosthetic torque absorber component can be provided that will allow up to a 40-degree range of internal and external rotation between the socket and foot. Although multiaxial ankles offer some rotational movement, a separate torque-absorbing component performs this most effectively. There are many torque-absorber options commercially available, but none can effectively match or be adjusted to the asymmetrical internal and external torque seen in able-bodied individuals.[31] Given the importance of minimizing transverse plane shear stress on vulnerable soft tissue, this component should still be considered even though it can match exactly to characteristics of the sound side.

Hafner et al[32] suggest that the development and recommendation of prosthetic feet without supporting evidence of their performance may be the result of conflicting or inconclusive results in the reported literature. There is a missing link between the scientific evidence and clinical experience of the medical providers. Although subtle changes in gait and performance parameters are not statistically significant, these differences are perceived by amputees to affect their preferences and perception of foot performance. Later studies do suggest that variations in prescription may allow for benefits such as greater propulsive impulses by the residual leg that contribute to limb symmetry.[33,34]

TRANSTIBIAL RUNNING

Prior to performing running activities, it is helpful to understand the running goals of the service member. If the primary desire of the individual is to jog for cardio-vascular endurance, a slow jog occurs at about 140 m/min. At this speed, the heel has minimal effect because the middle portion of the foot becomes the primary initial contact point. Because the heel is minimally used or virtually eliminated as speeds increase to approximately 180 m/min in running, a specific running foot without a heel component may be advantageous (Figure 21-4).[35] Prosthetic limb kinematics have been shown to mimic this able-bodied data.[36] The running foot is very light and highly responsive. There is a significant amount of deflection on weight bearing that adds to the shock-absorbing qualities. A running shoe tread is adhered to the plantar surface to further reduce weight. If a

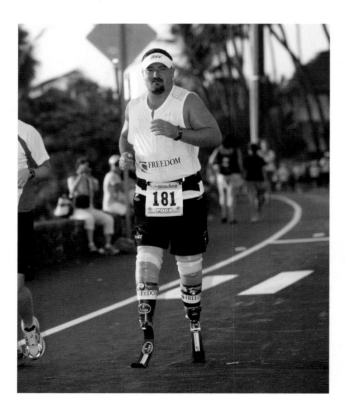

Figure 21-4. Running-specific foot modules are used to mimic natural running biomechanics.
Photograph: Reproduced with permission from ASI PHOTOS, Fort Worth, Texas.

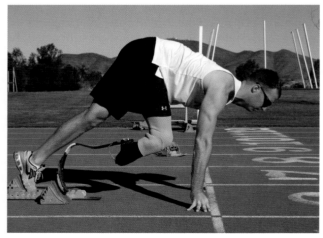

Figure 21-5. Track-and-field sprint-specific feet are used for quick acceleration and high cadence speed.
Photograph: Courtesy of Peter Harsch.

decrease in speed occurs (eg, when jogging with intermittent walking), the heel will become more important and a more versatile utility foot should be chosen. If the amputee desires to sprint and short bursts of speed are the goal, a sprint-specific foot should be considered (Figure 21-5). In general, the sprint foot is designed with a much longer shank that attaches to the posterior of the socket. This gives a longer lever arm for increased energy storage and return. For sprinting, the socket/limb interface should be a more intimate fitting that will maximize the transfer of motion from the limb to the socket. As with any running, use of gel liner interfaces is recommended. Choosing a thinner, 3-mm-thickness liner will reduce the motion of the tibia in the socket. If jogging, the liner should be 6-mm thickness or 9-mm thickness to maximize the shock-absorbing capabilities over a longer duration of the activity. Because suspension is a key factor in movement and shear reduction on the limb, an airtight sleeve and expulsion valve can give the best limb stability.[37]

TRANSFEMORAL RUNNING

Design of a transfemoral running limb follows the same guidelines as previously discussed for the transtibial running limb. Component choices are based on defining the goal of jogging and sprinting. Foot choices and use criteria are identical for both transtibial and transfemoral limbs. The next decision involves whether to incorporate a knee or begin with a nonarticulated limb. Beginning without a knee is

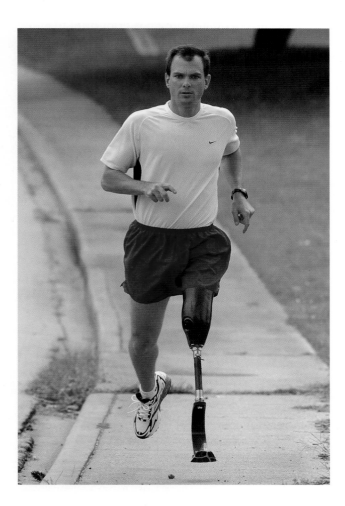

Figure 21-6. Transfemoral runners can use a nonarticulating limb with a circumducted gait to increase stance stability and energy efficiency.
Photograph: Courtesy of Thomas F. Martin, Jr, and Anderson Independent-Mail, Anderson, South Carolina.

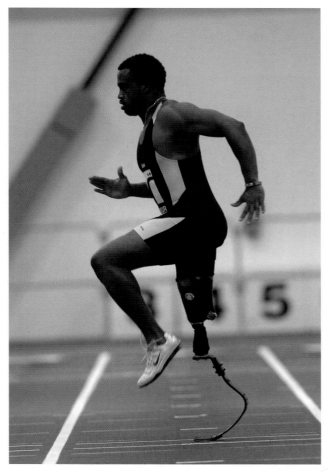

Figure 21-7. Transfemoral runner exhibiting a knee flexion running gait using a hydraulic single axis knee, sprint foot, and 20-degree angle bracket.
Photograph: Courtesy of Prosthetic Innovations LLC, Eddystone, Pennsylvania.

a viable option when stability is a concern or when suitable cardiovascular endurance has not yet been attained. Training begins with a circumducted gait to allow foot clearance in swing. If a patient intends to participate in distance running, a nonarticulated system eliminates the mental concern of inadvertent knee flexion and seems to be significantly less demanding for a longer run (Figure 21-6). When sprinting is the goal, use of a knee is generally recommended. There are several good choices available that use hydraulic control of flexion and extension resistance and that

interface well with the sprint feet (Figure 21-7). The knees and overall alignment must be fine-tuned to the individual needs of the patient. Interlimb asymmetry has been shown to increase significantly when the transfemoral amputee runs. Therefore, special attention to alignment, component adjustments, and training is particularly important.[36,38] Maximum sports performance may require modified or even specialized components or significant deviations from standard alignment techniques to help improve interlimb symmetry and running velocity.[39]

CYCLING

Cycling is an excellent exercise that is nonweight bearing and indicated for those who may have closed-chain impact restrictions. Once proper fitting of the bicycle has been completed, the prosthesis will need some accommodations if more than recreational cycling is intended (Figure 21-8). For the transtibial amputee, knee flexion restriction must be minimized. Suspension systems that cross the knee, such as suction with

gel sleeves, can be replaced with distal pin-and-lock options. If the sleeve is still preferred by the patient, choosing one that is preflexed and just tight enough to maintain a suction seal is adequate. The posterior socket brim is typically restrictive in full knee flexion. Providing an adequately low posterior brim to allow full knee flexion often will not comfortably support the limb during ambulation. This can be overcome by

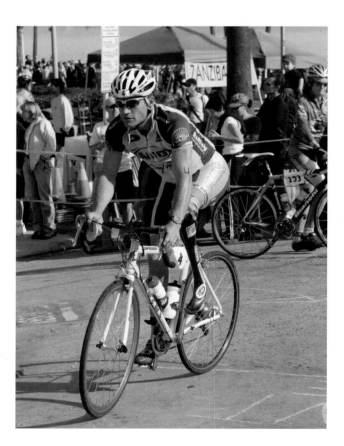

Figure 21-8. Paralympic cyclist with a direct attached carbon fiber foot and shin system to enhance aerodynamic efficiency. Photograph: Reproduced with permission from Brightroom, Inc, Fort Worth, Texas.

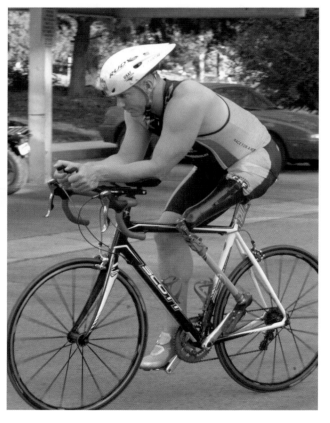

Figure 21-9. Transfemoral amputee exhibiting free swing from a seven axis knee with a direct attached carbon foot system.
Photograph: Courtesy of Coyote Design, Boise, Idaho.

designing a posterior brim that is removable for biking and replaced for ambulation.

The transfemoral amputee must be provided adequate clearance between the ischial tuberosity and the cycle seat. Careful socket adjustments in this region can usually provide a limb that is comfortable for limited ambulation and extended seat time (Figure 21-9). The knee choice will be based on the type of cycling that is intended. Typically, a knee that allows free motion on the bike will be easier to use. Choosing a knee component that is safe to walk on in a free swing mode will be helpful. For both levels of amputation,

the foot stiffness can be increased to ensure maximum transfer of energy to the pedal. This will leave the foot excessively stiff for comfortable ambulation, but more efficient for cycling. The sole of the biking shoe can be removed and attached directly to the prosthetic foot if additional weight and control are needed. Unilateral transtibial amputee cyclists have been shown to exhibit more pedaling asymmetry than the able-bodied population. This may be also related to foot stiffness, but was not shown to be statistically significant in preliminary data (Childers WL, Kistenberg RS, Gregor RJ, unpublished data, 2007).

ROCK CLIMBING

Rock climbing has increased in popularity in the past years. No longer does one have to travel to the natural outdoors to enjoy the exhilaration of this experience. Local indoor and outdoor climbing systems are available in many locales. Commercially produced prosthetic feet are unsuitable for rock climbing because the toe must be rigid enough to support the full body weight when only that portion of the prosthesis is in contact with the rock face (Figure 21-10). The foot should be shortened to decrease the torque and rotation that occur with a longer lever arm. The shape of the foot should be contoured to

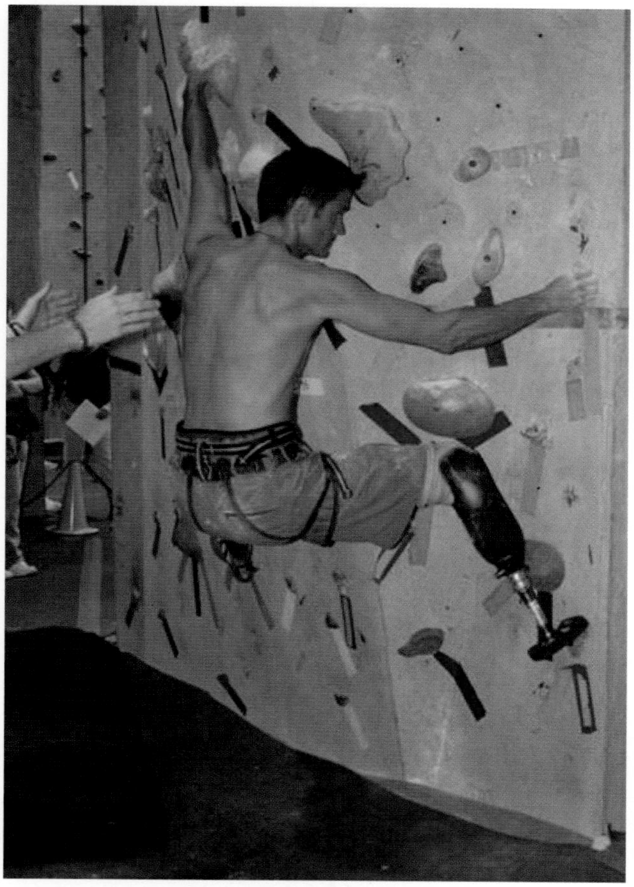

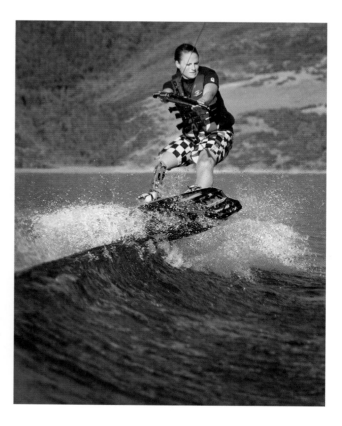

Figure 21-10. Custom foot module with spikes and Kevlar (Du Pont de Nemours and Company, Wilmington, Delaware) is used to increase traction while scaling an indoor rock-climbing wall.
Photograph: Courtesy of College Park Industries, Fraser, Michigan.

Figure 21-11. Wake boarding is made possible with sports-specific knees that provide stability with flexion- and extension-assisted support.
Photograph: Courtesy of Ed Rosenberger.

take advantage of small cracks, crevices, and contours of the climbing surface. Once an acceptable shape has been obtained, completely covering the foot with the soling from climbing shoes will give the texture needed

for optimum performance. Making the prosthesis easily height adjustable allows the user to optimize limb length for different types of climbs. If no prosthesis is used, limb protection should be provided.

<h2 style="text-align:center">WATER SPORTS</h2>

After running sports, water sports are the next most popular activities. Depending on geographical location, water sports may be more or less a part of the culture. Most prostheses will tolerate occasional and nominal exposure to moisture, particularly when protected under a layer of clothing. The everyday prosthesis should be made resistant to splashes that occasionally occur,

especially when living in a wet climate. A specialized, waterproof design is necessary when the amputee will have regular exposure to salt water or freshwater, especially if complete immersion is intended (Figure 21-11). For the bilateral transfemoral patient, prosthetic devices are usually bypassed in favor of specialty seating systems that allow participation at the highest levels.[40]

<h2 style="text-align:center">WINTER SPORTS</h2>

The amputee interested in winter sports currently has an unprecedented opportunity for participation. For those interested in downhill skiing, most individuals with unilateral transtibial amputation continue to use a prosthesis (Figure 21-12). Although a walking limb can be adapted and used, a ski-specific alignment should be performed for the duration of the activity. Additional foot dorsiflexion and external knee support should be added. For advanced users, specialty feet that eliminate the boot are available. The plantar surface of the ski foot is modeled after the

boot sole and will attach directly to the ski bindings, thus eliminating the boot altogether. This eliminates excess weight, but, more importantly, enhances energy transfer to the sporting equipment for more efficient performance. Unilateral transfemoral skiers will usually opt to use a single ski with bilateral forearm outriggers (Figure 21-13). The immense popularity of snowboarding has accelerated developmental designs for the transfemoral amputee. A recently released knee has been designed specifically for sports that require a loaded, flexed knee position. Snowboarders are in bilateral dynamic hip, knee, and ankle flexion as they negotiate the hill (Figure 21-14). This knee is adjustable and produces the weighted knee flexion necessary to snowboard successfully. The transtibial snowboarder needs additional dorsiflexion range and flexibility in the prosthetic foot.

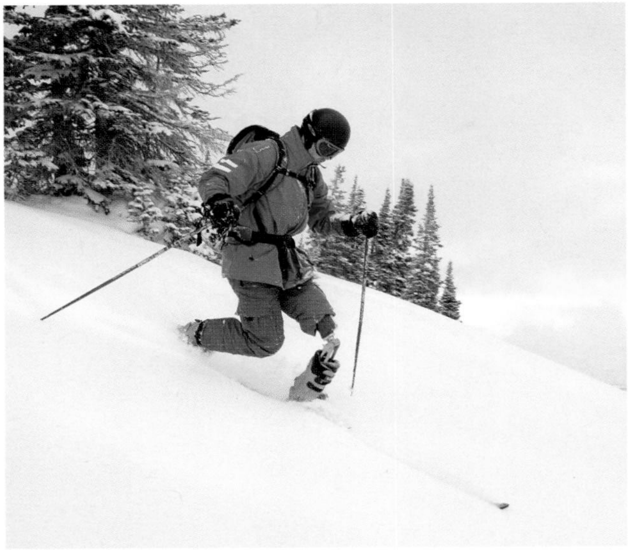

Figure 21-12. Advanced dynamic sport knee builds energy during flexion and returns energy in extension to provide superior control for the transfemoral skier. Photograph: Courtesy of SymbioTechs, USA LLC, Amity, Oregon.

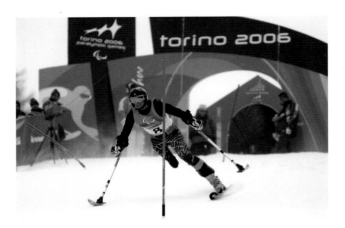

Figure 21-13. Adaptive ski poles for the downhill skier replaces the need for a sports-specific prosthesis. Photograph: Courtesy of Byron Hetzler.

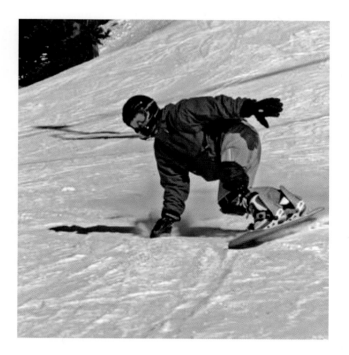

Figure 21-14. No additional adaptive gear is necessary for this transfemoral snowboarder when using this energy-storing prosthetic knee.
Photograph: Courtesy of Symbiotechs, USA LLC, Amity, Oregon.

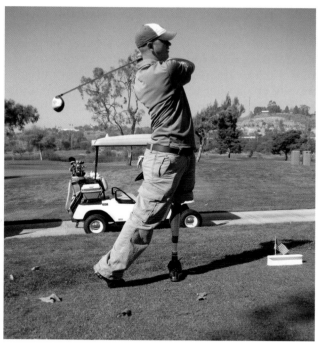

Figure 21-15. Torsion control systems allow for proper swing mechanics for the amputee golfer.
Photograph: Courtesy of Michael Pack, Artificial Limb Specialists, Phoenix, Arizona.

GOLF

The longevity of potential participation in this sport may be a major factor in its popularity. Golf is a sport that can be entered into when one is quite young and often followed throughout a lifetime. A correct golf swing requires triplanar movements at the ankle, hip, and shoulder joints. Because prosthetic feet cannot duplicate the three-dimensional movement of the ankle, torque absorbers or rotational adapters can be introduced (Figure 21-15). Amputee golfers report that these components can help them achieve a smooth swing and follow-through, and can reduce the uncomfortable rotational shear that would otherwise occur between the skin of the residual limb and the socket. Studies have confirmed this fact and show improved hip and shoulder rotations, particularly in the left-sided amputee.[41,42]

HIKING

Activity that includes traversing uneven terrain (eg, hiking) requires consideration of a multiaxial ankle. This type of ankle allows the prosthetic foot to conform to irregular surfaces, thus reducing the forces transferred to the residual limb.

As the amputee enters midstance on the prosthesis, the foot should accommodate uneven terrain and help control advancement of the tibia. If tibial advancement is too abrupt, the amputee will resist this knee flexion moment, increasing the forces on the residual limb within the socket. When aligning and adjusting a new prosthesis, the amputee should be evaluated on surfaces similar to those that will be encountered in the athletic activity limb. Perhaps even more significant than multiaxial feet and torque absorbers is the recent release of a motorized ankle. This type of ankle does not generate propulsive power, but rather senses electronically when the user is on an incline or decline. The ankle requires two strides to sense the orientation, then it will consequently plantarflex or dorsiflex the foot to ease the moments that are induced on the knee and the forces that act on the residual limb.

INJURIES AND LONG-TERM EFFECTS

With this focus on sports as an aspect of rehabilitation for the limb amputee comes an inherent increased risk of injury. Injuries for the disabled sporting community are similar to those for athletes without disabilities. Locations of the injury seem to be sports- and disability-dependent. Ambulatory amputee athletes more commonly have lower extremity injuries (eg, abrasions, strains, sprains, and contusions).[43] Spine and intact limb injuries are also common to the amputee.[44] Additional attention must be focused on the issue of depressive symptoms that are seen so commonly in conflict amputations. A correlation has been noted between depression and prediction of pain intensity and bothersomeness.[45] Amputees have also been shown to suffer from various comorbidities associated with biomechanical abnormalities.[46–49]

OTHER CONSIDERATIONS

Prescribing component recommendations that facilitate higher activities is typically based on the experience of the prosthetist primarily because of the lack of conclusive scientific evidence on these applications.[18] It is useful to clearly understand the functional and biomechanical demands of a specific sport when forming a prescription recommendation so that the functional characteristics of the components match these criteria. Participation in most sports can be facilitated by adaptations of conventional socket designs combined with commercially available components, but some activities are best accomplished with unique custom-designed components.

SUMMARY

The needs and preferences of the amputee should be clearly understood, and the functional demands of the activity should be determined prior to generating the prescription. Physical training status should be evaluated before intensive participation, particularly in sports unfamiliar to the participant. Early in the rehabilitation process, the prosthesis can usually be adapted to the activity and still be used effectively in therapy. As the amputee progresses and the demands of participation increase, a specialized prosthesis can be provided. A properly designed prosthesis can substantially expand the opportunities for participation in sports and augment the overall goals of the rehabilitation plan for each patient.

REFERENCES

1. Page SJ. Exploring competitive orientation in a group of athletes participating in the 1996 Paralympic trials. *Percept Mot Skills.* 2000;91:491–502.

2. Pasquena PF. National Disabled Veterans Winter Sports Clinic. *J Rehabil Res Dev.* 2006;43:xi–xv.

3. US Public Health Service, US Department of Health and Human Services. *Healthy People 2000: National Health Promotion and Disease Prevention Objectives.* Washington, DC: DHHS; 1991. DHHS Pub No. PHS 91-50212.

4. US Public Health Service, NIH Consensus Development Panel on Physical Activity and Cardiovascular Health. Physical activity and cardiovascular health. *JAMA.* 1996:276:241–246.

5. Kochersberger G, McConnell E, Kuchibhatla MN, Pieper C. The reliability, validity, and stability of a measure of physical activity in the elderly. *Arch Phys Med Rehabil.* 1996;77:793–795.

6. US Public Health Service, US Department of Health and Human Services. *Physical Activity and Health: A Report of the Surgeon General.* Atlanta, Ga: US Department of Health and Human Services, Centers for Disease Control and Prevention, National Center for Chronic Disease Prevention and Health Promotion, The President's Council on Physical Fitness and Sports; 1996.

7. Hahn RA, Teutsch SM, Rothenberg RB, Marks JS. Excess deaths from nine chronic diseases in the United States, 1986. *JAMA.* 1990;264:2654–2659.

8. Hicks AL, Martin KA, Ditor DS, et al. Long-term exercise training in persons with spinal cord injury: effects on strength, arm ergometry performance and psychological well-being. *Spinal Cord.* 2003;41:34–43.

9. Wettenhahn KA, Hanson C, Levy CE. Effect of participation in physical activity on body image of amputees. *Am J Phys Med Rehabil.* 2002;81:194–201.

10. Mezghani-Masmoudi M, Guermazi M, Feki H, Ennaouai A, Dammak J, Elleuch MH. The functional and professional future of lower limb amputees with prosthesis. *Ann Readapt Med Phys.* 2004;47:114–118.

11. Kegel B. Physical fitness: sports and recreation for those with lower limb amputation or impairment. *J Rehabil Res Dev Clin Suppl.* 1985;1:1–125.

12. Legro MW, Reiber GE, Czerniecki JM, Sangeorzan BJ. Recreational activities of lower-limb amputees with prostheses. *J Rehabil Res Dev.* 2001;38:319–325.

13. Chin T, Sawamura S, Fujita H, et al. Physical fitness of lower limb amputees. *Am J Phys Med Rehabil.* 2002;81:321–325.

14. Mizuno N, Aoyama T, Nakajima A, Kasahara T, Takami K. Functional evaluation by gait analysis of various ankle-foot assemblies used by below-knee amputees. *Prosthet Orthot Int.* 1992;16:174–182.

15. Stepien JM, Cavenett S, Taylor L, Crotty M. Activity levels among lower-limb amputees: self-report versus step activity monitor. *Arch Phys Med Rehabil.* 2007;88:896–900.

16. Donatelli R. *The Biomechanics of the Foot and Ankle.* Philadelphia: F. A. Davis Company; 1990: 9–27.

17. Coleman KL, Smith DG, Boone DA, Joseph AW, del Aguila MA. Step activity monitor: long-term, continuous recording of ambulatory function. *J Rehabil Res Dev.* 1999;36:8–18.

18. Bennet L, Kavner D, Lee BK, Trainor FA. Shear vs pressure as causative factors in skin blood flow occlusion. *Arch Phys Med Rehabil.* 1979;60:309–314.

19. Sanders JE, Daly CH, Burgess EM. Interface shear stresses during ambulation with a below-knee prosthetic limb. *J Rehabil Res Dev.* 1992;29:1–8.

20. Sanders JE, Lam D, Dralle AJ, Okumura R. Interface pressures and shear stresses at thirteen socket sites on two persons with transtibial amputation. *J Rehabil Res Dev.* 1997;34:19–33.

21. Dudek NL, Marks MB, Marshall SC. Skin problems in an amputee clinic. *Am J Phys Med Rehabil.* 2006;85:424–429.

22. Salawu A, Middleton C, Gilbertson A, Kodavali K, Neumann V. Stump ulcers and continued prosthetic limb use. *Prosthet Orthot Int.* 2006;30:279–285.

23. Meulenbelt HE, Geertzen JH, Dijkstra PU, Jonkman MF. Skin problems in lower limb amputees: an overview by case reports. *J Eur Acad Dermatol Venereol.* 2007;21:147–155.

24. Sanders JE, Zachariah SG, Baker AB, Greve JM, Clinton C. Effects of changes in cadence, prosthetic componentry, and time on interface pressures and shear stresses of three trans-tibial amputees. *Clin Biomech.* 2000;15:684–694.

25. Sanders JE, Zachariah SG, Jacobsen AK, Fergason JR. Changes in interface pressures and shear stresses over time on trans-tibial amputee subjects ambulating with prosthetic limbs: comparison of diurnal and six-month differences. *J Biomech.* 2005;38:1566–1573.

26. Sanders JE, Jacobsen AK, Fergason JR. Effects of fluid insert volume changes on socket pressures and shear stresses: case studies from two trans-tibial amputee subjects. *Prosthet Orthot Int.* 2006;30:257–269.

27. Sanders JE, Nicholson BS, Zachariah SG, Cassisi DV, Karchin A, Fergason JR. Testing of elastomeric liners used in limb prosthetics: classification of 15 products by mechanical performance. *J Rehabil Res Dev.* 2004;41:175–186.

28. Klute GK, Berge JS, Segal AD. Heel-region properties of prosthetic feet and shoes. *J Rehabil Res Dev.* 2004;41:535–546.

29. Gard SA, Konz RJ. The effect of a shock-absorbing pylon on the gait of persons with unilateral transtibial amputation. *J Rehabil Res Dev.* 2003;40:109–124.

30. Berge JS, Czerniecki JM, Klute GK. Efficacy of shock-absorbing versus rigid pylons for impact reduction in transtibial amputees based on laboratory, field, and outcome metrics. *J Rehabil Res Dev.* 2005;42:795–808.

31. Flick KC, Orendurff MS, Berge JS, Segal AD, Klute GK. Comparison of human turning gait with the mechanical performance of lower limb prosthetics transverse rotation adapters. *Prosthet Orthot Int.* 2005;29:73–81.

32. Hafner BJ, Sanders JE, Czerniecki J, Fergason J. Energy storage and return prostheses: does patient perception correlate with biomechanical analysis? *Clin Biomech.* 2002;17:325–344.

33. Graham LE, Datta D, Heller B, Howitt J, Pros D. A comparative study of conventional and energy-storing prosthetic feet in high-functioning transfemoral amputees. *Arch Phys Med Rehabil.* 2007;88:801–806.

34. Zmitrewicz RJ, Neptune RR, Walden JG, Rogers WE, Bosker GW. The effect of foot and ankle prosthetic components on braking and propulsive impulses during transtibial amputee gait. *Arch Phys Med Rehabil.* 2006;87:1334–1339.

35. Lehmann JF, Price R, Fergason J, Okumura R, Koon G. Effect of prosthesis resonant frequency on metabolic efficiency in transtibial amputees: a study in progress (abstract 035). *Rehabilitation R&D Progress Reports.* 1999.

36. Buckley JG. Sprint kinematics of athletes with lower limb amputations. *Arch Phys Med Rehabil.* 1999;80:501–508.

37. Soderberg B, Ryd L, Persson BM. Roentgen stereophotogrammetric analysis of motion between the bone and the socket in a transtibial amputation prosthesis: a case study. *J Prosthet Orthot.* 2003;15:95–99.

38. Burkett B, Smeathers J, Barker T. Walking and running inter-limb symmetry for paralympic trans-femoral amputees, a biomechanical analysis. *Prosthet Orthot Int.* 2003;27:36–47.

39. Burkett B, Smeathers J, Barker T. Optimising the trans-femoral prosthetic alignment for running, by lowering the knee joint. *Prosthet Orthot Int.* 2001;25:210–219.

40. Buckley M, Heath G. Design and manufacture of a high performance water-ski seating system for use by an individual with bilateral trans-femoral amputations. *Prosthet Orthot Int.* 1995;19:120–123.

41. Nair A, Heffy D, Rose D, Hanspal RS. Use of two torque absorbers in a trans-femoral prosthesis of an amputee golfer. *Prosthet Orthot Int.* 2004;28:190–191.

42. Rogers JP, Strike SC, Wallace ES. The effect of prosthetic torsional stiffness on the golf swing kinematics of a left and a right-sided trans-tibial amputee. *Prosthet Orthot Int.* 2004;28:121–131.

43. Ferrara MS, Peterson CL. Injuries to athletes with disabilities: identifying injury patterns. *Sports Med.* 2000;30:137–143.

44. Klenek C, Gebke K. Practical management: common medical problems in disabled athletes. *Clin J Sport Med.* 1999;17:55–60.

45. Ephraim PL, Wegener ST, MacKenzie EJ, Dillingham TR, Pezzin Le. Phantom pain, residual limb pain, and back pain in amputees: results of a national survey. *Arch Phys Med Rehabil.* 2006;86:1910–1919.

46. Royer T, Koenig M. Joint loading and bone mineral density in persons with unilateral, trans-tibial amputation. *Clin Biomech.* 2005;20:1119–1125.

47. Rabuffetti M, Recalcati M, Ferrarin M. Trans-femoral amputee gait: socket-pelvis constraints and compensation strategies. *Prosthet Orthot Int.* 2005;29:183–192.

48. Kulkarni J, Adams J, Thomas E, Silman A. Association between amputation, arthritis and osteopenia in British male war veterans with major limb amputations. *Clin Rehabil.* 1998;12:348–353.

49. Norvell DC, Czerniecki JM, Reiber GE, Maynard C, Pecoraro JA, Weiss NS. The prevalence of knee pain and symptomatic knee osteoarthritis among veteran traumatic amputees and nonamputees. *Arch Phys Med Rehabil*. 2005;86:487–493.

Chapter 22

UPPER LIMB AMPUTATION AND PROSTHETICS EPIDEMIOLOGY, EVIDENCE, AND OUTCOMES

SANDRA L. HUBBARD WINKLER, PhD[*]

[*]*Research Health Scientist, Rehabilitation Outcome Research Center Research Enhancement Award Program, Malcolm Randall VA Medical Center, 1601 SW Archer Road, 151-B, Gainesville, Florida 32608, and Assistant Professor, Department of Occupational Therapy, University of Florida, College of Public Health and Health Professions, PO Box 100164, Gainesville, Florida 32610; formerly, Research Associate, Predoctoral Fellow, Department of Rehabilitation Science and Technology, University of Pittsburgh, 5044 Forbes Tower, Pittsburgh, Pennsylvania*

INTRODUCTION

The hand has been described as the most individual and personal part of the human being.[1] However, in the civilian sector, research, funding, and access to specialized care for upper limb amputees have been overshadowed by the substantial increase in lower limb amputation because of dysvascular disease.[2–5] The prosthetic and rehabilitation needs of injured service members from Operation Enduring Freedom and Operation Iraqi Freedom have brought upper limb amputation to the forefront of current debate and attention. As of July 2008, over 800 individuals have sustained major limb amputations as a result of military operations in Iraq and Afghanistan, 20% of which were upper limb amputations. At the same time, an unprecedented number of upper limb amputees are returning to active duty military service.[6] This has led to a resurgence of research to improve the lives of individuals with upper limb loss both in the civilian and military communities.

Relying on the prevalence of upper limb amputation in the general US population to plan rehabilitation for all upper limb amputees is problematic for three reasons. First, most amputation epidemiological research in the general population has been funded by diabetes research dollars, and thus focuses on dysvascular-disease–related (and primarily lower limb) amputations. Second, results vary depending whether amputees, amputations, or amputation-related hospitalizations are counted.[7] Finally, most disability survey data are more than 10 years old. "Prevalence" is determined by the number of people living with amputations and looks at how many people are affected, and most estimates of amputation prevalence are derived from the 1996 National Health Interview Survey–Disability (NHIS-D).[8] "Incidence" refers to the number of new cases, usually per year, per population at risk. Sources of incidence data include community hospital and hospital emergency room discharge data and employment-related data. When interpreting incidence data, it is important to consider whether amputations or amputees are being counted and to identify the population at risk. For example, incidence rates of lower limb amputation for a population of individuals with dysvascular disease will be different than incidence rates for the US population. Frequently, statistical techniques are used to standardize the incidence rates to the US population by age, sex, and geographical region.[9]

Prevalence

According to analyses of the NHIS-D, there are 1.2 to 1.9 million people in the United States living with limb loss (data excludes finger tip and toe amputations), or about one in every 200 people. The 1.2 million figure was derived from analyses of 1996 NHIS-D data,[10] and the 1.9 million figure is a 2005 estimate based on 1996 NHIS-D data and US population growth.[8,11] One limitation of 1996 NHIS-D data is that only amputees are counted; the numbers of amputations were not considered. Also, upper and lower limb amputees were not distinguished from one another. Thus, the prevalence of upper limb amputation cannot be found in NHIS-D data. A third limitation of 1996 NHIS-D limb loss data is that fingers and toes are excluded from the count; though loss of a finger or toe may not be as disabling as loss of a limb, amputation of a finger can be more expensive than amputation of a limb (paid for by workers compensation funds).[12]

Incidence

According to a report published online by the Limb Loss Research and Statistics Program, a collaboration between the Johns Hopkins Bloomberg School of Public Health and the Amputation Coalition of America, 185,000 Americans undergo amputation each year.[13] Using community hospital discharge data from the Healthcare Cost and Utilization Project, Nationwide Inpatient Sample, Dillingham et al identified 1,199,111 hospital discharges that involved amputation or congenital limb deficiency from 1988 through 1996, averaging 133,235 amputations per year, and a 1996 annual rate of 52 amputations per 100,000 US population.[14] Unlike the NHIS-D data, the data from the Healthcare Cost and Utilization Project, Nationwide Inpatient Sample are categorized by upper limb amputation versus lower limb amputation. Dillingham et al[14] identified 166,464 community hospital discharges related to upper limb amputations over the 9-year period (14% of all discharges). During this time, there was an average of 18,496 upper limb discharges per year.[14,15] The 1996 incidence rate for discharges related to upper limb amputation was 5 per 100,000 US population, as opposed to a rate of 47 per 100,000 US population discharges related to lower limb amputations. These numbers include hospital discharges and not amputations; however, more than one amputation can occur during one hospitalization, and an amputee can be hospitalized more than once during a 9-year period. Of the upper limb amputation rate, 3.8 in 100,000 were trauma related, 1.3 in 100,000 were dysvascular related, and less than 1 in 100,000 were cancer related.

Emergency room visits, tracked by the National Electronic Injury Surveillance System All Injury Program, are another source of incidence data. According to analysis of 2001–2002 National Electronic Injury Surveillance System data, approximately 30,000 people with non-work–related amputations were treated in emergency rooms each year, an annual rate of 10 per 100,000 US population.[16] Most (91%) were treated for finger amputation. Work-related amputation data is tracked both at the national and state levels.[16] The

Bureau of Labor Statistics reported a 1999 work-related amputation rate of 15 per 100,000 population (the results did not differentiate upper from lower limb amputations).[17] For example, in Kentucky between 1994 and 2003, 96% of the Kentucky worker's compensation amputation claims were for upper limb amputation.[12]

UPPER LIMB RESEARCH: OUTCOMES

When designing any effective research program, it is imperative to reach some consensus on the best way to measure outcomes in various domains, such as functional performance, independence, quality of life, and cost. Research focused on upper limb amputation presents its own unique challenges. Recently, the Limb Loss Research and Statistics Program performed a survey to understand how both upper limb and lower limb amputation impact the outcomes of daily living and quality of life. Although the sample included 109 upper limb amputees (11% of the sample), results did not distinguish between upper and lower limb amputees. The results indicated 30% of the sample experienced difficulty with bathing and 7% required help with activities of daily living. It is possible that an upper limb amputee could have more difficulty with activities of daily living than a lower limb amputee because of the fine motor component of activities of daily living. Additionally, 81% of the sample used assistive technology (AT) other than prosthetic devices; for example, canes, walkers, and wheelchairs. AT needs of upper limb amputees remain unknown, though understanding an amputee's need for AT is an important consideration for reimbursement policy and best practice guidelines (ie, what type of equipment should be made available to amputees to maximize function when they are not able to use their prostheses). For example, 41% of lower limb amputees have dermatologic conditions associated with the amputation, regardless of prosthetic use.[18–20] Frequently, lower limb amputees are unable to use their prostheses during dermatologic episodes and must rely on mobility-related AT. No studies were found that addressed dermatologic conditions and AT needs for upper limb amputees.

An amputee's access to care is another important ideological factor to consider. The Limb Loss Research and Statistics Program study found 10% of amputees surveyed did not receive medical care when needed, and 20% did not receive rehabilitation when needed.[13] An earlier study (1979–1993) of acute inpatient data found the mean acute length of hospital stay was nearly double for lower limb versus upper limb amputees.[21] This is likely because most lower limb amputations are for dysvascular disease, a condition

that may have associated comorbidities that may also require inpatient care. Another finding of the Dillingham et al[21] study was that only 3% to 4% of upper limb amputees were discharged from acute care to rehabilitation, as opposed to 20% to 23% of lower limb amputees. It remains unknown if upper limb amputees fail to undergo inpatient rehabilitation because they do not use prostheses.[21]

Cost of care is another important consideration when designing a research program. In a 2004 study of both upper limb and lower limb amputees, Pezzin et al found the mean out-of-pocket expense for trauma-related amputation was $890, versus $485 for dysvascular-disease–related amputations.[22] Other important cost-related factors to consider include the costs of amputation in the United States (including the cost of hospitalization and the cost of a prosthetic device) and whether or not the cost is considered over the continuum of care. When considered across the entire continuum of care, the cost of a prosthetic device may appear more reasonable to third-party payers.

As technology becomes more sophisticated and prostheses become more expensive, the decision as to who is eligible for which technology becomes more complicated. The US military provides service members with upper limb amputations with a myoelectric prosthesis, a body-powered prosthesis, and a cosmetic prosthesis. This level of care is rare in the civilian community, where third-party payers typically fund only one prosthesis unless there is evidence that additional devices will increase function. The Limb Loss Research and Statistics Program study found most amputees wore their prostheses all day if satisfaction with the fit was high, and associated the highest level of satisfaction with ease of use. These results, however, include satisfaction with both upper limb and lower limb prostheses, so they do not accurately describe patient happiness with upper limb prosthetics, alone. One of the main problems in research investigating satisfaction with and use of prosthetic devices is inconsistency in the definitions of "use" and "satisfaction." Use has been measured with both continuous scales (ie, counting days per week and hours per day the prosthesis is worn) and categorical scales (ie, whether the prosthesis is worn regularly, a lot of the time, all the time, occasionally, not at all, or never).[13, 22–25] The Limb Loss Research and Statistics Program study found 95% of participants used their prostheses regularly; however, only 21% of the participants were upper limb amputees. Studies of upper limb amputees performed in England found 72% of participants used their prostheses "regularly."[23] A study performed in Australia found 18% of participants used their prostheses "all the time," and 13% used their prostheses "a lot of the time."[26] Additionally, Davidson measured the extent to which upper limb amputees used the grasp feature of their prostheses; 7% used the grasp feature "all the time" and 29% "never" used the grasp feature. A limitation of the satisfaction and use studies is that measurement has not been standardized. Additionally, the type of prosthesis used was not typically mentioned. In order to determine what factors account for variability in use of devices, future studies need to use consistent, standardized scales to evaluate "use" per type of device. For example, a study performed in Ireland by Graham et al found 56% of upper limb amputee participants used their prostheses functionally, and 34% used their prostheses cosmetically (however, participants could only select one of the two use responses).[24] Future studies should consider that participants may have more than one prosthesis, each used for a different purpose. In addition, studies should also account for other comorbidities that may affect outcomes. The Graham study was the only study found to include posttraumatic stress disorder (PTSD) as a factor related to use; 69% of the participants reported having PTSD. Most studies of upper limb amputation, including the Graham study, provide only descriptive analyses. Future studies could use PTSD as a variable in a regression model to more robustly determine the relationship between PTSD and use of a prosthesis.

A study published in 1989 used descriptive statistics to find an association between successful use of a prosthetic device and having a high school diploma, being employed or rapidly returning to work, accepting the amputation, perceiving that the prosthesis was expensive, and exhibiting less than two comorbidities.[27] Factors cited as unrelated to successful use of a prosthesis included age, hand dominance, rehabilitation, training in use of the prosthesis, and use of a temporary prosthesis. Forty participants with upper limb amputations were classified as successful users if they used a prosthesis every day, partially successful if they used a prosthesis for certain tasks, and unsuccessful if they did not use a prosthesis or did not use it functionally (ie, wore it only for cosmetic purposes). Forty-six percent of the successful users (n=12), 70% of the partially successful users (n=7), and 57% of the

unsuccessful users (n=3) had received rehabilitation.[27] Whether or not a participant had access to rehabilitation was not considered. One problem with this study is that descriptive statistics were used to explain multivariate relationships. However, this study could be helpful if it was repeated using a regression model design and current technology.

Time and error have been employed to measure successful prosthetic use with a motor learning approach. For example, in a 1993 study by Edelstein and Berger, children with traumatic upper limb amputation randomized to either a body-powered or myoelectric prosthesis were able to perform some tasks faster with a myoelectric prosthesis (donning socks, cutting paper, applying bandage) and other tasks faster with a body-powered prosthesis (playing cards, using form board) following a 3-month training period.[28]

Satisfaction with prostheses has also been inconsistently defined. In Australia, Davidson used a survey to measure the following: satisfaction with the ability to perform specific activities (ie, unsatisfied, just satisfied, or very satisfied), overall satisfaction with the prosthesis (ie, very satisfied, quite satisfied, okay, quite unsatisfied, or very unsatisfied), and satisfaction with the characteristics of the prosthesis (ie, not acceptable, fair, good, very good, or excellent).[26]

In 2004 Pezzin et al[22] used multivariate regression to examine use and satisfaction of prosthetic devices. Seventy-six percent of respondents were satisfied with the overall performance of their prostheses; however, data were not presented separately for upper limb and lower limb amputees. Other outcomes investigated by Pezzin et al included the relationship between satisfaction and use with time interval between amputation and receipt of prosthesis, level of amputation, geographic location, gender, race, ethnicity, insurance coverage, comorbidity, and age.[22]

Studies by Pezzin et al[22] and Pinzur et al[29] have shown a positive relationship between early fitting of a prosthesis and satisfaction and use. Early fitting is problematic for many service member amputees injured in Operations Enduring Freedom and Iraqi Freedom because of the extent of upper limb damage. Multiple surgeries may be necessary before a temporary prosthesis can be fitted. The Otto Bock MyoBoy (Otto Bock HealthCare, Minneapolis, Minn) computer-based technology enables upper limb amputees to train to use myoelectric prosthetic devices while waiting to be fitted for prostheses. This allows early muscle strengthening and retraining. A second reported benefit of myoelectric prosthetic use is reduced phantom limb pain.[30]

In a 1988 study by Melendez and LeBlanc,[31] upper limb amputees who did not use prostheses attributed their choice to lack of education and information on prosthetic devices.[31] Providing consistent delivery of prosthetic information and resources to both rural and urban populations remains a challenge.

Research on the effect of upper limb amputation on the outcomes of employment, driving, and participation in society is sparse. In a study of upper limb amputees in England, Datta et al found that 73% of upper limb amputees became employed or reemployed following their amputations, although 67% had to change jobs.[23] The study descriptively characterized the sample according to amputation level and type of prosthetic device used. Similarly, Pinzur et al found 72% of upper limb amputees in the United States were employed following amputation.[29] Future studies could use multivariate methods to associate amputation site and type of prosthetic device with employment-related factors. Predictors of return to work have been identified for lower limb amputees, but not for upper limb amputees.[32]

Jones and Davidson investigated the driving patterns and vehicle modifications of upper limb amputees in Australia.[25,26] The only US study of driving involved lower limb amputees. Boulias et al found 81% of lower limb amputee participants returned to driving

an average of 4 months after their amputations. However, in the United States, the percentage of drivers with upper limb amputations who return to work, and the modifications they use, remains unknown. It is also unclear how these drivers are assessed for safety and how their need for modifications is determined.[33]

Participation in society is an important outcome of rehabilitation according to the World Health Organization's *International Classification of Functioning, Disability, and Health*.[34] The US Centers for Disease Control and Prevention and Bureau of Labor Statistics measure participation by counting days missed from work as a result of a work-related amputation. Methods developed by the World Health Organization, Centers for Disease Control and Prevention, and Bureau of Labor Statistics to measure participation could be applied to study the degree to which upper limb amputees are able to participate in society.

Evidence for effectiveness of training in the use of upper limb prosthetics is necessary for third-party reimbursement of rehabilitation, but cannot currently be found in the literature. Models of prosthetic training should also be investigated (eg, peer training, inpatient, outpatient, and telerehabilitation).[35]

UPPER LIMB RESEARCH: MEASURES

From a health-services perspective, outcome measures monitor the extent to which invested resources contribute to desired results.[36] From a clinical perspective, outcome measures predict the relationship between doses of therapy and patient responses.[37] From a rehabilitation perspective, outcomes to be measured are functional health status and patient satisfaction.[38] Thus, outcomes can be measured at the system and patient levels. A challenge to measuring upper limb amputee and prosthetic outcomes is the interaction between the technology and the patient—a relationship that complicates AT research. Finally, once desired outcomes and appropriate measures have been identified, robust analyses must also be conducted.

Informal measures typically include using checklists developed by clinicians for assessment, developing an intervention plan, and monitoring progress. There are several informal checklists available. Occupational therapist Diane Atkins developed informal measures for upper limb amputees using body-powered prostheses. Occupational therapists at Otto Bock have developed the Occupational Therapist Upper Extremity Functional Evaluation and the Upper Extremity Prosthetic Functional Activity Checklist, both available on the Otto Bock Web site.

Formal measures have resulted in published psychometric properties; that is, reliability and validity

have been tested. Reliability measures the consistency or repeatability of the measurement with the intent of separating true score from error. Validity is the strength of the inference or the extent to which the construct was measured, minus the threats and biases that can undermine results and generalizations. One problem with upper limb amputation and prosthetic research is the inconsistency in operational definitions of prosthetic "use" and "satisfaction," resulting in the vast range (7%–88%) discussed earlier in this chapter.[39–43] Without a valid, reliable, and preferably standard measure of use, the relationship between use and functional status cannot be established. Without a valid, reliable and preferably standard measure of satisfaction, the quality of care provided to amputees cannot be established. In this context, a standard measure is one that may be considered the goal and used in a variety of environments so study results can be compared. For example, there are many measures of quality of life. For many, the Short Form-36 Health Survey remains the subjective standard that is conducive to comparison of health status across populations.[44,45] The Short Form-36 Health Survey has been used in at least one study of lower limb amputees.[44]

Three valid and reliable formal measures used in upper limb amputee and prosthetic research are the Disabilities of the Arm Shoulder Hand (DASH) questionnaire, the Orthotics and Prosthetics User Survey-Upper Extremity (OPUS-UE) scale, and the Trinity Amputation and Prosthetic Experience Scales (TAPES).[36,46–49] The DASH is a 30-item questionnaire developed by the Canadian Institute for Work & Health and the American Academy of Orthopaedic Surgeons. It measures the physical and social impact of upper limb disorders. Scoring is done on a 5-point Likert scale, with a lower score indicating less disability. Davidson used the DASH to determine disability of patients with upper limb amputations and to compare those to other upper limb injuries.[41] According to her findings, patients with brachial plexus injuries, Complex Regional Pain Syndrome, and bilateral upper limb amputations demonstrated significantly higher levels of disability compared to patients with unilateral upper limb amputations. Additionally, partial hand amputees reported a higher level of disability than major unilateral upper limb amputees.[41]

The OPUS-UE is a Rasch scale that measures activity limitations (23 items), quality of life (23 items), and patient satisfaction with services and devices (20 items). A lower score indicates higher function. The OPUS-UE is commonly used in lower limb amputation research; no studies were found that used the upper limb version.

The 54-item TAPES is designed to examine the psychosocial processes involved in adjusting to a prosthesis. There are four sections: (1) psychosocial (general adjustment, social adjustment, and adjustment to limitation subscales), (2) activity restriction (functional, social, and athletic restriction subscales), (3) satisfaction with the prosthesis (functional, aesthetic, and weight characteristics), and (4) exploration of phantom limb pain, residual limb pain, and other medical conditions not related to the amputation. The only known study using the TAPES with upper limb amputees was a study of the psychometric properties of the TAPES.[50]

ANALYSIS OF OUTCOMES

The majority of studies cited previously in this chapter used a survey design with descriptive statistical analyses that yield measures of central tendency. More recent studies use more robust study designs, such as logistic regression, that adjust for confounding factors such as marital status, employment status, educational level, and location of amputation.[43,50] These studies control for factors that vary from one amputee or one prosthetic device to another. In addition, these studies can identify interactions between the amputee and the device, amputee factors that are present only when certain device factors are present, and vice versa. From these studies, the conditions under which a device will benefit an amputee can be predicted.

Deathe et al studied formal versus informal outcome measures used in Canada.[51] Doffing and donning a prosthesis was informally assessed by 90% of respondents, dressing by 78%, bath transfers by 81%, and car transfers by 56%. Informal home visit assessments were performed by 29% of respondents. Formal assessments were categorized according to whether they were used in the academic or clinic environments. The Functional

Independence Measure (the most widely accepted functional measure in the research community; an 18-item, 7-level ordinal scale intended to be sensitive to change in an individual over the course of a comprehensive inpatient medical rehabilitation program), the Prosthetic Profile of the Amputee (a clinical follow-up questionnaire that measures both actual prosthetic use and factors potentially related to prosthetic use by individuals with lower limb amputation), and the walking speed, walking distance, repetitive chair rise, and timed up-and-go tests were performed in both environments.[52,53] The Barthel Index, a 10-item measure commonly used in rehabilitation medicine, measures functional outcome, including factors like mobility and self-care, and was only used in the clinic.[54] The Minimal Data Set (which evaluates the functional capabilities of residents in Medicare- and Medicaid-certified residential facilities), the Short Form-36 Health Survey (which produces a physical and mental component summary score), and goal attainment scaling (in which clinician and patient set individualized goals on a five-point scale) were only used in research.[45,55–58]

SUMMARY

Epidemiology and evidence-based research studies in upper limb amputation are few and outdated. There are potential upper limb amputation and prosthesis

outcome measures that have yet to be used in research. Studies that pilot these measures, from surgery to community reintegration, are needed.

REFERENCES

1. Baumgartner R. Upper extremity amputation and prosthetics. *J Rehabil Res Dev.* 2001;38(4):vii–x.

2. Bethel A, Sloan FA, Belsky D, Feinglos MN. Longitudinal incidence and prevalence of adverse outcomes of diabetes mellitus in elderly patients. *Arch Intern Med.* 2007;167(9):921–927.

3. Collins TC, Beyth RJ, Nelson DB, et al. Process of care and outcomes in patients with peripheral arterial disease. *J Gen Intern Med.* 2007;22(7):942–948.

4. Ephraim PL, Dillingham T, Sector M, Pezzin L, MacKenzie EJ. Epidemiology of limb loss and congenital limb deficiency: a review of the literature. *Arch Phys Med Rehabil.* 2003;84(5):747–761.

5. Kurichi JE, Stineman MG, Kwong PL, Bates BE, Reker DE. Assessing and using comorbidity measures in elderly veterans with lower extremity amputations. *Gerontology.* 2007;53(5):255–259.

6. Zucchino D. Amputee Marine returns to combat duty. *Los Angeles Times.* August 6, 2008. Available at: http://www.latimes.com/news/nationworld/world/la-fg-amputee6-2008aug06,0,1297101.story?page=1. Accessed October 8, 2008.

7. van Houtum WH, Lavery LA. Methodological issues affect variability in reported incidence of lower extremity amputations due to diabetes. *Diabetes Res Clin Pr.* 1997;38(3):177–183.

8. Centers for Disease Control and Prevention. *National Health Interview Survey on Disability (NHIS-D).* Washington, DC: CDC; 1997.

9. Koepsell TD, Weiss NS. Disease frequency: basics. In: Koepsell TD, Weiss NS, eds. *Epidemiologic Methods: Studying the Occurrence of Illness (Medicine).* New York, NY: Oxford University Press; 2003: 37–62.

10. Adams PF, Hendershot GE, Marano MA. Current estimates from the National Health Interview Survey, 1996. *Vital Health Stat 10.* 1999;200:1–203.

11. Esquenazi A, Meier R. Rehabilitation in limb deficiency. *Arch Phys Med Rehabil.* 1996;77(Suppl):S18–S28.

12. McCall BP, Horwitz IB. An assessment and quantification of the rates, costs, and risk factors of occupational amputations: analysis of Kentucky workers' compensation claims, 1994–2003. *Am J Ind Med.* 2006;49(12):1031–1038.

13. People with amputation speak out. Amputation Coalition of America, Limb Loss Research and Statistics Program Web site. Available at: http://www.amputee-coalition.org/people-speak-out/index.html. Accessed August 3, 2008.

14. Dillingham TR, Pezzin LE, MacKenzie EJ. Limb amputation and limb deficiency: epidemiology and recent trends in the United States. *South Med J.* 2002;95(8):875–883.

15. Esquenazi A. Amputation rehabilitation and prosthetic restoration. From surgery to community reintegration. *Disabil Rehabil.* 2004;26:831–836.

16. Conn JM, Annest JL, Ryan GW, Budnitz DS. Non-work–related finger amputations in the United States, 2001–2002. *Ann Emerg Med.* 2005;45(6):630–635.

17. Centers for Disease Control and Prevention, National Institution for Occupational Safety and Health. *Fatal and Nonfatal Injuries, and Selected Illnesses and Conditions.* Atlanta, Ga: NIOSH; 2004.

18. Dudek NL, Marks MB, Marshall SC. Skin problems in an amputee clinic. *Am J Phys Med Rehabil.* 2006;85(5):424–429.

19. Dudek NL, Marks MB, Marshall SC, Chardon JP. Dermatologic conditions associated with use of a lower-extremity prosthesis. *Arch Phys Med Rehabil.* 2005;86(4):659–663.

20. Meulenbelt HE, Geertzen JH, Dijkstra PU, Jonkman MF. Skin problems in lower limb amputees: an overview by case

reports. *J Eur Acad Dermatol Venereol.* 2007;21(2):147–155.

21. Dillingham TR, Pezzin LE, MacKenzie EJ. Incidence, acute care length of stay, and discharge to rehabilitation of traumatic amputee patients: an epidemiologic study. *Arch Phys Med Rehabil.* 1998;79(3):279–287.

22. Pezzin LE, Dillingham TR, Mackenzie EJ, Ephraim P, Rossbach P. Use and satisfaction with prosthetic limb devices and related services. *Arch Phys Med Rehabil.* 2004;85(5):723–729.

23. Datta D, Selvarajah K, Davey N. Functional outcome of patients with proximal upper limb deficiency—acquired and congenital. *Clin Rehabil.* 2004;18(2):172–177.

24. Graham L, Parke RC, Paterson MC, Stevenson M. A study of the physical rehabilitation and psychological state of patients who sustained limb loss as a result of terrorist activity in Northern Ireland 1969–2003. *Disabil Rehabil.* 2006;28(12):797–801.

25. Jones LE, Davidson JH. The long-term outcome of upper limb amputees treated at a rehabilitation centre in Sydney, Australia. *Disabil Rehabil.* 1995;17(8):437–442.

26. Davidson J. A survey of the satisfaction of upper limb amputees with their prostheses, their lifestyles, and their abilities. *J Hand Ther.* 2002;15(1):62–70.

27. Roeschlein RA, Domholdt E. Factors related to successful upper extremity prosthetic use. *Prosthet Orthot Int.* 1989;13(1):14–18.

28. Edelstein JE, Berger N. Performance comparison among children fitted with myoelectric and body-powered hands. *Arch Phys Med Rehabil.* 1993;74(4):376–380.

29. Pinzur MS, Angelats J, Light TR, Izuierdo R, Pluth T. Functional outcome following traumatic upper limb amputation and prosthetic limb fitting. *J Hand Surg [Am].* 1994;19(5):836–839.

30. Lotze M, Grodd W, Birbaumer N, Erb M, Huse E, Flor H. Does use of a myoelectric prosthesis prevent cortical reorganization and phantom limb pain? *Nat Neurosci.* 1999;2(6):501–502.

31. Melendez D, LeBlanc M. Survey of arm amputees not wearing prostheses: implications for research and service. *J Assoc Child Prost Orthot Clin.* 1988;23(3):62–69.

32. Hebert JS, Ashworth NL. Predictors of return to work following traumatic work-related lower extremity amputation. *Disabil Rehabil.* 2006;28(10):613–618.

33. Boulias C, Meikle B, Pauley T, Devlin M. Return to driving after lower-extremity amputation. *Arch Phys Med Rehabil.* 2006;87(9):1183–1188.

34. World Health Organization. *International Classification of Functioning, Disability and Health.* Geneva, Switzerland: WHO; 2001.

35. Lake C. Effects of prosthetic training on upper-extremity prosthesis use. *J Prost Orthot.* 1997;9(1):3–9.

36. Heinemann AW, Fisher W, Gershon R. Improving healthcare quality with outcomes management. *J Prost Orthot.* 2006;18(1S):46–50.

37. Granger CV. Quality and outcome measures for rehabilitation programs. eMedicine from WebMD. Available at: http://www.emedicine.com/pmr/TOPIC155.HTM. Accessed August 5, 2008.

38. Ware JE Jr, Phillips J, Yody BB, Adamczyk J. Assessment tools: functional health status and patient satisfaction. *Am J Med Qual.* 1996;11(1):S50–S53.

39. Datta D, Selvarajah K, Davey N. Functional outcome of patients with proximal upper limb deficiency—acquired and congenital. *Clin Rehabil.* 2004;18:172–177.

40. Davidson J. A survey of the satisfaction of upper limb amputees with their prostheses, their lifestyles, and their abilities. *J Hand Ther*. 2002;15(1):62–70.

41. Davidson J. A comparison of upper limb amputees and patients with upper limb injuries using the Disability of the Arm, Shoulder and Hand (DASH). *Disabil Rehabil*. 2004;26(14-15):917–923.

42. Pezzin LE, Dillingham TR, MacKenzie EJ. Rehabilitation and the long-term outcomes of persons with trauma-related amputations. *Arch Phys Med Rehabil*. 2000;81(3):292–300.

43. Pezzin LE, Dillingham TR, MacKenzie EJ, Ephraim PL, Rossbach P. Use and satisfaction with prosthetic limb devices and related services. *Arch Phys Med Rehabil*. 2004;85:723–729.

44. Ware JE. Conceptualizing and measuring generic health outcomes. *Cancer*. 1991;67(3):774–779.

45. Ware J. *SF-36 Health Survey Manual and Interpretation Guide*. Boston, Mass: Nimrod Press; 1993.

46. Heinemann AW, Gershon R, Fisher W. Development and application of the orthotics and prosthetics user survey: applications and opportunities for healthcare quality improvement. *J Prost Orthot*. 2006;18(1S):80-85.

47. Heinemann AW, Bode RK, O'Reilly C. Development and measurement properties of the Orthotics and Prosthetics Users' Survey (OPUS): a comprehensive set of clinical outcome instruments. *Prosthet Orthot Int*. 2003;27:191–206.

48. Hudak PL, Amadio PC, Bombardier C. Development of an upper extremity outcome measure: the DASH (disabilities of the arm, shoulder and hand). The Upper Extremity Collaborative Group (UEGC). *Am J Ind Med*. 1996;29(6):602–628.

49. Beaton DE, Katz JN, Fossel AH, Wright JG, Tarasuk V, Bombardier C. Measuring the whole or parts? Validity, reliability, and responsiveness of the Disabilities of the Arm, Shoulder and Hand outcome measure in different regions of the upper extremity. *J Hand Ther*. 2001;14(2):128–146.

50. Desmond DM, MacLachlan M. Factor structure of the Trinity Amputation and Prosthesis Experiences Scales (TAPES) with individuals with acquired upper limb amputations. *Am J Phys Med Rehabil*. 2005;84(7):506–513.

51. Deathe AB, Miller WC, Speechley M. The status of outcome measurement in amputee rehabilitation in Canada. *Arch Phys Med Rehabil*. 2002;83(7):912–918.

52. Gauthier-Gagnon C, Grisé MC. Prosthetic profile of the amputee questionnaire: validity and reliability. *Arch Phys Med Rehabil*. 1994;75(9):1309–1314.

53. Hershkovitz A, Brill S. Get up and go—home. *Aging Clin Exp Res*. 2006;18(4):301–306.

54. McGinnis GE, Seward ML, DeJong G, Osberg JS. Program evaluation of physical medicine and rehabilitation departments using self-report Barthel. *Arch Phys Med Rehabil*. 1986;67(2):123–125.

55. Hurn J, Kneebone I, Cropley M. Goal setting as an outcome measure: a systematic review. *Clin Rehabil*. 2006;20(9):756–772.

56. Uniform Data System for Medical Rehabilitation. The FIM System Web site. Available at: http://www.udsmr.org/WebModules/FIM/Fim_About.aspx. Accessed August 5, 2008.

57. Ware J. SF-36 health survey update. *Spine*. 2000;25(24):3130–3139.

58. Forbes DA. Goal attainment scaling. A responsive measure of client outcomes. *J Gerontol Nurs*. 1998;24(12):34–40.

Chapter 23

UPPER EXTREMITY PROSTHETICS

JOHN MIGUELEZ, CP, FAAOP[*]; DAN CONYERS, CPO[†]; MACJULIAN LANG, CPO[‡]; AND KRISTIN GULICK, OTR/L, BS, CHT[§]

[*]President and Senior Clinical Director, Advanced Arm Dynamics, Inc, 123 W Torrance Boulevard, Suite 203, Redondo Beach, California 90277
[†]Upper Extremity Specialist, Advanced Arm Dynamics, Inc, 10195 SW Egret Place, Beaverton, Oregon 97007
[‡]Clinical Specialist, Advanced Arm Dynamics, Inc, 123 W Torrance Boulevard, Suite 203, Redondo Beach, California 90277
[§]Occupational Therapist; formerly, Director of Therapy Services, Advanced Arm Dynamics, 123 West Torrance Boulevard, Suite 203, Redondo Beach, California

INTRODUCTION

Recent improvements in body armor, battlefield medicine, speed of evacuation, and surgical techniques have resulted in a high incidence of survival from blast wounds sustained during armed conflict (Figure 23-1). The mechanisms of injury include explosively formed projectiles, improvised explosive devices (IEDs), mobile IEDs, rocket-propelled grenades, suicide vehicle-borne IEDs, and gunshot wounds. Those individuals who survive are frequently polytraumatized and challenged with hearing or vision impairment, burns, traumatic brain injury (TBI), upper and lower extremity injuries, and/or amputations. Service members with well-irrigated, but open, wounds are rapidly transferred from the battlefield to a rehabilitation hospital, which requires an organized approach to prosthetic rehabilitation. To enable a young and motivated amputee population to return to highly active military and civilian lifestyles, the military healthcare system has implemented a comprehensive, multidisciplinary model of rehabilitative care.

The entire rehabilitation process is accelerated because of the superior premorbid physical status and goal-oriented mindset of the service member, both of which have been fostered in the military environment. Wounded service members approach rehabilitation with focused determination to reach the initial goal of returning to active duty or reintegrating into civilian life. They place high expectations on themselves and on the care they receive. Prosthetic rehabilitation for these individuals is also complemented by their previous training in the manipulation of external devices, including weaponry and computer systems, as well as the excellent hand-eye coordination developed through military training, recreational pursuits, and electronic gaming. Harnessing these characteristics, through the protocols discussed in this chapter and throughout this book, provides the military amputee with the best opportunity to achieve and maintain high levels of function, productivity, and quality of life. This chapter reviews amputation-level nomenclature, upper

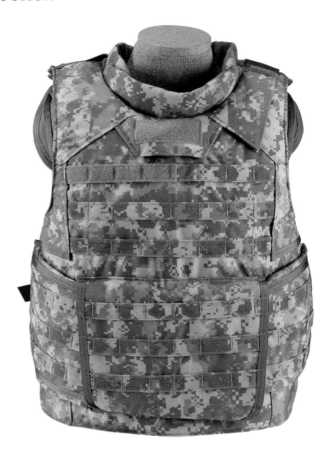

Figure 23-1. The Improved Outer Tactical Vest (IOTV) accommodates Small Arms Protective Inserts (SAPIs), Enhanced Small Arms Protective Inserts (ESAPIs), and Enhanced Side Ballistic Inserts (ESBIs).
Photograph: Courtesy of BAE Systems, Farnborough, Hampshire, United Kingdom.

limb prosthetic classifications, and treatment protocols for the three distinct phases of prosthetic rehabilitation: (1) the Preprosthetic Phase, (2) the Interim Prosthetic Phase, and (3) the Advanced Prosthetic Phase.

NOMENCLATURE AND CLASSIFICATIONS

Amputation Level Nomenclature

Historically, there has been varied nomenclature that describes amputations and amputation levels. In this chapter, level-specific language was adopted to describe amputations (Figure 23-2). Other terminology may be used throughout this book that is based on local variations in descriptive wording.

Prosthetic Options

There are five principal prosthetic options to consider for the upper limb amputee:

1. electrically powered prosthesis,
2. body-powered prosthesis,
3. hybrid prosthesis,

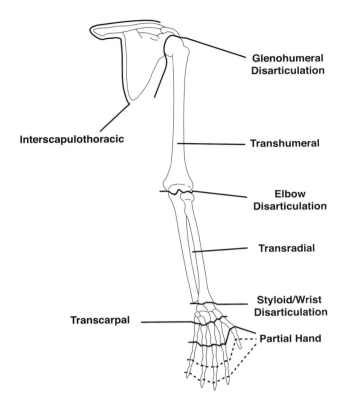

Figure 23-2. Upper limb amputation levels.
Illustration: Adapted with permission from Otto Bock HealthCare, Minneapolis, Minnesota.

4. passive/cosmetic restoration, and
5. task-specific prosthesis.

The types of prostheses recommended/selected are based on many factors, including level of amputation, condition of the residual limb, individual goals, and work requirements. Often, more than one option is required for an individual to accomplish all of his or her goals.

Electrically Powered Prosthesis

This category of prosthesis uses small electric motors in the terminal device [TD (hand or hook)], wrist, and elbow to provide movement. The motors are powered by a rechargeable battery system. There are several means of controlling this type of prosthesis, the most common of which is myoelectric control. (Figure 23-3). Myoelectric signals are derived from the contraction of voluntary control muscles in the residual limb and are recorded by surface electrodes implanted in the prosthetic socket. Electrodes must maintain contact with those particular muscles from

which the control signals are derived. The recorded myoelectric signal is first amplified and then processed into a control signal governing the electric motors that operate the prosthesis. The magnitude of the processed signal is roughly proportional to the isometric force exerted by the muscle, and the microprocessor calculates actions based on the strength of the myoelectric signal.[1,2] Proportional control allows the patient to control the speed and force of the TD and wrist and elbow movements by varying the strength of the muscular contraction/signal input. For example, the larger the myoelectric signal, the greater the grip force or speed of opening and closing. This provides a more natural response with less effort than the traditional on/off action of a purely digital control system. The programmable microprocessor enables a recent amputee with relatively weak or unbalanced electromyographic (EMG) signals to control the prosthesis effectively. As the amputee's EMG signals improve, further programming occurs to optimize control. The biophysics of myoelectric control and many of the technical considerations regarding signal extraction have been explained in detail previously.[3–6]

For amputees lacking adequate dual EMG output or control, or for prosthetic systems that require additional inputs to control more degrees of freedom, other potential methods of control include the following:

- single-site electrode control schemes,
- servo control,
- linear potentiometers,
- linear transducers,
- force-sensing resistors,
- push-buttons, and
- harness switch control mechanisms.

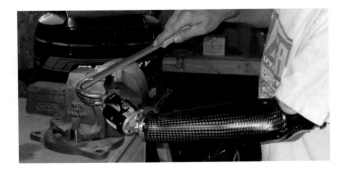

Figure 23-3. Transradial-level myoelectric prosthesis.
Photograph: Prosthesis provided by Advanced Arm Dynamics, Inc, Redondo Beach, California.

Several control schemes may be used on the same prosthesis to provide expanded function. The authors have presented technical considerations regarding these control options in other articles.[2,6] One of the unique characteristics of an electrically powered prosthesis is its ability to provide superior grasping force and wrist rotation capabilities without exerting excessive force on the fragile and acutely healing residual limb. Often, an electric prosthesis can be fit effectively within 24 hours of suture removal for rapid return to function. By contrast, the tissue traction and pressure applied to the distal end during actuation of a body-powered elbow or TD can significantly stress a suture line in the early stages of healing.

Inherent in the design of a myoelectric prosthesis is the elimination of external cabling needed for control of a body-powered prosthesis. Because electric motors are used to operate hand or hook function rather than a conventional cable and harness, grip force of the hand or hook is significantly increased, often in excess of 20 to 32 pounds per square inch. A cosmetic cover can also be applied to the prosthesis so that the prosthesis is not only highly functional, but also aesthetically superior. For amputations above the elbow, current prosthetic components allow simultaneous control of elbow flexion and extension while opening or closing the electric TD or while rotating the wrist. Historically, prosthetic options at and above the transhumeral level required the wearer to control one function at a time, also referred to as *sequential control*.

Unlike other prosthetic categories, the electrically powered prosthesis uses a battery system that requires regular maintenance (charging, discharging, eventual disposal, and replacement). Because of the battery system and the electrical motors, electrically powered prostheses tend to be heavier than other prosthetic options, although advanced suspension techniques can minimize this sensation. When properly fitted

and fabricated, electrically powered prostheses do not require excessive maintenance. However, when repairs are required, they are often more complex than other options because of their sophistication. Additionally, an electrically powered prosthesis is susceptible to damage when exposed to moisture (Table 23-1).

Body-Powered Prosthesis

A body-powered prosthesis, sometimes referred to as a conventional or cable-driven prosthesis, is powered and controlled by gross body movements. These movements—usually of the shoulder, upper arm, or chest—are captured by a harness system and used to pull a cable that is connected to a TD (hook or hand). For some levels of amputation or deficiency, an elbow system can be added to provide additional motion. For a patient to control a body-powered prosthesis, the individual must be capable of producing at least one or more of the following gross body movements:

- glenohumeral flexion,
- scapular abduction or adduction,
- shoulder depression and elevation,
- chest expansion, and
- elbow flexion.

Additionally, a patient must possess sufficient residual limb length for leverage, sufficient musculature to allow movement and excursion, and sufficient range of motion for operation and positioning of the prosthesis. Thus, it is often difficult for the humeral neck, glenohumeral disarticulation, and interscapulothoracic amputation levels to control a body-powered prosthesis effectively (Figure 23-4).

Because of its simple design, the body-powered prosthesis is highly durable and can be used for

TABLE 23-1

ADVANTAGES/DISADVANTAGES OF ELECTRICALLY POWERED PROSTHESIS

Advantages	Disadvantages
Proportional grip force	Battery maintenance
Ease of electric TD/wrist operation	Overall weight consideration
Can be fit early in rehabilitation	Repairs may be more complex
Natural appearance	Susceptible to damage from moisture or excessive vibration
Can be applied to high amputation levels	
Simultaneous control of elbow and TD or wrist	
Larger functional work envelope than body-powered prosthesis	

TD: terminal device

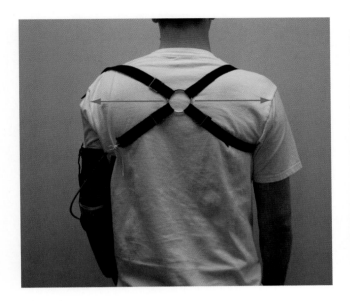

Figure 23-4. Figure-of-eight harness. *Arrows* indicate directional pull of biscapular abduction or glenohumeral flexion. Photograph: Prosthesis provided by Advanced Arm Dynamics, Inc, Redondo Beach, California.

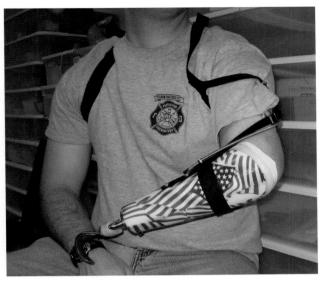

Figure 23-5. Definitive transradial-level, body-powered prosthesis.
Photograph: Prosthesis provided by Advanced Arm Dynamics, Inc, Redondo Beach, California.

tasks that involve water, dust, and other environments that could damage an electric prosthesis. Many patients who wear a body-powered prosthesis comment that they have a unique spatial awareness because of cable tension proprioception, which gives the wearer feedback on the position of the TD through the harness system. Maintenance costs for a body-powered prosthesis are also relatively low (Figure 23-5).

The most common complaint reported by wearers of this type of prosthesis is that the control harness is often uncomfortable, restrictive, and wears out clothes. Although new materials aid in reducing discomfort, the harness must fit tightly to capture the movement of

the shoulders and to suspend the prosthesis. This can restrict proximal joint range of motion and the effective envelope of the prosthesis. The harness and cable system also limits the possible grip force of the hook or other TD. Other patients dislike the appearance of the hook and control cables, and request a prosthesis that is more "lifelike." Lastly, because of the inherent forces exerted on the residual limb during actuation of a body-powered prosthesis, careful consideration is required for those patients who have fragile, healing tissues about the residual limb. If a body-powered prosthesis is fit too early in the rehabilitation process, patients can experience breakdown around the suture line (Table 23-2).

TABLE 23-2

ADVANTAGES/DISADVANTAGES OF BODY-POWERED PROSTHESIS

Advantages	Disadvantages
Durable and can be used in tasks or environments that could damage an electric prosthesis (ie, conditions involving excessive water, dust, or vibrations created by some motorized vehicles and power tools) Secondary proprioceptive feedback Lower maintenance costs than electric options	Restrictive harness Decreased grip force compared with electric options Forces exerted on residual limb Difficult to control for high amputation levels Limited function of typical body-powered hands Appearance of hook and cables

Hybrid Prosthesis

A hybrid prosthesis incorporates body-powered and electrically powered components in a single prosthesis. The hybrid prosthesis often uses a body-powered elbow and a myoelectrically controlled TD (hook or hand). If desired by the wearer, an electric wrist rotator can also be included. Another type of hybrid prosthesis combines an electrically powered elbow with a body-powered hook or hand. Most commonly, hybrid prostheses are used for individuals with transhumeral and humeral neck amputations. Glenohumeral and interscapulothoracic level amputations may also be fit with hybrid prostheses. However, these cases require precise interface design because of the amount of gross body movement needed to operate this type of prosthesis and the EMG signal interference potentially created in the socket of the myoelectrically controlled hybrid during such movement. It is important for the electrodes to remain in a constant relationship with the best EMG signal that is discovered throughout the patient's range of motion (Figure 23-6).

There are several advantages to a hybrid prosthesis. Most important is the ability to simultaneously control elbow flexion or extension while opening or closing the electric TD or while rotating the wrist. Some prosthetic options require the wearer to control one function at a time (sequential control). The hybrid prosthesis also weighs less than a prosthesis with an electrically powered elbow while maintaining ease of operation and increased grip force of electric TDs (Table 23-3).

Passive/Cosmetic Restoration

Passive/cosmetic restoration is a popular prosthetic option. This involves replacing what was lost from amputation with a prosthesis that is similar in appearance to the nonaffected arm or hand and aids in stabilizing

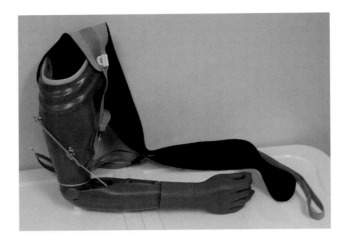

Figure 23-6. Transhumeral-level hybrid prosthesis with cable-driven elbow and myoelectric TD.
TD: terminal device
Photograph: Prosthesis provided by Advanced Arm Dynamics, Inc, Redondo Beach, California.

and carrying functions. A cosmetic prosthesis is sometimes called a passive prosthesis because it is a static device that does not provide active grasping capability. Cosmetic restoration is typically achieved using one of three materials: (1) flexible latex, (2) rigid PVC (polyvinyl chloride), or (3) silicone. These types of prostheses are often lighter weight than other prosthetic options and require less maintenance because they have fewer moving parts. Cosmetic restoration using silicone often goes unnoticed because it so closely resembles the nonaffected hand. Silicone does not stain like latex, and it provides the highest cosmetic restoration quality, with a longevity of 3 to 5 years, depending on usage patterns. These highly detailed silicone restorations are also commonly used to create a covering for the electric hands and body-powered hands in the previously discussed sections about those options (Figures 23-7 and 23-8; see also Table 23-4).

TABLE 23-3

ADVANTAGES/DISADVANTAGES OF HYBRID PROSTHESIS

Advantages	Disadvantages
Simultaneous control of elbow and TD or wrist	Requires a harness for elbow control
Lighter than fully electric elbow prosthesis	The force needed to fully flex the elbow may be difficult to
Increased grip force compared with body-powered options	generate for short transhumeral and higher amputation
Ease of electric TD/wrist operation	levels

TD: terminal device

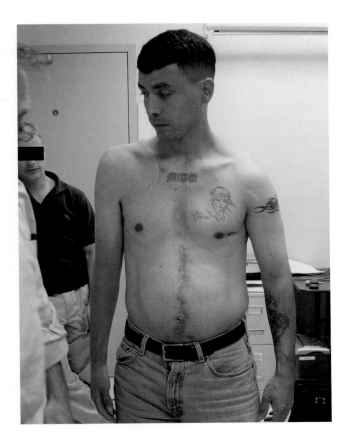

Figure 23-7. Glenohumeral disarticulation amputee wearing a cosmetic silicone restoration.
Photograph: Prosthesis provided by Advanced Arm Dynamics, Inc, Redondo Beach, California.

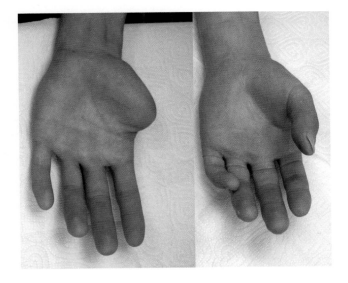

Figure 23-8. Silicone partial hand prosthesis.
Photographs: Prosthesis provided by Advanced Arm Dynamics, Inc, Redondo Beach, California.

TABLE 23-4

ADVANTAGES/DISADVANTAGES OF PASSIVE PROSTHESIS

Advantages	Disadvantages
Lightweight	Difficult to perform activities that require mechanical grasp
Minimal harnessing	Latex and PVC products stain easily
Low maintenance	
No control cables	
Cosmesis, positive body image	
Silicone products resist staining	

PVC: polyvinyl chloride

Task-Specific Prosthesis

Task-specific prostheses are designed particularly for an activity in which the use of a passive/cosmetic, body-powered, electrically powered, or hybrid prosthesis would place unacceptable limitations on function or durability. Often, this type of prosthesis is recreational in nature for activities such as fishing, swimming, golfing, hunting, bicycle riding, weight lifting, playing musical instruments, etc. Task-specific prostheses can also enhance work-related function involving the use of various tools. For more information regarding task-specific devices, see Chapter 24 on Upper Limb Prosthetics for Sports and Recreation (Table 23-5).

The current military prosthetic rehabilitation practice is to provide each service member an electric or

TABLE 23-5

ADVANTAGES/DISADVANTAGES OF TASK-SPECIFIC PROSTHESIS

Advantages	Disadvantage
Enhanced function in particular activity	Not appropriate for a broad range of functions
Minimal harnessing	
Limited or no control cables	
Durable, low maintenance	
Protects primary prosthesis from damage	

hybrid prosthesis, a body-powered prosthesis, and a passive silicone restoration prosthesis. As the service member progresses through prosthetic rehabilitation and his or her skills develop—allowing for exploration of sport activities and other specialized high-level skills—the team will address the need for a task-specific device. In most cases, the service member self-selects which prosthesis to use throughout the day for different tasks. Most service members routinely use all of their prosthetic options at some point while performing activities of daily living (ADLs). In the course of the rehabilitation process, a "primary" prosthesis will be identified, and this prosthetic option will often be duplicated to provide a backup device in the event that the primary prosthesis needs maintenance or repair.

Prosthetic Componentry

Upper extremity prostheses incorporate componentry from one or more of the following four categories, depending on the level of amputation:

1. TDs,
2. wrist units,
3. elbow systems, and
4. shoulder joints.

Terminal Devices

A large variety of TDs are available. TDs from all of the various manufacturers can be integrated into the rehabilitation plan to provide a variety of grip patterns, functional uses, and adaptations for specific tasks and appearances. Many service persons have identified useful TDs that can be interchangeable on a given prosthesis and some TDs that are best applied to a separate prosthesis for a unique application. Considerable ongoing research is being pursued to improve body-powered and electric TDs, as well as adaptive, task-specific TDs[2(p52),7-14] (Figure 23-9).

Two common categories of TDs include (1) the hook and (2) the hand. Hooks are useful for both fine prehension and rugged tasks. Hands provide a more anthropomorphic appearance, particularly with myoelectric TDs. Power to operate the body-powered TD is derived from body movements through a cable system, and electric TDs use electric motors from a battery-powered system. Body-powered TDs typically produce a voluntary opening, with rubber bands or springs providing the closing force. There are a number of body-powered TDs that provide voluntary closing functions. Service members with an amputation at the transradial level and longer

are given the option to try both voluntary opening and voluntary closing styles, and to self-select one or both, depending on the activity. Most amputees with amputations proximal to the transradial level find voluntary closing to be quite difficult because of the amount of cable excursion required to operate both an elbow and a TD.[15-17] In the United States, all body-powered hooks and hands have the same ½-inch, 20-thread stud for attachment to wrist units. This allows ease of TD interchangeability.[15]

Most hook-style TDs are made from high-density plastics, aluminum, stainless steel, or titanium. Plastics are used as coatings or as housings for electric motors. Aluminum is appropriate for lightweight/light-duty applications. Titanium is strong and lightweight, and stainless steel is used where weight is less of a consideration than the overall strength of the TD material. One or all of these materials may be present in a single TD.

The prosthetic treatment protocols detailed in the section on the Interim Prosthetic Phase recommend a combination of TD technologies for both the externally powered and body-powered prostheses. This methodology accommodates the broadest range of prehension patterns and functional applications in daily living activities. Users of externally powered prostheses are able to interchange microprocessor-controlled electronic hand TDs and different microprocessor-controlled electric work hook-type configurations.

The microprocessor-controlled electric hand provides a natural appearance and can produce a grip

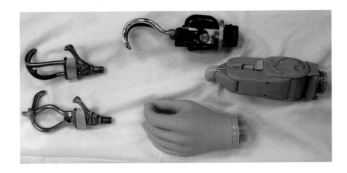

Figure 23-9. Examples of TDs: (*top center*) Motion Control ETD, (*right*) Otto Bock Greifer, (*bottom center*) Otto Bock SensorHand SPEED, (*bottom left*) Hosmer Dorrance 7LO work hook, and (*top left*) Hosmer 5XA hook.
ETD: Electric Terminal Device
TDs: terminal devices
Photograph: Product images used with permission from Motion Control, Inc, Salt Lake City, Utah; Otto Bock HealthCare, Minneapolis, Minnesota; and Hosmer Dorrance Corporation, Campbell, California.

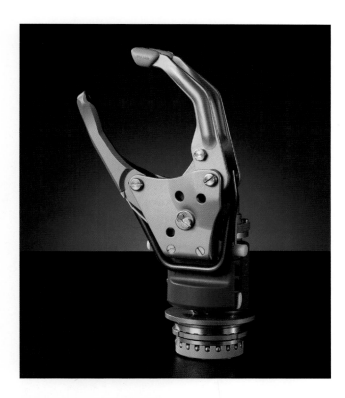

Figure 23-10. The Otto Bock SensorHand SPEED responds twice as quickly as other electric hands and offers an automatic grasp feature.
Photograph: Courtesy of Otto Bock HealthCare, Minneapolis, Minnesota.

be positioned at various angles of wrist flexion and extension, enhancing the functional envelope. Featuring water- and dust-resistant housings, the electric hook TD can be used in harsher environments without increasing the maintenance and servicing required. The lyre-shaped fingers allow the user to easily see what is being held for safe and accurate usage of tools and machinery. In an emergency, these hook fingers can be opened instantly by a patented safety release feature (Figure 23-11).

Another prehensor-type microprocessor-controlled TD offers a grip force of up to 32 pounds per square inch and is one of the widest opening electric TDs. This version is durably constructed with a protective coating and built-in friction-controlled wrist deviation. The grip surfaces are adjustable in all planes to allow multiple gripping and holding functions (Figure 23-12).

The electric hands and work hook-type TDs can be programmed to optimize prosthetic function. The programming systems provide the patient and the prosthetist with visual feedback of EMG signal strength and electronic adjustments on a computer screen. Once programming is complete, the patient-specific data settings are stored and can be uploaded to the specific TD after maintenance and repair. This prevents repetitive programming sessions and creates a comparative data cache for analysis of changes in muscle strength and muscle differentiation.

force of up to 24 pounds per square inch (Figure 23-10). The cylindrical grasp and palmar pinch patterns effectively handle cylindrical objects of various sizes, such as steering wheels, handlebars, control knobs, liquid containers, and many tools. Upgraded EMG processing capability enables one of these hands to respond to (myoelectric) muscle signals more than twice as quickly as standard electric hands. The sensory feedback technology and microprocessor allow the hand to react rapidly to changing situations. The automatic grasp feature of this hand monitors shear force and grip force, and automatically adjusts grip strength so that an object remains securely in the hand even when its center of gravity changes. Another microprocessor-controlled electric hand provides locking wrist flexion without the auto-grasp feature. The fingers of this hand can be opened instantly using the patented safety release feature. It is quite effective in all of the wrist positions.

One microprocessor-controlled hook-style TD combines powered pinch force with a tip-pinch grasping pattern to provide better purchase on small objects. The locking flexion wrist feature allows the wrist to

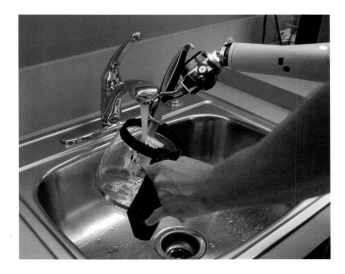

Figure 23-11. Motion Control ETD offers lyre-shaped fingers with water-resistant housings.
ETD: Electric Terminal Device
Photograph: Product image used with permission from Motion Control, Inc, Salt Lake City, Utah.

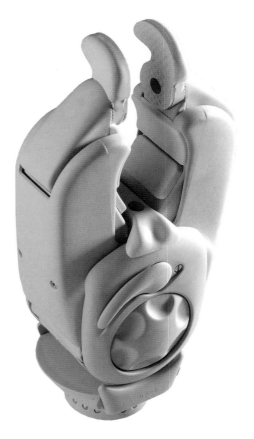

Figure 23-12. The Otto Bock Greifer provides up to 32 pounds of pinch force.
Photograph: Courtesy of Otto Bock HealthCare, Minneapolis, Minnesota.

Wrist Units

Wrist units connect the TD to the prosthesis. They are designed to position the TD for function and to provide the mechanism to interchange TDs. The appropriate selection of a wrist unit can greatly improve the functionality of a wearer by enhancing the range of TD positioning. There are essentially three capabilities of wrist units: (1) rotation (supination/pronation), (2) flexion and extension (or ulnar deviation/radial deviation), and (3) quick disconnection. Using these functions requires use of the contralateral limb or an object in the environment to manually rotate the unit unless an electric rotator is used. These three capabilities are sometimes combined into one unit. Rotation can be controlled by friction and optional locking positions. The quick disconnect ability allows wearers to easily interchange TDs based on the demands of their activities. Wrist units with flexion and extension allow the user to set the TD in some degree of flexion or extension. In many situations, a combination

of these features improves a wearer's ability to perform ADLs, vocational activities, and avocational activities by accommodating demanding positions and achieving access to midline tasks. Historically, these combination units were predominantly used for bilateral amputees. However, unilateral amputees also benefit from the use of combination wrist units that enhance the ability to perform tasks with the prosthesis and the contralateral limb simultaneously (Figure 23-13).

These combinations can be found not only on body-powered prostheses, but also on electrically powered prostheses. An electrically powered wrist offers active rotation and should be used in all situations, provided that symmetry is preserved and length considerations are addressed. In the preprosthetic treatment phase, communication of surgical considerations should include the residual limb length needed to accommodate this componentry and maintain the appropriate overall length of the prosthesis. There are several methods to actuate an electric wrist rotator, but many amputees

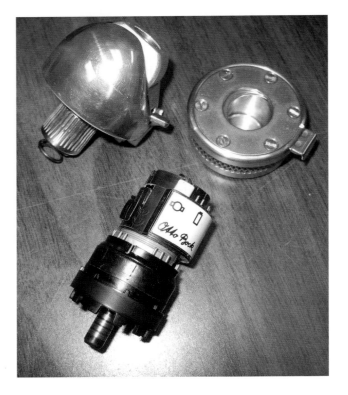

Figure 23-13. Example of wrist units: (*top right*) Hosmer Dorrance quick disconnect wrist unit; (*bottom*) Otto Bock four-channel processor and electric wrist rotator; and (*top left*) Sierra Wrist Flexion Unit.
Photograph: Product images used with permission from Hosmer Dorrance Corporation, Campbell, California, and Otto Bock HealthCare, Minneapolis, Minnesota.

prefer a method referred to as "quick-slow" or "fast access." This scheme interprets the speed of a muscle contraction in a myoelectric system and immediately directs control to the wrist or the TD, depending on the speed of contraction. Another common control scheme used to switch between wrist and TD control is co-contraction. This method requires the patient to quickly co-contract the antagonist and agonist muscle groups to alternate between control of the wrist and TD. This creates a delay and is more cognitively taxing because it requires a patient to do the following:

- co-contract to select the wrist,
- position the wrist,
- co-contract to select the TD, and
- operate the TD.

As a result, co-contraction control switching can lead to frustration and the potential to lose track of which function is active at a given point in time. One variation in co-contraction uses a method to simplify the process by creating an automatic return to TD function after a preset time has elapsed, with no EMG input to the prosthesis. Amputees tend to prefer a high level of predictability when selecting a control scheme, and our experience has shown that quick-slow schemes are typically well-accepted.

Elbow Systems

Elbow systems allow the wearer to flex or extend the elbow to a desired position and lock it when necessary. Most body-powered and electrically powered elbow systems also provide passively controlled humeral rotation (Figure 23-14).

Body-powered elbow systems require up to 4½ inches of cable excursion to fully flex the elbow and operate the TD. This significant amount of excursion often precludes use by patients with reduced strength, limited range of motion, or shorter residual limbs. By incorporating flexion assist in their elbow systems, several manufacturers mitigate the amount of force needed to flex the elbow. Spring lift assists or forearm-balancing units will help to overcome some of the weight of the TD and assist in flexing the elbow. Whenever possible, elbow flexion assists should be used to reduce not only the effort required by the wearer, but also the shear forces applied to the residual limb so as to prevent irritation and tissue breakdown. Elbow flexion assists are particularly important in hybrid systems because of the additional weight of the electric wrist and TD. At the elbow disarticulation level, various manufacturers' outside locking hinges are used in combination with lift assist mechanisms and/or automatic forearm-balancing units (Figures 23-15 and 23-16).

Electrically powered elbows provide motorized positioning of the forearm, reducing or eliminating the need for glenohumeral range of motion or strength required to operate body-powered systems. Microprocessors in the electric elbow can use a variety of control inputs, including electrodes, force sensors, touch pads, and various types of linear potentiometers. The functional advantage of an electric elbow system comes at the cost of increased weight. Therefore, it is important to factor this into preprosthetic occupational therapy training and into the patient's expectations.

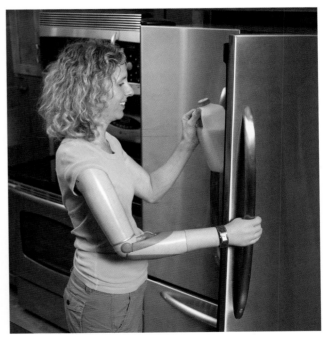

Figure 23-15. Otto Bock Dynamic Arm.
Photograph: Courtesy of Otto Bock HealthCare, Minneapolis, Minnesota.

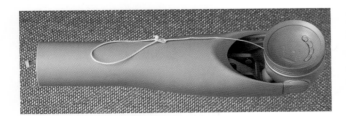

Figure 23-14. Otto Bock Ergo Arm.
Photograph: Courtesy of Otto Bock HealthCare, Minneapolis, Minnesota.

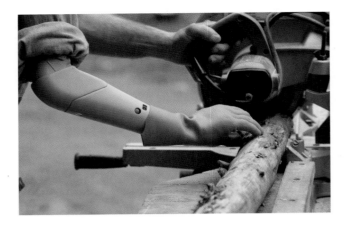

Figure 23-16. The Motion Control Utah 3 Arm.
Photograph: Courtesy of Motion Control, Inc, Salt Lake City, Utah.

Shoulder Joints

Currently, the only commercially available shoulder joints must be passively positioned for flexion, extension, abduction, and adduction. The motions of abduction and adduction are friction based, whereas flexion and extension can be either friction based or locking (Figure 23-17).

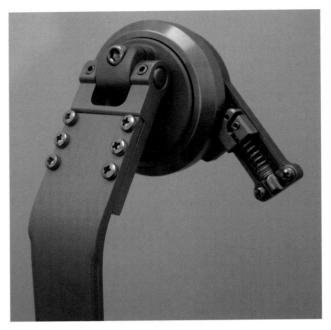

Figure 23-17. LTI Locking Shoulder Joint.
LTI: Liberating Technologies, Inc
Photograph: Product image used with permission from Liberating Technologies, Inc, Holliston, Massachusetts.

PREPROSTHETIC PHASE

Rehabilitation Team

Successful upper extremity prosthetic rehabilitation must fully address the unique constellation of clinical and functional requirements presented by the patient and is, therefore, dependent on the coordinated efforts of a multifaceted care team. This team must include, but is not limited to, the following:

- patient;
- family, friends, and significant other;
- surgeon;
- physician/physiatrist—physical medicine and rehabilitation;
- psychologist/psychiatrist;
- occupational therapist;
- physical therapist;
- case manager;
- prosthetist; and
- nursing staff.

The treatment plan must be tailored to the specific needs and goals of the injured service person. Each of the team members will contribute critical information and experience to develop a cohesive, individualized

treatment plan. During the Preprosthetic Phase, the Interim Prosthetic Phase, and the Advanced Prosthetic Phase, the prosthetist will consult with various members of the patient's rehabilitation team. The surgical team will use the prosthetist's input to identify an ideal amputation level and wound closure, and the occupational therapist will work closely with the prosthetist as the limb is prepared for prosthetic management, and the prosthetic devices are created and fit. During and following the Advanced Prosthetic Phase of initial rehabilitation, the prosthetist and other team members will work together to maintain consistent contact with the service member and address any subsequent prosthetic or medical issues.

Surgical Considerations for Optimal Prosthetic Rehabilitation

Although there are many issues for the military surgeon to consider in treating blast injuries, it is important to communicate the requirements of current prosthetic technology as they relate to residual limb length, shape, and musculature reattachment. The surgical considerations that will be described allow for optimal prosthetic rehabilitation for each level of amputation. As prosthetic technology evolves and different components are developed, surgical guidelines might require modification. Concomitant injuries might also take priority and affect the subsequent plan. The historical approach to "save as much as possible" can sometimes present difficult issues for the service person, particularly considering that residual limb length revisions may be necessary after closure so that a more functional solution for prosthetic rehabilitation can be achieved. If carefully planned in advance, surgery to close the amputation site can include any necessary length modifications and minimize the number of surgical procedures. In addition to the following general guidelines for residual limb length, muscle attachment, skeletal shaping, and soft-tissue closure, also see Chapter 8 (General Surgical Principles for the Combat Casualty With Limb Loss).

Guidelines for Residual Limb Length

The length of the residual limb can limit the prosthetic componentry options and therefore might affect functional potential. In determining the ideal length for amputation, it is essential that the surgeon and the patient understand how the individual's prosthetic options might be affected by the length of the residual limb. It should also be carefully explained that a residual limb that is too long might present complications when using a prosthesis in tight spaces or as it relates to cosmetic symmetry with the other arm/hand.

The following guidelines have proven helpful to support upper extremity prosthetic rehabilitation. For the transradial and transhumeral levels, formulas to determine optimal residual limb length have been suggested. These calculations were developed based on the sizes of an average individual and currently available mechanical and powered elbow, wrist, and TD units. In addition, patients will not use a prosthesis 100% of the time, and they might benefit from variations on these recommendations. Formulas to determine limb length for each amputation level should be developed after careful consideration of available componentry as it relates to leverage of the residual limb, both with and without a prosthesis.

Transcarpal and Transmetacarpal Levels. If at least two digits remain that are sensate and innervated (movable by patient), retain as much length as possible and minimize graft and scar tissue surface areas. If digits are insensate, lack an active range of motion, or are heavily grafted/scarred, revise the length to carpal level or styloid disarticulation, depending on the amount of graft and scar tissue present distal to the center of wrist articulation.

Styloid Level. Disarticulate at the wrist, keeping the radius, ulna, and interosseus membrane intact. A transradial-level amputation should be considered if supination and pronation are severely limited or absent secondary to injury of the forearm musculature and interosseus membrane.

Transradial Level. To determine optimal length that will accommodate current prosthetic componentry, the following steps are recommended (Figure 23-18):

1. Measure the contralateral/noninvolved limb from the lateral epicondyle to the thumb tip (with the elbow flexed at 90 degrees). This is X.
2. Subtract 8¾ inches or 22.5 cm (average length of prosthetic TD and wrist unit) from X, which will be the optimal final residual limb length for the affected side (or Y). A slightly larger value may be substituted for Y without a material decrease in functional levers.
3. Measure from the lateral epicondyle on the involved side marking the desired residual limb length (Y) determined in step 2. This should be the finished residual limb length, including soft-tissue padding. The ulna will be $^1/_4$ to $^1/_2$ inches (0.8 cm–1.25 cm) shorter than Y, and the radius will be $^1/_8$ to $^1/_4$ inches (1.25 cm–2.5 cm) shorter than overall length of the ulna.

Elbow Disarticulation Level. Disarticulation should be performed at the elbow, thus keeping the shape of the epicondyles intact.

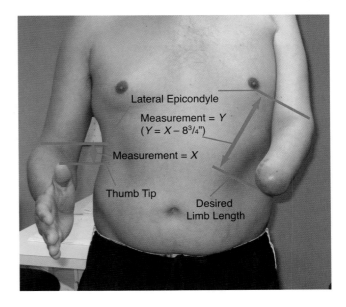

Figure 23-18. Procedure to determine preferred transradial residual limb length.

Transhumeral Level. To determine optimal limb length using current prosthetic componentry, the following steps are recommended:

1. Measure the contralateral/noninvolved limb from the acromion process to the distal olecranon (with the elbow flexed at 90 degrees). This is *X*. Subtract 5½ inches or 14 cm (the average length of the prosthetic elbow unit) from *X*, which will be the optimal final residual limb length for the affected side (or *Y*). A slightly larger value may be substituted for *Y* without a material decrease in functional levers.
2. Measure from the acromion process on the involved side marking the optimal residual limb length (*Y*) determined in step 1. This should be the finished residual limb length, including soft-tissue padding. The humerus will be $^1/_2$ to $^3/_4$ inches (1.25 cm–2.0 cm) shorter than *Y* (Figure 23-19).

Humeral Neck, Glenohumeral, and Interscapulothoracic Levels. Follow the general surgical principles for residual limb length.

Guidelines for Muscle Attachment

Myoplasty. Attaching the transected muscles to themselves or others increases the incidence of co-contraction of antagonistic muscles, thereby greatly diminishing myoelectric control potential. Myoplasty limits prosthetic options.

Myodesis. Attaching the transected muscle directly to bone creates a solid anchor for each muscle to pull against during contraction. This creates a clear and distinct EMG signal, which is useful for differentiating electromyography from multiple muscles and optimum myoelectric control potential (Table 23-6).

Guidelines for Skeletal Treatment

General surgical principles apply to the treatment of bone. The cut end of bone should not present any unnecessary sharp edges, rough prominences, or splintering (Table 23-7).

Soft-Tissue Closure/Distal Suture Line

Note these four points:

1. Finished amputation should have ¼ to ½ inches (0.8 cm–1.25 cm) of soft-tissue padding over the skeletal distal end.
2. Nerves are transected sharply under tension to prevent future formation of neuromas without negatively impacting sensation and innervation of associated muscles.
3. Distal suture/staple line should run medial/lateral when the patient's residuum is in the standard anatomical position.
4. Conical shape is preferred, with a smooth contour of the distal end taking care to eliminate or minimize both invagination of tissue and "dog ear" formation (note: dog ear usually refers to excess tissue at the ends of the skin closure

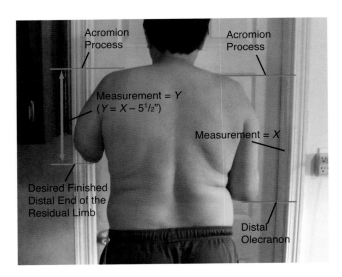

Figure 23-19. Procedure to determine preferred transhumeral residual limb length.

TABLE 23-6

GUIDELINES FOR MUSCLE ATTACHMENT

Level	Action
Transmetacarpal/transcarpal	Follow general surgical principles
Transradial Styloid disarticulation	Attach wrist flexors and extensors, and supinator and pronator muscle groups to radius and ulna
Transhumeral Elbow disarticulation	Attach biceps and triceps tendons to the humerus
Humeral neck, glenohumeral disarticulation, interscapulothoracic	Follow general surgical principles

TABLE 23-7

GUIDELINES FOR SKELETAL TREATMENT

Level	Action
Transmetacarpal/transcarpal	Follow general surgical principles
Transcarpal/transmetacarpal Styloid disarticulation	Do not bevel styloid prominence because this skeletal prominence will be used for suspension of the prosthesis
Transradial	Bevel and remove sharp edges from radius and ulna; radius should be ¼ to ½ inch (0.8 cm–1.25 cm) shorter than the ulna
Elbow disarticulation	Do not bevel epicondylar prominences because this skeletal prominence will be used for suspension of the prosthesis
Transhumeral	Bevel and remove sharp edges from the humerus
Humeral neck, genohumeral disarticulation, interscapulothoracic	Follow general surgical principles

that tend to be everted/protruding—somewhat triangular and pointed like a dog's ear).

Prosthetic Assessment and Rehabilitation Plan Formation

Once the residual limb length has been surgically established and the wound is initially closed, a comprehensive prosthetic assessment is performed. This occurs prior to suture or staple removal and is often initiated at the bedside in the intensive care unit or orthopaedic ward. The evaluation may span multiple visits to accommodate the physical, cognitive, and emotional status of the patient. Often, the initial visits are limited because the patient is heavily medicated or receiving medical attention for concomitant injuries. The prosthetic assessment includes the following:

- medical history,
- premorbid activities (vocational and avocational),
- psychosocial considerations,
- residual limb status,
- concomitant injuries, and
- patient functional requirements.

It is also important to consider the family/support system available to the patient and the potential discharge plan. The information gathered during the assessment is then used to develop a prosthetic recommendation that is used by the multidisciplinary team to create an individualized rehabilitation plan.

Patient Education

The prosthetic assessment also marks the beginning of the patient's education on prosthetic rehabilitation and the options available to him or her. Individuals who sustain blast wounds undergo myriad physical and psychological changes over the first weeks postinjury. Creating an open dialogue with service members and their families at this stage is essential to facilitate progression through the rehabilitation process. It is an opportunity to reconcile any preconceptions about prosthetic technology because exposure to popular films and media can create unrealistic prosthetic expectations. During this time, the service member and his or her family must process a significant amount of information regarding the injury, recovery, and implications for the future. Therefore, pertinent information should often be reiterated to ensure that it has been properly assimilated. Meetings with a trained peer visitor who has successfully completed prosthetic rehabilitation can also be beneficial in providing accurate information, as well as a user's perspective.

The anticipated timeline for prosthetic rehabilitation over the subsequent 12 to 18 weeks postinjury should be discussed during the assessment. Rehabilitation begins with residual limb management and preparation for prosthetic fitting, and continues beyond delivery of the definitive prostheses to the point wherein the patient is comfortable reintegrating into the community (see Interim Prosthetic Phase for level-specific protocols).

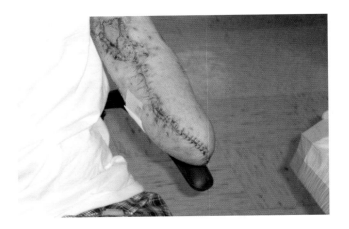

Figure 23-20. Healing residual limb.

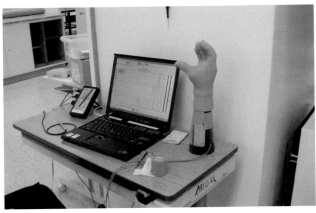

Figure 23-21. Otto Bock 757M11 MyoBoy for preprosthetic training with demonstration myoelectric hand and wrist. Photograph: Product image used with permission from Otto Bock HealthCare, Minneapolis, Minnesota.

Residual Limb Management

The first step in residual limb management is to address edema control. Blast injuries and multiple irrigations and debridements prior to wound closure can produce significant edema. Compressive dressings and garments are applied immediately following wound closure for the purpose of reducing swelling. Proper edema management using elastic bandages, presized tubular compressive fabrics, or silicone/urethane roll-on liners is necessary. Use of silicone liners has been particularly effective at edema reduction, but must not be implemented until drainage has ceased because of concerns regarding skin integrity and infection (Figure 23-20).

During the Preprosthetic Phase, the occupational therapist concentrates on desensitization, range of mo-

tion, myosite training, and limb loading in preparation for prosthetic fitting. This phase gives the prosthetics team valuable information on control schemes that are most likely to be immediately successful with the patient. This also allows the patient to develop a rapport with various members of the rehabilitation team who will be seen daily in the Interim Prosthetic Phase of rehabilitation. Finally, patients are encouraged to build confidence in their own abilities by controlling simulators and demonstration components, and working through challenging situations prior to early postoperative prosthesis (EPOP) fitting (Figure 23-21). Within 24 hours of suture and staple removal, residual limb impressions are taken to initiate the Interim Prosthetic Phase.

INTERIM PROSTHETIC PHASE

Military amputees, who are typically young and motivated, benefit from early prosthetic intervention because it offers greater independence, self-esteem, and long-term success.[18] As previously noted, the protocol established by the military healthcare system is to sequentially provide each service member with an electric or hybrid prosthesis, a body-powered prosthesis, a passive restoration prosthesis, and task-specific adaptations or prostheses. One of the goals during this stage of initial prosthetic device delivery is to minimize the time between suture removal and functional prosthetic use. Delivery of EPOP ideally occurs within 24 hours of suture removal. Often, the residual limb of these individuals presents multiple problems with healing, related to complicated suture lines, skin grafts, muscle flaps, or the presence of frag-

ments or other foreign bodies. Therefore, a myoelectric EPOP device offers the safest approach to introducing a prosthesis to the individual in a way that minimizes excessive forces on the often fragile and healing distal residuum. The electric prosthesis is well-suited for this application because it does not require a restrictive harness and gross body movements for control that can exert unwanted forces on the healing residual limb or other healing areas that would be in contact with the harness. Myoelectric control of the EPOP also offers the advantages of immediate functionality, proportional grip strength, and TD positioning at initial delivery. Prior to EPOP fitting, it is important for the patient to have developed basic myoelectric control skills in occupational therapy during the Preprosthetic Phase.

The EPOP is fit during this initial healing period

and is modified during rehabilitation until swelling is stabilized and wound closures are complete. The patient is fit with an EPOP using an expedited fitting protocol. A typical expedited fitting requires 1 to 3 days and allows the patient to begin occupational therapy with a functioning, but modifiable, device that can be used to address changes during initial rehabilitation and therapy for increased efficiency. EPOP procedures include adjustments for alignment, length, suspension, pressure distribution, functional performance, and programming of all electronics for system optimization and positioning of electrodes, batteries, access openings, and components.

The prosthetist must be prepared to accommodate the often dramatic volumetric changes in the residual limb for individuals who have sustained blast wounds. It is not uncommon during the first 4 to 8 weeks after EPOP delivery to perform multiple socket adjustments each week. A myoelectric prosthesis requires consistent skin-to-electrode contact to retain function. Therefore, it is imperative that adjustments for proper fit be performed in an expeditious manner. This is best accomplished using a thermoplastic flexible socket and rigid frame that can be modified several times during the Interim Prosthetic Phase.

EPOP methodology was developed to address military protocols for early fitting while minimizing the stresses on the healing residuum. Early in Operation Enduring Freedom and Operation Iraqi Freedom, it was found that the amount of residual limb edema was significant secondary to methods of irrigation and maintenance of open wounds prior to transferring patients to stateside medical care facilities. Many amputees had also sustained injuries to the chest wall, shoulder areas, and axillary regions that would preclude the use of a harness for control of a body-powered TD or elbow during the healing phase. Traditional immediate postoperative prosthesis (IPOP) has been bypassed because of the evolution of EPOP and because IPOP treatments cannot accommodate these rapid volume changes and preclude visual assessment of the healing limb, which is crucial immediately following closure. Closure of the amputated limb without the application of an IPOP allows the team to observe the healing wounds and begin preprosthetic therapy with shrinkers and myotraining as soon as the patient is cognitively and physically able. In preparation for the EPOP and Interim Prosthetic Phase, the surgeon is able to ensure that wound closure has matured to a point at which the mild pressures applied from a prosthetic socket that uses flexible thermoplastics against the skin can be tolerated. Fitting of the EPOP then provides the positive results of "instant gratification" and broad functional applications with minimal stress

to the healing anatomy. The ability to make significant, frequent changes to volume, alignment, componentry, and programming during the EPOP Phase allows the rehabilitation team to keep pace with the highly motivated amputee.

At the time of EPOP delivery, focus in the patient's therapy shifts to prosthetic training. When a prosthetic device is fit and delivered to a service member, thorough instruction on the system is given by the prosthetist. This instruction often takes place with the occupational therapist present so that various specifics can be noted for subsequent training sessions. Information is typically covered in a routine order, starting with donning and doffing. Common application techniques include the use of limited friction donning pull socks, evaporative moisture, or roll-on liners, as required by the design of the prosthesis. The following procedures are then taught from distal to proximal, dependent on amputation level:

- TD on-off and positioning;
- wrist controls;
- elbow on-off and lock-unlock;
- shoulder joint movements, lock-unlock;
- harness donning, doffing, and adjustment; and
- battery insertion, charging and care.

These functions are later practiced in occupational therapy. It is also necessary to review these functions periodically as the use of multiple prostheses and the interchangeability of TDs require slight variations in control. Consistent communication between prosthetist and occupational therapist is indispensable to ensure that any changes that impact the fit or programming of the prosthesis are immediately addressed. This relationship continues throughout the rehabilitation process to facilitate problem-solving as the patient is challenged to higher degrees.

There will come a time when the wounds have adequately healed and can sustain more aggressive pressures from the prosthetic socket interface. At this point, a transition is made from the EPOP approach to a preparatory version of the prosthesis. This preparatory phase still retains the adaptability of the EPOP for ongoing volume changes, but allows the socket to become tighter for improved suspension, electrode contact, and overall control of the prosthesis in space. By this time, the alignment, length, and basic structure should be well defined. The preparatory prosthesis provides the rehabilitation team with the opportunity to test the prosthesis and its components in real-world applications outside the clinic setting. Further modifications in volume, alignment, length, and structure can be made easily during this phase as the team prepares to progress to the definitive prosthesis (Figure 23-22).

Once the residual limb has reached volumetric stabilization, usually within 8 to 14 weeks after suture or staple removal, fabrication of the definitive prostheses begins. A goal for this stage is to ensure that at no point is the user left without a prosthesis. To accomplish this, it is often necessary to fabricate the definitive body-powered device prior to fabrication of the definitive myoelectric. Typically, both definitive devices are delivered within 7 to 10 days of each other.

Completion of the definitive silicone restoration/passive prosthesis and silicone restoration covering for the electric hand should coincide approximately with the fitting of the definitive electric and body-powered devices. This process typically takes 12 to 16 weeks from first impressions to definitive prosthesis. These remarkably life-like replications are custom painted on the inside of a clear silicone glove that is fabricated using a sculpted reversal of the amputee's sound limb. An impression of the sound side (if present) is taken in the Preprosthetic Phase. In bilateral upper extremity loss, the patient will often choose a family member as a model or even detailed photos of their own hands prior to the injury from which the artists can sculpt the restoration (Figure 23-23).

Evaluation for task-specific devices to support the service member's vocational and avocational interests occurs throughout the rehabilitation process. Not only are individuals returning to preinjury pursuits but also, through programs sponsored for wounded service members, they are developing new interests and challenges with their prosthetic devices. As described previously, this patient population is driven, competitive, and willing to test the limits of current prosthetic technology to reach their goals.

It is important to teach service members to perform

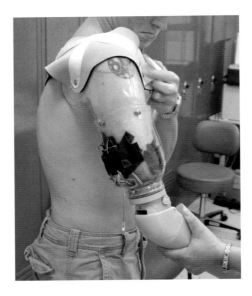

Figure 23-22. Preparatory transhumeral-level electric prosthesis.
Photograph: Prosthesis provided by Advanced Arm Dynamics, Inc, Redondo Beach, California.

basic maintenance on the various prostheses that they have received. Simple tasks (eg, cleaning, minor electrode adjustment, and cable and harness servicing) can be taught during the Interim Prosthetic Phase and reinforced in therapy as part of the treatment protocols. Service members are also taught to describe problems with their prostheses in a way that allows the prosthetist to diagnose and repair items that have broken or failed. In cases in which the service member has returned to active duty or is not near a service facility, the ability to describe a problem accurately will often help the rehabilitation team determine whether the service member should send a prosthesis to the center

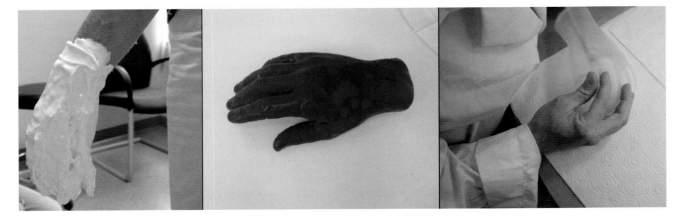

Figure 23-23. Steps in the silicone restoration process: (*left*) impression, (*center*) wax model, and (*right*) custom painting.

or directly to a component manufacturer for diagnosis and repair. This is especially important for the service member who requires a rapid turn-around of repairs because of essential job duties, whether military or civilian in nature.

The following section will address the specific and unique prosthetic requirements for each upper limb amputation level. Level-specific timelines, socket designs, components, and special considerations are discussed.

Level-Specific Recommendations

Finger, Thumb, and Partial Hand Amputations

Finger, thumb, and partial hand amputations comprise a portion of the military amputee population. Current prosthetic treatment approaches have been to create silicone restorations and to explore other mechanical and powered products. Typically, silicone restoration gives the service member some limited function for opposition against any remaining digits. The cosmetic nature of the restoration also gives the service member the appearance of wholeness in public, thus less attention is drawn to the injury. There have been some creative solutions to provide mechanical and powered function for finger and thumb prostheses. The current powered units are disadvantaged by the bulk of battery and controller shapes, as well as by the fragile nature of the components themselves. There are, however, some promising advances being made in this realm. A wide variety of task-specific adaptations for

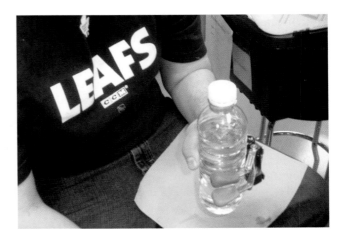

Figure 23-25. Advanced Arm Dynamics powered fingers. Photograph: Prosthesis provided by Advanced Arm Dynamics, Redondo Beach, Inc, California.

both the environment and a prosthesis have also been created to facilitate functioning for this population in ADLs, vocational activities, and avocational activities (Figures 23-24 to 23-26).

Styloid Disarticulation

The styloid disarticulation level has the benefit of an intact distal radial-ulnar joint, which preserves pronation and supination. Generally, the length of the residual limb will preclude the use of an electric wrist rotator or quick disconnect-style wrist unit to maintain length symmetry between the electric prosthesis and the noninjured limb. Because a quick disconnect wrist unit cannot be used, separate electric prostheses must

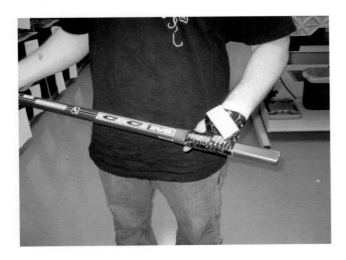

Figure 23-24. Custom-fabricated, task-specific hockey prosthesis.
Photograph: Prosthesis provided by Advanced Arm Dynamics, Inc, Redondo Beach, California.

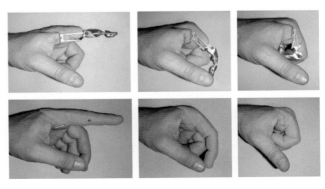

Figure 23-26. (*Top*) Body-powered X-Finger without silicone covering and (*bottom*) body-powered X-Finger with silicone covering (patent pending).
Photographs: Courtesy of Didrick Medical, Inc, Naples, Florida.

be fabricated for each TD. Without electric wrist rotation, it is imperative for the socket to allow anatomical rotation. This is best achieved through the use of a self-suspending suction socket that terminates distal to the olecranon and epicondyles. Suction is achieved through purchase over the styloids, with donning aided by the use of an evaporative moisture technique. In the case of a styloid-level, body-powered prosthesis—with the socket design's inherent suspension qualities—most often a figure-of-nine harness is used for control of the TD (Figure 23-27). There are occasions when heavy lifting will require an auxiliary figure-of-eight, with triceps cuff and flexible hinges to assist in load bearing. There are also cases in which a silicone suspension sleeve worn over the outside of the prosthesis has proven useful. Significant challenges exist if the styloid-level amputee lacks the ability to supinate and pronate or if the prominence of the styloids is insufficient to achieve suspension and rotational control. Therefore, it is important for the styloid disarticulation-level amputee to be carefully evaluated for appropriate suspension in the prosthetic design (Table 23-8).

Transradial Amputations

Transradial amputations are the most common level for upper extremity amputations proximal to the hand. Absence of the styloids creates the need for additional suspensory elements in the design of the prosthesis. This is most commonly achieved through self-suspending socket designs that use the bony anatomy of the elbow and proximal forearm contours to suspend the

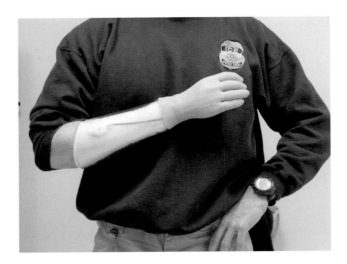

Figure 23-27. Preparatory styloid-level myoelectric prosthesis.
Photograph: Prosthesis provided by Advanced Arm Dynamics, Inc, Redondo Beach, California.

prosthesis. The surgical considerations covered earlier in this chapter define the optimal length of transradial level residual limb for use of componentry. Because of the shorter radius and ulna and damage to the interosseus membrane, anatomical pronation and supination are absent. To compensate for this deficiency, active or passive rotation must be provided for the amputee to preposition the TD.

For the electric prosthesis, an anatomically suspended dynamic muscle-contoured interface design—utilizing compression anterior to the epicondyles and superior to the olecranon and through the cubital fold—is often used. There are specific contours to allow hypertrophy of the remaining musculature in the residual limb. This socket design provides the best methodology to ensure superior suspension and skin to electrode contact throughout the range of motion.[19] To enhance comfort and range of motion, a window (referred to as a ¾ modification) can be removed from the socket about the olecranon. Residual limbs that are not suited for this type of prosthetic interface can, in some cases, be treated with silicone roll-on liners. Production and custom versions of these liners can be considered for short or irregularly shaped limbs.

Patients may prefer to use the same socket design for all of their prostheses. When the dynamic muscle-contoured socket is preferred, it is typically used with a figure-of-nine harness in the body-powered application. It is more common, however, to incorporate a silicone/urethane suction liner with a pin-lock system for the body-powered prosthesis. A figure-of-nine harness can also be used with this socket design, although there are occasions when heavy lifting will require an auxiliary figure-of-eight harness with triceps cuff and flexible hinges to assist in load bearing (Table 23-9).

Elbow Disarticulations

Amputations at the elbow disarticulation level have a unique advantage for suspension and natural humeral rotation countered by the loss of any powered prosthetic elbow options. The remaining humeral epicondyles can be used to achieve anatomical/suction suspension. Suction is achieved through purchase over the epicondyles, with donning aided by the use of an evaporative moisture technique or a reduced friction pull sock. Suspension is achieved by a combination of a bony lock proximal to the condyles and suction, generally eliminating the need for an auxiliary suspension harness. In the case of an elbow disarticulation-level, body-powered prosthesis with the socket design's inherent suspension qualities, a figure-of-eight harness is most often used for control of the elbow, elbow

TABLE 23-8

PROSTHETIC RECOMMENDATIONS FOR THE STYLOID DISARTICULATION LEVEL

Phase	Styloid Level
1	**EPOP Electric*** Flexible thermoplastic inner socket, one-way mini-expulsion valve, rigid thermoplastic frame Anatomically contoured, self-suspending suction/evaporative moisture donning technique Myoelectric control, dual-site with two viable EMG outputs (other control options are used for patients who do not have two myo-sites) EPOP used until the residual limb can sustain greater pressures from the tighter fitting preparatory prosthesis Due to the lack of quick disconnect capability, terminal devices must be associated with separate sockets and frames, ie, microprocessor-controlled hand prosthesis, microprocessor-controlled powered prehensor prosthesis, microprocessor-controlled work hook prosthesis
2	**Preparatory Electric*** Similar fabrication as EPOP with more aggressive suspension design Multiple socket adjustments/replacements continue until residual limb volume has stabilized
3	**Body-Powered** Fit concurrent with definitive fabrication of electric prosthesis Flexible thermoplastic inner socket, one-way mini-expulsion valve, carbon fiber frame Anatomically contoured, self-suspending suction/evaporative moisture donning technique Titanium VO hook, VO hand, titanium VC hook, stainless-steel quick disconnect locking wrist, limited friction cable
4	**Definitive Electric*** Flexible thermoplastic inner socket, one-way mini-expulsion valve, carbon fiber frame Anatomically contoured, self-suspending suction/evaporative moisture donning technique
5	**Silicone Passive** Fit and deliver definitive custom silicone passive prosthesis with suction suspension
6	**Evaluate for Task-Specific Needs**

EMG: electromyographic
EPOP: early postoperative prosthesis
VC: voluntary closing
VO: voluntary opening
*Multiple socket/frames required because of a lack of quick disconnect capability: microprocessor-controlled hand prosthesis; microprocessor-controlled powered prehensor prosthesis; and microprocessor-controlled work hook prosthesis.

lock, and TD. A shoulder saddle and chest strap can be integrated to assist with load bearing and comfort as needed, and is commonly used for the hybrid prosthesis as well (Figure 23-28).

The lack of space for a traditional elbow unit is a challenge at this level of amputation. An elbow unit will typically provide humeral rotation through a turntable mechanism, but the outside locking hinges required for this level do not. Additionally, if the elbow disarticulation-level amputee lacks sufficient prominence of the humeral epicondyles, suspension and rotational control are difficult to achieve anatomically. An externally powered prosthesis at the elbow disarticulation level is, therefore, a hybrid approach because there is insufficient room for an electric prosthetic elbow. Utilization of locking hinges limits the number of elbow-locking positions and often adds significant

medial-lateral width, which can be problematic with use of long-sleeved clothing. Specifically, patients have difficulty finding jackets and outerwear that fit over the prosthesis (Table 23-10).

Transhumeral Amputations

At this level of amputation, an elbow system is required. Although there are many elbow systems available, they can be broadly categorized as either mechanical or electrical (Figure 23-29).

A mechanical elbow system requires the amputee to use gross body motions of the shoulder, creating excursion through the harness system to flex the elbow. Electric elbow units provide powered flexion with myoelectric, linear potentiometer, linear transducer, force-sensing resistor, or switch control.

TABLE 23-9

PROSTHETIC RECOMMENDATIONS FOR THE TRANSRADIAL LEVEL

Phase	Transradial Level
1	**EPOP Electric**
	Flexible thermoplastic inner socket, rigid thermoplastic frame
	Anatomically contoured self-suspension with reduced friction donning sock technique, dynamic muscle-contoured interface with ¾ modification for transradial level
	Myoelectric control, dual-site, TD/electric wrist rotator switching (other control options are used for patients who do not have two myo-sites)
	Multiple interchangeable TDs through quick disconnect collar: microprocessor-controlled hand; microprocessor-controlled prehensor; microprocessor-controlled work hook with locking wrist flexion
	EPOP used until the residual limb can sustain greater pressures from the tighter fitting preparatory prosthesis
2	**Preparatory Electric**
	Similar fabrication as EPOP with more aggressive suspension design
	Multiple socket adjustments/replacements continue until residual limb volume has stabilized
3	**Body-Powered**
	Fit concurrent with definitive fabrication of electric prosthesis
	Flexible thermoplastic inner socket, carbon fiber frame
	Anatomically contoured self-suspension with reduced friction donning sock technique, dynamic muscle-contoured interface with ¾ modification for transradial level
	OR
	Silicone suction suspension using roll-on liner with pin-lock system
	Titanium hook, VO hand, titanium VC hook, stainless-steel quick disconnect locking wrist, limited friction cable (with wrist flexion unit for bilateral)
	Traditional flexible hinges/triceps cuff and figure-of-eight harness applied for load-bearing applications
4	**Definitive Electric**
	Flexible thermoplastic inner socket, carbon fiber frame
	Anatomically contoured self-suspension with reduced friction donning sock technique, dynamic muscle-contoured interface with ¾ modification for transradial level
5	**Silicone Passive**
	Fit and deliver definitive custom silicone passive prosthesis with suction suspension
6	**Evaluate for Task-Specific Needs**

EPOP: early postoperative prosthesis
TD: terminal device
VC: voluntary closing
VO: voluntary opening

Both electric and mechanical units provide passive humeral rotation. Socket design is critical and must allow as much range of motion of the glenohumeral joint as possible while eliminating any socket movement on the residuum. This can be achieved by using a dynamic, muscle-contoured socket that does not encapsulate the shoulder girdle.[20] Suspension of the electric prosthesis is achieved most often with suction suspension and an auxiliary dynamic shoulder saddle and chest strap. Suspension for the body-powered prosthesis can be accomplished in a variety of ways,

including a silicone suction and pin-lock system, a figure-of-eight harness and Bowden cable system, or a system similar to that used with the electric design (Figure 23-30).

It is important to note that the force required to flex the mechanical elbow of a body-powered transhumeral-level prosthesis increases significantly, with only a small additional weight in the TD. Therefore, the amputee's residual limb must be carefully evaluated for readiness to accept the increased forces inherent in a body-powered design (Table 23-11).

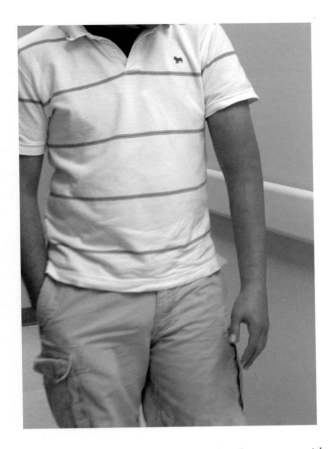

Figure 23-28. Elbow disarticulation-level amputee with custom silicone restoration.
Photograph: Prosthesis provided by Advanced Arm Dynamics, Inc, Redondo Beach, California.

Humeral Neck, Glenohumeral Disarticulation, and Interscapulothoracic Amputations

Humeral neck, glenohumeral disarticulation, and interscapulothoracic amputations present the most difficult challenges for upper extremity prosthetic rehabilitation. At these amputation levels, there is little if any lever arm available to produce sufficient excursion for control of a body-powered prosthesis. Humeral neck amputations that do not leave sufficient humeral length to control a prosthesis must be fit in the same manner as a complete disarticulation of the glenohumeral joint. Scapular abduction and shoulder elevation can be captured to provide some of the control motions required, but this is often insufficient to provide the excursion required to flex the body-powered elbow joint or open the TD fully. Glenohumeral abduction, flexion, and extension are achieved using a prosthetic shoulder joint. Shoulder joints provide friction-resisted passive abduction/

adduction and flexion/extension. Some shoulder joints permit multiple locking positions in the flexion-extension plane. This feature is particularly useful to enable patients to position the TD when operating the prosthesis over their heads.

Stability of the socket on a patient of this level is critical because slight movements between torso and socket are magnified into large motions at the TD. Myoelectrically controlled prostheses require consistent skin-to-electrode contact that is difficult, if not impossible, to achieve when the socket lacks stability. An infraclavicular interface design is the best methodology to provide enhanced stability while reducing surface area coverage, therefore resulting in a lighter weight prosthesis that reduces heat buildup. The infraclavicular design compresses anteriorly through the delto-pectoral region, posteriorly through the spine of the scapula, and inferiorly along the intercostal region.[21] The infraclavicular design is stabilized using a custom synthetic elastic harness.

The elbow joints used in these prostheses are the same as the units used in transhumeral prostheses and are controlled in similar ways. However, as noted previously, many patients have difficulty in achieving sufficient cable excursion to fully operate a body-powered prosthesis at this level. Adaptive devices designed to assist with this limitation include excursion amplifiers, elbow lift assists, and nudge control switches. Often, the prosthetist will resort to powered systems at this level for improved control and functional outcome (Table 23-12).

Bilateral Considerations

Bilateral amputees face a much more difficult rehabilitation process to become fully independent. The amputee does not have a sound limb to rely on or to provide fine prehension and sensory feedback. This creates an immediate need to learn how to operate prostheses to accomplish virtually all ADLs. Although the challenge is greater for bilateral amputees, they generally are also the most motivated because they rarely achieve full independence without mastering the use of prostheses.

The design of the prostheses is crucial because it must allow the patient to perform all ADLs as independently as possible. There is a tendency for the longer residual limb to become dominant in the bilateral amputee, and selecting the appropriate control scheme and prosthetic design for the now dominant side is critical for functionality. Design of the prostheses must allow the patient to bring the TDs to midline and operate them in that position. To achieve this positioning, the prosthetic

TABLE 23-10

PROSTHETIC RECOMMENDATIONS FOR THE ELBOW DISARTICULATION LEVEL

Phase	Elbow Disarticulation Level
1	**EPOP Hybrid** Flexible thermoplastic inner socket, one-way removable expulsion valve, rigid thermoplastic frame, outside locking hinges Anatomically contoured self-suspension (if epicondyles are present) with reduced friction donning sock technique or evaporative moisture technique Shoulder saddle/chest strap harness Myoelectric control, dual-site, TD/electric wrist rotator switching (other control options are used for patients who do not have two myo-sites) Multiple interchangeable TDs through quick disconnect collar: microprocessor-controlled hand; microprocessor-controlled prehensor; and microprocessor-controlled work hook with locking wrist flexion EPOP used until the residual limb can sustain greater pressures from the tighter fitting preparatory prosthesis
2	**Preparatory Hybrid** Similar fabrication as EPOP with more aggressive suspension design Multiple socket adjustments/replacements continue until residual limb volume has stabilized
3	**Body-Powered** Fit concurrent with definitive fabrication of electric prosthesis Flexible thermoplastic inner socket, one-way removable expulsion valve, carbon fiber frame, outside locking hinges Anatomically contoured self-suspension (if epicondyles are present) with reduced friction donning sock technique or evaporative moisture technique Shoulder saddle/chest strap harness Titanium VO hook, VO hand, stainless-steel quick disconnect locking wrist, limited friction cable, wrist flexion unit
4	**Definitive Hybrid** Flexible thermoplastic inner socket, one-way removable expulsion valve, carbon fiber frame, outside locking hinges Anatomically contoured self-suspension (if epicondyles are present) with reduced friction donning sock technique or evaporative moisture technique Shoulder saddle/chest strap harness
5	**Silicone Passive** Fit and deliver definitive custom silicone passive prosthesis with suction suspension
6	**Evaluate for Task-Specific Needs**

EPOP: early postoperative prosthesis
TD: terminal device
VO: voluntary opening

components may be angulated in relationship to the socket, creating preflexion for the TD. Flexion wrist units also improve midline accessibility by bringing the TD toward the head and mouth, which is essential for feeding and grooming activities. Many bilateral patients prefer a myoelectric prosthesis with an electric wrist rotator on at least one side for independent prepositioning of the TD. The body-powered prosthetic wrist unit will require manual positioning of the TD using the environment or another aspect of the body.

Bilateral amputees will also face challenges in donning and doffing their prostheses because they do not have a sound side to aid in the donning of the prosthesis. Rather, they must use their residual limbs to help position the prostheses to be donned. In the case of higher level amputations, it is often helpful to supply a donning stand or tree. The stand provides a place to store the prostheses while not being worn and to position one or both prostheses for donning. For prostheses that require a reduced friction donning

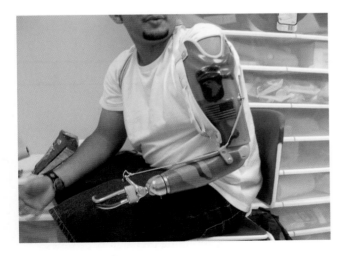

Figure 23-29. Transhumeral-level amputee wearing a definitive, body-powered prosthesis.
Photograph: Prosthesis provided by Advanced Arm Dynamics, Inc, Redondo Beach, California.

sock, the patient will often use his or her lower extremity to assist in pulling the limb into the socket.

When fitting an electric prosthesis, there are some additional componentry options that require consideration. Bilateral patients often prefer internal battery systems because they do not have to remove and replace the battery—a task requiring a higher degree of dexterity. The internal battery system allows the amputee to simply plug the prosthesis into the charger without removing a battery. When removable batteries are used, it can be beneficial to add on/off or remote power switches to the prostheses. Power switches enable the patient to turn the prosthesis off without having to remove a battery. As previously described, electric wrist rotators offer enhanced function by allowing efficient prepositioning of the TD and should be included as often as possible. Wrist flexion units should also be considered whenever there is room (Figure 23-31).

Sometimes the right and left backup prostheses are harnessed independently for use of one or both prostheses as desired by the patient. This allows for maximum flexibility in combining different types of prostheses, including electric and body-powered devices, as well as use of only one prosthesis at a time. For the combat amputee who often has concomitant injuries, both residual limbs may not be ready for prosthetic intervention at the same time. By harnessing the prostheses independently, the patient may begin prosthetic rehabilitation at the earliest opportunity. Conversely, at higher amputation levels, including

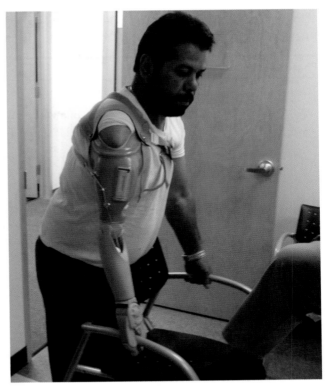

Figure 23-30. Transhumeral-level amputee wearing a hybrid prosthesis with myoelectric wrist and TD and body-powered elbow unit.
TD: terminal device
Photograph: Prosthesis provided by Advanced Arm Dynamics, Inc, Redondo Beach, California.

bilateral humeral neck or glenohumeral disarticulation levels, amputees may benefit from a socket and harness design that is integrated to facilitate donning, doffing, and suspension. This integration often creates a blending of prosthetic devices and harnessing that is donned and doffed much like a shirt or coat would be, often with the aid of a donning stand or dressing tree.

It is important to include input from members of the interdisciplinary team to design or recommend a variety of assistive devices and modifications to adapt the environment of the bilateral patient for maximum functional independence. It is not unusual to fabricate or provide a custom prosthesis for a specific ADL. An example would be a prosthesis designed specifically for bathing. Home, workplace, and vehicular adaptations are commonly used to promote function and independence in a variety of activities both with and without the use of the prostheses. Complete independence becomes more challenging at higher levels of amputations. Refer to Chapter 18 (Occupational

TABLE 23-11

PROSTHETIC RECOMMENDATIONS FOR THE TRANSHUMERAL LEVEL

Phase	Transhumeral Level
1	**EPOP Electric** Flexible thermoplastic inner socket, one-way removable expulsion valve, rigid thermoplastic frame Anatomically contoured interface with reduced friction donning sock technique Shoulder saddle/chest strap harness Microprocessor-controlled electric elbow unit; linear transducer control of elbow allows simultaneous control with myoelectric TDs or wrist rotator Myoelectric control, dual-site, TD/electric wrist rotator switching (other control options are used for patients who do not have two myo-sites) Multiple interchangeable TDs through quick disconnect collar: microprocessor-controlled hand; microprocessor-controlled prehensor; and microprocessor-controlled work hook with locking wrist flexion EPOP used until the residual limb can sustain greater pressures from the tighter fitting preparatory prosthesis
2	**Preparatory Electric** Similar fabrication as EPOP with more aggressive suspension design Multiple socket adjustments/replacements continue until residual limb volume has stabilized
3	**Body-Powered** Fit concurrent with definitive fabrication of electric prosthesis Flexible thermoplastic inner socket, one-way removable expulsion valve, carbon fiber frame Anatomically contoured interface with reduced friction donning sock technique Shoulder saddle/chest-strap harness Lift-assist enhanced elbow unit Titanium VO hook, VO hand, stainless-steel quick disconnect locking wrist, limited friction cable, wrist flexion unit
4	**Definitive Electric** Flexible thermoplastic inner socket, one-way removable expulsion valve, carbon fiber frame Anatomically contoured interface with reduced friction donning sock technique Shoulder saddle/chest strap harness
5	**Silicone Passive** Fit and deliver definitive custom silicone passive prosthesis with suction suspension or skin traction suspension
6	**Evaluate for Task-Specific Needs**

EPOP: early postoperative prosthesis
TD: terminal device
VO: voluntary opening

Therapy for the Polytrauma Casualty) for specific recommendations regarding therapeutic techniques and modifications for rehabilitation of the bilateral amputee.

Concomitant Considerations

Combat-wounded service members sustaining amputations often have concomitant injuries that can complicate rehabilitation. The following section describes some of the challenges encountered. See Chapter 1 (Developing a System of Care for the Combat Amputee) and Chapter 10 (Medical Issues) for more details.

Loss of Sight

The loss of sight in one or both eyes can significantly challenge a patient's ability to use a prosthesis. In the case of total blindness, the patient cannot use visual feedback that compensates for limited sensory feedback of prosthetic devices to develop prosthetic control skills. Typically, an amputee can observe an object being grasped and/or deformed by the TD and create an impression of the grip force being applied. At the transhumeral level or above, learning to operate an elbow system is also complicated by visual impairment

TABLE 23-12

PROSTHETIC RECOMMENDAITONS FOR THE HUMERAL NECK, GLENOHUMERAL DISARTICU-LATION, AND INTERSCAPULOTHORACIC LEVELS

Phase	Humeral Neck, Glenohumeral Disarticulation, Interscapulothoracic
1	**EPOP Electric** Flexible thermoplastic inner socket, rigid thermoplastic frame Infraclavicular interface Custom synthetic elastic harness Microprocessor-controlled electric elbow unit; linear transducer control of elbow allows simultaneous control with myoelectric TDs or wrist rotator Myoelectric control, dual-site, TD/electric wrist rotator switching (other control options are used for patients who do not have two myo-sites) Multiple interchangeable TDs through quick disconnect collar: microprocessor-controlled hand; microprocessor-controlled prehensor; and microprocessor-controlled work hook with locking wrist flexion EPOP used until the residual limb can sustain greater pressures from the tighter fitting preparatory prosthesis
2	**Preparatory Electric** Similar fabrication as EPOP with more aggressive suspension design Multiple socket adjustments/replacements continue until residual limb volume has stabilized
3	**Hybrid Prosthesis** Fit concurrent with definitive fabrication of electric prosthesis Flexible thermoplastic inner socket, carbon fiber frame Infraclavicular interface Custom synthetic elastic harness Lift assist-enhanced elbow unit Myoelectric control dual-site, TD/electric wrist rotator switching Multiple interchangeable TDs through quick disconnect collar: microprocessor-controlled hand; microprocessor-controlled prehensor; and microprocessor-controlled work hook with locking wrist flexion
4	**Definitive Electric** Flexible thermoplastic inner socket, carbon fiber frame Infraclavicular interface Custom synthetic elastic harness
5	**Silicone Passive** Fit and deliver definitive custom silicone passive prosthesis with suction suspension or skin traction suspension
6	**Evaluate for Task-Specific Needs**

EPOP: early postoperative prosthesis
TD: terminal device

because it is difficult to ascertain the position of the forearm without visual confirmation. Therefore, it may be necessary to provide additional training on creating feedback through environmental awareness techniques or the use of other body surfaces for proprioception.

Loss of Hearing

Many electrically powered prostheses provide auditory or vibratory feedback for mode changes and low battery warning. Amputees report that, with experience, they learn to use the sounds and/or vibrations produced by the motors of the elbow, wrist rotators, and TDs to provide positional feedback. Whereas both of these techniques take time to learn, they can develop into viable feedback. Auditory feedback may not work for the amputee with hearing loss; but, if vibratory feedback is strong enough to be noticed, it can assist. Generally the amputee with hearing loss, if vision is not affected, will rely on visual feedback for prosthesis position and function.

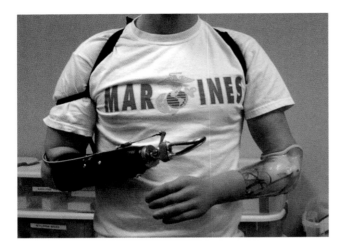

Figure 23-31. Bilateral upper limb amputee with right styloid-level body-powered prosthesis and left transradial-level myoelectric prosthesis.
Photograph: Prosthesis provided by Advanced Arm Dynamics, Inc, Redondo Beach, California.

Traumatic Brain Injury

It is not uncommon for a blast exposure to result in some level of TBI. Manifestations of TBI are diverse and individually unique based on the area of the brain that is affected. Some symptoms may include personality changes, loss of attention, changes in processing skills, changes in motor function, and frustration intolerance. Expeditious diagnosis of brain injury will allow more effective formulation of the individualized prosthetic and therapeutic rehabilitation plan. This may take the form of specific therapies for information processing, speech, motor control, and behavior modification. Sometimes a center specializing in TBI will be accessed prior to or during the other phases of rehabilitation. Depending on the outcome of more intensive treatments, some severe TBI amputees have successfully reintegrated into the prosthetic rehabilitation setting during or after TBI-specific treatment. It is useful to consider activating and training for one prosthetic component at a time to reduce frustration and encourage repetitive pattern formations. Introducing all of the possible functions of a given prosthesis in one visit may be overwhelming for a patient who has suffered TBI.

Lower Extremity Injury/Loss

Impaired lower extremity function or lower extremity amputation places further demands on the upper extremities for both stability and mobility needs. For amputees sustaining both upper and lower extremity amputations, gait training with a lower extremity prosthesis often requires the upper extremity prosthesis to be fit for safe balance with walking aids. Even those amputees who choose to wheelchair ambulate for a time will often benefit from the assistance of the upper extremity prosthesis to assist in propelling and controlling the manual or powered wheelchair. An upper extremity prosthesis is also useful for donning and doffing a lower extremity prosthesis (Figure 23-32).

Burns/Grafting

Thermal damage to the skin may require grafting and result in significant scar formation. Loss or change of the skin integrity creates range of motion and socket interface tolerance challenges. Silicone or urethane liners are often used to provide a protective barrier between the sensitive healing skin and the prosthetic

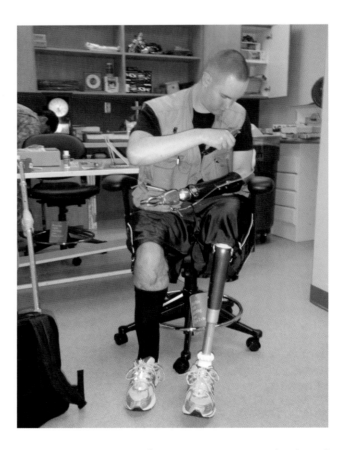

Figure 23-32. Patient with concomitant injuries (unilateral transfemoral-level and styloid-level amputations and shrapnel injuries to the right leg).
Photograph: Prosthesis provided by Advanced Arm Dynamics, Inc, Redondo Beach, California.

and external environment. Caution should be used with these liners if the wounds are open. These liners can trap bacteria and moisture, thus creating a breeding ground for infection that negatively impacts healing graft and scar tissue. Specific occupational therapy modalities for this amputee population may include ultrasound, massage, adherent scar treatments, and graft integrity management (Figure 23-33).

ADVANCED PROSTHETIC PHASE

Team members, including the patient, work together to formulate and execute a comprehensive rehabilitation plan beginning with the patient assessment and concluding with a long-term follow-up plan. Careful coordination and timing of the provision of services among team members result in seamless rehabilitation. Successful prosthetic intervention, combined with therapy protocols, contributes to the highest level of success for all amputation levels. When a rehabilitation plan is carefully executed as detailed in this chapter, it is imperative that functional gains and independence are not lost to follow-up.

Advanced prosthetic care is initiated after all definitive prostheses have been provided to the individual. Traditionally, this has been the end of initial prosthetic intervention; however, given our experience with service members rapidly returning to their previous lifestyles or attempting new vocational and avocational goals, advanced prosthetic protocols must be initiated sooner during the rehabilitation process. It is recommended that each service member be assigned a case manager or patient care coordinator who should contact the patient on a regular basis to ascertain his or her satisfaction with prosthetic function, fit, and overall condition. Specific issues that must be addressed include the following:

- volumetric changes resulting from residual limb maturation and/or weight fluctuation;
- repair or replacement of worn components;
- availability of new technology, as indicated for improved function;
- ongoing needs for therapeutic intervention; and
- new vocational and avocational requirements (Figure 23-34).

Advanced Prosthetic Phase Considerations

Residual Limb Stabilization

Because of the nature of the blast wound, and the progressive care model implemented by the military following wound closure, the amputee's residual limb is often extremely edematous. Throughout the Preprosthetic and Interim Prosthetic Phases, significant focus is therefore placed on reducing residual limb edema. Once residual limb edema stabilizes and the muscles cease to atrophy, the patient is ready to receive the definitive versions of the prostheses. After prolonged use of the definitive prostheses and full reintegration back into an active lifestyle with resolution of concomitant injuries, it is not uncommon for the muscles in the residual limb to hypertrophy. This is particularly notable in the myoelectric system, as prolonged use of EMG control results in muscle hypertrophy. The patient is also likely to gain weight as he or she returns to a normal diet, further changing residual limb size. Consistent communication with the service member following the delivery of the definitive prostheses is essential to ensure that volume changes secondary to hypertrophy or weight gain can be addressed in a timely manner. It is therefore

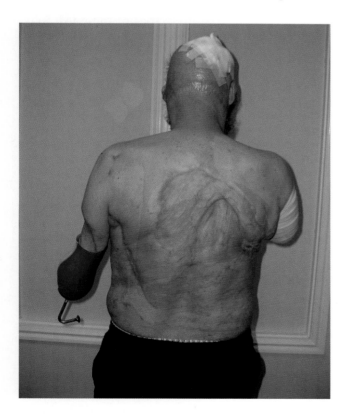

Figure 23-33. Patient with burn scar.

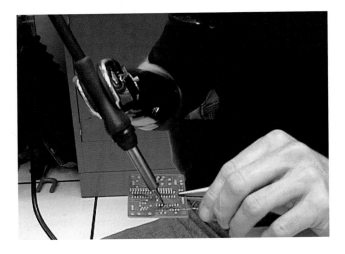

Figure 23-34. Advanced skills using a prosthesis.

important for the service member to have access to timely prosthetic care. The patient care coordinator should be able to arrange care in an expeditious manner so that prosthetic use is not interrupted. Significant lapses in care may lead to discontinuing prosthetic use because of comfort and control problems.

Self-Selection

The military model provides amputees with electric/hybrid, body-powered, and passive prostheses. Thorough training is absolutely essential to successful use of all three prostheses. Once competency has been reached, it is common for the service member to select which prosthesis will be used for certain activities. Often, the service member will alternate use of all three prostheses to meet the functional demands of daily life. Each amputee is unique, and it is not possible, nor is it prudent, to try to predict which single device will meet each amputee's current and evolving needs. Should an amputee self-select one type of prosthesis for a majority of activities, provision of a backup prosthesis should be considered to prevent discontinuation of prosthetic use when regular maintenance is required.

Challenges to Rehabilitation

Interruptions to the Rehabilitation Process

Prosthetic rehabilitation of the military amputee is often challenged by various interruptions. These interruptions may include convalescent leave, wound breakdown because of graft failure or infection, and the frequent need of additional surgeries to the residual limb or for other comorbid injuries. Additionally, problems such as the formation of heterotopic ossification (HO) or migrating retained fragments within the limb may impair prosthetic training. Concomitant injuries may take precedence over prosthetic interventions and delay rehabilitation until they are adequately resolved. Depending on the length of absence from prosthetic rehabilitation and the point at which the interruption occurs, the patient may require review and relearning of previously learned skills. Members of the rehabilitation team should make every effort to minimize delays and promote consistent communication to all members of the team, including patients and their families.

Residual Limb

The nature of blast wounds results in a residual limb that presents unique challenges. As discussed previously in this chapter, the resultant residual limb has significant edema that often contributes to pain issues. Proper edema management using ace wrap, elastic tubular sock, and silicone/urethane roll-on liners is necessary. Suture line breakdowns can be prevented with careful and regular monitoring. There may be times when prosthetic use must be temporarily suspended if the healing suture line is at risk. In addition, progression from an electric prosthesis to a body-powered prosthesis should be predicated on soft-tissue healing, especially surrounding the suture line.

In some cases, traditional socket designs may not provide effective suspension if the transradial limb is too short or irregularly shaped. At this level, custom silicone liners can often resolve challenging fitting issues. When used with specifically designed electrodes, custom liners can be helpful in providing a secure foundation on which to build the EPOP. If successful, this design can be carried forward into the preparatory and definitive phases. Custom silicone liners without electrodes can also be used for other types of prostheses. Very short transhumeral or humeral neck residual limbs are often best fit using infraclavicular interface techniques normally applied to glenohumeral disarticulation and higher amputation levels.[21]

Neuroma

Following nerve transection, neuromas typically occur as axons at the nerve ending attempt to regenerate. Symptomatic neuromas can often interfere with prosthetic use and function. They are usually identifiable by palpating or tapping the residual limb and replicating symptoms. If suspected, neuromas should be evaluated by a physician on the team, because treatment strategies should be used. Some common treatment approaches include oral medication and local steroid and anesthetic injections. Surgical resection may be necessary if there is no resolution of functionally limiting pain.[2(p61),22,23]

Heterotopic Ossification

HO seems to be more prevalent in amputees who have sustained a blast injury, and its presence may significantly impact the prosthetic rehabilitation process. HO is characterized by rapid and excessive bone growth throughout the residual limb. Bone growth is random and often so extensive that protrusions through the skin are not uncommon. Use of three-dimensional imaging technology and computed tomography scan can provide the rehabilitation team with an accurate three-dimensional model of HO formation and skeletal structure change. The three-dimensional model can be particularly useful in solving prosthetic socket-fitting issues resulting from the development of HO. Some amputees may require additional surgery to remove the bony growth should it affect range of motion or cause increased pain[24,25] (Figure 23-35).

Surfacing Shrapnel

Similar to the challenges associated with HO, blast wound injuries can also exhibit surfacing shrapnel. Dependent on the size and location of the fragments that are surfacing, socket modification may be needed, minor surgeries may be necessary, or prosthetic use may be temporarily suspended until the shrapnel is removed and the residual limb has healed.

Emotional Stressors (Psychosocial)

The less physical, but deeply important, aspect of amputation sustained in military action involves the psychosocial and emotional effects on the amputee. It is critical that each member of the team be aware of the status and treatment of the amputee from the psychological services team professionals. This will facilitate awareness of how service members best learn, what might unnecessarily frustrate them, and how the effects of their personal combat experience might compromise the aggressive rehabilitation plan.

FUTURE INNOVATIONS

Currently, there is a tremendous focus by independent research groups, DARPA (Defense Advanced Research Projects Agency), innovative prosthetic clinicians, and manufacturers to advance technology specific to the upper extremity amputee population. Areas of technological promise are aimed at increasing the degrees of freedom in componentry, as well as on the mechanisms for control, including:

- compliant hands,
- powered wrist units,
- powered shoulder and elbow joints,
- pattern recognition,
- targeted muscle reinnervation, and
- implantable electrodes.

Compliant hands allow for enhanced prehension patterns by powering independently articulating digits that can close around objects of various sizes and shapes. Powered wrist units that duplicate the complex movements of the human wrist (including rotation, flexion/extension, and radial/ulnar deviation) are currently being created and tested. Electrically powered elbow and shoulder joints that provide additional degrees of freedom will add functional capability for higher level amputees.

Although the evolution of these components is exciting and promising, the benefits of this technology will not be fully realized without advances in control schemes. Pattern recognition is an approach that uses the unique EMG signal patterns produced by specific muscle group contraction within the residual limb. Currently, between six and eight reproducible patterns can be captured and trained to control up to six degrees of freedom. Pattern recognition is limited by the number of surface electrodes that can remain in contact with the skin and the amount of processing power currently available within an electric prosthesis. One approach to address these challenges is targeted muscle reinnervation (Figure 23-36). This is a surgical technique that separates muscle tissue within the residual limb and reinnervates newly created sections of the muscle bellies with nerves previously used to control (innervate) the now amputated limb.[26] In another effort to address the limitations of surface electrodes, implantable electrodes are being developed that will use telemetry to transfer control information to the prosthesis. These exciting developments will undoubtedly benefit patients both now and in the future. It is the responsibility of rehabilitation team members to advance their knowledge, skills, and practices to apply these technologies effectively.

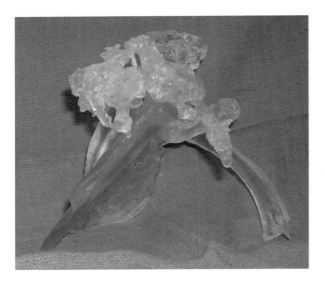
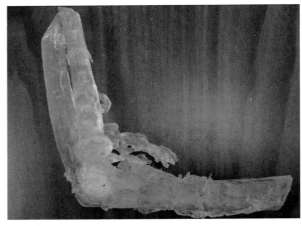

Figure 23-35. (*Left*) Model of heterotopic ossification in the area of the scapula and clavicle. (*Right*) Model of heterotopic ossification from a transradial-level amputation.

SUMMARY

The lifesaving benefits of body armor and battlefield medicine are unprecedented. In response to the increasing rate of survival with limb loss, upper extremity prosthetic treatment protocols have advanced to a new level of comprehensive care (Figure 23-37). The unique requirements and challenges presented by the military amputee population also influence the rehabilitation approach to prosthetic management (as outlined in this chapter). Preprosthetic Phase, Interim Prosthetic Phase,

and Advanced Prosthetic Phase management using state-of-the-art prosthetic technology and techniques combined with aggressive therapy enable the amputee to reintegrate into a fulfilling life as successfully and rapidly as possible. Treatment protocols call for expedited care and the delivery of electric, body-powered, and passive prosthetic options with thorough training to maximize rehabilitation potential. A review of prosthetic categories with specific recommendations for socket design and component integration for each amputation level has been presented. It must also be understood that this young and motivated patient

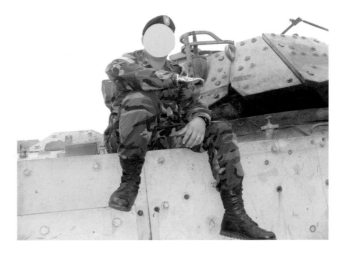

Figure 23-36. Captain Katie Yankosek, MS, OTR/L, CHT, at Walter Reed Army Medical Center with Jesse Sullivan, a research volunteer who has undergone targeted muscle reinnervation and is wearing a prototype prosthesis.

Figure 23-37. Through progressive military prosthetic rehabilitation, some service members can return to active duty.

group is helping to drive the field of upper extremity prosthetics forward. Many military amputees are participating actively in cutting-edge research and development projects, exploring (independently) alternative prosthetic solutions, becoming involved in the political arena, and pursuing careers in related fields. Their contributions in these areas will continue to challenge and inspire not only the interdisciplinary rehabilitation teams involved in their care, but also the prosthetic industry as a whole.

REFERENCES

1. Winter DA. *Biomechanics of Human Movement*. New York: John Wiley and Sons, Inc; 1979.

2. Dillingham TR. Rehabilitation of the upper limb amputee. In: Dillingham TR, Praxedes VB, eds. *Rehabilitation of the Injured Combatant*. Vol 1. *Textbook of Military Medicine*. Washington, DC: Department of the Army, Office of The Surgeon General, Borden Institute; 1998: 65.

3. Scott RN. Feedback in myoelectric prostheses. *Clin Orthop Relat Res*. 1990;256:58–63.

4. Scott RN. Myoelectric control systems research at the Bio-Engineering Institute, University of New Brunswick. *Med Prog Technol*. 1990;16:5–10.

5. Kelly MF, Parker PA, Scott RN. The application of neural networks to myoelectric signal analysis: a preliminary study. *IEEE Trans Biomed Eng*. 1990;37:221–230.

6. Lake C, Miguelez J. Comparative analysis of microprocessors in upper-extremity prosthetics. *J Prosthet Orthot*. 2003;15:48–65.

7. Michael JW, Gailey RS, Bowker JH. New developments in recreational prostheses and adaptive devices for the amputee. *Clin Orthop Relat Res*. 1990:256:64–75.

8. Meeks D, LeBlanc M. Preliminary assessment of three new designs of prosthetic prehensors for upper limb amputees. *Prosthet Orthot Int*. 1988;12:41–45.

9. Kruit J, Cool JC. Body-powered hand prosthesis with low operating power for children. *J Med Eng Technol*. 1989;13:129–133.

10. Sensky TE. A simple and versatile driving appliance for upper-limb amputees. *Prosthet Orthot Int*. 1980;4:47–49.

11. Chappell PH, Kyberd PJ. Prehensile control of a hand prosthesis by a microcontroller. *J Biomed Eng*. 1991;13:363–369.

12. Lewis EA, Sheredos CR, Sowell TT, Houston VL. Clinical application study of externally powered upper-limb prosthetics systems: the VA elbow, the VA hand, and the VA/NU myoelectric hand systems. *Bull Prosthet Res*. 1975; Fall:51–136.

13. Bergman K, Ornholmer L, Zackrisson K, Thyberg M. Functional benefit of an adaptive myoelectric prosthetic hand compared to a conventional myoelectric hand. *Prosthet Orthot Int*. 1992;16:32–37.

14. Almstrom C, Herberts P, Körner L. Experience with Swedish multifunctional prosthetic hands controlled by pattern recognition of multiple myoelectric signals. *Int Orthop*. 1981;5:15–21.

15. Bender LF. Upper-extremity prosthetics. In: Kottke F, Lehmann JF, eds. *Krusen's Handbook of Physical Medicine and Rehabilitation*. 4th ed. Philadelphia: WB Saunders; 1990.

16. Shurr DG, Cook TM. Upper-extremity prosthetics. In: Shurr DG, Cook TM, eds. *Prosthetics and Orthotics*. East Norwalk, Conn: Appleton and Lange; 1990.

17. Muilenburg AL, LeBlanc MA. Body-powered upper limb components. In: Atkins DJ, Meier RH, eds. *Comprehensive Management of the Upper-Limb Amputee*. New York: Springer-Verlag; 1989.

18. Malone JH, Childers SJ, Underwood J, Leal JH. Immediate post-surgical management of upper extremity amputation: conventional, electric and myoelectric prosthesis. *Orthot Prosthet*. 1981:35:1–9.

19. Miguelez J, Lake C, Conyers D, Zenie J. The transradial anatomically contoured (TRAC) interface: design principles and methodology. *J Prosthet Orthot.* 2003;15:148–157.

20. Andrews JT. Principles of prosthetics. In: Bowker JH, Michael JW, eds. *Atlas of Limb Prosthetics.* 2nd ed. St Louis, Mo: Mosby-Year Book, Inc; 1992: 255–265.

21. Miguelez J, Miguelez MD. The microframe: the next generation of interface design for glenohumeral disarticulation and associated levels of limb deficiency. *J Prosthet Orthot.* 2003;15:66–71.

22. Schnell MD, Bunch WH. Management of pain in the amputee. In: Bowker JH, Michael JW, eds. *Atlas of Limb Prosthetics: Surgical, Prosthetic, and Rehabilitation Principles.* 2nd ed. St Louis, Mo: CV Mosby; 1992.

23. Vaida G, Friedmann LW. Postamputation phantoms: a review. *Phys Med Rehabil Clin North Am.* 1991;2:325–353.

24. Potter BK, Burns TC, Lacap AP, Granville RR, Gajewski DA Heterotopic ossification following traumatic and combat-related amputations: prevalence, risk factors, and preliminary results of excision. *J Bone Joint Surg Am.* 2007;89:476–486.

25. Greenwell G, Pasquina P, Luu V, Gajewski D, Scoville C, Doukas W. Incidence of heterotopic ossification in the combat amputee. *Arch Phys Med Rehabil.* 2006;87:e20-e21.

26. Lipschutz RD, Kuiken TA, Miller LA, Dumanian GA, Stubblefield KA. Shoulder disarticulation externally powered prosthetic fitting following targeted muscle reinnervation for improved myoelectric prosthesis control. *J Prosthet Orthot.* 2006;18:28–34.

Chapter 24

UPPER LIMB PROSTHETICS FOR SPORTS AND RECREATION

ROBERT RADOCY, MSC[*]

INTRODUCTION

ADVANCES IN PROSTHETIC TECHNOLOGY

THE BALANCE BETWEEN PHYSICAL, PSYCHOLOGICAL, AND PROSTHETIC REHABILITATION

PREPROSTHETIC EXERCISE

BIOMECHANICS AND HUMAN MOVEMENT

PROSTHETIC DESIGN FOR SPORTS AND RECREATION
Archery and Weight Training
Golf and Baseball
Canoeing and Kayaking
Basketball, Volleyball, and Soccer
Swimming
Steering, Vehicle Control, and Other Activities with Similar Upper-Extremity Demand
Fishing
Firearms
Hockey
Water-Skiing
Snow Skiing and Snowboarding
Windsurfing
Scuba Diving
Mountaineering and Technical Climbing

SUMMARY

*Chief Executive Officer and President, TRS Incorporated, 3090 Sterling Circle, Studio A, Boulder, Colorado 80301

INTRODUCTION

The expansion and sophistication of technology, services, and communications in the 21st century is creating many new lifestyle opportunities for adults. Improved lives and lifestyles resulting from this expansion provide additional leisure time that can be directed at sports and recreational endeavors. Experts from the Centers for Disease Control and Prevention report that both physical and mental well-being are enhanced by physical activity.[1] In January 2007, the US government established the first federal medical classification code for upper limb prosthetic attachments for sports and recreation.[2] Sports and recreation activities have been linked to successful rehabilitation, and games and sports encourage socialization within selected micro and macro-social systems.[3] Therapeutic recreation and adaptive physical education programs help implement these avocational components into comprehensive rehabilitation programs.

There has been a growing demand for sports-specific (activity- or task-specific) prosthetic devices since the 1970s. In 1970, only a couple of simple adaptations were available for baseball and bowling. Today, a growing selection of adaptive prosthetic accessories are available that enable combat amputees to participate competitively in sports and task-specific activities. Most of today's combat veterans dealing with the challenges of a traumatic upper limb amputation are 20 to 30 years old and have the same dreams, drives, and needs as others their age. Through comprehensive rehabilitation, these amputees can participate in the same sports and recreational activities they enjoyed before they were injured. As survival rates continue to rise for traumatically injured service members, so will the demand for activity-specific prostheses. Knowledge of prosthetic sports and recreation equipment that is currently being developed in active military medical centers will eventually be incorporated into the care at national Veterans Administration hospitals, ensuring that combat amputees will continue to pursue specialized high-performance activities into the future.

ADVANCES IN PROSTHETIC TECHNOLOGY

The last 25 years have given rise to significant improvements in prosthetics materials and designs. Aerospace materials, such as carbon fiber and titanium, are now commonly incorporated into high-performance prosthetic limbs. High-strength resins and innovative suspension designs (with more intimate anatomical interfaces), combined with high-efficiency, body-powered systems or electromechanical components, provide better control, energy transfer, and delivery of biomechanical forces through prostheses. Roll-on silicone liners can augment suspension for better control throughout greater ranges of motion. Silicone liners excel in aqueous environments, where water lubricity makes it difficult to secure adequate suspension; however, they are not appropriate for all patients or environments. Myoelectric and electromechanical arms are not used in sports and recreation activities as often as traditional body-powered prostheses, probably because of the myolimb's inherent construction and more fragile, environmentally sensitive components. An externally powered arm is best used for activities and in environments that ensure its prolonged function and lifespan. The high impact and environmental exposure that result from many sports and recreational activities dictate that only a very durable, reliable, and functional prosthesis be constructed and used for these purposes.

Improved self-suspending socket designs[4] and a variety of new thermoplastics and thermoplastic elastomers are available to build uncompromising, strong, and comfortable prostheses. These improved suspension systems and strong, lightweight materials allow for the use of terminal devices, or "end effectors" (ie, accessories specifically designed to accomplish particular activities). The approach that appears to be the most successful focuses on activity-specific prosthetic attachments that are designed to emulate the biomechanics of the human hand and arm in that particular activity. This has led to the development of products that allow many amputees to perform not only recreationally but competitively with their two-handed peers. The pursuit of rigorous sports activities may further advance prosthetic science, bringing about new conditions or requirements that drive prosthetic revision and innovation.

THE BALANCE BETWEEN PHYSICAL, PSYCHOLOGICAL, AND PROSTHETIC REHABILIATION

Today's combat amputee may be faced with multiple amputation injuries compounded by tissue damage from explosions and burns. Patient assessment is comprehensive and includes efforts to evaluate future sports and recreation demands. The rehabilitation process can be significantly improved when amputee patients realize that sports and recreational pursuits are real possibilities for their futures.

It is important for the rehabilitation team serving the combat amputee in both the inpatient and outpatient settings to provide the most comprehensive rehabilitation program possible. Physical, psychological, and prosthetic rehabilitation must be balanced in order to foster success. Amputees cannot expect high performance from a prosthesis if they do not exhibit adequate range of motion, muscle hypertrophy, and strength. Conversely, they cannot be expected to perform at a high level if the prosthetic technology they receive does not complement their physical capabilities. Additional therapeutic intervention may be useful at this point in rehabilitation. The rehabilitation team should always endeavor to instill a positive attitude in the amputee and set realistic goals for accomplishing higher performance tasks. The combat amputee needs to be aware of the rehabilitation balance to focus perspective and direct rehabilitation. A direct involvement in rehabilitation decision making helps patients visualize the goals that need to be achieved. Specialty prostheses are prescribed and applied later in the rehabilitation cycle, following preliminary training and successful use of myoelectric and basic body-powered prostheses. Sports and recreation challenges are incorporated into the combat amputee's rehabilitation goals as soon as is realistically possible.

PREPROSTHETIC EXERCISE

Preprosthetic exercise should be considered in all cases where a definitive prosthesis cannot be applied or tolerated because of the severity of the injuries, tissue damage, skin grafts, or the like. In these cases, a padded, weighted harness may provide the patient with the ability to stimulate the muscles of the arm and shoulder, improving strength and range of motion. On a weighted harness with a transradial design, a triceps cuff is attached with flexible hinges to a padded cuff. The padded cuff is equipped with D-rings and a strap onto which disc weights can be added. The triceps cuff should strap above and below the biceps to prevent the harness from slipping off without inhibiting flexion. The padded cuff helps reduce abrasion to the tissues of the forearm while it supports the weights. The cuff should be placed as distally as possible to maximize resistance, but should not slide off the end of the arm. A weighted harness with a transhumeral design should replicate a standard figure-eight harness, padded as necessary to help reduce abrasion. Instead of terminating into a triceps cuff on the affected arm, a padded cuff, similar to that described for the transradial vest, can be applied. Weights can be added, and the therapist can create a variety of exercises to stimulate the musculature of the shoulder and remnant upper limb. A padded, weighted harness is an alternative to elastic-band or rubber-tube resistance exercise systems and can offer physiological benefits that those systems cannot provide.

BIOMECHANICS AND HUMAN MOVEMENT

In the past decade, there have been significant improvements in the design and function of activity-specific prosthetic devices. A focus on human movement and biomechanics has led to the development of prosthetic devices that integrate with the human body's biomechanics, allowing for improved movement and energy transfer through the torso and into the prosthesis. This is important for activities that require the dynamic (gross motor) use of the upper body, such as golfing and baseball. Improved range of motion throughout the forearm and at the wrist allow for two-handed function, more accurate control, and higher performance with a prosthesis than before.

Altering the design focus away from "one-model-fits-all" to activity specific has allowed for an evolution of products that may only excel in particular tasks and environments. Because of their specificity in function, these products harmonize with the physical demands of a particular activity, providing amputees with improved potential for performance and success. These new "focused" designs can help combat amputees meet the challenges of being actively involved and competitive in sports and recreation in a two-handed world.

PROSTHETIC DESIGN FOR SPORTS AND RECREATION

Understanding the biomechanics involved in performing a particular sport is the first step in providing a prosthetic solution. Certain activities, such as basketball, volleyball, and soccer, rely on bilateral hand function (volar hand surface control) that essentially ignores traditional opposed thumb (three chuck pinch) prehension. Other activities, such as baseball and golf, are successfully accomplished only when there are multiple degrees of freedom in the torso and arms and when efficient energy transfer is possible. The hand prehension aspects that may be required for a sport are not as important for performance; thus, analyzing and understanding an activity's demands is the primary concern, followed by an effort to duplicate those characteristics in a prosthesis. In certain circumstances, it is not feasible to easily duplicate what is required and innovative solutions are developed.

Another important element that must be considered is safety. Sheathing the hard exterior shell of a prosthesis with a stretchable, soft, padded cover helps protect the user and other players from injury. A 5-mm thick neoprene wetsuit material (fabric both sides or a variant) can be made into a sports cover that looks good and provides a safety cushion from impact. A variety of new sports-specific prosthetic accessories are designed to minimize or eliminate the potential for injury.

Archery and Weight Training

It may appear odd to group these two radically different activities together, but they have prosthetic design commonalities. Most prostheses are designed with a preflexion angle between the socket's center line and the forearm center line, so the face can be reached with a terminal device, prehensor, or hand. This type of preflexion alignment is counterproductive to many sports activities because it inhibits full arm extension when compared to an anatomical limb.

In archery and weight training, proper prosthetic alignment is critical to performance. A neutral alignment that allows for even loading of distally applied forces is necessary for control and performance. An improperly aligned prosthesis under load would be difficult to control, especially for the amputee with a short- to medium-length forearm (much like balancing a heavy weight on the end of a long stick). A preflexed socket inhibits performance in these activities because the alignment creates forces in and on the prosthesis that cannot be easily controlled.

In archery, the successful drawing of the arrow and its accurate release and true flight are impacted by prosthetic alignment (Figures 24-1 and 24-2). An improperly aligned prosthesis makes it impossible to accurately draw and release an arrow, especially when dealing with bows that have a draw weight in excess of 45 lb. Custom attachments have been developed to connect to a bow or attach to the bow string. Voluntary closing terminal devices with a prehensile configuration conform to most bow risers when a soft cushion is wrapped around the handle. The cushion allows the handle and bow to center in the device's grasp, helping eliminate torque when the arrow is released. Simple locking systems allow the bow to be held without concentration on cable tension (Figure 24-3). Another prosthetic accessory is designed to allow an archer to clip on to the bowstring and release

it mechanically with a lever that can be triggered by a chin nudge or other movement (Figure 24-4). Shooting a bow involves eye and hand dominance, so in many cases it is best to develop a solution that conforms to existing eye dominance traits.

Some other techniques and devices make archery accessible to those with hemiplegia or high-level limb absence. Mouth tabs and chest-suspended or chest-supported triggering systems help single-handed archers effectively and accurately shoot a bow and arrow.

The proper alignment of a prosthesis may dictate a user's ability to safely control weights while performing some weight-lifting exercises, such as bench press or dumbbell flies (Figures 24-5 and 24-6). Without a properly aligned and securely suspended prosthesis, an amputee with a medium or short residual limb will struggle to balance and control a barbell or dumbbell throughout the exercise's range of motion. A prosthesis built with a neutral (not preflexed) alignment is best for weight lifting. Carbon fiber can be added into the socket and forearm for strength. A self-suspending design may prove useful when combined with a roll-on liner and integral locking system for added suspension. If a thin roll-on liner is used, an additional partial liner of foam fabricated into the prosthesis will provide protection for the olecranon and elbow condyles (Figure 24-7). Such padding helps mitigate the pressure points created when the prosthesis sustains torque from a heavy load. Harnessing should be kept at a minimum because it typically restricts range of motion. Depending on the activity and the design of the prosthesis, a harness may not be necessary.

Conventional voluntary opening, split-hook technology, commonly used in prosthetics for simple ADLs, has proven ineffective for these types of high-performance activities. The prehension requirements of the activities, especially weight lifting, supersede the capabilities of almost all split-hook designs. Certain voluntary closing prehensors are designed and constructed to perform in both archery and weight lifting. The prehensile configuration includes opposed thumb grasp, which conforms to cylindrical shapes and handles, improving stability and control. These devices operate best when they are modified with a simple accessory locking system that eliminates the need to maintain cable tension in the body-powered harness for grasping and holding (Figures 24-8 and 24-9).

One system designed specifically for weight training is intended for light or moderate weight exercise (Figure 24-10). Another system includes two models. One is capable of withstanding extreme loads, including those used in Olympic events. The second model is more compact, lighter, and is designed for general gym weight training and conditioning (Figures 24-11 and 24-12). Both provide solid, stable control of barbells, dumbbells, and other weight-training equipment.

Golf and Baseball

Golf club and bat swinging require prostheses that provide appropriate degrees of freedom and control to allow for the efficient transfer of energy from the torso and body through the arms and prosthesis into the club or bat. Traditional or conventional prosthetic wrist components and terminal devices do not provide these capabilities.

Additionally, the site of the hand absence (right or left) and hand and swinging dominance dictate different solutions. There are a variety of prosthetic golf accessories; in the 1980s, most were custom made, single-use designs (devices built for use by a single individual and not intended for mass manufacturing). Experimentation was conducted to design a device that could duplicate the biomechanics in the wrist and forearm and produce a smooth swing and energy transfer. A flexible power coupling has evolved to be the best solution that fits the needs of most golfers. The length and stiffness of the coupling varies based on hand absence, swing-side dominance, and level of amputation. One golf device is designed primarily for right-handed individuals with left hand absence (Figure 24-13). The device can also be used by right-hand amputees who golf left handed, but a crossover grip is required. Although a second hand with normal gripping capability is required to use it, the device is versatile and can be easily adjusted to fit onto any golf club, adapting to the grip's diameter and taper.

Another alternative prosthetic golf system has models for both right and left hands to accommodate the differences (Figures 24-14 and 24-15). It uses a flexible coupling design similar to the device previously described, but the coupling stiffness is variable and the club attachment designs are different, dictating that uniform club grips be used. These devices are suitable for golfers with compromised strength, dexterity, or prehension in their second hand; they require only minimal assistance from another hand for club engagement. The application for bilateral amputees is viable. Typically, it is best to apply this device to the natural leading arm and allow the amputee golfer to experience and develop a controlled, one-handed swing using the prosthesis or residual arm for guidance and stability. Unique and individual solutions evolve for the second prosthesis, if required, as experience grows.

It is also possible, with the help of custom golf clubs modified with adapters, to directly and rigidly attach a golf club to a prosthesis. Although it is less convenient, this alternative may solve some control problems for amputee golfers.

Golf prostheses for individuals with transhumeral absence have evolved significantly since the 1990s. High-performance designs now use short sports prostheses that terminate in a wrist component, which is mounted anatomically close to where the normal elbow exists. A custom, lightweight, energy-storing, power-coupling device can entirely eliminate the need for a traditional prosthetic elbow or forearm. These couplings are designed to terminate into one of the previously described attachments. Prosthetic suspension can take advantage of roll-on locking liners to ensure unrestricted range of motion or use more traditional harnessing. Lightweight, carbon-reinforced prosthetic sockets help ensure that these short sports prostheses can tolerate the loads involved in the activity.

Swinging a bat has many of the same biomechanical challenges as swinging a golf club. In the past, many amputees batted single-handed, but being able to swing a bat two-handed using a prosthesis can improve performance. An innovative device for bat swinging is molded entirely from a strong, energy-storing, flexible polymer and is designed to quickly pry on and off the bat handle for convenience and safety (Figure 24-16). It uses a threaded mounting stud to fit any standard screw in a friction or disconnect wrist, and is designed to be grasped with an overhand grip from the sound hand. The device is versatile enough to allow function for either right or left hand absence and right or left hand swing preference.

Catching a ball adds additional challenges and choices for the amputee. Some prefer to play single handedly, transferring the glove on and off the sound hand as required. Others prefer to function with a prosthesis. Catching a ball below the waist requires that the forearm and glove are supine; catching above the waist requires pronation. For mid- or short-transradial amputees, these movements are impossible; merely placing a baseball glove on a prosthesis does not account for all the dynamic action involved. One prosthetic device made for baseball is designed to fit into a first-baseman's glove (Figure 24-17). The device is cable operated and functions like a large, voluntary opening split hook that is pulled and held open, then released to catch. Manual pronation and supination are required using the sound hand.

Another design replaces the traditional glove with a large mesh pocket so a ball can be caught forehanded or backhanded, eliminating the need to pronate or supinate the forearm (Figure 24-18). This lightweight, high-performance alternative meets the surface area requirements for gloves in regulated play.

Canoeing and Kayaking

Canoeing and kayaking require full range of motion and upper body coordination and strength. Manipulating handles and shafts requires different hand grasping configurations. Canoeing typically involves alternating paddling from starboard to port, complicating the situation for the amputee canoeist using a prosthesis because of the different grasps required.

A prosthetic finger or thumb can be inserted into a large-diameter hole drilled through a canoe handle..The improved articulation created with this modification is usually sufficient to allow the paddle to be controlled through a wide range of motion. The shaft is usually easy to grasp with a voluntary closing prehensor. Voluntary opening split hooks do not perform well because of their configuration and limited prehension, and have a tendency to pry off paddles under load. Padding or wrapping the shaft can improve control with most devices. Myoelectric prostheses can be useful for general recreational paddling; however, accidental immersion is a factor and must be considered. These factors usually preclude the use of myoelectric prostheses in river and white-water boating.

A new kayak and water sports prosthetic accessory attempts to meet the performance demands of river and whitewater kayaking, but also functions in flat water environments (Figure 24-19). It employs a quick connect and disconnect power strap to secure the kayak paddle shaft or canoe oar. The power strap stores energy as it is stretched from side to side, duplicating a radial–ulnar type of wrist articulation. A standard prosthetic wrist provides the additional adjustable, rotational friction needed for smooth paddling. The energy storage and return action allow for comfortable, forceful propulsion with a double-ended kayak or canoe paddle.

Basketball, Volleyball, and Soccer

Duplicating the volar (palmar) surface of the hand is important for activities that require coordinated bimanual function. A flexible interface that conforms to the large spherical surfaces of soccer balls, volleyballs, and basketballs also enhances control, improves performance, and provides some protection and safety. Several prosthetic accessories were specifically designed to emulate these hand characteristics and provide function and performance in these activities (Figures 24-20, 24-21, and 24-22). They are constructed of strong and flexible polymers that store and return energy, which helps duplicate certain wrist-like functions for improved ball handling and control.

Swimming

Swimming also requires the use of the volar hand surfaces, but for propulsion rather than manipulation. Prosthetic paddles or fins can enhance resistance during the power phase of a swimming stroke, improving propulsion but possibly impeding efficiency because often the amputee cannot pronate or "feather" the paddle or fin while swimming. This drag can be eliminated with a flexible or folding fin system. One swimming accessory with a folding fin is designed to be used on a custom, lightweight, short sports prosthesis specifically built for the water environment (Figure 24-23). Polypropylene, polyethylene, or copolymer materials are appropriate for use in the socket. A roll-on locking liner counteracts the water's natural lubricity, improving suspension for better control and higher loads during the power stroke. The fin collapses during retrieval, reducing or eliminating the water drag that a flat, rigid fin would create.

Amputees can swim without a prosthesis, but a prosthesis provides better propulsion and performance. The added resistance of a swimming fin or paddle is also therapeutic to the muscles of the upper arm, shoulder girdle, and upper torso, creating stimulation for growth and hypertrophy.

A prosthetist can use a kit to fabricate a flexible swimming paddle that is designed to fit directly onto a residual limb (Figure 24-24). This device can be a good introductory aid for therapeutic physical exercise before an amputee is fit with a prosthesis, or for amputees who cannot tolerate a normal prosthetic limb.

Steering, Vehicle Control, and Other Activities with Similar Upper Extremity Demands

Bimanual capability and rapid and reflexive grip and release are functions that enable safe and effective vehicle control, whether the vehicle is body powered or motor driven. Road and mountain bicycles, motorcycles, all terrain vehicles, watercraft, and automobiles emphasize the need for coordinated bimanual function. High grasping forces may be required for control in certain circumstances. Quick release may also be required to avoid or mitigate injury. Manipulating handlebars, steering wheels and other steering controls, shifts, and levers requires accurate, variable prehension from a prosthesis and is enhanced by the natural, directly proportional feedback generated by active or positive-grasping, voluntary closing prosthetic prehensors. Devices equipped with polymer gripping surfaces provide better control in these types of activities than devices with smooth metal or serrated surfaces. Driving and steering usually involve glenohumeral flexion, and voluntary closing devices harmonize with that biomechanical motion (Figures 24-25 and 24-26). Myoelectric hands and control systems also perform well and are reliable for activities that involve driving and steering, although direct positive feedback is not available with this technology.

Split hooks are actuated and controlled by a body harness in such a way that gripping control and stability can be compromised while driving or riding. Additionally, the split-hook configuration does not lend itself to handling the cylindrical shapes and curved or rounded surfaces that are often encountered with these activities. Split hooks produce a gripping feedback that is inversely proportional and therefore counterproductive to progressive gripping control.

Handlebars can be padded or cushioned to improve their frictional coefficients for better handling. Controls can be clustered together for easier, safer one-handed operation. Motorcycle controls can be grouped and integrated. The motorcycle twist throttle grip is easily combined with a lever action clutch and can be controlled simultaneously with the sound hand while the prosthesis is used primarily for handlebar control. Front and rear hydraulic brake systems can be integrated together to be operated independently with a single foot pedal or lever.

Similarly, front and rear mountain bike brake cables can be integrated to operate off a single lever, freeing the prosthesis to be used for handlebar stability and control (Figure 24-27). The progressive and powerful gripping capabilities of the voluntary closing prehensor easily withstand the bouncing and jarring conditions typical in off-road terrain. Should a fall occur, relaxation of cable tension in the system automatically releases the voluntary closing device from the handlebars, freeing the rider from the bike. Myoelectric prostheses also have the gripping capacity and control to meet these riding challenges. Rough off-road use creates significant shock and vibration that can be harmful to the function of electromechanical prostheses.

Two models of recreational-grade prosthetic bicycle accessories are available to suit different ages, abilities, and riding styles (Figure 24-28). These devices are constructed of flexible polymers and operate like rubber cleats, snapping on and off the handlebars. They are safe, lightweight, and easy to use.

Fishing

Handling fishing reels and rods for sport fishing requires bimanual function and coordination. It is important to manipulate handles and gears with a terminal device that provides controlled and adequate grasp. A simple, functional approach is to hold and control the fishing rod when possible with the sound hand and reel with the prosthesis (Figure 24-29). Accurately controlling a fishing rod in an activity like casting requires wrist action that prosthetic wrists do not provide.

One alternative prosthetic accessory consists of a rod system directly attached into the prosthesis (Figure 24-30). Another adapter is used to cradle and stabilize the rod in the prosthesis, but is not practical for casting (Figure 24-31). These systems are appropriate for anglers who prefer to use a prosthesis for rod handling or who cannot control a fishing rod with a sound hand and limb.

Most fishing reels can be easily modified to be more functional with a prosthetic terminal device. Slip-on rubber grips can stretch over most reel handles, making them easier to grasp with a prosthetic device (Figure 24-32). Myoelectric hands and externally powered hooks, as well as voluntary closing prehensors, can be used for reeling. Split hooks do not typically provide enough grasping force to be effective and tend to pry off the fishing reel handle under load. Most standard bait-casting and spinning reels, either open or closed face, can be easily manipulated. Reeling-specific prosthetic devices are also available (Figure 24-33). However, these products leave the angler single-handed for performing the other activities that are required while fishing (ie, changing lures, flies, and bait; netting fish; handling boating equipment; etc).

Fly-fishing requires coordination, bimanual dexterity, and gross motor upper limb involvement. The prosthesis should be capable of handling the fly line or the fly rod. Controlling the rod with the prosthesis is difficult in most cases because of the lack of freedom in most prosthetic wrists. Fly-fishing requires that the line be cast (instead of just the lure or fly). The fly line can be handled accurately with a prosthesis that provides controlled gripping force and some type of sensory feedback (eg, a voluntary closing prehensor with polymer gripping surfaces provides traction to control the line without damaging it; Figure 24-34). Fly-fishing is different than other types of fishing in that the line is not usually retrieved by reeling, but is pulled in by hand when a fish is caught and reeled up after the fish is netted. An individual who has experience with a voluntary closing prosthesis can potentially develop the technique, dexterity, and control to fly-fish. A few general accessories that help with holding small flies, dealing with fine leaders, and tying knots are also useful tools for creating a positive, successful fly fishing experience. Advances in myoelectric technology may make it possible to fly-fish with an electric hook prosthesis. The myoelectric hand will not have the dexterity to control the fly line, but the electric hook with narrow, rubber-lined, hook fingers can meet these challenges. Water immersion is a risk to consider when using a myoelectric limb for fly-fishing.

Firearms

Firearms expertise is an integral part of any military experience and rehabilitation program. Service members and veterans with an amputation may find it rewarding to return to shooting as a pastime or for sport. Firearms Training Simulation facilities have been created to help amputee soldiers regain and retune their firearms skills during rehabilitation and prepare for live-fire experiences. Firearms Training Simulation facilities feature laser-fired weapons and simulated combat scenarios.

Safely handling and controlling a firearm with a prosthesis is the primary concern when engaging in shooting activities. Most pistols can be modified and retrofit with oversized, compliant grips that improve control (Figure 24-35). If myoelectric prostheses are used, the shock and stress that result from firing guns with high recoil must be considered. Some voluntary closing prehensors and myoelectric hands have an opposed thumb design that conforms to the shape of a pistol handle and can generate the level of gripping force required to safely control the firearm. An overhand grip is typically used with the sound hand to help aim and trigger the pistol.

Long guns, such as rifles, carbines, and shotguns, can be safely controlled with prostheses. The shooter must decide whether or not to modify the firearm. A variety of pistol grip attachments can be added to the fore end of a gun to allow for improved control (Figures 24-36, 24-37, and 24-38). Prosthetists should rely on trained, certified gunsmiths for modifications instead of doing them themselves. In certain cases, a simple military strap added to the gun provides enough flexibility to shoot with a prosthesis. A stainless steel or brass ring can also be added to a gun's fore end and attached into a modified post used for a normal gun sling. The ring can be grasped by a prosthetic finger or thumb.

Another alternative avoids modifying the firearm altogether (Figures 24-39, 24-40, and 24-41). This device, designed initially to safely handle an M-16 firearm, is versatile enough to shoot almost any rifle, carbine, or shotgun, including pump-action and side-by-side double barrel guns. A flexible, strong, polymer yoke contains tapered rubber fins that allow the fore end of the gun to be snapped down into place. Pulling the firearm back towards the shoulder tightens the gripping action of the yoke so that the firearm can be locked onto the shoulder for stability and control. The device has a friction-lockable, stainless steel ball and socket, and a friction-adjustable swiveling mechanism allows for a broad range of motion. The barrel can be carried up or down, and the firearm can easily be swung to the shoulder for tracking, aiming, and firing. The device's yoke firmly grasps the gun's fore end but will not mar even finely checkered walnut stocks. The gun can be loaded and reloaded while secured in the prosthesis's hold. However, this type of a device is only useful for handling firearms, leaving shooters single-handed for other activities.

Another option is a plastic-covered steel yoke, into which the fore end of a gunstock can be positioned for support (Figure 24-42). This device offers another simple alternative to the amputee shooter, but provides less total control over the firearm.

Depending on eye dominance, the shooter may wish to fire a gun with the prosthesis. This takes a lot of practice to be safe and proficient. The lack of tactile finger sensation and fine dexterous movement in prostheses make triggering a firearm with a prosthetic finger problematic. Additionally, when a human hand triggers a gun, it also operates safety mechanisms and provides support for the stock, functions that are difficult to perform with a prosthesis while triggering.

Hockey

Ice and street hockey require bimanual upper extremity involvement and coordination. A jointed or flexible coupling at the end of the prosthesis connected to a hockey stick is important for safety. A 4-ft long hockey stick will create forces of leverage that can be transferred back into the prosthesis and injure the player's residual limb if some type of flexible linkage is not used.

Handedness and playing style (right or left) can dictate whether an amputee wishes to control the stick with the prosthesis at the top or down on the shaft (trial and error may help determine the best solution). A variety of custom prosthetic attachments attempt to make handling a hockey stick easy and efficient; some try to meet the needs of either stick-handling situation (Figure 24-43). The flexible coupling on these attachments bends enough to help eliminate injury when a player is forced into the rink's walls or falls. The coupling is stiff enough to allow handling the puck with just the prosthesis when necessary.

Water-Skiing

Water-skiing, especially slalom skiing, single-handed without a prosthesis is possible but tiring and physically demanding on the muscles of the remaining arm. Custom quick-detach mechanisms can be incorporated into a water-ski rope, but they must be controlled by the skier. A custom plastic water-ski hook used in conjunction with a floating, self-suspending prosthesis can be helpful. The hook creates enough grip to engage the rope handle so the skier can ski even single-handedly with a prosthesis. If the hook fails to twist off the handle during a fall, the skier can twist out of the prosthesis, avoiding injury.

A simpler alternative is to modify the ski rope handle. A small cup or tube (sized to slide over one end of a ski rope handle) and flexible line can be attached to the prosthesis or directly to a body harness. The attachment provides leverage so the arm and prosthesis can be used to resist the pulling load of launching and control the ski rope handle. When the sound hand releases the handle, the tube pops off the other end and releases the skier. Another way to use this technique is to attach a strip of polypropylene webbing (1.5–2 in. wide) securely to the end of the prosthesis, removing the standard terminal attachment. Six to eight inches of webbing should be left loose off the end of the prosthesis and can be wrapped once or twice around the rope handle and over-grasped with the sound hand. During a fall or to release the rope, the sound hand drops the handle and the web strap pulls free, releasing the prosthesis from the tow-rope handle.

Snow Skiing and Snowboarding

Snow skiers usually rely on ski poles, while snowboarders depend primarily on their upper limbs for balance. The snowboarder or rider can use almost any type of prosthesis that provides this function and is safe to wear, considering the rider might unexpectedly fall onto the prosthesis. A prosthesis often pulls heat from the residual limb, decreasing circulation and leaving the limb colder than the rest of the body. Wearing a thin, moisture-transferring liner sock under a wool-blend sock helps keep the residual arm dry and at a more consistent temperature.

One commercially available snow skiing tool is a skiing and fishing terminal device that operates without a cable (Figure 24-44). It is fabricated from flexible silicone polymers and accepts a pole that has been stripped of the standard grip. The ski pole is forced into the device and held in place by friction. The skier thrusts the pole forward using glenohumeral flexion (arm extension), and the pole rotates forward with a pendulum action. The natural elastomeric action of the device returns the pole to its original position.

Another device can be either cable driven or used like a simple pendulum, depending on the user's preference (Figures 24-45 and 24-46). The ski pole's

grip is removed and the bare tube fits into a cylindrical receiver attached to a shock-absorbing mounting system. An elastic retraction system keeps the pole flexed back out of the way until it is needed. The pole is easily removed. Natural glenohumeral flexion is used to pull on the cable, rotating the pole forward for a pole plant. A shock-absorbing module is built in to absorb the torque and stress created by using a ski pole. The device transfers upper limb power into the pole and provides the propulsion needed for Nordic skiing, yet is responsive enough to be used in moguls and for downhill pursuits.

Windsurfing

Windsurfing is a demanding activity for amputees. Windsurfers must be capable of quickly grasping and releasing the boom, sail, and control ropes. The grip required to engage and hold on is significant, and spontaneous release is important to avoid injury. A modified voluntary closing prehensor provides sufficient gripping force to control the mast and boom, and streamlined inner gripping surfaces allow for the prosthesis to be released smoothly or twisted off the boom when necessary during sailing.

The prosthesis needs to be waterproof and constructed with corrosion- and salt-resistant hardware. Leather will not survive long when repeatedly exposed to water. Roll-on silicone or similar liners, if used, should employ only strong plastic or stainless locking components. Cables have a tendency to foul with repeated exposure to saltwater; rinsing and flushing the cable system is important for efficient, reliable function. Synthetic cables constructed of polyethylene with an ultra-high molecular weight may be useful because they are strong, flexible, and naturally lubricious.

Scuba Diving

A prosthesis is not required for scuba diving and most amputee divers can become skilled enough to pass mandatory diver's certification courses single-handed. However, a prosthesis can be useful when handling gear and equipment underwater, and significantly aids climbing out of the water via a ladder. A scuba prosthesis should be designed to operate in both freshwater and saltwater environments. A voluntary opening split hook equipped with enough elastic bands will operate under a tight wetsuit, providing grasping function. The hook shape helps the diver climb ladders, get back onto the boat, and handle equipment and gear. Shorter, specially designed, lightweight prostheses that are passive and not cable operated may also be considered. A simple, strong, plastic terminal device can be designed to assist with basic functions, including ladder climbing and manipulating weight-belt buckles and other gear.

Mountaineering and Technical Climbing

Mountaineering and technical climbing require participants to be in top physical condition, possessing both strength and endurance. Good upper limb coordination, range of motion, and positive gripping force are necessary to handle equipment and meet the rigors of these activities. A stainless steel, voluntary closing device with an opposed thumb design can be used for mountaineering and climbing activities

(Figure 24-47). Custom modified split hooks have also been used (Figure 24-48). Two custom climbing and mountaineering devices were designed and built with the input of amputee climbers and several other experienced able-bodied climbers (Figures 24-49 and 24-50). These designs use standardized, chromium molybdenum ("chrom-moly") climbing aids integrated into custom pedestals designed to fit onto a prosthesis. They are specific to an individual climber's requirements and capabilities, and therefore have not been made commercially available. These devices represent an example of what an amputee climber might consider using to succeed in this challenging sport.

SUMMARY

Research in upper limb prosthetics is advancing as a result of funding from the federal government. The majority of this research is oriented toward high-tech, mostly externally powered, solutions to sophisticated problems and objectives. These solutions and technology have not historically been successfully applied to sports and recreation. Performance in sports and recreation for those with upper limb prostheses has improved with sports-specific mechanical designs and innovative materials. Future developments in upper limb prosthetics for sports will most likely continue to arise from engineered, mechanical solutions that focus on duplicating the sometimes complex biomechanics involved in the performance of a specific activity.

Applying energy-storing elastomers and other lightweight yet strong materials into sports-specific prostheses will improve performance. Focusing designs on the specific limitations created by various levels of amputation will also improve the capabilities and performance for a broader range of consumers. Future research and product development will be enhanced and accelerated by new financial input and resources that can be directed into this specific area of prosthetics. These resources, complemented by the innovative thinking, input, and demands of a new, young population of prosthetic users, will drive ideas and improve technology for even better performance in sports and recreation activities.

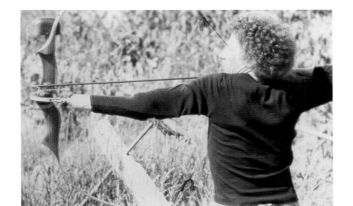

Figure 24-1. Incorrect prosthetic alignment. An improperly aligned prosthesis makes it impossible to accurately draw and release an arrow.
Photograph: Courtesy of TRS Inc, Boulder, Colo.

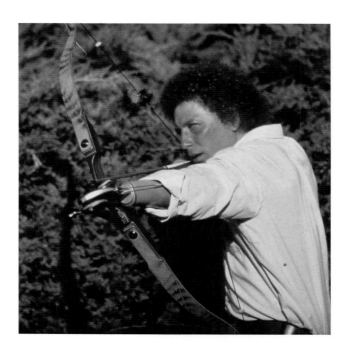

Figure 24-2. Correct prosthetic alignment, allowing for accurate arrow draw and release.
Photograph: Courtesy of TRS Inc, Boulder, Colo.

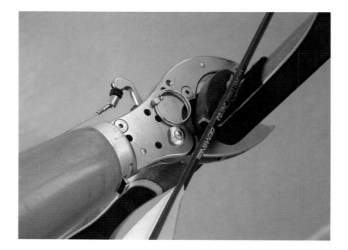

Figure 24-3. TRS GRIP 2S Prehensor with locking pin holding recurve bow and arrow.
Photograph: Courtesy of TRS Inc, Boulder, Colo.

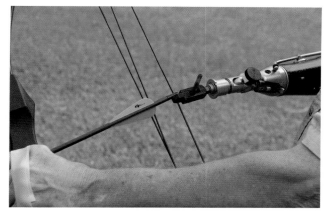

Figure 24-4. Quick Release Gripper archery trigger with N-Abler (Texas Assistive Devices LLC, Brazoria, Tex). Photograph: Courtesy of Texas Assistive Devices LLC, Brazoria, Tex.

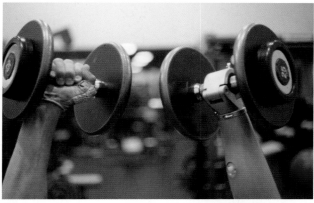

Figure 24-5. Bench press with dumbbells using a weight-lifting prosthesis. Photograph: Courtesy of TRS Inc, Boulder, Colo.

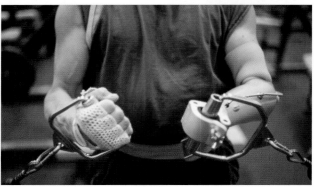

Figure 24-6. Biceps curls with dumbbells using a weight-lifting prosthesis. Photograph: Courtesy of TRS Inc, Boulder, Colo.

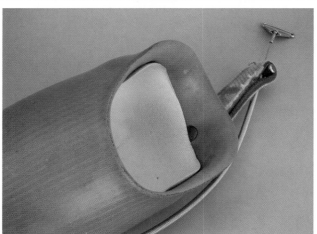

Figure 24-7. Weight-lifting prosthesis with partial liner padding. Photograph: Courtesy of TRS Inc, Boulder, Colo.

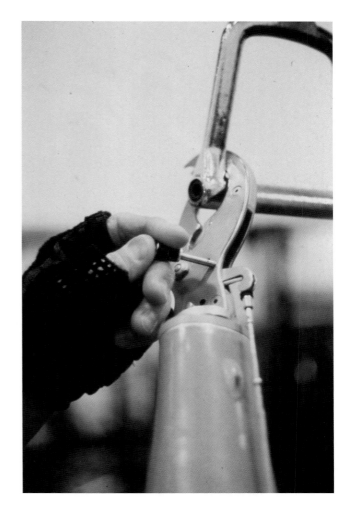

Figure 24-8. Prehensor with locking pin being used on weight equipment handle.
Photograph: Courtesy of TRS Inc, Boulder, Colo.

Figure 24-9. Prehensor with locking pin modification for weight lifting.
Photograph: Courtesy of TRS Inc, Boulder, Colo.

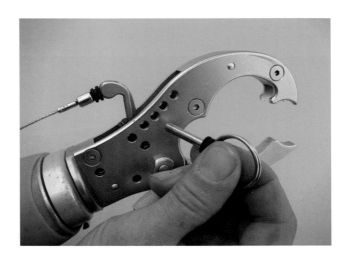

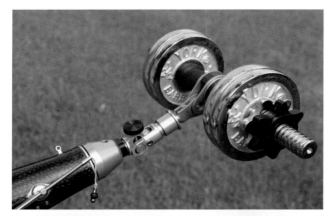

Figure 24-10. Weight-lifting device.
Photograph: Courtesy of Texas Assistive Devices LLC, Brazoria, Tex.

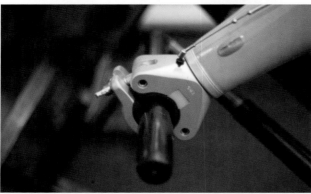

Figure 24-11. Heavy-duty weight-lifting device.
Photograph: Courtesy of TRS Inc, Boulder, Colo.

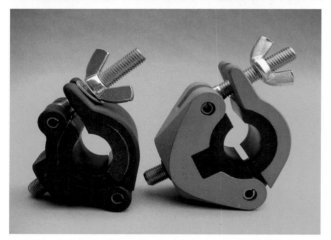

Figure 24-12. Weight-lifting devices.
Photograph: Courtesy of TRS Inc, Boulder, Colo.

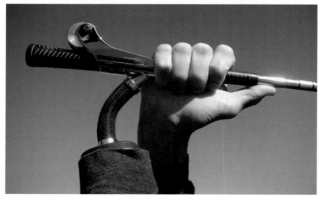

Figure 24-13. Golf prosthesis.
Photograph: Courtesy of TRS Inc, Boulder, Colo.

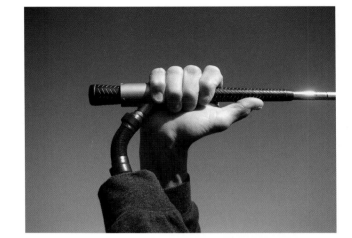

Figure 24-14. Golf prosthesis, left model.
Photograph: Courtesy of TRS Inc, Boulder, Colo.

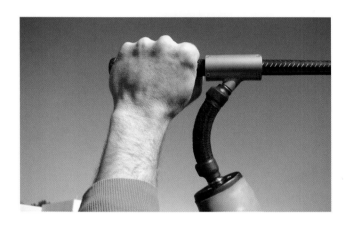

Figure 24-15. Golf prosthesis, right model.
Photograph: Courtesy of TRS Inc, Boulder, Colo.

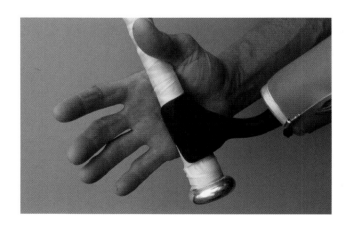

Figure 24-16. Baseball bat prosthesis.
Photograph: Courtesy of TRS Inc, Boulder, Colo.

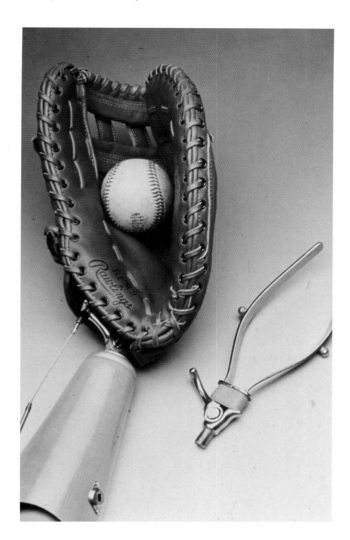

Figure 24-17. Baseball glove adapter split hook.
Photograph: Courtesy of TRS Inc, Boulder, Colo.

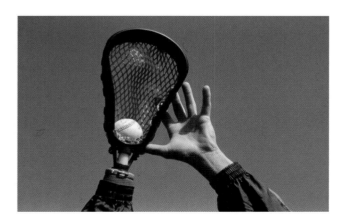

Figure 24-18. Baseball catching prosthesis.
Photograph: Courtesy of TRS Inc, Boulder, Colo.

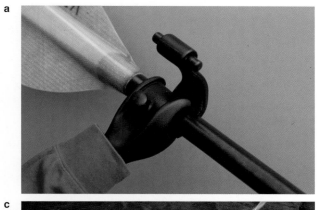

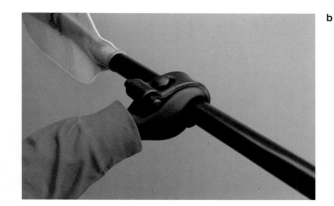

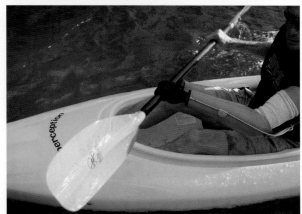

Figure 24-19. Kayak accessory. **(a)** Closed. **(b)** Open. **(c)** In use. Photograph: Courtesy of TRS Inc, Boulder, Colo.

Figure 24-20. Basketball accessory. Photograph: Courtesy of TRS Inc, Boulder, Colo.

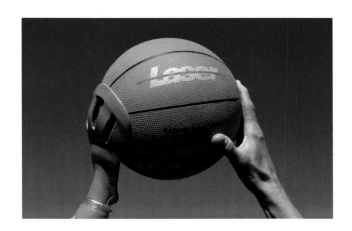

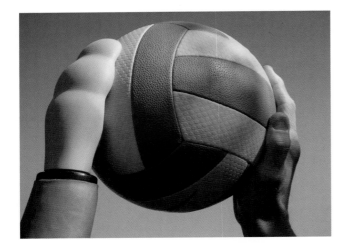

Figure 24-21. Volleyball handling device.
Photograph: Courtesy of TRS Inc, Boulder, Colo.

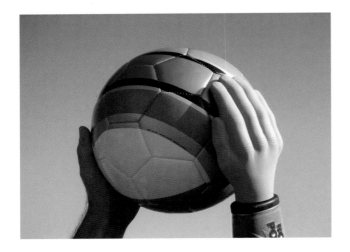

Figure 24-22. Soccer ball handling device.
Photograph: Courtesy of TRS Inc, Boulder, Colo.

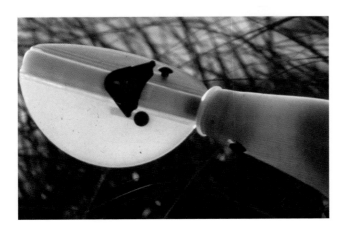

Figure 24-23. Freestyle swimming prosthesis.
Photograph: Courtesy of TRS Inc, Boulder, Colo.

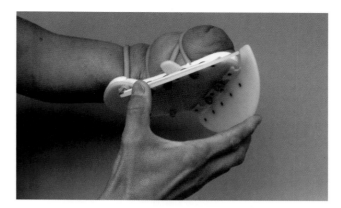

Figure 24-24. Swim fin kit (assembled).
Photograph: Courtesy of TRS Inc, Boulder, Colo.

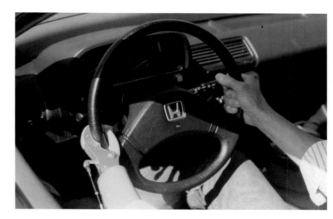

Figure 24-25. Prehensor used with a steering wheel.
Photograph: Courtesy of TRS Inc, Boulder, Colo.

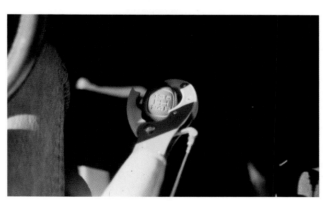

Figure 24-26. Prehensor used with stick shift.
Photograph: Courtesy of TRS Inc, Boulder, Colo.

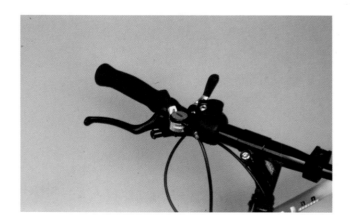

Figure 24-27. Dual bike brake lever.
Photograph: Courtesy of TRS Inc, Boulder, Colo.

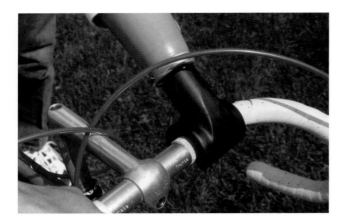

Figure 24-28. Bicycle accessory.
Photograph: Courtesy of TRS Inc, Boulder, Colo.

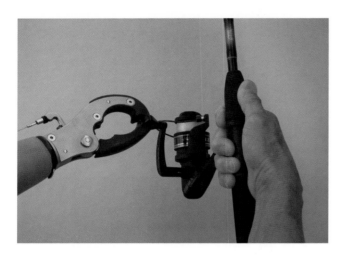

Figure 24-29. Prehensor with spinning reel.
Photograph: Courtesy of TRS Inc, Boulder, Colo.

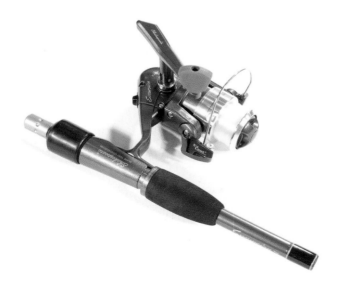

Figure 24-30. Fishing rod prosthetic adaptor.
Photograph: Courtesy of Texas Assistive Devices LLC, Brazoria, Tex.

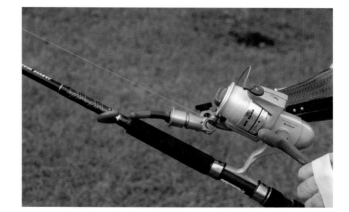

Figure 24-31. Universal Handle Holder (fishing rod application; Texas Assistive Devices LLC, Brazoria, Tex).
Photograph: Courtesy of Texas Assistive Devices LLC, Brazoria, Tex.

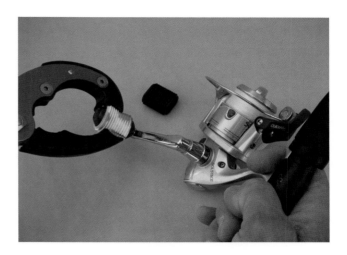

Figure 24-32. Rubber slip-on reel handle grip accessories.
Photograph: Courtesy of TRS Inc, Boulder, Colo.

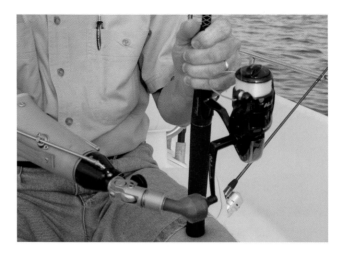

Figure 24-33. Crank adaptor.
Photograph: Courtesy of Texas Assistive Devices LLC, Brazoria, Tex.

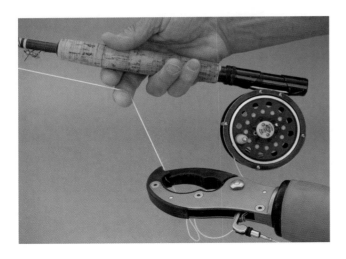

Figure 24-34. Prehensor with fly fishing rod, reel, and line. Photograph: Courtesy of TRS Inc, Boulder, Colo.

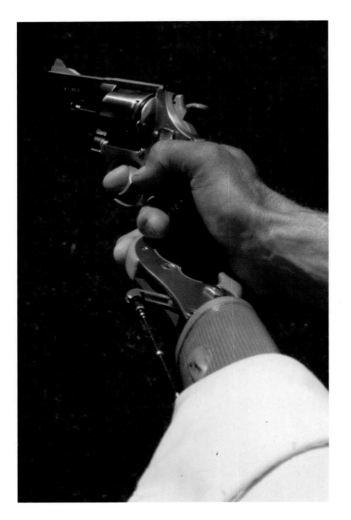

Figure 24-35. Prehensor with 44-magnum pistol. Photograph: Courtesy of TRS Inc, Boulder, Colo.

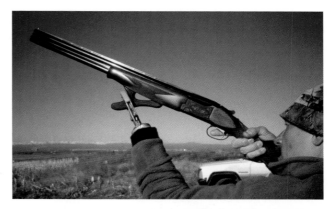

Figure 24-36. Over and under shotgun with fore-end modification and prehensor.
Photograph: Courtesy of TRS Inc, Boulder, Colo.

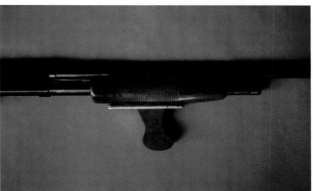

Figure 24-37. Pump style shotgun fore-end modification.
Photograph: Courtesy of TRS Inc, Boulder, Colo.

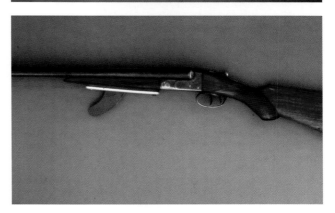

Figure 24-38. Side-by-side style shotgun with fore-end modification.
Photograph: Courtesy of TRS Inc, Boulder, Colo.

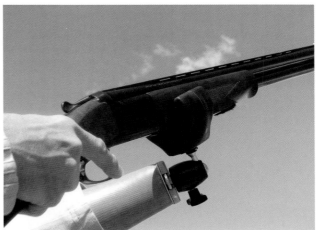

Figure 24-39. Gun turret prosthesis with over-and-under shotgun.
Photograph: Courtesy of TRS Inc, Boulder, Colo.

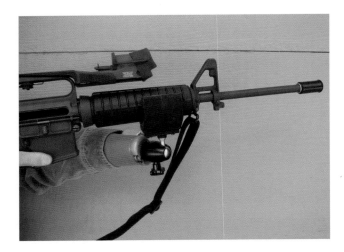

Figure 24-40. Gun turret used with an M-16.
Photograph: Courtesy of TRS Inc, Boulder, Colo.

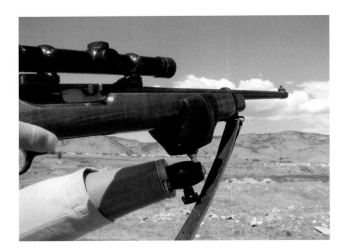

Figure 24-41. Gun turret used with a carbine.
Photograph: Courtesy of TRS Inc, Boulder, Colo.

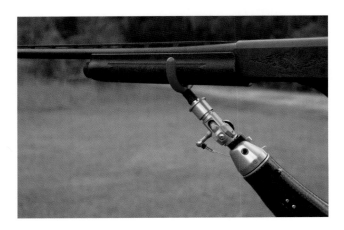

Figure 24-42. Tool/gun cradle adaptor.
Photograph: Courtesy of Texas Assistive Devices LLC, Brazoria, Tex.

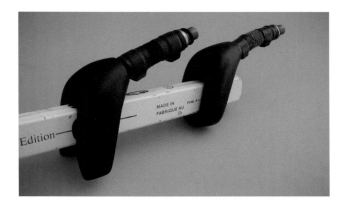

Figure 24-43. Prosthetic hockey accessories.
Photograph: Courtesy of TRS Inc, Boulder, Colo.

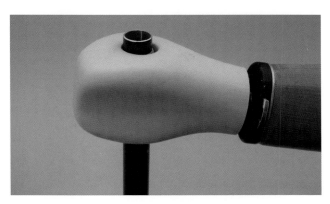

Figure 24-44. Ski/fishing prosthesis.
Photograph: Courtesy of TRS Inc, Boulder, Colo.

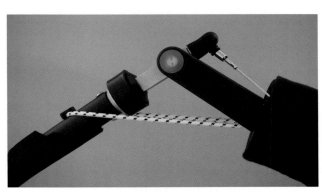

Figure 24-45. Ski accessory (extended for pole plant).
Photograph: Courtesy of TRS Inc, Boulder, Colo.

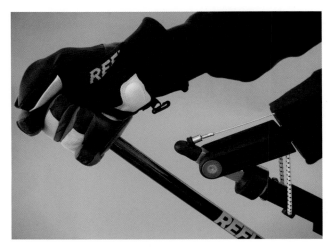

Figure 24-46. Nordic and alpine ski prostheses.
Photograph: Courtesy of TRS Inc, Boulder, Colo.

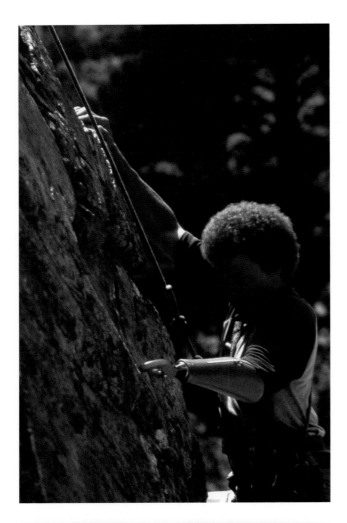

Figure 24-47. Prehensor used for technical climbing.
Photograph: Courtesy of TRS Inc, Boulder, Colo.

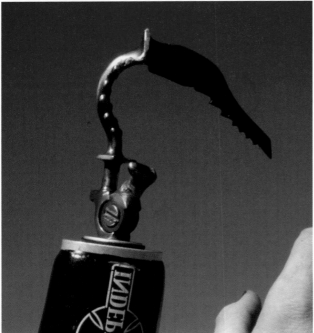

Figure 24-48. Modified split hook for climbing by Pete Davis,
accomplished amputee climber.
Photograph: Courtesy of TRS Inc, Boulder, Colo.

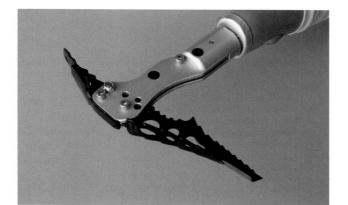

Figure 24-49. Mountaineering device custom built for Aron Ralston, who gained notoriety after amputating his lower arm that had become trapped by a boulder while he was climbing in Blue John Canyon, Utah.
Photograph: Courtesy of TRS Inc, Boulder, Colo.

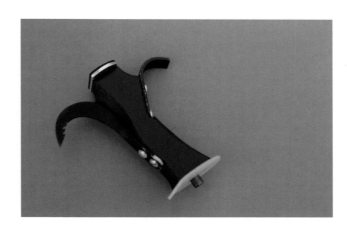

Figure 24-50. Technical climbing prosthesis custom built for Aron Ralston.
Photograph: Courtesy of TRS Inc, Boulder, Colo.

REFERENCES

1. Pate RR, Pratt M, Blair SN, et al. Physical activity and public health. Recommendation from the Centers for Disease Control and Prevention and the American College of Sports Medicine. *JAMA*. 1995;273(5):402–407.

2. DMECS Durable Medical Equipment Coding System. *Code: L6704: Terminal Device, Sport/Recreational/Work Attachment, Any Material, Any Size*. Available at: www.hcpcs@cms.hhs.gov. Accessed June 11, 2009.

3. Rarick GL. *Physical Activity, Human Growth and Development*. New York, NY: Academic Press; 1973: 257–332.

4. Miguelez JM, Lake C, Conyers J, Zenie J. The Transradial Anatomically Contoured (TRAC) Interface: design principles and methodology. *J Prosthet Orthot*. 2003;15(4):148–157.

Chapter 25

SPORTS AND RECREATION OPPORTUNITIES

ANDY KRIEGER[*]; FRANK BRASILE, PhD[†]; CAIBRE McCANN, MD[‡]; AND RORY A. COOPER, PhD[§]

INTRODUCTION

THERAPEUTIC BENEFITS

CLASSIFICATION

ASSISTIVE TECHNOLOGY

ACTIVITIES

SUMMARY

ATTACHMENT: ORGANIZATIONS PROMOTING SPORTS AND RECREATION FOR PERSONS WITH DISABILITIES

[*]Director, Department of Sports and Recreation, Paralyzed Veterans of America, 801 18th Street, NW, Washington, DC 20006; formerly, Adapted Athletic Specialist, Wright State University, 3640 Colonel Glenn Highway, Dayton, Ohio
[†]Professor, University of Nebraska, 6001 Dodge Street, Omaha, Nebraska 68182
[‡]Physiatrist-in-Chief (Retired), Department of Rehabilitation Medicine, Maine Medical Center, Portland, Maine
[§]Senior Career Scientist, US Department of Veterans Affairs, and Distinguished Professor, Department of Rehabilitation Science and Technology, University of Pittsburgh, 5044 Forbes Tower, Pittsburgh, Pennsylvania 15260

By participating in the Hawaii Ironman World Championships, I was accomplishing several things at multiple levels. As an example to all amputees, I was able to highlight the great things that anyone can accomplish through training and dedication to fitness. To my soldiers, I showed that heart and determination can serve you through the toughest challenges and as an Ironman, I was fit to fight. Most importantly, I was proving to myself that I could achieve more as an amputee than I had ever done in my able-bodied life.

—*US Army Major David M Rozelle, the first war amputee to ever complete the grueling Ironman World Championship triathalon in Hawaii, on the impact of sports and recreation to his rehabilitation. The event, held in October 2007, included 2.4 miles of swimming, 112 miles of biking, and 26.2 miles of running.*

INTRODUCTION

In spite of their traumatic injuries, individuals who incur amputations as a result of their military service have access to sports and recreation opportunities that enable them to lead active, healthy, and productive lives. Sports and recreation for Americans with disabilities was introduced in the 1870s, when deaf athletes competed in the sport of baseball at a school for the deaf in Ohio. In the late 1940s, at the close of World War II, famed neurosurgeon Sir Ludwig Guttmann of Stoke Mandeville, England, introduced wheelchair sports as a means to rehabilitate veterans with disabilities, including those with amputations.[1] Since then, sports and recreation for the disabled has proved to be a powerful tool in the rehabilitation process, providing a number of significant therapeutic benefits.[2]

Wheelchair Sports, USA (WSUSA), originally known as the National Wheelchair Athletic Association, was established in 1956 to accommodate athletes with disabilities who wanted to participate in sports other than basketball. Many of the athletes who helped create the organization were World War II veterans, as well as individuals with quadriplegia. WSUSA now offers sporting events to youth with disabilities, having hosted its first youth competition in 1984.[3]

The National Veterans Wheelchair Games, with 16 events, is the largest annual wheelchair sporting event in the world. It now includes an amputee clinic, developed with emphasis on amputees competing on prostheses in various track and field events and facilitated by athletes and coaches of the US Paralympic team. The US Paralympics is the highest caliber sporting event for elite athletes with disabilities.

THERAPEUTIC BENEFITS

Guttmann stated, "…the aims of sport embody the same principles for the disabled as they do for the able-bodied; in addition, however, sport is of immense therapeutic value and plays an essential part in the physical, psychological, and social rehabilitation of the disabled."[1(p12)] Coyle et al[4] cite a number of studies documenting the following therapeutic benefits related to sports and recreation for the disabled:

- Improvement in physical health status: participation in various exercise and fitness activities resulted in significant improvements in cardiovascular and respiratory functioning, and increased strength, endurance, and coordination for persons with disabilities including paraplegia, cystic fibrosis, and asthma.
- Reduction in complications related to secondary disability: physical activity has been demonstrated to reduce secondary medical complications arising from spinal cord injury and other physical disabilities.

- Improvement in long-term health status and reduction in health risk factors: lowered cholesterol levels, reduced heart disease risk, and improved ability to manage chronic pain were reported for persons with physical disabilities.
- Improvement in psychosocial health and well-being: decreased depression, improved body image, and increased acceptance of disability have been reported for physically disabled participants in fitness and athletic activities.
- Reduction in reliance on the healthcare system: participation in exercise and other physical recreation interventions by persons with disabilities resulted in reduced use of asthma medication, and in decreased anxiety and stress of a magnitude equal to or greater than that accomplished through medication. A group of wheelchair athletes demonstrated a rehospitalization rate that was one-third that of a matched group on nonathletes.

CLASSIFICATION

Classification for disabled athletes including amputees is a concept that applies to competitive sports and not to the wide range of recreation and sport activities encompassed in therapeutic, recreational, or fitness sport. The element of competition introduces such factors as rules and regulations for the sport, fairness, and equal opportunity for success despite great difference in individual impairments. Examples of this concept in able-bodied sport include grouping of participants by gender or age, and in certain sports such as weight-lifting, by body weight. When this concept is applied to amputee sports, it seems obvious, for example, that the competitor with an above-knee level of limb loss will be disadvantaged in competition with a below-knee amputee in a sport in which lower limb function is a factor.

From the earliest days of amputee sport, the process of determining the individual's degree of limb loss, or conversely the degree of residual limb function, was quite familiar in trauma surgery, so the first step in classification was considered a medical one. The language of amputee classification has not changed, based as it is on the anatomical facts of limb loss or preservation. Anatomical details, such as extremity or extremities involved and the level of loss within an extremity, represent the basic first step in grouping amputees in fair sport competition. This is sometimes described as "general classification."

Organized amputee competitive sports and classification was created and developed within the International Sports Organization for the Disabled (ISOD), founded in 1964. The ISOD classification system changed over time. Originally, amputee competitors internationally were divided into 27 classes according to their individual physical deficits. However, this approach led to insufficient numbers of competitors in each class and was unworkable. A decision to reduce the number of classes to 12 was made after the Toronto Olympiad in 1976, and in the 1992 Barcelona Paralympics the number was further reduced to nine, as follows[1,5]:

Class A1: double above-knee (A/K)
Class A2: single above-knee (A/K)
Class A3: double below-knee (B/K)
Class A4: single below-knee (B/K)
Class A5: double above-elbow (A/E)
Class A6: single above-elbow (A/E)
Class A7: double below-elbow (B/E)
Class A8: single below-elbow (B/E)
Class A9: combined lower and upper limb amputations

As disability sport has developed, the role of the individual sports federations has become more prominent, and the classification process has become incorporated into the rules of individual sports. In sitting volleyball for lower extremity amputation, for example, the regulations allow all eligible competitors to participate as one class. In wheelchair sports, lower extremity amputees are governed by the rules of the wheelchair sports organization that pertains primarily to spinal paralysis. Winter sports classification is based on the amount of technical device assistance used to allow the amputee to ski, such as the use of one or two adapted ski poles or sitting position for sledge racing. As the rules in specific sports change, classification may become more complex, but the anatomical details of amputation have remained the key determinant in amputee sports classification.

ASSISTIVE TECHNOLOGY

Today, the number of sports and recreation opportunities for veterans with disabilities is extensive, due in large part to advances in assistive technology that compensates for impairments. The Department of Veterans Affairs (VA) Veterans Health Administration is exemplary within the United States in the provision of adaptive recreational and sports equipment. The VA provides a variety of *adaptive* sports and recreation equipment to facilitate healthy living. Devices include sports wheelchairs, handcycles, skiing equipment, bowling equipment, and adaptations for archery, just to name a few. The Clinical Practice Recommendations for Issuance of Recreational and Sports Equipment, written by an interdisciplinary team with the VA Prosthetics Clinical Management Program and approved by the under secretary for health, outlines the recommended approach for providing adaptive equipment to beneficiaries. Key concepts are summarized below. The entire document, including comprehensive information about recreation and sports equipment provided by the VA and the process for purchasing equipment, see www.prosthetics.va.gov.

Each veteran is entitled to an individualized assessment for adaptive recreation and sports equipment. The evaluation includes examining the veteran's medical diagnoses, prognosis, functional abilities, and goals. Veterans and active duty service members enrolled for VA care with loss or loss of use of a body part or function for which an adaptive recreation device is appropriate may be prescribed and provided equipment. Adaptive sports or recreation technology may be issued to veterans seeking to enhance or maintain their health and attain a higher rehabilitation goal through sports or recreation and who meet eligibility criteria. Eligibility criteria includes (but is not limited to):

- medical clearance to perform the activity;
- completed education on appropriate activity and equipment options;
- demonstrated commitment to the activity through regular participation;
- opportunity to participate in the activity consistently (for example, snow must be adequate for cross-country skiing);
- trial of appropriate equipment options configured for specific needs and abilities;
- sports and recreation goals supported by the device; and
- demonstrated ability to use, transport, and store the equipment.

The VA defines "recreational leisure equipment" as any specialized equipment intended for recreational activities that does not inherently exhibit an athletic or physical rehabilitative nature. Examples include adaptive devices for hobbies and crafts or adaptive fishing or hunting devices. The VA defines "recreational sports equipment" as any specialized equipment intended to be utilized in a physically active or competitive environment. Examples include sports wheelchairs, handcycles, sit skis, and artificial limbs for recreational or sports applications. Powered devices for sport participation can potentially be provided to individuals whose activities are severely limited without their use when the individual meets general criteria for power mobility. An example of powered sports equipment is an electric-powered wheelchair for powered wheelchair soccer. Recreation and sports technologies provided by the VA must be adaptive in nature to specifically compensate for loss of or loss of use of a body part or body function. Standard nonadaptive equipment such as skis, boats, and two-wheeled bicycles are not provided by VA.

Accessories for adaptive equipment can also be provided when justified. For example, a car carrier to transport the device to a safe training area or indoor rollers for handcycles or racing wheelchairs in areas with inclement weather may be considered. Seating interventions for postural support and skin protection or specific adaptations for limited hand function may also qualify. The VA Prosthetics and Sensory Aids Service covers repairs and service on sports and recreation equipment per standard policy and procedure. A knowledgeable clinical professional (recreation therapist, rehabilitation engineer, kinesitherapist, physical therapist, or occupational therapist) must be involved in the comprehensive physical evaluation, equipment trials, selection and modification of devices, and education and training. The clinician works closely with the athlete, other equipment experts, and coaches to support the long-term goals of sports and recreation participation.

ACTIVITIES

The information provided below is intended to be a general introduction to sports and recreation opportunities available to amputees in the United States.[6–8]

Aerobics/Physical Fitness

Aerobics is a system of exercise designed to improve respiratory and circulatory function. Disabled Sports, USA (DSUSA) has developed a series of aerobic and strength training videotapes for amputees, paraplegics, quadriplegics, and those with cerebral palsy. DSUSA also has established fitness clinics in several cities across the United States.

Air Guns/Shooting

Air rifle and pistol shooting came onto the US competitive sports scene when WSUSA created a program in 1982. Competition requires shooting from three positions, using a specially designed shooting table or a wheelchair attachment on the athlete's wheelchair. These positions are in accordance with the International Shooting Committee for the Disabled. The sport is organized nationally through the National Wheelchair Shooting Federation/WSUSA. Shooting is a Paralympic sport (Figure 25-1).

Archery

Archery is organized by Disabled Archery USA, in accordance with Fédération Internationale Tir à l'Arc rules. Archers shoot 72 arrows from a distance of 70 m at a target of 122 cm. The National Archery Association has made a commitment to the US Olympic Committee/US Paralympics to act as the national governing body on behalf of archers with disabilities. Archery is a Paralympic sport (Figure 25-2).

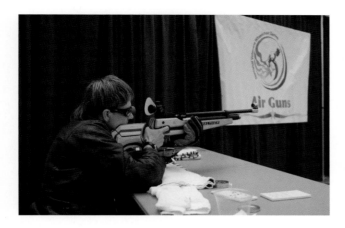

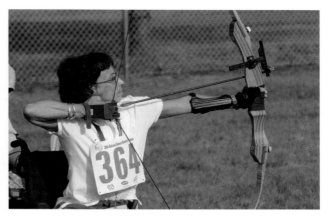

Figure 25-1. Air rifle shooting, 28th National Veterans Wheelchair Games, 2008, Omaha, Nebraska.
Photograph: Courtesy of National Veterans Wheelchair Games.

Figure 25-2. Archery, 28th National Veterans Wheelchair Games, 2008, Omaha, Nebraska.
Photograph: Courtesy of National Veterans Wheelchair Games.

Basketball

The National Wheelchair Basketball Association, which organizes the sport nationally, currently consists of 185 teams competing in 21 conferences. Conference play culminates in annual men's, women's, youth, and collegiate national tournaments held each spring. Wheelchair basketball rules are a slightly modified form of the National Collegiate Athletic Association rules to accommodate the use of a wheelchair. Wheelchair basketball is a Paralympic sport (Figure 25-3).

Bicycling/Handcycling

Handcycling is a form of adaptive cycling that enables athletes of all abilities to ride a "bike" exclusively using the upper body. Bicycle adaptations for hand propulsion include tandem cycles, units that attach to a wheelchair, and some true bicycles. Some models are designed for children. Handcycling follows the rules of the US Handcycling Federation and is governed by WSUSA. Both cycling and handcycling are Paralympic sports; handcycling, which made its first appearance in Athens, Greece, in 2004, is one of the newest competitions at the Paralympic Games (Figure 25-4).

Billiards

Billiards is regulated by the Wheelchair Poolplayers Association. All players must use a wheelchair for pool competition and must remain seated at all times while at the table (Figure 25-5).

Bowling

Wheelchair bowling is regulated by the American Wheelchair Bowling Association using modified American Bowling Congress rules. The Association hosts an annual national tournament and sanctions numerous other tournaments and local league play (Figure 25-6).

Camping

The Office of Special Populations of the National Park Service maintains up-to-date information on accessible parks and offers an individualized search

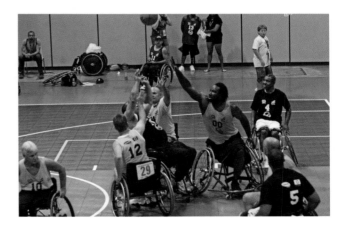

Figure 25-3. Basketball, 28th National Veterans Wheelchair Games, 2008, Omaha, Nebraska.
Photograph: Courtesy of National Veterans Wheelchair Games.

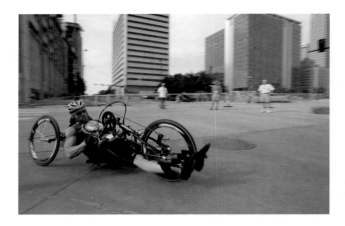

Figure 25-4. Handcycling, 28th National Veterans Wheelchair Games, 2008, Omaha, Nebraska.
Photograph: Courtesy of National Veterans Wheelchair Games.

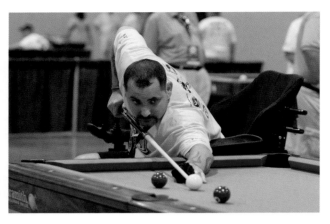

Figure 25-5. Billiards, 28th National Veterans Wheelchair Games, 2008, Omaha, Nebraska.
Photograph: Courtesy of National Veterans Wheelchair Games.

service for a particular geographic area. Many groups organize camping trips into the wilderness for individuals with disabilities.

Canoeing

Canoeing offers freedom to explore areas where a wheelchair will not go. Open canoes offer easy entry and exit and provide room for friends and gear, including wheelchairs.

Curling

Wheelchair curling is a game of great skill and strategy. The first World Cup in Curling for wheelchair players was held in January 2000 in Crans-Montana, Switzerland. Wheelchair curling had its debut at the Torino 2006 Paralympic Winter Games. The sport is open to male and female athletes with a physical disability in the lower part of the body, including athletes with significant impairments in lower leg/gait function (eg, spinal injury, cerebral palsy, multiple sclerosis, double leg amputation) who require a wheelchair for daily mobility. Each team must include male and female players. The game is governed by and played according to the rules of the World Curling Federation, with only one modification—no sweeping (Figure 25-7).

Fencing

Through the sport of wheelchair fencing, athletes practice the centuries-old art of swordsmanship. Wheelchair fencing was developed by Sir Ludwig

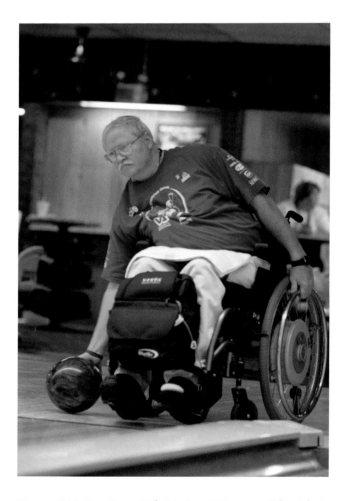

Figure 25-6. Bowling, 28th National Veterans Wheelchair Games, 2008, Omaha, Nebraska.
Photograph: Courtesy of National Veterans Wheelchair Games.

Guttmann at the Stoke Mandeville Hospital and introduced at the 1960 Paralympic Games in Rome. In 2006, 24 countries practiced wheelchair fencing. Requiring a combination of agility, strength, and concentration, fencers compete on one or more of the three weapons, foil, epee, or saber. Athletes compete in wheelchairs that are fastened to the floor. The official governing body is the International Wheelchair and Amputee Sports Federation. Wheelchair fencing is a Paralympic sport.

Fishing

Fishing is a sport that can be fully enjoyed by people with disabilities; a variety of assistive devices are available to meet their needs. Competitive bass fishing tournaments for anglers with physical disabilities are held throughout the United States, including the Paralyzed Veterans of America (PVA) Bass Tour (Figure 25-8).

Flying

Hand-controlled flying has grown in popularity since the Federal Aviation Administration approved the use of portable hand controls.

Football

Although it is a fledgling sport in terms of national organization, wheelchair football has been played for many years. Only a few modifications of the National Collegiate Athletic Association rules have been made for the sport. These include a 60-yard surface playing field with 8-yard end zones, six-person teams, two-hand touch tackles, down-field throws to simulate kicks, and 15 yards for a first down.

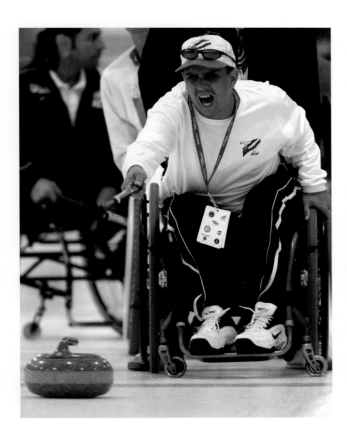

Figure 25-7. Curling, 27th National Veterans Wheelchair Games, 2007, Wisconsin.
Photograph: Courtesy of National Veterans Wheelchair Games.

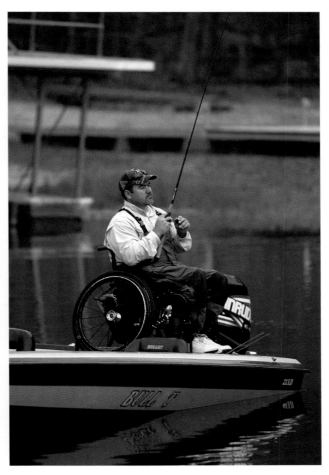

Figure 25-8. Southeastern Paralyzed Veterans of America BASS Tournament, 2008.
Photograph: Courtesy of National Veterans Wheelchair Games.

Golf

Golf is easily adapted for people with disabilities through the use of modified golf equipment. Instructional clinics are popular throughout the United States.

Hockey

Sled hockey is played at the regional, sectional, national, international, and Paralympic levels. Ice sled (sledge) hockey was invented at a Stockholm, Sweden, rehabilitation center in the early 1960s by a group of Swedish men who, despite their physical impairment, wanted to continue playing hockey. The group modified a metal-frame sled, or sledge, with two regular-sized ice hockey skate blades that allowed the puck to pass underneath. Just as in ice hockey, sled hockey is played with six players (including a goalie) at a time. Players propel themselves on their sledge by using spikes on the ends of two 3-foot-long sticks, which also allow the player to shoot and pass ambidextrously. Rinks and goals are regulation Olympic-size, and games consist of three 15-minute stop-time periods. Sled hockey is a Paralympic sport.

Horseback Riding

Horseback riding for the disabled is a popular therapeutic activity offered at a number of stables throughout the United States. Equestrian is a Paralympic sport.

Hunting

Hunting with either a bow-and-arrow or gun is regulated by state law. Many states and organizations have programs designed specifically for the disabled. For more information, contact individual state wildlife management services.

Kayaking

Opportunities for competitive kayaking—both whitewater and flat water—are expanding. The sport demands primarily upper-body strength, and athletes with lower level disabilities can compete equally with nondisabled competitors. The Disabled Paddlers Committee of the American Canoe Association governs the sport.

National Disabled Veterans Winter Sports Clinic

The National Disabled Veterans Winter Sports Clinic is currently the largest rehabilitative program of its type in the world and includes adaptive physical activities as well as workshops and educational sessions that aid in the rehabilitation of severely disabled veterans. Activities such as Alpine and Nordic skiing, snowmobiling, scuba diving, fly fishing, wheelchair golf, wheelchair self-defense, rock wall climbing, sled hockey, trapshooting, blues harmonica instruction, dog sledding, goal ball for the visually impaired, curling, wheelchair fencing, and amputee volleyball are only a small sampling of adaptive sports and activities that have been offered over the past 20 years. Set in the Rocky Mountains in Colorado, the Winter Sports Clinic targets disabled veterans with spinal cord injuries, amputations, neurological disorders, and visual impairments to improve physical well-being, mental health, and self-esteem. Copresented by the VA and Disabled American Veterans, the event hosts over 400 disabled veterans each year.

National Veterans Wheelchair Games

Developed by the VA in conjunction with the International Year of Disabled Persons, the National Veterans Wheelchair Games made its debut on the grounds of the McGuire VA Hospital in Richmond, Virginia, in 1981. There, 74 veterans participated in track, field, swimming, table tennis, slalom, bowling, and billiards. With each successive year, the number of competitors has grown, and now more than 500 veterans compete annually. In 1985 PVA became a copresenter, lending expertise in sports management and fundraising.

The National Veterans Wheelchair Games is now the largest annual wheelchair sporting event in the world, with 16 core events, including archery, basketball, bowling, handcycling, nine ball, quad rugby, softball, swimming, track and field, and weightlifting, conducted in a 4-day meet. Athletes range in experience from novice to master (age 40 and up), and seven physical classification levels ensure equal competition. In 2006 the VA and the US Olympic Committee signed a memorandum of understanding pledging mutual cooperation on training opportunities for veterans to qualify for future Paralympic teams. In 2007 an amputee clinic emphasizing amputees competing on prostheses was held for the first time, with various track and field events conducted and demonstrated by athletes and coaches of the US Paralympic team.

The National Veterans Wheelchair Games is open to all veterans eligible for healthcare through VA who have a physical disability requiring the use of a wheelchair for sports competition. The secretary of Veterans Affairs can and has made exceptions to this requirement to include active duty service members in their initial stages of rehabilitation who may not have been officially discharged from the service. This could include men and women who served in Operation Iraqi Freedom, Operation Enduring Freedom, or other conflicts. Veterans and service members attending the National Veterans Wheelchair Games for the first time receive an opportunity to gain knowledge from other veteran athletes and to acquire sports skills.[9]

Paralympic Games

The Paralympic Games is an international competition among each nation's elite athletes with physical disabilities, including amputees, and is second in size only to the Olympic Games. The Paralympic Games and the Paralympic Winter Games follow the Olympic Games and Olympic Winter Games at the same venues and facilities. The Paralympic Games have been played since 1960 and now feature competition in 19 sports. The Paralympic Winter Games, which showcase four sports, were first held in 1976. The following Paralympic sports include competition for amputees: archery, basketball, curling, cycling, equestrian, fencing, powerlifting, rowing, rugby, sailing, shooting, skiing (Alpine and Nordic), sled hockey, swimming, table tennis, tennis, track and field, and volleyball.

The Paralympic Games has three guiding principles: quality, quantity, and universality. The principle of quality is associated with the Games' grade of excellence, accomplishment, and attainment, achieved by the exciting and inspirational showcasing of elite athletes. Quantity is ensuring that athletes have the support and tools necessary for success, and universality is establishing conditions that reflect the diverse nature of the athletes, including gender and disability types.[10,11]

Power Soccer

With the growth of wheelchair sports, power chair users now have a competitive sport of their own. Power soccer is played with four players on a team trying to push an 18-in physio-ball over the end line of a regulation basketball court for a score. Thick plexiglas guards protect the players' feet and wheelchairs and allow the player to control the ball (Figure 25-9).

Quad Rugby

Quad rugby is a unique, competitive sport for quadriplegics. The game is played on a basketball court by four-member teams using a volleyball. The objective is to carry the ball across the opponent's goal line. WSUSA is the national governing body for this sport. Quad rugby is governed by the US Quad Rugby Association and is a Paralympic sport (Figure 25-10).

Road Racing

Wheelchair road racing is generally run in conjunction with established road races, and wheelchair athletes compete in a separate division against other wheelchair athletes.

Sailing

New designs in sailboats and adaptive equipment allow sailors with disabilities to get on and off and maneuver around sailboats with no or minimal assistance, enabling them to handle a boat much as a nondisabled person would. Sailing is a Paralympic sport.

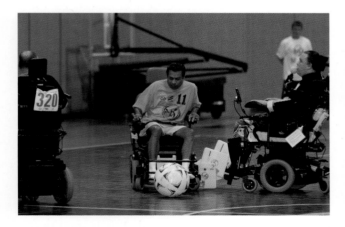

Figure 25-9. Power soccer, 28th National Veterans Wheelchair Games, 2008, Omaha, Nebraska.
Photograph: Courtesy of National Veterans Wheelchair Games.

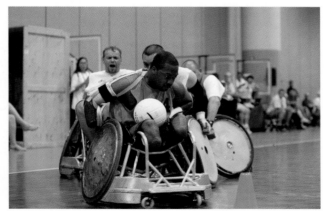

Figure 25-10. Quad rugby, 28th National Veterans Wheelchair Games, 2008, Omaha, Nebraska.
Photograph: Courtesy of National Veterans Wheelchair Games.

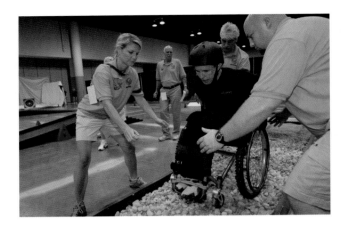

Figure 25-11. Slalom, 28th National Veterans Wheelchair Games, 2008, Omaha, Nebraska.
Photograph: Courtesy of National Veterans Wheelchair Games.

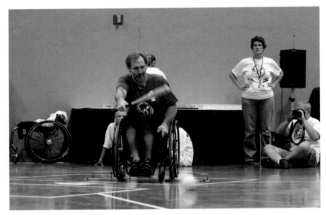

Figure 25-12. Softball, 28th National Veterans Wheelchair Games, 2008, Omaha, Nebraska.
Photograph: Courtesy of National Veterans Wheelchair Games.

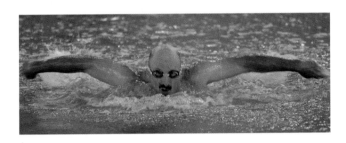

Figure 25-13. Swimming, 23rd National Veterans Wheelchair Games, 2003, Long Beach, California.
Photograph: Courtesy of National Veterans Wheelchair Games.

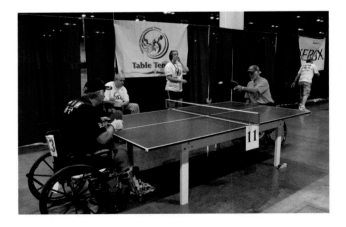

Figure 25-14. Table tennis, 28th National Veterans Wheelchair Games, 2008, Omaha, Nebraska.
Photograph: Courtesy of National Veterans Wheelchair Games.

Scuba Diving

Scuba diving has become readily available to people with disabilities as instructors become more aware of these divers' capabilities.

Skiing

Both competitive and recreation skiing is available for people with disabilities. Athletes can compete in downhill racing, slalom, and giant slalom. Amputees compete standing up in either three- or four-track (ie, with outriggers skis) competition or use a sit-ski or mono-ski, depending on their disability. Nordic and Alpine skiing are governed by DSUSA and are Paralympic sports.

Slalom

Slalom is a unique wheelchair sport that does not parallel an established able-bodied sport. It is a timed test of speed, dexterity, and maneuverability in which competitors follow an obstacle course clearly marked by arrows, flags, and gates. Slalom competition is governed by Wheelchair Athletics of the USA and WSUSA (Figure 25-11).

Softball

Competitive wheelchair softball is played under the official rules of 16-inch slow-pitch softball as approved by the Amateur Softball Association (Figure 25-12).

Swimming

Competitive and recreational swimming can be enjoyed by those with disabilities. Swimmers compete in a variety of distances in the standard strokes of freestyle, backstroke, butterfly, and breaststroke. Swimming is governed by USA Swimming and is a Paralympic sport (Figure 25-13).

Table Tennis

Singles and doubles competition for men and women is played regionally, nationally, and internationally, in accordance with US Table Tennis Association rules. Quadriplegics and others with impaired hand function play table tennis by strapping or taping the paddle to their hand. Table tennis is governed by the American Wheelchair Table Tennis Association and is a Paralympic sport (Figure 25-14).

Tennis

Wheelchair tennis can be enjoyed with nondisabled family and friends. The sport follows the rules of the US Tennis Association with one exception: the wheelchair tennis player is allowed two bounces instead of one. Athletes are classified according to their performance in competition. Introductory lessons are often available at community tennis programs. Wheelchair tennis is a Paralympic sport.

Track and Field

Track events are run on a hard surface, 400-m oval tack, ranging from 100 m to 10,000 m. Field events include the javelin, shot put, and discus. Track and field is governed by Wheelchair Track & Field, USA, and is a Paralympic sport (Figures 25-15 and 25-16).

Trap and Skeet Shooting

Trap and skeet shooting are two sports that allow wheelchair users to compete alongside nondisabled shooters under the same rules. Tournaments are held throughout the United States, including the PVA National Trapshoot Circuit (Figure 25-17).

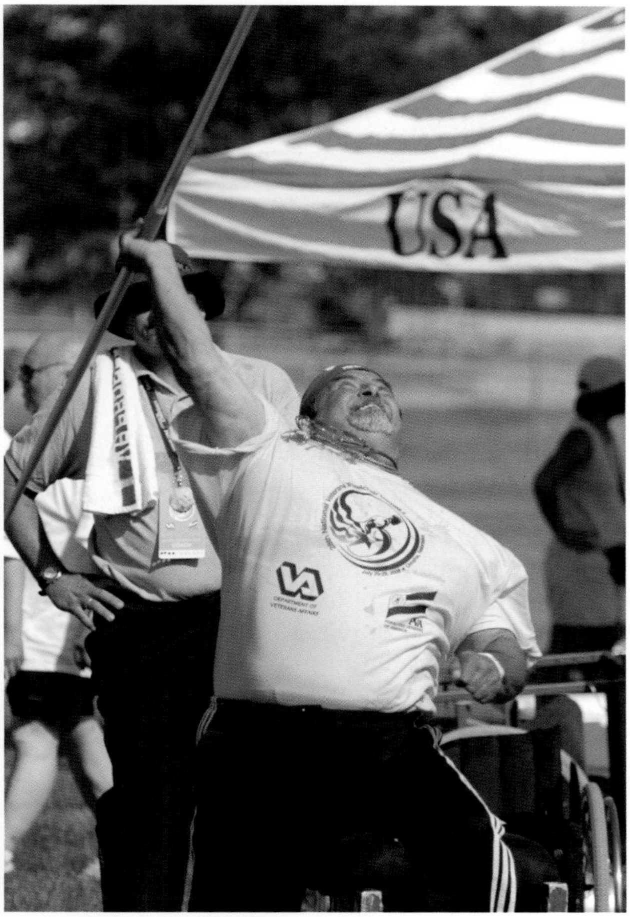

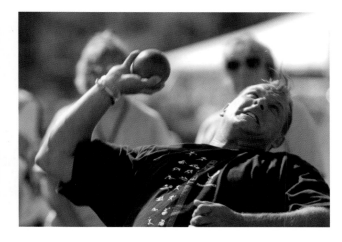

Figure 25-15. Javelin, track and field, 28th National Veterans Wheelchair Games, 2008, Omaha, Nebraska.
Photograph: Courtesy of National Veterans Wheelchair Games.

Figure 25-16. Shot put, track and field, 28th National Veterans Wheelchair Games, 2008, Omaha, Nebraska.
Photograph: Courtesy of National Veterans Wheelchair Games.

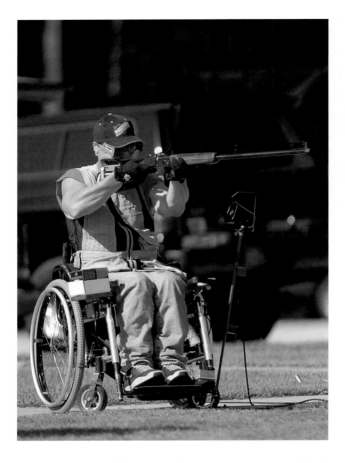

Figure 25-17. Trapshooting, 27th National Veterans Wheelchair Games, 2007, Wisconsin.
Photograph: Courtesy of National Veterans Wheelchair Games.

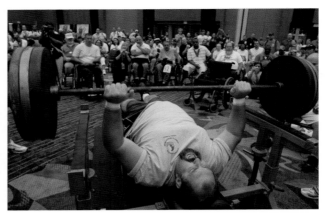

Figure 25-18. Weightlifting, 28th National Veterans Wheelchair Games, 2008, Omaha, Nebraska.
Photograph: Courtesy of National Veterans Wheelchair Games.

Waterskiing

People with disabilities who have the desire to learn to water ski can do so using a modified ski or technique.

Weightlifting

Athletes competing in the conventional bench press are placed in divisions based on body weight. Weightlifting is governed by US Wheelchair Weightlifting Association, and powerlifting is a Paralympic sport (Figure 25-18).

SUMMARY

Originating in the wheelchair games developed by World War II veterans, a wide variety of sports and recreational opportunities are available today to veterans and others with disabilities. Both recreational and competitive activities have documented therapeutic benefits for participants. Athletes participate in competitive sports according to classification systems based on the extent of their disabilities. Ongoing development of assistive technology increases the capabilities of amputees to engage in recreational as well as practical activities. An extensive list of organizations dedicated to promoting access to these activities for all Americans follows in the attachment to this chapter

REFERENCES

1. Guttmann L. *Textbook of Sport for the Disabled*. Aylesburg, England: HM&M Publishers; 1976.

2. Winnick JP, ed. *Adapted Physical Education and Sport*. 4th ed. Champaign, Ill: Human Kinetics Publishers; 2005.

3. About Wheelchair Sports, USA. Wheelchair Sports, USA Web site. Available at: http://www.wsusa.org/. Accessed January 4, 2008.

4. Coyle CP, Kinney WB, Riley B, Shank JW, eds. *Benefits of Therapeutic Recreation: A Consensus View*. Philadelphia, Pa: Temple University; 1991.

5. Scruton J. *Stoke Mandeville: Road to the Paralympics.* Aylesbury, England: Peterhouse Press; 1998.

6. Paralyzed Veterans of America. *A Guide to Wheelchair Sports and Recreation.* Waldorf, Md: PVA Distribution Center; 1997.

7. Sports associations. *Sports 'N Spokes.* 2007;33(1):40.

8. Sports & recreation programs. *Active Living.* 2007; 5(1):87–88

9. National Veterans Wheelchair Games face sheet. National Veterans Wheelchair Games Web site. Available at: http://www1.va.gov/vetevent/nvwg/2008/default.cfm. Accessed January 6, 2008.

10. Paralympic Games principles. Paralympic Games Web site. Available at: http://www.paralympic.org/release/Main_Sections_Menu/Paralympic_Games/Games_Principles/. Accessed January 4, 2008.

11. Steadward R, Peterson C. *Paralympics: Where Heroes Come.* Edmonton, Alberta, Canada: One Shot Holdings; 1997.

ATTACHMENT: ORGANIZATIONS PROMOTING SPORTS AND RECREATION FOR PERSONS WITH DISABILITIES

In addition to the activities described in this chapter, a number of organizations provide sports and recreation programming for individuals with disabilities. The information provided is a general introduction to organizations that offer sports and recreation programs for amputees in the United States.

Access to Sailing
6475 E Pacific Coast Highway
Long Beach, CA 90803
(562) 433-0561
www.accesstosailing.org

Access to Sailing provides therapeutic rehabilitation to disabled and disadvantaged children and adults through interactive sailing outings.

AccessSportAmerica
Acton, MA
(978) 264-0985
www.accessportamerica.org

AccesSportAmerica, a national nonprofit organization, is dedicated to the discovery and achievement of higher function and fitness for children and adults of all disabilities through high-challenge sports.

Achilles Track Club
New York, NY
(212) 354-0300

Achilles is a worldwide organization, represented in 60 countries. Its mission is to enable people with all types of disabilities to participate in mainstream athletics, to promote personal achievement, enhance self-esteem, and lower barriers between people.

Adapted Adventures
Evergreen, CO
(877) 679-2770
www.adaptiveadventures.org

Founded by a group of physically challenged individuals in 1999, Adaptive Adventures saw a need to increase awareness and participation in disabled sports and recreation for people of all ages. The organization improves the quality of life of individuals with disabilities through year-round adaptive sports and recreation programs.

Adapted Sports Association
Durango, CO
(970) 259-0374
www.asadurango.org

The Adaptive Sports Association (ASA) was founded in 1983 by Dave Spencer, a ski instructor who lost a leg to cancer as a young man. Spencer believed that skiing could challenge and increase the self-esteem of all individuals with disabilities. ASA helps to enrich and transform the lives of people with disabilities through sports. Through sports and recreation, participants meet positive role models, increase socialization skills, improve body image, and combat depression. Through the use of state-of-the-art equipment, ASA is able to offer its services to individuals with every type of disability. Over 50 ASA ski and snowboard instructors are nationally certified through Professional Ski Instructors of America and the American Association of Snowboard Instructors. ASA is also a member of DSUSA. Quality instruction and safety are primary concerns of ASA.

Adapted Sports Center
Crested Butte, CO
(866) 349-2296
www.adaptivesports.org

The Adaptive Sports Center is a nonprofit organization that provides year-round recreation activities for people with disabilities and their families.

Adaptive Aquatics
Wilsonville, AL
(205) 807-7519
www.adaptiveaquatics.org

Each year from April to October, Adaptive Aquatics provides nationwide water skiing instruction through comprehensive clinics and workshops. With the use of specialized equipment and expert instruction, Adaptive Aquatics opens avenues to greater independence and allows people with disabilities to experience the excitement of water sports.

Adventure Pursuit
Parkersburg, WV
(304) 485-0911
www.adventurepursuit.org

Adventure Pursuit is a nonprofit corporation that offers adventures in boating, biking, and swimming.

All Out Adventures
Easthampton, MA
(413) 527-8980
www.alloutadventures.org

All Out Adventure's mission is to provide individuals of all abilities unlimited opportunities to build confidence, foster independence, and promote wellness while exploring new environments. It offers summer and winter recreation programs throughout the New England area.

America's Athletes With Disabilities
Silver Spring, MD
(301) 589-9042
www.americasathletes.org

Founded in 1985, America's Athletes With Disabilities is a consortium of both single and multiple disability groups, organizations, individuals, and corporate sponsors who passionately advocate both single and multiple sport activities and programs to better serve persons with physical disabilities. The organization improves the quality of life for children, young people, and adults with physical disabilities and their families through sports, recreation, leisure, and fitness programs.

American Canoe Association
7432 Alban Station Boulevard, Suite B-232
Springfield, VA 22150
(703) 451-0141
www.acanet.org

Established in 1980, the American Canoe Association has a strong commitment to making all aspects of canoe sports—canoeing, river kayaking, and sea kayaking—accessible. The organization serves as a clearinghouse for information on paddling, as well as with paddlers on a one-to-one basis to recommend specific adaptations, instruction sites, and trip opportunities.

American Dancewheels Foundation, Inc
Bala-Cynwyd, PA
(215) 588-6671
www.americandancewheels.org

The foundation provides wheelchair dancing instruction to the disabled community.

American Wheelchair Bowling Association
PO Box 69
Clover, VA 24534
(434) 454-2269
www.awba.org

The American Wheelchair Bowling Association was formed in 1962 to organize and coordinate wheelchair bowling and provide national competition. Local and sectional tournaments are held across the country. Members receive a newsletter, rulebook, and a how-to guidebook on wheelchair bowling.

American Wheelchair Table Tennis Association
23 Parker Street
Port Chester, NY 10573
(914) 937-3932

American Wheelchair Table Tennis Association, a member organization of WSUSA, sanctions and conducts wheelchair table tennis tournaments throughout the United States. Membership entitles the individual to a quarterly newsletter, rulebook, and liability insurance, plus other benefits. The association organizes the American wheelchair table tennis team each year and also maintains a national athlete ranking system.

BlazeSports America
Atlanta, GA
(770) 850-8199
www.blazesports.com

BlazeSports America is a direct legacy of the 1996 Paralympic Games held in Atlanta, Georgia, the first Paralympic Games held in the United States. In 1993 the Atlanta Paralympic Organizing Committee established the US Disabled Athlete's Fund (USDAF) to develop a national program making community-based adaptive sports a reality for children and adults with physical disabilities. Following the 1996 Paralympic Games, USDAF, in partnership with the Georgia Recreation and Parks Association, introduced BlazeSports Georgia in 1997. BlazeSports America provides sports training, competitions, summer camps, and other sports and recreational opportunities for youth and adults who use wheelchairs or have a visual impairment, amputation, or neurological disability such as cerebral palsy or spina bifida.

Breckenridge Outdoor Education Center
PO Box 697
Breckenridge, CO 80424
(970) 453-6422
www.boec.org

Breckenridge Outdoor Education Center offers year-round wilderness adventure programs throughout the Rocky Mountains. Activities include backpacking, rock climbing, rafting, downhill and cross-country skiing, winter camping, and mountaineering.

Challenge Aspen
Aspen, CO
(970) 923-0578
www.challengeaspen.com

Established in 1995, Challenge Aspen provides access for all to a wide variety of seasonal sports and recreational and cultural activities for adults and children. Thanks to Challenge Aspen and a dedicated volunteer staff and board of directors, those with physical and mental challenges have access to recreational sports such as downhill and cross-country skiing, whitewater rafting, horseback riding, swimming, gymnastics, hiking, and fishing. Seasonal camps include a mono-ski camp and a rock climbing camp for paraplegics and amputees and a ski festival for the visually impaired. Based in Snowmass Village, with access to the area's four ski mountains, Challenge Aspen currently serves more than 400 participants each year, with over 2,100 participant days.

Challenged Athletes Foundation
San Diego, CA
(858) 866-0959
www.challengedathletes.org

It is the mission of the Challenged Athletes Foundation to provide opportunities and support to people with physical disabilities so they can pursue active lifestyles through physical fitness and competitive athletics. The Foundation believes that involvement in sports at any level increases self-esteem, encourages independence, and enhances quality of life.

Colorado Discover Ability Integrated
Outdoor Adventure
Fruita, CO
(970) 858-0200
www.coloradodiscoverability.com

Colorado Discover Ability is a nonprofit organization whose mission is to promote increased independence and self-worth through outdoor recreation for individuals with disabilities, as well as their families and friends. Its programs have been serving the disabled in the Grand Valley area of Colorado for over 20 years.

Cooperative Wilderness Handicapped Outdoor Group
Idaho State University
Box 8128
Pocatello, ID 83209
(208) 282-3912

Cooperative Wilderness Handicapped Outdoor Group offers a year-round calendar of whitewater rafting, camping, all-terrain vehicle trips, waterskiing, and Alpine skiing in rugged Idaho terrain. Activities span a half-day to a week.

Courage Center
Minneapolis, MN
(763) 520-0262
www.courage.org

Since 1928, Minneapolis-based Courage Center, a nonprofit rehabilitation and resource center, has improved the lives of people experiencing barriers to health and independence. Its continuum of care includes rehabilitation therapies; transitional rehabilitation; pain management; vocational and community-based services; and camping, sports, and recreation programs, including fitness centers and aquatic therapy, for people of all ages and abilities. Courage Center specializes in pain management, brain injury, spinal cord injury, and congenital disabilities.

Department of Veterans Affairs
810 Vermont Ave, NW
Washington, DC 20420
www.va.gov

The VA is the second largest cabinet department in the US government. The VA strives to meet the needs of America's veterans and their families in a responsive, timely, and compassionate manner in recognition of their service to the nation. With 220,000 employees, more than 160 hospitals, hundreds of outpatient clinics, and 58 regional offices, the department responds to the healthcare and benefits needs of the nation's 25 million veterans.

Wheelchair sports originated after World War II when disabled veterans began playing wheelchair basketball in VA hospitals throughout the United States. Wheelchair recreation and competition soon spread to other sports, such as track and field, bowling, swimming, and archery. The National Veterans Wheelchair Games, along with the VA's three other national rehabilitation special events (the National Disabled Veterans Winter Sports Clinic, the National Veterans Golden Age Games, and the National Veterans Creative Arts Festival) are outgrowths of VA's historical involvement in wheelchair sports. Since they were founded, these events have been on the cutting edge of innovative rehabilitative programs.

Disabled Archery, USA
PO Box 698
Langley, WA 98260
(360) 321-5979
www.da-usa.org

Disabled Archery USA's mission is to discover, develop, and support disabled men and women in the United States in their pursuit of world-class archery. As a part of this mission, and in coordination with USA Archery, Disabled Archery USA names athletes to the US national disabled archery team each year. Members from this national pool of athletes are then eligible for selection to various national archery teams that compete in events such as the International Paralympic Committee World Championships and the Paralympic Games. The selection process for these teams is a coordinated effort among Disabled Archery USA, USA Archery, and US Paralympics.

Disabled Sports, USA
451 Hungerford Drive, Suite 100
Rockville, MD 20850
(301) 217-0960
www.dsusa.org

A national, nonprofit, 501(c)(3) organization established in 1967 by disabled Vietnam veterans to serve the war injured, DSUSA now offers nationwide sports rehabilitation programs to anyone with a permanent disability. Sports and recreational activities include snow and water skiing, aerobics, canoeing, river rafting, biking, and horseback riding. Participants include those with visual impairments, amputations, spinal cord injury, dwarfism, multiple sclerosis, head injury, cerebral palsy, and other neuromuscular and orthopedic conditions.

In most cases, instruction and use of equipment are offered free of charge or at minimal cost. DSUSA organizes regional and national ski competitions from which the US disabled ski team is selected. DSUSA also organizes regional and national competitions for amputees, as well as fitness clinics for people with a wide range of disabilities. DSUSA members receive a newsletter three times each year and a reduction in program fees.

Like WSUSA, DSUSA is a member of the US Olympic Committee and therefore responsible for the sanctioning and conduct of competitions and training camps to prepare and select athletes to represent the United States at Summer and Winter Paralympic Games. Both groups function as umbrella organizations for their national governing bodies. DSUSA oversees Alpine and Nordic skiing, track and field, volleyball, swimming, cycling, and powerlifting.

In partnership with the Wounded Warrior Project, DSUSA conducts the Wounded Warrior Disabled Sports Project, which aims to work with wounded service members as soon as they enter occupational and physical therapy. With the proper adaptive equipment and trained instructors, patients can successfully learn the basics of almost any sport in just 1 day. This immediate success provides a foundation for the development of a positive self-image and outlook on life, key factors leading to an independent, full, and productive life. Even those suffering from the most severe injuries (eg, triple amputee, blindness, paralysis) are able to compete in the most extreme of sports. Rock climbing, kayaking, snow skiing, snowboarding, water skiing, golf, basketball, track and field, cycling, sailing, outrigger canoeing, scuba, wheelchair basketball, sled hockey, hunting and fishing are just a small sample of the different types of sports that the project offers. The project provides wounded service members and their families and friends these opportunities free of charge, including transportation, lodging, adaptive equipment, and individualized instructions. Family members are taught the sport as well. Programs take place at sites throughout the United States.

Eastern Amputee Golf Association
Bethlehem, PA
(888) 868-0992
www.eaga.org

The Eastern Amputee Golf Association was formed by Bob Buck, retired National Amputee Golf Association's eastern trustee, and others. The organization was formed with the same guidelines as the National Amputee Golf Association but has its own officers, constitution, bylaws, and membership dues. Its prime purpose is to organize and conduct amputee golfing events and "learn to golf" clinics for any physically challenged individual, provide communication between its members, and act as a bridge between its members and the National Association.

Electric Wheelchair Hockey Association
Minneapolis, MN
(763) 535-4736
www.powerhockey.com

Electric Wheelchair Hockey's mission is to provide a quality hockey program for persons requiring the use of an power wheelchair in daily life. Power Hockey is based on basic hockey rules with a few adaptations to allow everyone in a power wheelchair the ability to participate.

Fishing Has No Boundaries
Hayward, WI
(800) 243-3462
www.fhnbinc.org

Fishing Has No Boundaries provides recreational fishing opportunities for all anglers with disabilities regardless of age, race, gender, or disability. A resource for information on adaptive fishing equipment and accessibility, the organization promotes research and development of specialized adaptive equipment to enhance fishing experiences for anglers with disabilities.

Freedom's Wings International
P.O. Box 7076
East Brunswick, NJ 08816
(800) 382-1197
www.freedomswings.org

Freedom's Wings International is a nonprofit organization run by and for people with physical disabilities that provides the opportunity for those who are physically challenged to fly in specially adapted sailplanes, either as a passenger or as a member of the flight training program. For an annual membership fee, Freedom's Wings International provides flight training with certified instructors, hand-control–equipped aircraft, and support equipment for those who wish to become sailplane pilots.

Handicapped Scuba Association
1104 El Prado
San Clemente, CA 92672
(949) 498-4540
www.hsascuba.com

Since 1974 the nonprofit Handicapped Scuba Association has held diving classes pairing nondisabled with disabled divers. It also operates as a dive club, offering refresher courses and coordinating excursions. The organization can provide lectures and video presentations to any group. A videotape on scuba diving for people with disabilities is available. Dedicated to improving the physical and social well-being of people with disabilities through the exhilarating sport of scuba diving, the organization has become the worldwide authority in the field.

International Wheelchair Aviators
PO Box 2799
Big Bear Lake, CA 92314
(909) 585-9663
www.wheelchairaviators.org

Members of International Wheelchair Aviators, open to anyone interested in learning to fly, receive a monthly newsletter plus a roster of the group and are encouraged to participate in monthly fly-ins.

John's Golf Course
Eureka, MT
(406) 889-3685
www.johnsgolfcourse.com

John's Golf Course is a nonprofit course for the handicapped with no greens fees.

Kayak Adventures
Jacksonville Beach, FL
(904) 249-6200
www.kayakadventuresllc.com/disable.htm

With specialized paddling skills, technical knowledge, and adaptive equipment, Kayak Adventures offers kayaking to people with disabilities.

National Ability Center
Park City, UT
(435) 649-3991

Founded in 1985, the National Ability Center is a nonprofit, tax-exempt organization offering activities for the disabled at an affordable rate, with scholarships available, to ensure participation for all applicants. Programs are supported through special events, grants from private corporations and foundations, individual donations, and program fees.

National Alliance for Accessible Golf
Reston, WA
(703) 234-4136
www.accessgolf.org

Formed in 2001 by leaders of the golf industry and representatives of organizations serving people with disabilities, the National Alliance for Accessible Golf works to increase participation of people with disabilities in the game of golf.

National Amputee Golf Association
11 Walnut Hill Road
Amherst, NH 03031
(800) 633-6242
www.nagagolf.org

Begun in 1947, the National Amputee Golf Association is open to anyone who has lost a hand or foot at a major joint. It conducts learn-to-golf clinics for any physically disabled individual in the country. Members receive an annual magazine, newsletters, and tournament information.

National Rifle Association Disabled Shooting Services
11250 Waples Mill Road
Fairfax, VA 22030
(703) 267-1495
www.nrahq.org/compete/disabled.asp

The programs offered by the National Rifle Association's Disabled Shooting Services department have enabled thousands of Americans with physical disabilities to enjoy a variety of shooting activities, including competitive events and hunting. The organization has also worked to ensure that many shooting facilities are wheelchair-accessible.

National Sports Center for the Disabled
Winter Park, CO
(970) 726-1548
www.nscd.org

The National Sports Center for the Disabled began in 1970 as a one-time ski lesson for children with amputations for the Children's Hospital of Denver. Today it is one of the largest outdoor therapeutic recreation agencies in the world. Each year, thousands of children and adults with disabilities take to the ski slopes, mountain trails, and golf courses to learn more about sports, and themselves. With specially trained staff and its own adaptive equipment laboratory, the Center teaches a variety of winter and summer sports and activities to individuals with almost any physical, cognitive, emotional, or behavioral diagnosis.

National Wheelchair Basketball Association
8245 Charles Crawford Lane
Charlotte, NC 28262
(704) 547-0176
www.nwba.org

Founded in 1948, the National Wheelchair Basketball Association (NWBA) is the nation's oldest and largest disability sport organization. Based in Colorado Springs, Colorado, the NWBA is a nonprofit organization that serves as the national governing body for men's, women's, intercollegiate, and youth wheelchair basketball in the United States. The NWBA's mission is to provide persons with permanent lower limb disabilities the opportunity to play, learn, and compete in wheelchair basketball. Today over 2,000 member athletes compete on more than 185 teams throughout the United States.

In 1978 the NWBA established the Central Intercollegiate Conference—the only collegiate conference for disabled sport—to provide student-athletes with disabilities the opportunity to compete at the collegiate level. Since then, Conference member teams and their players have consistently competed at the sport's highest competitive levels while adhering to National Collegiate Athletic Association academic and eligibility standards. Today, the NWBA continues to be a major force in wheelchair basketball with the development of players and the dedication of a group of highly respected professionals in the areas of coaching and organization.

National Wheelchair Poolplayers Association
4370 Majestic Lane
Fairfax, VA 22033
(703) 817-1215
www.nwpainc.org

Established in 1994, the National Wheelchair Poolplayers Association is the governing body for all organized wheelchair pool. The association has nearly 400 members worldwide, including players of all ages and disability. All players must use a wheelchair for pool competition and must remain seated at all times while at the table.

National Wheelchair Shooting Federation
102 Park Avenue
Rockledge, PA 19046
(215) 379-2359

A member of WSUSA, the National Wheelchair Shooting Federation conducts and sanctions air rifle and pistol shooting in the United States. Members receive WSUSA services, the constitution and bylaws, and a bimonthly newsletter. Each year the Federation selects and organizes the US Wheelchair Shooting Team, which competes in international competition.

National Wheelchair Softball Association
6000 West Floyd Avenue #110
Denver, CO 80227
(303) 936-5587
www.wheelchairsoftball.org

Founded in 1976, the National Wheelchair Softball Association is the national governing body for wheelchair softball in the United States. Membership is open to competing teams and associate members. Members receive newsletters and other information throughout the year. The National Wheelchair Softball Tournament, held each year in September, is a double elimination tournament of 10 or more teams.

North American Riding for the Handicapped Association
PO Box 33150
Denver, CO 80233
(800) 369-RIDE
www.narha.org

North American Riding for the Handicapped Association has chapters nationwide, with specially trained teachers and horses available for use by riders with disabilities. Several types of membership are available, and the association provides a bimonthly newsletter, an annual journal, and discounts on related publications.

Northeast Passage
Durham, NH
(603) 862-0070
www.nepassage.org

Northeast Passage, founded in 1990, is a nationally recognized leader in the provision of innovative therapeutic recreation services. The organization delivers disability-related health promotion and adapted sports programs throughout New England. It is a program of the University of New Hampshire's School of Health and Human Services and an affiliate of DSUSA. Based at the University of New Hampshire's Durham campus, Northeast Passage runs six core programs for people with disabilities, their families, and friends.

Paralyzed Veterans of America
801 Eighteenth Street, NW
Washington, DC 20006
(800) 424-8200
www.pva.org

The PVA was founded in 1946 with the vision of a better life for paralyzed veterans and others with disabilities. In pursuing this goal, PVA has been instrumental in achieving significant advances in the areas of accessibility, employment, spinal cord injury/dysfunction research, and sports and recreation, so that people with disabilities have opportunities for full participation in society. Since its earliest days, PVA has been a leader in the development of wheelchair sports in the United States. Today PVA sponsors many major national wheelchair sports championship events and supports such organizations as the National Wheelchair Basketball Association, US Quad Rugby Association, National Wheelchair Softball Association, American Wheelchair Bowling Association, and the National Wheelchair Poolplayers Association. PVA also publishes *Sports 'n Spokes,* a full-color magazine that covers exciting events, personalities, training, and equipment in wheelchair sports. PVA and VA annually copresent the National Veterans Wheelchair Games.

PVA's boating and fishing program introduces people to recreational and competitive fishing. Its hallmark event is the PVA Bass Tour, an event sanctioned by the Bass Anglers Sportsman Society (BASS), through which PVA chapters across the country host fishing tournaments for people with disabilities. Anglers may fish from a boat or from shore, paired with able-bodied boat partners or volunteers on shore to provide any necessary assistance with fishing tasks. Each year an angler of the year earns a coveted spot in the BASS Federation Nation National Championship and the opportunity to qualify in the Bassmasters Classic.

The PVA shooting sports program has activities ranging from recreational and competitive shooting to big- and small-game hunts. The cornerstone of the program is the PVA National Trapshoot Circuit, which consists of tournaments throughout the country that give individuals with disabilities a chance to participate in the recreational and competitive sport of trapshooting. Trapshooting is one of the few sports where there are no rule distinctions between competitors using wheelchairs or standing.

In 2004 PVA implemented the Operation Iraqi Freedom/Operation Enduring Freedom Injured Troop Support program to provide outreach to Walter Reed Army Medical Center and financially support the participation of recently injured troops from the conflicts in Iraq and Afghanistan in the National Veterans Wheelchair Games, PVA Bass Tour, PVA National Trapshoot Circuit, Vermejo Park Ranch-PVA Elk Hunt, assorted hunting opportunities, and the Outdoor Channel Offshore Classic Sailfish Tournament. In 2007 PVA partnered with the National Wheelchair Poolplayers Association and the American Wheelchair Bowling Association to implement a billiards tournament series and a bowling tournament series, hosted by PVA chapters.

As part of its outdoor sports development program, PVA provides adaptive sporting equipment to military installations and state wildlife agencies. Such equipment provides a critical bridge of accessibility, enabling those with disabilities to participate in outdoor sports. For example, Huntmasters, wheelchair-accessible compartments that elevate to 20 ft, afford occupants a vantage point for hunting or wildlife viewing. PVA's commitment to wheelchair sports and recreation is recognized by the sporting industry, government agencies, and other organizations dedicated to providing outdoor experiences, sports, and recreational activities for their members.

Physically Challenged Bowhunters of America, Inc
New Alexandria, PA
(724) 668-7439
www.pcba-inc.org

Founded in 1993, the nonprofit Physically Challenged Bowhunters of America Inc has opened the outdoor sports of target archery, competitive archery, and bowhunting to tens of thousands of physically challenged people across the United States and Canada.

US Adaptive Recreation Center
Big Bear Lake, CA
(909) 584-0269
www.usarc.org

The US Adaptive Recreation Center was founded in 1983 (as California Handicapped Skiers) to ensure that access to skiing is available to people with all types of disabilities. The Center believes people are empowered when they undertake and succeed at challenging outdoor recreation. In 1989 the Center established the first full-time on-site adaptive ski school in southern California at Bear Mountain Resort. Adaptive watersports and summer camping programs were added in 1993.

US Disabled Alpine Ski Team
PO Box 100
Park City, UT 84060
(435) 649-9090
www.usskiteam.com

Begun after World War II, the US Disabled Alpine Ski Team is composed of athletes with disabilities who receive training with the US Ski Team.

US Fencing Association
1 Olympic Plaza
Colorado Springs, CO 80909
(719) 866-4511
www.usfencing.org

Wheelchair fencing in the United States is governed by the WSUSA. US Fencing Association wheelchair fencers are chosen to compete at the Paralympic and international levels.

US Golf Association
Colorado Springs, CO
(719) 471-4810, ext 15
www.resourcecenter.usga.org

The US Golf Association believes that golf's enjoyment should be accessible to all. The Association's Resource Center for Individuals with Disabilities, created to make golf more accessible for the growing population of individuals with disabilities, gathers and makes available information vital to potential or current golfers with disabilities and other interested members of the golf and medical communities.

US Handcycling Federation
PO Box 3538
Evergreen, CO 80439
(303) 459-4159
www.ushf.org

The US Handcycling Federation, governed by WSUSA, was formed in 1998 by wheelchair athletes, coaches, and supporters to promote integration of athletes with and without disabilities in the sport of cycling. The Federation is an association of individuals and organizations who share a common goal of health, fitness, and well-being for cyclists of all ages, abilities, and backgrounds. Handcycling is a form of adaptive cycling that enables athletes of all abilities to ride a "bike" exclusively using the upper body. Handcycling is also one of the newest competitions at the Paralympic Games, where it made its first appearance in Athens, Greece, in 2004.

US Olympic Committee/US Paralympics
One Olympic Plaza
Colorado Springs, CO 80909
(719) 632-5551
www.usoc.org

The US Olympic Committee, composed of 72 member organizations, is the coordinating body for Olympic-related athletic activity in the United States. The Committee's vision is to assist in finding opportunities for every American to participate in sport, regardless of gender, race, age, geography, or physical ability. US Paralympics is a division of the US Olympic Committee, formed in 2001 to increase support for Paralympic sport.

The Paralympic military program is conducted in coordination with the VA and Department of Defense. Under a current proposal, the US Olympic Committee would coordinate Paralympic sport activities for service members at Walter Reed Army Medical Center, Brooke Army Medical Center, and US Navy Medical Center–San Diego, including daily coaching in multiple sports, on-site coordination of sport activities, and transition assistance to service members being discharged to home installations or civilian life. Existing activities are listed below.

Military Sport Camps

Paralympic military sports camps, held twice a year, provide opportunities for injured service members and veterans to demonstrate their abilities through clinics and low-impact competition. There is no cost to the service member.

World-Class Athlete Programs

The Army and Air Force world-class athlete programs allow a military athlete full-time training for up to 3 years prior to an Olympic Games. In 2005 both the Air Force and the Army programs became available for Paralympic-eligible athletes on active duty. Paralympic-eligible service members are identified by the Paralympic coaching staff at various qualification events across the country.

Veterans' Paralympic Performance Program

The Veterans' Paralympic Performance Program (VP3) is a new venture to cultivate and support Paralympic-eligible military veterans at upcoming Paralympic Games. VP3 is being created primarily to serve veterans under the age of 35 who have been injured in current overseas military actions, but the program will be open to any Paralympic-eligible, athletically qualified veteran with an honorable discharge who meets the other requirements and commitments of the program.

US Quad Rugby Association
1702 Lincoln Drive
Voorhees, NJ 08043
(856) 491-4210
www.quadrugby.com

In 1988, the US Quad Rugby Association was formed to help promote and regulate the sport of quad rugby on both a national and international level. Since its organized inception, the sport has grown from an original four teams to more than forty-five teams in the United States today! In addition to the growth of the sport in the United States, it has grown internationally as well. It is now played in more than 24 nations.

US Sled Hockey Association
710 N Lake Shore Drive, 3rd Floor
Chicago, IL 60611
(312) 908-4292
www.sledhockey.org

The US Sled Hockey Association organizes and sanctions sled hockey competition in the United States.

US Tennis Association
70 W Red Oak Lane
White Plains, NY 10604
(914) 696-7000
www.usta.com

Wheelchair tennis is one of the fastest growing and most challenging of all wheelchair sports. To meet this demand, the US Tennis Association offers programs geared toward the wheelchair player. Rules are the same as stand-up tennis, except the wheelchair player is allowed two bounces of the ball. A wheelchair tennis player must have a medically diagnosed, mobility-related disability, with a substantial or total loss of function in one or more extremities. In wheelchair tennis, the player must master the game and the wheelchair. Learning mobility on the court is exciting and challenging, and helps build strength and cardiovascular ability. Proficient wheelchair users can actively compete against stand-up players. Wheelchair tennis provides persons with disabilities the opportunity to share in activities with their peers and family, whether able-bodied or disabled.

USA Volleyball
Colorado Springs, CO
(719) 228-6800
www.usavolleyball.org

USA Volleyball offers sitting and standing volleyball.

US Wheelchair Swimming, Inc
PO Box 5266
Kendall Park, NJ 08824
(732) 422-4546
www.wsusa.org

This member organization of WSUSA conducts and sanctions swimming competition for individuals with disabilities in the United States. Members receive a quarterly newsletter, rulebook, and other benefits. US Wheelchair Swimming selects and organizes swimmers with disabilities for international and Paralympic competition.

US Wheelchair Weightlifting Federation
PO Box 5266
Kendall Park, NJ 08824
(732) 422-4546
www.wsusa.org

This member organization of WSUSA conducts and sanctions weightlifting in the United States.

Universal Wheelchair Football Association
UC Raymond Walters College
Disability Services Office
9555 Plainfield Road
Cincinnati, OH 45236-1096
(513) 792-8625

The Universal Wheelchair Football Association promotes a version of wheelchair football for individuals with all types and levels of disabilities. Association football is played indoors or outdoors with a foam football.

Veterans on the Lake Resort
161 Fernberg Road
Ely, MN 55731
(800) 777-7538
www.veterans-on-the-lake.com

Veterans on the Lake Resort, a not-for-profit organization, provides a barrier-free setting for outdoor recreation experiences for disabled veterans, veterans, their families, friends, and supporters.

Water Skiers With Disabilities Association
1251 Holy Cow Road
Polk City, FL 33868
(800) 533-2972
www.usawaterski.org

The Water Skiers With Disabilities Association was created in 1949 as an official sport division of the American Water Ski Association (now USA Water Ski). Its purpose is to organize, promote, and direct water skiing for individuals with disabilities from learn-to-ski clinics to international competition. The US Olympic Committee and the International Water Ski Federation recognize USA Water Ski as the national governing body for the sport of water skiing in the United States.

Wheelchair Dancesport USA Association
Irvington, NY
(212) 245-0004
www.wheelchairdancesportusa.org

The mission of the nonprofit Wheelchair Dancesport USA is to promote, initiate, and stimulate the growth and development of wheelchair "dancesport" in the United States. The organization provides wheelchair dance programs and organizes classes, performances, training camps, and seminars for those serving children and adults with disabilities, as well as supporting recreational and competitive wheelchair dancers and able-bodied dancers, while emphasizing the healthful physical, mental, and social benefits of wheelchair ballroom dancing. Wheelchair Dancesport prepares wheelchair athletes and coaches to participate in regional, national, and international competitions.

Wheelchair Sports, USA
PO Box 5266
Kendall Park, NJ 08824
(732) 422-4546
www.wsusa.org

WSUSA and DSUSA are disabled sports organizations that function as umbrella organizations for their respective national governing bodies. Both are members of the US Olympic Committee and therefore responsible for the sanctioning and conduct of competitions and training camps to prepare and select athletes to represent the United States at summer and winter Paralympic Games. WSUSA was established in 1956, and oversees the following national governing bodies: Wheelchair Archery, USA; Wheelchair Track & Field, USA; National Wheelchair Shooting Federation; USA Swimming; American Wheelchair Table Tennis Association; and US Wheelchair Weightlifting Association.

Wheelchair Track & Field, USA
2351 Parkwood Road
Snellville, GA 30039
(770) 972-0763

This member organization of WSUSA conducts and sanctions track and field in the United States.

Wilderness Inquiry
808 14th Avenue, SE
Minneapolis, MN 55414-1586
(800) 728-0719

Headquartered in Minneapolis, Wilderness Inquiry conducts integrated outdoor adventures throughout North America for people with a wide range of physical abilities.

Wilderness on Wheels
Wheat Ridge, CO
(303) 403-1110
www.wildernessonwheels.org

The Wilderness on Wheels Foundation was established as a not-for-profit corporation in 1986. Its mission is to improve access for disabled persons to natural outdoor environments by constructing a model wilderness-access facility consisting of an 8-ft boardwalk starting at 9,100 ft and extending to the top of a 12,300-ft mountain. To date, over 116,000 hours have been invested in the project by some 3,500 volunteers. The boardwalk is just over a mile long. Wilderness on Wheels has provided advice and counsel to entities nationwide including the US Forest Service and the National Park Service.

World Curling Federation/US Curling Federation
1100 Center Point Drive
Suite 102, Box 866
Stevens Point, WI 54481
(715) 344-1199

The World Curling Federation is the world governing body for curling accreditation. It was formed out of the International Curling Federation during the campaign for Olympic winter sport status for the sport.

Chapter 26

ASSISTIVE DEVICES FOR SERVICE MEMBERS WITH DISABILITIES

RORY A. COOPER, PhD[*]; ROSEMARIE COOPER, MPT, ATP[†]; ERIK J. WOLF, PhD[‡]; KEVIN F. FITZPATRICK, MD, CPT[§]; GARRETT G. GRINDLE, MS[¥]; AND JOHN J. COLTELLARO, MS, ATP[¶]

[*]*Senior Career Scientist, US Department of Veterans Affairs, and Distinguished Professor, Department of Rehabilitation Science and Technology, University of Pittsburgh, 5044 Forbes Tower, Pittsburgh, Pennsylvania 15260*

[†]*Assistant Professor, Department of Rehabilitation Science and Technology, University of Pittsburgh, Center for Assistive Technology, Forbes Tower, Suite 3010, 3600 Forbes Avenue, Pittsburgh, Pennsylvania 15213*

[‡]*Research Engineer, Department of Physical Medicine and Rehabilitation, Walter Reed Army Medical Center, Building 2A, Room 146, 6900 Georgia Avenue, NW, Washington, DC 20307*

[§]*Major, Medical Corps, US Army; Physiatrist, Department of Othopaedics and Rehabilitation, Walter Reed Army Medical Center, 6900 Georgia Avenue, NW, Washington, DC 20307*

[¥]*Research Associate, Department of Rehabilitation Science and Technology, University of Pittsburgh, Human Engineering and Research Labs, 7180 Highland Drive, Building 4, Second Floor East Wing 151R7-H, Pittsburgh, Pennsylvania 15206*

[¶]*Clinical Instructor, Department of Rehabilitation Science and Technology, University of Pittsburgh Center for Assistive Technology, Forbes Tower, Suite 3010, 3600 Forbes Avenue, Pittsburgh, Pennsylvania 15213*

INTRODUCTION

Assistive devices provide essential support for people with disabilities, allowing them to participate in community, vocational, and recreational activities and to perform activities of daily living (ADLs). A service member with a severe disability will likely rely on a variety of assistive devices to maximize function and independence. It is critical to properly fit the technology to the individual and train the user to effectively manipulate it. The availability of transportation (personal or public), accessible housing, personal assistance services, and assistive technology (AT) are among the most critical factors to be addressed once the acute rehabilitation phase has been completed.

A team approach is most effective when assessing an individual for AT. Ideally, the clinical team includes a physiatrist, therapists (physical, occupational, and speech), a rehabilitation engineer, a vocational rehabilitation counselor, and a rehabilitation technology supplier. The service member and family should be at the center of the team and ultimately decide on the most appropriate technology. This will often require patient education, but eventually many people with disabilities gain considerable knowledge about their AT needs.

The goal of AT is to allow the individual with the disability to perform activities as independently as possible in a variety of situations and environments. A thorough AT assessment includes evaluating the individual's physical abilities (eg, strength, endurance, flexibility), cognitive abilities (eg, decision making, information processing, comprehension), sensory function (eg, vision, hearing, sensation), living environment (eg, home, work, school), support systems (eg, family assistance, paid assistance), and affect (eg, acceptance of disability, participation in process).

AT has been shown to be associated with successful rehabilitation outcomes. As injuries become more severe and the resulting disabilities greater, an individual's need for AT grows. Social support becomes more important as the severity of the injury and disability increases. Although there are methods for severely injured service members to receive paid personal assistance, it is often family members who provide the bulk of their care, especially in the early years. AT provides independence and reduces the exertion placed on others. For example, powered wheelchair seating functions can allow an individual with a disability to change position to increase comfort or alter pressure without relying on the assistance of others.

When making recommendations for AT, consideration must be given to the home environment and fixed and movable features.[1–3] Ramps, stair lifts, and widened doorways may be needed to allow effective use of some devices within the home. Moveable features, such as furniture, can be rearranged to allow access pathways through the home and, in some cases, may need to be replaced. For example, it is more difficult to get in and out of a soft low couch than a higher recliner with armrests. Community activities also need to be included in a thorough evaluation. Community-based tasks, such as shopping, using automated teller machines, and eating in restaurants, all provide important insight into AT needs and associated training. It is also important to provide exposure to integrated activities, such as skiing, hand cycling, swimming, and playing billiards, because they build self-confidence and help individuals adjust to a new self-image. It is easy to forget that travel is also an important community activity. Individuals with disabilities should be taken to events during their rehabilitation that require an overnight stay in a hotel so they can learn to perform tasks outside the structure of their homes.

Very severely injured soldiers and their families present with some unique needs and situations. Typically, severely injured soldiers must adjust to loss at a young age. These losses may include limbs, bodily functions, friends, and separation from the military unit that has served as a source of support. Losses may be complicated by the service members' duty status (National Guard, reserve, active duty) and proximity to their duty stations or homes. Soldiers and their families have unique social support systems, such as their units, other soldiers, veterans' service organizations, various Department of Defense programs, and the Department of Veterans Affairs. Each can make important contributions and bring resources to the severely injured soldier. It is also important to consider the preinjury socioeconomic status of the severely injured soldier, because this may impact the ability of the family to provide support and therefore influence the living environment. Soldiers have a unique occupation and even after sustaining severe injury, some want to return to active duty. AT may help some individuals pursue this career choice, while others may need to be guided toward other occupations.

Individuals with lower limb loss are likely to use multiple assistive devices, and the types of devices they use are likely to change over the individual's course of rehabilitation and lifespan. Nearly all service members with lower-extremity amputations will start out using wheelchairs, often in combination with prosthetic limbs. The wheelchair will serve as their source of mobility as they learn prosthetic ambulation skills. Some people will progress to the point where they will only require the wheelchair on rare occasions (eg, people with unilateral transtibia amputations), whereas others may decide to use their wheelchairs as their primary means of mobility (eg, those with short bilateral transfemoral amputations). Over a lifetime, comorbid conditions may make it necessary to rethink the individual's technology needs. For example, a manual wheelchair user may transition to an electric-powered wheelchair (EPW) because of severe shoulder pain from repetitive strain injury,[4-9] or a prosthetic-limb user may transition to a manual wheelchair because of reduced metabolic capacity.[10-14] A substantial challenge for service members to overcome is their own perceptions of disability and their potential to reintegrate into society, including active duty, and to return to an active lifestyle. Few service members have experience with disability, and many may base their views on popular perceptions and stereotypes. One goal of rehabilitation is to help the wounded, injured, or ill service member adapt and objectively evaluate the pros and cons of AT in pursuing their life goals.

Like other areas of rehabilitation, AT services are best provided using a team approach.[2,15-17] Individuals with disablties and their families are critical members of the rehabilitation team, and they should set the goals. The ideal prescription process includes six steps:

1. The clinical team assesses the user's impairments, diagnosis, prognosis, residual abilities, extent of social participation, goals of wheelchair use, financial resources, priorities (trade-offs will invariably be necessary), and dimensions.
2. The clinical team and user develop a generic list of ideal AT features.
3. The ideal-feature list is compared with items available from a reputable manufacturer and that can receive reliable service.
4. The user tests the device under consideration in the presence of a member of the clinical team.
5. Once the appropriate AT has been selected, the user is trained in its optimal use (including static indoor and outdoor challenges, or simulations thereof) and the results of training are documented.
6. After the AT has been used for a few months (and periodically thereafter), the situation should be reviewed and adjustments made.

Ideally, an AT team includes a physician, therapist, AT supplier, and rehabilitation engineer. Each professional has a unique but complementary role and, in cooperation with the end user, provides a comprehensive view of the AT needs. Physiatrists make the best

physicians on AT teams because of their residency training and the opportunities that AT provides to benefit people with disabilities. The increasing complexity of AT selection, justification, fitting, tuning, and training requires specialized knowledge. Physical therapists are well qualified to assess physical capacities and limitations, especially as they affect mobility. Occupational therapists can assess functional capacity and deficits in performance of basic and instrumental ADLs. It is important to know how people perform tasks, where they are deficient, and how AT can compensate for the deficits in order to augment task performance. Rehabilitation engineers have an important role in understanding the capabilities and application of various technologies to assist in the selection process and product design. It is also important to include a qualified equipment supplier early in the rehabilitation process because the supplier will be familiar with the available devices and how they can be applied to solve problems.

The Rehabilitation Engineering and Assistive Technology Society of North America (RESNA) acknowledged the need for consumers and insurers to recognize individuals with relevant experience and specialized knowledge. RESNA has created three levels of credentials to help enssure that consumers and insurers receive reliable information about AT. The AT supplier credential is intended for distributors and manufacturer representatives of AT. This is the most important credential offered by RESNA because it has started to bring order to an area of AT that was previously largely unregulated; before RESNA created the certification, there was no reliable credential for a supplier or manufacturer representative to demonstrate competency, and no way for consumers to readily identify qualified suppliers. The AT professional credential is geared toward therapists (physical, occupational, speech–language, counselors, and special educators). This credential recognizes qualified clinicians for their specialized knowledge and expertise. For decades, rehabilitation engineers provided clinical services without formal recognition of their expertise and, in many cases, their services were not reimbursed by insurance agencies. The rehabilitation engineering technology credential addresses the needs of rehabilitation engineers and provides other professionals and consumers a way to recognize them. To obtain the rehabilitation engineering technology credential, the engineer must also have obtained the AT professional credential. All of the RESNA credentials require proof of relevant experience and a passing score on a comprehensive examination. The credentials appear to have improved the quality of available AT services.

WHEELCHAIRS: SELECTION, FITTING, AND SKILLS TRAINING

Mobility devices, in particular wheelchairs and scooters, make up a significant portion of the assistive devices in use today.[2] Manual wheelchairs are mainly used by individuals who have the necessary upper body strength, function, and stamina for everyday propulsion.[7,10,14,18] Comorbid conditions, such as excessive body weight, overuse of the upper limbs, long time living with a disability, and poor health and nutrition, can impair a user's ability to independently propel a manual wheelchair, making EPWs more functional. For individuals who cannot use power wheelchairs, a manual wheelchair is prescribed and mobility is facilitated by an attendant or caregiver.

Only wheelchairs that comply with RESNA or International Standards Organization standards should be recommended. These criteria are intended to ensure minimal quality.[19] Best results are often obtained through independent testing conducted within a reputable testing laboratory.

Manual Wheelchairs

Design is critical to a manual wheelchair user's mobility because upper body strength needs to be sufficient to bear the load of the wheelchair in addition to the individual's bodyweight.[4,5,7,9,19] Standard manual wheelchairs (typically used in hospitals and nursing homes) tend to be bulky, heavy, and generically sized. They have the benefit of folding, which allows for simple storage and transportation. However, the seat and backrests are sling upholstery, which provides little comfort and does not relieve pressure. These wheelchairs are not intended for long-term use, but rather for temporary use of less than a few hours a day. Strong, ultralight wheelchairs have been designed for individuals requiring long-term use.[2,19–21] These wheelchairs can be customized to fit the user, allowing for better comfort and mobility. They are typically made of materials such as aluminum and titanium rather than the heavy steel used in standard wheelchairs (Figures 26-1 and 26-2). Ultralight manual wheelchairs are often appropriate for soldiers, who tend to be very active.

The basic features of an ultralight wheelchair include adjustable seat height, width, and depth; backrest height; armrest height; seat and back angles; rear wheel camber; and rear axle position (Figure 26-3). Lightweight wheelchairs have limited adjustability and standard wheelchairs have no adjustability. Manual wheelchair frames are made of aluminum, high-strength steel alloy tubing, titanium, and lightweight composite materials. The frame structure affects durability, transportability, and storage. For example, rigid

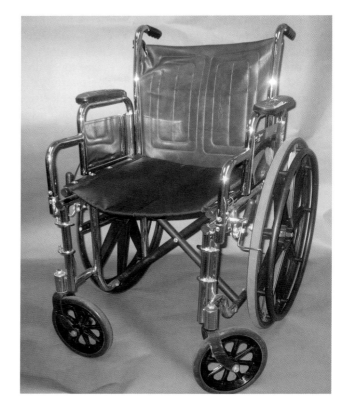

Figure 26-1. A standard manual wheelchair with a folding steel frame and sling seat.

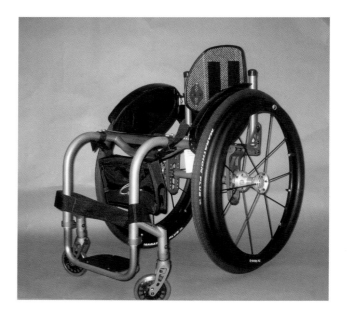

Figure 26-2. An ultralight manual wheelchair with a rigid titanium frame.

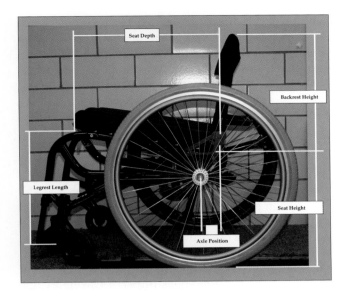

Figure 26-3. Key dimensions of an ultralight manual wheelchair: axle position, seat height, seat depth, backrest height, and footrest length.

frame chairs are one piece with removable wheels and foldable back supports for transport and storage, while cross-brace frames allow the wheelchair to collapse in the middle for storage. Some frames have suspension elements to decrease shock and vibration and make for a smoother overall ride.[22]

In some instances, none of the previously mentioned wheelchairs meets the needs of the user. For example, obese or overweight individuals need a larger, stronger wheelchair to support their weight. This class of wheelchairs is called heavy-duty or bariatric. They can support individuals ranging from 300 to 1,000 pounds.

Seat Height

Seats should be positioned so that leg length is accommodated, leaving about 50 mm under the footrest for obstacle clearance. Seat height needs to be at a level that allows the individual the necessary knee clearance to fit under tables, counters, and sinks.

Seat Depth

Seat depth provides support for the thighs. There should be about 50 mm behind the popliteal area of the knees. Improper depth may cause increased pressures on the thighs or buttocks. Shallow-depth seats increase sitting pressure because there is less contact between the thighs and seat, which may decrease the overall pressure distribution. If the seat depth is too

great, pressure behind the knees and on the calves is increased.

Seat Width

The width of the wheelchair seat should be slightly larger than the user's buttocks (about 25 mm). The hands should be able to just slip between the hips and the side guards or armrests. If the seat is too narrow, pressure increases on the sides of the hips, which may result in pressure sores. If the seat is too wide, the user will be forced to use a more abducted arm position for propulsion and will have more difficulty negotiating doorways and narrow passages.

Back Height

A wheelchair's back height depends on comfort and the amount of postural support needed. The backrest should be low enough that it does not impede the range of motion of the arms during propulsion. If the backrest is too high, the user will not be able to contact as much of the pushrim; if it is too low, the user will not have the necessary postural support and may experience discomfort or long-term deformity.

Seat and Back Angles

Seat angle is the horizontal angle between the seat and back, and back angle is the vertical angle between the seat and back with respect to vertical. Both are selected or adjusted to provide the most comfort and support for the user. Increasing the seat dump (declining the seat toward the rear) can help stabilize the pelvis and spine, which may improve propulsion. However, too much dump may increase the sitting pressure on the ischial tuberosities and make it more difficult to transfer from the wheelchair. Increasing the back angle is another way to ensure user comfort. If an individual has difficulty with hip flexion, the back can be opened to alleviate discomfort. However reclining too far can shift the center of gravity, making the chair unstable.

Armrests and Footrests

There are a variety of armrest lengths and styles. The armrest should be positioned at a comfortable height so the arm lies parallel to the ground. Armrests that are too high or too low may cause discomfort in the user's neck and shoulders. Many ultralight wheelchair users prefer not to have armrests because they tend to increase the overall width of the wheelchair, cause the arms to abduct more during propulsion, and may inhibit access to desks and tables. Cross-brace framed chairs typically have foot rests that can flip up or down, swivel, are angle-adjustable, or can be removed, while rigid-framed chairs have the footrest built into the frame. Although these footrests cannot typically be removed, they can be slightly adjusted to accommodate various leg lengths.

Wheels and Tires

A typical manual wheelchair has four wheels, two large rear wheels and two small front wheels called "casters." The casters are usually solid rubber, but can be polyurethane, pneumatic, or a combination. Caster size varies from 50 mm to 200 mm in diameter, depending on the wheelchair type and user preference. The standard rear wheel is a pneumatic 24-inch (0.6096 m) tire. Different tire types are available, such as solid insert tires, semipneumatic, or synthetic. Ultralight wheelchairs have quick release axles so the wheels can be easily removed for repair, storage, and transport.

Rear Wheel Camber

Camber is the amount of rear wheel vertical angle. At 0° camber, the wheels are vertical. To increase camber, the top of the wheel is tilted inward, moving the bottom of the wheel outward. Ultralight wheelchairs have up to 8° of camber, but about 3° camber is typical. Increasing camber provides more stability at the cost of increased wheelchair width. More than 8° camber is seen on many special-purpose sport wheelchairs.

Rear Axle Position

The rear axle position can be adjusted or selected horizontally and vertically. Horizontal positioning affects propulsion ability and technique. Placing the axle position forward allows users to grasp more of the wheel during propulsion. Moving the position further back limits the amount of pushrim that the individual can reach. Moving the axle forward increases the tendency of the wheelchair to tip backward. Users can take advantage of this feature to perform wheelies (when a manual wheelchair user lifts the front wheels from the ground by applying forward force to the pushrims and maintains balance on the rear wheels by forward and backward forces on the pushrims) and traverse obstacles more easily. Antitippers can be added to reduce the risk of tipping backward. Forward axle position also decreases the number of strokes and amount of effort used for propulsion.

Vertical axle adjustments can provide similar propulsion advantages. Moving the axle position up

with respect to the seat lowers the seat height, which improves stability. However, if the seat is too low, arm abduction can lead to poor propulsion patterns. An appropriately placed axle can lower the stress on the arms that results from everyday wheelchair propulsion.

Manual Wheelchair Propulsion and Skills

Various features of a manual wheelchair can affect a user's overall propulsion capability.[6,13,21,23] Wheelchair propulsion can be broken down into two components: the propulsion phase and the recovery phase. The propulsion phase begins with the initial hand contact on the pushrim and ends with the release of hand contact from the pushrim. The recovery phase begins with the release of hand contact from the pushrim and ends with the hand contact onto the pushrim.[21] Individual propulsion styles impact push frequency (the number of times the pushrim is contacted over a given distance or for a given time), push length (the distance the hand travels while in contact with the pushrim), push force (the magnitude of force applied to the pushrim in multiple dimensions), and the speed (the distance the wheelchair moves over a given time). Understanding and recognizing the effects of these key components in an individual's wheelchair propulsion style reduces the risk of secondary repetitive strain injuries associated with wheelchair prolusion.[5,6,21,24] Ultimately, the user should be trained to use a smooth, long stroke; a semicircular pattern that corresponds to a decreased push frequency with more time spent on the pushrim; decreased forces; and increased propulsion efficiency.[21,25]

Manual wheelchair skills further enhance the user's safety, efficiency, and independence. Maneuverability and adaptability in multiple environments are key goals of wheelchair skills training. Training may begin with basic skills, such as negotiating obstacles, turning in tight areas, and opening and closing doors—skills needed to allow a person to conduct all mobility-related ADLs within their homes. Eventually, training advances to higher-level skills, including wheelies. The wheelie position is useful for transiently reducing the loads on the ischial tuberosities, decreasing neck discomfort when talking to a standing person, turning in tight spaces, and negotiating obstacles, such as rough or soft ground, inclines, and curbs.

Although engaging in an active lifestyle is beneficial for maintaining quality of life, a majority of wheelchair users are inactive. Using a custom logging device, Tolerico et al studied the wheelchair activity patterns of 52 veterans at the National Veterans Wheelchair Games and in their home communities for a period of 13 to 20 days.[12] They found that individuals traveled

2,457 m/d, at an overall average speed of 0.8 m/s, over 8.3 h/d. Veterans who were employed covered more distance, accumulated more minutes of movement, and traveled a greater distance between consecutive stops than those who were unemployed. Cooper et al examined the activities of two groups of power wheelchair users over a 5-day period.[26] Results indicated that the group of individuals who attended the National Veterans Wheelchair Games was more active in terms of distance and speed traveled compared to a group of subjects monitored in their home environments (Pittsburgh, Pennsylvania). Fitzgerald et al tracked the activities of community-dwelling manual wheelchair users who used pushrim-activated, power-assisted wheelchairs and personal wheelchairs.[13] No significant differences were found in the distance and speed traveled using either wheelchair. Hoover et al[27] collected data from both the National Veterans Wheelchair Games participants and those in their home environments. The speed at which the power and manual wheelchair users traveled was 0.711 m/s and 0.3092 m/s, respectively.

A properly fitted manual wheelchair used by a well-trained and skilled individual can provide a high degree of mobility. Many service members with lower limb amputations can develop remarkable wheelchair skills. Tasks such as negotiating curbs, escalators, stairs, uneven terrain (sand, grass, and gravel), slopes, and narrow spaces are all teachable skills. Wheelchair skills training is a critical component of the rehabilitation and mobility training of individuals with lower limb amputations. Individuals with lower extremity amputations should be thoroughly assessed for wheelchairs and provided training in their use (Figure 26-4).

Electric-Powered Wheelchairs

EPWs are indicated for a wide range of individuals with disablities.[28–30] For some individuals with severe sensory–motor impairments (eg, individuals with high-level tetraplegia, traumatic brain injury, or multiple amputations), EPWs are the only functional mode of mobility.[28,29,31] Sensory–motor impairments can limit functional motor control to individual parts of the user's body. In these cases, EPW input devices must be customized to take advantage of the user's intact motor function.[26,29,32] Microswitching mechanisms that can be activated with the mouth (sip-and-puff) or other parts of the body (feet, head, etc) must be used as controller input. EPWs are also indicated for people who are at risk of falling or in pain when ambulating and who cannot safely or functionally propel a manual wheelchair. For these individuals, the EPW represents a safe and pain-free means of mobility.[33] For all users,

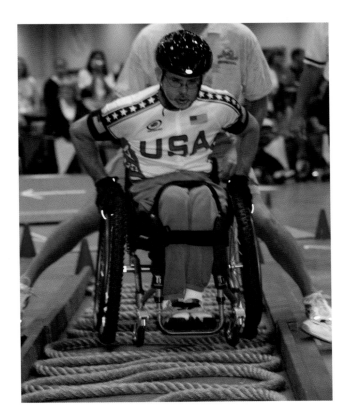

Figure 26-4. Wheelchair athlete demonstrating advanced mobility skills.

the goal of the EPW is to provide greater independence and quality of life.[2,30,34,35] As EPWs have become more technologically advanced, they have been able to serve this need for a broader range of people with disabilities.[30,31,34,35] Because people with disablities have diverse and complex needs to achieve independence, customizable EPWs can reach a larger proportion of the population with disabilities.[19,36] The technological advances of controller programmability, special seating systems, and integrated control units (with augmentative communication devices, environmental control units, etc) have allowed a wider population of people with disabilities to become independent.

There are two types of EPW frame designs: traditional (based on a manual wheelchair design) or power-base. Because the manual wheelchair design predates the power wheelchair, the first designs for power wheelchairs included simple power devices added on to manual wheelchairs (Figure 26-5). These devices still exist, especially for portable EPWs that can be easily disassembled, but the majority of EPWs are power-base styles. The conventional frame design was an easy first step in EPW development, but adding special seating features (eg, tilt and recline) made

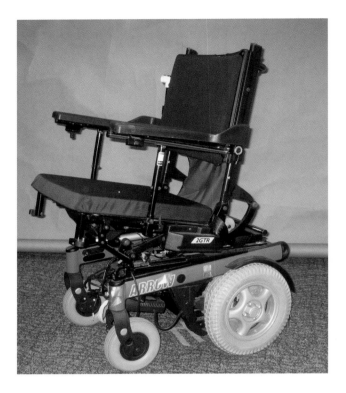

Figure 26-5. A traditional power wheelchair.

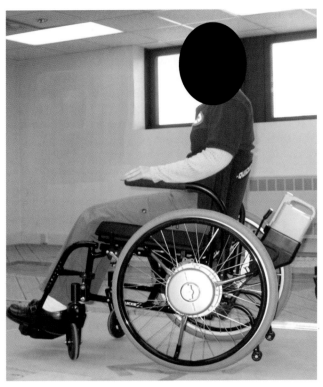

Figure 26-6. A pushrim-activated, power-assist wheelchair.

the wheelchair heavy and unstable. To accommodate these additional features, the EPW was redesigned in a two-component power-base style. The bottom power-base component houses the batteries, motors, and, in most cases, the controller. The seat component attaches to the power base, and thus can be swapped for whatever style of seat best meets the user's needs. A secondary benefit of separating the seating and power and control system is that the power-base design can be optimized nearly independently of the user's seating requirements. Consequently, power-base designs have progressed rapidly to include complex suspension systems, a low center of gravity, and excellent maneuverability. Likewise, seating technology has advanced to meet the needs of a wide range of users.

An EPW seating system can be as low-tech as a captain's chair or as complex as a power-actuated seat, which has any combination of the following features: tilt (changing the whole seat angle relative to the horizontal), recline (changing the seat-back to seat-bottom angle), elevating leg rests (leg-rest-to-seat-bottom angle), seat elevator (changing the height of the seat), and a standing mechanism (raising the person into a standing posture). Depending on the user's pressure management needs and musculoskeletal system state, any combination of the above motions may be pre-

scribed. Seat tilt is one of the most common features because it allows pressure to be shifted from the buttocks to the back, which can prevent the pressure ulcers common to wheelchair users with sensory loss.

Power-Assisted Wheelchairs

Power-assist devices include standalone-powered units external to the wheelchair that the wheelchair user holds onto, power add-on devices that attach to the wheelchair and have steering mechanisms or input devices for control, or pushrim-activated systems (PASs) with motors in the wheelchair hubs (Figure 26-6).[14,36,37] A PAS operates much like a manual wheelchair but requires less effort,[11,14] making it suitable for people with, or at risk for, upper extremity joint degeneration, reduced exercise capacity, and low upper-extremity strength or endurance.

One type of PAS measures pushrim forces using a linear compression spring and a simple potentiometer that senses the relative motion between the pushrim and the hub. A microprocessor uses these signals to control a permanent magnet direct current motor attached to each rear wheel. Each motor is connected to a ring gear, resulting in a 27:1 gear reduction. The PAS controller provides the feel of a traditional manual wheelchair by simulating inertia and compensating for discrepancies between the two wheels (eg, differences in friction), and increases user safety with an automatic speed limiting and braking system through the use of regenerative braking. Power is supplied by either a single, custom-designed, nickel–cadmium battery or a nickel–metal hydride battery.

Multifunctional Wheelchairs

Multifunctional wheelchairs are capable of changing drive configurations to adapt to environmental changes or challenges.[31,38–41] An example of this is the iBOT transporter, which uses a two-wheel cluster design (Figure 26-7).[38,40,41] With this design, the iBOT transporter can assume five different drive configurations: standard, four-wheel, balance, stair, and remote. In standard function, the transporter resembles a rear-wheel–drive wheelchair by raising the foremost drive wheels and lowering the front casters. In four-wheel configuration, all four drive wheels are in contact with the ground and the front castors are elevated. This configuration enables the user to climb curbs (up to 10 cm high) and easily traverse uneven and sloped terrain. The stair-climbing ability is achieved by controlling the cluster rotation on the basis of the position of the center of gravity. The device strives to keep the system's center of gravity above the ground-contacting wheels and between the front and rear wheels at all times, regardless of disturbances and forces operating on the system. Pitch-and-roll motion, recorded with gyroscopes, is used by a closed-loop control algorithm to drive motors to keep the seat level. The joystick is deactivated during stair climbing to prevent unintentional deflection. Users can initiate the function on their own and can maintain stability by holding the stair handrails, or assistants can control the rate of climbing through the assist handle. When a user or assistant leans forward or backward, shifting the center of gravity, the device rotates the wheel cluster, allowing the device to climb down or up one stair. The control system requires the device to dwell on each step for a few seconds before allowing another cluster operation. This hiatus helps keep the device from going out of control on stairs. The stair configuration performs well in descending and ascending stairs that are standard height, width, and depth.

In balance configuration, the clusters are rotated so that one set of drive wheels is positioned directly over the other set, leaving only two wheels in contact with the ground. The gyroscopes and closed-loop control

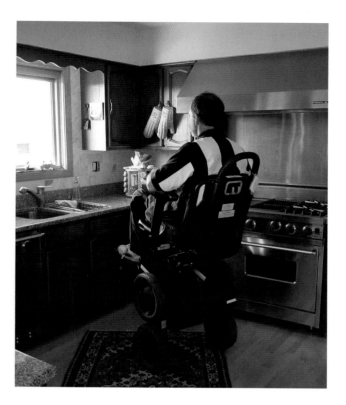

Figure 26-7. The iBOT transporter in standing mode.

system enable the user to remain balanced even during perturbations. For example, if a user shifts forward to reach something off a shelf, the transporter responds by bringing the wheels forward to compensate for the change in the occupant's center of gravity and to keep the occupant balanced. Although driving is possible in this configuration, the main purpose of the balance mode is to enable users to interact at eye level with their able-bodied peers and to extend their reaching height. Remote configuration allows users to detach the joystick and drive the device into a vehicle for easier transport. The iBOT can be connected to a computer so system logs, errors, and software updates can be downloaded and uploaded. This feature allows a remote technician to connect to the transporter and determine and potentially fix problems related to its operation or perform software updates.

The iBOT is the first stair-climbing device to appear on the market that does not use a track-based design. The major advantage of tracked-based stair-climbing wheelchairs is simple control and robustness in operation on irregular stairs. However, a disadvantage is the high pressure exerted on the stair edges and the difficulties associated with everyday use (it tends to be bulkier, heavier, and less maneuverable).

SEATING SYSTEMS

The human body is not designed to sit in the same position for prolonged periods of time.[39] It alters its position frequently from various lying, sitting, and standing positions, depending on the task being performed. For people with disabilities who are unable to walk and require wheeled mobility and seating devices, sitting is necessary, and identifying the most effective seating system for a specific individual's needs can be challenging.

The human body is a dynamic structure that is designed to perform and engage in a number of tasks in a variety of positions. Even while in a lying position, the body frequently (and subconsciously) changes position. The same applies in a standing or seated position. In a standing position, the body is a constantly dynamic structure, able to change its base of support frequently depending on movement and placement of the feet (base of support) in relation to the torso. The same applies to the body in a seated position, where the pelvis and thighs act as the base of support and the hip joints are placed in a flexed position, resulting in a potentially unstable base of support. In a seated posture, the pelvis is free to tilt and rotate in multiple directions, ultimately affecting the position and posture of the rest of the upper body (including the spine, trunk, upper extremities, and head). The seated body is therefore dynamic but also unstable.

Before providing a seating system, an individual's muscle strength, joint range of motion, coordination, balance, posture, tone, endurance, sitting posture, cognition, and perception must be assessed to obtain a basic understanding of the individual's capacity and needs. These assessments should be performed by a qualified professional with specialty training, certification, and knowledge of wheelchair seating and mobility applications. A proper assessment begins with listening to the user's needs, concerns, and goals for a device. Realistic goal setting fosters discussion related to the technology's capabilities.

The physical–motor assessment begins by observing and noting the person's seated posture; this provides a baseline of the seated postures the user may assume. A person may sit in a particular position because of preference, limitations, or the design of the seating system. It is therefore necessary to move the person from the existing system to an unsupported seated position on a flat surface, such as a therapy mat table, to observe the individual's posture without postural supports. If the user's unsupported sitting balance is limited, the examiner may need to provide support. Careful attention should be paid to the individual's pelvic and spinal alignment. While the person is sitting on the mat table, the examiner should apply appropriate forces (with the hands) to determine if observed deformities of the pelvis and spine are fixed or flexible. A fixed deformity cannot be corrected by a seating system and needs to be accommodated by the system. A flexible deformity can be corrected in varying degrees, depending on complexity, and needs to be supported by the seating system.

The user should then be asked to transition or be assisted to a supine position, where pelvic and spinal alignment can be reassessed with the pull of gravity working in a different plane on the body. Range of motion at the hips and knees should be assessed in this position. Limitations in hip flexion will affect the seat-to-back angle configuration of the seating system. With the hip flexed, knee range of motion (especially extension) needs to be assessed, considering the hamstrings cross the hip and knee joints. This will determine the optimal angle of the leg rests and position of the feet. In either a seated or supine position, upper extremity strength and range of motion need to be examined using commonly accepted measures and procedures. During this assessment, it is also necessary to note the quality of movements related to coordination because it is affected by tone, spasticity, tremors, and primitive reflexes.

Seating systems can be classified in three general categories: prefabricated, modular or adjustable systems, and custom contoured systems. Every user should be given a seating system designed and provided specific to the individual's medical, functional, and personal needs. A system should address issues of soft tissue management, comfort, orthopaedic deformities, and maintaining vital organ capacity. Functionally, the system should address the movements the user needs to perform, such as reaching or accessing objects, transferring, getting under tables, and completing ADLs. This requires carefully matching critical chair dimensions to body dimensions, user ability, and intended use. The user's goals and priorities need to be primary considerations; for example, a user may forgo pressure relief and comfort for a firmer system that provides greater stability and allows sliding off the seat for transfers.

The simplest form of prefabricated or premanufactured seating system is a linear seating system. A linear seating system refers to a planar seat and back with fixed angles and orientations. These types of systems may not provide a great deal of contour or support; however, they may be indicated for users who need more freedom of movement or who will experience rapid changes in size. Generically contoured systems are indicated for people who have minimal to moderate postural support needs and who have body shapes and dimensions that fit within these generic contours. Modular systems are composed of components that can be adjusted, added, or removed to address a specific postural need, such as lateral trunk supports and thigh guides. These systems are ideal for people with progressive conditions, such as multiple sclerosis, whereby postural needs may increase over time. They are also indicated for conditions that might improve, such as stroke or brain injury. Modular components are also ideal when a user's needs change throughout the day or activity. For example, a person may fatigue toward the end of the day and need more lateral trunk support added to the backrest, but may want these supports removed because they interfere with reaching activities or transferring out of the wheelchair.

Custom molded and contoured systems are more complicated to design and apply clinically. These systems are indicated for people with moderate to severe fixed or semifixed postural deformities, including curvatures of the spine, pelvic obliquities, and windswept postures of the lower extremities. A disadvantage of custom seating is it may limit function and movement because the system is specific to body shape. There are also concerns with people who might grow, change, gain or lose weight, or have seasonal variations in the thickness of their clothing. Designing these systems requires liquid foam, molding bags, and computer-aided design or computer-aided manufacturing technologies. Seating systems should not attempt to overcorrect postural deformities, but should accommodate them. Reduction or correction of postural deformities and joint contractures is best addressed through other interventions, including surgery, controlled passive stretching, or orthotic devices.

Seating systems are composed of several components, including at least a seat and back support. Other components often include supports for the arms, legs, and head. Adjustable features may include a reclining backrest, tilt-in-space ability, elevating seats, and standing capabilities.

Seat Support

The seat interface should balance pelvic stabilization and pressure distribution, allow for some degree of movement, and be functional to the individual's needs. The seat is the base of support for the pelvis, which supports the rest of the upper body. A seat should have an underlying, rigid base of support. Sling seats, commonly found on standard manual wheelchairs, provide limited postural support and are intended to allow easy folding. Sling upholstery tends to stretch and bow over time, and may contribute to adduction and internal rotation of the hips as well as a posterior pelvic tilt and kyphotic posture. The angle and shape of the seat contributes to pelvic stabilization. Without stabilization, the pelvis tends to rotate posteriorly, causing the buttocks to slide forward in the seat. This can result in shearing forces in the buttocks and may lead the spine to further collapse into a slouched posture. Providing a posterior slope to the seat angle, wedging the seat, or designing an ischial shelf in the shape of the cushion can provide greater pelvic stabilization and a better sense of balance, but may not always be ideal. It could make it more difficult to slide forward out of the seat for transfers, increase pressure in the ischial tuberosity and coccyx regions, or promote greater posterior pelvic tilt if the back support is not adequate. A posterior slope may also be inappropriate for people who self-propel with their feet. However, wheelchair users sometimes want to slide forward in their seats, slouch to relax, and change position because sitting upright continuously is difficult and fatiguing.

Back Supports

Long-term collapsing deformities of the spine, including kyphosis and scoliosis, can compromise breathing and other vital organ functions. Properly applied back supports can slow the onset of these problems. Back supports can be categorized by their shape, height, and stiffness. The preferred backrest provides posterior and lateral support but does not inhibit movement in the trunk and upper extremities (which may be needed for the propulsion of a manual wheelchair or other activities, such as reaching). A contoured or curved back should accommodate the width of the user and follow the natural curves of the spine to provide enough trunk support without compromising movement or function. Standard sling-back upholstery also tends to stretch over time, which can result in a posterior pelvic tilt and contribute to a kyphotic posture. Flat or planar backs allow for more movement, but might be uncomfortable and less stable because they do not provide lateral stabilization or conform to natural spinal curves. A high back provides greater support through the spine, but may interfere with trunk rotation and shoulder movements. Back supports below the scapulae and thoracic spine allow for greater freedom of movement, but may result in long-term spinal deformities. Fabric backs with adjustable tension straps are now more common, especially in manual wheelchairs, and tend to be lightweight compared to rigid, shell-back supports. They can be adjusted for varying needs and shapes; however, they stretch and wear out over time and do not provide rigid stabilization.

Current trends in backrest design focus on styles with taller backs, lateral curves around the thoracic-lumbar regions, and cutouts in the scapular region to provide spinal support while allowing for shoulder movements. Attention is also being focused on using adjustable, durable, carbon-fiber materials to construct back supports.

Arm Support

Arm supports may be necessary to rest the arms, provide a greater sense of lateral trunk stability, and decrease pressure loads in the buttocks by bearing weight through the upper extremities. They may also provide a place to hold onto with one hand while reaching with the other, and to push off of for weight shifts or transfers. Armrest assemblies can also contain the pelvis and thighs to keep the thighs in alignment, and can protect clothing and skin from rubbing on the tires of a manual wheelchair. However, armrests add weight to manual wheelchairs and can get in the way of accessing the pushrims for effective propulsion. Therefore, many active manual wheelchair users choose to forgo arm supports. If arm supports are used, they should be removable or capable of swinging out of the way. They should also be set at an optimal height for the user or be adjustable.

Foot Supports and Leg Supports

Foot supports and leg supports can be classified by the angle at which they position the knees and where they place the feet. Traditional swing-away footrests are designed to keep the user's feet out in front, with about 60° to 70° of knee flexion, to avoid interference with caster swivel and rotation. This is not necessarily a natural seated position; it promotes slouching by pulling the hamstrings and the pelvis into a posterior pelvic tilt.

Elevating leg rests pose an even greater problem. A perceived purpose of elevating leg rests is to help manage edema (swelling) in the lower extremities. However, being seated in an upright position with the hips flexed and the knees extended does little to reduce edema unless the feet and legs can get to or above heart level, which can only be accomplished by tilting the seat back and reclining the backrest. Elevating leg rests without these features will also likely place greater pull on the hamstrings, promote a slouched posture, and cause significant problems for people with limited knee extension (Figure 26-8).

Some people (eg, active manual wheelchair users)

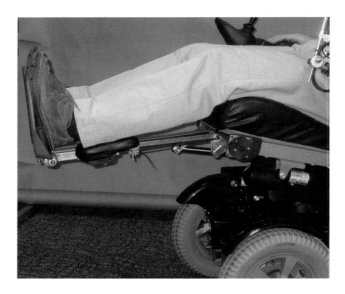

Figure 26-8. Elevating leg rests.

prefer to sit with their knees at a more natural, 90° (or greater) flexed position, with their feet tucked under the seat to provide greater postural stability and shorten the length of the wheelchair for maneuverability. This position also warrants tapering the footrests inward to keep the feet from interfering with front caster swivel. In a power wheelchair, a front- or mid-wheel drive configuration positions the feet so the knees are flexed at 90° because front casters are not needed. Some active wheelchair users also prefer to have the foot supports fixed in a one-piece structure to add rigidity and durability. However, removable or swing-away foot supports should not be eliminated for people who stand for transfers out of the wheelchair or propel a manual wheelchair with their feet.

Head Support

The head can be difficult to position because of its size and movements in the cervical spine or neck. A head support is warranted for those with poor head control. Prior to positioning the head, the pelvic and spinal support and balance should be addressed because the head is more distal to these structures and will tend to position itself based on their position. A head support is also almost always indicated in wheelchairs that include tilt and reclining backrests because the head needs to be supported in these positions. A head support may be warranted if the user needs to rest in the wheelchair and if the wheelchair is to be used as a seat in a vehicle (to provide support in the event of a collision).

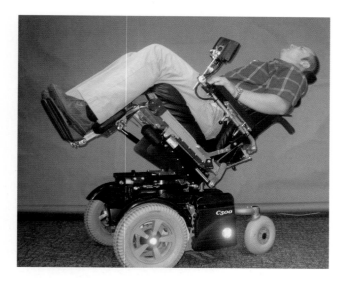

Figure 26-9. A powered tilt seating system.

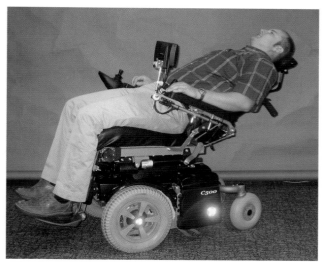

Figure 26-10. A powered reclining backrest system.

Like all other seating components, head supports come in various shapes and sizes to address different needs and preferences. Some people prefer to go without head support because it interferes with head movement and can reduce field of vision. Flat head supports provide a surface to rest against, while curved supports provide some degree of lateral stability. Wide head supports allow for greater area to place the head, but tend to interfere with field of vision. Head supports can be aggressive for people with poor head control (eg, those with amyotrophic lateral sclerosis), and may include lateral head and suboccipital supports. Head supports should be mounted to the seating system using adjustable hardware so they can be moved, adjusted, and removed as needed.

Tilt Frames and Reclining Backrests

Because it is unnatural to sit in one position for prolonged periods of time, tilt frames and reclining backrest systems are options that benefit those unable to move or reposition themselves effectively. These options redistribute pressure, manage posture and tone, provide comfort, and help with personal care activities. Tilt frames and reclining backrests are available for both manual and power wheelchairs and can be operated by the wheelchair user as a powered feature or manually by an attendant.

Tilt allows the entire seating system to pivot posteriorly while keeping the hip and knee joints in the same position. This helps redistribute pressure away from the buttocks region and into the back support. It is also useful in repositioning because people tend to slouch and slide forward when sitting upright for

prolonged periods of time. The trunk is able to extend in a tilted position, countering a kyphotic posture and potentially reducing or slowing the development of trunk and spinal deformities (Figure 26-9).

A reclining backrest allows the hip flexors to stretch and opens the hip angle to assist with attending to catheters, toileting, dressing, and dependent transfers. However, reclining the backrest creates shear forces in the seat and back because the user tends to slide down in the seating system. The addition of a tilt-in-space feature will counter this tendency and should be considered when recline is warranted. Both systems also allow a person to rest in the wheelchair without having to be transferred to a bed. Research supports use of combined tilt and reclining backrest interventions to optimally distribute pressure (Figure 26-10).

Standing Systems

Wheelchairs that allow the user to passively stand benefit individuals who would typically be unable to do so otherwise. The benefits of passive standing may include decreased bladder infections, reduced osteoporosis, and decreased lower extremity spasticity. In addition, there are likely psychological benefits resulting from the sensation of upright posture and the ability to interact at eye level, and functional benefits associated with being able to reach objects in higher locations. It is critical to carefully assess a person's posture and range of motion prior to considering a standing device because those with range-of-motion limitations and postural deformities cannot stand upright. A candidate for a standing wheelchair should be carefully assessed by a physician or other qualified practitioner before standing to address concerns with orthostatic hypotension in cases where people have not stood for a prolonged period of time.

Seat Elevation Systems

Some of the benefits obtained from a standing system, such as reaching objects in higher locations, accessing high surfaces, and being at eye level with standing people, can be accomplished through the use of a seat-elevating system (Figure 26-11). This is a feature typically available only on power wheelchairs. Raising the seat is also sometimes critical to facilitate safer and more efficient transfers. For a person using a sliding board or performing a lateral transfer, a seat elevator allows for transfers in a downhill direction, which has been shown to require less strain on the upper extremities as compared to transferring to a level or higher surface. In other cases, the seat elevator can facilitate transfers for people who stand to transfer but have difficulty rising from a low seat to floor height.

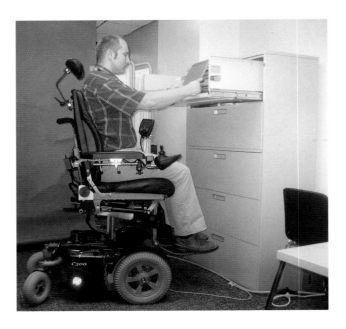

Figure 26-11. A seat elevator can be used to reach higher objects.

SPORTS AND RECREATION EQUIPMENT

The human need for recreation is especially important in the presence of physical, sensory, or cognitive impairment that affects the ability to function in everyday activities and environments. Primary rehabilitation interventions emphasize self-maintenance, education, and employment activities. Recreation allows humans to challenge their physical limits in a setting that accepts new participants, provides instruction and emotional support for learning, includes social participation, and promises fun and escape from the realities of everyday life. Recreation puts humans in touch with their imagined self (eg, a person who is adventurous, strong, or graceful) and does not need to be justified in the same way as work and self-maintenance activities; it is chosen just because it is appealing to the participant.[42] Healthy competition with self and others through sports and recreation creates an arena for continuing the gains of medical rehabilitation, challenging personally held ideas about disability and handicap learned from culture, and testing out a new self-concept that can include acceptance of disability.[43]

Basketball wheelchairs are similar to typical manual wheelchairs but incorporate features to enhance stability and maneuverability. They are lightweight to allow for speed, acceleration, and quick braking. Although wheelchair basketball is not a contact sport, some incidental contact is inevitable, so spoke guards cover the rear wheel spokes to prevent damage. Spoke guards

made of high-impact plastic provide several additional benefits. They allow players to pick the ball up from the floor by pushing it against the spoke guard and rolling it onto the lap, they protect hands and fingers from aggressive play when reaching for the ball, and they provide space to identify team affiliations and sponsor names. Stability comes from the camber in the wheels, which creates a broader wheelbase; it brings the top of the wheel closer to the body, making the wheelchair more responsive to turns, and protects a player's hands during collision because hands are located away from the plane of contact. To gain an advantage for shooting baskets, forwards usually try to make wheelchair seats as high as possible within the 53-cm limit. Seats typically angle toward the rear, creating "squeeze" or seat bucketing of 0.085 radians to 0.255 radians (5°–15°) to increase the player's pelvic stability. Guards prefer lower seat heights, which, combined with increased seat angle, makes chairs faster and more maneuverable for ball handling. Cushions may be used if made of flexible material the same size as the seat of the wheelchair and no higher than 10-cm thick, unless a player is classified as being restricted to a cushion that cannot exceed 5 cm. Because equipment can be used to create competitive advantage, it is carefully regulated. Equipment cannot completely equalize player performance, so modified rules and classification work to create functional equivalence between teams. These parameters work together to create a sport that is equal in challenge and excitement to stand-up basketball.

Wheelchair rugby differs from basketball in that players must have both an upper and lower extremity impairment to be eligible to participate. The object of wheelchair rugby is to cross the opponent's goal line with two wheels while in possession of the ball. While the offensive team tries to advance the ball, the defense works to halt its progress with turnovers. Players tend to use extreme wheelchair configurations, elastic binders, foam arm protectors, and special tacky gloves to improve performance. As in basketball, players become extremely proficient in adapting their equipment to promote balance and speed, so much that they often appear to possess more functional capacity than their diagnoses would suggest. Wheelchair styles are strictly regulated to ensure fairness, but vary considerably depending on a player's preferences, functional level, and role on the team. Rugby chairs have extreme amounts of camber (16°–20°), significant bucketing, and antitip bars. Camber provides lateral stability, hand protection, and ease in turning. Bucketing helps with trunk balance and ball protection.

Serious tennis players use special wheelchairs that are equipped with three wheels—two large for propulsion, and a single, 5-cm caster in the front under the feet that allows for quick turning. The large wheels are typically 61 cm to 66 cm (24–26 in.) in diameter and use high-pressure tires (8.4 k/cm–14.1 k/cm, or 120–200 psi) to reduce rolling resistance on the court. Wheels are set with extreme camber to maximize mobility and stability on the court, especially when making shots. Players with high-level spinal cord injury play with power wheelchairs and with longer rackets to compensate for length taken up by strapping the racket to the hand.

The track and field sports have been adapted to disability since the Stoke Mandeville Games, and include throwing and racing events.[44] The throwing events allow competitors to use specially designed throwing chairs attached to holding devices because they offer greater stability and support. Throwing chairs are taller and eliminate the large wheels that could potentially interfere with the dynamic upper body movements required in throwing events. When a wheelchair is used, the seat and cushion must not exceed 75 cm in height.[45] The chair design is important because it can significantly enhance performance, depending on how well it matches the thrower's body and functional abilities. Consequently, athletes select chairs of different configurations to optimize their throwing performance.

Wheelchair racers and others with physical impairments compete in events from short distance sprints through marathons. Wheelchairs used in racing are customized and designed to fit the body of each user. The design of a racing wheelchair optimizes the abilities of each user, incorporating features such as three-wheeled design, use of high-pressure tubular tires, lightweight rims, precision hubs, carbon disc or spoked wheels, compensator steering, small push rings, ridged frame construction, and 2° to 15° of camber. The fit of the racing chair to one's body and abilities is critical to overall performance.[46] Racing chair manufacturers require many body measurements when a chair is ordered because the frame and seat cage are made to fit each individual.[47] Individuals with upper transradial amputations may use cosmetic prosthetic hands that have been positioned into a fist or ball with a high-friction surface to simulate racing gloves.

Wheelchairs have also been redesigned for use in backcountry and wilderness. Athletic individuals with a desire to hike, camp, and go where conventional wheelchairs cannot have designed adaptations to make rough terrain navigable. They use 66-cm (26-in.) knobby tires like those on mountain bikes to gain traction on soft, wet, or difficult terrain. Front casters are significantly larger to decrease the chance of getting stuck on obstacles. Larger casters require frame redesign, so an off-road wheelchair looks more like a four-wheel buggy than a typical wheelchair.

Cycling using adaptations to typical bicycles, tandem cycles, or hand cycles opens this recreational and competitive sport to individuals with many types of impairments. Using toe clips, altering the size of the arc of the pedals, or modifying the handlebars, handgrips, or placement of the gears and brake levers are the only modifications some need.[48]

For those with lower extremity impairment, such as spinal cord injury, multiple sclerosis, hemiplegia, and amputation, hand cycles substitute use of the upper extremities and provide the greater stability of three wheels and placement close to the ground.[49] Cuffs can be mounted to the arm crank handles for those with reduced grip strength. Two types of hand cycle designs are typically used: upright and recumbent. In an upright hand cycle, the rider is in a vertical position, as in a wheelchair. Upright hand cycles use a pivot steer in which only the front wheel turns while the rear wheels of the cycle follow.

It is easier to transfer into and balance an upright cycle. In the recumbent hand cycle, the rider's torso is semireclined and the legs are positioned in front of the pelvis. Steering occurs in one of two ways. In one, as the rider leans toward the turn, force is transferred through a linkage bar, causing the frame to pivot and turn, which is challenging for riders without trunk stability. A pivot-steering, recumbent hand cycle uses the rider's arms and shoulders to execute turns like a typical bike. Recumbent hand cycles are ideal for racing because they are light and fast.[50] Individuals with upper limb amputations require modifications to the pedal handle and to the terminal device to facilitate a firm interface that promotes pushing and pulling on the handle throughout the pedal cycle (over 360°).

Water sit skis can compensate for trunk instability and hand weakness and incorporate a variety of adaptive features to suit a wide range of functional levels. Some skis adjust vertically, horizontally, and diagonally at the fin, allowing users to fine-tune their equipment to meet various skiing styles, body weights, and boat velocities. At the competitive level, sit-skiing events include men's and women's slalom, tricks, and jumping.[50]

Adaptive ski equipment (eg, outriggers, monoskis, and biskis) emerged from analyzing the physics of skiing and applying mechanical concepts to compensate for a skier's movement limitations. Veterans with limb loss learned stand-up methods that added outriggers. Originally, outriggers were made from the tips of outriggers from damaged skis mounted to the ends of forearm crutches. The Austrians used outriggers with the ski tips in a continuous running position, but flip-skis use a spring-loaded mechanism to allow the tip to either parallel the snow in running position or, when released, to flip up on the heel of the ski tip so outriggers can function more like poles or crutches. A claw bolted to the heel of the tip provides traction in icy lift lines. The monoski combines a fiberglass, form-fitting cab with a suspension mechanism attached to a single ski. A lever mechanism allows the skier to raise the height of the cab to the level of a chairlift. Once up, monoskiers can push forward in the lift line, using outriggers in pole position, and allow the chairlift and its momentum to scoop them up. To dismount, the skier leans forward as the lift reaches the dismount down slope, creating the momentum to drop off the lift.

In sled hockey, typical ice hockey rules apply, with some changes because of the nature of the game and its participants. The ice surface, goal net, and pucks are all the same as in stand-up hockey.[51] The primary piece of equipment used in sled hockey is the sledge, a metal-framed oval sled with two blades and a small runner; a seat with a backrest; leg straps; and optional push handles. A typical hockey stick is shortened to 73.6 cm (29 in.) and modified with two picks (metal pieces with a minimum of three teeth, measuring a maximum of 4 mm) attached to the end.[51] Picks provide traction to move the player down the ice and give the player leverage for shooting the puck with the blade end of the stick. With a quick flip of the wrist, players are able to propel themselves using the spikes, then play the puck with the blade end of the stick. Players generally use two sticks with blades to facilitate both propulsion and shooting with either hand.

TRANSPORTATION

Transportation is a key component of full integration into the community. Accessible public transportation is necessary to provide persons with disabilities the same opportunities as others: employment, education, religious worship, and recreation. In the United States, the Individuals with Disabilities Education Act[52] and the Americans with Disabilities Act of 1990[53] have provided people with disabilities the opportunity to access schools and public transportation. The Americans with Disabilities Act transportation requirements mandate accessible fixed-route vehicles, as well as complementary paratransit services for those unable to use the fixed-route service. A subset of the disabled population is the wheelchair user, who may not be able to transfer to a vehicle seat and might, therefore, remain seated in a wheelchair.

The wheelchair user should be afforded the same level of safety as passengers sitting in vehicle seats that meet federal safety standards. However, the wheelchair-seated passenger is usually at increased risk of injury in event of a vehicle collision or emergency maneuver. Currently, there are no federal safety standards for devices used to transport wheelchair-seated passengers. However, there is a national and international effort to develop product safety standards for wheelchairs used as seats in motor vehicles. The standards establish the severity of vehicular crashes the wheelchair should withstand, as well as set the design criteria for securing the wheelchair in a vehicle.[54,55] They evaluate the complete wheelchair, frame, base, and seating system; however, seating systems are often added aftermarket. Wheelchairs using aftermarket seating systems are not likely to be tested to evaluate their ability to withstand crash forces, or they may invalidate some testing. Because the seating system directly interfaces with the user, it is critical that these systems do not fail during a vehicular crash.

Motor vehicle seats must be effectively anchored to the vehicle floor to ensure that their mass does not add to the restraint loads on the occupant. When an occupant remains seated in the wheelchair, the wheelchair becomes the vehicle seat. Aftermarket securement systems must be used to anchor a wheelchair to the vehicle floor. Again, due to the lack of federal safety standards for devices used to transport wheelchair-seated passengers, national and international efforts strove to develop voluntary product safety standards for wheelchair tie-down and occupant restraint sys-

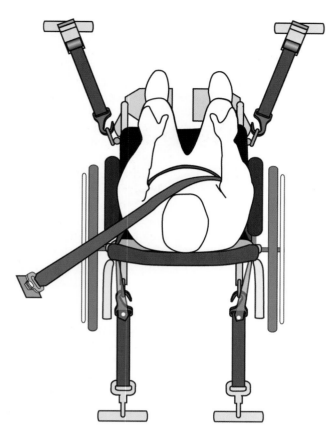

Figure 26-12. A four-point tie down system for wheelchair transportation.

tems. In the United States, the Society of Automotive Engineers' Adaptive Devices Subcommittee developed *SAE J2249: Wheelchair Tie-Downs and Occupant Restraint Systems for Use in Motor Vehicles*.[55] Shortly after, an international standard was published.[56] The most common securement system found in public transportation is the four-point tie-down system (Figure 26-12). This system consists of four tie-down straps that anchor to the vehicle floor and four points on a wheelchair (two front and two rear). The end fittings that attach to the wheelchair can be hooks or loops that wrap around the wheelchair frame. The main advantage of this type of system is that it can be used with a wide variety of wheelchairs and does not require special hardware to be added to the wheelchair.

A second method of securement is an automatic docking system, which uses a wheelchair adaptor—special hardware mounted on the wheelchair—to engage with a docking station or receptacle mounted to the vehicle floor or sidewall. The advantages of wheelchair docking technology have been seen with proprietary systems that have been used for independent securement of wheelchairs in private vans.

Driving Controls

Adaptive driving controls for an individual's vehicle are prescribed after the individual completes a comprehensive driving evaluation and education and training program provided by a certified driving rehabilitation specialist. The evaluation assesses the individual's basic skills necessary for driving, such as vision, perception, cognition, physical functioning, and knowledge of driving, and an on-road assessment that evaluates actual driving skills. After completing the program, the certified driving rehabilitation specialist and the individual can determine if the person will be able to drive with the recommended equipment.

Adaptive driving controls may include modified steering devices, accelerators, and a variety of secondary vehicle controls. A steering device, such as a spinner knob attached to the steering wheel, can allow for one-handed steering (Figure 26-13). A left-sided accelerator can be used if the individual's right foot cannot operate the gas or brake pedals. A turn signal crossover, which relocates the turn signal indicator from the left side of the steering wheel to the right, can be used to allow individuals to access the turn signal using only the right hand if the left is impaired. Other secondary vehicle controls, such as windshield wipers, lights, and horns, can be relocated to provide timely and accurate access with the functional or dominant hand.

Positioning straps (eg, chest harnesses), used in combination with the seatbelt, provide additional trunk control if sitting balance is compromised and interferes with functional operation of the vehicle. A strap or other modification for seatbelt retrieval is helpful if grasp or reach is limited. A parking brake extension allows access to floor-mounted parking or

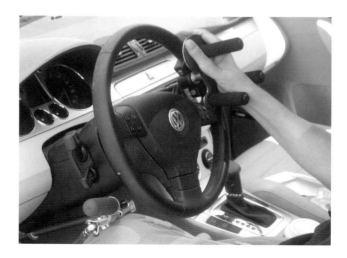

Figure 26-13. A steering knob can aid in driving.

emergency brake pedals. Mirrors may compensate for partial loss of visual fields or the presence of scotomas. As with all adaptive equipment, specialized education and training is required to assure correct placement and proper use of the additional mirrors.

Vehicle Access Technology

A variety of adaptive equipment and vehicle modifications can be used for vehicle ingress and egress. Automatic car door openers (ie, keyless entry), built-up key holders, or key turners are recommended if hand function is impaired. To ease the transfer for driver or passenger from the wheelchair into the vehicle seat, a power base seat can swivel out, glide out of the vehicle, and lower to a desired level. Portable wheelchair ramps are available to load and unload unoccupied mobility equipment, such as manual or power wheelchairs or scooters, into the vehicle without significant vehicle modifications (Figure 26-14). Car topper lifts attach to the top of a sedan and lift and store a manual wheelchair on top of the vehicle. Wheelchair or scooter users may require a vehicle ramp or lift to get into their vehicles or to lift their mobility devices into their

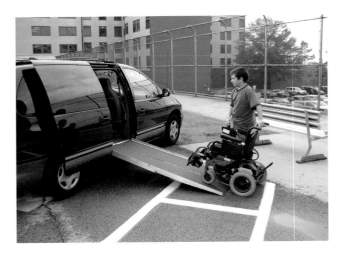

Figure 26-14. A portable wheelchair ramp can be used to access vehicles.

vehicles. Before the recommendation and installation of any adaptive equipment in a vehicle, the individual, mechanical device, and vehicle compatibility should be verified.

REHABILITATION ROBOTICS

Rehabilitation robotics can be categorized into three main categories: mobility aids, manipulation aids, and therapeutic robots. The use of robots in rehabilitation is quite different from industrial applications, where robots operate in structured environments with predefined tasks and are usually separated from human operators. Many tasks cannot be preprogrammed in rehabilitation robots, such as picking up a newspaper or opening a door. Although some evaluations and studies have looked at rehabilitation robots, the benefits and disadvantages of systems in service need to be further analyzed to better understand the users and their needs. Many individuals with disabilities can be satisfied with traditional mobility aids (eg, canes, walkers, manual wheelchairs, power wheelchairs, scooters). However, for some people with disabilities, it is difficult or impossible to use current mobility devices without assistance.[58] Individuals with low vision, visual field neglect, spasticity, tremors, or cognitive deficits may benefit most from "intelligent" mobility aids that have evolved from mobile robots. People with these conditions often lack independent mobility and rely on a caregiver to provide mobility. Intelligent mobility aids often consist of either a wheelchair or walker, to which a computer and a collection of sensors have been added, or a mobile robot base to which a seat or handlebars have been attached. Intelligent mobility aids have been designed based on a variety of traditional mobility

aids and provide users with navigation assistance (eg, assuring collision-free travel, aiding the performance of specific tasks, and autonomously transporting the user between locations). Smart wheelchairs are ideal devices to test novel input methods because, unlike standard wheelchairs, the interface can be implemented on their onboard computers. More importantly, smart wheelchairs can avoid obstacles, providing a safety net for input methods that are inaccurate or that have limited bandwidth. For example, voice control has proven difficult to implement on standard wheelchairs; however, obstacle avoidance capabilities built into control software may protect a user from the consequences of unrecognized (or misrecognized) voice commands and can "fill in" the small, rapid navigation commands that are much easier on a high-bandwidth input device, such as a joystick.

Robotic manipulation aids provide people with disablities tools to perform ADLs and vocational support tasks that would otherwise require assistance. Operators usually control manipulation aids with joysticks, keypads, their voices, or other input devices. Robotic manipulation aids can be classified into three groups:

1. Task-specific devices: electromechanical devices used to perform simple tasks, such as powered feeders and page turners.

2. Workstation robots: the robotic manipulator may be built into a workstation and can be used in a vocational environment.
3. Wheelchair robots: a manipulator arm mounted on the electric-powered wheelchair that augments mobility and manipulation, allowing the user to accomplish ADLs and vocational tasks.

Both the interface between the user and the robot and the interface between the robot and the objects being manipulated affect the functionality of a robot manipulation aid. A robot's operation sophistication is limited because users are only able to exert so much control. The interface between the robot and the objects being manipulated is usually a simple pincer-like gripper; however, a large portion of activities performed in school, work, and daily living involve pick-and-place tasks that may be carried out with this simple end effector.

AUGMENTATIVE AND ALTERNATIVE COMMUNICATION

Augmentative and alternative communication (AAC) refers to any communication approach that supplements or replaces natural speech or writing. Effective communication is desired for individuals to be able to participate in work, school, leisure, and entertainment activities. Although a range of AAC interventions are possible to engineer solutions for improved function and participation, the demands of communication should be analyzed in terms of language requirements.

AAC endeavors to optimize the communication of individuals with significant communication disorders.[59] The basic elements of a comprehensive AAC assessment and the role of rehabilitation engineers in making decisions about AAC technology are critical to achieving successful outcomes. The significance of language issues and AAC language representation methods must be understood before evaluating solutions, emphasizing the need for AAC technology to support the spontaneous generation of language to optimize communication function and participation. Only by understanding the language issues can rehabilitation engineering professionals appreciate the technology, device features, and human factors associated with AAC interventions.

AAC interventions can be classified by the methods used to transmit messages (ie, aided or unaided).[60] Unaided symbols do not require an external device or apparatus; nothing other than an individual's body parts are needed to transmit a message (eg, using one's hands to gesture). Aided symbols, on the other hand, require an external device. Technology for aided AAC can be further classified into low, light, or high performance. High-performance technology solutions can then be delineated into nondedicated or dedicated AAC systems. Nondedicated technology generally refers to computers that are running AAC software, but the primary application of the technology is computer based. Conversely, dedicated AAC devices have been designed and evaluated specifically for communication, but frequently have secondary features that provide computer or environmental controls. The range of aided technology increases as the availability of power, voice output, electronics, and computer chips become part of the system.

Comprehensive Assessment

The AAC assessment may be the most important event in the life of an individual with a severe communication disorder that limits functional use of natural speech. For the beginning communicator, the AAC assessment process should establish AAC interventions to build communication competence to maximum potential across the individual's life span. However, for an adult with a degenerative neurological disorder, an AAC assessment should consider the individual's changing communication needs throughout the course of the disease.

An AAC assessment improves an individual's communicative functioning and participation in various activities and environments. The assessment is a client-centered, multidisciplinary team process.[61,62] Various AAC assessment models have been proposed that contain feature-match components, including the predictive assessment model[63,64] and the participation model.[65] With these AAC assessment models, data are collected and information is gathered to make intervention and management decisions.[66] The three primary objectives of an AAC assessment are to determine functional communication needs, identify (match) interventions to increase or maintain interactive communication, and monitor or measure the effectiveness of intervention.[65–67] The principles of evidence-based practice should be reflected in comprehensive AAC assessment.[59,68]

Language Representation

Three basic methods are used to represent language in AAC systems and are termed "AAC language representation methods" (LRMs). Evaluating the effectiveness of each method starts by considering the nature of a language. To be effective, AAC LRMs used with technology need to have the characteristics of natural language, such as being generative, recursive, and polysemous, in order to achieve maximum performance. Rehabilitation engineers systematically evaluate the performance of various methods against the characteristics of natural language.

The three common LRMs are based on single-meaning pictures or univocal pictures (intended to have only one meaning), semantic compaction or polysemous pictures (intended to have more than one meaning), and traditional orthography (the alphabet). Studies have shown that univocal LRMs, polysemous LRMs, and alphabetic LRMs have differential effects upon performance.

COMPUTER ACCESS

Client-side AT helps disabled users access computers. Computer operating systems and applications coevolved with the mouse, and some software cannot be used without one. This is problematic because the operations that are most troublesome for individuals with physical disabilities are often those that involve button presses. However, pointing devices come in a variety of shapes and sizes. The most familiar pointing devices are the mouse and the trackpad (most often seen on laptop computers). Other frequently seen pointing devices include the trackball and the trackpoint. Pointing devices more commonly associated with individuals with disabilities include touch screens, head-mounted mouse emulators, and mouse keys. Each pointing device requires a different set of skills, which a clinician can match to an individual's abilities.

ELECTRONIC AIDS TO DAILY LIVING

Electronic aids to daily living (EADLs; also referred to as "environmental control units") are specialized AT designed to enable individuals to operate household appliances and electronics if they cannot use the standard controls (eg, light switches, television, cable box, DVD player, stereo, heating and air conditioning, fans, doors, draperies or blinds, etc; Figure 26-15).

The user display and user control interface constitute the human–technology interface.[69] The user control interface is the selection method used to control other AT (eg, direct selection, scanning, directed scanning, auditory scanning, voice recognition, and coded access). The user display is usually a visual feedback system that helps the individual operate the device; though auditory feedback systems can be used to help the visually impaired. The central processing unit is generally a microprocessor-based system designed to process input signals and direct output signals. The output signals may include infrared, radio, telephone, and electrical signals transmitted over house wiring (via an X-10 system). Typically, X-10 modules and receivers provide power control of household appliances (eg, lights, fans, etc). Additional control, such as channel changing and raising and lowering volume, requires infrared signals.

The ideal assessment for an EADL would include the client, an occupational therapist, and a rehabilitation engineer, and the evaluation would be conducted in the client's home. The occupational therapist can help establish the best user control interface, and the rehabilitation engineer can help choose the appropriate technology. The advantage of conducting the evaluation in the client's home is that all the options can be explored in the environment in which the system will be used.

Factors to consider when performing an evaluation for an EADL include:

- client's goals (ie, what controls are desired?);
- client's physical abilities and ability to use a control interface;
- other AT the individual uses;

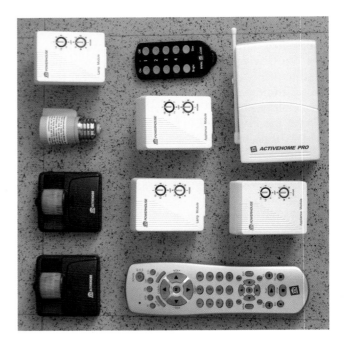

Figure 26-15. The principle components of an electronic aid to daily living.

- client's prognosis (ie, is the condition stable or expected to get progressively worse?);
- client's cognition;
- the system's purpose (ie, for use in the home or at work, in one room or throughout the house, etc);
- system reliability, flexibility, and ease of operation;
- local technological support for installation, configuration, service, and updates; and
- expense of the system and the funding source.

Some EADLs are available commercially, either as stand-alone systems (ie, they only perform environmental control unit functions) or systems integrated with other AT. Voice-activated systems have recently made progress. Once a system is identified and purchased, it is important that it is properly set up and configured in the home, and that the client is provided proper training in its use. Setup, configuration, and client training should be provided by the vendor or local representative. In addition, a local vendor should be able to provide the client with follow-up service and support (Exhibit 26-1).

VETERANS WITH DISABILITIES AND RECREATIONAL SPORTS EQUIPMENT

Today, the number of sports and recreation opportunities for veterans with disabilities is seemingly endless, due in large part to advances in AT that compensate for impairments. The Veterans Health Administration (VHA) provides adaptive recreational and sports equipment.

The *Clinical Practice Recommendations for Issuance of Recreational and Sports Equipment*, written by an interdisciplinary team with the Veterans Affairs Prosthetics Clinical Management Program, outlines the recommended approach for providing adaptive equipment to beneficiaries.[70] According to the published recommendation, each veteran is entitled to an individualized assessment for adaptive recreation and sports equipment. The evaluation includes examining the veteran's medical diagnosis, prognosis, functional abilities, and goals. The VHA defines "recreational leisure equipment" as any specialized equipment intended for recreational activity that does not inherently exhibit an athletic or physical rehabilitative nature. Examples include adaptive devices for hobbies and crafts or adaptive fishing or hunting devices. The VHA defines "recreational sports equipment" as any specialized equipment intended to be used in a physically active or competitive environment. Examples include sports wheelchairs, hand cycles, sit skis, and artificial limbs for recreational or sports applications. Powered devices for sport participation can potentially be provided to individuals whose activities are severely limited without their use when the individual meets general criteria for power mobility. An example of powered sports equipment is an EPW for powered wheelchair soccer. Recreation and sports technologies provided by the VHA must be adaptive in nature to specifically compensate for loss of or loss of use of a body part or body function. Standard nonadaptive equipment, such as skis, boats, and two-wheeled bicycles, are not provided by the VHA.

Veterans and active duty service members enrolled for VHA care who have lost or lost use of a body part or function for which an adaptive recreation device is appropriate may be prescribed and provided equipment. Adaptive sports or recreation technology may be issued to veterans seeking to enhance or maintain their health and attain a higher rehabilitation goal through sports or recreation and who also meet eligibility criteria. In order to qualify for adaptive sports and recreation equipment, the veteran must have (among other criteria):

- medical clearance to perform the activity;
- completed education on appropriate activity and equipment options;
- demonstrated commitment to the activity through regular participation;
- the opportunity to participate in the activity consistently (eg, must have regular access to snow for cross-country skiing);
- tried the appropriate equipment options configured for specific needs and abilities;
- selected a device that supports the veteran's sports and recreation goals; and
- demonstrated the ability to use, transport, and store the equipment.

Accessories for adaptive equipment can also be provided when justified (eg, a car carrier to transport the device to a safe training area, indoor rollers for hand cycles or racing wheelchairs in areas with inclement weather). Seating interventions for postural support and skin protection or specific adaptations for limited hand function may also qualify. The Veterans Affairs Prosthetics and Sensory Aids Service covers repairs and service on sports and recreation equipment. A knowledgeable clinical professional (ie, a recreation therapist, rehabilitation engineer, kinesio-therapist, physical therapist, or occupational therapist) must be involved in the comprehensive athlete evaluation, equipment trials, selection and modification, and education

EXHIBIT 26-1

CASE PRESENTATION

While serving in a combat zone, a 26-year-old male US Army officer was injured by an improvised explosive device. As a result of the blast, the patient sustained multiple injuries, including a right transtibial amputation, right transradial amputation, and massive soft tissue wounds and defects to the right posterior thigh and gluteal region. After evacuation from the combat zone to the continental United States, the officer underwent a prolonged hospital course that included multiple surgical procedures to the right upper and lower extremities for amputation revisions, wound washouts, and split-thickness skin grafting to his soft-tissue defects; multiple wound and blood-borne infections with multidrug-resistant organisms; acute renal failure induced by antibiotic medications; malnutrition; and sacral skin breakdown.

Once medically stable, rehabilitation was initiated to address the soldier's impaired functioning. Therapy initially focused on regaining independence with bed mobility and activities of daily living in the hospital bed, as well as a preprosthetic preparation. The patient quickly regained the ability to transfer from his bed to his hospital-provided manual transport wheelchair, and the importance of addressing his seating and mobility needs was immediately evident. While simultaneously being fitted for and training with his upper and lower extremity prostheses, the patient began wheelchair training. He consistently refused to use a power wheelchair, and he reported that he viewed a manual wheelchair as a tool to regain the strength and endurance that had been lost.

By 6 weeks after his injury, the patient was functioning at a level suitable for discharge to outpatient rehabilitation. His rehabilitation, including upper and lower extremity prosthetic fitting and training, continued on an outpatient basis. A few weeks after discharge, the patient was seen in a seating and mobility clinic for a customized wheelchair prescription. The weeks spent in a hospital-provided wheelchair allowed him to develop preferences and experience regarding his seating and mobility needs. With input from the patient as well as the rehabilitation and seating teams, the patient was prescribed an ultralight, folding wheelchair with an air-filled, adjustable volume cushion; removable, adjustable height, desk-length arm rests; 18-inch seat-to-floor height; spoke wheels with a quick-release mechanism; aluminum handrims; and push handles.

Because of right upper extremity amputation, the patient propels his wheelchair with his left arm and his left leg. After being successfully fitted with an upper extremity prosthesis, he was able to use his prosthesis to assist with wheelchair propulsion. His prosthetic device does not afford him the strength, agility, and coordination to grip, push, and release the handrim in a manner compatible with efficient wheelchair propulsion; however, he is able to create enough friction between his silicone prosthetic hand and the aluminum handrim to assist with propulsion. Even with this assistance, the patient chooses to propel with his left leg more than 90% of the time. A relatively low seat-to-floor height allows him to easily use his intact left lower extremity for propulsion.

The patient admits to having difficulties climbing hills in his wheelchair. He ascends hills with the wheelchair facing down the hill, locks the brakes for rest periods, and allows his wife or other companion to assist by pushing his wheelchair. He insists that he prefers to use these strategies rather than a powered wheelchair.

The patient opted for a folding frame because of the relative ease with which he could fold and maneuver the chair into small spaces. With trials of rigid framed chairs, he found the process of removing the wheels while suspending the weight of the chair in the opposite arm cumbersome, given his amputation and the limitations of his prosthesis. Given his limited upper extremity strength and function, an ultralight wheelchair was necessary to ensure efficient propulsion and ease of transport (ie, placing it in a vehicle).

The history of sacral skin breakdown, multiple wounds in the patient's right posterior thigh and gluteal regions, and insensate regions at the sites of his skin grafts necessitated the use of a pressure-reducing, air-filled, adjustable-volume seat cushion. By 6 months after his injury, his sacral pressure ulcer had fully healed, but his right lower extremity soft tissue wounds and skin grafts still needed to be monitored, requiring him to continue using this cushion.

The patient prefers ambulation with a prosthetic device as his primary means of mobility. Because of the extensive and severe soft tissue wounds and skin defects in his residual right lower extremity, he has a limited tolerance for weight bearing in a prosthetic leg. In addition, his prosthetic components frequently require maintenance, resizing, and other adjustments. For these reasons, the patient realizes the need to have an efficient and reliable secondary mode of mobility, and his wheelchair fills this need effectively.

and training. The clinician works closely with the athlete, other equipment experts, and coaches to support the long-term goals surrounding sports and recreation participation.

SUMMARY

AT has an important role in the rehabilitation, community reintegration, and vocational success of veterans with disabilities. Many veterans with major limb amputations use multiple forms of AT daily, including wheelchairs for mobility. In order to obtain maximal benefit and to minimize the risk of abandonment, a proper assessment by a qualified, multidisciplinary, veteran-centered rehabilitation team is necessary.

REFERENCES

1. Hubbard SL, Fitzgerald SG, Reker DM, Boninger ML, Cooper RA, Kazis LE. Demographic characteristics of veterans who received wheelchairs and scooters from Veterans Health Administration. *J Rehabil Res Dev*. 2006;43(7):831–844.

2. Cooper RA, Boninger ML, Spaeth DM, et al. Engineering better wheelchairs to enhance community participation. *IEEE Trans Neural Syst Rehabil Eng*. 2006;14(4):438–455.

3. Ding D, Cooper RA, Kaminski BA, et al. Integrated control and related technology of assistive devices. *Assist Technol*. 2003;15(2):89–97.

4. Koontz AM, Yang Y, Boninger DS, et al. Investigation of the performance of an ergonomic handrim as a pain-relieving intervention for manual wheelchair users. *Assist Technol*. 2006;18(2):123–145.

5. Mercer JL, Boninger M, Koontz A, Ren D, Dyson-Hudson T, Cooper R. Shoulder joint kinetics and pathology in manual wheelchair users. *Clin Biomech*. 2006;21(8):781–789.

6. Koontz AM, Cooper RA, Boninger ML, Yang, Y, Impink BG, van der Woude LH. A kinetic analysis of manual wheelchair propulsion during start-up on selected indoor and outdoor surfaces. *J Rehabil Res Dev*. 2005;42(4):447–458.

7. Boninger ML, Koontz AM, Sisto SA, et al. Pushrim biomechanics and injury prevention in spinal cord injury: recommendations based on CULP-SCI investigations. *J Rehabil Res Dev*. 2005;42(3 suppl 1):9–20.

8. Boninger ML, Impink B, Cooper RA, Koontz AM. Relation between median and ulnar nerve function and wrist kinematics during wheelchair propulsion. *Arch Phys Med Rehabil*. 2004;85(7):1141–1145.

9. Boninger ML, Dicianno BE, Cooper RA, Towers JD, Koontz AM, Souza AL. Shoulder magnetic resonance imaging abnormalities, wheelchair propulsion, and gender. *Arch Phys Med Rehabil*. 2003;84(11):1615–1620.

10. Hunt PC, Boninger ML, Cooper RA, Zafonte RD, Fitzgerald SG, Schmeler MR. Demographic and socioeconomic factors associated with disparity in wheelchair customizability among people with traumatic spinal cord injury. *Arch Phys Med Rehabil*. 2004;85(11):1859–1864.

11. Arva J, Fitzgerald SG, Cooper RA, Boninger ML, Spaeth DM, Corfman TJ. Mechanical efficiency and user power reduction with the JWII pushrim activate power assisted wheelchair. *Med Eng Phys*. 2001;23(12):699–705.

12. Tolerico ML, Ding D, Cooper RA, et al. Assessing mobility characteristics and activity levels of manual wheelchair users. *J Rehabil Res Dev*. 2007;44(4):561–572.

13. Fitzgerald SG, Arva J, Cooper RA, Dvorznak MJ, Spaeth DM, Boninger ML. A pilot study on community usage of a pushrim-activated, power-assisted wheelchair. *Assist Technol*. 2003;15(2):113–119.

14. Algood SD, Cooper RA, Fitzgerald SG, Cooper R, Boninger ML. Impact of a pushrim-activated power-assisted wheelchair on the metabolic demands, stroke frequency, and range of motion among subjects with tetraplegia. *Arch Phys Med Rehabil*. 2004;85(11):1865–1871.

15. Cooper RA, Cooper R, Tolerico M, Guo SF, Ding D, Pearlman J. Advances in electric-powered wheelchairs. *Top Spinal Cord Inj Rehabil*. 2006;11(4):15–29.

16. Fitzgerald SG, Collins DM, Cooper RA, et al. Issues in maintenance and repairs of wheelchairs: a pilot study. *J Rehabil Res Dev*. 2005;42(6):853–862.

17. Chaves ES, Boninger ML, Cooper R, Fitzgerald SG, Gray DB, Cooper RA. Assessing the influence of wheelchair technology on perception of participation in spinal cord injury. *Arch Phys Med Rehabil*. 2004;85(11):1854–1858.

18. Fay BT, Boninger ML, Fitzgerald SG, Souza AL, Cooper RA, Koontz AM. Manual wheelchair pushrim dynamics in persons with multiple sclerosis. *Arch Phys Med Rehabil*. 2004;85(6):935–942.

19. Cooper RA. Engineering manual and electric powered wheelchairs. *Crit Rev Biomed Eng*. 1999;27(1–2):27–73.

20. Fitzgerald SG, Cooper RA, Boninger ML, Rentschler AJ. Comparison of fatigue life for 3 types of manual wheelchairs. *Arch Phys Med Rehabil*. 2001;82(10):1484–1488.

21. Boninger ML, Souza AL, Cooper RA, Fitzgerald SG, Koontz AM, Fay BT. Propulsion patterns and pushrim biomechanics in manual wheelchair propulsion. *Arch Phys Med Rehabil*. 2002;83(5):718–723.

22. Kwarciak AM, Cooper RA, Ammer WA, Fitzgerald SG, Boninger ML, Cooper R. Fatigue testing of selected suspension manual wheelchairs using ANSI/RESNA standards. *Arch Phys Med Rehabil*. 2005;86(1):123–129.

23. Sawatzky BJ, MacDonald HM, Valentine N. Healing on wheels. *Rehab Management*. 2003.

24. Kaminski B. *Application of a Commercial Datalogger to Electric Powered and Manual Wheelchairs of Children* [master's thesis]. Pittsburgh, Pa: University of Pittsburgh; 2004.

25. Paralyzed Veterans of America Consortium for Spinal Cord Medicine. *Preservation of Upper Limb Function Following Spinal Cord Injury: A Clinical Practice Guideline for Health-Care Professionals*. Washington, DC: Paralyzed Veterans of America; 2005.

26. Cooper RA, Thorman T, Cooper R, et al. Driving characteristics of electric-powered wheelchair users: how far, fast, and often do people drive? *Arch Phys Med Rehabil*. 2002;83(2):250–255.

27. Hoover A, Cooper RA, Ding D, Dvorznak MJ, Cooper R, Fitzgerald SG, Boninger ML. Comparing driving habits of wheelchair users: manual vs power. Paper presented at: 26th Annual RESNA Conference; September 2003; Atlanta, Ga.

28. Dicianno BE, Spaeth DM, Cooper RA, Fitzgerald SG, Boninger ML, Brown KW. Force control strategies while driving electric powered wheelchairs with isometric and movement-sensing joysticks. *IEEE Trans Neural Syst Rehabil Eng*. 2007;15(1):144–150.

29. Dicianno BE, Spaeth DM, Cooper RA, Fitzgerald SG, Boninger ML. Advancements in power wheelchair joystick technology: effects of isometric joysticks and signal conditioning on driving performance. *Am J Phys Med Rehabil*. 2006;85(8):631–639.

30. Pearlman JL, Cooper RA, Karnawat J, Cooper R, Boninger ML. Evaluation of the safety and durability of low-cost nonprogrammable electric powered wheelchairs. *Arch Phys Med Rehabil*. 2005;86(12):2361–2370.

31. Simpson R, LoPresti E, Hayashi S, et al. A prototype power assist wheelchair that provides for obstacle detection and avoidance for those with visual impairments. *J Neuroeng Rehabil*. 2005;2:30.

32. Dan D, Cooper RA. Review of control technology and algorithms for electric powered wheelchairs. *IEEE Contr Sys Magazine*. 2005;25(2):22-34.

33. Corfman TA, Cooper RA, Fitzgerald SG, Cooper R. A video-based analysis of "tips and falls" during electric powered wheelchair driving. *Arch Phys Med Rehabil*. 2003;84(12):1797–1802.

34. Fass MV, Cooper RA, Fitzgerald SG, et al. Durability, value, and reliability of selected electric powered wheelchairs. *Arch Phys Med Rehabil*. 2004;85(5):805–814.

35. Rentschler AJ, Cooper RA, Fitzgerald SG, et al. Evaluation of selected electric-powered wheelchairs using the ANSI/RESNA standards. *Arch Phys Med Rehabil.* 2004;85(4):611–619.

36. Cooper RA, Fitzgerald SG, Boninger ML, et al. Evaluation of a pushrim-activated, power-assisted wheelchair. *Arch Phys Med Rehabil.* 2001;82(5):702–708.

37. Algood SD, Cooper RA, Fitzgerald SG, Cooper R, Boninger ML. Effect of a pushrim-activated power-assist wheelchair on the functional capabilities of persons with tetraplegia. *Arch Phys Med Rehabil.* 2005;86(3):380–386.

38. Cooper RA, Boninger ML, Cooper R, Kelleher A. Use of the Independence 3000 IBOT Transporter at home and in the community: a case report. *Disabil Rehabil Assist Technol.* 2006;1(1–2):111–117.

39. Crane BA, Holm MB, Hobson D, Cooper RA, Reed MP, Stadelmeier S. Development of a consumer-driven Wheelchair Seating Discomfort Assessment Tool (WcS-DAT). *Int J Rehabil Res.* 2004;27(1):85–90.

40. Cooper RA, Boninger ML, Cooper R, Fitzgerald SG, Kellerher A. Preliminary assessment of a prototype advanced mobility device in the work environment of veterans of spinal cord injury. *NeuroRehabilitation.* 2004;19(2):161–170.

41. Cooper RA, Boninger ML, Cooper R, et al. Use of the Independence 3000 IBOT Transporter at home and in the community. *J Spinal Cord Med.* 2003;26(1):79–85.

42. Kielhofner G. *A Model of Human Occupation: Theory and Application.* Baltimore, Md: William & Wilkins; 1985.

43. Schlein SJ, Ray MT, Green FP. *Community Recreation for People with Disabilities: Strategies for Inclusion.* 2nd ed. Baltimore, Md: Brookes Publishing Co; 1997.

44. Scruton J. *Stoke Mandeville Road to the Paralympics: Fifty Years of History.* Aylesbury, Buckinghamshire, England: The Peterhouse Press; 1998.

45. Wheelchair Track & Field, USA. *2008 Competition Rules for Track & Field and Road Racing.* Available at: http://www.wsusa.org/index.php?option=com_docman&Itemid=39. Accessed August 27, 2008.

46. Cooper RA, Boninger ML, Cooper R, Robertson RN, Baldini FD. Wheelchair racing efficiency. *Disabil Rehabil.* 2003;25(4–5):207–212.

47. Cooper RA. Wheelchair racing sports science: a review. *J Rehabil Res Dev.* 1990;27(3):295–312.

48. Buning ME. Recreation and play technology. In: Hammel J, ed. *Assistive Technology and Occupational Therapy: a Link to Function, a Study Course.* Bethesda, Md: American Occupational Therapy Association; 1996.

49. Cooper RA, Cooper R. Design of an arm-powered general purpose tricycle for use by people with mobility impairments. *Saudi J Disabil Rehabil.* 2003;9(2):92–96.

50. Rice I, Cooper RA, Cooper R, Kelleher A, Boyles A. Sports and recreation for persons with spinal cord injuries. In: Sisto SA, Druin E, Sliwinski MM, eds. *Spinal Cord Injuries: Management and Rehabilitation.* Saint Louis, MO: Mosby/Elsevier; 2009:455–477.

51. United States Sled Hockey Association. *What is Sled Hockey?* Available at: http://www.usahockey.com/Template_Usahockey.aspx?NAV=PL_05_06&ID=17202. Accessed February 10, 2009.

52. 34 CFR, Part 300.

53. 49 CFR, Part 37.

54. International Standards Organization. *Wheelchairs—Part 19: Wheeled Mobility Devices for Use in Motor Vehicles.* Geneva, Switzerland: ISO; 2000. ISO Standard 7176-19.

55. American National Standards Institute and Rehabilitation Engineering and Assistive Technology Association of North America. Wheelchairs used as seats in motor vehicles. In: *Requirements and Test Methods for Wheelchairs (Including Scooters)*. Vol 1. Arlington, Va: RESNA.

56. Society of Automotive Engineers Adaptive Devices Subcommittee. *SAE J2249: Wheelchair Tie-Downs and Occupant Restraint Systems for Use in Motor Vehicles*. Warrendale, Pa: SAE; 1999.

57. International Standards Organization. *Part 1: Requirements and Test Methods for All Systems*. Geneva, Switzerland: ISO; 2000. ISO Standard 10542-1.

58. Rentschler AJ, Cooper RA, Blasch B, Boninger ML. Intelligent walkers for the elderly: performance and safety testing of the VA-PAMAID robotic walker. *J Rehabil Res Dev*. 2003;40(5):423–432.

59. American Speech-Language-Hearing Association. *Evidence-Based Practice in Communication Disorders: An Introduction*. Rockville, Md: ASHA; 2004. Available at: http://www.asha.org/docs/pdf/TR2004-00001.pdf. Accessed August 27, 2008.

60. Lloyd LL, Fuller DR, Arvidson HH. *Augmentative and Alternative Communication: A Handbook of Principles and Practices*. Boston, Mass: Allyn and Bacon; 1997.

61. Parette HP, Huer MB, Brotherson MJ. Related service personnel perceptions of team AAC decision-making across cultures. *Education and Training in Mental Retardation and Developmental Disabilities*. 2001;36(1):69–82.

62. Rose J, Alant E. Augmentative and alternative communication: relevance for physiotherapists. *S Afr J Physiother*. 2001;57(4):18–20.

63. Yorkston K, Karlan G. Assessment procedures. In: Blackstone S, ed. *Augmentative Communication: An Introduction*. Rockville, Md: American Speech-Language-Hearing Association; 1986.

64. Glennen S, DeCoste DC. *The Handbook of Augmentative and Alternative Communication*. San Diego, Calif: Singular Publishing Group; 1997.

65. Beukelman DR, Mirenda P. *Augmentative and Alternative Communication: Management of Severe Communication Disorders in Children and Adults*. Baltimore, Md: PH Brookes Publishing; 1992.

66. Wasson CA, Arvidson HH, Lloyd LL. AAC assessment process. In: Lloyd LL, Fuller DR, Arvidson HH. *Augmentative and Alternative Communication: A Handbook of Principles and Practices*. Boston, Mass: Allyn and Bacon; 1997.

67. Swengel K, Varga T. Assistive technology assessment: the feature match process. Paper presented at: Closing the Gap Conference: 1993; Minneapolis, Minn.

68. Hill K. Augmentative and alternative communication and language: evidence-based practice and language activity monitoring. *Top Lang Disord*. 2004;24:18–30.

69. Cook AM, Hussey SM. *Assistive Technologies: Principles and Practice*. 2nd ed. St Louis, Mo: Mosby; 2002.

70. US Department of Veterans Affairs, Veterans Health Administration. *Clinical Practice Recommendations for Issuance of Recreational and Sports Equipment*. Available at: http://www.prosthetics.va.gov/docs/Recreational_and_Sports_Equipment.pdf. Accessed February 12, 2009.

Chapter 27

THE FUTURE OF ARTIFICIAL LIMBS

JONATHON SENSINGER, PhD[*]; PAUL F. PASQUINA, MD[†]; AND TODD KUIKEN, MD, PhD[‡]

[*]*Assistant Research Professor, Neural Engineering Center for Artificial Limbs, Rehabilitation Institute of Chicago, Room 1309, 345 East Superior Street, Chicago, Illinois 60611*

[†]*Colonel, Medical Corps, US Army; Chair, Integrated Department of Orthopaedics and Rehabilitation, Walter Reed Army Medical Center and National Naval Medical Center, Section 3J, 6900 Georgia Avenue, NW, Washington, DC 20307*

[‡]*Director of Amputee Services, Department of Physical Medicine and Rehabilitation, Rehabilitation Institute of Chicago, Room 1309, 345 East Superior Street, Chicago, Illinois 60611*

INTRODUCTION

In recent years a remarkable convergence of new science, technology, public awareness, and funding have instigated the development of advanced artificial limbs. For the sake of discussion, research into artificial limbs can be broadly grouped into three different areas: (1) limb interface systems, (2) control systems, and (3) mechatronics. This chapter will document recent developments in these fields, discussing future directions of various innovations as well as areas in need of further research.

LIMB INTERFACE SYSTEMS

Arguably the most important part of any prosthesis is the limb interface system, which must provide both function and comfort. In terms of function, the limb interface system must transfer loads between the prosthesis and the user, and it must allow the user to control the position of the prosthesis. In terms of comfort, the system must allow expedient donning and doffing and be reasonably comfortable while worn, or else the device will not be used.

Sockets and Liners

Advancements have been made to both upper and lower extremity prosthesis sockets and liners, primarily through enhanced materials. Carbon graphite sockets now offer greater durability at a lighter weight. The incorporation of flexible materials within the socket may offer a more adaptable and comfortable socket.

Custom fitting can be enhanced by the use of computer-aided design and computer-aided manufacturing (CADCAM). Computer-aided design has the potential to transform socket fitting from an art to a science. As the understanding of tissue compliance, loading, and force transfer improves, socket-fitting performance and reliability should also improve. In the future, fitting may be completely automated using three-dimensional imagining techniques such as magnetic resonance imagery or computed tomography. Computer-aided manufacturing (CAM) technology also holds promise for improving prostheses because it could reduce fabrication errors and inconsistencies, thereby increasing quality. CAM could also greatly reduce socket fabrication time, allowing amputees the ability to be trained with a custom prosthesis sooner. Finally, CAM could reduce fabrication costs. "Squirt Shape," a technique under development at Northwestern University, is an example of promising CAM research.[1] Unlike many other CAM products that create a socket by removing material from a blank, Squirt Shape places material only where it will be used in the socket. As a result, no material is wasted in the process of extruding the socket from a block, resulting in increased efficiency and decreased waste, and material cost of only $1 per socket. Squirt Shape also uses an automated process to acquire the model of the residual limb, resulting in an accurate and precise model in a short time.

Advances in custom fitting techniques and materials have allowed better suction suspension systems. The Vacuum-Assisted Socket System has been introduced by TEC Interface Systems (St Cloud, Minn) and Otto Bock HealthCare (Minneapolis, Minn). The principle behind this design is to create negative pressure within the socket for suspension, particularly during the swing phase of gait, which may improve residual limb perfusion, reduce limb volume changes, and improve fit and comfort.[2,3] Although objective clinical trials of this technology are lacking, it clearly shows promise for lower limb amputees. Reductions in size and mass will be beneficial. The application for dynamic vacuum suspension systems in upper limb amputees is also being investigated. A simpler means to achieve suction suspension has been introduced by Ossur (Reykjavik, Iceland) in the Iceross Seal-In liner.[4] This system incorporates a membrane lip placed circumferentially around the distal aspect of the liner to cause a "plunger" effect and create negative pressure when moving from stance to the swing phase of gait.

Advances in upper extremity sockets allow self-suspension at the long transradial and wrist disarticulation level and minimize restriction of elbow flexion as well as pronation and supination. Additionally, inventive ways have been developed to incorporate myoelectric sensors and metal connections within silicone and elastomeric liners to improve the consistency of electromyogram (EMG) signal acquisition and improve control of myoelectric prostheses.[5,6]

Artificial Condyles

There are significant advantages to joint disarticulation amputation, including improved suspension from remaining condyles, fixation of the condyles (an important feature in fleshy limbs), rotational stabilization, better weight bearing through the end of the residual limb, and preservation of distal muscle attachment (eg, the adductors in a knee disarticulation). However, joint disarticulations are not commonly performed because when a socket and hinges are placed over the residual limb, the socket is bulky, the limb is functionally too long, cosmesis is poor, and the hinges cause problems with clothing (although some polycentric designs can minimize these effects).

Alternative surgical approaches have been used to preserve the advantages of a joint disarticulation and mitigate the disadvantages. Bone modification can sometimes be done surgically. A midhumeral or midfemoral osteotomy can be done in conjunction with an elbow or knee disarticulation, respectively. This preserves the condyles (for suspension), rotational control, and distal muscle insertions while providing room for a prosthetic joint. Similarly, a humeral angulation osteotomy can sometimes be performed to create a bony element for suspension and rotational control of a transhumeral prosthesis. Unfortunately, these options are rarely available for traumatic amputees due to the inability to perform a disarticulation or lack of bone available for an angulation osteotomy.

Another approach under development is implantation of artificial condyles. Termed "subfascial implant supported attachments," these implants have been inserted in seven patients with transhumeral amputations.[7] This concept presents a viable alternative for individuals whose amputation was caused by trauma, leaving them without sufficiently long bone to undergo other surgical approaches. Initial implants have met with success in five out of the seven subjects, and future refinements of the condyle geometry should provide improved success.

Osseointegration

All the systems described above rely on some type of socket interface. The inherent problem with socket interfaces is that soft tissues are between the load-bearing skeletal structures and the rigid socket systems. These soft tissues are very compliant and thus not efficient in transferring loads. Soft tissues are ill suited for localized high pressure and load bearing, which generally leads to some level of discomfort and frequently causes skin breakdown. Finally, socket systems encase the residual limb, retaining heat and moisture and providing an environment conducive to bacterial growth.

An appealing alternative is the concept of directly attaching prostheses to the skeletal structure, called "osseointegration." Direct skeletal attachment could alleviate the inherent problems of sockets and provide a very efficient mechanical interface for a prosthesis. The first successful model for osseointegration was the dental implant method developed by Swedish bioengineer Per-Ingvar Brånemark. Today, the integration of titanium dental implants is used worldwide. Dr Brånemark's laboratory also performed the first successful osseointegration procedure for artificial limbs, with direct skeletal attachment of prostheses in amputees with short transfemoral amputations.[8] Osseointegration has now been performed in many levels of both upper and lower limb amputations. Clinical trials are ongoing in Sweden, England, Australia, Germany, and Spain, and animal studies are being performed in the United States.

Osseointegration surgery is performed in two stages. First, a metallic fixture is inserted into the medullary cavity of the bone, and the skin is closed over the fixture. Bony ingrowth occurs around the fixture over 3 to 6 months. A pin-line "abutment" is placed into the fixture during the second surgery. An opening through the skin allows the abutment to protrude and serve as the interface for the prosthetic device. A progressive weight-bearing schedule is started soon after surgery. The benefits reported include a secure and rigid attachment that allows excellent mechanical control. Osseointegration systems eliminate the problems with prosthesis sockets described above, providing greater comfort. Additionally, recipients report improved sensory feedback from their directly skeletally attached limb. "Osseoperception" and proprioception are improved because stiffness between the residual limb and the prosthesis is greatly increased, giving more accurate sensing of the endpoint of the prosthesis. A number of technical challenges remain to be solved before widespread acceptance and use can be expected. The fairly high incidence of infection at the percutaneous interface is of significant concern. Bone resorption, osteomyelitis, and abutment failures are additional complications. Although this procedure is not being performed in the United States because of the relatively high complication rate,[9] the potential benefits are enormous and have inspired ongoing basic science research.

CONTROL SYSTEMS

The lack of control in upper limb prostheses is a severely limiting factor for function, especially for high-level amputees in whom disability is greatest. Current devices use primarily shoulder motion transmitted through Bowden cables or myoelectric control. Body-powered systems allow control of only one degree of freedom at a time with shoulder motion. Myoelectric prostheses also allow operation of only one joint at a time. Myoelectric prostheses are intuitive for transradial amputees to use because hand flexion and extension muscles are present to operate the motorized hand. With higher levels of amputation, however, control is less intuitive because proximal muscles are now used to control distal arm functions. With both body-powered and myoelectric systems the hand, wrist, and elbow must be controlled sequentially, which is cumbersome and slow. Body-powered and myoelectric control can be combined in a hybrid approach that allows simultaneous operation of two joints, although the cognitive burden is high. Finally, existing prostheses provide very little sensory feedback. Body-powered devices give some sensory feedback because the user can feel how hard they are pulling the cable, but no current device provides touch feedback or sensation during object interaction.

The control of lower limb prostheses is also an important issue. Although significant dexterity and multiple degrees of freedom are not required, as with the upper limb, excellent control is required for maximal mobility and safety. Once again, the higher the amputation level, the greater the challenge and need. Significant advances have been made in recent years with computerized knee systems that attempt to predict the intent of the user and adapt to different gait patterns. These systems acquire information only from sensors in the prosthesis, however, and so must rely on other control sources, such as push buttons or key fobs, to allow the user to switch gait modes.

Neural–Machine Interfaces

To address all the above problems, a neural–machine interface that can provide motor commands to operate the prosthesis and serve as a conduit to provide sensory feedback is needed. Three types of neural interfaces are currently being investigated: (1) brain–machine interfaces, (2) peripheral nerve interfaces, and (3) targeted reinnervation. Most limb control signals originate in the brain. As a result, it seems intuitive to tap directly into the source of this information (Figure 27-1), rather than capture it en route (peripheral nerve interfaces) or translate by-products of its endpoint (myoelectric control and targeted reinnervation). A recent increase of encouraging work in this field, termed "brain–machine interfaces," involves individuals with spinal cord injury who are able to control a pointer on a computer screen.[10–12]

Two roadblocks must be overcome before this technology can be considered for prosthetic use. The first involves the complexity of the brain's information structure, and our ignorance of how it works. Although understanding of the brain has grown exponentially in recent decades, very little is understood, from a neuron-to-neuron basis, about how the brain trans-

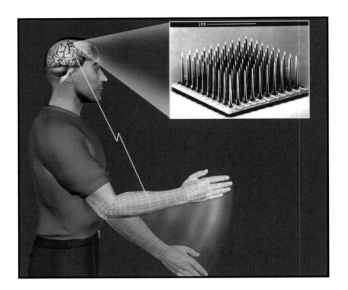

Figure 27-1. The University of Utah's cortical array (inset) records activity from individual neurons in the brain and transmits the signals to a processor outside of the brain. These signals may be used to stimulate muscles of a paralyzed limb, or to control a prosthesis if the limb is missing.
Drawing: Courtesy of John Hopkins University Applied Physics Laboratory and the University of Utah.

mits control signals to execute complex movements. Debate remains over the mechanisms involved (eg, force control, position control, synergies). These concepts must be much better understood to bridge the gap between simple control of a cursor and intuitive control of complex trajectories. The second roadblock involves physical connection of the sensor to the brain. Infection around implanted sensors is still a concern, as is heat dissipation for wireless systems. Fixation of sensors to a finite neuron for a long period of time is also difficult. These roadblocks are substantial, but a great deal of basic science research is currently devoted to surmounting them. Brain–machine interfaces might not be used in prostheses for some time, but they are likely to be adopted much earlier for patients with spinal cord injuries.

In peripheral nerve interfaces, electrodes are directly connected to the residual nerves of the amputee, and the electric signal from the nerve is used to control the artificial limb[13–16] (Figure 27-2). Although this concept offers the potential for improved control, it has several inherent problems such as the fragility of nervous tissue and permanence of electrode array fixation.[17] In addition, the neuroelectric signal is very small, difficult to record, and difficult to separate from EMGs of the surrounding muscle.[18] Additional challenges arise in transmitting signals from the nerve to an external device, which requires either persistent percutaneous

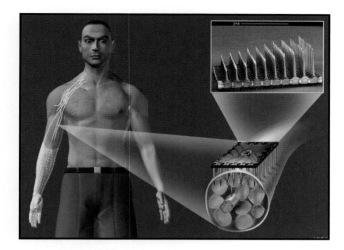

Figure 27-2. The Utah slant array (inset) records activity from individual nerve fascicles of a peripheral nerve. It is implanted into the muscle adjacent to the nerves, as shown in the image in the lower right quadrant of the figure. The slanted tips ensure that nerve fascicles at different depths of the nerves are probed. These signals may then be transmitted to a controller, which in turn controls a prosthesis.
Drawing: Courtesy of John Hopkins University Applied Physics Laboratory and the University of Utah.

wires (which tend to become infected) or complex transmitter–receiver systems. Finally, the durability of the implanted hardware is a critical issue. Prosthetic control systems must function for decades, and implanted neuroelectric control systems may require surgery to repair. At this time several laboratories are making progress toward solving these problems. As a result, peripheral nerve interfaces may one day be widely used, allowing intuitive, finely tuned control.

Targeted muscle reinnervation (TMR) is a new technique that improves the function of myoelectric upper limb prostheses by creating new myosites[19,20] (Figure 27-3). TMR transfers residual nerves from an amputated limb onto alternative muscle groups that are not biomechanically functional due to the amputation. The target muscles are denervated prior to the nerve transfer. The reinnervated muscle then serves as a biological amplifier of the amputated nerve motor commands.[14] TMR thus provides physiologically appropriate surface EMG control signals that are related to functions in the lost arm. TMR with multiple nerve transfers provides simultaneous, intuitive control of multiple degrees of freedom via the motoneuron activity originally associated with the amputated muscles. Great success has been achieved in clinical practice for myoelectric prosthesis control.

Using simple myoelectric control paradigms based on amplitude measurement of the EMG signal de-

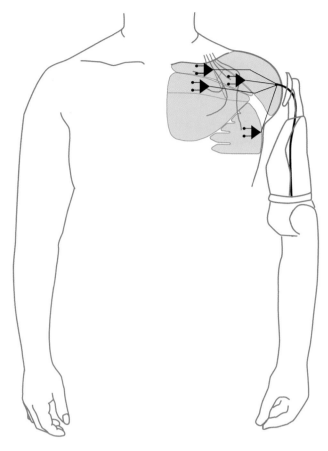

Figure 27-3. Targeted muscle reinnervation reroutes nerves to remaining, nonfunctional muscles. Instead of using artificial implantable sensors, this technique allows the muscles themselves to act as biological amplifiers. Conventional surface electrodes may then be used to sense these new control signals. Signals from these electrodes are transmitted to a microcontroller, which controls the prosthesis.

veloped from each discrete target muscle region, the first four successful TMR patients have demonstrated the ability, for the first time, to control two degrees of freedom simultaneously using only EMG signals. Functional task performance has been evaluated using the box and block test and clothespin test. The subjects have shown a 2.5- to 7-fold increase in speed for task completion. Subjectively, they have reported significantly easier and more natural control of their prostheses.[20–23]

More recent research combines TMR with advanced signal processing techniques to further improve the control of artificial arms. Using pattern recognition classification algorithms, control of advanced prosthetic arms has been demonstrated, including the operation of powered elbows, two-function wrists, and multifunction hands. Targeted reinnervation can also provide physiologically appropriate cutaneous sensation feedback. The afferent fibers in the residual nerves can be directed to reinnervate different residual limb skin, for example, the chest skin of a shoulder disarticulation patient. When this reinnervated skin is touched, it feels like the missing hand is being touched. Studies[23–25] show that the patient can feel very light touch, graded pressure, heat, cold, sharp and dull sensations, and pain—all as if it were in the missing hand.

Current research is being performed to integrate sensors in the artificial hand and tactors (devices that appropriately stimulate the reinnervated skin) into advanced limb systems to provide patients with useful sensory feedback. Broader clinical trials are in progress with current arm systems. Laboratory trials with advanced arm systems are also in progress, and clinical trials with advanced arm systems are planned for the near future. Targeted reinnervation with the potential to improve the function of lower limb prostheses is in the very early stages of development.

Artificial Intelligence

Humans adjust their grasp or gait based on many low-level, unconscious control decisions. If a glass is about to slip, people instinctively tighten their grasp; likewise, as water is poured into a cup, the hand reflexively tightens the grasp. When people start to walk faster, their muscles fire more strongly to prevent the leg from jerking to a stop. This same type of low-level control, termed "artificial intelligence," is even more beneficial in the field of prosthetics, where there is a paucity of control channels. With so few ways to control a prosthesis, it would be ideal for the user to direct only the highest level of control, allowing the prosthesis to provide lower level decisions. Several implementations of this concept have been introduced into prostheses. Examples include the following:

- the Otto Bock SensorHand Speed hand (Otto Bock Healthcare), which senses when an object is about to slip and tightens its grasp;
- the Otto Bock C-Leg (Otto Bock Healthcare), which changes knee resistance depending on the activity required as determined by the prosthesis; and
- the Ossur RHEO KNEE (Ossur, Aliso Viejo, California), which continuously adapts to provide better low-level control of the prosthetic knee throughout the entire life span of the prosthesis.

Future artificial intelligence technology may play a crucial role in orchestrating the control of prosthetic hands with multiple actuated fingers, the interaction of powered lower limb prostheses with the environment to provide proper dynamics, the low-level coordination of prostheses for subjects with bilateral amputation, and many other areas of control.

MECHATRONICS

Powered prostheses consist of three general components: (1) a power source, (2) an actuator and transmission system, and (3) some form of feedback. These components largely parallel the human body. The human arm has two sources of power: (1) the complex network of energy in the form of sugars and fats, and (2) tendons (often forgotten), which absorb and transmit energy during various phases of activities. The actuator in the human arm is muscle, which generates an incredible amount of force but contracts only a minute amount. To move the arm great distances, a transmission is needed, which is found in the bones and muscle insertions. Arm bones and muscle act as lever arms to convert large forces and small movements into smaller forces and larger movements. Finally, the feedback system consists of various layers of sensors and neurons with complex decisions made at various levels, including the spinal cord and brain. In a robotic prosthesis (Figure 27-4) the energy source is typically a battery, the actuator is typically an electric motor, the transmission is usually a gear drive, and types of feedback vary, from simple wires to microprocessors.

Power

The most important characteristic of a power source is its energy-to-weight density. Other important characteristics include maximum discharge and recharge rate, the ease of recharging, and the safety of the power source in the event of a failure.

Nickel cadmium batteries are slowly being replaced by lithium ion batteries, which offer triple the amount of energy for the same weight. Lithium ion batteries are standard for applications such as power drills. Lithium polymer batteries offer even better densities than lithium ion batteries because they require less packaging. They also conform more easily to a given space (they aren't required to be rectangular boxes and can follow limb contours), and so represent an ideal

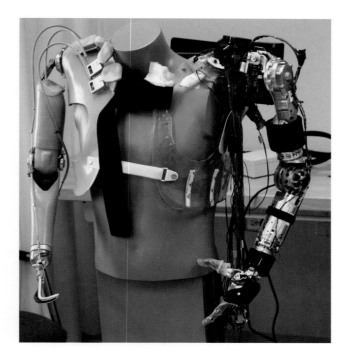

Figure 27-4. The left arm of the mannequin is an initial prototype of a robotic prosthetic arm designed to provide greater function to people who have had amputations at the shoulder, whereas the right arm is a traditional body-powered prosthetic arm. The robotic prosthetic arm was made by DEKA Research & Development Corporation (Manchester, NH) for the Defense Advanced Research Projects Agency (DARPA). It uses lithium ion batteries for power, brushless DC motors, and a variety of sensors including encoders, Hall effect sensors, and load cells.
Photograph: Courtesy of DEKA Research & Development Corporation.

power source for cosmetically appealing prostheses. Several recent nanoscale advances are now commercially available, and will likely be accepted into prosthetic use in the next 5 to 10 years. These batteries offer increased efficiency and hold the promise of increased power density. Methanol fuel cells, which have over ten times the density of lithium ion batteries, may soon be used to power laptops and could be inserted into prostheses in the near short term. However, they require improvement in several areas before commercial implementation, including temperature management, water management, and flow control.

The elbow flexion assist in the Otto Bock Ergo Arm (Otto Bock HealthCare) is an excellent example of a power supply that counteracts the power lost to gravity. Likewise, clutches resist gravity without consuming power, and so may be thought of as a power source. Human tendons are extremely efficient at storing and

releasing energy, much more so than electrical regenerative systems such as those found in hybrid cars. A biomimetic advancement in prostheses is the introduction of artificial tendons, typically through a spring.[26] Denser power sources, however, have implications for other components. For example, the power density of lithium ion batteries makes the added complexity and weight of a clutch a detriment; the same result may be achieved with less added weight merely by using a slightly larger battery. If fuel cells become an option in prosthetics, other items such as elbow flexion assists may likewise become disadvantageous.

Actuators and Transmissions

As with the power source, the most important characteristic of an actuator is its power density. Several technologies such as hydraulic, pneumatic, and electromagnetic motors actually have greater power density, and therefore better performance, than human muscle. Other cutting-edge technologies, such as nitinol, artificial muscles, and piezoelectric motors have significantly lower power density than human muscle. As those technologies improve, they may provide new avenues of discovery for prosthetics (Figure 27-5).

Hydraulic motors have long been advocated as a better actuator than the more conventional electromechanical motor because they have triple the power density. Commonly used in large construction equipment such as cranes, hydraulic motors lose much of their advantage, however, when they are miniaturized to fit into a hand, and recent miniature hydraulics have been unable to perform as well as equivalent electromechanical motors.

A possible alternative for prosthetics is the "cobot," a concept developed for the automotive industry[27,28] in which a central motor spins continuously, and additional, tiny motors tap into the power created by the central motor to actuate numerous joints simultaneously. This setup is appealing because it allows for fast, independent movement of multiple joints, as well as power grasps by all the joints acting in unity, similarly to the human hand. Electromechanical motors waste a substantial amount of energy speeding up and slowing down for each individual movement, and cobots solve this problem. They are likely to be useful only for actuation of the fingers for patients with transhumeral amputation.

The most important characteristic of a transmission component is its efficiency, which in prosthetic devices ranges from 30% to 95%. Planetary gears offer the highest efficiency rates, often over 90%, but are unable to withstand large torques in a small package. Helical

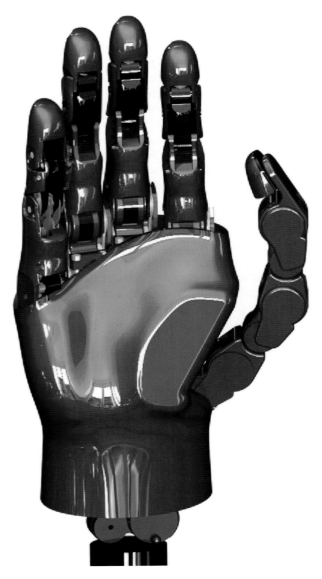

Figure 27-5. Intrinsic hand design, which allows such functions as the pinch-grip, created by the John Hopkins University Applied Physics Laboratory for the Defense Advanced Research Projects Agency (DARPA). All of the actuators are intrinsic within the space of the hand, allowing the device to be fit to patients with a long transradial amputation (actuator technologies such as hydraulics and cobots are excluded due to their large space requirements). 15 brushless DC motors are used to actuate 18 degrees of freedom.
Drawing: Courtesy of John Hopkins University Applied Physics Laboratory.

teeth and ceramic materials improve efficiency and reduce noise, although increasing cost. Harmonic drives, used in the LTI Boston Digital Arm System (Liberating Technologies Inc, Holliston, Mass) provide significant speed adjustment in a single stage. However, they are not as efficient (70% maximum) as planetary gears, and they are noisier, although recent developments have made them significantly quieter in the Touch Bionic elbow (Touch Bionics, Livingston, United Kingdom). Other concepts, such as Ikona gears (Ikona Gear International Inc, Coquitlam, British Columbia, Canada) and cycloid gears, face similar problems.

A promising development is continuously variable transmission (CVT), which can optimize the gear ratio to achieve maximum performance or efficiency in a variety of situations. The Otto Bock DynamicArm (Otto Bock Healthcare) uses a CVT, as does the cobot. CVTs typically involve increased cost and complexity, and often necessitate an additional motor. Several suggestions for CVTs in prostheses without the need for additional motors and electronics have recently been proposed.

Sensors and Controls

The ability to sense various torques allows such features as CVT, auto-grasp during a slip, advanced control schemes such as impedance control or minimum jerk trajectories, maximum power efficiency, and adaptive stance control of the knee. Sensor-based control is what transforms robotics into mechatronics, and it is in this area that the field of prosthetics will likely grow in the next 10 years. Microcontrollers are becoming increasingly small—many powerful microcontrollers are now smaller than a nickel—allowing for precise control schemes to optimize any feature. As microprocessors become more integrated, different components may be able to communicate and provide feedback; for example, feedback in the socket–residual limb interface could allow adaptation of the socket shape based on the type of gait or phase of the gait cycle.

Mechatronic technology in which power transmission is isolated from signal acquisition is readily available. As researchers and industry alike continue the paradigm shift from conventional robotics to mechatronics, prostheses will exhibit increased power and dexterity without increases in weight. Although prostheses will admittedly become more complex, and in some ways more fragile, mechatronics, coupled with new power sources such as fuel cells, will provide a platform for a new surge of innovation in the field of prosthetics.

SUMMARY

Many advances in the last 20 years have had a remarkable impact on the function of prostheses, more so for lower limb than upper limb prostheses. Significant recent advances, including the shrinking size of microprocessors and new types of batteries, have created a new level of technology, now standard in the commercial sector, that should have a substantial impact on the future of prosthetics. The one area where success has been limited is socket suspension. Although commercial companies have devoted attention to this area, prosthetic interfacing requires substantial investigation and innovation to be part of an entire system superior to today's prostheses. The future of artificial limbs will certainly be both challenging and exciting, and should lead to improved quality of life for end users.

REFERENCES

1. Rolock JS, Tucker K. Squirt shape—development of an automated fabrication technique to enhance prosthetics CAD/CAM. Paper presented at: Second National VA Rehabilitation Research & Development Conference; February 20–22, 2000; Arlington, Va.

2. Otto Bock HealthCare Web site. Available at: http://www.ottobock.com/cps/rde/xchg/ob_com_en/hs.xsl/601.html. Accessed December 30, 2008.

3. Beil TL, Street GM, Covey SJ. Interface pressures during ambulation using suction and vacuum-assisted prosthetic sockets. *J Rehabil Res Dev*. 2002;39:693–700.

4. Ossur Web site. Available at: http://www.ossur.com/pages/11836. Accessed December 30, 2008.

5. Dietl H. New developments in upper limb prosthetics. In: Smith DG, Michael JW, Bowker JH, eds. *Atlas of Amputations and Limb Deficiencies*. Rosemont, Ill: American Academy of Orthopaedic Surgeons; 2004: Chap 28.

6. Daly W. Clinical application of roll-on sleeves for myoelectrically controlled transradial and transhumeral prostheses. *J Prosthet Orthot*. 2000;12:88–91.

7. Witsø E, Kristensen T, Sivertsen S, et al. Improved comfort and function of arm prosthesis after implantation of a humerus-T-prosthesis in transhumeral amputees: the subfascial implant supported attachment (SISA) project. Paper presented at: 12th World Congress of the International Society for Prosthetics and Orthotics; July 30–August 3, 2007; Vancouver, British Columbia, Canada.

8. Brånemark R, Brånemark PI, Rydevik BL, Myers RR. Osseointegration in skeletal reconstruction and rehabilitation: a review. *J Rehabil Res Dev*. 2001;38:175–191.

9. Marks LJ, Michael JW. Science, medicine and the future: artificial limbs. *BMJ*. 2001;323:732–735.

10. Musallam S, Corneil BD, Greger B, Scherberger H, Andersen RA. Cognitive control signals for neural prosthetics. *Science*. 2004;305:258–262.

11. Hochberg LR, Serruya MD, Friehs GM, et al. Neuronal ensemble control of prosthetic devices by a human with tetraplegia. *Nature*. 2006;442:164–171.

12. Taylor DM, Tillery SI, Schwartz AB. Direct cortical control of 3D neuroprosthetic devices. *Science*. 2002;296:1829–1832.

13. De Luca CJ. Control of upper-limb prostheses: a case for neuroelectric control. *J Med Eng Technol*. 1978;2:57–61.

14. Hoffer JA, Loeb GE. Implantable electrical and mechanical interfaces with nerve and muscle. *Ann Biomed Eng*. 1980;8:351–360.

15. Edell DJ. A peripheral-nerve information transducer for amputees: long-term multichannel recordings from rabbit peripheral-nerves. *IEEE Trans Biomed Eng*. 1986;33:203–214.

16. Andrews B. Development of an implanted neural control interface for artificial limbs. Paper presented at: 10th World Congress of the International Society of Prosthetics and Orthotics; July 2–6, 2001; Glasgow, Scotland.

17. Childress D, Weir RF. Control of limb prostheses. In: Smith DG, Michael JW, Bowker JH, eds. *Atlas of Amputations and Limb Deficiencies*. Rosemont, Il: American Academy of Orthopaedic Surgeons; 2004: 173–195.

18. Upshaw B, Sinkjaer T. Digital signal processing algorithms for the detection of afferent nerve activity recorded from cuff electrodes. *IEEE Trans Rehabil Eng*. 1998;6:172–181.

19. Kuiken TA. Consideration of nerve-muscle grafts to improve the control of artificial arms. *J Tech Disabil*. 2003;15:105–111.

20. Kuiken TA, Dumanian GA, Lipschutz RD, Miller LA, Stubblefield KA. The use of targeted muscle reinnervation for improved myoelectric prosthesis control in a bilateral shoulder disarticulation amputee. *Prosthet Orthot Int*. 2004;28:245–253.

21. Lipschutz RD, Miller LA, Stubblefield KA, Dumanian GA, Phillips ME, Kuiken TA. Transhumeral level fitting and outcomes following targeted hyper-reinnervation nerve transfer surgery. In: *Proceedings of the Myoelectric Control Symposium*. Fredericton, New Brunswick, Canada: University of New Brunswick; 2005: 2–5.

22. Ohnishi K, Weir RF, Kuiken TA. Neural machine interfaces for controlling multifunctional powered upper-limb prostheses. *Expert Rev Med Devices*. 2007;4:43–53.

23. Kuiken TA, Marasco PD, Lock BA, Harden RN, Dewald JP. Redirection of cutaneous sensation from the hand to the chest skin of human amputees with targeted reinnervation. *Proc Natl Acad Sci U S A*. 2007;104:20061–20066.

24. Hijjawi JB, Kuiken TA, Lipschutz RD, Miller LA, Stubblefield KA, Dumanian GA. Improved myoelectric prosthesis control accomplished using multiple nerve transfers. *Plast Reconstr Surg*. 2006;118(7): 1573–1578.

25. Kuiken TA, Miller LA, Lipschutz RD, et al. Targeted reinnervation for enhanced prosthetic arm function in a woman with a proximal amputation: a case study. *Lancet*. 2007;369:371–380.

26. Paluska D, Herr H. The effect of series elasticity on actuator power and work output: implications for robotic and prosthetic joint design. *Robot Auton Syst*. 2006;54:667–673.

27. Peshkin MA, Colgate JE, Wannasuphoprasit W, Moore CA, Gillespie RB, Akella P. Cobot architecture. *IEEE Trans Robot Autom*. 2001;17:377–390.

28. Gillespie RB, Colgate JE, Peshkin MA. A general framework for cobot control. *IEEE Trans Robot Autom*. 2001;17:391–401.

Chapter 28

ROAD MAP FOR FUTURE AMPUTEE CARE RESEARCH

JENNIFER COLLINGER, BSE[*]; GARRETT G. GRINDLE, MS[†]; CHRISTINE HEINER, BA[‡]; BRADLEY IMPINK, BSE[§]; AMOL KARMARKAR, MS[¥]; MICHELLE SPORNER, MS, CRC[¶]; PAUL F. PASQUINA, MD[**]; AND RORY A. COOPER, PHD[††]

INTRODUCTION

PROGRAMMATIC GOALS AND OPPORTUNITIES

CONSENSUS PROCESS

RESEARCH PRIORITIES
Outcomes Research and Cost-Effectiveness Studies
Rehabilitation and Therapeutic Interventions
Advancement of Surgical Interventions
Advancement of Medical Interventions
Support Programs
Technology
Amputee Care Center of Excellence

SUMMARY

[*]Bioengineer, Department of Physical Medicine and Rehabilitation, University of Pittsburgh, Human Engineering Research Laboratories, 7180 Highland Drive, Building 4, Floor 2, 151R1-H, Pittsburgh, Pennsylvania 15206; formerly, Graduate Student Fellow, Bioengineering, University of Pittsburgh, Pittsburgh, Pennsylvania

[†]Research Associate, Department of Rehabilitation Science and Technology, University of Pittsburgh, Human Engineering and Research Labs, 7180 Highland Drive, Building 4, Second Floor East Wing 151R7-H, Pittsburgh, Pennsylvania 15206

[‡]Communications Specialist, Human Engineering Research Laboratories, VA Pittsburgh Healthcare System/University of Pittsburgh, 7180 Highland Drive, 151RI-HD, Building 4, 2nd Floor East, Pittsburgh, Pennsylvania 15206

[§]Predoctoral Fellow, Human Engineering Research Laboratories, VA Pittsburgh Healthcare System, 7180 Highland Drive, 151R1-H, Building 4, 2nd Floor East, Pittsburgh, Pennsylvania 15206; formerly, Graduate Student Researcher, Department of Bioengineering, University of Pittsburgh, Pittsburgh, Pennsylvania

[¥]Research Associate, Human Engineering Research Laboratories, VA Pittsburgh Healthcare System/University of Pittsburgh, 7180 Highland Drive, 151RI-H, Building 4, 2nd Floor East, Pittsburgh, Pennsylvania 15206; formerly, Research Assistant, Department of Rehabilitation Science, State University of New York at Buffalo, Buffalo, New York

[¶]Research Assistant, Human Engineering Research Laboratories, VA Pittsburgh Healthcare System/University of Pittsburgh, 7180 Highland Drive, Building 4, 2nd Floor, 151R1-H, Pittsburgh, Pennsylvania 15206

[**]Colonel, Medical Corps, US Army; Chair, Integrated Department of Orthopaedics and Rehabilitation, Walter Reed Army Medical Center and National Naval Medical Center, Section 3J, 6900 Georgia Avenue, NW, Washington, DC 20307

[††]Senior Career Scientist, US Department of Veterans Affairs, and Distinguished Professor, Department of Rehabilitation Science and Technology, University of Pittsburgh, 5044 Forbes Tower, Pittsburgh, Pennsylvania 15260

INTRODUCTION

The global war on terror, like many previous conflicts, has brought about tremendous advances in amputee care, as well as revealing areas in need of further investigation. Although much can be learned from the care of individuals with major limb amputation among the civilian population, the military population is unique in many ways. Current injury patterns among wounded military service members involve complex amputations with often multiple complex comorbid injuries, such as burns, paralysis, traumatic brain injury (TBI), hearing and vision loss, mental health disorders such as posttraumatic stress disorder, and a multitude of soft tissue wounds and bony fractures. Combat wounds are often infected, requiring multiple debridements and extensive reconstruction. Fortunately, most members of the armed forces are young and highly active, often considered to be "tactical athletes." With the advances in acute combat casualty care, protective gear, and rehabilitation, in conjunction high premorbid levels of fitness, injured service members are often able to recover from wounds that were heretofore thought to be fatal, and, impressively, many return to very high levels of activities.

Many young service members have not yet established their long-term professional goals; for those who sustain a severe combat injury, this situation presents a significant challenge for recovery. Although some service members seek a professional military career, many individuals join the military as a means of exploring possibilities for future careers. Because much of the success for recovery and rehabilitation is accomplished through goal-driven behavior, it is helpful to have a clear idea of the goals and aspirations of each injured service member. Great success can be achieved by harnessing the military spirit of mission accomplishment, which may be translated to returning to active duty or regaining maximal functional recovery.

It is not uncommon, however, for young service members to equate "physical recovery" to "functional recovery," which are two independent goals. Physical recovery is important, but functional recovery involves much broader challenges, including behavioral health, socioeconomic and educational status, family and community support systems, vocational interests, and return to active participation in the community. It is the responsibility of the military and Department of Veterans Affairs (VA) medical and rehabilitation teams to assist all injured service members in establishing both short- and long-term goals with the overall objective of helping them reach their full potential.

The last time the US military healthcare system handled a large number of war injuries was in the 1970s, following combat actions in Vietnam. Although much of the knowledge gained and programmatic changes of this era were not thoroughly documented, significant advances in combat casualty care were achieved, particularly in medical and surgical resuscitation and medical evacuation techniques. During the intervening time, however, the focus of research within the Department of Defense (DoD) and VA shifted toward chronic care, secondary injury prevention, noncombat conditions, and health services research. All of these areas remain important; however, current conflicts in the global war on terror have brought about the need to refocus those research priorities. This chapter is an attempt to report on priorities that have been identified by experts in the field who have been providing ongoing combat casualty amputee care for the past 6 years. Although this chapter is not meant to be all encompassing, some of the broader policy issues are indirectly addressed, such as balancing the VA and DoD portfolios in bench science, clinical studies, engineering science, and heath services research. Furthermore, the contributors to this textbook believe strongly that injured service members (and their families) must play a pivotal role in research and developing research priorities. Therefore, their participation was solicited whenever possible in formulating the recommendations within this chapter.

PROGRAMMATIC GOALS AND OPPORTUNITIES

The military healthcare system has the obligation to provide expert, world-class combat healthcare delivery and rehabilitation. An active research program is essential to this mission. Unfortunately, most military clinical departments lack the research infrastructure typically available at major academic medical facilities. Despite this situation, many military healthcare providers and scientists are extremely productive researchers. Success is often achieved through collaboration within and among institutions, including military, VA, and civilian organizations. Conducting research within the military offers many unique opportunities, including its relative insulation from commercial and financial bias. Therefore, the military is well positioned to create and support programs seeking new knowledge and translating knowledge into practice to improve the lives of service members and their families.

Numerous mechanisms are available for supporting research to ultimately improve the medical and rehabilitative care of injured service members and to facilitate successful community reintegration, including return to duty. This chapter does not attempt to provide a comprehensive listing of all of the funding opportunities available, only noting that both private and public organizations provide research support. Each mechanism has its advantages. Private agencies tend to award smaller grants, but are able to assume more risk of failure and rely less on pilot data. Federal research funding agencies are typically more capable of making larger long-term investments concerning broader public health issues. The DoD is somewhat unique in that it can provide needed funding to address unique military problems that often benefit civilian populations. A key to making the greatest positive impact in research is to establish collaborative partnerships. Often a team approach works best; clinicians who have patient care responsibilities frequently struggle to maintain a productive research program. Conversely, basic or engineering scientists benefit from working closely with clinicians to gain a greater understanding of clinical and medical questions.

The challenges of current research include the many unknowns of treating injured or ill service members, in addition to limited research funding across the board, significant regulatory barriers and delays, restricted contact with study participants, and the severely limiting requirements of institutional review boards. One strong recommendation by this workgroup is for military treatment facilities and the Veterans Health Administration to establish cross-organizational centralized institutional review boards to allow submission to one board for multisite studies.

Both the VA and DoD need to invest greater resources over the long term in building research capacity. The area of greatest need is increasing the number of active and effective clinician-scientists, which is especially challenging to the military given frequent deployments, changes in duty assignments, and lack of a formal mechanism for protected long-term research time. Also, too few funds are available for education and research career development awards. Members of the Medical Corps, Nurse Corps, and Medical Service Corps have limited time and funding to participate in research training. The military and VA must grow a cadre of clinician and nonclinician scientists to address the problems facing this generation of veterans, as well as future generations. It is critical for students, residents, and fellows participating in military graduate medical educational programs and for junior attending physicians to build research relationships and experience. The offices of the Army, Navy, and Air Force surgeon generals should strongly consider creating career scientist awards for senior uniformed officers who are successful clinician-scientists, similar to the programs within other federal agencies.

CONSENSUS PROCESS

To ensure optimal treatment and rehabilitation of combat-related amputees, the medical and rehabilitation community has been in need of a "road map" to provide focus for efforts and priorities. With this mission in mind, Colonel Paul F Pasquina, MD, and Dr Rory A Cooper organized a 3-day symposium titled "Rehabilitation of the Combat Amputee—Consensus Conference and Creating a Roadmap for the Future," held at the Center for the Intrepid/Brooke Army Medical Center in Fort Sam Houston, Texas, on September 17–19, 2007. The event brought together VA, civilian, and military experts in amputee care, rehabilitation, and community reintegration to help establish consensus on standard-of-care issues, as well as to help identify areas most in need of further clinical, technical, translational, and developmental research. A total of 18 experts presented on current practice and knowledge during the symposium, including engineers, physiatrists, therapists, surgeons, historians, psychiatrists, neuropsychologists, neurologists, prosthetists, audiologists, and experts in pain management and veterans benefits. The speakers came from the VA, DoD, and universities, as well as private companies and institutions. The 100 to 120 symposium attendees formed five small discussion groups:

- programs and systems practices,
- surgical management and planning,
- special medical considerations,
- physical rehabilitation and therapeutic interventions, and
- prosthetic devices and assistive technologies.

Prior to the conference, attendees were asked to prepare manuscripts within their area of expertise that would be the basis for the chapters within this textbook. Each group was challenged to come to a consensus on critical items and management plans as outlined in each chapter. Furthermore, each group was tasked with forming a consensus for the most critical areas of investigation and research needed within their discipline to better meet the challenges of combat-related injuries, particularly those resulting in limb loss. The results are presented in the following section.

RESEARCH PRIORITIES

Outcomes Research and Cost-Effectiveness Studies

Consensus opinion highlighted the importance of outcome-related research. Specific outcomes of interest included programmatic issues, vocational rehabilitation, return-to-duty demographics, and the effects of therapeutic interventions. Participants identified the lack of well-designed longitudinal and retrospective epidemiological studies analyzing the incidence rates of amputation in combat casualties and the impact that etiologic and demographic data have on short- and long-term outcomes. In particular, factors such as level of amputation and extent of comorbidities should be examined to establish their impact on functional performance, quality of life, depression, return to duty/work/community, and healthcare costs, as well as acute and chronic pain. To effectively quantify the success of the treatment programs available to service members, better tools, especially for functional measures, must be designed. Additionally, the extent to which other comorbidities, especially cognitive or behavioral problems, have on outcome measures must be fully investigated. Because existing literature on best care practices is scarce, a process for making clinical decisions based on evidence-based studies must be better established.

The group also agreed that more research on vocational rehabilitation (VR) is needed. Although all healthcare professionals recognize the importance of recovery to the point of meaningful vocation, the best approach to VR intervention, as well as when during the recovery phase VR should begin, remain unclear. Additionally, tools to measure the effectiveness of VR interventions, as well as validated tools to evaluate community reintegration, should be developed. These tools will provide a framework for researchers to assess predictors of successful VR interventions. VR-related research should also investigate the effectiveness of rehabilitation technologies and explore barriers that may exist to return to military duty.

When an injured service member returns to active duty, it is important to establish a longitudinal registry to track information such as how long he or she remains on active duty and both the successes and difficulties that individuals experience. Data elements should include promotions, military awards, performance in military schooling, and attainment of advanced degrees, as well as possible subsequent related physical or psychological health problems. Keeping such a longitudinal registry of these individuals, including those who change military occupations, will allow further analysis of effective and ineffective

paths to success. Furthermore, initial qualitative studies should be conducted to identify issues surrounding acceptance of an injured service member back into his or her unit and the perceptions of those in the recipient unit. These studies will help future generations determine who is more likely to return to successful active duty and what interventions could be made to help support greater success.

The consensus panel concluded that effective outcome research could not be conducted without a more uniformly standard way of providing case management to injured service members and their families. It was agreed that military and VA institutions have been inconsistent in counseling individuals. These inconsistencies have been compounded by the rapidly changing benefits system, which has made it increasingly more difficult for accurate and complete information to reach those who need it. More consistent case management should include appropriate structural organization within the DoD and VA, as well as standardization of the competencies required by each case manager. Educational materials also must be regularly updated and readily available for patients, families, and providers. Research studies should be conducted on evaluating the effectiveness of case management programs, and model programs should be replicated across the country.

As with other outcomes of interest, tools to measure the effectiveness of interventions, particularly in multimodal pain management, role of regional anesthesia, and integrated rehabilitation strategies for polytrauma care still need to be developed. Lastly, better outcome measures to assess the effectiveness of prosthetic components and technology, particularly as they relate to individuals with upper limb amputation, are needed to help physicians, therapists, and prosthetists better determine the device best suited for a particular individual.

Rehabilitation and Therapeutic Interventions

Very few longitudinal studies have been conducted on individuals with amputation, which has left significant gaps of knowledge for professionals attempting to determine how factors (such as demographics, health, and environmental factors) influence the use of a prosthesis and other mobility devices after amputation. This knowledge gap is especially wide for the cohort of active young service members with traumatic amputations, since most studies have focused on older, civilian patients with amputation related to vascular disease or diabetes. Significant challenges also exist in examining the effectiveness of continually advancing technology. It is generally believed that advances in technology, particularly in prosthetic devices and wheelchairs, improve function, preserve the musculoskeletal system, and decrease energy expenditure over time, but it has been difficult to prove this scientifically. Recent studies advocate the use of prosthetic prescription models that take into consideration factors such as age, demographic characteristics, health, and behavioral-related factors in predicting successful prosthetic rehabilitation. These studies, however, do not take into consideration the functional performance levels often observed in young, otherwise healthy injured military service members. Nor do these studies take into account the importance attributed to a prosthetic device by the user, which undoubtedly has an impact on use and overall patient satisfaction.[1,2] Therefore, dedicated research is needed to inform innovative therapeutic approaches and advanced rehabilitation techniques for higher functioning younger amputees with the goal of returning to sports and military duty.

Consensus panel members identified the need to examine the impact of long-term prosthetic use in this unique patient population. To date, data has been lacking on overuse and repeated injuries related to prosthetic use. Unlike research on wheelchair-related technology, which has generated literature that strongly supports clear prescription guidelines for manual wheelchairs that preserve upper limb functioning,[3] similar data is lacking for prosthetic prescriptions. It is essential to look for findings of cumulative traumatic and overuse changes, both during the first year of prosthesis use as well as over subsequent years of long-term prosthetic use. This information will contribute to the development of early therapeutic and technological interventions to prevent excessive stresses on joints and the occurrence of chronic painful conditions such as low back and limb pain, which may lead to significant functional impairment and disability. It is equally important to objectively assess any occurrence of pathological changes on the nonamputated side from overuse, abnormal posture, or gait deviations to develop intervention protocol for preventing these secondary injuries.

Rehabilitation has traditionally been considered to involve a patient and his or her provider; however, interdisciplinary teamwork is becoming increasingly important for success, as has been demonstrated in the stroke literature.[4] Also, anecdotal evidence has been observed by the consensus group that family members, friends, and peer supporters have both positive and negative effects on rehabilitation outcomes. At each DoD amputee care program, family members are able to obtain local lodging, which allows them to participate directly in their loved one's care. In addition, a formal peer visitation program is well established at each DoD site, and all staff support and contribute to the therapeutic milieu. Further investigation, however, is needed to better understand the dynamics of recovery and how to best incorporate all parties into improving outcomes. Qualitative analyses, through interviews and focus groups with family members, could help in understanding their perspectives and potentially optimize their role in the recovery process of each service member.

Rehabilitation research on upper limb amputation was noted to be significantly lacking, particularly as compared to that on lower limb amputation. This is in part due to the complex nature of the rehabilitation process after upper limb amputation and the higher rejection and abandonment rate of upper limb prostheses. Research determining probabilities of upper limb prosthesis rejection, based on level of amputation and amputation of dominant versus nondominant upper limb, could be crucial for determining the course of the rehabilitation process and the prescription of particular prosthetic devices. The use of novel techniques such as metronome-based intervention was specifically mentioned as a potential means of improving body symmetry and postural control to aid in upper limb prosthetic rehabilitation. A study on differences of upper limb prosthesis acceptance based on hand dominance might drive protocols that address the inherent differences in a patient's acceptance and accommodation to use of a prosthetic device. With increasing use of functional magnetic resonance imaging and positron emission tomography, such a study could also include cortical scans to explore any difference in brain hemispheric activity based on hand dominance and prosthetic use. Other areas of potential research that may provide further insight on user preferences include investigating the effect of training variables, the patient's perceived benefit of the device, the quality and durability of components, and level of amputation. In summary, many research avenues should be explored within this new generation of upper limb amputees. Therapists working with this patient population should be diligent in seeking new knowledge to improve efficiency and minimize variability within care delivery methods.

As technology progresses, rehabilitation techniques and the sophistication of outcomes measurement tools must advance as well. All panel members agreed that systems such as motion analysis, kinematic and kinetic assessment techniques, and virtual-reality–based assessment and treatment modalities all warrant further development and clinical research funding.

Furthermore, systems that are able to acquire more real-time data on prosthetic usage, function, and effects on quality of life will be much more useful than the traditional patient recall methodology.

Advancement of Surgical Interventions

The consensus panel identified research priorities related to both acute and long-term medical and surgical care. Among those considered most important in the acute phase of care are optimizing surgical approaches and wound management strategies. Improving surgical techniques during the initial combat wound care as well as during the definitive amputation will have an impact on an individual's short-term recovery and likely positively influence his or her quality of life. Specific research emphasis should focus on techniques to improve peripheral nerve management associated with limb amputation to maximize sensory and motor function of the residual limb. Research is needed to evaluate the optimal way to manage sectioned nerves—for example, targeted reinnervation (see Chapter 27, The Future of Artificial Limbs)—which may reduce acute and chronic pain as well as improve future prosthetic control strategies. Also, data must also be collected to establish infection rates and investigate new methods of infection prevention and treatment. Furthermore, research is required to develop novel methods for wound management at all echelons of care. This should include investigation of various biomarkers and wound matrix analyses to better predict wound healing and optimize timing of surgical debridement, closure, or use of any bio-healing products.

Panel members reported a particular concern with the formation of prevalence of heterotopic ossification seen in war extremity trauma. Heterotopic ossification is the abnormal formation of bone that can limit joint range of motion and cause pain. A better basic science understanding of what turns on and off bone matrix formation is needed. Additionally, surgeons strive to optimize limb length, limb shape, and muscle/soft tissue balance. While a longer residual limb may provide increased function when an individual is not using a prosthesis, current prosthetics technology often requires extra space to accommodate more sophisticated components, and therefore in some circumstances a shorter residual limb may be desirable. Additionally, the residual limb shape needs to conform to the intended prosthetic device, adding another confounding factor. Likewise optimizing muscle length during attachment with either a myodesis or myoplasty may have a significant effect on residual limb muscle balance, strength, and function.

Considering residual limb bone management, participants did not reach a consensus about when bone-bridging techniques should be used in transtibial amputations. Some patients present with a divergent fibula because of injury to the syndesmosis or the proximal tibia–fibula joint, which may result in pain and/or hypermobility of the residual limb. Many bone-bridging techniques exist, but none have been proven superior because limited research data on functional outcomes following surgery is available. Additionally, the effect of timing (acute or revision) for bone-bridging procedures must be explored.

Panel members recommended that further research be conducted to explore the potential for and safety of osseointegration. Osseointegration is the direct skeletal attachment of a prosthesis to the residual limb, by implanting a metallic pin/buttress to the distal bone and allowing it to extend through the skin to connect with a prosthetic device. Current challenges include proper design, materials, surgical intervention techniques, and postoperative rehabilitation techniques. Emphasis should be placed on discovering methods to achieve direct skin growth/adherence to the metal implant to avoid infection, because combat wounds have an increased susceptibility to infection. Panel members agreed that if this technology becomes available it will likely revolutionize prosthetic fitting and require surgeons to change their current approach to residual limb-shaping procedures.

Advances in regenerative medicine may also have a significant impact on the medical and surgical management of amputees. Further investigation of composite tissue allografts and limb regeneration is necessary to explore the limits of this science and its application for injured service members. Additionally, further advances in peripheral vessel and nerve regeneration, grafting, and transplants may allow severely mangled limbs to heal to a point where amputation is not indicated.

Advancement of Medical Interventions

Polytrauma care for the combat amputee requires a complex medical treatment plan. Panel members noted that little is currently known about the neuroendocrine aspects of polytrauma care. Although the majority of combat-wounded soldiers are male, it is important to understand the effect of gender in healing and recovery. Specifically, research should be conducted to investigate the role that hormones, particularly testosterone, play in behavioral tendencies as well as healing following polytraumatic injuries.

Pain management was also cited as an important aspect of management needing further investigation.

Opioid use, in particular, which is often prescribed for pain management related to polytrauma, remains controversial because little is known about its short- and long-term effects on combat-wounded soldiers. Issues such as opioid-induced hyperalgesia have been reported, but little is understood about the pathophysiology of this phenomenon. Therefore, the safety and effectiveness of prescribing opioids for pain management needs to be assessed. Likewise, further investigation is needed to evaluate the effectiveness of other pain management techniques, including pharmacological and nonpharmacological treatments such as mirror treatment, acupuncture, therapeutic modalities, biofeedback, and electrical stimulation.

Residual and phantom limb pain often significantly impact the lives of combat-wounded amputees; however, little is known about what causes these phenomena or how to best treat them. Research efforts should focus on improving knowledge of the etiology and pathophysiology of residual and phantom limb pain. Further investigation should evaluate genetic predisposition to such pain syndromes as well as advanced neuroimaging and biological measures to achieve a more objective measurement of pain. Interventions such as regional anesthesia have been cited by the symposium's expert panel as extremely helpful in managing extremity pain syndromes and minimizing opioid use; however, further documentation is needed to translate these findings into everyday practice.[5] New diagnostic tests as well as novel treatments must be developed for these complex pain syndromes, and better data is needed to capture the incidence and etiologies of residual limb and phantom pain in this patient population.

Further needs identified include improved medical prevention and treatment of conditions such as venous thrombosis, pulmonary embolism, heterotopic bone formation, osteoporosis, and osteoarthritis. Additionally, treatment and prevention of other causes of long-term morbidity and mortality associated with major limb loss such as cardiovascular disease, hyperlipidemia, hypertension, peripheral vascular disease, and diabetes should be fully investigated. Such advances would benefit not only the combat-wounded amputee, but the general population as well. An additional area of research that has not yet been examined is the effect that comorbid TBI has on the rehabilitation and recovery of an individual with limb loss. Panel members reported up to a 60% incidence of brain injury in the combat amputee population. Although the majority of these cases are classified as "mild" TBI, it is likely that sequencing and training regiments could be optimized for these patients.

Support Programs

Multiple support groups and programs have been developed for injured service members. Programs such as Navy Safe Harbor, Marine Corps Wounded Warrior Regiment, Military Severely Injured Center, and Army Wounded Warrior (AW2) program have all been designed to assist wounded service members and their families. It remains unclear, however, how effective each of these programs are or how that effectiveness is being measured. Moreover, it is possible that multiple programs, while well-intended, may be adding to the confusion of patients and their families. Similar opportunities exist for recreational and sporting participation; however, it is unclear how to maximize the impact of these programs. Scientific methodology must be applied to these interventions to better understand their effect and document outcomes.

Technology

Advances in prosthetic design have led to greater emphasis on technology, which in turn has produced research priorities in this area. One of the most important of these questions is validation of these advanced designs. Research is needed to determine the best methods for validation. Once validation methods have been established, the efficacy of technologies can be objectively considered.

Future prosthetic research should include developing performance standards for prosthetic components and devices. The combat amputee population tends to be more active and is likely to participate in rigorous recreational activities, which must be considered when establishing these performance criteria. Another important consideration is that some members of this population will return to active duty. Prosthetic devices, therefore, must be able to perform at extremely high levels of function, reliability, and durability to prevent failure in the field or tactical environment.

Despite the great advances in prosthetic technology, more research and development is needed. Specific areas of interest include powered prosthetics, advanced robotics for manipulation, incorporation of artificial intelligence, and improved prosthetic–body interfaces. In addition to advancing the technology of prosthetic devices themselves, research should also focus on developing devices that may enhance the rehabilitation process. Specifically, systems that incorporate real-world simulations or virtual reality have great potential in this area. Novel systems such as the Computer-Assisted Rehabilitation Environment (CAREN [MOTEK Medical, Amsterdam, Netherlands]) should be further explored as a means of providing multisystem rehabilitation training in a highly user-engaging fashion.

Efforts should also be made to incorporate advanced rapid prototyping technologies to the assistive technology (AT) prescription process. Technologies such as stereolithography, selective laser sintering, and three-dimensional scanners may allow for cost-effective manufacturing of small numbers of custom components. The ability to readily procure custom components would enable individualized solutions that may increase the usefulness of commercially available AT or fill a gap where no commercial product exists.

AT advancement may also help prevent secondary injuries. Studies examining the use of prosthetics in combination with wheeled mobility as a means of preserving intact joints, or the development of techniques to mitigate overuse of the upper extremities over time, may have a significant long-term impact on quality of life. Initial studies should examine current AT usage within the combat amputee population. This line of research would provide the answer to key questions, such as what types of AT are in use, how often these technologies are used, and whether AT is being used to it fullest potential.

Lastly, longitudinal studies should be conducted to assess how a user's need for technology changes over time. In all likelihood the types of AT used will change as this population faces decreasing function associated with aging. Research should be conducted to identify strategies for transitioning between types of AT. Studies of this nature could facilitate predictions for technology needs of this population, as well as provide insight into device adaption as users age. Additionally, methods of increasing access to AT must be established; programs should be established to increase awareness of available AT among both the end users and the clinicians who prescribe them.

Amputee Care Center of Excellence

A central lesson learned through the care of military service members during the global war on terror is the need to provide a coordinated system of care. At the core of this system should be an amputee "center of excellence" (ACoE), with a critical mass of healthcare professionals, research scientists, benefits coordinators, and strong leadership, including collaboration between VA and DoD and strong ties to academic institutions. Adequate resources are necessary to ensure the ACoE's success during war and in peace. These resources should include, but not be limited to, state-of-the-science research equipment and facilities, state-of-the-art clinical tools, diverse and talented staff, inclusion of activities for families, and a supportive environment for patients.

It is crucial that ACoE expertise be maintained as deployment and high operational tempos diminish. Although much has changed since earlier military conflicts, the experiences gained during World War II and Vietnam provided important insights. The postwar decision to disband and decentralize services should not be repeated. An ACoE would allow patients to continue being treated in sufficiently large groups to maintain interaction, provide a large enough cohort to advance research, and preserve an environment for clinical excellence. Ultimately, an ACoE will improve military and VA medicine while helping veterans with major limb amputations, who deserve the best that medicine and science have to offer.

SUMMARY

Armed forces' recruiting advertisements and slogans are designed to attract individuals of courage, commitment, and patriotism. Nowhere are these characteristics more evident than in the military amputee population. Hundreds of stories have been presented throughout the media across the globe illustrating the dedication and courage of injured American soldiers. In addition to the multiple stories in the press praising the work of the military medical community, the US DoD and VA are in unique positions to lead other countries and universities in the research and care of traumatic amputees. The ability of military and VA healthcare providers to pursue cutting-edge research in amputee care will foster a climate of enhanced job satisfaction across multiple medical, healthcare, and engineering disciplines. National and international recognition of the military and VA in this unique area of medicine and rehabilitation will also likely improve recruitment of medical specialists within the DoD medical departments and VA, but most importantly greatly contribute to the continued improvements in care delivery to the nation's heroes.

REFERENCES

1. Kurichi JE, Kwong PL, Reker DM, Bates BE, Marshall CR, Stineman MG. Clinical factors associated with prescription of a prosthetic limb in elderly veterans. *J Am Geriatr Soc.* 2007;55(6):900–906.

2. Kurichi JE, Stineman MG, Kwong PL, Bates BE, Reker DM. Assessing and using comorbidity measures in elderly veterans with lower extremity amputations. *Gerontology.* 2007;53(5):255–259.

3. Consortium for Spinal Cord Medicine. *Preservation of Upper Limb Function Following Spinal Cord Injury: A Clinical Practice Guideline for Health-Care Professionals.* Washington, DC: Paralyzed Veterans of America; 2005. Available at: http://www.guideline.gov/summary/summary.aspx?doc_id=7197&nbr=004300&string=Preservation+AND+Upper+AND+Limb+AND+Function+AND+Following+AND+Spinal+AND+Cord+AND+Injury. Accessed December 19, 2008.

4. DeJong G, Horn SD, Conroy B, Nichols D, Healton EB. Opening the black box of post-stroke rehabilitation: stroke rehabilitation patients, processes, and outcomes. *Arch Phys Med Rehabil.* 2005;86(12 suppl 2):S121–S123.

5. Ford RP, Gerancher JC, Rich R, et al. An evaluation of immediate recovery after regional and general anesthesia: a two year review of 801 ambulatory patients undergoing hand surgery. *Reg Anesth Pain Med.* 2001;26(Suppl):41.

ABBREVIATIONS AND ACRONYMS

A

AAC: augmentative and alternative communication
AAROM: active assistive range of motion
ABC: *Acinetobacter baumannii-calcoaceticus* complex
ABC: American Board for Certification in Orthotics, Prosthetics & Pedorthics
ACoE: amputee center of excellence
ACS: abdominal compartment syndrome
ACL: anterior cruciate ligament
AD: assistive device
AD: autonomic dysreflexia
ADL: activity of daily living
AIS: ASIA Impairment Scale
AOC: area of concentration
AR: Army regulation
ARDS: acute respiratory distress syndrome
AROM: active range of motion
ASA: Adaptive Sports Association
ASIA: American Spinal Injury Association
ASP: Adaptive Sports Program
AT: assistive technology
AW2: Army Wounded Warrior program

B

BAMC: Brooke Army Medical Center
BAS: basic allowance for subsistence
BOC: Board for Orthotist/Prosthetist Certification
BOS: base of support
BPPV: benign paroxysmal positioning vertigo

C

CAAHEP: Commission on Accreditation of Allied Health Education Programs
CAD: computer-aided design
CAM: computer-aided manufacturing
CAP: central auditory processing
CAP: Computer and Electronic Accommodation Program
CAREN: Computer-Assisted Rehabilitation Environment
CARF: Commission on Accreditation of Rehabilitation Facilities
CDC: Centers for Disease Control and Prevention
CFI: Center for the Intrepid
CIP: combat-related injury and rehabilitation pay
CK: creatine kinase
CKC: closed kinetic chain
COAD: continuation on active duty
COAR: continuation on active reserve
COM: center of mass
COX: cyclooxygenase
CNS: central nervous system
CPM: continuous passive motion
CPNB: continuous peripheral nerve block
CR: concurrent receipt
CRC: Certified Rehabilitation Counselor
CRSC: combat-related special compensation
CSH: combat support hospital
CT: computed tomography
CWT: compensated work therapy
CVT: continuously variable transmission

D

3-D: three-dimensional
DARPA: Defense Advanced Research Projects Agency
DASH: disabilities of the arm, shoulder, and hand
DAV: Disabled American Veterans
DES: disability evaluation system
DEXA: dual-energy X-ray absorptiometry
DIP: distal interphalangeal
DNS: Dragon Naturally Speaking
DoD: Department of Defense
DSUSA: Disabled Sports, USA
DVBIC: Defense and Veterans Brain Injury Center
DVT: deep venous thrombosis

E

EADL: electronic aid to daily living
EMEDS: expeditionary medical support
EMG: electromyogram or electromyography
EPOP: early postoperative prosthesis
EPW: electric-powered wheelchair
ESAR: energy storage and return
ESBL: extended-spectrum beta-lactamase

F

FCE: functional capacity evaluation
FDS: flexor digitorum superficialis
FIM: functional independence measure
FM: frequency modulation
FTE: full-time equivalent
FY: fiscal year

G

GME: graduate medical education
GS: government service
GWOT: global war on terror

H

H2H: Heroes to Hometowns program
HIV: human immunodeficiency virus
HL: hearing loss
HO: heterotopic ossification
HUDVET: US Department of Housing and Urban Development Veteran Resource Center

I

IAD: instrumental activity of daily living
ICES: Infection Control and Epidemiology Service
ICR: instantaneous center of rotation
ICRC: International Committee of the Red Cross
ICU: intensive care unit
IDT: interdisciplinary team
IED: improvised explosive device
IP: interphalangeal
IPOP: immediate postoperative prosthesis
ISOD: International Sports Organization for the Disabled
IU: international units
IV: intravenous

J

JAG: judge advocate general

L

LBD: low back pain
LRM: language representation method
LCL: lateral collateral ligament
LPN: licensed practical nurse

LEAP: Lower Extremity Assessment Project

M

MCP: metacarpophalangeal
MCPJ: metacarpophalangeal joint
MDRO: multiple drug-resistant organism
MEB: medical evaluation board
MET: metabolic equivalent
MHS: Military Health System
M4L: Marine for Life program
MMRB: medical MOS retention board
MOI: mechanism of injury
MOS: military occupational specialty
MRI: magnetic resonance imaging
MRSA: methicillin-resistant *Staphylococcus aureus*
MTBI: mild traumatic brain injury
MTF: medical treatment facility
MWWR: Marine Wounded Warrior Regiment

N

NARSUM: narrative summary
NCA: National Cemetery Administration
NGO: nongovernmental organization
NHIS-D: National Health Interview Survey-Disability
NMDA: *N*-methyl-D-aspartate
NPO: non per os
NSAID: nonsteroidal antiinflammatory drugs
NWB: nonweight bearing
NWBA: National Wheelchair Basketball Association

O

OEF: Operation Enduring Freedom
OH: orthostatic hypotension
OIF: Operation Iraqi Freedom
OIH: opioid-induced hyperalgesia
OPUS-UE: Orthotics and Prosthetics User Survey-Upper Extremity
OT: occupational therapy
OWF: Operation Warfighter program

P

PACT: Preservation-Amputation Care and Treatment
PAS: pushrim-activated system
PCA: patient-controlled analgesia
PCWP: pulmonary capillary wedge pressure
PDES: physical disability evaluation system
PDR: permanent disability retirement
PEB: physical evaluation board
PEBLO: physical evaluation board liaison officer
PIP: proximal interphalangeal
PLP: phantom limb pain
PMP: Preventive Medical Psychiatry Service
PM&R: physical medicine and rehabilitation
PNB: peripheral nerve block
PNS: polytrauma network site
PPOC: polytrauma point of contact
PRAA: perioperative regional anesthesia and analgesia
PRC: polytrauma rehabilitation center
PROM: passive range of motion
PSAS: Prosthetic and Sensory Aids Service
PSC: Polytrauma System of Care
PSCT: polytrauma support clinic team
PTB: patella tendon bearing
PTN: polytrauma telehealth network
PT/BRI: polytrauma and blast-related injuries

PTSD: posttraumatic stress disorder
PVA: Paralyzed Veterans of America
PVC: polyvinyl chloride

Q

Q-TFA: questionnaire for persons with a transfemoral amputation
QUERI: Quality Enhancement Research Initiative

R

REE: resting energy expenditure
RESNA: Rehabilitation Engineering and Assistive Technology Society of North America
ROM: range of motion
RN: registered nurse

S

SACH: Solid Ankle Cushion Heel
SBA: US Small Business Administration
SCD: sequential compressive device
SCI: spinal cord injury
SC/SCSP: supracondylar/supracondylarsuprapatella
SFAC: Soldier Family Assistance Center
SGLI: Servicemembers' Group Life Insurance
SM: service member
SSI: surgical site infection
SSWV: self-selected walking velocity
STSG: split-thickness skin graft

T

TA line: line connecting the trochanter and ankle
TAPES: Trinity Amputation and Prosthetic Experience Scales
TBI: traumatic brain injury
TBSA: total-body surface area
TD: terminal device
TDRL: temporary disability retirement list
TENS: transcutaneous electrical nerve stimulation
TFA: transfemoral amputation
TM: tympanic membrane
TMR: targeted muscle reinnervation
TSA: Transportation Security Administration
TSB: total surface bearing
TSGLI: Traumatic Servicemembers' Group Life Insurance
TTA: transtibial amputation

U

UBE: upper body ergometer
USAISR: US Army Institute of Surgical Research
USPDA: US Army Physical Disability Agency
UTI: urinary tract infection

V

VA: Veterans Administration
VA: Department of Veterans Affairs
VAC: vacuum-assisted closure
VACO: Veterans Affairs central office
VASRD: Veterans Affairs Schedule for Rating Disabilities
VBA: Veterans Benefits Administration
VERIS: Veterans Examination Request Information System
VETS: Veterans'Employment and Training Service
VHA: Veterans Health Administration
VICTORS: Visual Impairment Center to Optimize Remaining Sight
VISN: veterans integrated service network
VISOR: Visual Impairment Services Outpatient Program

VP3: Veterans' Paralympic Performance Program
VR: virtual reality
VR: vocational rehabilitation
VRE: vancomycin-resistant enterococcus
VR&E: Office of Vocational Rehabilitation and Education
VTE: venous thromboembolism

W

WRAMC: Walter Reed Army Medical Center
WSUSA: Wheelchair Sports, USA
WTU: warrior transition unit
WWBN-E: Wounded Warrior Battalion East
WWBN-W: Wounded Warrior Battalion West

Z

ZOI: zone of injury

INDEX

A

AAC. *See* Augmentative and alternative communication
AAROM. *See* Active assisted range-of-motion exercises
ABC. *See Acinetobacter baumannii-calcoaceticus;* American Board for Certification in Orthotics, Prosthetics and Pedorthics
Able-bodied ("normal") gait
    energy conservation and, 539, 540
    gait cycle, 540
    six determinants of gait, 540
Access to Sailing
    contact information, 682
AccessSportAmerica
    contact information, 682
Accreditation Council for Graduate Medical Education
    pain management recommendations, 13
Accufuser pumps, 244
Acetaminophen
    burn casualties and, 297
    mechanism of action, 248
    phantom limb pain treatment, 248
    residual limb or stump pain treatment, 233
Achilles Track Club
    contact information, 682
    Paralympics sponsor, 15
Acinetobacter baumannii-calcoaceticus
    battle wounds and, 194
    heterotopic ossification and, 210
    prevalence of multidrug-resistant form, 194
    soldiers returning from Operation Enduring Freedom/Operation Iraqi Freedom and, 197
ACL. *See* Anterior cruciate ligament
Active assisted range-of-motion exercises
    considerations for use of (exhibit), 329
Active duty service
    benefits delivery at discharge, 82
    financial assistance for purchasing a vehicle, 82
    fitness criteria, 61
    healthcare benefits, 82
    home loan guaranty benefits, 82
    individuals with major limb amputations and, 2, 54–55
    insurance programs, 81–82
    Medal of Honor pension payments, 82
    MHS healthcare services mission, 4
    need for longitudinal studies to track injured service members who return to active duty, 734
    phase four of the physical therapy rehabilitation program and, 479–482, 489–490
    recommendations for daily use prosthesis, 578–579
    retirement and disability compensation and, 61–62
    specially adapted housing grants, 82
    Veterans Benefits Administration benefits for, 81–82
    vocational rehabilitation and employment, 82
Active range-of-motion exercises
    burn edema and, 301, 302, 304
    considerations for use of (exhibit), 330
    heterotopic ossification and, 329
    safety of, 329
    skin grafts and, 315
Active reserve service
    retirement and disability compensation, 61–62
Activities of daily living
    acute phase of burn casualty rehabilitation, 333–335
    adaptations for self-care, 333, 496, 497, 500, 522
    aids for dressing, 337–338
    avoiding trauma or shearing the skin surface, 336

bathing safety aids, 337
benefits of independent performance of, 333
bilateral upper extremity activity of daily living task sample technique options and considerations (table), 501–502
bilateral upper limb amputees and, 500–503
burn casualties and, 319, 333–338
circulatory changes and, 336
classifications of, 333
communications, 335, 338
donning pressure garments, 337
electronic aids to, 335, 426, 714–715
factors influencing outcome of functional activity programs, 333
family involvement and, 333
home accessibility aids, 338
home management responsibilities, 335
housekeeping aids, 338
independence and, 333
intermediate phase of burn casualty rehabilitation, 319, 335–336
kitchen modifications, 338
long-term phase of burn casualty rehabilitation, 336–338
one-handed, 514
phase one of the upper limb amputee protocol of care and, 496–497
phase two of the upper limb amputee protocol of care and, 500–503
phase three of the upper limb amputee protocol of care and, 511–514
prosthetic training, 511–514
reading and writing, 335, 338
safety and, 333
self-feeding and, 333–334, 336, 496, 500
self-grooming, 334, 336
speed of performance and, 333
spinal cord injuries and, 425–426
toileting skills, 335, 337, 496
work-hardening programs, 336
Activity-based therapy
    locomotor training, 423–424
    spinal cord injuries and, 423–424
Actuators
    characteristics, 727
    "cobot," 727
    hydraulic motors, 727
Acupuncture
    phantom limb pain treatment, 249
Acute abdomen
    spinal cord injury and, 432–433
Acute rehabilitation programs
    description, 46
Acute respiratory failure
    spinal cord injuries and, 428
AD. *See* Autonomic dysreflexia
Adapted Adventures
    contact information, 682
Adapted housing
    home accessibility aids, 338
    kitchen modifications, 338
    specially adapted housing grants, 81, 82
    VA Prosthetic and Sensory Aids Service and, 72
Adapted Sports Association
    contact information, 682
Adapted Sports Center
    contact information, 682
Adaptive Aquatics

Care of the Combat Amputee

contact information, 683
Adaptive sports program. *See also* Sports and recreation opportunities
    description, 524
ADLs. *See* Activities of daily living
Adult day healthcare
    Veterans Health Administration and, 73
Advanced phase of upper limb prosthetic rehabilitation. *See also* Phase four of the upper limb amputee protocol of care
    challenges to rehabilitation, 636–637
    heterotopic ossification and, 637
    interruptions to the rehabilitation process and, 636
    neuromas and, 636–637
    patient care coordinators and, 635
    psychosocial/emotional issues, 637
    rehabilitation plan formulation, 635
    residual limb and, 635–636
    surfacing shrapnel and, 637
Adventure Pursuit
    contact information, 683
Advisory Committee of the Secretary of Veterans Affairs on Prosthetics and Special Disability Populations
    creation of, 7–8
    mission and vision statements, 8
Aerobic training. *See* Strength training and cardiovascular conditioning
Aerobics/physical fitness
    description, 672
    opportunities available to amputees, 672
Afghanistan. *See* Operation Enduring Freedom/Operation Iraqi Freedom
Age factors
    disease-related amputations, 7
Agent Orange
    presumptive conditions considered for disability compensation for veterans exposed to, 76
Ahrenholz, D.H.
    creatine kinase as an indicator of muscle damage from electrical burns, 282
Air Force rehabilitation center, Pawling, NY
    specialty amputee rehabilitation program, 5–6
Air Force Wounded Warrior Program
    description, 107
Air guns/shooting
    opportunities available to amputees, 672
Alcohol and substance abuse
    posttraumatic stress disorder and, 349
All Out Adventures
    contact information, 683
Allografts
    burn casualties and, 313
Amateur Softball Association
    competitive wheelchair softball regulation, 678
AmbIT pumps, 244
Ambulation. *See also* Gait analysis and training
    arm swing and, 476
    assistive devices and, 461–462, 477–478
    average energy costs of prosthetic ambulation (table), 546
    backward walking, 479
    contraindications, 423
    evaluation of the amputee's potential for, 461
    goals for spinal cord injuries, 423
    in parallel bars, 461
    pelvic rotation and, 476
    phase one of the physical therapy rehabilitation program and, 461–462
    phase three of the physical therapy rehabilitation program and, 476
    sidestepping, 479

    stride length, width, and cadence, 476–477
    swing-through gait, 423
    trunk rotation and, 476
American Academy of Physical Medicine and Rehabilitation
    VA collaboration with, 49
American Board for Certification in Orthotics, Prosthetics and Pedorthics
    prosthetist certification, 554
American Burn Association
    morphine recommendation, 298
American Canoe Association
    contact information, 683
    Disabled Paddlers Committee, 676
American College of Sports Medicine
    amount of exercise guidelines, 332
American Dancewheels Foundation, Inc.
    contact information, 683
American Legion
    present-day role, 29
    support programs, 111
American Medical Association
    Guides to Evaluation of Permanent Impairment, 63
American Medical Rehabilitation Providers Association
    VA collaboration with, 49
American Red Cross
    relaying information to families, 349
    support programs, 111
    tours of government buildings for amputees, 523
American Society of Anesthesiologists
    "Practice Guidelines for Acute Management in the Perioperative Setting," 233–234
    Task Force on Preoperative Fasting guidelines, 299
American Society of Plastic Surgery
    reconstructive surgery definition, 358
American Society of Regional Anesthesia
    central neuroaxis blockade guidelines, 238
    Web site, 238
American Spinal Injury Association
    Impairment Scale, 418
    spinal cord injury classification, 418–419
    standard neurological classification of spinal cord injury worksheet (figure), 419
American Wheelchair Bowling Association
    contact information, 683
    regulations for disabled players, 673
American Wheelchair Table Tennis Association
    competitive table tennis regulation, 679
    contact information, 683
Americans with Disabilities Act
    provisions, 710
America's Athletes With Disabilities
    contact information, 683
Amitriptyline
    phantom limb pain treatment, 247, 248
Ampicillin
    surgical site infection treatment, 196
Amputation Coalition of America
    Limb Loss Research and Statistics Program, 598
Amputee care programs. *See also* Individuals with limb amputations; US Department of Orthopaedics and Rehabilitation; *specific programs*
    advances in prosthetics and, 14
    continuing education program element, 12
    database element, 12
    graduate medical education and research element, 11
    historical background, 5–7, 20–37
    interdisciplinary teams, 10–11, 608
    key elements of, 8–15
    medical management element, 12–13

xxviii

M

O

U

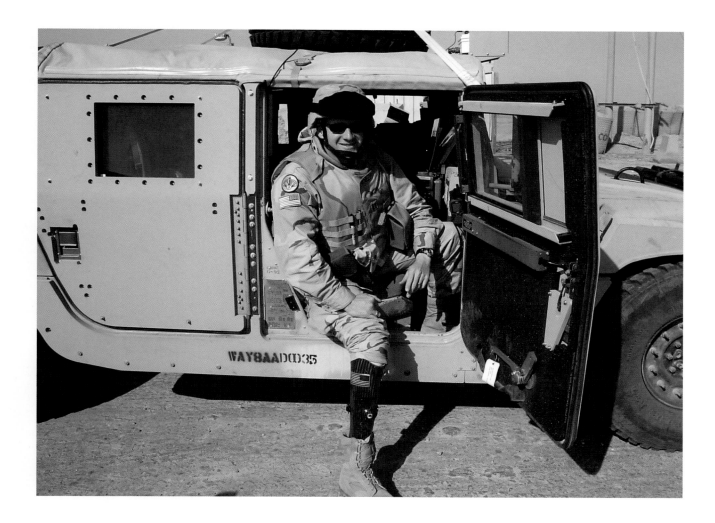

Major David Rozelle had his foot amputated due to injuries incurred from an improvised explosive device blast that struck his Humvee while he was serving as a company commander in Iraq. After undergoing surgery and rehabilitation at Walter Reed Army Medical Center (WRAMC), Major Rozelle asked to continue on active duty and return to Iraq to complete his tour. His request was granted, and this photograph was taken on his second tour. Major Rozelle was the first soldier with a major limb amputation to return to the theater of combat operations. After completing his tour in Iraq, Major Rozelle returned to WRAMC to work within the Armed Forces Amputee Care Program, helping other service members injured in Iraq or Afghanistan to maximize their potential. He also helped lead the design and construction of the Military Advanced Training Center at WRAMC. After completing this assignment, he served as aide-de-camp for the Surgeon General of the Army, and later attended the Marine Corps University. At the time of printing, Major Rozelle had returned to the Cavalry Corps and was once again assigned to a combat unit. In addition to Major Rozelle's many military accomplishments, he has also completed the Iron Man Triathlon and several marathons.

Photograph: Courtesy of Major David Rozelle.

ISBN 978-0-16-084077-7

90000